$82.95

D0164550

Maternity Nursing Care

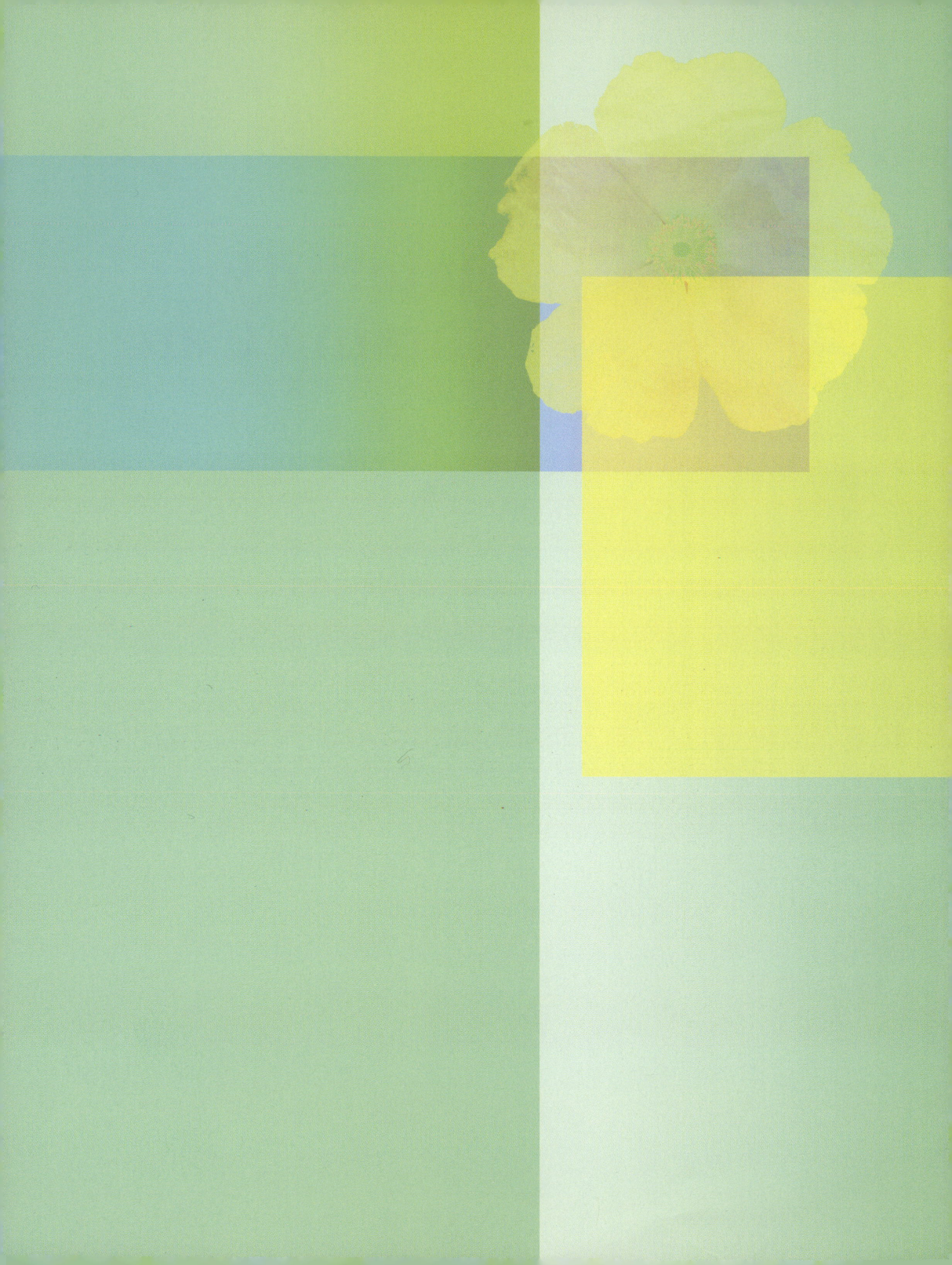

Maternity Nursing Care

Lynna Y. Littleton, RNC, PhD

Director of the Women's Health Care Nurse Practitioner Program
Women's Health Nurse Practitioner
Associate Professor of Clinical Nursing
University of Texas Health Science Center at Houston
Houston, Texas

and

Joan C. Engebretson, RN, HNC, DrPH

Professor
Nursing for Target Populations/Head of Division of Women
  and Childbearing Families
University of Texas Health Science Center at Houston
Houston, Texas

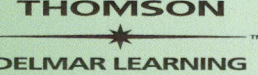

THOMSON

DELMAR LEARNING

Australia   Canada   Mexico   Singapore   Spain   United Kingdom   United States

618.2
LIT
2005
C.3

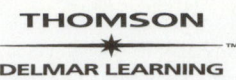

THOMSON
DELMAR LEARNING

Maternity Nursing Care
by Lynna Y. Littleton and Joan C. Engebretson

Vice President, Health Care Business Unit:
William Brottmiller

Editorial Director:
Cathy L. Esperti

Senior Acquisitions Editor:
Matthew Kane

Senior Developmental Editor:
Elisabeth F. Williams

Editorial Assistants:
Erin Silk, Michelle Leavitt

Marketing Director:
Jennifer McAvey

Marketing Coordinator:
Karen Summerlin

Technology Director:
Laurie K. Davis

Technology Project Manager:
Victoria Moore

Technology Coordinators:
Sherry Conners, Carolyn Fox

Senior Production Editor:
James Zayicek

Project Editor:
David Buddle

Art and Design Specialist:
Robert Plante

COPYRIGHT © 2005 Thomson Delmar Learning, a part of the Thomson Corporation. Thomson, the Star logo, and Delmar Learning are trademarks used herein under license.

Printed in Canada
1 2 3 4 5 6 7 XXX 08 07 06 05 04

For more information, contact Delmar Learning, 5 Maxwell Drive, Clifton Park, NY 12065

Or find us on the World Wide Web at http://www.delmarlearning.com

ALL RIGHTS RESERVED. No part of this work covered by the copyright hereon may be reproduced or used in any form or by any means—graphic, electronic, or mechanical, including photocopying, recording, taping, Web distribution or information storage and retrieval systems—without the written permission of the publisher.

For permission to use material from this text or product, contact us by
Tel (800) 730-2214
Fax (800) 730-2215
www.thomsonrights.com

Library of Congress Cataloging-in-Publication Data

Littleton, Lynna Y.
    Maternity nursing care / Lynna Y. Littleton, Joan C. Engebretson.
        p. ; cm.
    Includes bibliographical references and index.
    ISBN 1-4018-1192-2
    1. Maternity nursing. 2. Gynecologic nursing. 3. Obstetrical nursing. 4. Pediatric nursing.
    [DNLM: 1. Maternal-Child Nursing. 2. Holistic Nursing. 3. Women's Health. WY 157.3. L781ma 2005] I. Engebretson, Joan. II. Title.
    RG951.L565 2005
    618.2'0231—dc22
                                2004051667

NOTICE TO THE READER

Publisher does not warrant or guarantee any of the products described herein or perform any independent analysis in connection with any of the product information contained herein. Publisher does not assume, and expressly disclaims, any obligation to obtain and include information other than that provided to it by the manufacturer.

The reader is expressly warned to consider and adopt all safety precautions that might be indicated by the activities described herein and to avoid all potential hazards. By following the instructions contained herein, the reader willingly assumes all risks in connection with such instructions.

The publisher makes no representations or warranties of any kind, including but not limited to, the warranties of fitness for particular purpose or merchantability, nor are any such representations implied with respect to the material set forth herein, and the publisher takes no responsibility with respect to such material. The publisher shall not be liable for any special, consequential, or exemplary damages resulting, in whole or part, from the reader's use of, or reliance upon, this material.

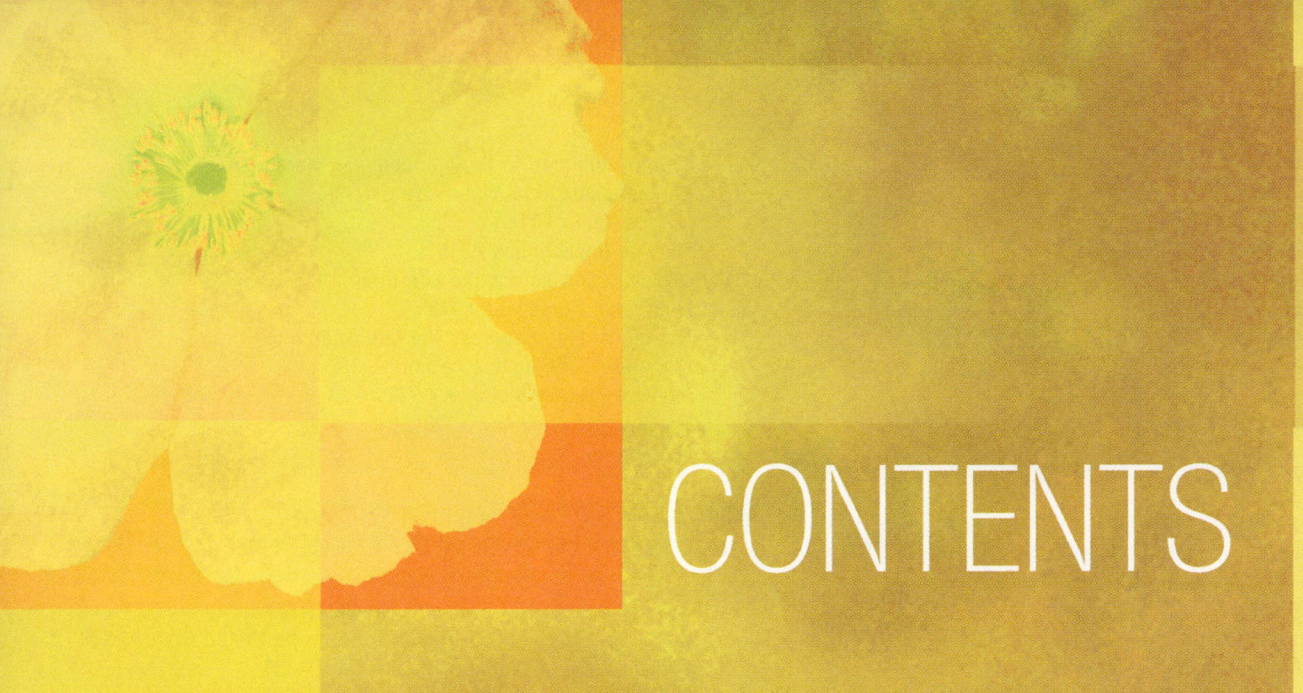

CONTENTS

Unit I: Foundations of Maternal, Neonatal, and Women's Health Nursing

114455

CHAPTER 12   FETAL DEVELOPMENT
AND WELL-BEING 397

Unit 5:   Childbirth

CHAPTER 13   PROCESSES OF LABOR
AND DELIVERY: ANALGESIA AND
ANESTHESIA 453

Unit 6:   Postpartum Nursing Care

Unit 7:   Newborn Development and Nursing Care

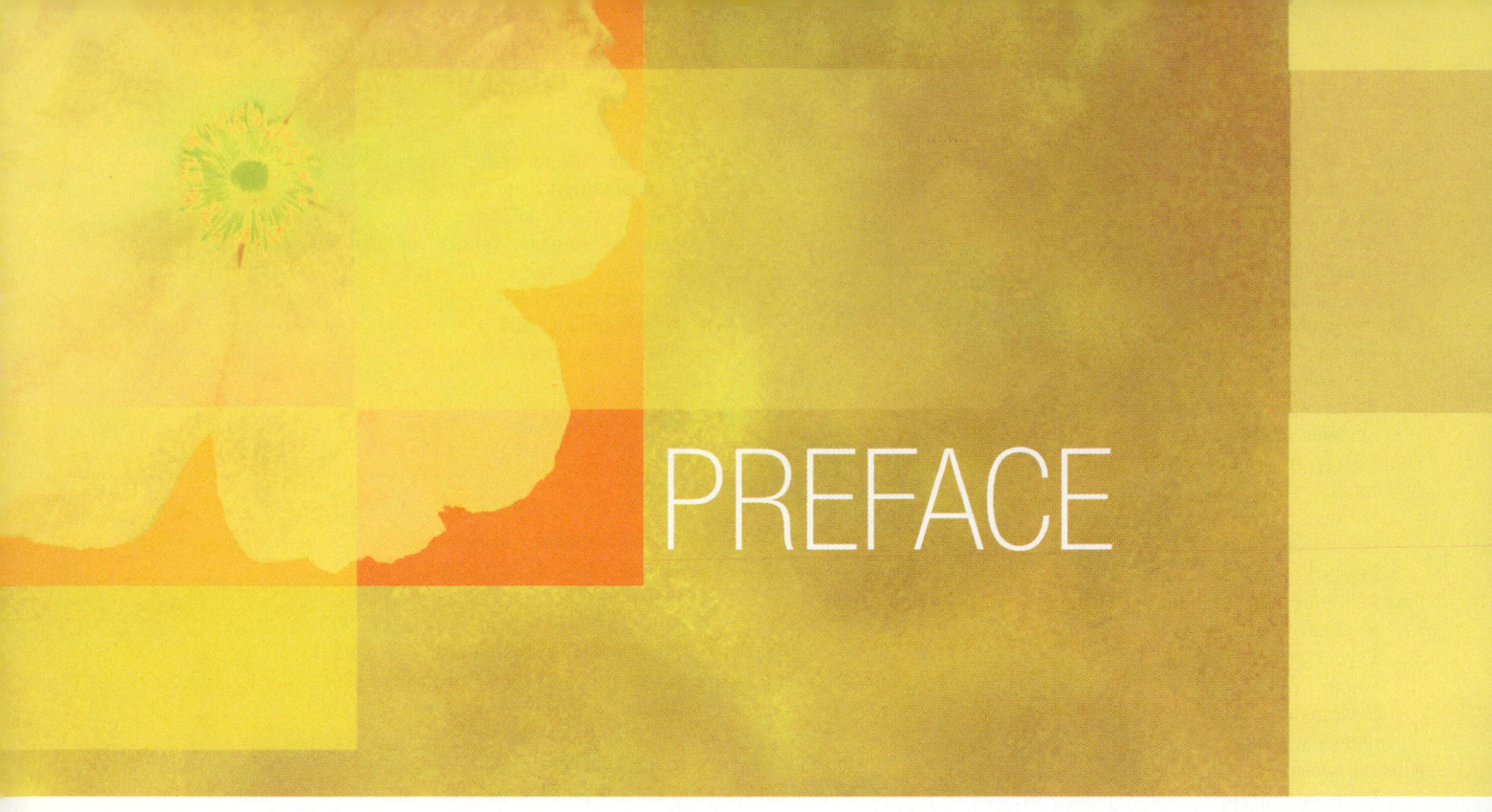

PREFACE

Being a nurse in today's world is a rewarding and at times challenging endeavor. The health care system is changing and evolving rapidly, clients are becoming more educated about their health care, and population diversity makes sensitive nursing care more important than ever. Undertaking a nursing course of study requires attention to all these aspects, along with a solid foundation in basic knowledge and skills.

Maternity Nursing Care offers a holistic perspective to the study of women's health, and emphasizes the nurse-client relationship as part of the caring approach. Content is presented within the framework of the changing health care system, with an emphasis on the nurse's role and responsibilities. Teaching clients about their own health and encouraging them to be proactive in maintaining wellness are threads that underlie this entire text. Embracing clients as complete individuals with emotional, spiritual, and cultural needs in addition to physical needs is a cornerstone of this approach. Understanding that teaching and classroom time is often limited, the focus of this text is to provide the reader with all the essential information required to deliver competent and sensitive care.

Recent changes in the licensing examination have placed greater emphasis on a broader competency base, expanding the scope of knowledge to include a more holistic (physically, mentally, and emotionally) approach to evaluating and delivering nursing care to clients and their families. The revised examinations have also en-

dorsed a shift toward the use of technology in the classroom: *Maternity Nursing Care* supports this movement with an impressive line-up of electronic student and instructor resources.

ORGANIZATION

Maternity Nursing Care consists of 22 chapters organized into seven units. **Unit 1: Foundations of Maternal, Neonatal, and Women's Health Nursing**, introduces the topics and lays the foundation for study. The contemporary health care system is discussed, as are theoretical perspectives on the childbearing family, so that the reader will have a clear understanding of the environments in which care takes place. Current topics of emphasis, such as complementary and alternative therapies, and ethics, laws, and standards of care, round out the foundation of understanding for the maternal, neonatal, and women's health course of study.

Unit 2: Health Care of Women across the Life Span takes a holistic approach to care by encouraging readers to understand women and their families across the life span. Promoting health during all age brackets is emphasized, as are health care issues and reproductive concerns that are specific to women.

The entire reproductive cycle is explored in **Unit 3: Human Reproduction**. Related topics of concern to clients and their families, such as sexuality, infertility, and family planning, are also discussed. Of growing concern to potential parents as well as health care providers is the risk of inborn anomalies; therefore, a separate chapter that covers genetics and genetic counseling is included.

Unit 4: Pregnancy walks through each trimester of a pregnancy and the physical, social, emotional, and psychological adaptations that the pregnant woman and her family will be facing. The progression of a normal pregnancy is examined in detail, as is the nursing care appropriate to the pregnant woman and her family. High-risk pregnancies are discussed next, along with the associated nursing care and interventions. The unit closes with in-depth coverage of fetal development and well-being.

The birthing experience for the mother and family is the focus of **Unit 5: Childbirth**. Processes of labor and delivery, including analgesia and anesthesia, are covered in detail, with an emphasis on the nurse's roles and responsibilities. High-risk births and obstetric emergencies are covered in a separate chapter.

Unit 6: Postpartum Nursing Care emphasizes nursing care of the mother and family following childbirth. Complications that may occur in the postpartum period, such as neonatal loss, are discussed in a caring manner. Breast- and bottle-feeding are given thorough coverage in a separate chapter devoted to newborn nutrition.

The final unit, **Unit 7: Newborn Development and Nursing Care**, will assist readers in grasping the many and potentially complex adaptations the newborn must make to the extrauterine environment. Nursing responsibilities are outlined for care of the healthy newborn. Care of newborns at risk related to birth weight, premature delivery, and birth anomalies is also presented.

FEATURES

Delivering safe, sensitive, and thoughtful care to clients and their families is a goal of every nurse. To this end, *Maternity Nursing Care* includes many special features to help you develop compassion and master skills and gain competence when caring for your clients.

- **Key Terms** are bolded in color and defined within the chapter, and highlight significant terminology for you as you read the chapter. A master listing of all terms with definitions is included in the Glossary.
- **Competencies** outline the targeted learning goals for each chapter to guide you in your reading and study.
- **Critical Thinking** boxes appear throughout the text at key spots. These features challenge you to analyze your understanding of the subject matter and consider how to apply this knowledge to your nursing practice.

- **Reflections from Nurses and Families** offer stories and anecdotes from nurses, clients, and their families. These reflections will help you keep in mind the different viewpoints that may be associated with various situations.
- **Collaborative Care** boxes emphasize the nurse's role as a member of the interdisciplinary health care team, and stress the importance of this relationship in delivering comprehensive, client-centered care.
- **Procedures** outline the step-by-step instructions for performing select skills. Rationales support the reasoning for nursing actions.
- **Drug Boxes** highlight specifics on medication administration related to a given drug, emphasizing the nurse's responsibilities.
- **Client Education** features underscore the critical role nurses play in teaching clients about self-care and health promotion.
- **Nursing Alerts** advise you of certain situations that may be dangerous to either you or your client.
- **Nursing Tips** include advice from experienced nurses that will benefit you as you begin your nursing career.
- **Photo Stories** are vivid photographic essays on select skills and procedures. Five step-by-step photo stories are included in Chapters 13, 14, and 20.
- **Case Study/Care Plans** feature real-life scenarios of actual client care situations. Each presentation follows the nursing process, and includes standardized wording from the Nursing Outcomes Classification (NOC) and the Nursing Interventions Classification (NIC).
- **Web Activities** appear at the end of each chapter and list suggested Internet exercises for you to increase your learning and knowledge base on the given topic.
- **Key Concepts** summarize the main points of the chapter and serve as a quick reference for study.
- **Review Questions and Activities** invite you to test your understanding of the chapter content by performing activities and responding to scenarios.
- **References, Suggested Readings, and Resources** close each chapter and emphasize the research base underlying the chapter content.

STUDENT RESOURCES

The **Online Companion** is a fun and highly interactive learning resource for users of *Maternity Nursing Care*. This free, Web-based offering includes self-study challenge activities to enhance learning and promote a deeper comprehension of the material presented in the text. Visit www.delmarhealthcare.com and look for Online Companions.

The **Student Study Guide** (order 1-4018-1193-0) is an accompanying workbook for self-paced learning. Organized by chapter, it consists of Competencies, Key Terms, Reading Assignments, Activities, Self-Assessment Quizzes, and Critical Thinking Exercises. Answers are found in the back of the manual to encourage a programmed approach to study and learning.

INSTRUCTOR RESOURCES

The **Electronic Classroom Manager** (order 1-4018-1196-5) is a complete teaching tool to aid instructors in preparing lessons, creating lectures, developing quizzes, and outlining presentations. This complementary item for adopters of *Maternity Nursing Care* includes:

- **Instructor's Manual**, which provides suggestions for the direction of classroom lecture. Chapter Competencies, Key Terms, Teaching Methods and Strategies, Lesson Plans, Learner Activities, and Web Resources are all offered on a chapter-by-chapter basis.

- **Computerized Test Bank** consists of 1,000 questions to aid in the development of quizzes and tests. Create new question banks or edit existing ones with this intuitive software that combines a word processor with unique menus and options to work with tests.

- **Microsoft PowerPoint Presentation** offers a visually appealing means of drawing on the key points in each chapter to enhance classroom discussion. This slide package includes 470 slides.

- **Image Library** is an extensive collection of art and photographs from the text. Copy and save any of the images on the CD to facilitate classroom presentations. You can also easily paste images into a Microsoft PowerPoint presentation.

- **Conversion Grids** are supplied to facilitate transition of lecture notes from competing texts to *Maternity Nursing Care*.

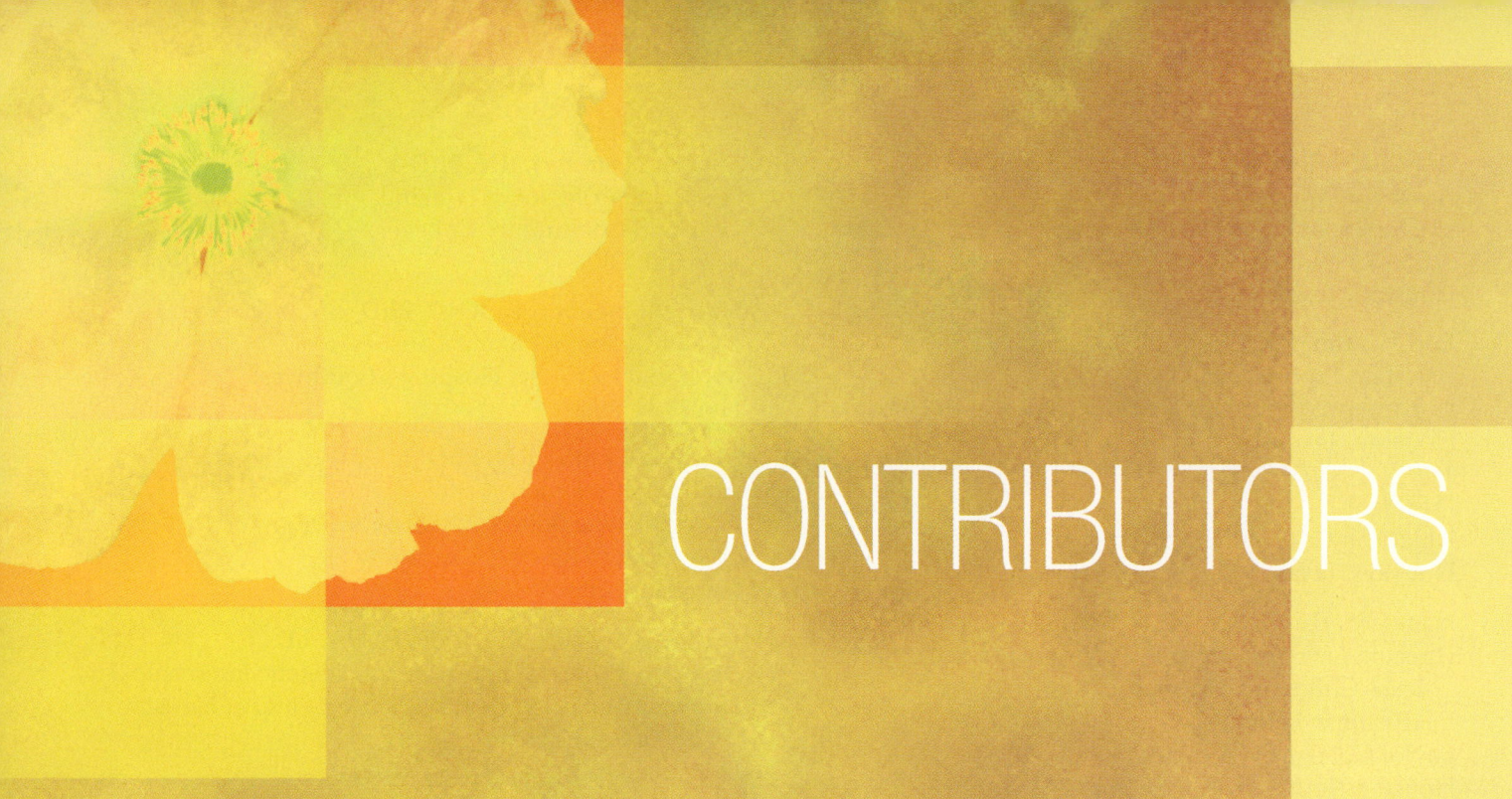

CONTRIBUTORS

Janet M. Banks, RN, PhD CPNP
Coordinator, Pediatric Nurse Practitioner Program
Assistant Professor, Department of Family Nursing Care
University of Texas Health Science Center at San
    Antonio School of Nursing
San Antonio, Texas

M. Colleen Brand, RNC, MSN, NNP
Clinical Instructor
Neonatal Nurse Practitioner Program
University of Texas Health Science Center at Houston
School of Nursing
Houston, Texas
and
Neonatal Nurse Practitioner
Neonatal Nurse Practitioner Program
Texas Children's Hospital
Houston, Texas

Nancy H. Busen, RN, PhD CFNP
Associate Professor
University of Texas Health Science Center at Houston
School of Nursing
Houston, Texas

Kathy Clarke, RNC, MS
Director, Women's Services
Memorial Hermann Hospital
Houston, Texas

Miguel F. da Cunha, PhD
Professor
University of Texas Health Science Center at Houston
School of Nursing
Houston, Texas

Diana Reyna Delgado, RN, MSN
Assistant Professor
Nursing Department
University of Texas Pan American
Edinburg, Texas

Judy Freidrichs, RN, MS
Death Educator and Grief Support Facilitator
Education and Quality Coordinator
Rush—Presbyterian—St. Luke's Medical Center
Chicago, Illinois

Patricia G. Grantom, RNC, MS, CNS, NP
Perinatal Nurse Practitioner
Private Practice
Pasadena, Texas

Chris Hawkins, RN, PhD
Associate Professor and M.S. Program Coordinator
College of Nursing—Houston Center
Texas Woman's University
Houston, Texas

Judith Headley, RN, PhD
Assistant Professor
University of Texas Health Science Center at Houston
School of Nursing
Houston, Texas

Lori Hinton, RN, DrPH
Assistant Professor
University of Texas Health Science Center at Houston
Houston, Texas
and
President
American Case Management
Houston, Texas

Nancy M. Hurst, RN, MSN, IBCLC
Director, Lactation Support Program and Milk Bank,
    Texas Children's Hospital
Instructor in Pediatrics
Baylor College of Medicine
Houston, Texas

Margaret H. Kearney, RNC PhD
Women's Health Nurse Practitioner
and
Associate Professor
Boston College School of Nursing
Chestnut Hill, Massachusetts

Bonnie Kellogg, RN, DrPH
Professor
California State University—Long Beach
Long Beach, California

Elizabeth King, CNS, PhD
Assistant Professor of Clinical Nursing
University of Texas Health Science Center at Houston
School of Nursing
Houston, Texas

Karren Kowalski, RN, PhD, FAAN
President, Kowalski and Associates
Maternal Child and Women's Health Consultants
Castle Rock, Colorado

Lynn L. LeBeck, CRNA, MS
DNSc student, Rush University
Chicago, Illinois
and
Assistant Director
Oakland University—Beaumont Hospital Graduate
    Program of Nurse Anesthesia
Royal Oak, Michigan

Terry Leicht, MSN, CNS, PNNP
Labor and Delivery
John Sealy Hospital
University of Texas Medical Branch at Galveston
Galveston, Texas

Dorothy Lemmey, RN, PhD
Associate Professor of Nursing
Lakeland Community College
Kirtland, Ohio

Harriet Linenberger, RNC, PhD
Vice President of Patient Care Sevices
Memorial Hermann Hospital—Southwest
Houston, Texas

Marilyn J. Lotas, RN, PhD
Associate Professor
Frances Payne Bolton School of Nursing
Case Western Reserve University
Cleveland, Ohio

Jeanne B. Martin, RD, PhD, FADA, LD
Associate Professor and Director, Dietetic Internship
University of Texas Health Science Center at Houston
School of Public Health
Houston, Texas

Yondell Masten, RNC, PhD, WHNP, CNS
Professor
Texas Tech University Health Sciences Center
School of Nursing
Lubbock, Texas

Barbara McFadden, RNC, MSN, NNP
Clinical Instructor
Neonatal Nurse Practitioner Program
University of Texas Health Science Center at Houston
School of Nursing
Houston, Texas
and
Neonatal Nurse Practitioner
Neonatal Nurse Practitioner Program
Women's Hospital of Texas
Houston, Texas

Cynthia L. Milan, RN, MSN, EdD
Assistant Professor
Nursing Department
University of Texas Pan American
Edinburg, Texas

Major Lourie R. Moore, RNC, MSN, CNS
Nurse Manager/Element Chief
Obstetrical Unit
56th Medical Group
Luke Air Force Base
Glendale, Arizona

Carol A. Norman, MEd, MSN
Instructor
University of Texas Health Science Center at Houston
School of Nursing
Houston, Texas

Jacquelyn Normand, RNC, MSN
Women's Health Care Nurse Practitioner
Southwest Clinic
Houston, Texas

Deborah A. Raines, RNC, PhD
Assistant Professor
College of Nursing
Florida Atlantic University
Boca Raton, Florida

Faun G. Ryser, RN, PhD, CNS
Assistant Professor of Clinical Nursing
University of Texas Health Science Center at Houston
School of Nursing
Houston, Texas

Janine Sherman, RNC, MSN
Instructor
University of Texas Health Science Center at Houston
School of Nursing
Houston, Texas

Maureen E. Sintich, RNC, MSN, CS, FNP
Administrator
Women's Health Service Line
North Carolina Baptist Hospitals, Inc.
Wake Forest University Baptist Medical Center
Winston-Salem, North Carolina

Jan Weingrad Smith, CNM, MS, MPH
Assistant Professor
Boston University School of Public Health
Department of Maternal and Child Health Program
Nurse Midwifery Education Program
Boston, Massachusetts

Lene Symes, RN, PhD
Texas Woman's University
College of Nursing
Houston Center
Houston, Texas

Karen Trierweiler, MS, CNM
Nurse Consultant
Women's Health Section
Colorado Department of Public Health and Environment
Denver, Colorado

Christine J. Valentine, RD, MD
Pediatric Resident, Neonatal Nutrition Consultant
Baylor College of Medicine
Houston, Texas

Elias Vasquez, PhD, NP, FAANP
Associate Professor of Clinical Nursing
Director, Neonatal Nurse Practitioner Program
University of Texas Health Science Center at Houston
School of Nursing
Houston, Texas

Marlene Walden, RNC, PhD, NNP, CCNS
Assistant Professor
School of Nursing
University of Texas Medical Branch at Galveston
Galveston, Texas

Pam Willson, RN, PhD, FNP-C
Veterans Affairs Medical Center
Houston, Texas

Anne Young, RN, EdD
Associate Professor and Doctoral Program Coordinator
Texas Woman's University
College of Nursing
Houston, Texas

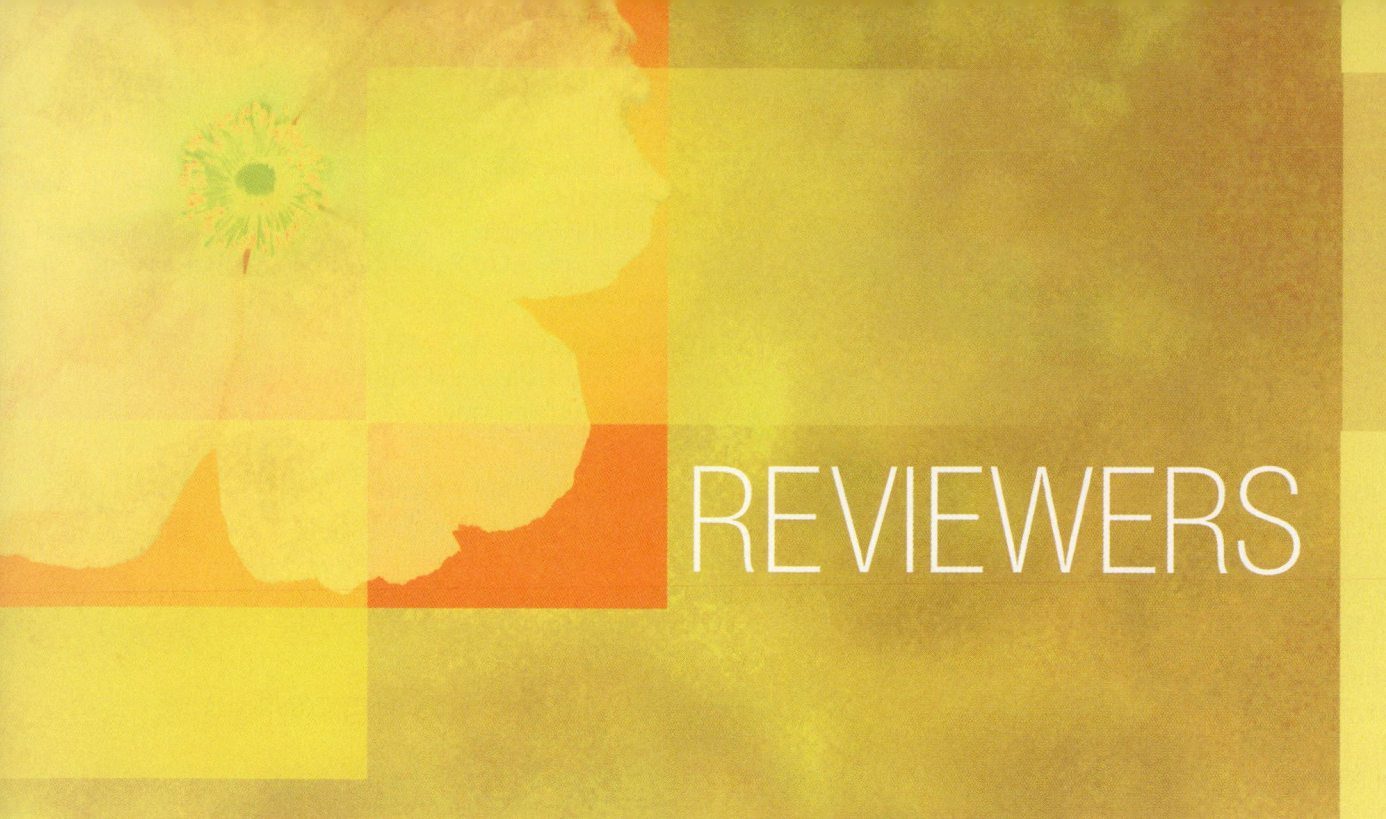

REVIEWERS

Brenda Gleason, RN, BSN
Nursing Instructor
Iowa Central Community College
Gowrie, Iowa

Sheryl L. Gray, RN, BSN
Associate Professor and Assistant Chair
Division of Nursing
Daytona Beach Community College
Daytona Beach, Florida

Margaret S. Hamilton, DNS, RN
Assistant Professor
Florida International University
School of Nursing
Miami, Florida

Susan A. Johnson, MS, RNC
Assistant Professor of Nursing
College of St. Catherine
White Bear Lake, Minnesota

Linda Jean Kapinos, RNC, MSN, MEd, IBCLC
Associate Professor of Nursing
Capital Community College
Chicopee, Massachusetts

Pat S. Kupina, RN, MSN
Professor in Nursing
Joliet Junior College
Crest Hill, Illinois

Maxine Lesser, MSN, ARNP
Associate Professor of Nursing
Daytona Beach Community College
Daytona Beach, Florida

Tamella P. Livengood, APRN, BC, MSN, FNP
Professor of Nursing/Faculty Member
Northwest Michigan College
Traverse City, Michigan

Linda Miedem, RN, MSN
Dean of Allied Health Division
Brevard Community College
Cocoa, Florida

Mary Tennies Moseley, EdD, MN, RN
Professor of Nursing
North Virginia Community College
Annandale, Virginia

Vicki Nees, RNC, MSN, APRN, BC
Associate Professor
Ivy Tech State College
Lafayette, Indiana

Vicky K. Parker, RN, MS, CNP
Assistant Professor, Associate Degree Program
Ohio University—Chillicothe
Chillicothe, Ohio

Linda Pehl, RNC, PhD
Associate Dean and Professor
Scott and White School of Nursing
University of Mary Hardin Baylor
Belton, Texas

Jane Peterson, PhD (c), RN, BC, ARNP, FNP-C
Assistant Professor
Fort Hayes State University
Hays, Kansas

Anita K. Reed, MSN, RN
Instructor of Nursing
St. Elizabeth School of Nursing
Lafayette, Indiana

Regina D. Reed, MSN, FNP-C
Assistant Professor, Associate Degree Nursing
Washington State Community College
Reedsville, Ohio

Alice Riddle, RN, MSN
Assistant Professor of Nursing
Brevard Community College
Titusville, Florida

Susan Sienkiewicz, MA, RN
Associate Professor
Community College of Rhode Island
Warwick, Rhode Island

Bobbie M. Smith, MSN, RNC, CFNP
Family Nurse Practitioner
Muskingum Emergency Physicians
Zanesville, Ohio

Margaret E. Souders, RNC, MS, CNS
Department Chair
Phoenix College
Phoenix, Arizona

Laura J. Wallace, CNM, MS
Instructor of Nursing
Georgia Perimeter College
Clarkston, Georgia

ACKNOWLEDGMENTS

The following individuals should be acknowledged because without their support and skill this book would not have been possible. We are eternally grateful to these people and many more.

Earl Littleton, my husband of 37 years, who supported, encouraged, and provided unconditional love. My sisters, Carla Funderburg, Dorris Petrey, and Melva Fizeseri and my brother, John Petrey, who have been patient with my work and kind in my absence. Wentworth Eaton MD, longtime friend and mentor.

—L.L.

David Cohen, my husband, who has patiently dealt with very late dinners and frenzied weekends, and still provided support for this project. My three sons, Andrew, Adam, and Ethan, who patiently appreciated the time and energy that has been diverted to this project. To my colleagues at UTHS School of Nursing who have heard the frustrations and elations, and steadily kept us afloat during the deadlines.

—J.E.

The many contributors to this text from all over the country. Harriett Linenberger for approving incredible photographic access. Carol Kanusky for making things happen at the hospital. Nancy Busen, Mary Brown, and Linda Shoene for their irreplaceable technical assistance. Matt Kane for his organizational ability. Tom Stock for his photographic skill. Bob Plante for his artistic design. David Buddle for his attention to detail. Joe Chovan for his incredible artistic talent. Jim Zayicek for his production skills. Erin Silk for her editorial skill and patience. The many students and faculty that provided input into the development of the book. And, finally, to Beth Williams, our developmental editor, who has nursed this project from beginning to end. She has demonstrated great patience and attentiveness to detail, and developed the vision of the completed product that was, at times, nebulous to us through the process.

—L.L. & J.E.

ABOUT THE AUTHORS

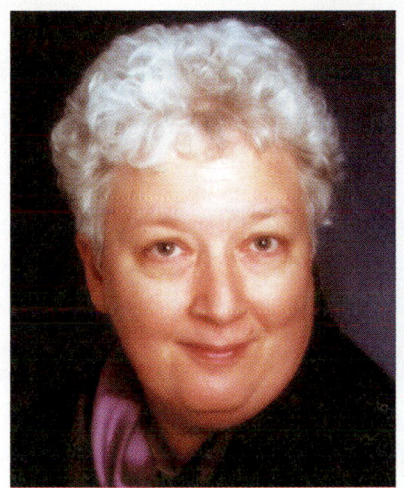

Lynna Y. Littleton

Lynna Y. Littleton has a diploma from City of Memphis Hospitals School of Nursing, with a BS, MS, and PhD in nursing from Texas Women's University. She has worked in numerous women's health care settings, including labor and delivery, postpartum, and antepartum units in hospitals. She has also worked in ambulatory care settings. She is a women's health care nurse practitioner, an Associate Professor of Clinical Nursing, and Program Director of the Women's Health Care Nurse Practitioner Program at University of Texas Health Science Center at Houston. She has taught both undergraduate and graduate courses related to maternal and child health as well as women's health. She maintains a clinical practice as a nurse practitioner. She has won numerous teaching and clinical awards.

Joan C. Engebretson

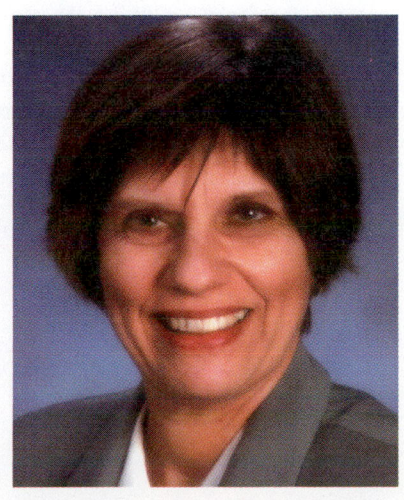

Joan Engebretson received a BSN from St. Olaf College in Northfield, Minnesota, an MS from Texas Women's University, and a DrPH at University of Texas Health Science Center at Houston School of Public Health. She is a Professor at University of Texas Health Science Center at Houston School of Nursing with an adjunct position at the School of Public Health. She has a clinical background in community health nursing, with a focus on maternal-child health. She has taught graduate and undergraduate courses in maternal-infant and women's health. She has conducted research on complementary therapies, touch therapies, and menopause. She also collaborated in the development of the Wee Thumbie, a pacifier for low-birth-weight infants. She is active in the Council of Nurse Anthropologists, the American Holistic Nurses Association, and the Holistic Nursing Credentialing board and other professional organizations.

HOW TO USE THIS TEXT

Special features in *Maternity Nursing Care* will help you master content and gain confidence in your skills in providing effective care to maternity clients and their families. Following are suggestions on how to use these special features.

CHAPTER OPENERS

Get a flavor for what is to come in the chapter by reading these thought-provoking scenarios. Question your preconceived notions on the topic at hand and challenge yourself to be open-minded about the material you are about to read.

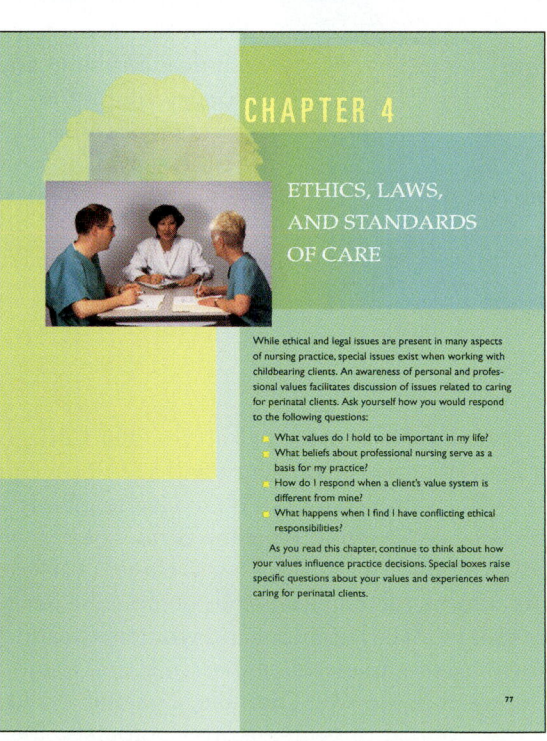

CHAPTER 4

ETHICS, LAWS, AND STANDARDS OF CARE

While ethical and legal issues are present in many aspects of nursing practice, special issues exist when working with childbearing clients. An awareness of personal and professional values facilitates discussion of issues related to caring for perinatal clients. Ask yourself how you would respond to the following questions:

- What values do I hold to be important in my life?
- What beliefs about professional nursing serve as a basis for my practice?
- How do I respond when a client's value system is different from mine?
- What happens when I find I have conflicting ethical responsibilities?

As you read this chapter, continue to think about how your values influence practice decisions. Special boxes raise specific questions about your values and experiences when caring for perinatal clients.

77

KEY TERMS

Pretest your knowledge of the subject matter by reviewing the list of key terms at the beginning of each chapter. Make a list of terms you need to learn, and watch for them as you read the material. Once you complete the chapter, revisit the list to gauge how your mastery of the terms has changed; then use the list of terms as you prepare to take your exams.

COMPETENCIES

Read this list of targeted objectives before you begin reading the chapter, so you have a grasp of the scope and depth of the content to be presented. Note any questions you may have about unfamiliar topics, then refer back to these questions as you study to test how well you have met these objectives.

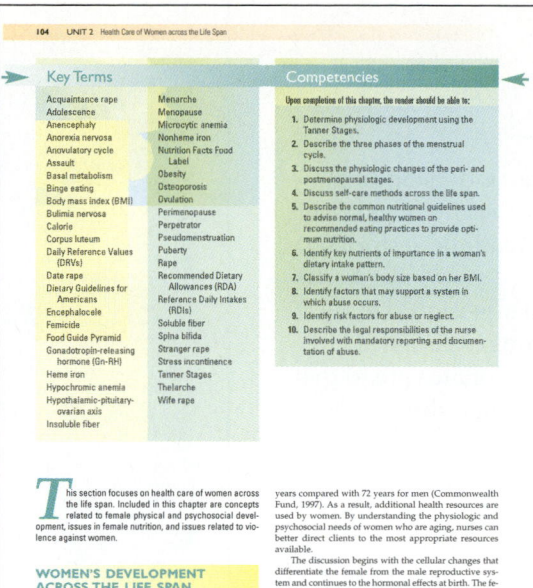

COLLABORATIVE CARE BOXES

Nurses are important members of an interdisciplinary health care team. Understanding how these various specialists function will improve overall client care. As you read each box, ask yourself what your understanding is of the different roles and responsibilities of the various care team members, and how nurses can best interact with these professionals to maximize positive client outcomes.

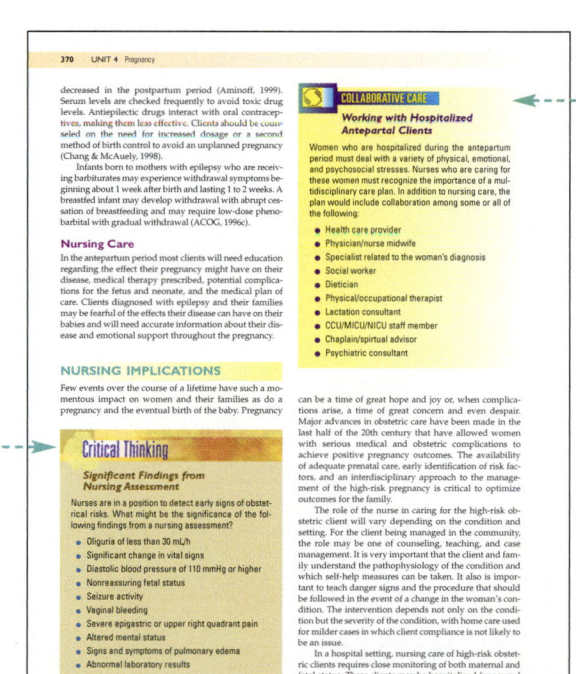

CRITICAL THINKING

Sprinkled throughout the text at key spots, these boxes encourage you to stop and ask yourself how well you have processed the material presented. Are you able to answer the questions or respond to the challenges? If you feel uneasy or unsure, reread the content until you can confidently respond to the critical thinking activities.

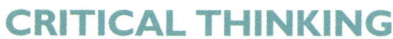

REFLECTIONS FROM NURSES AND FAMILIES

A significant aspect of nursing care is understanding how different situations affect the parties involved, both nurses and clients/families. As you read these stories, try and put yourself in the shoes of the storyteller to ask yourself, "How would I react in that situation? Do I understand the emotions and reactions experienced by this storyteller? Could I offer compassionate care to that individual, or can I grow from having had this experience?"

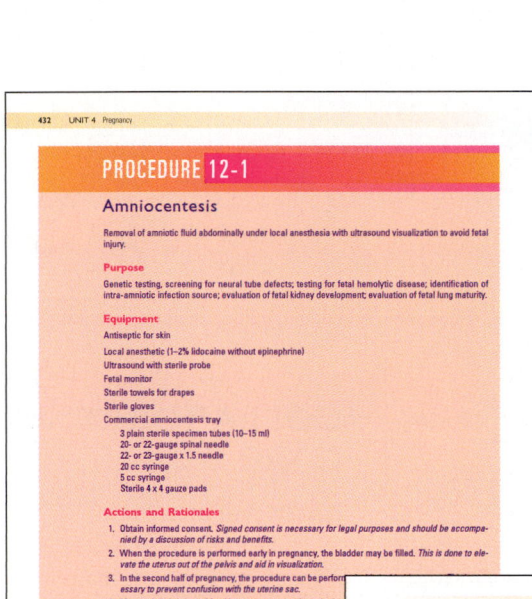

PROCEDURES

Learn to safely and effectively deliver client care by studying these step-by-step instructions for performing skills. Ask yourself if you understand the purpose, equipment, actions, rationales, and follow-up associated with each procedure.

DRUG BOXES

Delivering medications is a critical and potentially intimidating nursing responsibility. Carefully review each drug box to ensure that you have a thorough understanding of the effects, dosages, adverse reactions, contraindications, nursing considerations, and teaching responsibilities for each drug.

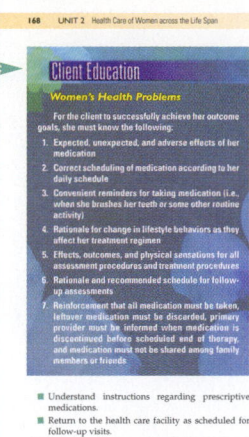

CLIENT EDUCATION

Clients often approach nurses first when they have health concerns. Read and understand these boxes to learn how to discuss difficult and sensitive topics, to offer sound clinical advice, and to help identify potential health problems or self-care measures for clients.

NURSING TIPS

Experienced nurses have a wealth of information that can benefit you as you begin your career in nursing. You will be better prepared and more efficient by taking to heart these helpful hints, tips, and strategies from skilled nurses.

NURSING ALERTS

Critical situations arise in health care, and nurses must be able to identify and respond accurately and, in some cases, rapidly. Make a list of these boxes in each chapter to ensure that you fully understand not only what the issue is, but also how to react to ensure the healthiest outcome for the client and family.

Administration of Spinal Anesthesia

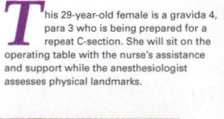

*T*his 29-year-old female is a gravida 4, para 3 who is being prepared for a repeat C-section. She will sit on the operating table with the nurse's assistance and support while the anesthesiologist assesses physical landmarks.

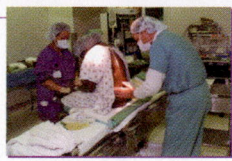

Upon identification of landmarks, preparations are made to cleanse the injection site.

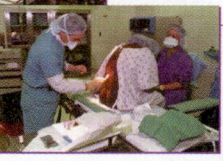

The nurse has the responsibility to promote client comfort and limit motion during the procedure.

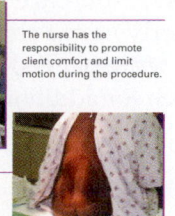

Once the area surrounding the injection site is cleansed, a sterile sponge is used to remove Betadine (povidone-iodine) from the injection site.

PHOTO STORIES

Five step-by-step photo stories are included in Chapters 13, 14, and 20. These visually stunning depictions of procedures and nursing care emphasize clinical excellence and the nurse-client relationship.

CASE STUDY/CARE PLAN

Real-world scenarios are included to walk you through the nursing process as applied to a particular client situation. As you read these, see if you agree with the nursing diagnoses, nursing interventions, and nursing outcomes, and challenge yourself to identify additional areas of client care that would be appropriate.

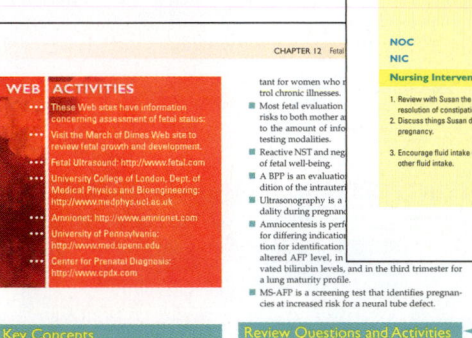

WEB ACTIVITIES

Continue and expand your learning by following the suggested activities in these boxes. Search the Internet for additional resources or to answer challenge questions to confirm your understanding of content.

KEY CONCEPTS

Use this listing of the main content points covered in the chapter as you study and prepare to take exams. Identify areas where your knowledge is not as strong as you would like it to be, and reread those sections of the chapter.

REVIEW QUESTIONS AND ACTIVITIES

Prior to reading the chapter, take a look at these activities and see how much you know about the content. Once you have read the chapter, revisit these questions to see how well you have mastered the material.

REFERENCES, SUGGESTED READINGS, AND RESOURCES

These resources emphasize the research base underlying the chapter content. Use them as you write papers, test your knowledge, or search for additional facts.

HOW TO USE THE ONLINE COMPANION

HOW TO USE THE STUDYWARE™ ONLINE COMPANION

The StudyWare™ Online Companion helps you learn terms and concepts in *Maternity Nursing Care*. As you study each chapter in the text, be sure to explore the activities in the corresponding chapter in the Online Companion. Use StudyWare as your own private tutor to help you learn the material in your *Maternity Nursing Care* textbook.

Getting started is easy:

- Go to www.delmarhealthcare.com/health.
- Click on the link for Online Companions, then on the link for Nursing.
- Click on *Maternity Nursing Care* in the alphabetized list.
- Click on the link for StudyWare. When the StudyWare program starts, enter your name so you can track your quiz scores.

Now you can choose a chapter from the menu and take a quiz or explore one of the activities.

Menus

You can access any of the menus from wherever you are in the program. The menus are organized by chapter and include quizzes, activities, and scores.

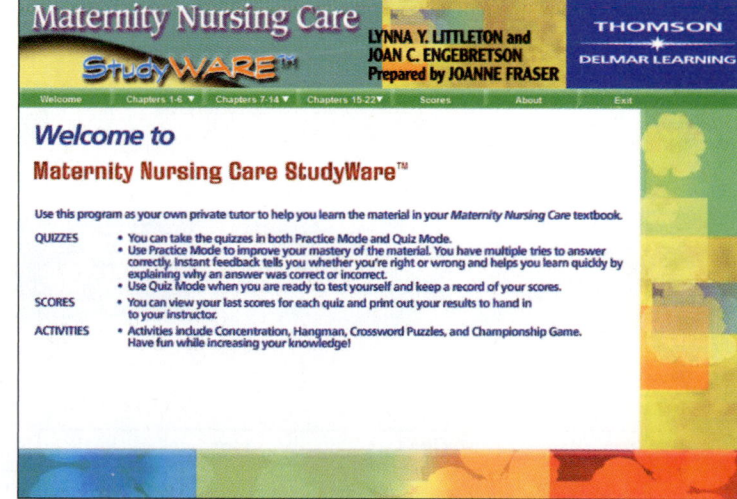

Quizzes. Quizzes include multiple choice, true/false, and fill in the blank questions. You can take the quizzes in both Practice Mode and Quiz Mode. Use Practice Mode to improve your mastery of the material. You have multiple tries to get the answers correct and are assisted by hints on wrong answers. Use Quiz Mode when you are ready to test yourself and keep a record of your scores. In Quiz Mode, you have one try to get the answers right before submitting them.

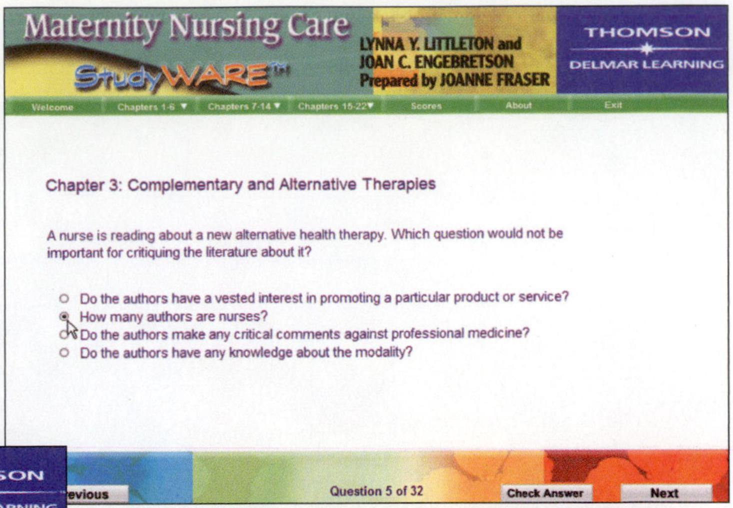

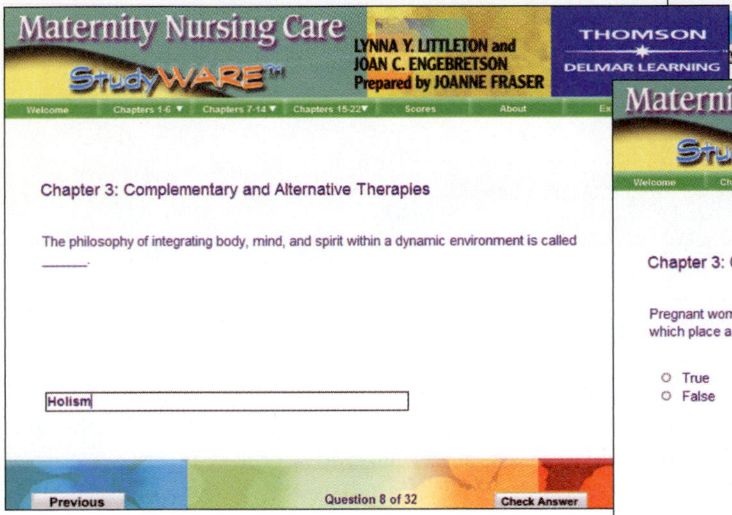

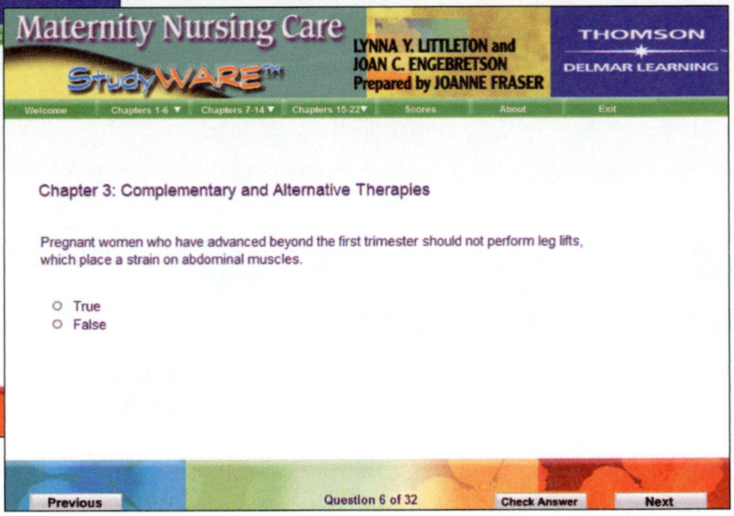

Scores. You can view your last scores for each quiz and print out your results to hand in to your instructor.

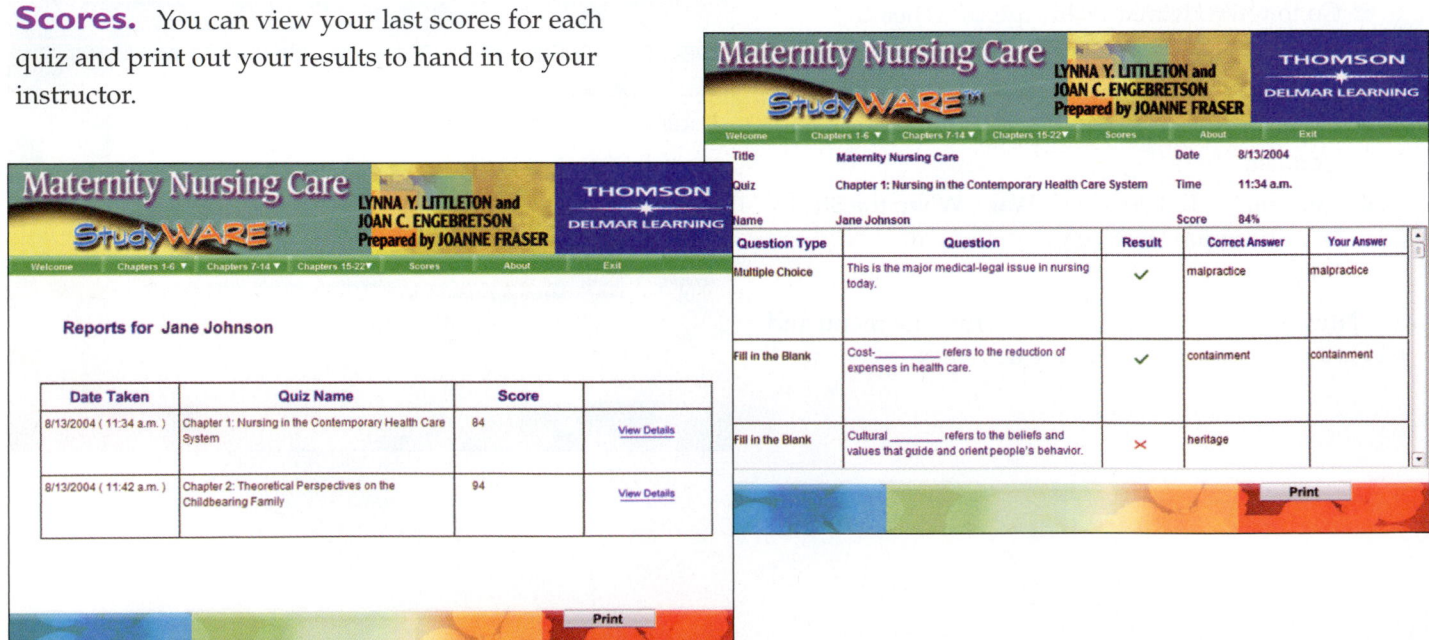

Activities. Activities include hangman, concentration, crossword puzzles, and a Jeopardy-style championship game. Have fun while increasing your knowledge!

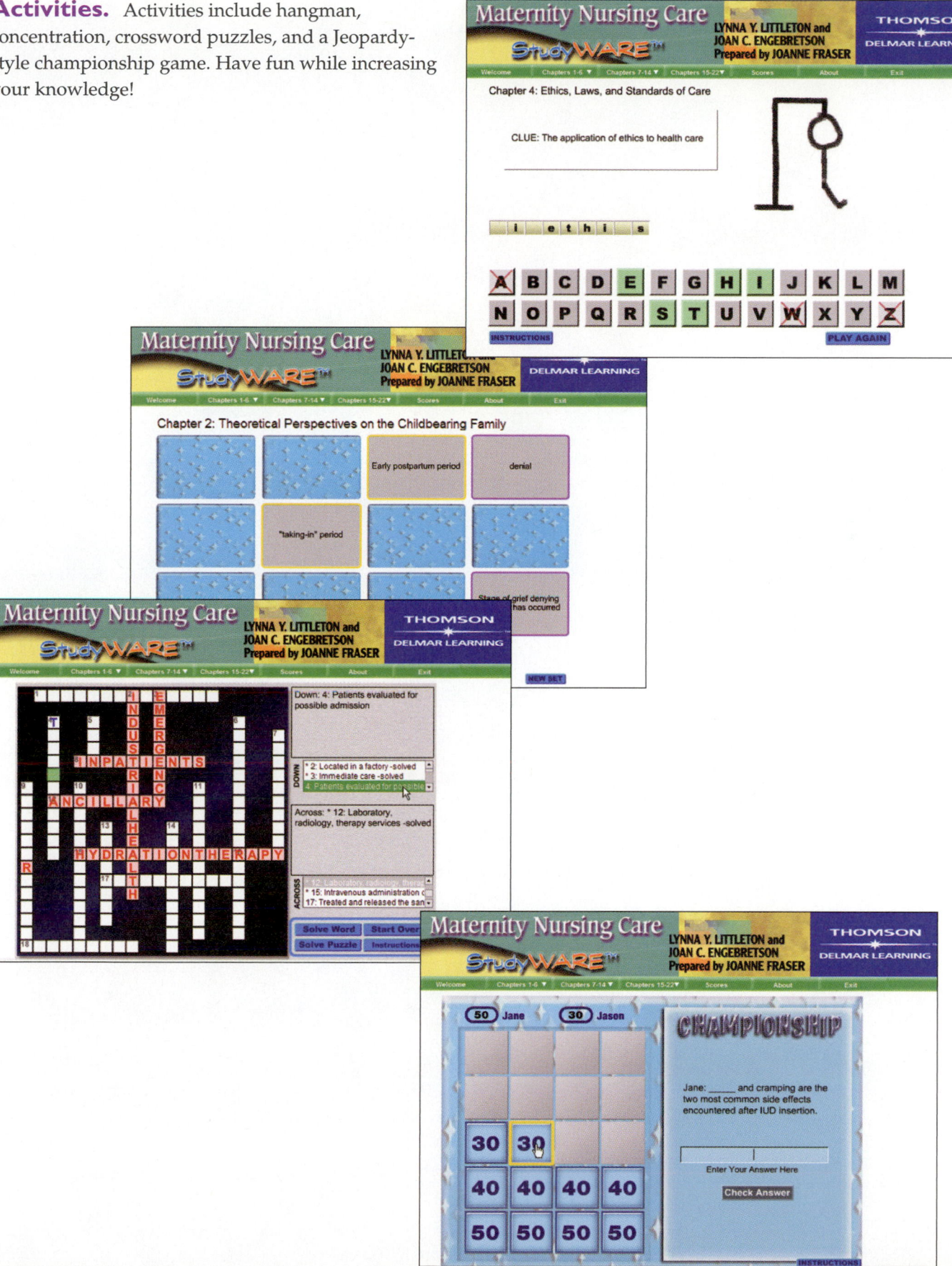

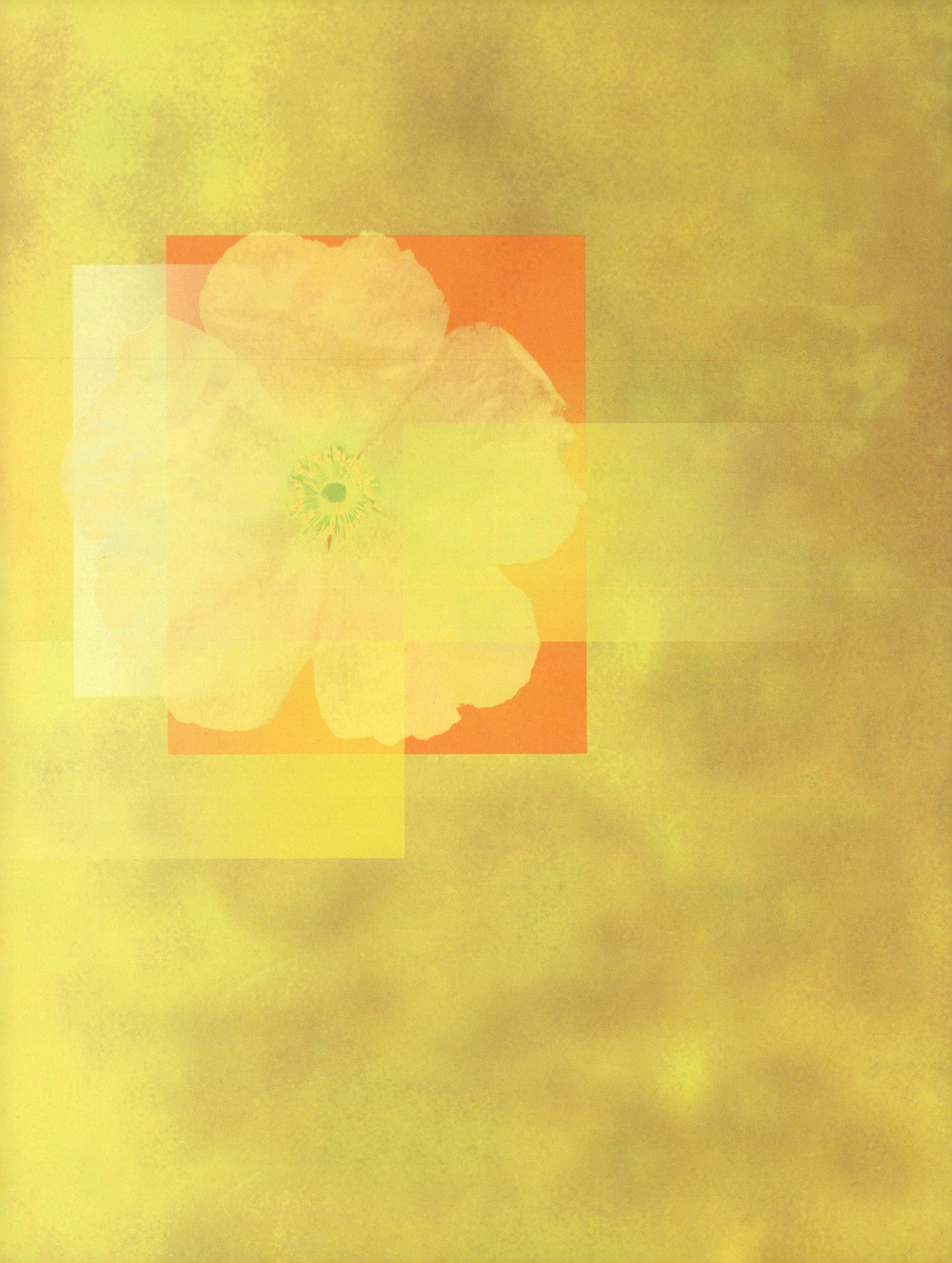

UNIT 1

Foundations of Maternal, Neonatal, and Women's Health Nursing

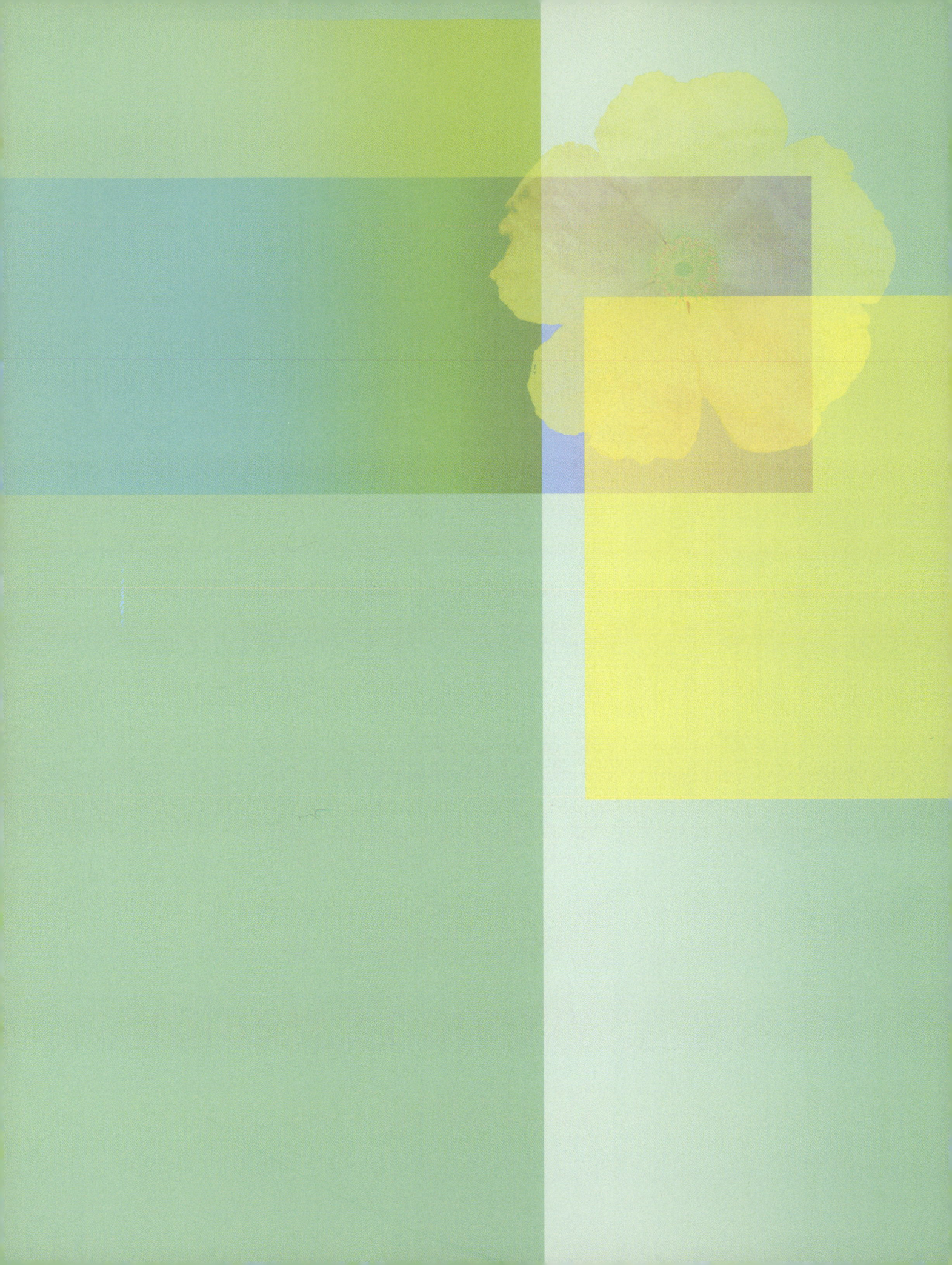

CHAPTER 1

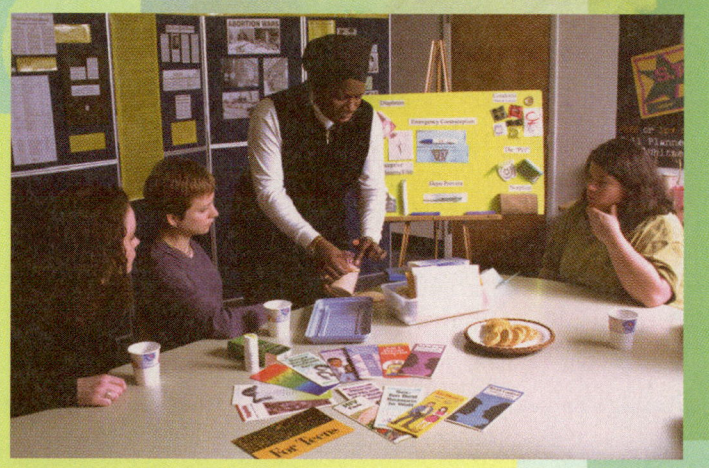

NURSING IN THE CONTEMPORARY HEALTH CARE SYSTEM

Understanding the contemporary health care system is vital to providing effective and appropriate nursing care. Understanding how your personal beliefs and values may influence your interpretation of the system is also important. Consider the following:

- Have I ever wondered what health means?
- How does the health care system help keep clients healthy?
- If I am sick and see a clinician in Idaho, would I receive the same quality of care as I would in Connecticut?
- What are the things that affect my health?
- Who pays for expensive methods of diagnoses and treatments?
- How do people in other cultures think about health, illness, and disease?

Key Terms

Cost containment
Cultural competence
Disease prevention
Early detection
Evidence-based practice
Goals

Health promotion
Interdisciplinary teams
Managed care
Position statement
Risk assessment

Competencies

Upon completion of this chapter, the reader should be able to:

1. Describe the shift in health care delivery to encompass health outcomes.
2. Identify national goals and guidelines that direct the health care industry.
3. Discuss measures that have been undertaken to contain health care costs.
4. Describe some contemporary challenges facing all health care providers.
5. List effective leadership strategies nurses use to promote collaboration on health care teams.
6. Discuss pertinent issues related to maternal, neonatal, and women's health.
7. Give examples of technologic advances in the field of maternal, neonatal, and women's health.
8. Analyze the importance of goals and guidelines for the practicing nurse.

Health care is affected by many factors both within the health care industry and external to it. Health care has expanded the focus beyond disease treatment to disease prevention and health promotion. A dual emphasis of cost containment and prevention has moved much of health care delivery into the community and even into client's homes. Nurses are now functioning on multidisciplinary teams.

In response to health care disparities, national objectives have been established and outcomes are being tracked. Guidelines are available to assist the clinician in providing the best care. A number of discoveries are changing our understanding of health, illness, disease, and treatment. These discoveries also have raised ethical issues and stirred controversy as they challenge some of the previous ideas about health. Nurses need specific skills to practice in the current health care system.

CURRENT STATE OF HEALTH CARE DELIVERY

Throughout history, most models of health care have been focused on diagnosis and treatment of diseases and disorders. In the late 20th century the delivery of health care, especially in the United States, underwent changes related to scientific and technologic advances. In addition to more sophisticated methods of diagnosing and treating disease, these advances expanded the focus of health beyond disease and treatment of the person to the broader concepts of health maintenance and the health of populations. The delivery of health care also was becoming very expensive, and, therefore, economics was a major factor in the changes made in health care.

Technologic Advancement for Diagnosis and Treatment

Technologic development has transformed the way diseases are diagnosed and treated; however, medical advances often increase the costs of health care. Computerized technologies and microtechnology have allowed for more accurate monitoring and for management of intricate dynamic physiologic systems. For example, diagnostic tests and surgery can be performed on a fetus in utero to determine and limit future health problems. The future holds unlimited technologies and microtechnology that will be applied to health care.

Focus on Health

The focus of health care has moved beyond specific diseases of individuals or public health concerns of containing or preventing epidemics. This broadened focus took three forms: early detection and treatment of disease, disease prevention, and health promotion.

Early detection allows for early intervention. More sensitive and specific screening techniques have become available to identify the early stages of a disease, when early treatment may reduce its development (Figure 1-1). Mammograms are an example of health screening.

Disease prevention consists of measures taken to prevent the onset of a disease or disorder. Immunizing nonpregnant women against rubella is an example of preventing complications from fetal exposure to the disease.

Health promotion is a broad concept and includes actions that enhance the quality of life and reduce the risk of disease such as developing good stress management skills.

The emphasis on disease prevention and health promotion has permeated most of health care. Government agencies and private foundations have been developing recommendations to move the health care system toward promoting better health for the entire population. Health indicators have been identified that allow more accurate evaluation of the health of the U.S. population and that identify risk factors that may be targeted for better health outcomes. Awareness of inequalities in the health of dif-

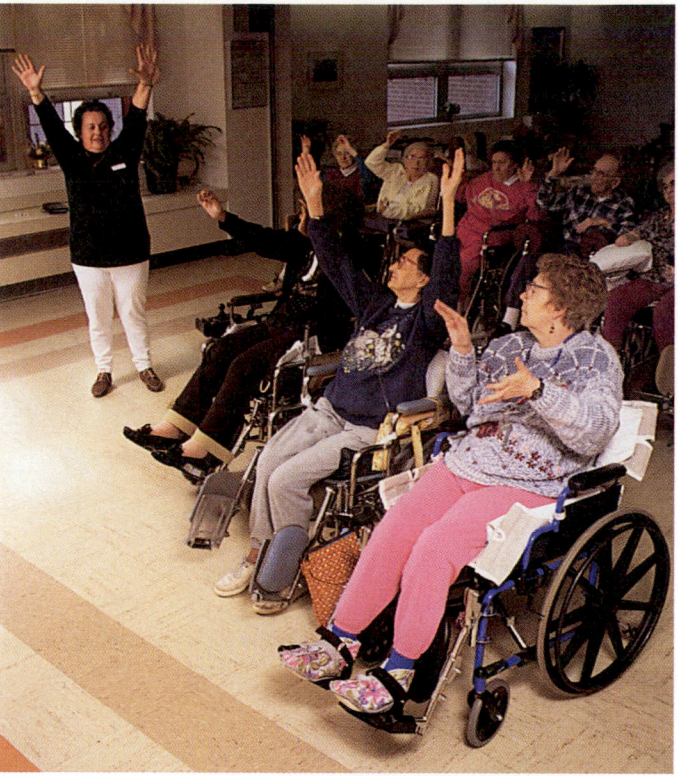

Figure 1-2   Health promotion activities may include exercises appropriate to the client's age and ability.

ferent groups of people has been the stimulus for developing programs to improve the availability and quality of health care for all (Figure 1-2). With the emphasis on health, health care services and programs are increasingly being provided in community settings, with individuals and communities engaged as partners in the pursuit of health. Healthy People 2010 has as a major goal to reduce health disparities.

Establishment of Health Goals

The emphasis on health was reflected in the 1979 publication of "Healthy People: The Surgeon General's Report on Health Promotion and Disease Prevention" (USDHHS, 1979). This document outlined goals and strategies to improve the health of the nation. These goals have been evaluated and new goals and specific objectives toward health are established each decade. The first "Healthy People" document outlined three broad strategies: disease prevention (activities that prevent a disease or disorder), health promotion, and health protection (USDHHS 1979).

The current goals (Healthy People 2010) support the elimination of health disparities and outline several health indicators in the goals for the nation (Box 1-1).

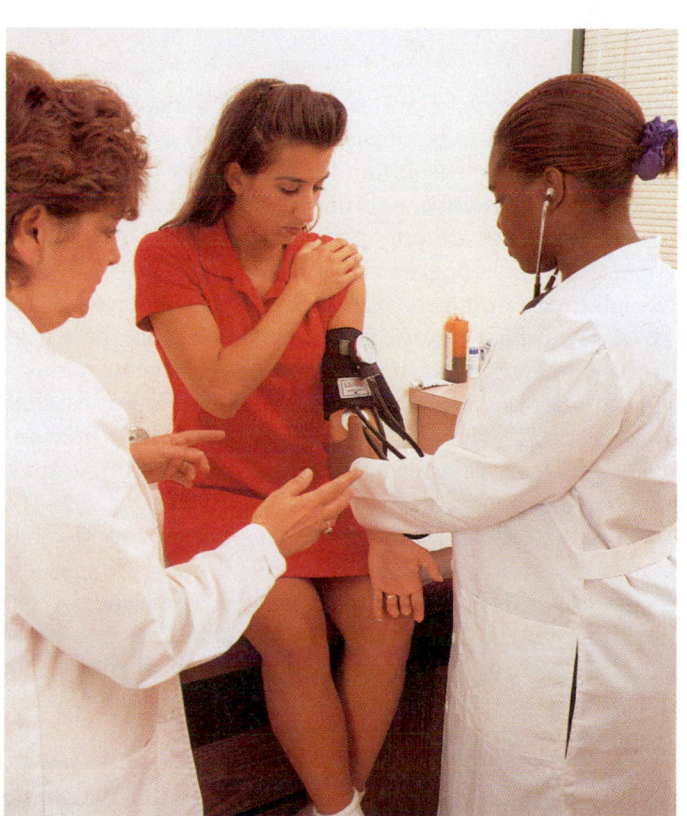

Figure 1-1   Routine blood pressure measurements are useful for early detection of some health problems.

Box 1-1

Leading Indicators for "Healthy People 2010"

- Physical activity
- Overweight and obesity
- Tobacco use
- Substance abuse
- Sexual behavior
- Mental health
- Injury and violence
- Environmental quality
- Immunization
- Access to health care

Risk Assessment and Management

Factors have been identified that could predict with some degree of probability that a person might develop a disease in the future. **Risk assessment** is the process of examining the risk factors that place a person at risk for disease.

Risk assessment and management are now part of basic clinical care. Some risk factors can be altered, thereby decreasing the probability of acquiring a disease. Changing dietary and exercise behaviors are examples of initiating change to lower cholesterol levels, thereby reducing the risks of coronary artery disease, the number 1 killer of women.

Nursing Tip *ANA Position Statement*

The American Nurses Association (ANA) issued a position statement supporting the promotion of health and prevention of disease and illness and disability. This position advocates comprehensive primary, secondary, and tertiary levels of prevention and engaging client participation. Prevention has long been within the scope of nursing as nurses work toward wellness with clients, families, and communities (ANA, 1995b).

Movement of Health Care to the Community

Consistent with the shift in emphasis toward health, interventions have also shifted from large hospitals into the community in which the holistic approach has come to be recognized as increasingly important. New types of care delivery are emerging, such as day hospitals, day surgery, and transitional care, to move clients from the hospital to the home or other community setting. Nurses are frequently providing both high-risk perinatal and neonatal care in the home as well as in hospitals and clinics. Nurses have had to incorporate interdisciplinary knowledge and cognitive skills to respond to this change in focus. As risk factors become better understood, psychologic, social, and environmental factors frequently are being implicated as contributors to health.

Cost Containment

The costs of health care have continued to increase. Much of the increase is related to the high cost of technology and the expense of educating and training personnel to operate and interpret this technology. More often today, nurses are being asked to consider the cost-benefit ratio of their actions.

Health Disparities

Ethnic, racial, gender, and socioeconomic disparities have been documented. Emphasis is placed on understanding the relationship of health and the effects of poverty. Currently, the large number of uninsured is an area of great concern. Differences among population groups exist even when racial and ethnic gaps in income and health insurance coverage are eliminated (Weinick, Zuvekas, & Cohen, 2000).

A second aspect of disparities in health is the variation in practice patterns and the gap between what is known scientifically about medical treatment and what is practiced. The inequalities in health care led to an evaluation of access to health care services and redirecting resources to expand access.

The Institute of Medicine also has issued a report that lays out a strategy to reduce medical errors that is directed toward government, industry, consumers, and health providers. The strategy was initiated because of reports of death and injury as a result of medical errors. The goal is to reduce medical errors by 50% in the next 5 years (Kohn, Corrigan, Donaldson, 2000).

A third aspect of reducing disparities is the move toward **evidence-based practice**, which is a systematic approach that uses existing research for clinical decision processes (Westhoff, 2000). Organizations are striving to provide cost-effective care based on the best evidence.

Health care administrators are increasingly monitoring the outcomes of delivery of care in their organizations. This process involves gathering data on the status of client outcomes. For example, an organization may want to look at outcomes of deliveries and then compare them (e.g., the rate of cesarean sections or postpartum infections) with other institutions that are of similar size and have similar clientele. This process is called benchmarking. The organizations would evaluate their practice with guidelines, standards, and the literature on evidence-based practice. The organizations would then attempt to implement these guidelines, standards, and recommended practices and may alter the way care is delivered to meet those standards and improve outcomes. Many hospitals hire nurses for positions as outcomes managers. These nurses gather and analyze data from outcomes and may be involved in problem-solving techniques, such as continuous quality improvement, to achieve or improve on the benchmark standards.

Managed Care

The advent of managed care has had a major impact on the U.S. health care delivery system in the last decade of the 20th century. **Managed care** refers to health care plans with a selective list of providers and institutions from which the recipient is entitled to receive health care that is reimbursed by the insurer (Committee on the Future of Primary Care, 1996). Typically, managed care plans also control the nature, amount, and site of services provided. Access to specialists may be restricted through the use of primary care providers as gatekeepers to the system (Mezey & McGivern, 1999).

Three types of managed care plans currently exist: preferred provider organizations (PPOs), health maintenance organizations (HMOs), and point-of-service plans (POS). PPOs allow the consumer to see any provider or use any health care institution. The rate of reimbursement, however, is better when a provider or institution within the network is used.

Health maintenance organizations offer the consumer fewer options. Consumers must identify a primary care provider from a list of providers. When specialist care is sought there must be a referral from the primary care provider or the expenses will not be reimbursed. The incentives for consumers to use this type of care usually are that the plan requires only a small copayment ($10 to $25) and all other expenses are covered by the plan. In HMO plans, hospitalization is usually covered by insurance, with a small copayment ($10 to $25).

Point-of-service plans are more flexible but more expensive for the consumer than are the other plans. PPOs allow the insured to be a member of an HMO but also seek health care outside the HMO at increased cost.

Initially, cost-containment measures focused on early discharge. Later, care maps, critical pathways, guidelines, and protocols were developed to streamline client care and make it cost-effective. Because nursing salaries are one of the major costs, many times hospital administrators choose to reduce staff or substitute licensed vocational nurses or technicians as a means of cost reduction. Later, administrators often realize the lack of wisdom in this decision and look at the necessity of having more advance-degree nurses on staff.

Development of Collaborative Teams

With the broader focus on health and the simultaneous concerns of improving effective care for all while containing costs, collaborative efforts from a variety of disciplines are necessary (Figure 1-3). *Multidisciplinary care* has been described as sequential provision of discipline-specific health care by various persons, whereas *interdisciplinary care* includes coordination, joint decision making, communication, shared responsibility, and shared authority (Dossey, Keegan, & Guzzetta, 2000).

The Pew Health Professions Commission (1998) proposed a set of 21 competencies for all health professionals; these are found in Box 1-2. These 21 competencies were further differentiated for various practice levels of nursing: Licensed Practical Nurse (LPN), Associate Degree in Nursing, (ADN), Bachelor of Science in Nursing (BSN), and those with a Master of Science in Nursing (MSN) degree (Brady et al., 1999).

Working closely on **interdisciplinary teams** (health care delivered by persons from various disciplines who share responsibility, authority, and decision making) has allowed professionals from different disciplines to understand other disciplines and appreciate their contributions

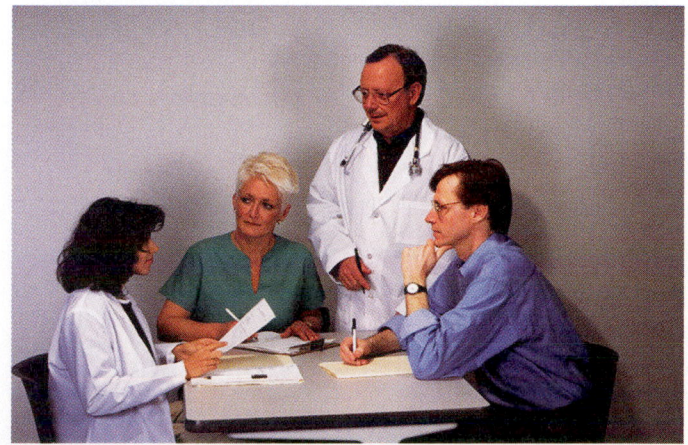

Figure 1-3   Multidisciplinary care involves coordination and joint decision making with members of other health disciplines.

Box 1-2

Twenty-one Competencies for the 21st Century

1. Embrace a personal ethic of social responsibility and service.
2. Exhibit ethical behavior in all professional activities.
3. Provide evidence-based, clinically competent care.
4. Incorporate the multiple determinants of health in clinical care.
5. Apply knowledge of the new sciences.
6. Demonstrate critical thinking, reflection, and problem-solving skills.
7. Understand the role of primary care.
8. Rigorously practice preventive health care.
9. Integrate population-based care and services into practice.
10. Improve access to health care for those with unmet health needs.
11. Practice relationship-centered care with individuals and families.
12. Provide culturally sensitive care to a diverse society.
13. Partner with communities in health care decisions.
14. Use communication and information technology effectively and appropriately.
15. Work in interdisciplinary teams.
16. Ensure care that balances individual, professional, system, and societal needs.
17. Practice leadership.
18. Take responsibility for quality of care and health outcomes at all levels.
19. Contribute to continuous improvement of the health care system.
20. Advocate for public policy that promotes and protects the health of the public.
21. Continue to learn and help others learn.

Note: From *Recreating Health Professional Practice for a New Century. The Fourth Report of the Pew Health Professions Commission,* by Pew Health Professions Commission, December 1998, San Francisco: Author.

 **COLLABORATIVE CARE**

Health Care Team for a Woman in Labor

In today's health care system, members of the team collaborate to meet the client's health care needs. A client in labor and delivery may have the following professionals participating in her care:

- Anesthesiologist/nurse anesthetist
- Laboratory professionals
- Nurse manager
- Nurse midwife
- Nurse practitioner/clinical nurse specialist
- Nutritionist
- Obstetrician/gynecologist
- Pediatrician
- Pharmacist
- Staff nurse

to client care, as well as better understand different perspectives. Ideally, this approach offers the most comprehensive care to clients; however, it also requires good communication skills. Most disciplines have developed their own language, perspectives, and unique body of knowledge. It may not be easy to understand the perspective of persons in another discipline or their contribution to care. Conversely, nurses sometimes find it challenging to articulate the perspective and contribution of nursing.

The Pew Commission made a number of recommendations on scope of practice and regulation of professions that would inform and protect the public against the actions of health care professionals outside of their scope of practice (Pew Charitable Trust Commission on Health Professions, 1995). Nurses often find that they are collaborating with other nurses and with nurses at other levels of practice. For example, an ADN-prepared nurse may be working with an advanced practice nurse (APN). It is important to be clear on the unique professional perspective of nursing and the scope of practice at each level to effectively collaborate.

Changing Demographics

The U.S. demographics are changing. Trends in ethnic distribution and the projected increases in the population of older persons have implications for health care provision.

A dramatic increase has occurred in U.S. ethnic and minority populations. The U.S. Census Bureau has classified people according to race as African American, Caucasian, other races, and people of Hispanic origin. According to Census Bureau projections, European Americans are the majority; however, African Americans, Hispanics, and other ethnic groups are increasing at a faster rate. Projections of the increase in population between 1995 and 2050 are as follows: Caucasians are expected to increase by 35.1%, African Americans by 82.8%, other races by 233.9%, and Hispanics by 258.3% (Administration on Aging, 2001). As a result, health care providers are providing care to clients who often do not speak the same language and have beliefs, values, and traditions that differ from their own. Cultural competence and linguistic competence are needed to respond effectively to health care encounters with these clients.

The Office of Minority Health (OMH) has published recommendations for national standards and an outcomes-focused research agenda regarding ensuring cultural competence in health (OMH, 2001). **Cultural competency** describes a process of integrating cultural awareness in the delivery of culturally appropriate clinical care. Cultural competency is becoming a more recognized skill for all health care providers.

NURSING SKILLS FOR PROFESSIONAL PRACTICE

In the current health care system, it is not sufficient for the practicing nurse to simply follow physician's orders. As an important member of the health care team, the professional nurse is required to participate in planning and implementing effective, cost-efficient health care. This role requires a nurse who has good cognitive abilities and who is able to reason and apply sound clinical judgment. As health care and information technology continue to advance, the nurse must have adept technical skills. Nurses also need effective communication skills for counseling and educating clients and communicating professionally with the interdisciplinary team. Self-reflection also is an important skill for the nurse to advance professional and personal development. These skills are learned throughout the nurse's career; however, the foundation must be laid during basic nursing education.

Cultural competency is a skill developed through continual exposure, reflection, and awareness of cultural differences. This process begins with a recognition of the importance that cultural heritage plays in any human interaction. An understanding of one's personal heritage provides a platform from which to understand the cul-

ture of others. Cultural heritage refers to those beliefs and values that guide and orient our behavior, many of which are so integrated into daily life that one is generally unaware of one's own cultural perspective. Nurses may focus on the culture of the client when it is different from their own but are unaware of the cultural heritage of their own beliefs. This lack of awareness then takes the form of prejudices, assumptions, and expectations. Decisions may be made from this cultural basis and may therefore create ethical conflicts. Thus, it is important for nurses to be aware of their own beliefs to avoid imposing them on others. Value clarification is a strategy to increase personal awareness and make some of the beliefs explicit.

CHANGES REFLECTED IN MATERNAL, NEONATAL, AND WOMEN'S HEALTH CARE

Many factors have affected the course and practice of women's health care over the past few years and decades. Some of the most important influences are discussed.

Advances in Diagnosis and Treatment

Many advances in diagnosis and treatment have been made in the 20th century. These advances have included use of new technology, improved methods of prenatal screening, more effective methods for management, and recognition of new entities affecting health. Examples of advances in women's health are the routine use of Pap tests, mammography, and the advent of laser technology for treatment of gynecologic conditions.

In the 1960s the use of $Rh_0(D)$ immune globulin (RhoGAM) made an important contribution to maternal and newborn health by greatly reducing the number of cases of Rh isoimmunization. Before the introduction of RhoGAM, women who were Rh-negative and pregnant with an Rh-positive fetus were at risk for having an infant with hydrops, and that risk increased with each succeeding pregnancy. Since the routine administration of RhoGAM, the incidence of this condition has decreased sharply, with the exception of women who have had an early spontaneous abortion and are unaware of the need for antibody testing and immunization.

Fetal monitoring first became available in the 1970s for general use. It was developed to reduce the incidence of fetal intrauterine hypoxic ischemic events that occur during labor. As a result, the number of children born with brain damage and the incidence of unnecessary

Reflections from a Nurse

I have been in nursing for almost 40 years and in maternal, neonatal, and women's health for most of that time. Expectations of nurses have changed radically during my career to the extent that the practice of nursing today requires much more responsibility and accountability for tasks that were not in the nursing domain when I went into practice. I wish I could predict how maternal, neonatal, and women's health nursing will change over the next 40 years. As I near retirement, if I were asked what advice I would give new graduates into the profession, I would say to never be afraid of taking risks or accepting change. In taking risks, however, be sure that you practice within your scope of practice, within the law, and within your personal ethics—and always consider the best interests of your clients.

cesarean sections decreased. Although the technology has flaws, it is still widely used (Figure 1-4).

In the 1970s, ultrasonography became an important tool in the diagnosis of maternal, neonatal, and women's health conditions (Callen, 1994). This technology has been important in identifying ectopic pregnancy before rupture. Ultrasonography has been instrumental in facilitating other tests such as amniocentesis and chorionic villus sampling. This technology has been widely accepted and performed in pregnancy to establish gestational age, fetal anomalies, and multiple gestation. In the neonatal arena, ultrasonography has become an important tool in assessing the infant for intraventricular hemorrhage. In the women's health arena, ultrasonography has been used to screen for ovarian cancer, uterine fibroids, and endometrial cancer. This technology has advanced to the degree that three-dimensional ultrasonography is now available. An expert nurse with special training may be the provider who conducts the ultrasound evaluation (Huffman & Sandelowski, 1997).

The biophysical profile (BPP) was developed to provide additional information about fetal well-being. The BPP uses ultrasonography in combination with fetal monitoring technology to increase the reliability of prediction of negative fetal outcome. The BPP has increased the likelihood that the health care provider will identify the fetus at risk. The incidence of negative fetal outcome, however, has still not been reduced to zero.

Endoscopy has been a major advance in the diagnosis and treatment of women's health problems and has eliminated the need for major surgery in many cases. The laparoscope has been used for salpingectomy, myomectomy, and oophorectomy (Schenk & Coddington, 1999). The hysteroscope has been used for menstrual ablation to treat intractable uterine bleeding with few risks and side effects. Most recently the endoscope has been used in a transcervical, transvaginal approach to visualize the fallopian tube from the uterotubal junction to the fimbria (Surrey, 1999).

Advancement in diagnosis and treatment has been made with the Human Genome Project. The advancement has significant implications for diagnosis and treatment. Two examples of application of knowledge obtained by the Human Genome Project follow. Research has been done on the Y chromosome. Until recently, scientists had great difficulty determining its role. It was thought that the Y chromosome played a limited role in fertility (Jegalian & Lahn, 2001). New findings demonstrate that the history of this sex chromosome has been strikingly dynamic. These findings have assisted in the explanation of some infertility problems in males. If deletions occur in any of three significant areas on the Y chromosome, infertility results. This type of azoospermia may be successfully treated with intracytoplasmic sperm injection.

Another example of application of knowledge discovered from the Human Genome Project is the technology in which gene and stem cell transplantations are used to treat disease. The earliest use of this technology was to treat genetic disorders such as cystic fibrosis and Duchenne muscular dystrophy (Kaji & Leiden, 2001). Geneticists

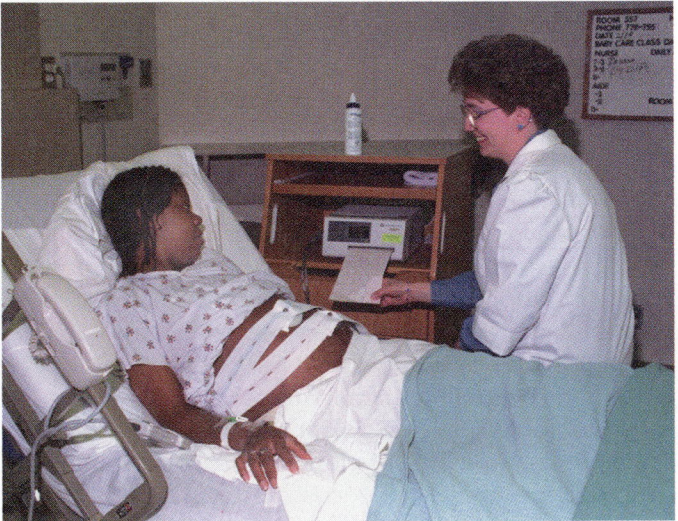

Figure 1-4 Fetal monitoring during labor is a good example of maternity care technology that has changed over the years.

Critical Thinking

Competencies in Genetics

The National Coalition for Health Professional Education in Genetics (NCHPEG, 2001) has put forth a set of core competencies in genetics essential for all health care professionals. All health care professionals should, at minimum, be able to:

- Appreciate the limitations of their expertise in genetics.
- Understand the social and psychologic implications of genetic services.
- Know how and when to make a referral to a professional in genetics.

  What do you think the role of a professional nurse is related to the criteria above?

  How would you prepare yourself to function responsibly in the area of genetics?

  How would you keep current in this area?

have identified human genes involved in many disorders involving single genes and some cancers.

Guidelines for working in the field of genetics are described in the above Critical Thinking box.

Risk Assessment and Management

Risk assessment, early identification, and prevention of complications are the essence of prenatal care. In the case of pregnant women, risk assessment is used to identify those women who have factors that contribute to having negative maternal or fetal outcomes. The risk can be biologic, behavioral, environmental, psychologic, or social. Assessments of maternal and fetal risks are completed and documented at the first visit and each additional client interaction with the health care system.

Providing neonatal care risk assessment is essential because the infant is unable to discuss signs and symptoms. Risk assessment may be the only tool available to the health care provider to predict adverse reactions and conditions. As we obtain more information about genetic makeup, risk assessment will become even more important as a tool.

Women's health care risk assessment is used to screen for cancer, domestic violence, eating disorders, and chronic diseases. Early identification and treatment can prevent illness, facilitate recovery, and prolong life.

Cost Containment and Professional Guidelines

Cost containment refers to the reduction of expenses by working more efficiently. Cost containment has come to the forefront as a factor in delivery of health care. Thus, it has become very apparent that it is no longer acceptable for individual health care providers to act without considering health care costs. Practice must become standardized, and a number of goals and guidelines have been established to guide health care providers.

Each profession sets forth guidelines for members of that profession. The American Nurses Association (ANA) sets forth policies and position statements to help guide nurses. For example, the ANA has set forth a **position statement** (formalized statement by a professional organization to express the opinion of its membership) on home care for the mother, infant, and family following birth (ANA, 1995a). This position statement strongly supports individualized postpartum care provided to the family in the home environment.

In a 1991 position statement, the ANA crafted a statement concerning physical violence against women (ANA, 1991). This statement formalized support for the education of nurses, health care providers, and women in the skills necessary to prevent violence against women.

Agencies have issued guidelines for care in maternal, neonatal, and women's health. Such agencies include the American Academy of Pediatrics (AAP); American College of Obstetricians and Gynecologists (ACOG); Association of Women's Health, Obstetric, and Neonatal Nurses (AWHONN); and National Association of Neonatal Nurses (NANN). It is important that nurses gain familiarity with these guidelines because a national standard of care is being developed based on them. This means that the individual nurse is expected to provide the same services with the same degree of skill as is any other nurse. Standardization of care is a way of protecting against negative outcomes and reducing costs.

TRENDS IN MATERNAL, NEONATAL, AND WOMEN'S HEALTH CARE

The nurse in maternal, neonatal, and women's health nursing must be aware of trends that affect practice. Whereas many trends are affecting today's health care system, some of the major factors are described in this chapter.

The past century of maternity care has been one of medicalization as physicians increasingly made decisions for women, and demedicalization as women decided they wanted control of this natural process (Figure 1-5). Today,

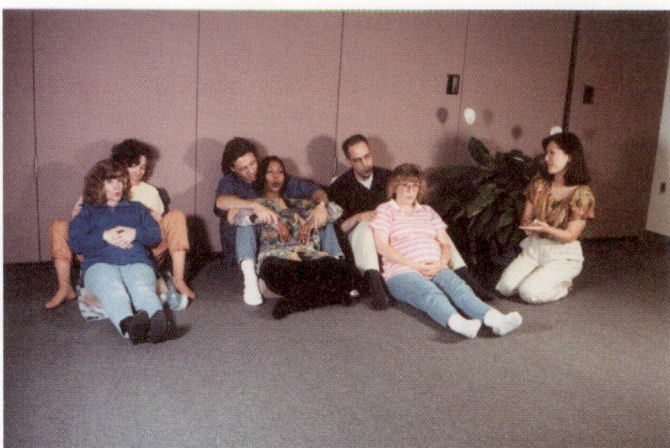

Figure 1-5   Childbirth education classes are a means for women and their partners to learn about pain management and the birth process.

more births outside of hospitals are occurring, and more women are choosing midwifery care as opposed to physician care for their childbirth experience.

Decreased Hospital Stay

Decreased hospital stays have been a major source of cost reduction in the past 10 years. In the 1980s, a 3-day hospital stay was standard for a normal delivery and a 5-day hospital stay was standard for major operative procedures such as a hysterectomy or cesarean section. In the 1990s, however, the 24-hour discharge of mother and newborn became common. After many complaints from health care professionals and clients and some tragic outcomes, Congress stepped in and federally mandated that insurance companies must cover a 48-hour hospitalization after delivery. Women may return home sooner if they request. If complications occur, the hospital stay may be extended past 48 hours. Clients having hysterectomy or cesarean section typically return home 3 to 4 days after surgery.

Reduction in Intervention

In the practice of maternal and child health care, reduction in intervention has been a major issue in the past decades. Many women consider birth a natural process. Yet historically, when they were admitted to the hospital, they had to experience childbirth under the control of physicians. Induction of labor was widespread, use of Lamaze was discouraged in many facilities, and forceps deliveries and cesarean sections were commonplace. Some of these interventions were undertaken as first choices under the advice of physicians. As women have become more verbal and cost-containment more of an issue, the first choice is now more often supportive of the natural process, with interventions used to promote maternal and fetal health.

Family-Centered Care

In 1994, Celeste Phillips, a maternity nurse, and Dr. Loel Fenwick worked together to develop the concept of family-centered maternity care. Family-centered maternity care is based on 10 principles that reverse many of the restrictive policies and practices and return choices about the childbirth process to families (Figure 1-6). This philosophy has been adopted across the country as women decide they want to be in control of their bodies and reproductive processes (Zwelling, 2000).

Community-Centered Care

There has been a trend to move maternity care away from major medical centers and to community-based facilities. The effect of this change has been twofold. Being in the community enables better family interaction in the birth process because of convenience. This practice also has caused the maternity facilities in major cities to gain a higher percentage of high-risk maternity clients, changing the client demographics of and increasing the costs to these facilities.

Evidence-Based Practice

As mentioned previously, evidence-based practice is a systematic approach to finding, appraising, and judiciously using research results as a basis for clinical decision making (Westhoff, 2000). This type of systematic approach to decision making is becoming more popular in health care in general but specifically in maternal,

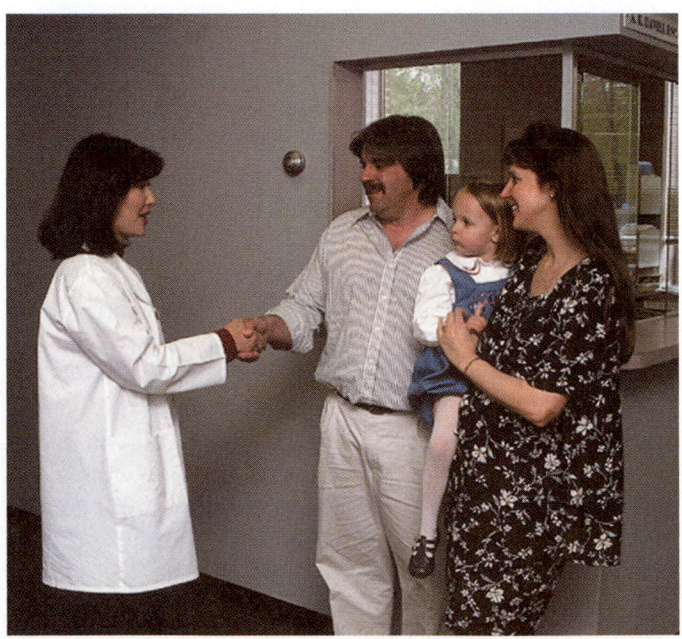

Figure 1-6   Family-centered care involves family members, in addition to the pregnant woman, in decision-making processes.

neonatal, and women's health. For example, the University of Texas Health Science Center at San Antonio, Texas, is studying management of chronic hypertension in pregnancy and management of chronic fatigue syndrome, a condition seen more commonly in women (AHRQ, 2000a and 2001).

UNDERSTANDING WOMEN'S HEALTH

The many elements that overall comprise women's health are discussed.

Biologic Issues

Until the 1990s it was assumed that the biology of men and that of women were identical and, therefore, what worked in the treatment of men should work for women. In the 1990s, the public began to question the validity of this assumption. As a result of this questioning, the Women's Health Initiative was begun to study parameters of women's health. It became apparent that women metabolize alcohol, experience heart disease, and metabolize medications differently than do men. The Women's Health Initiative currently is studying other biologic differences between men and women. One area of investigation is the interrelationship of hormones and mental health.

Behavioral Issues

Behavior is a very important component of health. It is becoming increasingly apparent that obesity is a particular problem in our society. Being overweight contributes to the development of chronic diseases such as diabetes, hypertension, and cardiovascular disease. The negative health effects of being overweight can be prevented by early identification and treatment. Overeating in pregnancy contributes to the development of gestational diabetes, increases the risks for negative fetal outcomes because of macrosomia and hypoglycemia, and increases the woman's risk of developing adult-onset diabetes later in life. Because gestational diabetes is a major health problem in the United States, the Centers for Disease Control and Prevention (CDC, 1986) issued guidelines for enhancing diabetes control through maternal and child health programs. Despite these guidelines the incidence of gestational diabetes has not decreased.

Environmental Issues

Rural women face unique and specific health challenges regarding health care access as a result of geographic and occupational circumstances. Many women in the United States are farmworkers. An estimated 313,000 farmworkers may suffer from pesticide-related illnesses each year and from 800 to 1,000 farmworkers die each year as a direct result of pesticide exposure (Gaston, 2001).

Women are exposed regularly to teratogens in the workplace, as are men. Manicurists are exposed to inhalants that may be toxic. Nurse anesthetists have a higher rate of spontaneous miscarriage than does the normal population. There may be numerous other examples of workplace exposure to teratogens; further discussion can be found in Chapter 12.

Social Issues

In the exploration of the differences between women's and men's health, a leading question is biologic compared with sociocultural determinants to explain these patterns. An attempt to differentiate between these factors was discussed in the Agenda for Research on Women's Health for the 21st Century (USDHHS, 1999). One suggestion was to use the terms *sex* and *gender*, respectively, to refer to biologic and sociocultural differences. This differentiation is similar to the one between race and ethnicity, which refer to biologic and sociocultural factors, respectively.

As we come to understand more about the effects of socioeconomic status on health, we find that many of the issues disproportionately affect women. Greater numbers of women live at low income or poverty levels, both in single-parent families and among older persons (Administration on Aging, 2001). Poverty affects not only access to health but also many of the resources needed to promote health such as a healthy diet and places to exercise. Lack of power and social status creates additional stressors that can be damaging to one's health over time. Women have different patterns of health care use than do men; women use health care services more than men and, on average, live longer than men.

Women's social roles and expectations also impact their health. Women's roles as mothers may make them more aware of health and more receptive to health education because they are eager to promote the health of their families (Loustaunau & Sobo, 1997). In many families, however, women may play a subservient role to their male partners. If the family is prone to domestic violence, women are more likely to be the victims. Women may be reluctant to leave an abusive relationship because of the role expectations of wife and mother. Women also may relate to their doctor or nurse practitioner in a different manner than do men relevant to their social roles.

In industrialized countries as women joined the labor force, generally their fertility rates declined. In developing countries, this relationship is much more complex

(Sargent & Brettell, 1995). In many cases women see clear, concrete advantages to reducing their own fertility; however, social pressures may make it impossible for them to do so. This contradiction between beliefs and reality may lead to physical and emotional overburdening of women, posing health threats to these women and their children.

Cultural Issues

Women's roles are determined by culture. In many cultures, women make decisions about their health and that of their family. Culture also determines many activities of women that have health implications. Cultural beliefs and values underlie the basic assumptions about biomedicine and the delivery of health care.

Women often are the decision-makers in the home regarding nutrition, daily health practices, and treatment of minor illnesses (Figure 1-7). These decisions arise from cultural heritages and the attendant beliefs, values, and practices related to health and health-seeking behaviors. For example, dietary habits, food choices, and food preparation are based on cultural practices. Pregnancy and birth are special transition times, with particular customs and beliefs that direct activities and behaviors. These beliefs direct behavior throughout a woman's life span.

Cultural beliefs will influence a woman's social roles and her relationship with her husband and other family members. Culture also influences lifestyle and health seeking behaviors.

In many cultures, women do not have social authority to access health care outside of the family (Sargent & Brettell, 1995). Other family members, generally the woman's husband, must make the decision to go to a health

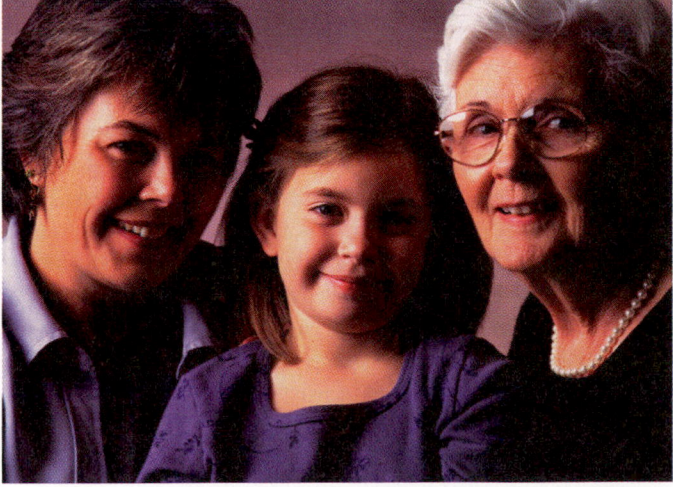

Figure 1-7 Women pass on knowledge of domestic health in many cultures.

care provider and whether to adhere to the provider's recommendations.

Complementary and Alternative Therapies

Women often use complementary and alternative therapies. Because of their use for health promotion and domestic health, these therapies may be particularly appealing to women. Women may be more inclined to use these therapies because women traditionally are in positions to nurture the health of their family members. Many of these therapies are gentle and nourishing and therefore more in keeping with women's social roles. Practice also suggests that many women use alternative therapies because of an inherent distrust of "the system."

ISSUES RELATED TO THE CARE OF WOMEN AND INFANTS

As trends in maternal, neonatal, and women's health have developed, issues have evolved that have affected practice in the field. Among those issues are access to care, medical errors, medical-legal issues, and issues related to the philosophy of care provision.

Access to Care

Access to care remains a very important issue related to maternal, neonatal, and women's health. An estimated 48 million Americans lack access to health care, and 44 million have no health care insurance (Gaston, 2001). Many of the uninsured are women. When a person does not have insurance, access to health care may be delayed and treatment may be less effective or ineffective. In addition, access to care involves the availability of appropriate health care services in the community, transportation, and childcare—and many other factors. Ensuring affordability of health care continues to be a major issue in the United States as is evidenced by public attention and congressional rhetoric.

Reduction of Medical Errors

Increasingly, medical errors have gained attention as being major causes of morbidity and mortality. The Institute of Medicine (IOM, 2000) indicates that errors usually represent plans in which the system failed and the breakdown resulted in harm. Further, the IOM suggests that errors depend on two kinds of failure: actions do not go as intended, or the intended action is not the correct one.

These two types of errors are commonly referred to as errors of execution or errors of planning, respectively. Contrary to popular belief, errors usually are not caused by incompetence (Dickenson-Hazard, 2001). In many instances, downsizing and re-engineering, which are facts of life in contemporary health care organizations, are found to be at the root of the problem (Knox et al., 1999). In some instances, organizational changes undertaken to increase productivity or cut operational costs result in systems that break down, and, often, client safety is not a primary consideration.

Nurses have been an easy target on whom to place blame for medical errors. In reality, nurses are doing their jobs in a health care system that is in turmoil. Individual nurses and nursing organizations across the country are committed to improving health care by developing practice standards, developing system improvements, and recruiting additional workers to the profession (Dickenson-Hazard, 2001).

Reducing the occurrences of medical errors must be a collaborative effort on the part of doctors, nurses, administrators, and all other health care workers (Underwood, 2001). Nurses are an important part of the solution (Figure 1-8). Client outcomes are better in hospitals with higher staffing levels and higher ratios of registered nurses in the staffing mix than in hospitals with lower levels and ratios. Nurses are fiercely committed to quality client care (Kincaide, 2001).

The Agency for Healthcare Research and Quality (AHRQ) recommends that clients become involved in their health care as a means to reduce medical errors. The AHRQ provides 20 tips in a client education fact sheet, an adaptation of which is included in the following Client Education box.

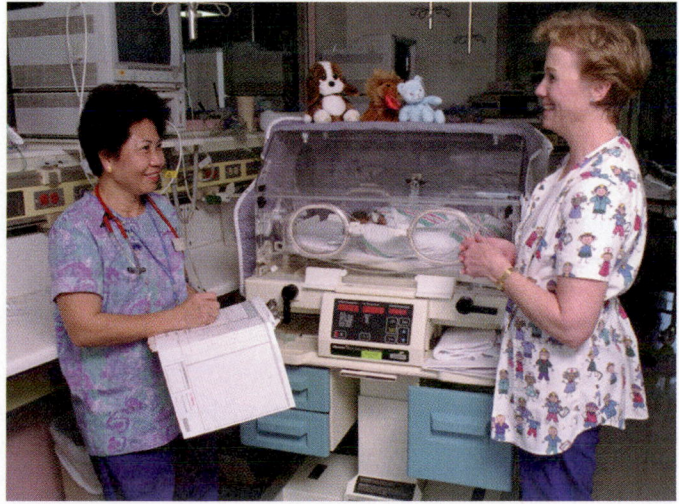

Figure 1-8   Charting is a responsibility of the entire interdisciplinary care team.

Medical-Legal Issues

The major medical-legal issue in nursing today is malpractice. *Malpractice* is a specific kind of negligence that occurs when the standard of care that reasonably can be expected is not performed (Aiken & Catalano, 1994). Four elements are required to prove liability for malpractice:

1. Duty
2. Breach of the standard of care
3. Proximate cause
4. Harm to the client

Further discussion of the concepts involved with proving malpractice will help clarify the meaning of these elements and make them more easily understood.

The concept of duty is a legal term that means that the nurse has or should have undertaken the care of the client in the capacity of a nurse. Duty may be independent of payment for services (Hall, 1996). For example, a nurse comes to the labor and delivery unit to deliver a message to another nurse. As she enters the unit, it is very apparent there is a crisis situation because the nurses are engaged in preparing for an emergency cesarean section. As the nurse passes a client's room, the client calls out: "Nurse. Can you help me?" The nurse is from the neonatal unit and has no experience in dealing with laboring women. She has no duty to assist this client. If the nurse enters the room, the care provided must meet the same standard of what a reasonable prudent nurse would do under the same or similar circumstances. If this standard is not met and harm to the client occurs as a result of the nurse's action or inaction, then malpractice can be proven.

If the nursery nurse, rather than entering the room, explained to the client that she was not a labor and delivery nurse and therefore was not qualified to deliver nursing care to the laboring client, she has not taken on the duty to provide such care. The ethical nurse, however, should find the appropriate nurse to assist the client.

Many of the malpractice cases in maternal, neonatal, and women's health nursing involve poor pregnancy outcomes. Some examples of negative outcomes are infants born with low Apgar scores in the face of nonreassuring fetal heart monitoring patterns and shoulder dystocia. Shoulder dystocia is an emergency condition in which the fetal shoulders become entrapped in the maternal bony pelvis after the head has been delivered. Immediate action is required to prevent permanent damage or death to the infant. Many times these infants experience nerve damage if there is too much traction placed on the neck in an attempt at vaginal delivery. The nerve damage can cause a paralysis of the affected upper extremity.

Client Education

Preventing Medical Errors

The AHRQ (2000) recommends these 20 tips for clients to help prevent medical errors.

1. The single most important way you can prevent errors is to be an active member of the health care team.

2. Make sure all doctors know about everything you are taking, including prescription medications, over-the-counter medications, vitamins, and herbs.

3. Make sure your doctor knows about allergies and adverse reactions you may have had to medications.

4. When your doctor writes a prescription, make sure you can read it.

5. Ask about your medications in terms you can understand at the time of prescription and the time of administration.

6. When you pick up your medications from the pharmacy, ask: Is this the medicine that my doctor prescribed?

7. If you have any questions about the directions on your medication label, be sure to ask them.

8. Ask your pharmacist for the best device to measure your liquid medicine.

9. Ask for written information about the side effects your medicine could cause.

10. If you have a choice, choose a hospital where many clients have had the procedure or surgery you need.

11. If you are in a hospital, consider asking all health care workers who have direct contact with you whether they have washed their hands.

12. When you are being discharged from the hospital, ask the doctor to explain the treatment plan you will use at home.

13. If you have surgery, make sure you, your doctor, and the surgeon agree and are clear on exactly what will be done.

14. Speak up when you have questions or concerns.

15. Make sure that someone, such as your personal doctor, is in charge of your care.

16. Make sure that all health professionals involved in your care have important health information about you.

17. Ask a family member or friend to be there with you and to be your advocate.

18. Know that "more" is not always better.

19. If you have had a test, do not assume that no news is good news.

20. Learn about your conditions and treatments by asking your doctor and nurse and by using other reliable resources.

Following these AHRQ recommendations does not guarantee that clients will avoid experiencing medical errors. By participating in their own care, however, clients can reduce this possibility.

In the past, physicians were the primary target of malpractice suits. As the status of nursing has evolved, however, professional responsibility has increased and so has legal accountability (Aiken & Catalano, 1994). Currently, when a malpractice action is taken, the nurse is usually involved as an employee of the hospital. The in-volvement may be as simple as not maintaining adequate documentation or as complex as failing to intervene on the client's behalf when the physician does not perform a timely cesarean section.

Hagedorn & Gardner (1997) suggest that there are several ways nurses can reduce their risks of being a de-

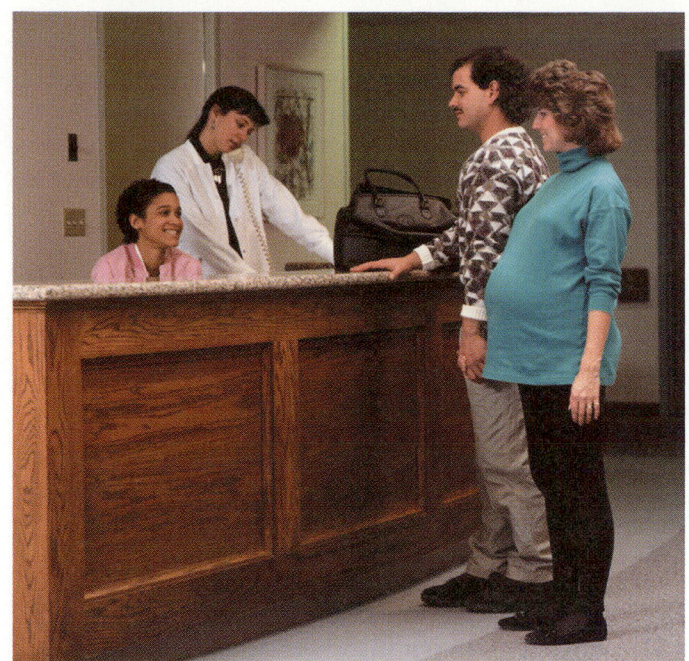

Figure 1-9   Most births in the United States today occur in a hospital setting and health care is more specialized, demanding good communication.

fendant in a lawsuit. Nurses must develop caring relationships with clients, because a failed relationship between a health care provider and the client and family is a major source of malpractice claims. The key to good relationships is good communication (Figure 1-9).

Nurses must maintain clinical competence (Hagedorn & Gardner, 1997). It is not acceptable to practice based on yesterday's knowledge. In this age of change, nursing is not the same profession it was 10 or even 5 years ago. The only way to remain clinically competent is to continue to practice and continue to learn.

Nurses must know their legal responsibilities (Hagedorn & Gardner, 1997). It is no longer safe to assume the nurse will not be sued because the physician and hospital have more financial resources. Knowing responsibility also refers to being familiar with standards, guidelines, and institutional policies and procedures.

The nurse must define appropriate assignments (Hagedorn & Gardner, 1997). As costs are being reduced, nurses are being asked to take on more responsibility with the aid of assistive personnel. The nurse is accountable for assignments given to assistive personnel and the outcome of that care. The nurse also should be cognizant of the fact that unsafe assignments can be declined.

Nurses must take action when the client's condition deteriorates (Hagedorn & Gardner, 1997). In the physician's absence, the nurse is responsible and accountable for attempting to provide the health care the client requires. If the client decompensates, it is the nurse's responsibility to call another physician if the client's physician is not available to provide the needed intervention or is unable to provide the needed intervention because of policy or condition. For example, if the hospital has a policy that a family physician may perform a delivery in a low-risk pregnancy, when the client's condition changes the nurse has a duty to discuss making a referral with the family physician. If the physician refuses to make the referral, the nurse has a duty to advocate for the client and institute action by what is called the chain of command. The chain of command is a method of providing care when the physician is not following policy or is placing the client in danger. The staff nurse usually notifies her immediate supervisor, who notifies the chief of obstetrics. The chief of obstetrics ordinarily will resolve the issue. In case of nonresolution, however, the chain of command further involves hospital administration and the chief of the medical staff. Any such intervention should be documented.

Nurses should defensively document client care, treatment, and intervention (Hagedorn & Gardner, 1997). Accuracy is of paramount importance. Additionally, all legally relevant material should be documented (Figure 1-10). In nursing documentation, several important considerations should be made (Box 1-3).

Moores (1997) indicates that proactive risk management begins with the nurse at the bedside. The nurse should feel empowered to be proactive. Organizations

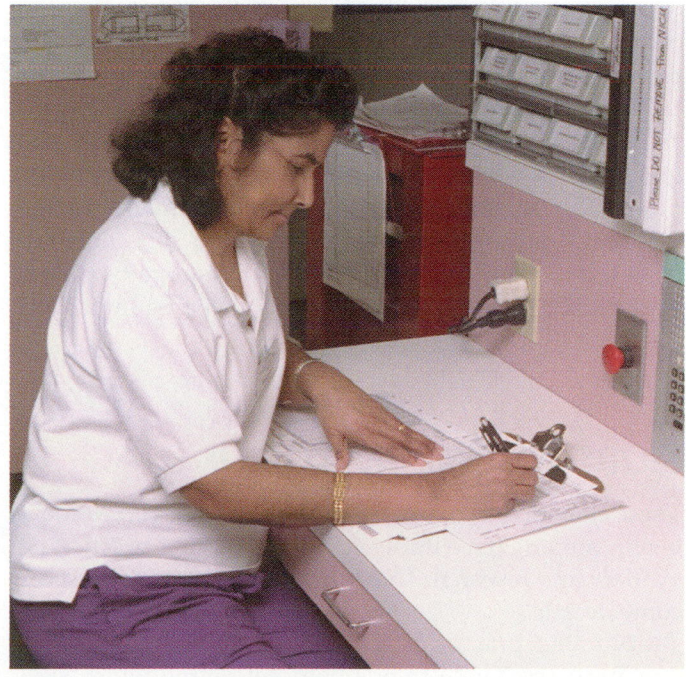

Figure 1-10   Accurate and timely documentation is a strong defense against legal action.

Box 1-3

Considerations in Nursing Documentation

- Accuracy
- Thoroughness
- Compliance with standards
- Individualized nursing care based on client need
- Appropriate goals and interventions that are timely in completion
- Discharge planning

that want to reduce their risks of being sued will empower nurses to work in a proactive manner to advocate for the client and prevent client dissatisfaction and harm.

Philosophy of Care

Philosophy of care refers to the values the nurse places on certain interventions regarding client care. For example, much discussion is occurring about whether it is more important for the nurse to ensure the technology is working correctly and the documentation is flawless, or whether it is more important for the nurse to concentrate on those aspects of practice that are related to touch. Touch in this context means communicating with the client, ensuring comfort, and ensuring the client's individual needs are met. Traditionally, nursing has been a high-touch discipline. Many nursing leaders insist that the concept of caring is what makes nursing different from other professions and why nurses are held in high esteem by the public. In maternal, neonatal, and women's health, the high-touch philosophy is very much required to meet the client's needs. The nurse in this specialty must be very skilled to manage the high-tech versus high-touch dilemma.

NURSING IMPLICATIONS

These changing trends in maternal, neonatal, and women's health nursing have implications for nursing practice, education, and research. These implications are discussed in some detail.

Nursing practice is affected by trends in the health care industry. These trends help determine which skills will be required of practicing professional nurses. The acquisition of these skills will determine successful licensure and credentialing.

Skills Required for Practice

As the profession continues to develop, the skills required to practice maternal, neonatal, and women's health care nursing will change. Nurses must know the parameters within which they can practice so as not to exceed that which is legal. To practice beyond one's scope of practice is illegal. The nurse in maternal, neonatal, and women's health nursing is required to have strong assessment skills. In this field, in particular, nurses are asked to care for the fetus in utero and the newborn in the nursery. Neither of these clients can communicate verbally to let their needs be known. Technologic skills are required to use fetal monitoring equipment, ultrasonography, and fetal pulse oximetry. Other technologic advances also are certain to occur.

Licensure and Credentialing

Licensure is a requirement by state law to perform the services of a registered nurse and to call oneself a registered nurse. To become licensed, the person must graduate from a school that is approved by the Board of Nursing in the state where the school is located. Licensure has been classified as defining the minimal acceptable standard for the practice of professional nursing. Each state has scope-of-practice guidelines.

Credentialing is a process that the individual nurse undertakes beyond basic education and licensure. Credentialing is sought to illustrate expertise in an area of practice. At this time in the United States, credentialing is required for advanced practice in nursing. There has been overture, however, to make certification more broadly applicable to the general practice of nursing. Certification is the process by which a nurse becomes credentialed as an expert. In maternal, neonatal, and women's health nursing there are a number of advanced practice specialties that require certification, including nurse midwife, women's health care nurse practitioner, clinical nurse specialist, and neonatal nurse practitioner. Each of these specialties requires a certification examination and specific criteria, which are designed to provide information about continued competency.

Collaborative Relationships

Collaboration within nursing will become a necessity for nursing practice. Nurses must collaborate with peers to ensure continuity of care. Collaboration among different levels of nursing is increasing; for example staff nurses with advanced practice nurses and maternity nurses with neonatal nurses.

Collaboration with other professions is equally important for nursing. The nurse brings very important skills to the team.

WEB ACTIVITIES

••• Use a search engine to look up a particular health-related topic.

••• Search a medical library site for evidence-based practice.

••• Visit the Web site of the American Nurses Association, and examine some of the position statements.

••• Visit the Web site of the Office of Women's Health at the National Institutes of Health, and explore the research agenda concerning women.

••• Visit the Web sites of the Centers for Disease Control and Prevention and the Agency for Healthcare Research and Quality, and search for guidelines for practice.

••• Using the Internet, which sites can you find that are related to maternal, neonatal, and women's health?

••• Which resources are available to the woman who cannot afford the expense of milk and dairy products during her pregnancy?

Key Concepts

■ An understanding of population health and the need to cut costs have shifted the emphasis of the health care delivery system from treatment of disease to prevention and health promotion. The concepts of risk assessment and management have pervaded all of health care.

■ This shift has moved much of health care to the community setting and engaged multidisciplinary teams of providers, with both individuals and communities as active partners in the pursuit of health.

■ The nursing profession historically has valued and described a holistic approach that is congruent with the changes in health care delivery.

■ The nurse needs not only to develop content knowledge but also cognitive skills, technical skills, communication skills, cultural competence, collaborative skills, and a practice of self-reflection to fully enact the professional role.

■ Nursing in maternal, neonatal, and women's health care is influenced by societal trends.

■ A number of professional organizations utilize research and set out guidelines based on the most cost-effective and beneficial interventions for the best practices in a given situation.

Review Questions and Activities

1. One of the most fundamental shifts in health care delivery in the United States in the late 1900s has been:
   a. Lowering of costs of providing care
   b. Expansion to a focus on health
   c. Emergence of nurses to positions of power in health care delivery
   d. Advancement of isolated specialties

   The correct answer is b.

2. Which of the following is a true statement regarding cultural competency?
   a. One can be certified by taking a short course
   b. One must go to foreign countries to learn this
   c. One must understand one's own culture
   d. One must learn this from certified experts

   The correct answer is c.

3. Holistic theories in nursing are most congruent with which of the following issues in contemporary health care?
   a. Managed care
   b. A focus on health promotion
   c. Multidisciplinary teams
   d. Alternative systems of health care

   The correct answer is b.

4. What is the origin of practice standards and guidelines? What is the purpose of standards and guidelines?

5. Why has great emphasis been placed on prenatal care for women?

6. What are the risks and benefits of managed care?

References

Administration on Aging. (2001). *Demographic changes*. Retrieved January 31, 2001; from http://www.aoa.dhhs.gov/aoa/aging/21 demography

Agency for Healthcare Research and Quality (AHRQ). (2000a). *Management of chronic hypertension during pregnancy*. AHRQ Publication No. 00-E011, August 2000. Retrieved from http://www.ahrq.gov/clinic/hyperinv.htm

Agency for Healthcare Research and Quality (AHRQ). (2000b). *Patient fact sheet: 20 tips to prevent medical errors*. Retrieved from http://www.ahcpr.gov/consumer/20tips.htm

Agency for Healthcare Research and Quality (AHRQ). (2001). *Defining and managing chronic fatigue syndrome.* AHRQ Publication No. 01-E061, September 2001. Retrieved from http://www.ahrq.gov/clinic/epcsums/cfssum.htm.

Aiken, T. D., & Catalano, J. T. (1994). *Legal, ethical, and political issues in nursing.* Philadelphia: F. A. Davis.

American Nurses Association (ANA). (1991). *Position statement: Physical violence against women.* Retrieved February 15, 2001, from http://www.nursingworld.org

American Nurses Association (ANA). (1995a). *Position statement: Home care of the mother, infant, and family following birth.* Retrieved February 15, 2001, from http://www.nursingworld.org

American Nurses Association (ANA). (1995b). *Position statement Promotion and disease prevention.* Retrieved February 13, 2001, from http://www.nursingworld.org/readroom/position

Brady, M., Leuner, J. D., Bellack, J. P., Loquist, R. S., Cipriano, P. F., & O'Neil, E. H. (1999). *A framework for differentiating the 21 Pew Competencies by level of nursing education.* The Center for the Health Professions. Retrieved February 6, 2001 from http://futurehealth.uscf.edu/pewcomm/competenciesRNs.htm

Callen, P. W. (1994). *Ultrasonography in obstetrics and gynecology* (3rd ed.) Philadelphia: W. B. Saunders.

Centers for Disease Control and Prevention (CDC). (1986). Perspectives in disease prevention and health promotion public health guidelines for enhancing diabetes control through maternal- and child-health programs. *Morbidity and Mortality Weekly, 35*(13), 201–208, 213.

Committee on the Future of Primary Care. (1996). *Primary Care: America's Health in a New Era.* Washington DC: National Academy Press.

Dickenson-Hazard, N. (2001). Wrongly blaming nurses: A response from Sigma Theta Tau, *Lifelines, 4*(6), 11.

Dossey, B. M., Keegan, L., & Guzzetta, C. E. (2000). *Holistic nursing: A handbook for practice.* Gaithersburg, MD: Aspen.

Gaston, M. H. (2001). 100% access and 0 health disparities: Changing the health paradigm for rural women in the 21st century. *Women's Health Issues, 11*(1), 7–16.

Hagedorn, M. I., & Gardner, S. I. (1997). Accountability for professional practice. In *Legal aspects of maternal-child nursing.* Menlo Park, CA: Addison-Wesley.

Hall, J. K. (1996). *Nursing ethics and law.* Philadelphia: W. B. Saunders.

Huffman, C., & Sandelowski, M. (1997). The nurse-technology relationship: The case for ultrasonography. *Journal of Obstetric, Gynecologic, and Neonatal Nursing, 26*(6), 673–682.

Institute of Medicine (IOM). (2000). *To err is human: Building a safer health system.* Washington, DC: National Academy Press.

Jegalian, K., & Lahn, B. T. (2001). Why the Y is so weird. *Scientific American, 284*(2), 56–61.

Kaji, E. H., & Leiden, J. M. (2001). Gene and stem cell therapies. *Journal of the American Medical Association, 285*(5), 545–550.

Kincaide, G. G. (2001). Create a responsible discussion: A response from AWHONN. *Lifelines, 4*(6), 11–12.

Knox, G. E., Kelley M., Hodgson S., Simpson K. R., Carrier, L., & Berry, D. (1999). Downsizing, reengineering and patient safety: Numbers, newness, and resultant risk. *Journal of Healthcare Risk Management, 19*(4), 18–25.

Kohn, L. T., Corrigan, J. M., & Donaldson, M. S. (2000). *To err is human: Building a safer health system.* Washington, DC: National Academy Press.

Loustaunau, M. O., & Sobo, E. J. (1997). *The cultural context of health, illness and medicine.* Westport, CT: Bergin & Garvey.

Mezey, M. D., & McGivern, D. O. (1999). *Nurses. Nurse practitioners: Evolution to advanced practice.* New York: Springer.

Moores, P. (1997). Empowering women in the practice setting. In M. I. Hagedorn & S. L. Gardner (Eds.), *Legal aspects of maternal-child nursing practice.* Menlo Park, CA: Addison-Wesley.

National Coalition for Health Professional Education in Genetics (NCHPEG). (2001). *Core competencies in genetics essential for all health-care professionals.* Retrieved February 7, 2001, from http://www.nchpeg.org/news-boxcorecompetencies000.html

Office of Minority Health (OMH). (2001). *Assuring cultural competence in health: Recommendations for national standards and an outcomes-focused research agenda.* Washington, DC: Public Health Service. Retrieved January 16, 2001, from http://www.omhrc.gov/CLAS

Pew Charitable Trust Commission on Health Professions. (1995). *Critical challenges in revitalizing the health care professions for the twenty-first century.* San Francisco: UCSF Center for Health Professions.

Pew Health Professions Commission. (1998). *Recreating health professional practice for a new century. The Fourth Report of the Pew Health Professions Commission.* San Francisco: Author.

Sargent, C., & Brettell, C. (1995). *Gender and Health: An international perspective.* New York: Prentice Hall.

Schenk, L. M., & Coddington, C. C. (1999). Laparoscopy and hysteroscopy. *Obstetric and Gynecology Clinics of North America, 26*(1), 1–22.

Surrey, E. S. (1999). Falloscopy. *Obstetric and Gynecology Clinics of North America, 26*(1), 53–62.

Underwood, P. (2001). Flawed care delivery system: A response from ANA. *Lifelines, 4*(6), 12–13.

U.S. Department of Health and Human Services (USDHHS). (1979). *Healthy people: The Surgeon General's report on health promotion and disease prevention.* Washington, DC: U.S. Government Printing Office.

U.S. Department of Health and Human Services (USDHHS). (1999). *Agenda for research on women's health for the 21st century.* Executive summary (NIH Publication No. 99-4385). Bethesda, MD: Author.

Weinick, R. M., Zuvekas, S. H., & Cohen, J. W. (2000). *Medical Care Research Review, 57*(Suppl. 1), 36–54. Racial and ethnic differences in access to and use of health care services, 1977–1996.

Westhoff, C. L. (2000). Evidence-based medicine: An overview. *International Journal of Fertility, 45* (Suppl. 2), 105–112.

Zwelling, E. (2000). Trendsetter: Celeste Phillips, the mother of family-centered maternity care. *Journal of Obstetric, Gynecologic, and Neonatal Nursing, 29*(1), 90–94.

Suggested Readings

Agency for Healthcare Research and Quality (AHRQ). (2000). *The National Guideline Clearinghouse. Fact sheet* (Publication No. 00-0047). Rockville, MD: Author. Retrieved from http://www.ahrq.gov/clinic/ngcfact.htm

Angier, N. (1999). *Woman: An intimate geography*. New York: Anchor Books.

The Center for the Health Professions. (2000). *Future health: Views from the Center*. San Francisco: University of California. Retrieved January 31, 2001, from http://futurehealth.ucsf.edu

Niesen, K. M., & Quirk, A. G. (1997). The process for initiating nursing practice change in the intrapartum: Findings from a multisite research utilization project. *Journal of Obstetric, Gynecologic, and Neonatal Nursing, 26*(6), 709–719.

Niessen, L., Grijseels, E. W. M., & Rutten, F. F. H. (2000). The evidence-based approach in health policy and health care delivery. *Social Science and Medicine, 51*(6), 859–869.

Olshansky, E. (2000). *Integrated women's health: Holistic approaches for comprehensive care*. Gaithersburg, MD: Aspen.

Resources

American College of Obstetricians and Gynecologists, 409 12th Street, SW, P.O. Box 96920, Washington, DC 20024-2188, http://www.acog.org

American Nurses Association, 600 Maryland Avenue, SW, Suite 100 West, Washington, DC 20024-2571, 800-274-4262, http://www.ana.org.

Association for Women's Health, Obstetric, and Neonatal Nurses, 2000 L Street, NW, Suite 740, Washington, DC, 20036, 800-673-8499, http://www.awhonn.org

The Center for the Health Professions, http://www.futurehealth.ucsf.edu

Centers for Disease Control and Prevention, http://www.cdc.gov

Medscape, http://www.medscape.com

National Association of Neonatal Nurses, 4700 W. Lake Avenue, Glenview, IL 60025-1485, 800-451-3795, http://www.nann.org

National Institutes of Health, http://www.nih.gov

Nursing index to journal articles, http://www.cinahl.com

Search medical and health related journals, http://www.pubmed.com

Office of Women's Health, http://www.4woman.gov

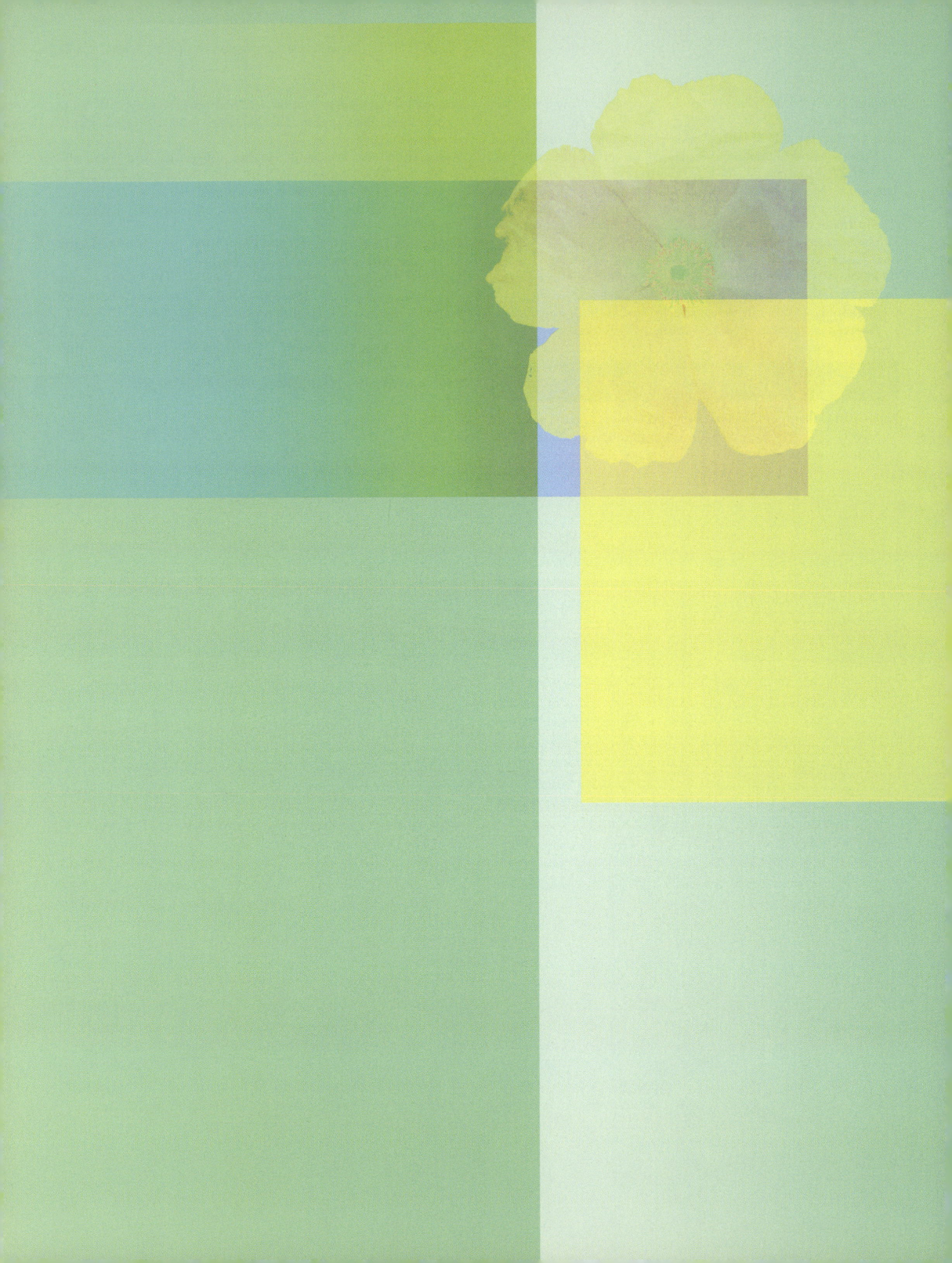

CHAPTER 2

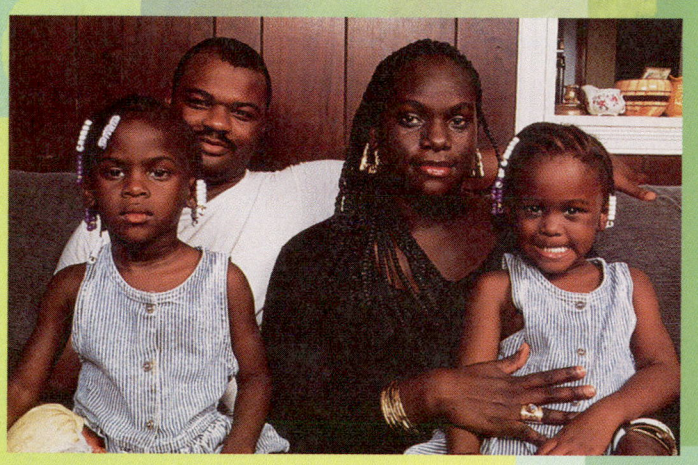

THEORETICAL PERSPECTIVES ON THE CHILDBEARING FAMILY

Working with childbearing families is one of the most rewarding challenges in nursing practice. Families are more open, receptive to education, and willing to make changes in their lives during the childbearing years. While assisting a family during pregnancy, labor, birth, and the immediate postpartum period, the nurse has an opportunity to examine the client's personal views, choices, and experiences.

Consider the following questions as you examine your personal feelings regarding birth.

- What are my personal experiences with birth?
- How do I feel about families that are different from mine?
- How can nurses include the family in their care?
- What communication techniques can be used to allow clients to express their personal views?

Key Terms

Blended family
Cohabitation
Communal family
Crisis
Cultural competence
    continuum
Developmental crisis

Dyad
Extended family
Family structure
Nuclear family
Reconstituted family
Situational crisis

Competencies

Upon completion of this chapter, the reader should be able to:

1. Identify various family structures.
2. Discuss the developmental theories of family as they pertain to the childbearing family.
3. Discuss how crisis theories apply to childbearing families.
4. Discuss the effect of an uncomplicated birth experience on mothers and fathers.
5. Describe the potential effect of a new birth on siblings.
6. Explain how to identify the needs of a family that is experiencing a complication of birth.
7. Apply the nursing process in the assessment of the family's response to birth, the identification of adaptive and maladaptive processes, the development of a plan of care that supports positive responses or assists the family in developing appropriate responses, and the evaluation of the care provided.

Maternal-child nursing has focused on family-oriented care beginning with the need to care for mother and infant together. Maternal-child nurses later expanded their sphere to care for the entire family unit as it prepared for and then incorporated a new member.

This chapter includes descriptions of the structure and function of the family system and concerns of the childbearing family.

FAMILIES ARE SYSTEMS OF FUNCTION AND STRUCTURE

Family units are systems that have a structure and that provide unique functions for the individual members of the family and for society in general. All cultures have family units, although the structure and roles that family members take may vary. Families have universal functions, which are to care for and protect their members and to socialize upcoming generations for productive participation in society.

Family Function

Functions are those things the family does to meet the needs of its members and of society. Friedman (1992) lists five family functions that are important in assessing and intervening with families:

1. **Affective Function:** Promotes the stability of family members by meeting their psychologic needs.
2. **Socialization and Social Placement Function:** Socializes children to become contributing members of society and gives social status to family members.
3. **Reproductive Function:** Allows the family to continue over generations and allows society to survive.
4. **Economic Function:** Allows the family to acquire and allocate adequate financial resources to meet its needs.

Critical Thinking

Definition of Family

Think of the families you know. Describe them to yourself.

- What do you think a typical family is?
- Do you know any typical families?

5. Health Care Function: Allows the family's physical needs to be met.

Family Structure

Family structure refers to the composition of the family and how the members are related to each other. For example, it can refer to the form (e.g., single- or two-parent family), marital partners (e.g., cohabitation, married, or homosexual partners), or composition (traditional nuclear family or communal). The most useful approach for the nurse is to accept clients' definition of who is in the family and their relationship (Figure 2-1). Some typical structural variations are discussed next.

Traditional or Nuclear Family

The traditional family is a **nuclear family** composed of two generations, parents and their children. Their **extended family** includes members of other generations, such as grandparents, great grandparents, aunts, uncles, nieces, and nephews, or perhaps even a second nuclear family. This structure is often thought of as the idealized family. Some people assume that the traditional structure is equated with idealized function. Families may assume that their family will succeed without work, and clinicians assume that there are no family concerns. Nurses must be sensitive to family concerns even in traditional structures.

Critical Thinking

Care of Families as Individuals or as a Unit

In *First, Do No Harm*, Lisa Belkin (1993) described 15-year-old Patrick, his family, and the hospital community where he had spent much of his life. Patrick was born with Hirschsprung disease. The severity of the disease and the more than 20 surgeries that gradually removed his intestine had left Patrick dependent on intravenous (IV) nutrients dripped directly into his heart. His veins were too damaged by numerous previous IV lines to be useful for the IV feedings. Patrick had survived longer than most children with this disease but was entirely dependent on this type of feeding. Patrick was on a ventilator and had a feeding tube. The feeding tube was intermittently clogged as a result of chronic infections.

Patrick's biologic family consisted of his mother, Oria, and his grandmother. His father had left his mother before he was born. When not at the hospital, Patrick slept at his grandmother's home, which was next door to his mother's home. His mother often worked three poorly paying jobs. To encourage her to spend more time with her son, social workers found her a job in the hospital cafeteria. They included her in meetings about his care, although often she was late or simply did not come. The nurses were angry with her because she often slept or sat silently during her short and infrequent visits to her son. The grandmother, who provided most of Patrick's care at home, did not visit the hospital.

In the hospital the play therapist, a primary nurse, and many others constituted Patrick's surrogate family. When the primary nurse who cared for him for the first 10 years of his life left the hospital to take another job, she "gave" Patrick to the primary nurse, Kay. Kay remained involved in Patrick's care until his death. Both Kay and the play therapist, Richard, took Patrick on outings. Patrick called Kay at home in the middle of the night when he was scared, anticipating surgical procedures. Celebrities visited Patrick, and he participated in hospital celebrations of major holidays.

Patrick was re-admitted to the hospital with another serious infection of his feeding tube. It was later discovered that Patrick had contaminated his line with feces and dirt to ensure that he would be admitted to the hospital. He had done this previously. Patrick admitted that he did not want to die but was fearful of being outside the hospital. After Patrick's death, his mother stated that she was "bone tired" and that she was not a bad mother, although she felt that the staff did not understand that Patrick had been seriously ill for 15 years and the whole family was tired.

Throughout Patrick's life the professionals who cared for him viewed him, not his family, as the focus of care. They did not ignore his mother but limited their assessments and interventions to attempts to change the ways she mothered. Patrick's mother had long ago decided that the doctors and nurses were better parents to Patrick than she could ever be. They were better educated, more sophisticated, wealthier, and could ease his pain better than she could.

- Did the nurse's role harm or help Patrick?
- Was it helpful for the staff to take Patrick on outings and allow him to call them at home?
- Do you think Patrick's family was addressed?
- Would viewing the family unit rather than Patrick as the focus of care have improved Patrick's life?
- How do you think the nurses viewed the mother's lack of response?
- How did it happen that the nurses gave competent care to the child but missed the family?

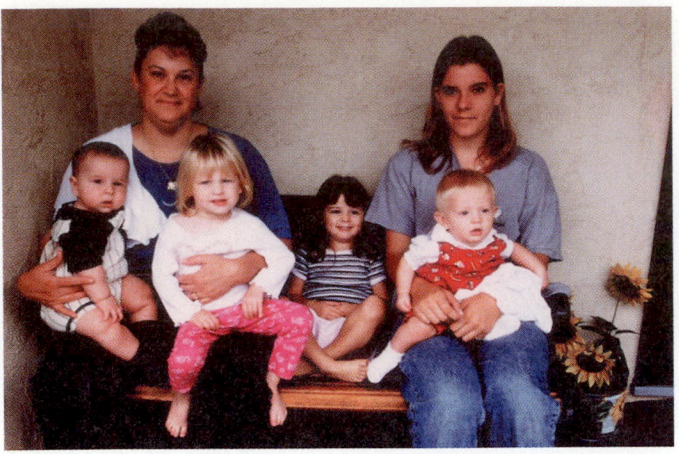

Figure 2-1 The nurse must understand a family's system and structure to provide appropriate care and guidance.

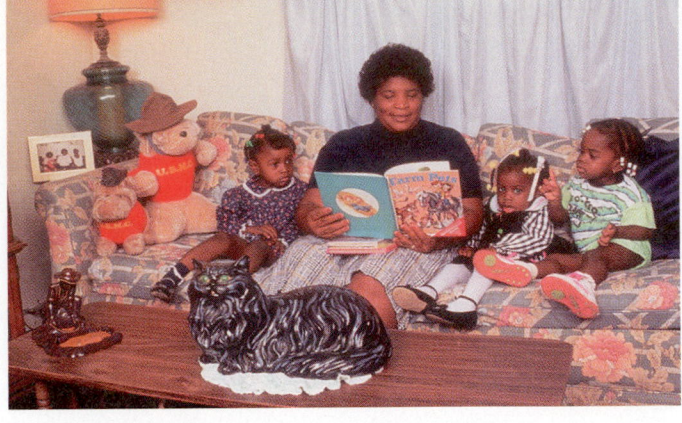

Figure 2-2 Grandparents often assume some childcare responsibilities in extended families.

Childless Dyads

Couples, also called **dyads**, may be childless by choice, because of infertility, or because of spontaneous abortions. Nurses should not assume they know why a couple is childless or what being childless means to a couple. A couple's decision not to have children is influenced by many cultural changes and personal circumstances. A woman may choose not to become a mother for many reasons. Women today have greater educational and professional opportunities. A woman may need to work for financial reasons or may not want to bear the responsibilities of parenthood.

Couples who are not childless by choice may be struggling with whether to accept being childless, pursue fertility treatments, or adopt a child. Nurses should remain sensitive to the feeling of the family and not act on preconceived ideas about childless couples.

Extended Family

Extended families are of two main types. Three, four, or even five generations may live in one household or two or more nuclear families may live in households located near each other (Figure 2-2). Even when members of the extended family do not live together, they may give and receive social support and exchange goods and services. Tensions may arise in extended families related to decision making over parenting issues. Issues of who has authority—the parent, grandparent—may create conflict.

Communal Family

A **communal family** forms when individuals, couples, or families live together and jointly carry out family functions. Couples may or may not be monogamous. Child-rearing responsibilities may be shared or parents, perhaps

particularly mothers, may retain responsibility for rearing their biologic children.

Unmarried Heterosexual (Cohabitation) Family

Many couples live together without entering into marriage. They may have children that they bring to the relationship or they may have children together. They may view **cohabitation** as a temporary stage, a trial period before entering a legal marriage.

Reflections from Clients

Tom and Jill pursued fertility treatments. When the treatments were unsuccessful, they decided to remain childless and now say, "We like having time for each other and feel very close. We also enjoy relationships with our nieces and nephews."

Philip and Sue pursued fertility treatments unsuccessfully and now are the proud parents of two adopted children. They say, "We wish we had decided to adopt right away because we love being parents."

Jamal and Mercedes thought about having children but have successful careers that bring them into daily contact with young adults whom they mentor. They say, "We are happy with our lives the way they are. We don't want to change a thing."

Homosexual Family

Homosexual families are diverse, as are all families. The household may be headed by a single parent or a couple. In either case the parent or parents may be gay or lesbian. The children may be adopted, biologic, foster, or some combination.

Parenting may bring forth issues in this structure related to acceptance in the general culture.

Single-Parent Family

The single-parent family has only one parent, mother or father. Single-parent families are formed in numerous ways: when adults without marital partners choose to

Nursing Tip   *Single-Parent Family*

After a death or divorce, the reorganized, single-parent family often bonds itself into a very close unit emotionally (Seibt, 1996).

Nursing Tip   *Single-Parent Support*

Nurses may refer single parents to support groups, such as Parents Without Partners, that provide help with parenting and also act as a source of social support for single parents.

Critical Thinking

Children in Single-Parent Families

"The children raised by single parents can be just as healthy and normal as those raised in the traditional two-parent family. In fact, despite the obstacles, children in most single-parent families are provided with the love and nurturing that all children need and deserve" (Seibt, 1996).

- What aspects of family function are met by this family structure?
- Which needs are met when a child is loved and nurtured?
- Can you think of ways to evaluate whether a child's needs for love and nurturing are being met?

Reflections from a Client

As a single mother, I often felt ambivalent about leaving household chores undone to spend time with my children or to take time for myself. As a solution, I decided to ask myself if the chore would matter in 50 years. When the answer was no, the chore could wait—and almost always did.

have a child, when teenagers become pregnant, when parents in traditional families divorce or separate, and when a spouse dies. Single-parent families are most likely to be headed by mothers and are more likely to be financially disadvantaged than are two-parent families. A higher incidence of poverty exists in families headed by women.

Reconstituted Family

A **reconstituted family** differs from a traditional family. Authors use various terms to label the reconstituted family, including remarriage family, stepfamily, and **blended family**. These terms are used interchangeably.

The reconstituted family forms because the earlier marriage or partnership of one or both of the parents ended. Usually the marriage ended in divorce or, less frequently, a spouse died. As members of the reconstituted family recover emotionally from the loss of the earlier marriage, they can begin planning for the new family. It will take time and patience for all the family members to take on new roles in the reconstituted family. There will

Nursing Tip   *Reconstituted Families: The Most Typical*

Following divorce about 75% of men and 65% of women go on to remarry. Remarried families have been predicted to become the predominant family form—the most normal, in the sense of typical (Walsh, 1993).

- One out of every 3 Americans is a member of a stepfamily.
- 52%–62% of all first marriages end in divorce, and 75% of all divorced persons remarry.
- 43% of all marriages are remarriages for one of the adults.
- 60% of all remarriages eventually end in divorce. This makes stepfamilies one of the more typical family structures (Stepfamily Association of America, 2001).

Critical Thinking

Establishing a Family Unit

Slowly, former alliances and ways of doing things become transformed, as stepfamily members move from having little or no emotional connections between them to the establishment of bonds that give them a sense of belonging together as a family unit (Visher & Visher, 1993).

As a nurse you understand that it may take time for members in a stepfamily to establish a strong sense of bonds. How would you respond to a mother who is holding a newborn and looking somewhat sad when she says, "I've never had these feelings for my stepdaughter. I love this baby so much"? Would the following statements by a nurse support the mother's bonds with both children? "This baby is so precious. Having a new baby can be an exciting time in a family. What is your stepdaughter's name? Will she see her baby sister soon?" What else could the nurse say?

Reflections from a Stepmother

Seth was 6 years old and had lived with his stepmother since he was 4 years old, when his biologic mother had died. He had known his stepmother since he was a toddler. He saw little of his biologic mother's mother. He called his stepmother's parents grandma and grandpa. His grandpa thought he was wonderful, and he and Seth loved being together. However, when his grandpa learned that his daughter, Seth's stepmother, was pregnant, he said, "Finally a real grandchild." His wife quickly turned to him and said, "Don't ever say that again. How do you think Seth will feel if he hears this?" Fortunately, Seth was not present, and his bond with his grandpa was not harmed. Years later, when Seth and his younger half-brothers were adults, his stepmother recounted that scene, saying, "There were so many feelings of guilt and anger, but we were enriched. It didn't just happen. Our lives have been so much richer than if we were just a nuclear family."

How could you respond if your client spoke of having "real" grandchildren? What makes a family relationship real?

be a period of confusion as they decide where to spend holidays and what their relation is to people to whom other members of the reconstituted family are biologically related (e.g., their stepfather's sister). They will have to work through the issues of who belongs where, who has authority for what, and how space and time will be apportioned to various members. They will need to deal with emotional issues, including guilt, loyalty conflicts, a desire for mutuality, and the fact that some past hurts may never be resolved. The family that successfully negotiates these tasks will develop a family that permits children to move from the household of one biologic parent to another, and engages in the ongoing work of keeping lines of communication open among the parents, grandparents, and children (Carter & McGoldrick, 1989). The family members also will have twice as many sources of support, and four sets of aunts and uncles and grandparents.

THE CHILDBEARING FAMILY

The moment of birth is a transition point, a line of demarcation between life before the baby and life with the baby. No matter how well prepared a woman or her family believes they are for this transition, the reality of the experience of birth is impossible to predict. Each birth is unique, each infant unlike any other. The congruence of the quality of the labor and the specific experiences of the birth and the characteristics of the infant with the expectations of the participants determines the response of family members to the birth (Maushart, 1999). Expectations of birth are influenced by cultural beliefs and personal experiences. The family members' exposure to birth in their own or other's families is important. One important family experience during the birth process is fear for the life or health of the mother and the infant. Assessment of the family member's immediate response to the birth experience sets the stage for nursing interventions during the postpartum period.

By using the nursing process and thoroughly understanding the diverse aspects of nursing, obstetric, psychological, sociologic, educational, and political theory that intersect during the time of birthing, the nurse can choose culturally competent interventions that assist the family in moving through the birth experience (Cross, Bazron, Dennis, & Isaacs, 1989).

Client Education

Working with Reconstituted Families

The following tips might be useful in working with a reconstituted family:

- All members of the family need to realize that establishing family rituals, traditions, and relationships will take time.

- Parents must take the time and energy to nurture their own relationship because it is pivotal for the health and stability of the family.

- All members of the family need to establish dyadic relationships and learn to function as a family unit (Figure 2-3).

- Parents need to work together to establish mutual rules related to discipline.

- Parents should help make noncustodial children feel they are a permanent part of the family. When they visit, make sure they have their own space to keep personal items.

- Parents should take extra time for holiday planning because there are additional relatives to consider.

- All members of the family must be flexible.

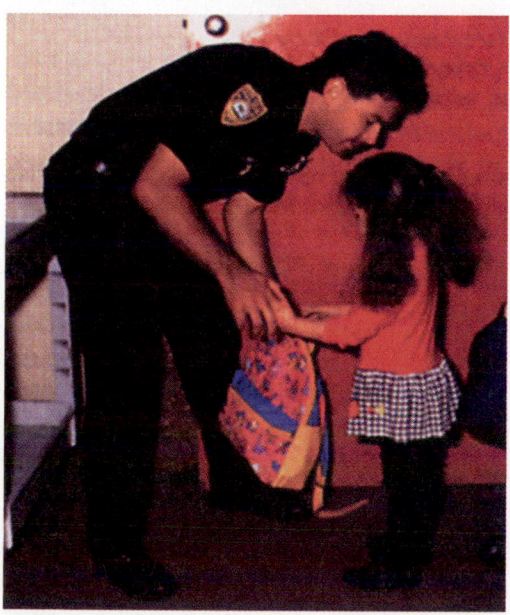

Figure 2-3   Family dynamics and role responsibilities will vary from family to family. Several dyadic relationships form within families.

Cultural Considerations in a Family's Response to Birth

Worldwide, pregnancy and birth are perceived from either a wellness or an illness viewpoint. Racial, religious, ethnic, political, economic, and technologic advancement all influence perspectives of childbirth. Over time, culturally specific practices have developed that enable family members to deal with this time of vulnerability for the mother and her child and of change for the family and community. The way a family experiences birth is influenced by the values of the culture that they are born into and the congruence of that orientation with the culture in which they birth (Esposito, 1999).

Birth sites and those individuals who staff them have their own orientation to childbearing, which is influenced by the same factors. Given the mobility available to individuals and families today, it is quite likely that a family from one culture gives birth in a place unlike their homeland and is cared for by attendants who come from still other environments. Based on the interactions of the individuals in these multicultural situations, the potential exists for powerful, positive, growth-enhancing outcomes for the family and the practitioners and also for negative, personally destructive outcomes.

A **cultural competence continuum** is a progressive description of the ability of an individual or institution to respond to the individual, culturally specific needs of people. Table 2-1 illustrates the layers of a cultural competence continuum from cultural incapacity through cultural competence (Cross et al., 1989). Individuals or agencies can fall anywhere on this continuum and therefore have a positive or destructive interaction with a family during the birth experience. Nursing professionals have a responsibility to assess where they fall on the cultural competence continuum and seek opportunities to move forward toward cultural competence.

Theoretical Approaches Applied to the Childbearing Family

A family's adaptation and response to a birth can be viewed through different frameworks. Systems theory, developmental theory, and crisis theory each provide a context for understanding a family's growth and change.

Systems Theory

Systems theory describes the relationship of the individual and the multiple forces with which the individual interacts throughout life. Each person is a part of multiple larger groups and contributes to the totality of those groups. The family is the primary group. As a system the family is influenced by its individual members and responds to

Table 2-1	A Cultural Competence Continuum
Cultural destructiveness	Attitudes, policies, and practices, including person interactions that are destructive to cultures and, consequently, to the individuals within the culture. For instance, belittling ritual practices and denying access to culturally acceptable healers.
Cultural incapacity	Attitudes, policies, and practices, including personal interactions that are not intentionally destructive but which reflect a lack of ability or capacity to help clients of other cultures. For instance, restricting a laboring woman to only one "helper" or stereotyping women based on their behavioral response to labor pains.
Cultural blindness	Functioning with the belief that skin color and culture make no difference at all and that all people are the same. Usually characterized by the belief that the helping approaches used by the dominant culture are universally applicable. This approach ignores the cultural strengths of a family, encourages assimilation, and blames the family for not "fitting in."
Cultural pre-competence	Individuals and agencies recognize their weaknesses in providing services to families of other cultures and seek to develop approaches to meet some of the needs of some of the families. Characterized by the ability to ask, "How can I help?" This level is indicative of beginning the process of becoming culturally competent but shows a lack of information and clear knowledge of how to proceed.
Cultural competence	Individuals and agencies that accept and respect the differences of the varied families they serve. They see the differences between cultures and within cultural subgroups, each distinct from each other and having important strengths. Such individuals are able to engage in self-assessment regarding culture, pay careful attention to the dynamics of difference between their cultural orientation and that of their clients, and are continually expanding their cultural knowledge and resources.
Cultural proficiency	Advanced cultural competence. Every culture is held in high esteem. Individuals and agencies conduct research and develop new therapeutic approaches based on culture. They advocate for cultural competence and improve relations in their own agencies and communities. For instance, the development of a culturally specific doula program would address the individual needs of families giving birth.

Note. Adapted from *Towards a Culturally Competent System of Care: Vol. 1,* by T. Cross, B. Bazron, K. Dennis, and M. Isaacs, 1989, Washington, DC: National Technical Assistance Center for Children's Mental Health, Georgetown University Child Development Center.

the feedback from other systems and the social network in which it is maintained. As both the individual member and the group interact with other organizations and individuals in the environment, adaptive changes occur. In this way, the family system responds and contributes to its environment. By balancing the needs of the individual and the collective group, the family dynamically progresses through life (Cox & Paley, 1997).

Family systems have four central functions that affect their members and the society of which the family is part. These functions are (1) family formation, which provides a sense of belonging, direction for life, and identity for its members; (2) economic provision for the basic needs of food, clothing, shelter, and other resources for its members; (3) nurturance, education, and socialization, which provide physical, psychological, social, and spiritual development and instills social values and norms; and (4) protection, which provides care for young and vulnerable members (Patterson, 1999). The ability of the family to fulfill these responsibilities for its members and for society depends to a large extent on its relationship with the macrosystem.

Birth represents a change in the family system—in its constellation and its internal communications—and challenges the family's ability to provide the basic necessities and protection for its members (Figure 2-4). This is a time when the family system interacts with the medical care

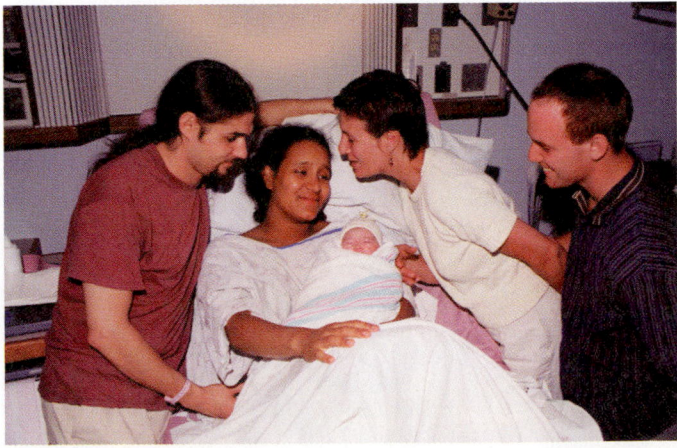

Figure 2-4 The birth of a child presents the extended family with new opportunities for growth and bonding.

system and other institutional systems and a time when the relationships with employment systems may change. At the time of birth, the nurse is in a unique position to facilitate the dynamic changes the family is going through by being sensitive to the cultural, economic, and physiologic issues confronting the family members; by assisting them in navigating the medical system; and by supporting them in making choices that improve their level of functioning.

Developmental Theory

Families, like individuals, go through developmental stages. Family structure changes with the addition of members during the childbearing cycle or through adoption, and when family members leave, such as a young adult leaving home or the death of a family member. Family functions change and family roles are negotiated as members move from dependency to contribution and then become more independent (Patterson, 1999) (Figure 2-5). At birth, the family is in the process of moving from one developmental stage to another. For instance, at this time a two-person family must move from the stage of independence to a stage of nurturance, with the addition of a totally dependent new member. This transition to parenthood disrupts the balance the family has achieved and requires learning new roles and strategies for coping. While working with families during labor and birth, the nurse has the opportunity to provide anticipatory guidance that will assist the family during this transition (Patterson, 1999).

Crisis Theory

A **crisis** can be defined as a situation in which a family or individual's balance is disrupted, requiring development of new coping strategies. Erikson first used the term

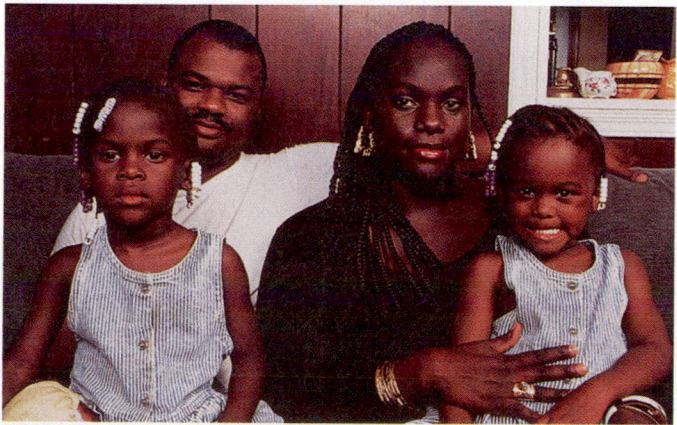

Figure 2-5   Families go through predictable growth stages as members are challenged to adapt to developmental transitions of the family unit combined with changing needs of individual members.

Nursing Alert

Family Developmental Tasks

Family members engage in individual developmental tasks simultaneously with family developmental tasks. Sometimes these tasks may create conflict. For example, meeting the family task of adapting to needs and interests of a preschool child may create tension with the needs of the young adults to establish intimacy.

developmental crisis in describing the adjustment of the individual to new stages of development (Erickson, 1963). In his work, Erikson describes the work involved in each developmental crisis, or turning point, as the individual moves from birth to death. The key to successfully resolving the crisis is reduction in the anxiety level generated by the person's move from homeostasis to disequilibrium and back to equilibrium, once the turning point is successfully negotiated (Maushart, 1999; Erickson, 1963; Elkind, 1994).

These same events can be viewed as situational crises in the life cycle. A **situational crisis** is an event or situation that occurs in a person or a family's life, which requires the adaptation or acquisition of new coping mechanisms. Using Erickson's theoretical framework, the adaptations that a 16-year-old needs to make in life to accommodate pregnancy and parenting are added to the adaptations necessary to work through the developmental stage of adolescence (Erickson, 1963). Health risks or other changes in the family such as job loss are additional situational crises.

Birth represents a crisis or turning point for the family. The family brings to the birth room all its baggage, hopes, expectations for the experience of birth, expectations for the baby, and projections for the future. As the birth unfolds, there is congruence or lack of congruence with family members' expectations (Cross et al., 1989; Esposito, 1999; Mercer, 1995). Perhaps the labor is longer than expected and the time commitment of the family is an issue, or perhaps there is more pain or noise than family members expected or can tolerate.

NURSING IMPLICATIONS

The nursing process is a valuable framework for working with families. Using the nursing process, the nurse gathers data and assesses the response of the family unit and of individual family members to birth. Based on these observations, decisions can be made about the level of positive or negative response and a specific plan can be developed in collaboration with the family to identify the goals of the individual members and of the family as a system. With an understanding of the needs and goals of the family, the nurse can choose appropriate interventions, which may include referrals to other health care professionals, and design a strategy for evaluating the progress of the family as they journey toward meeting their goals.

At the time of birth, the nurse must assess each family member's response to the experience. This is a time of heightened awareness, when potential risks to mother, infant, and family system can be identified, and a time when positive responses can be reinforced.

In promoting a positive response to the birth the nurse must validate the family's experience. Assessment of the family unit based on knowledge and understanding of family process and this particular family is the first step. Listening and then asking therapeutic questions is the process by which the professional nurse formulates a plan and interventions. The nurse must understand that, because most families have limited experience with the birth process and medical procedures, their own perceptions of the events are reality for them. Reinforcing positive responses to the birth, the infant, and the support of the family is an important strategy in helping a woman integrate the events that have occurred. Assisting the woman and her family in identifying those events that were consistent with their expectations and helping them to find honest adaptations to those events that were inconsistent with their expectations helps to promote a positive response to the birth.

Effect of Birth on the Family

Each member of the birthing family experiences a period of adaptation after the birth of a new member. An individual's response is shaped by personal experience, history, cultural background, and developmental stage.

Maternal Adaptation

Labor and birth encompass a proportionately short period in a woman's life. However, no other experience has the intensity of physical and emotional feelings or represents such a profound life change (Simkin, 1996; Rubin, 1984). A woman's self-concept is affected by the congruence of her birth experience and her expectations. Ego strength may be enhanced by a birth, leaving the woman with a sense of accomplishment, some sense of control, and positive reinforcement from family. In contrast, an experience that does not meet expectations or that leaves the woman with a sense of loss of control may foster feelings of frustration, disappointment, or shame (Mercer, 1995; Katz-Rothman, 1996).

The maternal response to an uncomplicated birth experience is colored by her previous birth experiences and her expectations for this birth. During a comparatively short period, the woman has an intense physical experience that is totally outside of her control. Her body acts on its own in ways she might not have anticipated. Choices in dress, food, and activity may be dictated by the stage of labor, institutional policy, and provider preference. The amount of control that a woman perceives that she has during the birth process and the degree of pain she feels both have direct relationships to her feelings about that experience and to her self-concept (Mercer, 1995).

The timing of the birth, whether at term or postterm, affects the mother's response to birth. For example, a woman experiencing the birth of an infant during the 2 weeks past her due date may be disappointed with herself and her body's inability to perform "correctly and on time" (Mercer, 1995). The fact that delivery within 42 weeks' gestation is within the realm of normal may not be reassuring enough for a woman who has been looking to the estimated date of delivery (EDD) as the marking point of the end of pregnancy.

The duration of labor has an effect on the woman's response to the experience. A long labor can leave a woman exhausted and depleted of resources at the birth. However, a precipitous birth experience may be frightening.

The difficulty of the delivery is another variable that influences the mother's response (Figure 2-6). A normal vaginal birth can be perceived to be difficult. A situation that requires manipulation by the birth attendant, for example, shoulder dystocia, may cause the mother to experience fear for herself, her baby, and her birth. Immediately after such an experience, the woman may feel relief that all is well, disappointment that this was not the birth experience she expected, or anger that she or her infant could have been hurt.

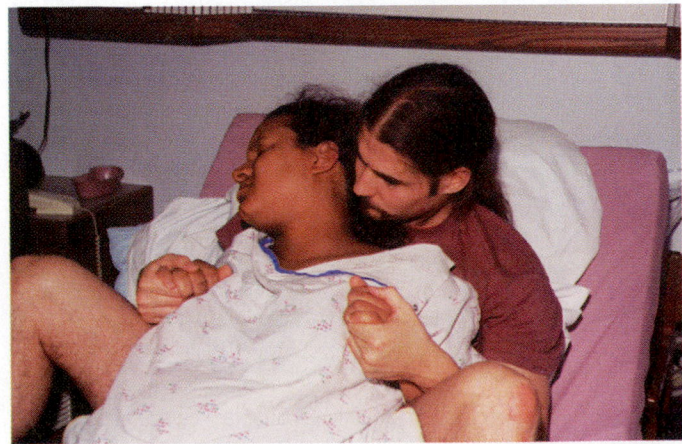

Figure 2-6   The difficulty of the delivery may influence a couple's response to the birth process.

A woman's relationship with her own mother, and her mother's attitudes about sexuality and body image, may also have a profound effect on a woman's view of the birth experience.

Theories of Maternal Adaptation

Rubin, Lederman, Mercer, and others have described the developmental tasks of pregnancy and have discussed how the completion or noncompletion of these tasks affects a woman's labor, birth, and parenting experience. Building one upon the other, the woman first accepts the reality of her pregnancy during the first trimester; second, develops a relationship with the unborn child during the second trimester; and third, prepares for the unknown experience of giving up the fetus and meeting her newborn. Women who do not complete these tasks before delivery may not be fully psychologically equipped to move into their role as mother (Mercer, 1995; Rubin, 1984; Lederman, 1984).

Rubin (1984) discusses the immediate response of the mother to her infant. After months of fantasizing, the woman meets her newborn at the moment of birth (Rubin, 1984). The match of that real infant with her fantasy affects her response and her incorporation of the child into her reality. From observation and client interviews, Rubin describes the stages of attachment between mother and child that the mother experiences. These stages are: "taking-in" describing the early postpartum period; "taking-hold" during the later postpartum period around a week after birth; and "letting go" the final incorporation of the maternal role. Moving from touching the infant with her fingertips to using finger pads and then palmar surfaces to encircle the infant, the woman brings the baby close to her body again. The "en face" position, in which the mother turns face to face with the baby, was found to occur in women who had a positive self-image (Mercer, 1995).

In her research describing women's birth experience, Simkin (1996) found that women remember their labor and birth with unusual clarity for up to 20 years after the event. The benefits of continuous labor support have been documented by several authors (Scott, Klaus, & Klaus, 1999; Fowles, 1998). Women who feel they were surrounded by supportive people in labor have been shown to have more positive feelings about their experience, use less pain medication, and be more likely to choose to breastfeed their baby and to breastfeed for a longer period of time. During the later postpartum period, these women are less likely to experience depression and more likely to exhibit higher levels of self-esteem and demonstrate increased sensitivity to the needs of their infants (Scott et al., 1999; Scott, Berkowitz, & Klaus, 1999; Hodnett, 2000).

Reflections from a Mother

Becoming a mother is the most life-altering and wonderful experience a woman can have. It becomes who you are, and everything you do in life becomes secondary to that, requiring extraordinary ability to balance it all. While pregnant or awaiting the arrival of a child through adoption, you can read and read about how your relationship with your spouse will change and how you need to maintain that relationship with your spouse. What I'd never read about and wish I'd known more about is that your spouse changes, too, from becoming a parent. And that in a sense, you will fall in love again with this new person, who is now a father and showing tenderness toward the child you carried for 9 months.

A pleasant surprise is how all of your relationships change as you evolve into a mother. Suddenly, to everyone in your life, you are someone's mother, with the expectations of that role in their eyes (and that's different for so many people). And then you are the other things around that—daughter, daughter-in-law, professional, friend, sister. All of the continuous emotional growth in my life that stems from being a mother has, in most cases, helped me be a more empathetic daughter, daughter-in-law, professional, friend, and sister, and to realize the powerful effect a mother's nurturing has on the entire world—in a way only a mother can do it.

Paternal Adaptation

The history of the participation of men in birth experiences has been affected by gender role definitions, cultural mores, economic status, politics, and social expectations. Some cultures have prescribed activities for fathers during pregnancy and childbirth. However, to a great extent throughout most of history, men have been excluded from participation in the childbearing process (Jordan, 1990a; Heggenhougen, 1980).

In industrialized societies, there is a common notion that, because conception is a shared experience, birth should be no less so. This perspective was influenced by the growth of the women's movement and the changing view of men's role in the family. Fathers were provided with specific tasks for labor by the prepared-childbirth movement. This ability to take an active part in birth is viewed by families and health professionals as an important step in consolidating the family unit (Nichols & Humenick, 2000; Pryia, 2000). Research also indicates that fathers who take an active role in the pregnancy and birth process are more likely to remain involved in the child's life.

Fathers may be anxious about loss of income when the woman stops working in a two-income family and his ability to provide for a new family constellation. He may have feelings of inadequacy in childcare activities because of lack of exposure and concern about the change in status he may experience in the relationship as he anticipates sharing his partner with the new family member (Jordan, 1990b). The level of anxiety for a father and his feelings of helplessness may be increased when the pregnancy is unplanned and he feels as though he was unable to prepare for these significant events (Clinton & Kelber 1993; Hall, 1995).

The decision to share the birth experience is one that fathers do not take lightly. This is one subject about which men have traditionally been deprived of information. Fear of the unknown, discomfort with "female" bodily processes, and inability to cope with his partner's pain all influence the man's decision to attend the birth. In some areas of Western society today, this trend is to almost demand the father's participation in labor and birth whether he is comfortable with it or not. It is important for the nurse to ensure that the family determine who should be present at birth and the role of the father.

Paternal Role Attainment

While the fetus becomes real to the mother as she feels it move, the father does not perceive the reality of the child until after the birth, when his perception moves from secondhand, or vicarious, to face-to-face, seeing and holding the baby after birth (Figure 2-7)

The experience of the father at birth may be a different one from that of the mother (Nolan, 1996). He must be a participant and an observer of the changes experienced by his partner. The early relationship of the father and his child and the father as parent with his partner in this new family constellation is significantly influenced by the emotional experience of birth (von Klitzing, Amsler, Schleske, Simoni, & Burgin, 1996).

The experience of fathers is also influenced by attitudes of the health care providers who interact with him during the birth experience. Jordan (1990b) found that

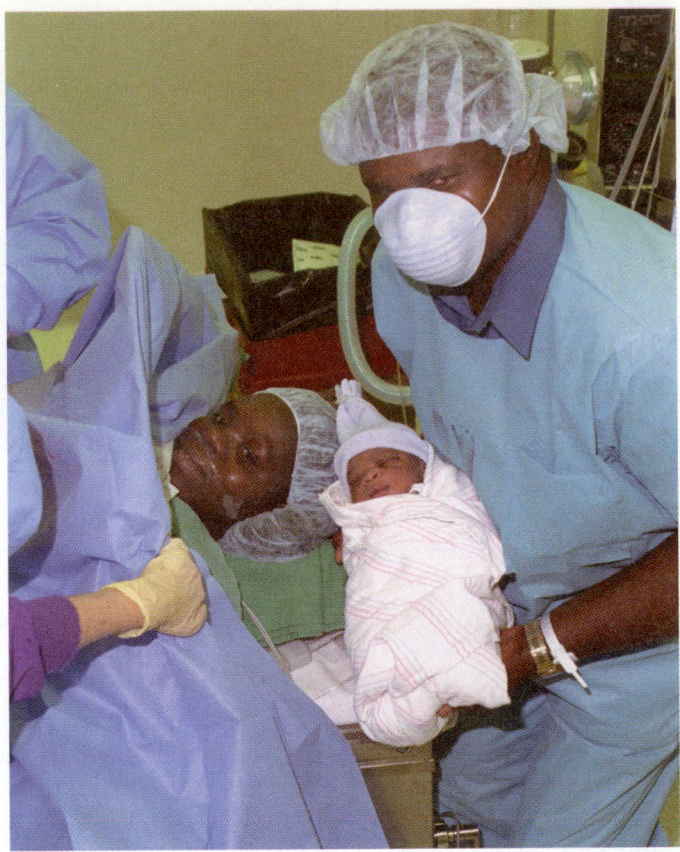

Figure 2-7   Immediately after his wife's cesarean delivery, this father begins to bond with his newborn son.

Reflections from a Father

Becoming a father is the greatest thing that ever happened to me. Children are an absolute blessing. It struck me, however, on the birth of my second daughter, how different the experience was from the birth of my first daughter. When Madeline was born (after 20 hours of labor, my wife would want pointed out), I couldn't stop crying. I was incredibly happy and relieved that everything went well, but I was simply overwhelmed with raw emotion. By contrast, when my second daughter was born (9 hours of labor), my wife and I couldn't stop laughing. We were both thrilled, relieved, and emotional, but this time we expressed it through laughter. It was so bad that, when my wife went into hard labor, she got the giggles. That has always struck me as an odd contrast.

fathers predominantly felt treated as peripheral to the mother by health care professionals. Their needs were addressed only as they related to the woman. In this way, the man felt excluded from active participation in the birth. Inclusion of the father as an active participant in the support system and provision of care to the laboring woman significantly increased the father's investment in the labor and birth. Nurses working closely with the laboring couple have an unparalleled opportunity to assist the father in having a positive birth experience, which can bolster his self-concept and help him lay the foundation for effective coping as a parent.

Nursing Implications

When working with families, it is important for the nurse to understand the father/partner's role, which may be evidenced by his participation in the prenatal course and previous birth experiences. While interacting with the father, the nurse should observe his physical relationship to his partner (does he physically soothe her, massage her back, or sit by the bed without touching her?) and listen to his interaction with the laboring woman (does he coach her, encourage her, and share her experience?). His coping strategies and desire to hold or touch his newborn may also be indicative of his view of his new parental role. Positive adaptations may be seen in the father's identifying ways in addition to feeding that he can participate in the care of his newborn, and the father's participation in identifying childcare options.

Nursing interventions that can assist the father in developing a realistic interpretation of his birth experience might be: including the father in discussions about the decisions being made with the laboring woman, providing the father with explanations about what is happening, encouraging the father to cut the umbilical cord, and encouraging the father to hold the baby with the mother, to enfold both of them in his arms (Figure 2-8).

Sibling Adaptation

The participation of siblings in birth has a history similar to that of fathers. The acceptance of children in the birth setting has been influenced by social attitudes regarding

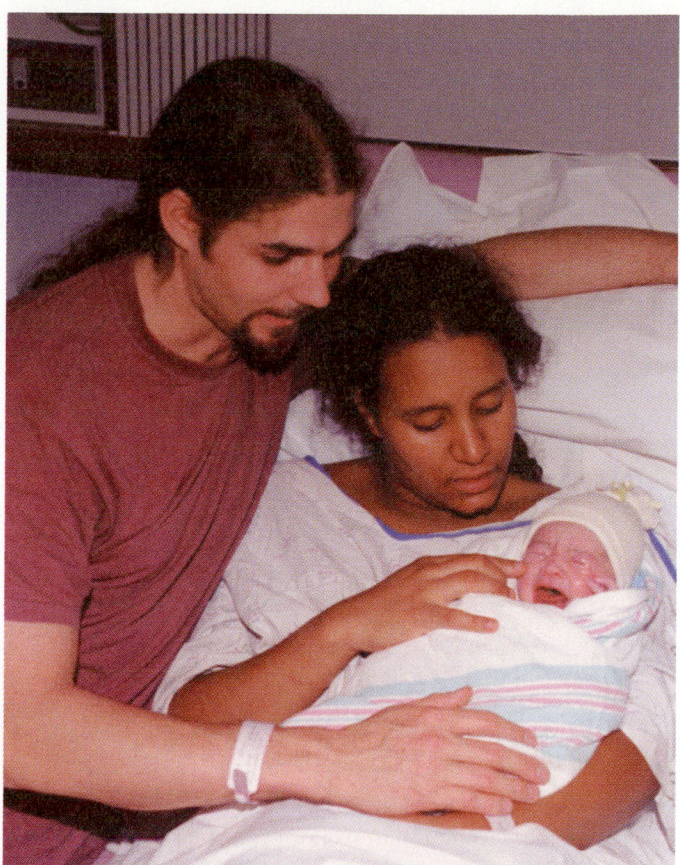

Figure 2-8   This father welcomes his daughter to the world by enfolding the mother and baby in his arms.

children, economics, cultural beliefs, and the politics of birthing institutions.

In cultures in which extended families live in close proximity and pregnancy is an accepted developmental rite of passage, children are more likely to be a part of the group experience of birth. The presence of alternative caretakers, such as older children or other family members, has also dictated whether children were sent away from the home when birth occurred.

Developmental Issues

Children's perceptions of birth are highly influenced by their developmental stage. Preschool children may not be attentive to the activities of the adults around them. In the birth setting, they may be focused on their dolls or toys, ignoring the adults. School-aged children may be bothered by the noise of a birth setting. They may perceive their mothers' pain and, in some way, take responsibility for not being able to relieve it. Adolescents may be able to be supportive or may identify with the bodily functions inherent in the birth process and personalize the events (Erickson, 1963).

Nursing Tip   *Father Attending a Birth*

The decision of the father being present at the birth needs to be made by the family. It is just as harmful to force a father to be present if he doesn't choose to be, as it is to deny a father who wishes to be present.

Nursing Alert

Children Attending a Birth

If children are present during labor and delivery, one adult (other than professional staff) must be present for each child to provide safe and adequate supervision.

Nursing Tip

Nursing Interventions that Can Assist Siblings at Birth

- Providing simple factual explanations of events at the level of the child's understanding
- Answering questions posed by the children as simply and honestly as possible
- Orienting the children to the birth environment as early as possible before the intensity of the experience clouds their vision
- Allowing the children to move in and out of the birth environment at will
- Ensuring that there is a competent adult present, other than the staff, whose only responsibility is to meet the needs of the children
- Encouraging the parents to interact with the children as much as possible so that the children see that the parents are safe
- Interacting with the child or children as much as possible
- Providing simple explanations to the children about procedures that they see their mother undergoing
- Creating a space for the child or children (perhaps at the head of the bed rather than at the foot of the bed) that allows them to interact with their mother but preserves her modesty
- Providing positive reinforcement for the decisions the child makes relative to his or her participation in the labor and birth and his or her response to the newborn

The participation or attendance at birth of older children is determined on the basis of the dynamics of the individual family and institutional and provider policy. In more traditional hospital birth settings, the children's presence is dictated by institutional and infection control policy. Most hospitals require some preparation for children who will attend a birth. This may take the form of a puppet show, a hospital tour, viewing a video, or attending a series of classes with parents. Parents are told of the need to be alert to health concerns, such as viral illnesses, that would prevent the older children's participation, and some institutions may require proof of health screening and up-to-date vaccination status of children who wish to attend.

Grandparent and Extended Family Adaptation

Adults view pregnancy, birth, and child rearing from the perspective of their own experience. "Birth baggage" refers to the feelings one has about one's own child birth experience. Included in this "baggage" are all the feelings about needs that were met or unmet. The expectations of birth held by grandparents are colored by the experiences they had during childbirth experiences. A woman who was not given a choice about the use of medication may not understand her daughter's desire for an unmedicated delivery. A man who waited in the waiting room during the birth of his children may not understand the desire of his son to be present at delivery (Figure 2-9). Alternatively, extended family members who were not able to birth as they would have liked or who may, for example, have had emergency operative deliveries may be strongly supportive of the choices made by the birthing family.

Grandparents who have successfully negotiated the life stages preceding having children will be ready to view the birth as an addition to their own lives (Figure 2-10).

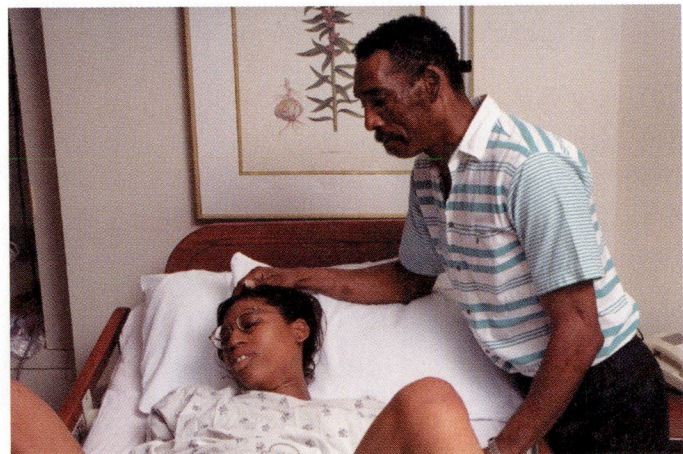

Figure 2-9   To help his daughter through her labor and delivery, this father, soon to be a grandfather, needed to be open-minded to the changes in practice that have occurred since his children were born.

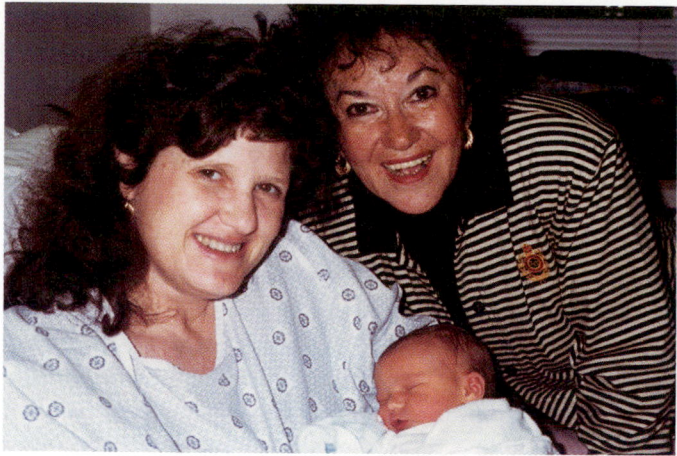

Figure 2-10   Birth: three generations.

Critical Thinking

A New Mother

J.L. is a 21-year-old primapara single woman who has just given birth to an 8 lb baby boy. Her pregnancy was obstetrically uncomplicated. However, her social situation was not stable during the last trimester. Her partner, the baby's father, moved to another state and refused to communicate with her; she moved in with her parents, who have been supportive of the pregnancy and her decision to continue as a single parent. Her parents accompanied her in labor; her mother was her primary support person. Because she had an uncomplicated labor and birth, J.L. will be discharged from the hospital after 48 hours.

- Discuss appropriate nursing assessments that will indicate the level of risk that J.L. has for difficulty in adjusting to her role as a mother.

- What are the strengths of this situation that will ultimately assist J.L. in adjusting to her role as a new mother?

- How can you assess the response of the grandparents to the birth of their grandson?

- What are two immediate and two long-term interventions that you can implement to assist this family?

Variations in the Birth Process: Impact on the Family

Birth, by its very nature, is an unpredictable experience. Any deviation from expectations can leave the woman and her family feeling unfulfilled or detract from their feelings of confidence and wholeness. For the birthing woman, a prolonged labor may indicate to her that her body won't work correctly. A delivery assisted by forceps, vacuum, or episiotomy may place her in a position of loss of confidence in her body, loss of integrity of her body boundaries, or a sense of unfulfillment or of ineptitude (Hawkins & Gorvine, 1985).

For a partner, a prolonged labor and difficult delivery may challenge his or her self-concept as a protector. The persistent feeling of helplessness in the face of the events of birth can influence the partner's response to the newborn. A partner who feels guilty about not protecting the woman from the difficulties of the birth may experience anger or frustration. The nurse is in a pivotal position to help partners come to terms with their feelings of disappointment and frustration and to avoid displacing these feelings on each other. By using communication skills to engage partners in a discussion about the experience and validating their frustrations and fears, the nurse can guide the partners to an understanding of their response and channel that energy into positive activities to assist the new mother, such as breastfeeding support.

Cesarean Delivery

Cesarean delivery may be perceived as the ultimate inability of the woman's body to perform the normal function of giving birth. Women delivered by cesarean section often felt less satisfied with their birth experience than those who delivered vaginally, and initially, cesarean-birth mothers viewed their babies in a less positive light (DiMatteo et al., 1996).

Response of the At-Risk Family

DeMeir, Hynan, Harris, and Manniello (1996) evaluated the incidence of post-traumatic stress disorder (PTSD) in mothers who experienced a high-risk birth. They found that mothers of premature and term infants who required neonatal intensive care reported significantly more symptoms of PTSD than mothers of term infants who were born without those stress factors present. Older children in a family who experienced a difficult birth may blame themselves for interfering or causing the problem. The extended family fears for the safety of both the mother and the baby. Maternal grandparents fear for their daughter and her infant. They may feel guilt for nonsupport or the level of support they gave their child. The experience may seem to confirm their fears that their child isn't normal and that there is some undiagnosed reason that she is not able to birth normally, for which they are responsible. They may feel they did not do enough. Alternatively, they may be angry with the partner or obstetric professionals for not protecting their daughter from harm or illness.

The family reaction to a difficult birth experience also has implications for the relationship with the new infant. In a family in which the infant is blamed for the pain or the type of delivery, the infant is potentially at risk for neglect or abuse; such an infant is termed a "vulnerable infant." Some families may become overprotective of the infant in an attempt to shield him or her from further trauma. Identification of negative responses to the mother or child in the birth setting may be the first sign of risk to the infant for neglect or abuse.

Response to Loss at Birth

Loss of an infant at birth can be viewed from several perspectives. One is the incongruity of the experience with the expectations of the parents: the loss, so to speak, of the perfect baby. The stillbirth of a fetus is another type of loss. Finally, the birth of an infant that is to be relinquished, either to adoption or because the woman cannot keep the child (for example, an incarcerated mother) is a different type of loss.

Any type of loss sets in motion a process of grieving in the parents and family. The value placed on the pregnancy and the newborn influences the depth and intensity of the emotions. The intensity of loss felt in the family who has labored through the process of infertility treatment may be stronger and more prolonged because they are forced to deal with the emotional rollercoaster of assisted fertility (Woods & Esposito-Woods, 1997).

Kübler-Ross (1969) identified stages of grieving, through which individuals move, as they try to come to terms with death and loss. These include denial that the event has occurred; anger directed at anyone deemed responsible, including self, God, the midwife or doctor; the hospital, other family members; bargaining by trying to find alternatives to accepting the reality of the event; resolution to the facts; and, finally, acceptance. In the birth setting, the most likely stages that the nurse sees and assists the family with are anger, denial, and bargaining. The entire process can take days, months, years, or, for some families, remain forever unresolved.

Even after an uncomplicated birth experience, a woman may grieve the loss of the fetus as a part of her body.

Another area of loss is that felt by parents who relinquish their birth child for adoption. Fathers in particular are left out of the literature. Loss of the child continues to be an unresolved issue of grieving for the mothers as well as the fathers many years later. There is a delicate balance that must be kept to address the needs of the father in this situation, along with the needs and rights of the mother, the child, and the adoptive family. Nurses as care providers in the birth setting are in a pivotal position to help birth fathers and mothers own the decisions they have made and develop coping strategies.

Response of Health Care Professionals

The professional and institutional response to loss at birth has changed dramatically over the years. Historically, in an effort to "spare" the mother and parents, women were anesthetized for delivery and stillborn babies were whisked out of sight. Infants slated for adoption were removed from the delivery room quickly to protect the mother from seeing or hearing the child and feeling the sadness of her decision. Today most institutions have perinatal grief teams, which are specially developed teams of nurses, social workers, and others who are available to assist families and staff with the issues of grieving. Rather than trying to brush the experience away, we know today that it is necessary for families and care givers to come to closure with the loss of the baby to develop effective coping strategies for continuing their lives.

NURSING IMPLICATIONS

When applying the nursing process to a family, the nurse follows the usual steps of the process but for the family as a whole and not for an individual client. During the assessment, information is gathered about the structure, interrelationships, and dynamics of the family. The strengths, resources, and concerns of the family also are assessed. A diagnosis is then made based on the assessments. A plan is developed through a mutual, ongoing process. For the plan to be successful, the family members must act as collaborators; the outcomes are on the level of the family and not on the level of the individual client.

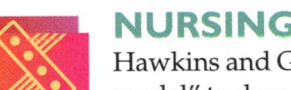 ### NURSING PROCESS

Hawkins and Gorvine (1985) used the "crisis model" to develop a framework for maternal newborn nurses to use in assessing family responses to birth and in planning appropriate interventions for postpartum women and their families. They discuss the risks to the postpartum woman in negotiating this time of crisis and how to develop the coping strategies required to enter the role of parent. Those women who meet this challenge experience a reduction in anxiety as they achieve equilibrium in the resolution of the pregnancy and birth. Those women unable to achieve equilibrium experience a continuing level of anxiety, which interferes with achieving the role of mother and the development of successful parenting skills (Hawkins & Gorvine, 1985).

Client Education

Self-Care for Postpartum Families

Recent work by Deborah Sichel and Jeanne Watson Driscoll (1999) describes the effects of birth on brain chemistry and the ability of the woman to adapt to the new family relationships postpartum. To enable women to address the emotional challenges of this period, these researchers have developed a self-care program that can maximize the woman's ability to develop effective coping strategies during the postpartum period. The program is called NURSE and provides the following guidelines to use in developing a plan with the woman:

- **N—Nourishment:** Maintain basic nutrition, using the food pyramid as a guide, to provide the brain with appropriate vitamins and basic nutrients. Discuss a multivitamin supplement with your midwife or physician. Be sure to include adequate amounts of alpha–3 omega fatty acids, such as those found in fish proteins, because they are important for nerve cell functioning and, through modulating chemical nerve transmission, may have mood-stabilizing effects.

- **U—Understanding:** Work with the new mother and family to develop strategies that provide support in the form of listening, validating feelings, and nurturing each other. Identify family resources for backup, such as the phone numbers of counseling services and community support groups.

- **R—Rest and relaxation:** Adequate rest and sleep are essential for the brain to restore itself biochemically. New parents may become sleep-deprived if they do not actively plan rest periods and sleep when the infant sleeps. Planning for rest periods and for taking turns at getting up with the infant may be important strategies to protect against sleep deprivation.

- **S—Spirituality:** Each woman and family has experiences and activities that nourish their souls. Planning to include such activities, which can be as simple as buying fresh cut flowers to place in a living space or listening to soulful music, addresses this need.

- **E—Exercise:** It is well-documented that physical exercise causes the release of endorphins, which cause a feeling of well-being. A daily exercise regimen can be as simple as taking the newborn out together for a walk.

Nursing interventions in this model are designed to enable postpartum women and their families to develop successful coping strategies for this new dimension of their lives by using what they bring to the experience with them as well as resources available through their extended family and community. Examples of resources that a woman brings to the childbirth experience may include: previous coping mechanisms, nutritional status (which influences her physiologic ability to adapt to birth), and belief system. Examples of external resources include family and friends, community support groups, social services, and religious organizations (Hawkins & Gorvine, 1985).

Assessment

Relevant clinical, demographic, and social data can be gathered from the medical record or the client herself, including:

- Cultural background
- Gravidity (number of pregnancies) and parity (number of pregnancies that reached viability)
- Prenatal course (complications or lack thereof)
- Social situation, including housing, income, presence of partner, gender of partner, and extended family
- Work situation, type, and job title
- Recorded plans for infant feeding and postpartum care

While interacting with the woman during labor and birth, the nurse should gather data, such as the following:

- Conduct and length of labor
- Type of birth, vaginal or operative
- If the mother holds the infant immediately after birth
- What the mother says to the infant, e.g., "I am so glad to see you" or "you nearly killed me"
- If the mother looks at the infant
- How the mother touches the infant (e.g., does she progress from fingertips to encircling the infant, or turn away or hold the infant away from her body?)
- How the mother interacts with her support network

Nursing Diagnoses

Nursing diagnoses represent the nurse's decision about the data gathered. Diagnoses commonly seen include impaired parenting related to inability to bond with the newborn, and anxiety about feelings of loss. The North American Nursing Diagnosis Association (NANDA) publishes a listing of standardized diagnosis language that is helpful to nurses developing care plans.

Outcome Identification

Outcomes can be described in terms of short- and long-term goals. For example:

- The mother demonstrates positive interaction with her newborn.
- The client discusses the difference between postpartum "baby blues" and the symptoms of depression.
- The client and her partner identify childcare options within their extended family and community for babysitting.

Standardized language exists for outcome identification; this is known as the Nursing Outcomes Classification, or NOC.

Planning

With the client, the nurse identifies those strategies that will assist the client in meeting short- and long-term goals. Strategies range from bedside education and reading materials to referral to a visiting nurse service or social services.

Nursing Intervention

Nursing interventions can assist the mother in developing a realistic interpretation of her birth experience and may include:

- Encouraging the mother to talk about what she experienced

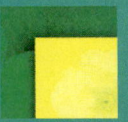

CASE STUDY/CARE PLAN
A GROWING FAMILY

G.P. is gravida 3, para 3 (G3, P3), a Native American woman who has delivered at the New Market Birth Center and is now 2 hours postpartum.

After a 15-hour labor and without the use of medications, Dahlia Louise was born over an intact perineum, weighing 8 pounds, with an Apgar score of 9 at 1 and 5 minutes. The baby breathed spontaneously and was delivered onto the mother's abdomen. M.P., the father, was present, providing labor support throughout, and cut the umbilical cord. During the labor and birth, specially recorded taped music was played; the family explained to the nurse that the pieces were special spiritual songs that promoted peacefulness and inner strength.

Also present during labor and for the birth were both sets of grandparents; Marc, the couple's 8-year-old son; and Jean, the couple's 4-year-old daughter.

During the labor and birth, Jean slept, colored, and roamed around the center, appearing unconcerned with the events in the birth room. Marc was actively involved, giving his mother ice chips and timing contractions, while his father provided physical support. The grandparents alternated sitting in the family room, visiting and observing activities in the birth room, and going out for provisions. Much of their conversation was about the changes in birth practices and worries about the safety of out-of-hospital birth. After the birth, they gathered in the birth room, cooing over the baby and praising G.P. and M.P. for their accomplishment.

Postpartum assessments have been within normal limits. The midwife has done a newborn examination that yielded results that were within normal limits. The mother has been to the bathroom and eaten. The baby has had a stool and passed urine.

The family plans to leave the birth center at 12 hours postpartum to return home. They live in a single-family dwelling with two flights of stairs. M.P. has to return to work in 2 days. G.P. plans to exclusively breastfeed her baby, as she did her first two children, and has already put the baby to breast, establishing a good latch-on. G.P. plans to return to work in 6 weeks and to place the infant in daycare with her 4-year-old daughter.

Assessment

- No contributory medical or surgical history
- Pregnancy at term without complications
- Postpartum recovery without complication
- Newborn examination (within normal limits), baby has passed urine and meconium
- Multiparous family, apparently prepared for the birth experience and comfortable with participation from all members, each member having a proscribed role
- Family does not have a plan for support after discharge

(continues)

Nursing Diagnosis

Interrupted family processes related to the birth experience

Expected Outcomes

1. The client and family will validate their experiences during labor and birth.
2. The family will list support strategies, using community and family support systems.
3. Before leaving the birth center, G.P. will discuss specific strategies that she can employ to help her organize life at home to reduce stress.
4. The client and family will discuss the warning signs of postpartum depression.
5. At 3 days and 1 week postpartum, the family will not exhibit signs of dysfunction related to the birth experience.

Planning

The nurse can include the family and siblings in planning care that will reflect the needs of the family as a whole.

NOC

Family functioning

NIC

Family process maintenance

Nursing Interventions

1. The nurse will encourage the individual members of the family to talk about how they felt during the labor and birth.
2. The nurse will provide referrals to home visiting nursing services for intervals at 24 hours postdischarge and 3 days postpartum to assess the mother, newborn, and family adjustment. The nurse will also provide a pediatric referral to the pediatrician of the mother's choice 48 hours postpartum for newborn assessment and relevant testing.
3. The nurse will discuss specific options, such as the NURSE program, to help the client manage stress.
4. The nurse will discuss the specifics of the signs of postpartum depression and suggest interventions.
5. The nurse will make follow-up phone calls to the client at 3 days and 1 week postpartum and document the success of the care plan for this family or identify problems needing resolution.

Rationales

1. At this time, the nurse will validate feelings and provide accurate information about events.
2. This assists the family in identifying community resources, such as church, to enlist in providing postpartum support services.

3. These strategies offer resources to the client to learn how to manage stress.
4. This helps the client become independent and assists the family in recognizing symptoms that should be addressed.
5. To assess family adjustment and offer assistance if needed.

Evaluation

Family adjustment is facilitated by actions of the nurse that foster maternal self-confidence and family support. By beginning with validation of the birth experience, the nurse can identify feelings of satisfaction or dissatisfaction and congruence or dissonance with actual events. Helping the family put the experience in perspective before they leave the birth site is a preventive measure. Assisting the family to identify and develop support systems after discharge is preventive and supportive. Evaluating the family at proscribed intervals allows the nurse to address developing issues before they lead to dysfunction.

- Describing the birth of the baby, if she was not able to see it in a mirror
- Helping the mother distinguish between what she thought happened and what actually occurred
- Assisting the woman to inspect the infant
- Encouraging the mother to hold her baby

Standardized intervention language also exists in the form of Nursing Intervention Classification, or NIC.

Evaluation

The ability of the nurse to evaluate the success of the interventions varies, depending on the length of interaction with the family. Observations of behaviors that meet stated goals may be possible. Additionally, referral to collaborative agencies or providers may be necessary to evaluate the progress toward long-term goals.

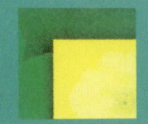

CASE STUDY/CARE PLAN
IMPLEMENTING THE NURSING PROCESS WITH A FOCUS ON THE FAMILY

The nurse who works in labor and delivery sees Joel nervously pacing in the waiting room. Earlier, during his wife's labor with their second child, he had left the room quickly if she seemed distressed or if a procedure was being carried out. He had chosen not to be present during the delivery of the couple's first child. Now, when his child is about to be born, he says, "I don't know anything about newborns. I've never even held one." The nurse says, "Lots of men have been in your shoes, and they did fine. Fathers are important people. I will help you the first time." The father quietly says, "Thank you." Later, the nurse from the newborn nursery wheels out the baby in the isolette. When the father reaches out to the baby, the nurse says, "You aren't allowed to walk with the baby. You might drop him." She then wheels the baby into the mother's room, with the father following some distance behind.

The labor and delivery nurse is in the room with the mother. As the father enters the room the mother turns to her and says, "What does he know about it? He didn't go through it." The nurse says, "No, he doesn't get to be a mother but I bet he'll be a great father. He is so concerned and anxious about the two of you." The father is standing awkwardly near the door. Turning to him the nurse says, "Sit down in that chair. Arrange your arm to make a cradle to hold your baby." She then places the baby in the father's arms, making sure the baby is well supported. Then, after making sure the baby is awake and alert, she says, "Look at him. He wants to see your face. Good. Now talk to him. Keep watching. Did you see him respond? Your baby knows you. He likes to hear your voice. He knows it." The baby had turned to the sound of his father's voice. The father then settled back more comfortably in the chair and smiled. He kept looking at the baby and started touching his face. The nurse turned to the mother and said, "You have a great family." The mother smiled.

Assessment

During her assessment of the family, the labor and delivery nurse noted the father's pacing, his comment about never having held a baby, and the mother's comment that suggested she did not think he knew much about parenting. The nurse's informal assessment was that the father was not sure how to father and the mother also was insecure and doubtful about his abilities.

Nursing Diagnosis

If she had formalized her diagnosis it might be the following: compromised family coping related to father's expressed lack of experience caring for infants.

Expected Outcomes	Family members will begin to understand and accept the differing roles they play and the unique attributes each brings to the family unit.
Planning	Throughout the process, the labor and delivery nurse collaborates with the family as she plans her intervention.
NOC	Family coping
NIC	Family support

Nursing Interventions	**Rationales**
1. The father shares his lack of experience with a newborn, and the nurse suggests a plan. She offers to help him; he accepts.	1. All the nurse's actions are geared to helping this family function as a unit.
2. The nurse acknowledges the mother's role in giving birth and her roles as wife and mother in this family. The nurse stresses the positive aspects of the father's behavior and, through teaching and encouragement, empowers him to become an active parent and partner with his wife.	2. This strengthens the family unit.

(continues)

Nursing Interventions	Rationales
3. The nurse does not side with either parent at the expense of the other.	3. This avoids splitting within the family and promotes the family as a unit.

Evaluation   The nurse needs to observe the interaction of the family unit. The manner in which the father interacts with the infant reveals a lot about his relationship with the infant, his wife, and their adaptations to the new infant. The way the couple interact with each other also is important. For example, when the father brings flowers to the wife and tells her how proud he is of her, this would be one indicator of a positive adjustment to the birth of a child.

WEB ACTIVITIES

• • •   Search the Web sites listed in the Resources section and explore resources and information for single parents and stepfamilies.

• • •   Search the Internet for support groups for various family concerns, such as families with a new baby or family caretakers of a chronically ill member.

• • •   Examine Internet sites for appropriate information based on the principles and theories discussed in this chapter.

Key Concepts

■ Many types of family structures exist: traditional, extended, single-parent, reconstituted, unmarried heterosexual, homosexual, and communal structures. These need to be understood to adapt nursing care to an individual family.

■ Family functions of providing for its members, child rearing, and transmitting cultural values are found across cultures. The beliefs, values, and manner in which the functions are carried out, however, are highly dependent on culture.

■ Nursing care of the birthing woman and her family is based on an understanding of the theoretical framework of the family's response to birth.

■ A family's response to birth reflects their culture, belief system, and style of coping with changing life circumstances.

■ Birth is a crisis, or turning point, in life that challenges the family to adapt their lifestyle coping mechanisms. This is an unprecedented time, during which the nurse has the opportunity to assist the family in moving into a new stage.

■ An understanding and acceptance of the nurse's personal experience and response to both the birth experience, and the loss of an infant at birth help ensure that these issues do not interfere with the nurse's ability to meet the needs of the client and family.

Review Questions and Activities

1. In general, health care providers tend to have expectations regarding families that are predicted on which family structure?
   a. Traditional
   b. Single-parent family
   c. Reconstituted family
   d. Communal

   The correct answer is a.

2. Describe theories of maternal response to birth.

3. Define birth as a "crisis," or turning point, for families.

4. Discuss the impact of birth on the father, siblings, and grandparents.

5. Discuss how personal unresolved feelings that a nurse may have about birth can interfere with his or her ability to assist the family in reaching their goals for birth.

6. In what specific ways can a normal, uncomplicated birth be an empowering experience for the woman, her partner, and her family?

7. Discuss the implications of the birth experience for older children. List nursing interventions that can assist children in appreciating the experience.

References

Belkin, I., (1993). *First, do no harm*. New York: Fawcett.

Carter, B., & McGoldrick, M. (Eds.), (1989). *The changing family life cycle* (2nd ed.). Boston, MA: Allyn and Bacon.

Clinton, J. F., & Kelber, S. T. (1993). Stress and coping in fathers of newborns: Comparisons of planned versus unplanned pregnancy. *International Journal of Nursing Studies, 30*(5). 437–443.

Cox, M. J., & Paley, B. (1997). Families as systems. *Annual Review of Psychology, 48,* 243–267.

Cross, T., Bazron, B., Dennis, K., & Isaacs, M. (1989). *Towards a culturally competent system of care: Vol I.* Washington, DC: National Technical Assistance Center for Children's Mental Health. Georgetown University Child Development Center.

DeMier, R., Hynan, M., Harris, H., & Manniello, R. (1996). Perinatal stressors as predictors of symptoms of posttraumatic stress in mothers of infants at high risk. *Journal of Perinatology, 16*(4), 276–280.

DiMatteo, M. R., Morton, S., Lepper, H., Damush, T., Carney, M., Person, M., & Kahn, K. (1996). Cesarean childbirth and psychosocial outcomes: A meta-analysis. *Health Psychology, 15*(4), 303–314.

Elkind, D. (1994). *Ties that stress: The new family imbalance.* Cambridge, MA: Harvard University Press.

Erickson, E. (1963). *Childhood and society* (2nd ed.). New York: W. W. Norton.

Esposito, N. (1999). Marginalized women's comparisons of their hospital and freestanding birth center experiences: A contrast of inner-city birthing systems. *Health Care for Women International, 20,* 111–126.

Fowles, E. (1998). Labor concerns of women two months after delivery, *Birth, 25*(4), 235–240.

Friedman, M. M. (1992). *Family nursing theory and practice* (3rd ed.). Norwalk, CT: Appleton and Lange.

Hall, E. O. (1995). From fun and excitement to joy and trouble—An explorative study of three Danish fathers' experiences around birth. *Scandinavian Journal of Caring Sciences, 9*(3) 171–179.

Hawkins, J., & Gorvine, B. (1985), *Post partum nursing: Health care of women.* New York: Springer.

Heggenhougen, H. K. (1980). Father and childbirth: An anthropological perspective. *Journal of Nurse Midwifery, 25*(6), 21–26.

Hodnett, E. D. (2000). Support from caregivers during childbirth. In J. P. Neilson, C. A. Crowther, E. D. Hodnett, G. J. Hofmeyr, & M. J. N. C. Keirse. (Eds.), *Pregnancy and childbirth module of the Cochrane database of systematic reviews.* Oxford, England: Cochrane Collaboration.

Jordan, P. (1990a). Laboring for relevance: Expectant and new fatherhood. *Nursing Research, 39*(1), 11–16.

Jordan, P. (1990b). First-time expectant fatherhood: Nursing care considerations. *NAACOGS Clinical Issues in Perinatal & Womens Health Nursing, 1*(3), 311–316.

Katz-Rothman, B. (1996). Women, providers, and control. *Journal of Obstetric, Gynecologic, and Neonatal Nursing 25,* 253–256.

Kübler-Ross, E. (1969). *On death and dying.* New York: Macmillan.

Lederman, R. P. (1984). Psychosocial adaptaton in pregnancy: Assessment of seven dimensions of maternal development. Upper Saddle River, NJ: Prentice-Hall.

Maushart, S. (1999). *The mask of motherhood: How becoming a mother changes everything and why we pretend in doesn't.* New York: W. W. Norton.

Mercer, R. T. (1995). *Becoming a mother: Research on maternal role identity from Rubin to the present.* Springer Series: Focus on Women. New York: Springer.

Nichols, F., Humenick, S. (2000). *Childbirth education: Practice, research, and theory.* New York: Harcourt Health Sciences.

Nolan, M. (1996). The birth of Natasha: One labour, two very different experiences. *Modern Midwife, 6*(2), 6–9.

Patterson, J. M. (1999). Healthy American families in a postmodern society: An ecological perspective. In H. Wallace, G. Green, K. Jaeos, L. Paine, & M. Story (Eds.), *Health and welfare for families in the 21st century.* Sudbury, MA: Jones & Bartlett.

Pryia, J. V. (2000). Birth traditions and modern pregnancy. In F. Nichols & S. Humenick (Eds.), *Childbirth education: Practice, research and theory.* New York: Harcourt Health Sciences.

Rubin, R. (1984). Maternal identity and the maternal experience. New York: Springer.

Scott, K., Berkowitz, G., & Klaus, M. (1999). A comparison of intermittent and continuous support during labor: A meta-analysis. *American Journal of Obstetrics and Gynecology, 180,* 1054.

Scott, K., Klaus, P., & Klaus, M. (1999). Obstetrical and postpartum benefits of continuous support during childbirth. *Journal of Women's Health and Gender-Based Medicine, 8*(10), 1257–1264.

Seibt, T. H. (1996). Nontraditional families. In M. Harway (Ed.), *Treating the changing family* (pp. 39–61). New York: John Wiley.

Sichel, D., & Driscoll, J. W. (1999). *Women's moods.* New York: William Morrow.

Simkin, P. (1996). The experience of maternity in a woman's life. *Journal of Obstetric, Gynecologic, and Neonatal Nursing 25,* 247–252.

Stepfamily Association of America. (2001). Retrieved March 2001, from http://www.stepfam.org.

Visher, E. B., & Visher, J. S. (1993). Remarriage families and stepparenting. In F. Walsh (Ed.), *Normal family processes* (2nd ed., pp. 235–253). New York: The Guildford Press.

von Klitzing, K., Amsler, F., Schleske, G., Simoni, H., & Burgin, D. (1996). Effect of psychological factors in pregnancy on the development of parent-child relations. 2. Transition from prenatal to postnatal phase. *Gynakologisch-Geburtshilfliche Rundschau, 36*(3), 149–155.

Walsh, F. (Ed.). (1993). *Normal family processes* (2nd ed.). New York: The Guildford Press.

Woods, J., & Esposito-Woods, J. (1997). *Loss during pregnancy or in the newborn period: Principles of care with clinical cases and analyses.* Pitman, NJ: Jannetti.

Suggested Readings

Dochterman, J. M., & Bulechek, G. M. (2004). *Nursing Interventions Classification (NIC).* St. Louis: Mosby.

Moorhead, S., Johnson, M., & Maas, M. (2004). *Nursing Outcomes Classification (NOC).* St. Louis: Mosby.

North American Nursing Diagnosis Association (NANDA). (2003). Nursing Diagnoses: Definitions & Classification, 2003–2004. Philadelphia: Author.

Wright, L. M., & Leahey, M. (2000). *Nurses and families.* Philadelphia: F.A. Davis.

Resources

American Association for Marriage and Family Therapy, http://www.aamft.org

American College of Nurse-Midwives, 818 Connecticut Avenue NW, Suite 900, Washington, DC 20006. 202-728-9860, Fax: 202-728-9897, info@acnm.org, http://www.midwife.org

Association of Women's Health, Obstetric, and Neonatal Nurses (AWHONN), 2000 L. St. NW Suite 740, Washington, DC 20036, 800-673-8499, http://www.awhonn.org

March of Dimes, Education Services, 1275 Mamaroneck Avenue, White Plains, NY 10605, 888-MODIMES, http://www.modimes.org

National Center for Education in Maternal and Child Health, 2000 15th St North, Suite 701, Arlington, VA 22201-2617, 703-524-7802, http://www.ncemch.org

Parents without Partners, http://www.parentswithoutpartners.org

Stepfamily Association of America, http://www.stepfam.org

U.S. Health Resources and Services Administration, 888-275-4772, http://www.ask.hrsa.gov

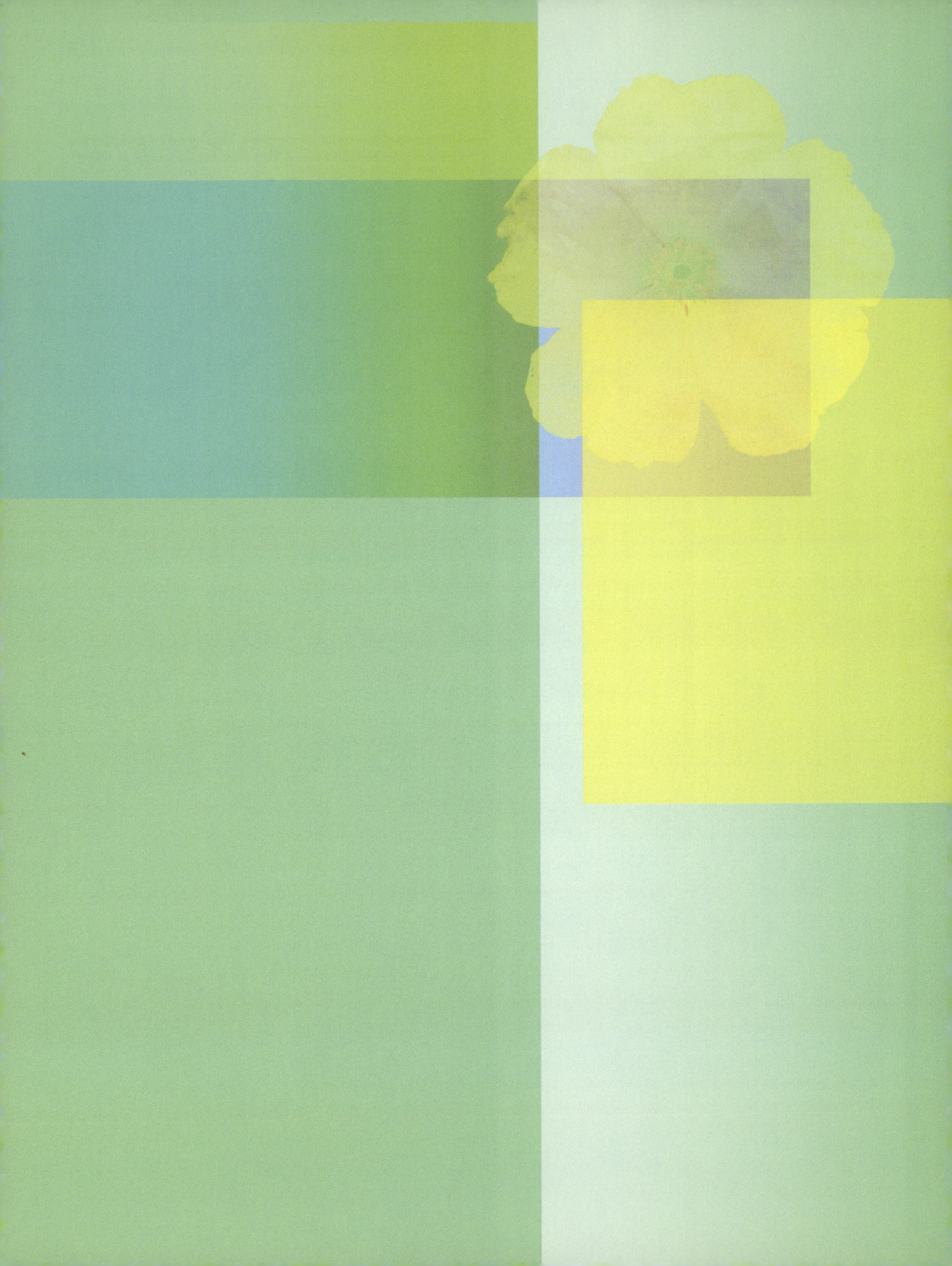

CHAPTER 3

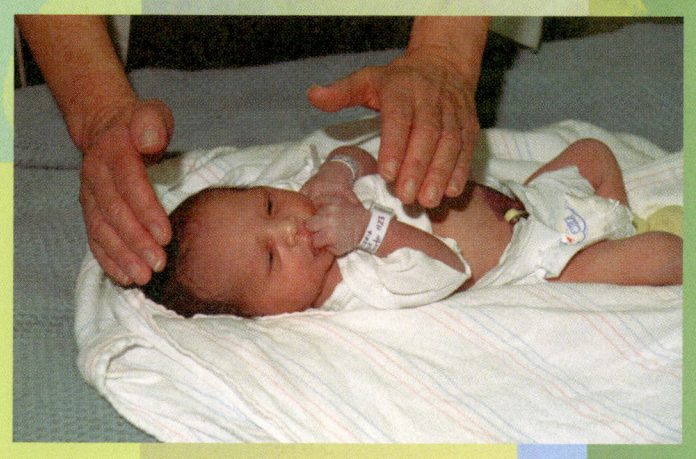

COMPLEMENTARY AND ALTERNATIVE THERAPIES

Kim is a 52-year-old nurse who was diagnosed with breast cancer. She was treated surgically with a modified radical mastectomy, followed by chemotherapy for 6 months and radiation therapy for 6 weeks. Having grown up on a farm, Kim felt that proper nutrition might reduce the side effects of chemotherapy and radiation and decrease the chance of a recurrence. She consulted a nutritionist, who put her on a diet of all organic foods, including a juice consisting of celery, carrots, parsley, lettuce, and beets. After her treatments, she continued to restrict her diet and incorporated yoga, exercise, writing in a journal, and meditation into her daily routine. Kim feels that the most difficult part of her experience was dealing with the fear of cancer recurrence.

Have you ever wondered how you would react to a life-threatening diagnosis? Engaging in complementary therapies (CTs) may improve one's sense of well-being and control throughout such an experience. Some CTs have been reported to decrease the side effects of standard treatments. However, CTs may be expensive in terms of time, energy, and money, and the degree to which they may interfere with standard biomedical therapy or yield toxicities of their own often is not known. Nurses can influence the decisions clients make regarding the use of CTs, which often are widely advertised and easily available.

Key Terms

Acupressure
Acupuncture
Allopathy
Alternative therapies
Ayurvedic medicine
Biomedicine
Chi
Chi gong
Complementary
  therapies

Culture
Dosha
Healing systems
Holism
Integrated medicine
Meridian
Moxibustion
Phytotherapy
Prana
Vitalism

Competencies

Upon completion of this chapter, the reader should be able to:

1. Differentiate between complementary and alternative therapies.
2. Discuss the evolution of traditional healing systems and their influence on healing approaches.
3. Identify possible influencing factors for the contemporary use of complementary therapies by clients and their families.
4. Describe a classification of complementary modalities of healing.
5. Discuss legal, regulatory, and ethical issues encountered by nurses with regard to complementary therapies.
6. Discuss the use of complementary therapies for health promotion.
7. Identify indications and contraindications for complementary therapies in women with health deviations.
8. Recognize resources for further education or certification to incorporate complementary therapies into the client's plan of care.

The popularity of complementary and alternative medicine (CAM) has increased since the 1990s. The terms *alternative*, *complementary*, and *unconventional medicines* have been used interchangeably in the literature and in health care practice. The term **alternative therapy** implies outside of or apart from **biomedicine** (the scientific-based professional medicine taught in medical schools and generally practiced in the United States and Canada) and is best reserved for the therapies used *instead of* biomedical treatment. Because many of these therapies are used as a complement to biomedical treatment or for health promotion, **complementary therapy (CT)** is a more appropriate term. These modalities are used *in addition to* standard treatments for comfort, pain reduction, and symptom relief. Many CTs also facilitate coping and promote or maintain general health.

Many health care providers, health maintenance organizations, and third-party payers are advocating **integrated medicine**, which combines biomedicine with CTs to provide holistic care. This change in health care delivery has come about largely because of consumer demand for holistic health care services. Consumers want emphasis on health promotion, self-care, and attention to the human experience of health and illness.

Many modalities currently identified as popular CTs have previously been described as independent nursing interventions (Snyder & Lindquist, 1998). Nurses are in a position to provide or help the client access many of these services. Nurses also should assess client interest in and use of such services to help clients safely integrate complementary modalities into their health care.

CONTEMPORARY USE OF COMPLEMENTARY THERAPIES

Surveys have indicated that CT use has increased since the 1990s. Many surveys indicate that about half the U.S. population uses some form of CT. The rate increases in clients with chronic diseases; for example, one survey in clients with cancer found the use rate was 83% (Richardson, Sanders, Palmer, Greisinger, & Singletary, 2000). Women account for two thirds of the use of CTs, which is consistent with their more frequent use of conventional health care services (Beal, 1998). Other surveys have described CT users as highly educated, relatively affluent, and often having a holistic orientation toward health (Astin, 1998; Eisenberg et al., 1998; McGuire, 1988). In

Reflections from a Nurse

As an oncology nurse caring for women with breast cancer, I became interested in complementary and alternative therapies as I noted that more and more clients were seeking these therapies. Many of these women had metastatic disease and were coming to the major comprehensive cancer center where I worked as a clinical nurse specialist with the hope of a cure, only to be disappointed that they had exhausted all treatment options. Other women who were without evidence of active disease wanted to do all that they could to prevent cancer from recurring. Women were consuming large doses of vitamins and herbs, sometimes with evidence of toxicity. One client was admitted for severe electrolyte imbalances resulting from coffee enemas, and another with thrombocytopenia and bleeding related to the combination of chemotherapy and ginseng. Young women receiving adjuvant chemotherapy were experiencing disabling hot flashes from the toxic effect of the drugs on the ovaries. This was particularly distressing because hormone replacement therapy is contraindicated in women with breast cancer, and there were no known effective alternatives. Little was known about CAM use and its effects in clients with cancer prior to the 1970s and 1980s. It was apparent, however, that women with breast cancer were desperate for anything that might offer some degree of hope and control over this ravaging disease.

many cases, consumers do not tell their physicians nor are physicians aware of the use of CTs. Problems can result from treatment contraindications, interactions, and poor communication patterns between client and provider.

Congress mandated the National Institutes of Health (NIH) to set up an Office of Alternative Medicine (OAM), which was started in 1992, and which was later upgraded to the National Center for Complementary and Alternative Medicine (NCCAM) to study non-conventional therapies and disseminate information to providers and the public. CAM practices have been cataloged into seven broad categories: mind-body interventions, bioelectromagnetic applications, alternative systems of medical practice, manual healing methods, pharmacologic and biologic treatments, herbal medicine, and diet and nutrition in the prevention and treatment of chronic disease (National Institutes of Health, 1994) (Box 3-1). Some modalities have been recommended for incorporation into general health care. For example, integration of behavioral and relaxation therapies such as meditation, hypnosis, and biofeedback into medical management of chronic pain and insomnia was recommend by an NIH consensus panel of experts (Chilton, 1996).

Several peer-reviewed journals have been established to focus exclusively on CAM therapies. A number of research studies and articles related to CAM also have been published in most medical and specialty journals across health care disciplines. According to one survey, 64% of medical schools have added courses covering CAM (Wetzel, Eisenberg, & Kaptchuk 1998).

The American Holistic Nurses Association, which focuses on incorporating select complementary modalities into nursing care, is one of the fastest growing nursing organizations. The American Holistic Medical Association is a comparable organization of physicians who advocate incorporating select CAM into holistic health care.

National commissions related to health care delivery have made recommendations related to CAM. Both the Robert Wood Johnson Foundation and the Pew Charitable Trust called for the following recommendations: cost containment, focus on health, use of innovative and diverse provisions for health care, and engaging the client as an active agent in health care (Marston & Jones, 1992; Pew, 1995). The Hastings Center for Bioethics established goals

Box 3-1

Classification of Complementary and Alternative Practices

- Mind-body control: art therapy, meditation, and music therapy
- Bioelectromagnetic applications: electromagnetic fields and electrostimulation
- Alternative systems of medical care: acupuncture and homeopathic medicine
- Manual healing: chiropractic and therapeutic touch
- Pharmacologic and biologic treatments: antioxidizing agents and chelation therapy
- Herbal medicine: echinacea and ginseng root
- Diet, nutrition, and lifestyle changes: macrobiotics and nutritional supplements

Nursing Alert

Cancer Recurrence

For women with a personal history of breast cancer, all exogenous hormonal preparations, including hormone replacement therapy (all oral, patch, vaginal, and injectable forms) and oral contraceptive agents, are contraindicated owing to the potential for such agents to stimulate recurrence of breast cancer. Some biologics are sold that contain ground animal ovaries and other hormonal agents. Phytoestrogens also should be avoided because their influence on cancer recurrence has not been validated scientifically.

for medicine in 1996, calling for more research on alternative therapies (Callahan, 1996). The Institute for Alternative Futures (1998) anticipates that two thirds of the population will use some form of CAM by 2010. Many of these complementary modalities are well-matched with the changing health care focus on health promotion and healthy lifestyles.

DIFFERENTIATING ALTERNATIVE FROM COMPLEMENTARY THERAPIES

This chapter focuses on CTs, which are used in conjunction with biomedicine as opposed to alternative therapies, which are used instead of biomedical treatments. These generally natural, noninvasive, holistic treatments are used as supplements to biomedical treatments or to enhance health and well-being. Many CTs are used to reduce stress, enhance coping, and engage the natural

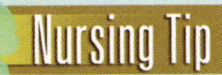 ## Nursing Tip — Disadvantages of Complementary and Alternative Medicine Therapy

Some disadvantages associated with some complementary and alternative therapies are the following:

- May be based on anecdotal evidence and testimonials
- Lack scientific data
- Lack standardization
- May be costly
- May interfere with the effectiveness of standard therapies

healing of the body. Although some clients may abandon biomedical treatment to pursue these treatments, most use these therapies in conjunction with biomedicine or to enhance their health and sense of well-being (Astin, 1998). It is therefore important for nurses to conduct thorough assessments related to the use of CTs.

BACKGROUND AND CLASSIFICATION OF MODALITIES

Many of these modalities have their origins in ethnic traditional healing or the historical healing practices of Europe and America. Many practices are part of the client's or family's actions toward health and reflect cultural orientations and understandings about health. Therefore, when caring for clients from diverse cultures, it is important to understand some of their traditional health beliefs and practices. Practices of traditional cultural systems of healing, such as acupuncture, traditional Chinese medicine (TCM), yoga, or traditional Indian Ayurvedic medicine, are becoming popular with clients of diverse backgrounds. As clients are exposed to health care modalities from other cultures, many are incorporating those practices into their own use.

Critical Thinking

Complementary and Alternative Medicine Literature

As a responsible health care provider, you search the literature related to alternative and complementary therapies. You find a variety of reports about a particular modality. Being a critical consumer of the literature, you ask yourself the following questions:

- Are the authors uncritically enthusiastic?
- Do they make unsubstantiated claims?
- Do they have a vested interest in promoting a service or product?
- Do they make general comments against biomedicine?
- Are the authors uncritically dismissive of the modality?
- Do they make unsubstantiated claims disapproving of the modality?
- Do they make general comments against complementary therapies?
- Do they have any knowledge about the modality?

Systems of Healing

Systems of healing generally employ several modalities under an organizing unified framework. For example, biomedicine is the system of scientifically based professional medicine taught in medical schools. It is the system of healing with which most persons are familiar. Biomedicine uses many modalities of physical manipulation, such as surgery, ingested and applied medications, therapeutic diets, and other therapies (such as psychotherapy) within one system. **Healing systems** reflect a way to classify disease, determine causes, and provide treatment based on an understanding of health and illness.

Healing systems are dynamic and culturally embedded. Many of these systems have developed over time and have incorporated techniques adapted from the environment and interaction with other cultures. (**Culture** is the knowledge, beliefs, art, morals, customs, laws, and other characteristics of persons and members of society [Andrews & Boyle, 1999]). All these systems have components of treatment, prevention, and wellness. Cultural beliefs, values, and worldviews are reflected in the way in which persons understand illness. Five traditional healing systems are discussed briefly: TCM, Ayurvedic medicine, yoga, shamanic healing, and ritual healing systems.

Traditional Chinese Medicine

Traditional Chinese medicine is a complete health system that is thousands of years old. It encompasses exercise, herbal medicine, massage, nutrition, and a holistic approach to healthy living. (**Holism** is the philosophy of integration of body, mind, and spirit within a dynamic environment.) TCM also includes treatments using herbs, acupressure, and acupuncture. The TCM system is based on the interrelatedness between the whole person and nature. Health is based on a balance of opposites. The popular symbol for the union of yin and yang in a circle reflects one aspect of this complex philosophy.

The concept of energy is described in Asian healing systems as chi, ki, or qi. **Chi** is best translated as the point at which matter converts to energy or energy to matter (Kaptchuk, 1983). Chi is understood to flow through various energy channels of the body called **meridians** that have been mapped out over centuries of Asian medical practice. Illness is a disturbance of chi within the body (Ergil, 1996). Treatment modalities aim to restore balance and the unimpeded flow of chi through the meridians. **Acupuncture** and **acupressure** are applied to specific points along the meridians to facilitate the smooth flow and balance of chi. In acupuncture, fine needles are inserted into the skin and rotated; in acupressure, physical pressure is applied to specific points along the meridians. **Moxibustion** is the application of heat, herbs, or both to the energy points. **Chi gong** ("working the chi"), tai chi, and other Asian movement techniques use breathing, movement, and meditation to cleanse, strengthen, and circulate the vital life energy and blood.

Several states have enacted legislation regulating and licensing acupuncturists, ensuring that sterile needles are used and practitioners have met certain standards. Use of Asian herbal medicine is not regulated, however, and caution should be used because these herbs do not necessarily conform to U.S. standards of preparation.

Ayurvedic Medicine

Ayurvedic medicine originated in India and means knowledge of life or science of longevity. These ancient teachings have been passed on through the Vedas, a body of ancient Sanskrit literature (Micozzi, 1996). This approach is holistic and based on the concepts of balance and a vital life force. Ayurvedic medicine in India is centered on the concept of **prana**, a type of vital energy. Health is based on well-being, prevention of disease, and aligning lifestyles with one's individual constitution and personal medical history. Harmony with the environment is sought through understanding and balancing circadian rhythms, seasons, behavior, emotions, and other sensory experiences. Diet, herbs, yoga, meditation, and internal cleansing preparations are addressed in the concept of health. Three **doshas** or metabolic types of people exist: kapha, pitta, and vata, with one being dominant. For optimal health, all doshas need to be in balance; however, the dominant dosha determines the types of foods and other lifestyle practices one should incorporate.

Yoga

Yoga is a classic Indian practice dating back 5,000 years. It is a philosophy of ethics and personal discipline. Although yoga is an entire system of life practice with a spiritual philosophy, many Westerners use the techniques without ascribing to the entire practice that includes a philosophy of living. Aspects of the practice of hatha yoga, which focuses on fitness, have become the most popular. Various stretches and postures are used to relieve mild aches and pains, increase flexibility and coordination, and reduce stress while promoting deep relaxation. Breathing, stretching, taking various body postures, and meditating are incorporated in yoga. These exercises are used to improve circulation, stimulate the internal organs, stretch the body and restore normal alignment, and facilitate proper breathing. Yoga has been shown to reduce blood pressure, reduce heart rate, improve circulation, enhance memory, and release endorphins, the body's natural opiates.

Shamanic Healing

Shamanic healing systems refer to many traditional cultural healing systems. Medicine and religion are fused in

Reflections from a Client

When I developed a nagging pain in my left thigh and hip in 1988, I went to many physicians in search of a cause and treatment. Finally, 17 doctors and 1 year later, a neurosurgeon, who insisted on a myelogram (despite the multiple MRI films I carried with me to the consultation with him), diagnosed a meningioma impinging on my thoracic spine. After a laminectomy to resect the benign tumor, my pain was partially relieved enough so that I was able to discard my cane and gradually wean myself off opioid analgesics. The pain did not go away entirely, however, despite extensive physical therapy, rehabilitation, and nerve blocks.

My long-established faith in the medical model as a health care practitioner was seriously challenged as I slowly realized that there was no cure for the pain. Once I accepted that fact, however, I was able to mobilize other resources for dealing with the pain. Over the past decade, I have engaged in a number of complementary therapies, including acupuncture, neuromuscular massage, yoga, biofeedback, and healing touch. I find that I am best able to manage the pain with regular massage, meditation, and yoga, and with healing touch sessions as needed. Having this experience with pain has enabled me to look beyond the biomedical community for self-care and holistic approaches to enhance my sense of health and well-being, even though the pain is still present.

these systems. The shaman's healing powers are related to the ability to communicate with the spiritual world for direction in healing. The shaman enters a controlled trance or altered state of consciousness. In this state, the shaman is able to transcend the physical body and sojourn into the spirit world, which is one of the most characteristic elements of shamanic systems (Kinsley, 1996). A shaman learns these skills through an apprenticeship with an elder shaman. A special marking at birth, exhibition of special healing skills as a child, or overcoming a personal illness or hardship identifies future shamans.

The calling is a lifelong commitment to healing the members of the community (National Institutes of Health, 1994; Micozzi, 1996). Shamanic systems most familiar to American nurses are Native American healing systems Curanderisimo, Espiritisimo, Santeria, and African folk healing systems such as hoodoo, voodoo, and rootwork (Gordon, Nienstedt, & Gesler, 1998).

Ritual Healing

Spiritual or religious healing has been part of most cultures. Laying on of hands, prayer, and other religious rituals are fairly universal parts of healing practice. Healing has been a strong emphasis in Judeo-Christian practice and beliefs. Numerous accounts of ritual or spiritual healing are recorded in the Bible and related literature (Kinsley, 1996). Recently, medical and scientific investigators have begun to look at the healing power of faith and religious ritual practices (Dossey, 1993; Koenig, 1999). Levin (1994) found positive health benefits associated with participation in church activities. Some religious ritual practices include penance, forgiveness, meditation, and prayer.

Nursing Implications

The traditional healing practices mentioned previously reflect cultural heritages and beliefs about health, illness, and life in general. Nurses should approach the use of these practices as part of culturally competent care. When the practices are not harmful and do not interfere with medical treatments, nurses should support and facilitate clients in their use and practice. Clients determine which practices are congruent with their belief system; nurses should never impose a ritual or symbolic healing system on clients.

Recently, many people in Western cultures have become very interested in varying systems of health and healing. Often the yoga teacher or the shamanic healer is a person of European-American descent who has developed an interest in this system without being from the traditional culture. Nurses should be cautious about making referrals because a certification process rarely exists in these healing systems and one does not usually know much about the individual practitioner. Some organizations, such as the American Holistic Nurses Association, may be useful in providing information and resources.

Healing Approaches Congruent with Self-Healing

Vitalism has been an underlying belief in many cultural healing practices and in many of the following popular healing approaches. Vitalism refers to a "vital energy" or spiritual force. This force or energy is necessary to explain life and health and cannot be reduced to physical and mechanical function. This describes many therapeutic techniques in Western cultures such as Christian Science, chiropractic medicine, osteopathy, naturopathy, homeopathy, hydrotherapy, acupuncture, hypnosis, crystals, and other types of psychic healing. Some of the more popular approaches are discussed: osteopathy, chiropractic medicine, homeopathy, and naturopathy.

Osteopathic Medicine

Osteopathy emphasizes the structural integrity of the body. The principles are holistic and include the unity and self-regulation of the body. When it is in normal structural relationship and has favorable environmental conditions and adequate nutrition, the body is capable of making its own remedies against disease and other toxic conditions (Wagner, 1996). Currently, there are 15 schools of osteopathy in the United States. Graduates earn a doctor of osteopathy degree, or DO. Doctors of osteopathy are licensed to practice all recognized branches of clinical medicine, having much the same education as do medical doctors. Doctors of osteopathy have additional training and emphasis in diagnosis and treatment of the musculoskeletal system and osteopathic manipulative therapy. Many of these techniques also are used in standard medical practice (American Osteopathic Association, 2003)

Chiropractic Medicine

Chiropractic medicine is a manual healing art that originated in 1895 based on two premises: vertebral subluxation (a spinal misalignment causing abnormal nerve transmission) is the cause of virtually all disease; and chiropractic adjustment or manual manipulation of the subluxated vertebra is the cure. Chiropractors treat primarily musculoskeletal conditions, principally back and neck pain and headaches. The Agency for Health Care Policy and Research (AHCPR) endorsed spinal manipulations for back pain in the 1994 Guidelines for Acute Lower Back Pain. Chiropractors are licensed and educated in accredited schools. Several research studies have shown chiropractic treatments to be effective in low back pain and headaches.

Homeopathy

Samuel Hahnemann, a German physician and chemist, developed homeopathy in the early 1800s (Jacobs & Moskowitz, 1996). He felt that symptoms were the body's attempt to self-heal. Based on these observations, he developed a process of provings in which a substance that produced the same symptoms in a well person could be used to augment the body's efforts in combating disease. This practice of using medications producing symptoms similar to those of the disease contrasts with the standard practice of **allopathy** (traditional or established medical or surgical procedures, both invasive and noninvasive, used in the diagnosis and treatment of mental or physical ill-

nesses), or using medicines to counteract the symptoms. Hahnemann believed that spirit was more powerful than matter; therefore, the essence (spirit) of the medicine was more important than the substance.

Homeopathy is practiced widely in Europe, India, Mexico, and other parts of the world; it flourished in the United States until the early 20th century. In the United States, practitioners of homeopathic medicine currently are adding homeopathic practice to an existing legal practice license. For example, many medical doctors and chiropractors also practice homeopathy under their professional licenses. Current research has demonstrated efficacy in a number of chronic conditions such as asthma, allergies, and other conditions not involving advanced tissue damage.

Naturopathy

Naturopathy is concerned with a philosophy of life rather than a particular type of disease treatment. Naturopathy is holistic and focuses on health by integrating osteopathic medicine, chiropractic medicine, hydrotherapy, and homeopathy. Naturopaths believe that most disease is the result of ignoring or violating the laws of nature. Naturopaths espouse natural treatment, healthy nutrition (primarily vegetarian), fresh air, and natural light as natural healing. The principles of naturopathy are holistic; the whole person is treated, with a focus on preserving health, preventing disease, avoiding harm, and using the inherent natural healing systems of harmony to correct the underlying cause of disease (Pizzorno, 1996). The practitioner is a teacher whose major focus is to educate the client toward natural health.

Naturopathic physicians are licensed in some states and practice as primary care providers. They use a variety of natural therapies and diagnostic methods.

COMPLEMENTARY MODALITIES

A host of complementary therapies and therapists currently is available. These are discussed in the following general categories: physical movement and manipulation, ingested and applied substances, energy-based therapies, psychologic or mind-body therapies, and spiritual healing.

Physical Manipulation

Manipulation of the physical body is a common type of modality both in biomedicine and CTs and includes those body movements a person performs and therapeutic manipulations performed by a therapist on the client. Physical manipulations in biomedicine include surgery, physical therapy, and other physical treatments. Complementary modalities include exercise and physical movements and various types of body work.

Exercise and Physical Movements

Exercise and physical movements have a well-established link to health and well-being. A number of specific techniques and approaches currently is available. Exercise programs are designed to do one or a combination of the following. Flexibility exercises are planned and deliberate actions taken to enhance range of motion using a combination of stretching and relaxation techniques, such as yoga and calisthenics. Endurance exercises are used to build stamina and general conditioning. They often are aerobic and are helpful in maintaining cardiovascular health and losing weight. Aerobic exercises aim to increase cardiac endurance and include fast walking, jogging, cycling, and swimming. Strengthening exercises often use weights or machines, with repetitions to build muscle. Sports and athletics often are good methods to achieve a variety of exercise benefits.

Exercise is important for women of all ages. The type of exercise, however, may need to be modified for age and physical condition (Figure 3-1). Exercise should continue during pregnancy to maintain strength and stamina. Stretching also is a good preparation for labor. Pregnant women should avoid leg lifts that may put strain on abdominal muscles after the fourth month. Women should engage in weight-bearing exercise throughout life to help prevent osteoporosis. Swimming and cycling are good aerobic and strengthening exercises but do not strengthen bone. In choosing an exercise program, women need to follow the type of activities they enjoy and to which they are able to adhere. For example, some women are motivated by the social aspects of sports and group exercises, whereas others find a solitary jog is a welcome time alone each day. Many sports and fitness clubs have trainers, kinesologists, or exercise physiologists available for individualized exercise programs.

Specific Exercise or Movement Techniques

A number of specific body techniques is available from teachers who have special training or certification in a particular technique. Some examples are found in Table 3-1.

Body Work

Body work techniques are types of physical manipulation that require a trained therapist. Some of the more popular techniques, such as craniosacral manipulations, massage therapy, myofascial release, Rolfing, and Trager, are described in Table 3-2. Some nurses have acquired additional training and can offer these types of body work to clients.

Nursing Implications

Body work and exercise are very popular and generally have few risks. Most body-work therapists are certified in their training and have been educated to avoid medical risks. It is generally a good practice to ask about certification or preparation of the provider. For women with chronic illnesses and the frail elderly, it is a good idea to consult the physician or nurse practitioner before having body work performed.

Ingested and Applied Substances

Pharmaceuticals are the most commonly applied and ingested substances and are the major focus of biomedical treatment. Many medical pharmaceuticals are derived from plants, and plant-derived products are found in all healing systems. Foods and dietary supplements along with *phytomedicines* (plant-based medicines) are among the most popular forms of CTs.

Numerous dietary plans to lose weight, improve health, and cure diseases are available by way of the popular media. Many diets have not been researched, and nurses should exercise caution in providing dietary advice that may interfere with a therapeutic diet or guidelines for healthy nutrition. Another popular health practice is fasting, which is relatively safe for healthy people for a short duration (less than 3 days). Frequent or long-term fasting may deprive the client of adequate nutrients.

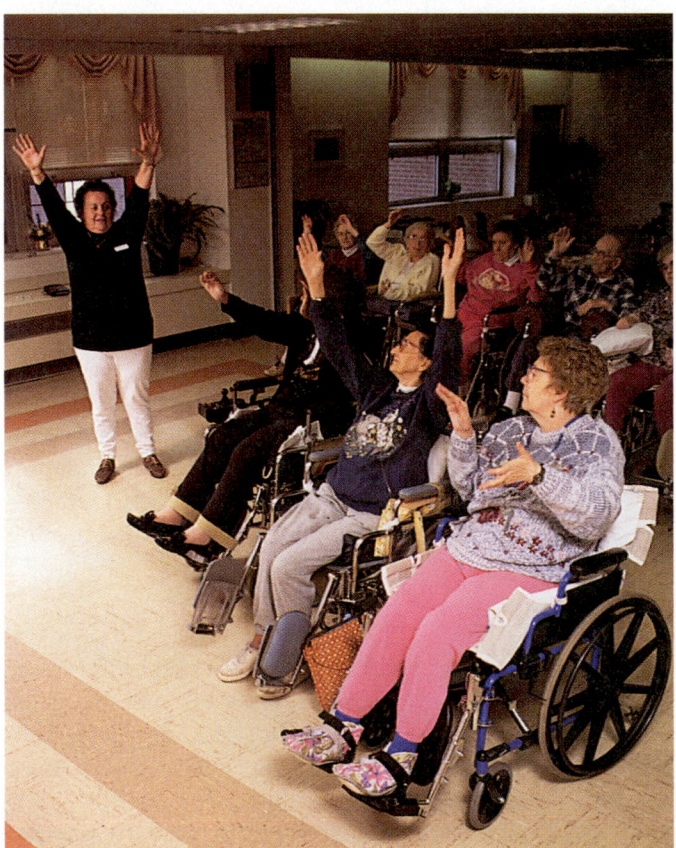

Figure 3-1 All exercise should be tailored to the individual's lifestyle and physical abilities.

Table 3-1	**Select Exercise and Movement Techniques**			
TECHNIQUE	**DESCRIPTION**	**USES AND HISTORY**	**PROVIDERS AND AVAILABILITY**	**INFORMATION**
Alexander technique	Form of body technique or postural therapy that works on proper alignment of head, neck, and spine. This alignment is thought to improve physical and psychologic well-being. Relearning better alignment and posture has been associated with reduction in chronic pain from previous injuries or poor posture.	Developed by Frederick Alexander, an actor, to help him project his voice. Became popular with dancers, singers, and other performers.	Classes are available in many cities taught by certified instructors who have completed a 3-year training program.	http://www.alexander technique.com
Feldenkrais	Awareness through movement, this method focuses on various parts of the body while sequencing simple movements. It has been helpful in clients with neuromuscular disorders, such as multiple sclerosis, musculoskeletal pain, cerebral palsy, and stroke, and in older persons and those with spinal injuries (Rosenfeld, 1996).	Developed by Moshe Feldenkrais who investigated various sciences to treat his knee injuries.	Certified Feldenkrais instructors have training throughout the country.	http://www.feldenkrais .com
Pilates	Method that aims to create balance, flexibility, and coordination by focusing on specific muscles. Very individualized technique. Also is useful for rehabilitation from injury.	Developed by Joseph Pilates in the early 1900s to assist dancers' performance and help recovery from injuries.	Local trainers and classes.	http://www.pilates.net

Dietary Supplements

Ingested or applied substances include various enzymes, hormones, and other biologic products. These generally are not recommended unless under a physician's direction. A number of products are sold for weight loss. The active ingredient in many of these products is *ephedra*, or ma huang, which acts as a stimulant, often in combination with caffeine. Some persons have suffered elevated blood pressure and strokes while using products that contain ephedra without medical supervision. Other effects that have been reported are seizures, kidney stones, myocarditis, vasculitis, and cardiovascular events. The Food and Drug Administration (FDA) has advised consumers to stop using dietary supplements containing ephedra. Producers are under a ban on the sale of dietary supplements containing ephedra.

Herbal Medicine or Phytotherapies

Phytotherapy refers to the therapeutic use of plants, often meaning herbal remedies. Fresh plant parts, including roots, leaves, seeds, and flowers, may be used in cooking or the preparation of foods. Plant parts, often the dried leaves or flowers, may be crushed and placed in gelatin capsules. Dried leaves, flowers, or roots may be loose or finely ground and used in infusions or teas. The plant parts may be prepared in tablets or liquids for ingestion or in poultices, lotions, salves, or oils for topical application.

Nursing Alert

Herbal Therapy Precautions

There are many species for one genus, which may have various therapeutic or side effects. Keep in mind the following:

1. Not all parts of the plant have medicinal action or similar effects.
2. The levels of active ingredients vary with growing conditions (e.g., soil and climate).
3. The amounts of active ingredients vary among and within brands.
4. A lack of standardized manufacturing exists, although the FDA has proposed regulatory standards.
5. Some plant ingredients are toxic.

Table 3-2   Select Body Work Techniques

TECHNIQUE	DESCRIPTION	USES AND HISTORY	PROVIDERS AND AVAILABILITY	INFORMATION
Craniosacral manipulations	Based on theory that unimpeded flow of cerebrospinal fluid (CSF) is key to good health. Gentle pressure applied on the client's head to lengthen spine and facilitate flow of CSF. Reported to help with cognition, concentration, and learning disabilities.	Originally described by William Sutherland, OD, in the early 1900s; further developed over the past 30 years by John Upledger, OD.	May be practiced by osteopaths, chiropractors, physical therapists, body workers, and some massage therapists.	http://www.upledger.com
Massage: may employ a variety of techniques. It is generally safe, except in cases of specific physical conditions, such as bleeding disorders, phlebitis, and some skin conditions.	Massage therapy has long been popular with athletes and recently has gained more general popularity. The American Massage Therapy Association (AMTA) endorses various techniques. ● Deep tissue and friction massages release chronic patterns of tension using slow strokes and deep finger pressure on contracted areas. ● *Effleurage*, a smooth gliding stroke used to relax soft tissues, is taught in childbirth classes as a relaxation technique for labor. ● Sports massage focuses on muscle groups related to particular sports. ● Swedish massage uses long strokes, kneading, and friction on superficial muscle layers. ● *Tapotement* incorporates percussion-type movements. ● Trigger-point massage applies pressure to active and latent trigger points in muscles; then muscles are stretched to help relaxation.	Various techniques of massage are used for health maintenance and relief of pain from muscle strain and stiffness. Massage is widely used to treat minor sports injuries because it reduces muscle spasms, increases circulation, and allows for elimination of lactic acid after physical activity. Massage also is useful in hospitalized or immobilized clients because it relieves pain and discomfort, increases circulation, and enhances relaxation. Infant massage has been introduced in many hospitals and often is taught to parents to soothe infants.	Massage therapists are registered and licensed as Registered Massage Therapists (RMT) by state or local boards or Nationally Certified in Therapeutic Massage and Body-work (NCTMB). Some nurses also are RMTs and certified to provide massage therapies.	http://www.amtamassage.org
Myofascial release	Form of body work that seeks to rebalance the body and facilitate inherent ability to correct soft tissue dysfunction. This interactive stretching technique uses feedback from client's body to determine force, duration, and direction of therapist's strokes. It releases tension in *fascia*, (web-like connective tissue within the body), allowing the body to realign to reduce future injury. It helps restore musculoskeletal function, relax contracted muscles, increase circulation, and increase venous and lymphatic drainage.	Originated in the osteopathic literature of the 1950s and is founded on neurophysiologic function.	Many physical therapists are trained in this technique.	http://www.myofascialrelease.com

Table 3-2 *(continued)*

TECHNIQUE	DESCRIPTION	USES AND HISTORY	PROVIDERS AND AVAILABILITY	INFORMATION
Rolfing	Rolfing, or structural integration, uses various body manipulations to work on fascia. Chronic stress and inactivity cause the normally loose, mobile fascia to become thick and fused. Muscles react by painful spasms. Rolfing stretches the fascia to re-establish proper alignment and thus improve function. Treatment usually involves a series of 10 2-hour sessions 1–2 wk apart.	Developed by Ida Rolf. Some studies have demonstrated efficacy in range of motion, general body movement, posture, and pain.	Certified Rolfers who have completed a course of classroom and practicums can be found through the institute. They are licensed in some states but requirements vary.	http://www.rolf.org
Trager	Approach that uses simple self-induced movements and passive movement, guided by a practitioner, to assist clients in recognizing and unlearning physical and mental habits that limit movement, cause pain, and prevent optimum function. It consists of gentle rhythmic body work to loosen stiff joints and muscles, and dancelike exercises to increase awareness of body movement.	Developed by Milton Trager, MD, an American physician, in the 1940s. It was used to release deep-seated physical and mental patterns to facilitate deep relaxation and improve function.	Certified by the Trager Institute.	http://www.trager.com

> ### Nursing Tip **Informed Consumers**
>
> Nurses can help clients be prudent consumers by teaching them to read labels carefully and avoid taking excessive doses of potentially dangerous products.

> ### Nursing Tip **Health History and Herbal Substances**
>
> You should always assess clients for use of other ingested and applied substances including over the counter (OTC) and dietary supplements, because clients often will not relate this information when asked about medications. Many herbs have biologic effects that may interfere with or add to the effect of medications and produce complications to medical treatment. Always ask clients directly about herbs, vitamins, or other dietary supplements they are taking. Neglecting to ask this question may subject clients to harmful drug interactions and side effects.

> ### Nursing Alert
>
> #### Restriction of Herbal Preparations
>
> Clients taking anticoagulants or antiplatelet agents should be cautioned against using certain herbal preparations. Bioflavonoids found in feverfew, ginkgo biloba, grape seed extract, and bilberry possess antiplatelet activity. These clients also should avoid herbal preparations of ginger, garlic, and ginseng (Glisson, Crawford, & Street, 1999).

There are few risks with the culinary use of herbs, other than individual sensitivities or allergic reactions; however, potentially harmful amounts may be ingested when herbs are concentrated in pill or capsule form. Many consumers think that because these are natural products, there are no risks. Thus, they will take exceptionally large amounts. Herbal products may have therapeutic effects but also can have toxic effects if taken at the wrong time, in the wrong amount, in the wrong combination, or by the wrong person.

An overview of the more popular herbs and their known actions and uses is given in Tables 3-3 and 3-4. Although nurses generally should not recommend herbs, it is important for nurses to be knowledgeable about them to advise clients of risks or alert other members of the medical team about potential problems. Because research information is being published rapidly, the nurse should look for updates on descriptions of herbs, official classifications, labeling statements, possible uses, dosages, preparation, research, and risks. Additional information may be found in *The Commission E Monographs* and *The Physician's Desk Reference (PDR) for Herbal Medicine*.

Regulatory Issues and Herbal Remedies

Currently, the FDA regulates most herbal products in the United States under the classification of food supple-

ments. The 1994 Dietary Supplement Health and Education Act (DSHEA) allows manufacturers to advertise benefits of the products as long as they do not claim the products cure or prevent specific illnesses. The products are regulated by safe handling and labeling; however, because they often are natural products, considerable dosage variation may occur. The current DSHEA regulation allows for labeling that includes structure and function claims without going through full FDA review. Labels can claim that the product affects the structure or function of the body but cannot make disease claims that involve treatment, cure, or diagnosis of a medical condition without FDA evaluation. The manufacturer needs to be able to substantiate all claims it makes, and the label needs to state that the product is a supplement and has not been evaluated by the FDA. The herbal industry has attempted to regulate itself. A classification system has been proposed by the American Herbal Products Association (AHPA) Botanical Safety Rating to address safety issues in the use of herbal products, ranging from Class 1 (no restrictions) to Class 4-4 (insufficient data on safety), that can be accessed on the AHPA Web site.

They are classified as follows:

Class 1 considered safe—no restrictions

Class 2 safe but with restrictions
> 2a external use only
> 2b avoid use in pregnancy
> 2c avoid use in lactation
> 2d miscellaneous restrictions

Class 3 recommend to be used only under guidance of an expert

Class 4 Insufficient data available.

(McGuffin, Hobbs, Upton, & Goldberg, 1997)

During pregnancy, a conservative approach is best, as many of the effects of herbal ingestion are unknown;

Table 3-3   Herbs of General Use for Women

NAME	ACTIONS AND USES	SIDE EFFECTS	CONTRAINDICATIONS	CLASSIFICATION	RESEARCH
Bilberry (*Vaccinium*)	Vasoprotective, antidiarrheal, and astringent actions. Used for circulatory and eye disorders and healthy eye function. Used for dyspepsia and diarrhea.	None known		Commission E-approved AHPA Class 1	
Capsicum (cayenne pepper, chili pepper)	**External:** acts as a counter-irritant, increasing blood flow; used for peripheral neuropathies and herpes zoster. **Internal:** acts as an antispasmodic and antiflatulent; used for GI disorders and hyperlipidemia.	Irritant and hypersensitivity	Do not use on injured skin.	Commission E-approved FDA-GRAS Approved as over-the-counter drug (capsaicin, Zostrix) AHPA Class 1 (Internal) AHPA Class 2d (External)	
Chamomile	**Internal:** digestive aid sometimes used for inflammatory bowel disease. **Oral:** used as mouthwash for mouth irritations. **Topical:** used for inflammatory eczema, insect bites, and poison ivy.	None known	Avoid if allergic to ragweed, asters, and chrysanthemums.	Commission E-approved	
Cranberry (*Vaccinium macrocarpon*)	Antibacterial and acidifier. Used for prophylaxis and treatment of UTIs.	Diarrhea (with large doses)		Not evaluated by Commission E Not rated by AHPA	Reduces bacteriuria and pyuria and lowers pH of urine.
Echinacea (*Echinacea angustifolia* and *E. purpurea*)	Immune stimulant, antibacterial, antiviral, and anti-inflammatory. **Internal:** used for colds, respiratory infections, and arthritis. **External:** used for eczema, herpes, and burns. **Oral:** used for vaginal yeast infections.	Tongue numbness Allergic reactions	Autoimmune diseases and some systemic disease, such as MS and TB. Avoid if allergic to daisies. Avoid in children.	Commission E-approved FDA-GRAS	Equivocal; some studies show efficacy and decreased incidence and severity of colds and flu, whereas others show little difference.
Evening Primrose (fever plant)	Essential fatty acid (omega-6) and prostaglandin precursor. Decreases inflammation and dilates coronary arteries. Used for eczema, PMS, menopausal symptoms, psoriasis, MS, asthma, diabetic neuropathy, and cancer.	GI disturbances Headaches		Not evaluated by Commission E FDA dietary supplement AHPA Class 1	Promising use of essential fatty acids in decreasing PMS symptoms, pain in mastalgia, symptoms of psoriasis, and cholesterol in hyperlipidemia.
Feverfew (*Tanacetum parthenium*)	Migraine prophylactic, anti-inflammatory, antipyretic, and antispasmodic. Used for prevention and treatment of migraine, fever, arthritis, and menstrual cramps. Long-term treatment required: 4–6 wk.	Rebound migraine Mouth ulcers GI irritation	Avoid if allergic to daisies. Avoid in pregnancy.	Not evaluated by Commission E FDA-GRAS AHPA Class 2b	Some studies indicate reduction in number of migraines.

(continues)

Table 3-3 (continued)

NAME	ACTIONS AND USES	SIDE EFFECTS	CONTRAINDICATIONS	CLASSIFICATION	RESEARCH
Garlic (Kwai)	Allicin is the active ingredient. Used for hyperlipidemia, prophylaxis of atherosclerosis, hypertension, and respiratory infection. Lowers cholesterol, triglycerides, and BP; decreases intermittent claudication; and increases resistance to infection and possibly stomach and colorectal cancers. Similar to dicyclomine (Benocol) and some of the new butter substitutes. Enteric coating enhances allicin availability.	Nausea and vomiting Flatulence GI burning	Use caution because of possible interaction with anticoagulants. Avoid in lactation. Avoid in pregnancy.	Commission E-approved FDA-GRAS AHPA Class 2c	Several studies found mild effectiveness in lowering low-density lipoprotein cholesterol; long-term protection against cardiovascular disease is inconclusive.
Ginger	Volatile oil promotes secretion of saliva and gastric juices. Used as antiemetic, especially for morning and motion sickness. Used in India for years as antiemetic and digestive aid.	In large doses, may cause heartburn	May interact with warfarin (antiplatelet). May interfere with anti-diabetic agents. Avoid with gallstones. Avoid prolonged and excessive use in pregnancy.	Commission E-approved FDA-GRAS AHPA Class 1	Inconsistent results.
Chinese ginseng (*Panax schinseng*)	Expensive. Has long history as general tonic, stimulant, and antioxidant. Used for stress, fatigue, debility, diabetes, depression, hyperlipidemia, and to improve physical performance and enhance immunity. **Note:** Be sure to distinguish from American ginseng (*P. quinquefolius*)	Hypertension Irritability Hypoglycemia Diarrhea	May interact with anti-psychotics, monoamine oxidase inhibitors, stimulants, and anticoagulants. Avoid with hypertension.	Commission E-approved FDA-GRAS AHPA Class 2d	Not effective as an exercise enhancer; in reviewing the literature be sure to clarify which type of ginseng was used.
Ginkgo biloba	Active ingredients 6% lactones and 24% glycosides. Improves circulation and acts as antioxidant. Used for dementia, memory enhancement, cardiovascular insufficiency, intermittent claudication, peripheral neuropathy, depression, tinnitus, retinopathy, and early Alzheimer's disease. Need to build up dosage over time for effects.	Nausea and vomiting Headache	May interact with anticoagulants.	Commission E-approved FDA-GRAS	Some efficacy in controlled trials for treatment of dementia and memory deficit.

(continues)

Herb	Uses	Side effects	Cautions	Rating	Efficacy
Goldenseal (*Hydrastis canadensis*)	Used for upper respiratory conditions, flu, and menorrhagia.	GI effects Uterine contraction Blood vessel contraction Hypoglycemia	Avoid with diabetes. Avoid with hypertension. Avoid in pregnancy.	Not evaluated by Commission E FDA-GRAS AHPA Class 2b	None for URIs.
Grape seed extract	Antioxidant and anti-inflammatory. Used for inflammatory conditions and circulatory disorders. Used as antioxidant for disease prevention.	None known		Not evaluated by Commission E FDA dietary supplement Not rated by AHPA	No human studies.
Kava kava (*Piper methysticum*)	Similar to valerian. Active ingredient is kava lactones (70% kava lactones in standard preparation). Used as antianxiety and tension-reducing agent. Currently very popular with teenagers.	Yellowing of skin Allergic reactions	Acts as sedative and may interfere with driving and other types of performance. May interact with antidepressants and barbiturates. Avoid with depression. Avoid in pregnancy.	Commission E-approved	
Milk thistle (*Silybum marianum*)	Used as liver tonic since the days of Pliny. Used to treat viral hepatitis, hepatitis C, and other liver diseases, and for exposure to environmental toxins.	Transient laxative		Commission E-approved	
St. John's wort (*Hypericum perforatum*)	Increases neurotransmitter levels of serotonin and norepinephrine. **Internal:** used for depression, anxiety, and dyspepsia. **External:** used for wounds and burns. May have mild antiviral activity.	GI disturbances Photosensitivity	Interacts with antidepressant drugs, and when used together could alter dosage. May require dietary restriction of tyramine. May interfere with AIDS medications. May increase size of cataracts. Avoid in pregnancy.	Commission E-approved FDA-GRAS AHPA Class 1	In a meta-analysis found to be effective in treating mild to moderate depression.
Valerian root (*Valeriana officinalis*)	Action of binding benzodiazepine receptors Used for insomnia, nervous excitability, hysteria, rheumatic pain, and dysmenorrhea.	Sedation and paradoxical reactions	Should not be paired with other drugs or herbal preparations with the same effects.	Commission E-approved FDA-GRAS AHPA Class 1	Some efficacy in clinical trials.

The authors thank the following persons for their advice and help with the preparation of this table: Sherri Konzem, PharmD, University of Houston, College of Pharmacy and Memorial-Hermann SW Family Practice Residency Program, Houston, Texas; and Roberta Anding, MS, RD/LD, CDE, Instructor, Section of Adolescent Medicine, Baylor College of Medicine and Texas Children's Hospital, Houston, Texas.

GI—gastrointestinal; UTIs—urinary tract infections; MS—multiple sclerosis; TB—tuberculosis; PMS—premenstrual syndrome; BP—blood pressure; URIs—upper respiratory infections.

American Herbal Products Association (AHPA) Botanical Safety Rating: Class 1, internal use. Class 2a, avoid with hypertension. Class 2b, avoid in pregnancy. Class 2c, avoid in lactation. Class 2d, external use. Commission E-approved. FDA-GRAS, Food and Drug Administration

Table 3-4 **Herb Use in Perimenopause**

NAME	ACTIONS AND USES	SIDE EFFECTS	CONTRAINDICATIONS	CLASSIFICATION	RESEARCH
Black cohosh (*Cimicifuga racemosa*), also called snakeroot and squawroot	Appears to reduce luteinizing hormone and may potentiate hormonal production with a mild estrogenic action and uterine tonic. Used for reduction in menopausal symptoms, such as hot flashes, sleep disturbances, and irritability. Was one of the primary ingredients in Lydia Pinkham's woman's tonic, popular remedy in the early 20th century.	Headaches Increased menstrual bleeding Central nervous system depressant	Avoid in pregnancy because may cause uterine contractions.	Commission E-approved	Some studies show effectiveness in reducing perimenopausal symptoms.
Chaste berry (*Vitex agnus-castus*) also called chaste tree	Assumed to increase progesterone if insufficient. Thought to act as hormonal balancing agent during hormonal fluctuations. May affect anterior pituitary and increase progesterone production in luteal phase. Used for premenstrual syndrome (PMS), menopausal problems, especially for heavy menstrual flow and to reduce hot flashes caused by high levels of follicle-stimulating hormone.	None known	Concomitant use with oral contraceptives may result in diminished effect. Avoid in pregnancy.	Commission E-approved	
Dong Quai (*Angelica sinensis* or *A. phymorpha maxim*)	Contains phytoestrogens (plant estrogens). Acts as coumarin and affects blood clotting and hematopoiesis. Is a uterine relaxant. Used for menopausal symptoms.	Photosensitivity May cause heavy menstrual bleeding May cause heart palpitations	Avoid in women with heavy menstrual periods, spotting, or uterine fibroids. Avoid taking blood thinners. Avoid during menstruation. Avoid in pregnancy.	Not evaluated by Commission E AHPA Class 2b	No more effective than placebo in some studies; more research needed.
Motherwort	Mild cardiotonic and aid to female reproductive system. Used for menopausal symptoms, PMS, menstrual cramps, and sleep disturbances.	May cause heavy menstrual bleeding	Avoid in pregnancy.	Commission E-approved	
Sage (*Salvia officinalis*)	Contains bioflavonoids and phytoesterols for weak estrogenic and progesteronic effects. Mild antibacterial and antifungal properties. Used for excessive perspiration and relief of hot flashes, night sweats, and mood swings.	May dry mucous membranes in mouth and vagina	Excessive use may cause kidney or liver problems. Avoid in pregnancy.	Commission E-approved	

Note. From "Harmonizing Herbs: Managing Menopause with Help from Mother Earth," by C. D. Learn and P. G. Higgins, October–November 1999, *Lifelines*, pp. 39–43; and from "Herbs of Special Interest to Women," by M. L. Hardy, 2000, *Journal of the American Pharmaceutical Association, 40*, (2) 234–242. American Herbal Products Association (AHPA) Botanical Safety Rating: Class 2b, avoid in pregnancy. Commission E-approved.

some herbs that should not be used in pregnancy and lactation are found in Box 3-2.

The Food and Drug Administration has a classification: Generally Regarded as Safe (GRAS). Commision E-approved means that they were reasonably safe when

Nursing Tip

FDA Proposes New Regulations for Dietary Supplements

In March 2003, the U.S. Food and Drug Administration (FDA) published proposed good manufacturing practices (GMPs) for dietary supplements. These regulations contain requirements regarding storage and manufacture of supplements, including production and process controls, testing, packaging, and labeling. Many responsible manufacturers in the herbal industry have supported and already meet the projected GMPs.

Box 3-2

Herbal Use in Pregnancy and Lactation

Pregnancy
The most conservative approach is to avoid all but ginger because the purity and dosages of products cannot be ensured.
   The following *should not* be used in pregnancy:

- Pennyroyal*
- Tansy*
- Rue*
- Black cohosh* and any of the herbs that cause uterine contractions
- Ma huang
- Cascara sagrada and other harsh laxatives

Lactation
A number of herbs have been used in folk culture to enhance or reduce milk flow. The following *should not* be used during lactation:

- Aloe
- Black cohosh
- Buckthorn
- Cascara sagrada
- Cocoa†
- Coffee†
- Kava kava
- Ma huang
- Sage
- Senna
- Tea†
- Wintergreen

*Abortifacients and should be avoided by childbearing women.
†Avoid excessive consumption.

Note. From "Herbs of Special Interest to Women," by M. L. Hardy, 2000, Journal of the American Pharmaceutical Association, 40(2), pp. 234–242.

Nursing Alert

Drug Reactions
If a client has an adverse effect or drug interaction to an herbal product, you should report it to the Food and Drug Administration's MEDWATCH (1-800-FDA-1088).

Client Education

Medical Supervision Required

The following herbs are considered dangerous and should not be used without medical supervision:

- Borage
- Coltsfoot
- Life root
- Germander
- Ma huang or ephedra
- Calamus
- Comfrey
- Chaparral
- Licorice (herbal, not the candy form)

Nursing Alert

Ephedra (MaHuang)
Many popular weight-loss dietary supplements contain ephedra. Use of ephedra, especially in combination with other stimulants such as caffeine, has been linked with cardiovascular health risks. Use of these products along with strenuous physical activity can be dangerous (U.S. FDA, 2003). Ephedra has recently been banned from dietary supplements, however some may still be available for consumers. It is important that nurses caution clients to carefully read the labels of any weight-loss preparation.

used according to the dosage: contraindications and other warnings are specified in the monographs. Efficacy was based on reasonable verification of historical use.

Applied Substances

Essential oils have been used for centuries and are used in perfumes and in body and bath products. Essential oils can be applied to the skin through lotions, salves, oils, poultices, plasters, or taken sublingually; these oils also are inhaled by placement in a diffuser. Essential oils are very concentrated and should not be used without dilution in a carrier oil. Once diluted, the oil may then be used directly on the skin, in bath water, or in a diffuser. Flower essences, such as Bach Flower Remedies often are diluted with brandy or an alcoholic base and taken by dropper sublingually. Lavender or tea tree oil can be used on burns and skin eruptions as long as one does not have extremely sensitive skin. Testing for sensitivities, with a patch test of a 2% dilution and observing for 12 hours, is recommended. Contact with the eyes and sensitive mucous membranes should be avoided when using certain oils, and most should not be ingested. Caution should be exercised when used in pregnancy because some oils may contribute to miscarriage. Oils that are considered safe in pregnancy are rose, neorli, lavender, ylang-ylang, chamomile, citruses, geranium, sandalwood, spearmint, and frankincense (Keville & Geeen, 2000). The American Holistic Nurses Association (AHNA) has endorsed educational programs in aromatherapy such as the Pacific Institute of Aromatherapy and the National Association for Holistic Aromatherapy.

Energy-Based Therapies

Energy is a concept that is used to explain forms of healing touch, therapeutic touch, Reiki, and laying on of hands. These treatments may involve actual touching or noncontact touch, such as placing the hands several inches from the body. The focus is the "energy field" rather than the physical body.

Nursing Alert

Drug Absorption

Another risk of using essential oils is an allergic reaction that can be severe because many oils are very concentrated. In addition, substances taken sublingually are absorbed into the bloodstream very quickly.

Magnetic Healing

Magnetic healing includes use of magnets for pain relief and the use of transcutaneous electrical nerve stimulation (TENS), which involves passing low-voltage current through pads applied to the skin. Some research has demonstrated efficacy in pain reduction. TENS has been used to aid in the start of healing of fractured bones, promote healing and tissue regeneration, and reduce pain. TENS has been used with some effectiveness in reducing labor pain (Kemp, 1996).

Touch Therapies

Touch therapies have been used historically and across cultures. The use of human touch for healing has been recorded in early records and archeological data across cultures. Healing by laying on of hands is a key element in many spiritual traditions, including Judeo-Christian scriptures. Touch has been shown to be vital to human development (Figure 3-2). Infants and young children may develop pathologies and may even stop eating and die if they do not receive caring touch. Nurses have embraced touch as integral to caring for clients.

Two groups have promoted touch therapies within the nursing profession: Therapeutic Touch (TT), founded by Dolores Krieger; and Healing Touch International (HTI), founded by Janet Mentgen. Both these groups provide education and training for nurses interested in practicing this modality. Reiki is another form of touch therapy that is practiced by both nurses and laypersons.

Therapeutic Touch

Therapeutic touch was brought into nursing by Dolores Krieger, PhD, RN. She had worked with healers Oskar Estebany and Dora Kunz. Kreiger's research on the increase of hemoglobin after therapeutic touch was one of the first studies conducted on this modality. In learning this technique, the practitioner is taught to enter a calm state

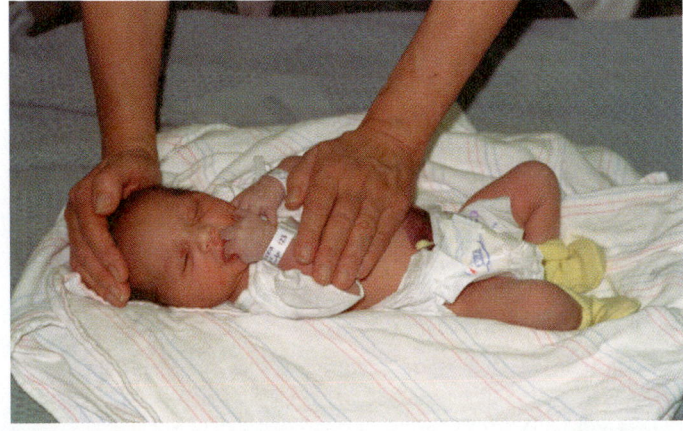

Figure 3-2 Laying on of hands is one means of touch therapy.

through a process of "centering" and to hold an "intention" of desiring to help the client. The practitioner is taught to assess the client's energy field and then modulate or correct the deficient, congested, or unbalanced areas. The practitioner's hands are placed a few inches above the physical body, which is felt to be the optimal area to work with the energy (Figure 3-3).

Healing Touch

Healing touch also uses touch to influence energy. Along with touch, it employs a number of additional techniques the practitioner can use in working with clients. These techniques are used to align and balance the energy field, thus facilitating the client's self-healing. Proponents claim that these techniques are healing in a holistic manner because they act on physical, emotional, and spiritual domains. This program is taught in a series of classes as the practitioner advances to different levels. The program is available to nurses as well as laypersons. HTI is one of the most rapidly growing healing organizations in this country.

Reiki

Reiki is based on the Tibetan Sutras (ancient sacred texts) and was reintroduced into Japan by Usui in the 1800s (Stewart, 1995). Takawa, a Japanese woman who moved to Hawaii, trained several healers who then brought the technique to the United States. Novice practitioners are initiated through a ritual involving ancient symbols. The healer channels universal healing energy through the hands, which can be placed directly on or held at a distance from the client. The healer does not direct the energy but holds the intent to heal. The energy then goes to where it is needed. This modality also uses a technique for distance healing. Preparation is through weekend seminars and work with a Reiki Master. The Master level involves a lifelong commitment to healing and to Reiki. Many nurses and non-nurses are Reiki healers.

Nursing Implications

Nurses and clients often cite anecdotal reports of the benefits of touch therapies; however, relatively few research studies have established their efficacy. Most nursing research into touch therapies has been conducted in therapeutic touch. Research supports decreased anxiety and increased relaxation; results on wound healing are equivocal. Some recent studies demonstrate that exposure to touch therapies may increase humoral immunity; however, results are preliminary (Wardell & Engebretson, 2001; Olsen et al., 1997). Touch modalities are of particular interest to the profession of nursing and are low-cost and low-risk strategies that many clients claim have benefit. Many hospitals have integrated these modalities into their care delivery and have sponsored nurses' preparation in them.

Although little research has been done on the use of touch therapies in pregnancy and labor, many nurses have used these techniques to aid in comfort and relaxation. Touch therapies also have been used in infants. Noncontact or light touch may be particularly useful in infants in the neonatal intensive care unit for whom rigorous physical contact, such as massage, may lead to overstimulation (Figure 3-4). These areas currently are under research.

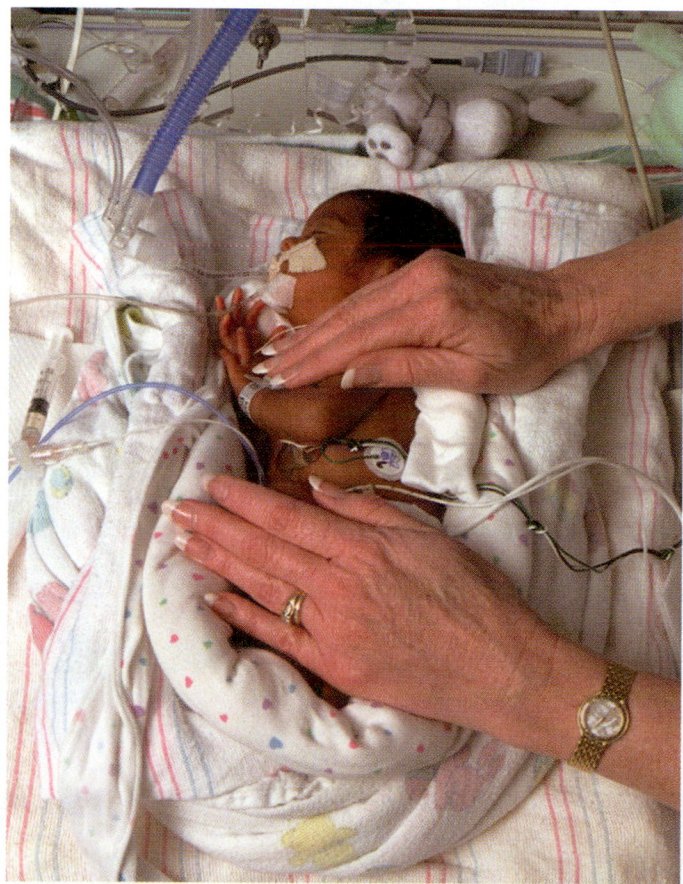

Figure 3-4 Infants in the NICU can benefit from calm, warm, nondisruptive touch therapy.

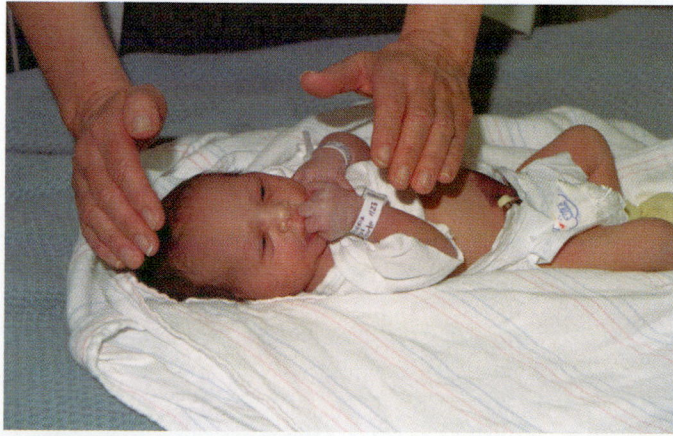

Figure 3-3 Therapeutic touch involves centering and assessing the client's energy by placing the hands a few inches above the client's body.

Psychologic or Mind-Body Therapies

Mind-body medicine has become established in health care. The recent understanding of psychophysiologic mechanisms has provided a firm base for many of these strategies to be well researched. Much of the research has been based on stress reduction and relaxation. Other strategies include cognitive repatterning, behavioral modification, psychotherapy, group therapy, and coping strategies. Many of these techniques are incorporated into the therapeutic relationship that nurses establish with clients and use in wellness counseling.

Relaxation strategies, such as autogenic training, progressive muscle relaxation, distraction techniques, and paced breathing, have been used in the care of women during pregnancy and in preparation for labor over the past 40 years (Figure 3-5). In addition to the relaxation strategies taught in childbirth preparation, some additional techniques that nurses can use to promote relaxation are biofeedback, mindfulness, self-reflection, mental imagery, affirmations, and music therapy. Research has demonstrated such techniques to be effective adjuncts in reducing pain and anxiety related to surgery or invasive procedures, and with symptom control related to specific treatment side effects. The AHNA has described several practices that are part of holistic nursing care, many of which are felt to facilitate stress reduction and relaxation. *Holistic Nursing: A Handbook for Practice* (Dossey, Keegan, & Guzzetta, 2000) is a good reference for additional guidance on how to develop and use these skills in clinical practice.

Mental imagery, a therapeutic process in which imagination and memory are used to mentally taste, smell, see, and hear images that suggest a state of health, is used for promoting both health and healing. AHNA endorses a program for learning the techniques of visual imagery, which is directed by nurses and offers certification.

Spiritual Healing

Spirituality is the essence of who we are as human beings and includes but is not limited to the process of discovering purpose, meaning, and inner strength throughout life's journey. Spirituality is experienced and expressed in many ways outside the context of *religion*, which can be identified as an organized system of beliefs and practices shared by a group of people. According to Burkhardt and Jacobsen (2000), elements of spirituality can include connectedness to an Absolute or Higher Power, to nature, to others, and to self.

Both illness and wellness activities have been derived from spiritual practices. Spiritual issues often concern suffering, redemption, forgiveness, faith, hope, grace, and love. Healing can imply a restoration of wholeness, establishment of internal and external resources, a sense of transcendence, or a feeling of interconnectedness (Burkhardt & Jacobsen, 2000). Many rituals and health practices have been described that focus on the attainment or restoration

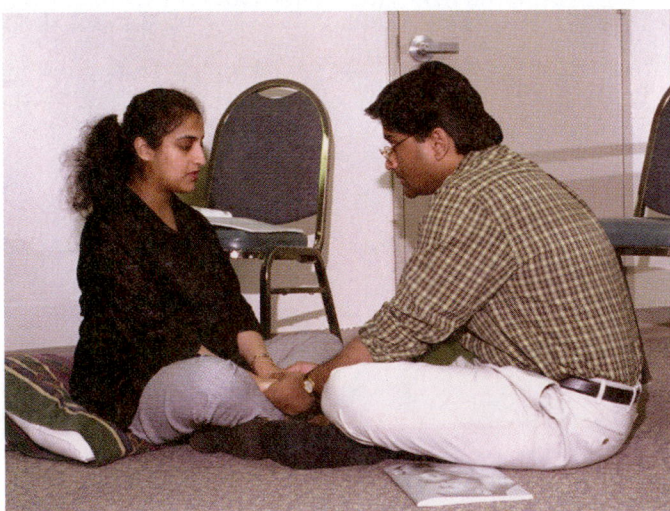

Figure 3-5   Childbirth preparation classes often include techniques wherein the partner helps the woman to relax, focus, and breathe deeply.

Client Education

Questions for Consideration for Clients Interested in Taking or Engaging in Complementary Therapies

- Do they make claims to cure cancer, enhance treatment, or relieve symptoms or side effects?
- What are the credentials of those supporting the therapy?
- Have they published or referenced trustworthy journals?
- What are the costs of the treatment?
- Is it widely used in the health care community, or is access limited?
- Is it used in place of standard therapies and if so will the delay affect a chance for effective treatment?

Note. Adapted from *Alternative vs. Complementary Therapies,* 1999 by the American Cancer Society. Retrieved October 17, 2003, from http://www.cancer.org.

of balance between mind, body, and spirit. Some of these may seem quite appropriate within Judeo-Christian traditions, such as worship and prayer; whereas others from Native American or Southwestern cultures, such as chanting or use of a medicine wheel, may be unfamiliar.

Religious practices, such as participating in church activities, have demonstrated positive health benefits (Levin, 1994). Meditation has been used in many spiritual traditions as a way of attaining balance both internally and with the environment. Meditation also has been researched for its efficacy in relaxation and stress reduction. Prayer and primal religious experiences are spiritual actions found in many cultures and are associated with healing. Many CTs have their roots in spiritual traditions and practices (Kinsley, 1996).

Because no consensus exists on the definition, scope, and measurement of spirituality, it is vital that nurses recognize all forms of spiritual expression to provide professional and holistic care. The connectedness inherent in the therapeutic nurse-client relationship is an avenue of nurturing spiritual awareness for both the nurse and client.

NURSING IMPLICATIONS

Nurses must be aware of the types of health-related activities in which their clients may be engaged. This awareness is important for the assessment of safety and the interaction of these activities with biomedical care. If the nurse is knowledgeable about complementary therapies, appropriate referrals may be made that can help clients augment their treatments, cope with symptoms and unpleasant side effects from treatments, and maintain and promote their health. A number of strategies that currently are labeled as CTs have been part of nursing care and are well documented in the nursing literature. Table 3-5 lists some of these interventions described by Snyder and Lindquist (1998) and listed in the *Nursing Interventions Classification* (Dochterman & Bulechek, 2004).

Implications for Women's Health

Women seek care more frequently than do men from both CTs and traditional medicine. In many cultures, women are central to the physical and emotional health of the family. Women prepare most of the food, purchase dietary supplements, and provide the majority of childcare. Women generally are the caregivers and tend to the sick of the family, both old and young. Many CTs are likely to be well received by women and meet many of their needs and those of their families. Promoting the health of women over the life span improves not only the client's health but also that of the entire family.

Client Education

Complementary Approaches for Women

Nausea in Pregnancy

- Acupuncture
- Sea bands
- Ginger
- Vitamin B$_6$
- Visualization
- Relaxation techniques

Premenstrual Syndrome

- Good nutrition: reduce intake of sugar, caffeine, dairy products, and animal fats
- Exercise
- Body work
- Herbal: chaste berry, black cohosh, wild yam, ginkgo biloba, and progesterone creme
- Supplements: vitamin B$_6$, vitamin E, magnesium
- Acupuncture

Menopause

- Good nutrition
- Exercise: strengthening, flexibility, weight-bearing, and mild aerobic
- Movement therapies: Pilates, Feldenkrais, Alexander technique, and yoga
- Body work: massage and various therapeutic techniques
- Mind-body: Stress reduction, relaxation, and biofeedback
- Spiritual: prayer, meditation, and religious rituals
- Social: connections with family, friends, and other groups
- Herbal: black cohosh, vitex, and other herbs, depending on symptoms
- Acupuncture and acupressure

Table 3-5 Complementary Modalities in the Nursing Literature

RELAXATION	RELATIONSHIPS	THERAPEUTIC USE OF SELF	EXERCISE	ENERGY-BASED TECHNIQUES	COGNITIVE THERAPIES	SPIRITUAL	OTHER
Anxiety reduction	Advocacy	Active listening	Body work techniques	Biomagnetic healing*	Decision-making support	Meditation	Aromatherapy*
Autogenic relaxation training*	Assertiveness training	Caring or healing presence*	Exercise promotion	Healing touch*	Guided imagery	Prayer*	Art therapy
Biofeedback training	Family support	Humor	Tai chi*	Therapeutic touch	(simple) Hypnosis	Spiritual counseling	Environmental management
Breathing techniques*	Group support	Presence	Yoga*	Touch	Self-awareness	Spiritual	Music therapy
support	Herbal remedies*				Self-esteem enhancement		Nutritional counseling
Progressive muscle relaxation	Pet or animal therapy				Self-reflection*		Pain management
					Storytelling		
					Values clarification		
					Writing in journal*		

*Interventions discussed in the literature but not officially recognized by the Nursing Interventions Classification Code.

Nursing Tip *Assessment for Use of CAM*

The nurse should assess all clients for their use of alternative/complementary therapies

Interview

One way to systematically assess for these therapies is to ask about the following:

- **Use of other healers:** Does the client see any type of healer or provider for health promotion or for any health condition?
- **Physical manipulation:** What type of exercise or physical activity does the client do? Does the client use any type of bodywork such as massage?
- **Ingested or applied substances:** What type of diet, dietary supplements, vitamins, minerals, herbs, nonprescription medication, or other preparations does the client take?
- **Energy work:** Does the client use magnets, touch therapies, acupuncture, or Eastern medicine?
- **Psychological:** What does the client use for stress management?
- **Spiritual:** Does the client engage in any spiritual practices?

Interpretation

Examine the assessment data for the following. The nurse may not have enough information to make a decision, in which case the information should be reported to the medical team.

- Is the client using other healers or healing activities instead of seeking biomedical care?
- Are any of the activities contraindicated by biomedical conditions?
- Could any activities or substances interact with medications or biomedical treatments?

Reporting to the Medical Team

All information should be reported to the medical team. The nurse should draw attention to the areas in which the activity might possibly be harmful.

Documentation in the Client Record

All the assessment data should be recorded in the client record in a concise and thorough manner.

Nursing Tip *Holistic Nurse-Certification*

Registered nurses with a baccalaureate degree (BSN) or higher can become certified as holistic nurses (HNC). This certification acknowledges nurses' knowledge of holistic practices and complementary therapies. This certification *does not* certify the nurse to practice specific modalities, which generally require separate certificates. More information may be obtained by calling American Holistic Nurses Certification Corporation headquarters at 1-877-284-0998 or by e-mailing AHNCC0@flash.net.

Implications for Practice

As they incorporate these complementary therapies into practice, nurses must ensure they have adequate education, training, and experience. Nurses attempting to engage in these interventions may need additional training or certification for some techniques. Nurses not educated in the technique have the professional responsibility to obtain the proper preparation, either from the literature or from continuing education. The AHNA Web site provides a current listing of endorsed educational and certificate programs. All clients should be assessed regarding supplements or substances they may be taking. Nurses must be very cautious in recommending herbal remedies. It is imperative that nurses be in compliance with the Board of Nurse Examiners scope of practice regulations of their state.

NURSING PROCESS

The nursing process can be applied to clients seeking or engaging in alternative and complementary therapies.

Assessment

In assessing clients, it is important to ask specifically what vitamins, minerals, herbs, and over-the-counter medications they are taking in addition to prescribed medications. Clients also should be asked about therapies that they are considering taking, their financial resources for such therapies, and modalities that they would consider acceptable or unacceptable.

Nursing Diagnoses

North American Nursing Diagnosis Association (NANDA)-approved nursing diagnoses for clients seeking or engaging in CTs might include the following (NANDA, 2003):

- Deficient knowledge regarding the potential benefits and applicability of CTs
- Deficient knowledge regarding the types and availability of CTs
- Deficient knowledge regarding the potential risks associated with CTs
- Decisional conflict related to the accessibility and efficacy of standard therapies and CTs
- Chronic pain
- Ineffective coping
- Hopelessness
- Powerlessness
- Anxiety
- Fear
- Spiritual distress
- Fatigue
- Ineffective health maintenance
- Interrupted family processes

Specific nursing diagnoses in women may include the following:

- Stress urinary incontinence
- Imbalanced nutrition
- Sexual dysfunction
- Disturbed sleep pattern
- Caregiver role strain

- Impaired parent-infant attachment
- Risk for constipation
- Rape-trauma syndrome
- Ineffective breastfeeding
- Ineffective thermoregulation

Outcome Identification

In partnership with the client, the nurse should outline the desired results of care and therapy. Targeted goals should be prioritized according to the client's physical and emotional state and needs and to the client's wishes. Family members and significant others can be included in the goal-setting as requested by the client.

Planning

In planning interventions, it is important to engage the client in mutual planning of appropriate use of CTs and discuss expected outcomes. Referral sources for certified practitioners of specific modalities with regard to the client's financial resources are crucial. Integration of selected CTs into the medical plan of care also is advised.

Nursing Intervention

Appropriately prepared nurses may provide the interventions, particularly for CTs, that relate to client education for self-care. Many nurses are able to guide clients in relaxation techniques or provide touch therapies. Nurses need to be knowledgeable about the risks, benefits, and indications of specific CTs. Clients should be informed that behavioral interventions take practice and lifestyle changes are most effective when accomplished gradually. Efficacy of such therapies, as well as those of ingested and applied substances, may not be apparent for several weeks.

Evaluation

Evaluation of the effectiveness of the intervention depends on the therapeutic indications and goals. Evaluation can be obtained by client follow-up reporting, although many self-reporting instruments are available for clients to document changes in symptoms in the interim and over time. Nurses should keep in mind that many behavioral interventions have therapeutic effects beyond symptom relief in that effectiveness of biologic response to medical treatments sometimes improved.

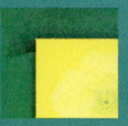

CASE STUDY/CARE PLAN
USE OF COMPLEMENTARY THERAPY

Mary is a 55-year-old married woman who is having mood swings, fatigue, insomnia, vaginal dryness, hot flashes, and muscular stiffness related to perimenopause. After discussing the issue with her health care provider, she has decided not to take hormone replacement therapy. Mary approaches you for advice regarding nondrug therapies for her symptoms, which are interfering with her daily living and ability to perform her work as a professional seamstress.

Assessment

- Mary has no difficulty in falling asleep but wakes up several times at night perspiring and tossing off her bed covers. She is often too tired to complete her usual workload or engage in social activities.
- Mary is taking no medications other than a daily multivitamin and occasionally an over-the-counter laxative. Her medical history is unremarkable, and she denies having allergies.
- Mary has numerous hot flashes daily, which interrupt her work and ability to concentrate.
- Mary states that she often is irritable about situations that previously would not have bothered her and has also had regular episodes of feeling "down."
- Mary is increasingly reluctant to engage in sexual intercourse owing to dyspareunia.
- Mary has noted increasing muscular stiffness, especially when the weather is cold; she denies joint pain.
- Mary is interested in therapies other than prescribed estrogens or progesterones, and a regular exercise routine.

Nursing Diagnosis

Disturbed sleep pattern related to night sweats, hot flashes, and muscular stiffness.

Expected Outcome	In 3 weeks, Mary will report decreased frequency and severity of hot flashes, decreased muscular stiffness, and decreased awakening during sleep.
Planning	Assist Mary in developing a plan for sleep and exercise activities that will fit into her routines and lifestyle.
NOC	Sleep
NIC	Sleep enhancement

Nursing Interventions	Rationales
1. Advise Mary to discuss the use of herbal preparations such as black cohosh, Evening Primrose oil, and vitamin E supplements, and soy-based dairy products with her health care provider.	1. Use of these preparations may relieve her hot flashes.
2. Instruct Mary in forms of exercises such as yoga, tai chi, or Pilates along with resources for certified instruction in such methods, if not medically contraindicated.	2. These exercises will reduce muscle tension and diminish muscle stiffness.
3. Assist Mary in planning daily activities to allow for intermittent rest periods.	3. Rest periods during the day will help diminish fatigue; they also can help make up for lost sleep at night, until Mary's nighttime sleep routine is reestablished.

Evaluation	Goal will be evidenced by client self-report on a list of menopausal symptoms, including symptoms for insomnia and hot flashes.

(continues)

Nursing Diagnosis

Ineffective role performance related to fatigue, irritability, decreased mental concentration, and diminished sexual activity.

Expected Outcomes In 2 months, Mary will report decreased irritability, reestablishment of usual work routine, and overall improved quality of life.

Planning Help Mary identify those areas in which she has positive role involvement and those areas (such as work and spousal relationship) where she feels there is a need to improve.

NOC Role performance

NIC Role enhancement

Nursing Interventions	Rationales
1. Instruct Mary in deep breathing exercises to use regularly and when feeling irritable.	1. Controlled breathing releases tension and has a calming effect.
2. Advise Mary of the need to continue social and other activities that are enjoyable for her.	2. Maintaining social contacts will reinforce a sense of normalcy and help Mary keep a balanced perspective on her life.
3. Advise Mary to use a water-based lubricant for sexual intercourse and as needed in between, and to engage in regular intercourse as desired.	3. Lubricant will reduce feeling of vaginal dryness.

Evaluation Progress will be evidenced by a self-report of fewer menopausal symptoms including irritability and fatigue, and by work productivity and client report of quality of life rating of 8 or more on a 1 to 10 scale.

WEB ACTIVITIES

• • • Search the Internet for alternative therapies for the discomforts of pregnancy. Critically analyze the source, information, and potential effect the information might have on clients.

• • • Go to the AHNA Web site. Explore the endorsed programs and other information.

• • • Choose a modality of interest to you, and search the Internet.

• • • Go to the National Institutes of Health's Center for Complementary and Alternative Therapies Web site and read about current research.

Key Concepts

- Complementary therapies are those used in conjunction with biomedical therapy, whereas alternative therapies are those used in place of standard biomedical therapy.
- Traditional healing systems are closely tied to cultural and religious influences and are generally thousands of years old.
- Biomedicine is an example of a healing system.
- Many complementary therapies are congruent with autonomous nursing interventions in that they support self-care and self-healing of the client.
- The complexity and technology of modern medicine, lack of effective standard therapies for chronic illnesses, the crisis in health care delivery in Western society, and increasing availability and advertising are factors contributing to the use of complementary therapies by clients and their families.
- Some complementary therapies have been accepted as nursing interventions, such as relaxation, therapeutic use of self, range-of-motion exercise, spiritual

support, touch therapies, cognitive therapies, and nutritional counseling. Other techniques may require additional training and certification. It is vital that nurses are in compliance with the Board of Nurse Examiners scope of practice regulations of their state.

■ Complementary therapies can be helpful and should be permitted if they are not harmful in general or do not interfere with standard biomedical treatment. It is important that nurses familiarize themselves with indications and contraindications before encouraging or recommending these therapies to clients.

■ Resources for further information include the American Holistic Nurses Association, National Institutes of Health Center for Complementary and Alternative Therapy, and American Botanical Council.

Review Questions and Activities

1. Which one of the following reasons might *best* explain the appeal of alternative therapy to women with chronic illnesses?
   a. Alternative therapies are generally aimed at treating the disease
   b. Alternative therapies are relatively inexpensive
   c. Alternative therapies usually are efficacious and nontoxic
   d. Alternative therapies generally involve self-care

   The correct answer is d.

2. Many clients use alternative and complementary therapies in addition to standard treatments. Which of the following clients who are using such therapies might you be most concerned about?
   a. A healthy perimenopausal woman who is taking black cohosh for relief of hot flashes
   b. A woman using acupuncture for control of nausea related to morning sickness
   c. A woman receiving standard chemotherapy for ovarian cancer who is taking weekly colonic irrigations
   d. A woman who has had an uncomplicated pregnancy continuing her yoga classes into her third trimester

   The correct answer is c.

3. Which is the nursing diagnosis *most* applicable to an adolescent girl who is concerned about her weight, although she is within normal range for her height, and is considering taking an ephedra-based herbal product to lose weight?
   a. Deficient knowledge related to risks and benefits of complementary therapies

   b. Imbalanced nutrition, more than body requirements
   c. Ineffective health maintenance related to adequate nutrition
   d. Deficient knowledge related to availability of complementary therapies

   The correct answer is a.

4. Which of the following statements is true regarding the role of the nurse in recommending or administering complementary therapies?
   a. Nurses should recommend only herbs and vitamin or dietary supplements that have been approved by the Food and Drug Administration
   b. Nurses should recommend or practice only those complementary therapies whose efficacy has been scientifically documented
   c. Nurses should encourage the use of alternative therapies that do not interfere with biomedical treatment
   d. Nurses should seek additional education or certification before recommending or practicing complementary therapies that are unfamiliar

   The correct answer is d.

5. How can the efficacy of mind-body therapies best be measured clinically?
   a. By measurement of biochemical markers of immune function
   b. By self-reporting of symptom relief
   c. By the absence of disease states
   d. By measurement of clients' performance accuracy for such therapies

   The correct answer is b.

6. Body work is most likely to be contraindicated in which women?
   a. Those with a history of degenerative joint disease
   b. Those with the human immunodeficiency virus
   c. Those with bleeding disorders
   d. Those with osteopenia

   The correct answer is c.

7. Which persons are most likely to use complementary and alternative therapies?
   a. Those with limited education
   b. Those with an acute life-threatening illness
   c. Those with access to practitioners of such therapies
   d. Those with higher income

   The correct answer is d.

8. Visit a local holistic health center, natural food store, or bookstore and explore the offerings for complementary or alternative health.

References

American Cancer Society. (1999). *Alternative vs. complementary therapies*. Retrieved October 17, 2003, from http://www.cancer.org

American Osteopatic Association. (2003). Retrieved October 17, 2003, from http://www.aoa.net.org

Andrews, M. M., & Boyle, J. S. (Eds.). (1999). *Transcultural concepts in nursing care* (3rd ed.). Philadelphia, J. B. Lippincott.

Astin, J. A. (1998). Why patients use alternative medicine. *Journal of the American Medical Association, 279*, 1548–1553.

Beal, M. (1998). Women's use of complementary and alternative therapies in reproductive health care. *Journal of Nurse Midwifery, 43*, 224–234.

Burkhardt, M. A., & Jacobsen, M. G. N. (2000). Spirituality and health. In B. M. Dossey, L. Keegan, & C. E. Guzzetta (Eds.), *Holistle nursing: A handbook for practice* (3rd ed.). Gaithersburg, MD: Aspen.

Callahan, D. (1996 November–December). The goals of medicine. *Hastings Center Report: Special supplement*, S1–26.

Chilton, M. (1996). Panel recommends integrating behavioral and relaxation approaches into medical treatment of chronic pain, insomnia. *Alternative Therapies in Health and Medicine, 2*, 18–28.

Dochterman, J. M., & Bulechek, G. M. (1996). *Nursing interventions classification (NIC)*. St. Louis, MO: Mosby.

Dossey, L. (1993). *Healing words: The power of prayer and the practice of medicine*. San Francisco: Harper.

Dossey, B., Keegan, L., & Guzzetta, C. E. (Eds.). (2000). *Holistic nursing: A handbook for practice* (3rd ed.). Gaithersburg, MD: Aspen.

Eisenberg, D. M., Davis, R. B., Etner S. L., Appel, S., Wilkey, S., Van Rompag, M., & Kessler, R. C. (1998). Trends in alternative medicine use in the United States, 1990–1997. *Journal of the American Medical Association, 280*, 1569–1575.

Ergil, K. V. (1996). Chinese Medicine/China's Traditional Medicine. In M. S. Micozzi (Ed.), *Fundamentals of complementary and alternative medicine*. New York: Churchill Livingstone.

Glisson, J., Crawford, R., & Street, S. (1999). Review, critique and guidelines for the use of herbs and homeopathy. *The Nurse Practitioner. 24*(4) 44–67.

Gordon, R. J., Neinstedt, B. C., & Gesler, W. M. (1998). *Alternative therapies: Expanding options in health care*. New York: Springer.

Hardy, M. L. (2000). Herbs of special interest to women. *Journal of the American Pharmaceutical Association, 40*(2), 234–242.

Institute for Alternative Futures. (1998). *Complementary and alternative approaches in U.S. health care*. Retrieved October 17, 2003, from http://www.altFutures.com

Jacobs J., & Moskowitz, R. (1996). Homeopathy. In M. S. Micozzi (Ed.), *Fundamentals of complementary and alternative medicine*. New York: Churchill Livingstone.

Kaptchuk, T. J. (1983). *The web that has no weaver: Understanding Chinese medicine*. New York: Congdon and Weed.

Kemp, T. (1996). The use of transcutaneous electrical nerve stimulation on acupuncture points in labour. *Midwives, 109*(1307) 318–320.

Keville, K., & Green, M. (2000). Aromatherapy: Guidelines for using essential oils and herbs. Retrieved July 2, 2000, from http://www.healthy.net

Kinsley, D. (1996). *Health, healing, and religion: A cross-cultural perspective*, Upper Saddle River, NJ: Prentice-Hall.

Koenig, H. G. (1999). *The healing power of faith*. New York: Simon & Schuster.

Learn, C. D., & Higgins, P. G. (1999 October–November). Harmonizing herbs: Managing menopause with help from mother earth. *Lifelines*, 39–43.

Levin, J. S. (1994). Religion and health: Is there an association, is it valid and is it causal? *Social Science and Medicine, 29*, 589–600.

Marston, R. Q., & Jones, R. M. (Eds.). (1992). *Medical education in transition*. Princeton, NJ: The Robert Wood Johnson Foundation.

McGuffin, M., Hobbs, C., Upton, E., & Goldberg, A. (Eds.). (1997). *American Herbal Products Association's botanical safety handbook*. Boca Raton, FL: CRC Press.

McGuire, M. B. (1988). *Ritual healing in suburban America*. New Brunswick, NJ: Rutgers University Press.

Micozzi, M. S. (Ed.). (1996). *Fundamentals of complementary and alternative medicine*. New York: Churchill Livingstone.

National Institutes of Health. (1994). *Alternative medicine: Expanding medical horizons*. A Report to the National Institutes of Health on Alternative Medical Systems and Practices in the United States (Publication No. 017-040-00537-7). Washington, DC: U.S. Government Printing Office.

North American Nursing Diagnosis Association (NANDA). (2003). *Nursing Diagnoses: Definitions and Classification 2003–2004*. Philadelphia: Author.

Olsen, M., Sneed, N., LaVia, M., Virella, G., Bonadonna, R., & Michel, Y. (1997). Stress-induced immunosuppression and therapeutic touch. *Alternative Therapies in Health and Medicine, 3*, 68–74.

Pew Health Professions Commission. (1995). *Critical challenges: Revitalizing the health profession for the twenty-first century*. San Francisco: Author.

Pizzorno, J. E. (1996). Naturopathic medicine. In M. S. Micozzi (Ed.), *Fundamentals of complementary and alternative medicine*. New York: Churchill Livingston.

Richardson, M. A., Sanders, T., Palmer, J. L., Greisinger, A., & Singletary, S. E. (2000). Complementary/alternative medicine use in a comprehensive cancer center and their implications for oncology. *Journal of Clinical Oncology, 18*, 2505–2514.

Rosenfeld, I. (1996). *Guide to alternative medicine*. New York: Random House.

Snyder, M., & Lindquist, R. (Eds.). (1998). *Complementary/alternative therapies in nursing* (3rd ed.). New York: Springer.

Stewart, J. C. (1995). *Reiki touch*. Atlanta, GA: The Reiki Touch.

U.S. Food and Drug Administration. (2003, February 28). HHS acts to reduce potential risks of dietary supplements containing ephedra. *FDA News* (PO3-13). Retrieved October 30, 2003, from http://www.fda.gov/bbs/topics/NEWS/2003/NEW00875.html.

Wagner, G. N. (1996). Osteopathy. In M. S. Micozzi (Ed.), *Fundamentals of complementary and alternative medicine*. New York: Churchill Livingstone.

Wardell, D., & Engebretson, J. (2001). Biological correlates of Reiki touch healing. *Journal of Advanced Nursing, 33*(4), 439–445.

Wetzel, M. S., Eisenberg, D. M., & Kaptchuk, T. D. (1998). Courses involving complementary and alternative medicine at US medical schools. *Journal of the American Medical Association, 280*, 784–787.

Suggested Readings

The Burton Goldberg Group. (1994). *Alternative medicine: The definitive guide*. Tiburon CA. Future Medicine.

Cassidy, C. M. (1996). Cultural context of complementary and alternative medicine systems. In M. S. Micozzi (Ed.), *Fundamentals of complementary and alternative medicine* (pp. 9–34). New York: Churchill Livingstone.

Collinge, W., & Duhl, L. (1996). *The American Holistic Health Association complete guide to alternative therapies*. New York: Warner Books.

Cox, H. (1995). *Fire from heaven*. Boston: Addison-Wesley.

Dossey, B. (Ed.). (1997). *Core curriculum for holistic nursing*, Gaithersburg, MD: Aspen.

Engebretson, J. (1996). Comparison of nurses and alternative healers. *Image: Journal of Nursing Scholarship, 28*, 95–99.

Engebretson, J. (1997). A multiparadigm approach to nursing. *Advances in Nursing Science, 20*, 22–34.

Goodwin, M. (1997). A health insurance revolution [Special edition]. *New Age Journal 1997–1998*, 66–69.

Kaptchuk, T.J. (1996). Historical context of the concept of vitalism in complementary and alternative medicine. In M. S. Micozzi (Ed.), *Fundamentals of complementary and alternative medicine*. New York: Churchill Livingstone.

Lovallo, W. R. (1997). *Stress and health: Biological and psychological interactions*. Thousand Oaks, CA: Sage.

Moore, N. G. (1997). The Columbia-Preshyterian complementary care center: Comprehensive care of the mind, body and spirit. *Alternative Therapies in Health and Medicine, 3*, 30–32.

Nurse's handbook of alternative and complementary therapies. (1999). Springhouse, PA: Springhouse.

Ray, P. H. (1997). The emerging culture. American demographics. Retrieved from http://www.demographics.com

Resources

Advances: The Journal of Mind-Body Health

Alternative Therapies in Health and Medicine

Herbalgram

Holistic Nursing Practice

Journal of Alternative and Complementary Medicine

Journal of Holistic Nursing

Acupuncture, http://www.acupuncture.com

Alternative Health News Online, http://www.altmedicine.com

American Botanical Council, http://www.herbalgram.org

American Holistic Health Association, http://www.ahha.org

American Holistic Nurses Association, http://www.ahna.org

Healing Touch International, http://www.healingtouch.net

National Center for Complementary and Alternative Medicine at the National Institutes of Health, http://www.nccam.nih.gov

National Center for Homeopathy, http://www.homeopathic.org

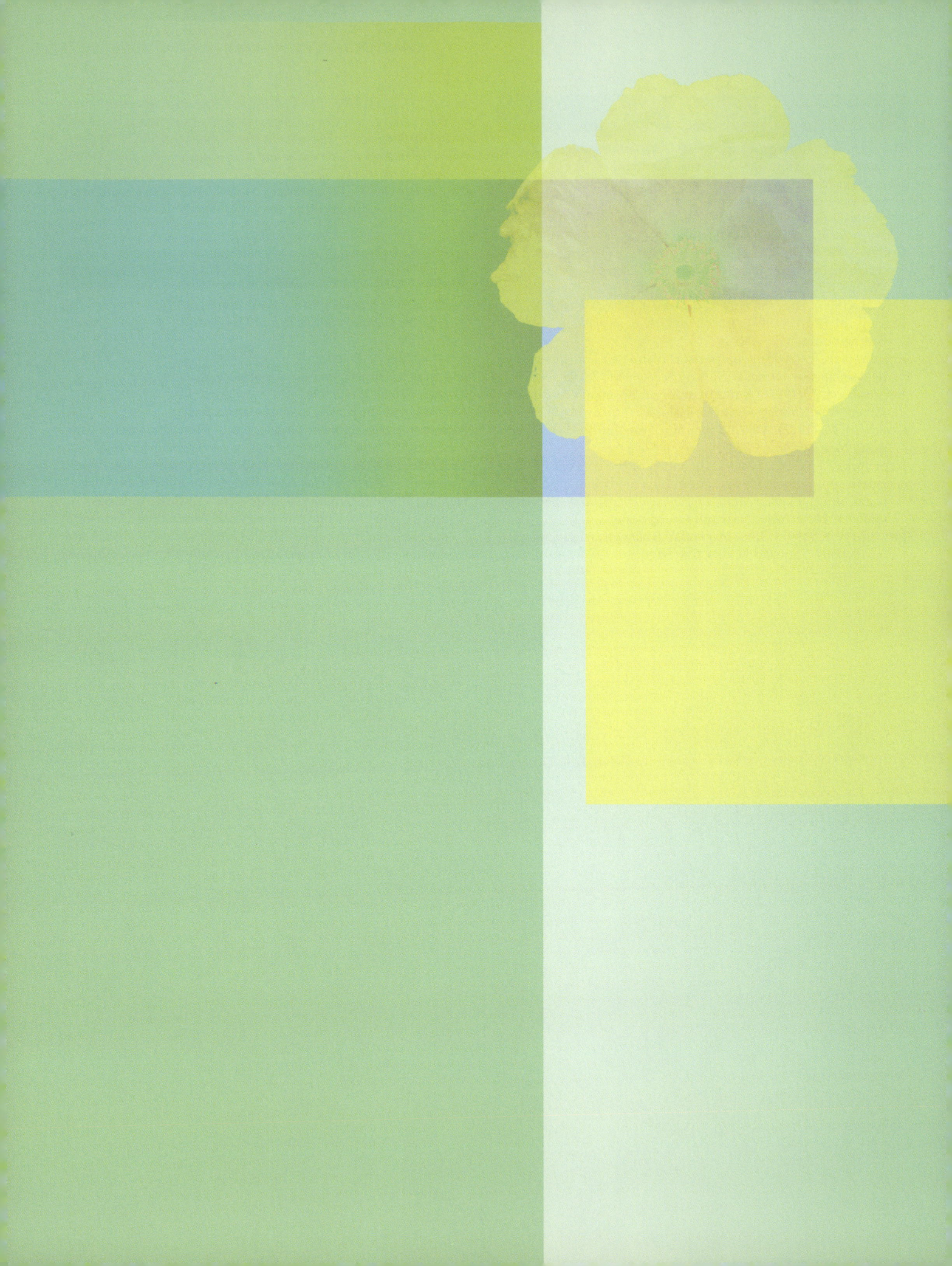

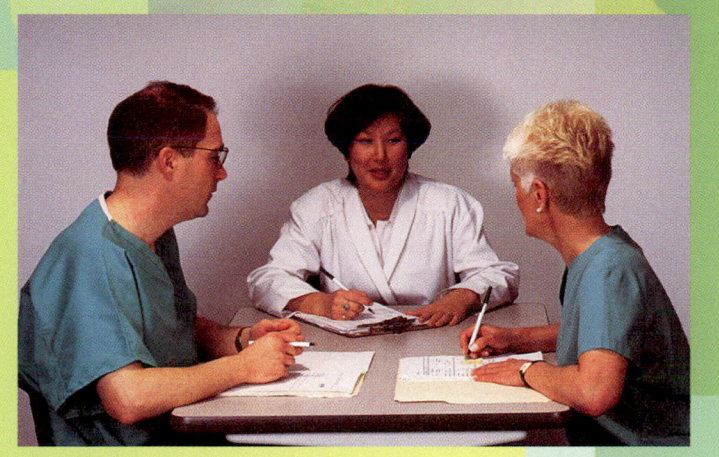

CHAPTER 4

ETHICS, LAWS, AND STANDARDS OF CARE

While ethical and legal issues are present in many aspects of nursing practice, special issues exist when working with childbearing clients. An awareness of personal and professional values facilitates discussion of issues related to caring for perinatal clients. Ask yourself how you would respond to the following questions:

- What values do I hold to be important in my life?
- What beliefs about professional nursing serve as a basis for my practice?
- How do I respond when a client's value system is different from mine?
- What happens when I find I have conflicting ethical responsibilities?

As you read this chapter, continue to think about how your values influence practice decisions. Special boxes raise specific questions about your values and experiences when caring for perinatal clients.

Key Terms

Autonomy
Beneficence
Categorical imperative
Civil law
Code
Criminal law
Deontology
Dilemma
Doctrine of the golden
    mean
Due care
Ethics
Ethic of care
Fidelity
Harm
Informed consent
Justice

Law
Liability
Malpractice
Material principles of
    justice
Negligence
Nonmaleficence
Paternalism
Prima facie
Standards of care
Tort
Universalizability
Utilitarianism
Veracity
Virtue
Virtue ethics

Competencies

Upon completion of this chapter, the reader should be able to:

1. Describe common ethical and legal issues in maternal-child nursing.
2. Discuss basic ethical theories that potentially guide decision making, including utilitarianism, deontology, virtue ethics, and nursing ethics.
3. Identify four ethical principles that can be applied in ethical thinking.
4. Outline the basic steps that lead to dilemma resolution.
5. Describe documentation safeguards that should be used to adequately document care for childbearing clients.
6. Discuss standards of care commonly used in maternal-child nursing.

Who has more rights during a pregnancy—the mother or the fetus? Can anything be legally done to make pregnant women stop using illicit drugs during their pregnancies? Do all women have a right to prenatal care? What measures should be taken so that care given to clients during the perinatal period is safe and appropriately documented? What care standards should guide care given during the perinatal period?

While ethical and legal considerations are a component of all aspects of nursing care, some unique issues exist in maternal-child nursing. Many of these issues occur because two parties, tightly linked, are involved—the mother and the developing fetus. This chapter focuses on basic concepts related to ethical and legal considerations, including relevant ethical theories and principles; a method for conflict resolution and specific dilemmas that nurses may encounter; legal concepts, standards of care for maternal-child nursing, and guidelines for practicing within legal boundaries. Readers will find guidance for practice issues that nurses face in maternity nursing.

What is meant when the term *ethics* or *laws* is used? Ethics refers to the branch of philosophy that provides rules and principles that can be used for resolving ethical dilemmas. Laws are rules that govern the behavior of individuals and represent the minimum standard of morality (Tschudin, 2003).

Since this chapter concerns both ethical and legal issues, a good beginning would be to examine the similarities and differences between law and ethics. Both laws and ethics identify social sanctions and provide guidance for actions. In fact, many laws are derived from ethical considerations. Both laws and ethics provide mechanisms through which disputes can be settled. However, laws and ethics can differ in important ways. Laws are rules that are external to an individual and that members of society must obey. On the other hand, ethics tend to be personal and involve values, beliefs, and interpretations to guide behavior. Laws are written with the interests of society as the major consideration, whereas ethics focus on the interests of an individual within the society. Laws are enforced through law enforcement agencies and the judicial system. Ethical decisions are more reflective, and ethics committees often serve as a forum for discussion, persuasion, and recommendations for action (Figure 4-1).

Some actions are both ethical and legal. For example, informed consent of clients is an ethical obligation for health care providers as well as a legal one. Some actions are legal but may not be considered ethical. One possible example of an ethical and legal conflict, depending on the individual's point of view, would be abortion; an individual who feels abortion is unethical may have difficulty with its legality. Finally, some actions that are illegal might be considered ethical. An example of this situation would be assisted suicide. Although some care providers consider assisted suicide to be within the realm of ethical behavior, such assistance is currently illegal.

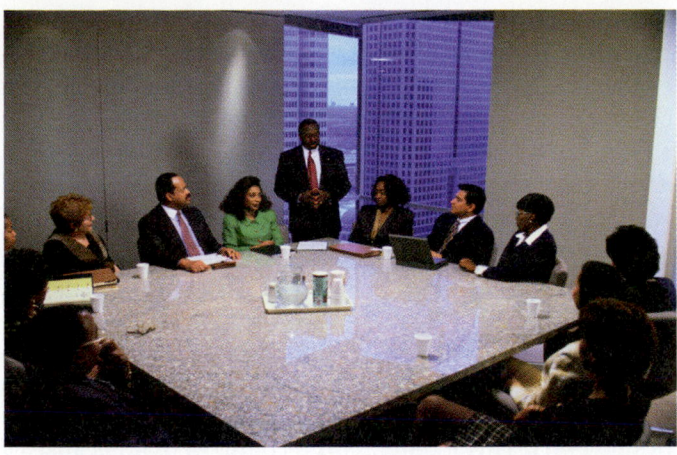

Figure 4-1 Many institutions have ethics committees designed to provide guidance and support in the critical issue of client care. (Photo courtesy of Photodisc)

ETHICAL ISSUES

Nurses frequently encounter ethical dilemmas. In a survey by the American Nurses Association Center for Ethics and Human Rights, 79% of nurses reported encountering ethical issues in practice on either a daily or weekly basis (Scanlon, 1994). Many of these issues were related to cost containment that jeopardized client welfare, end-of-life issues, breaches in confidentiality, and incompetent or unethical practices of colleagues. Unfortunately, 59% of the nurses surveyed indicated that their educational programs had not sufficiently prepared them for managing ethical issues found in practice. This section focuses on some basic ethical theories and principles and suggests a method that nurses can use for resolving ethical dilemmas in practice.

Bandman and Bandman (1999) suggest that ethics are concerned with doing good and avoiding harm. Certainly, nurses have opportunities to promote client welfare and prevent harm. However, just what constitutes good and what can be defined as harmful is open to interpretation. For example, is it better to promote fetal health at the expense of overriding the expectant mother's right to make decisions about her care?

Why are some dilemmas considered to be ethical dilemmas? Ethical dilemmas can arise out of a conflict in duties. For example, nurses have obligations to many parties—their clients, their employing institution, physicians, and most importantly, themselves. Unfortunately, these obligations sometimes conflict. Clients may demand one thing, a hospital or clinic another, and the profession of nursing another. It can be difficult to identify the obligation that is the most important and act on it.

Ethical dilemmas deal with human concerns. Making an ethical decision is different from determining what kind of car you might like to buy or which color is your favorite. A dilemma sometimes encountered in practice is how to protect the health and safety of a fetus while promoting a mother's right to make choices about her pregnancy. Perhaps the most apt description of a **dilemma** is that it is making a choice between two unsatisfactory alternatives (Davis, Aroskar, Liaschenko, & Drought, 1997). Regardless of the choice, the desired happy ending cannot occur. Nonetheless, ethical dilemmas are resolvable situations that demand attention and thoughtful reasoning. Understanding ethical theories and principles can be useful in helping to resolve dilemmas and in discussing the rationale for our actions with others. Each of the ethical theories presented below offers different perspectives about how a dilemma may be viewed and how right actions can be selected.

Basic Ethical Perspectives

The concept of bioethics, or the application of ethics to health care, was popularized in the late 1960s and early 1970s because care providers felt a need to have better methods to resolve dilemmas. Ethical conflicts have always existed, but increased use of technology in health care has increased the number and visibility of dilemmas. Initially, two major classes of theories, derived from existing studies of ethics, were used: utilitarianism and deontology. As the field of bioethics began to grow, providers were concerned that while these perspectives provided guidance for ethical decision making, they did not reflect the characteristics of care providers. Another class of ethics was revived: virtue ethics, an ancient theoretical perspective. Nursing theorists also began to explore the unique relationships that nurses have with clients and to examine the basis for their care. Out of this tradition, an ethic of care, linked to nursing ethics, was proposed to encompass some of the unique perspectives that nurses bring to the health care arena. Because nurses work collaboratively in health care, they must understand the perspectives that each of these theories brings to ethical decision making, because these perspectives can guide thinking and provide a mechanism for explaining and justifying actions. Although these theoretical perspectives can serve as a guide for action, each has some shortcomings.

Utilitarianism

Utilitarianism is a type of ethical theory focusing on the consequences of actions. Although ethical theories are not exactly identical, the overarching themes are similar. In utilitarianism, acts are right if they produce the greatest possible balance of good when everyone is considered

(Mappes & DeGrazia, 1996). No action in itself is considered to be right or wrong. Rather, right actions are those that produce the best possible outcomes.

Utilitarian thinking involves a certain amount of calculation. An individual tries to predict all of the possible good and bad consequences arising from each action that could potentially be taken. Once those are identified, the decision maker would weigh the outcomes and select the action that would produce the best results and the least number of bad results for everyone involved. Utilitarian theory requires that the decision maker be impartial and the decision not be based on personal interests. One difficulty with utilitarian theory is that it might permit the interests of the majority group to override the interests of a minority group (Beauchamp & Childress, 2001). A positive aspect of utilitarianism is that it works to promote good.

For example, it is good for women to receive prenatal care during pregnancy because it helps both mothers and their babies to be healthier. We also have technology available to provide care for low-birth-weight babies. However, resources are limited and there is not enough funding to pay for both prenatal care for all pregnant women and high-technology care for all low-birth-weight infants. From a utilitarian perspective, this problem would be weighed to find a solution that would promote the best outcomes for the greatest number of individuals. In this situation, would better outcomes for more people be produced by provision of early prenatal care to all expectant mothers or by provision of "high-tech" care to a smaller number of low-birth-weight infants? Based on the benefits to the greatest number of individuals, a utilitarian solution would be to provide prenatal care to all expectant mothers.

Deontology

Deontology is another type of ethical theory that is concerned with people doing the right thing. The word "deontology" is derived from *deon*, which means duty. Rather than focusing on whether or not actions bring about the best outcome, deontology strives to identify the best possible action directed by one's duty or obligations, without considering rather than based on the consequences of actions.

The utilitarian theory previously discussed had many critics. Immanuel Kant considered utilitarianism as providing a "wavering and uncertain standard" for action (Mappes & DeGrazia, 1996, p. 16). To remedy this situation, Kant proposed what is known as the **categorical imperative**, or supreme rule, that should govern actions. Simply expressed, the categorical imperative is to act only on that maxim (or rule) that can be willed to become universal law (Kant, 1981). In other words, the rule used to

guide actions should be one that could be followed in all other similar situations. This concept is called **universalizability** because it refers to the concept that the rule should be generalizable to other situations. For example: Is telling a lie to a client ever acceptable? To answer this question, an individual would have to decide if telling lies to clients was acceptable in other situations. Since telling the truth is better in most situations, lying would not be acceptable in any specific instance.

Kant identified several formulations of the categorical imperative. Another formulation that is of interest to health care providers is to always act to treat humanity, either yourself or others, as an end rather than as a means (Kant, 1981). This formulation recognizes that because of their rationality, human beings have inherent worth and dignity. Therefore, we should have respect for all persons, including ourselves. Also, we should never use others simply as a means to an end. For example, clients are a means to our livelihood as nurses. If we care for clients simply as a means to earn a paycheck, we are treating them as only a means. However, if we treat clients with the respect they deserve because they are human beings with inherent worth, then even though clients help us earn a living (means), we are also treating them as an end as well. While Kant's theory provides clear guidelines for action in many situations, it is sometimes criticized for offering such a rigid system of choice that it is difficult to follow.

Other deontologists feel that a supreme rule, such as the categorical imperative, is insufficient to guide decision making in all ethical situations, particularly when a conflict of duties exists. W. D. Ross (1994) proposed the concept of conditional duties, or *prima facie* duties, as a guide for correct action. Rather than asserting that there is a supreme duty, a *prima facie* duty is a conditional duty that can be overridden by a more stringent duty. Ross suggests that some duties are derived from previous acts, such as a promise; acts done by others for which we may owe an obligation; special relationships to families or employers; or acts that serve as a mechanism for personal growth or for benefit to others. From the perspective of Ross, the moral decision maker would decide which obligation or duty was the most important and then act accordingly. For example, as nurses, we have an obligation to follow hospital policies. However, we also have a professional obligation to render safe care for clients. When working in an understaffed environment, a nurse may feel that safe care cannot be given, potentially putting clients at risk for harm. The nurse would then have to choose which obligation was the most stringent, either following the institutional policy of accepting assignments given or rendering safe care to clients. The nurse would act on the basis of which obligation was perceived to be the most important.

Virtue Ethics

A **virtue** is a character trait that is valued; a moral virtue is a trait that is morally valued. **Virtue ethics** focus on the personal characteristics of the moral agent or person and the way in which these virtues guide moral action. Virtue ethics are attributed to Aristotle (Singer, 1994), the ancient Greek philosopher who believed that a virtuous life would be a happy one. According to Aristotle, all living things are endowed with certain capacities or potentialities. For human beings to live a happy life, they must live a life that is distinctive from other creatures through the development of intellectual and moral virtues. Intellectual virtues enable humans to discover and recognize rules of life that should be followed. Moral virtues deal with feelings, emotions, and impulses that make the effective use of intellect possible.

Virtues are not attributes that humans are born with but characteristics that are perfected. Aristotle proposed the **doctrine of the golden mean** as a guide for virtue development. This doctrine suggests that many virtues develop at the midpoint between extremes of less desirable characteristics. For example, one is not born brave but becomes brave by conquering fear. However, if fear is diminished too much, then dangerous risks may be taken. The virtue of courage demonstrates the doctrine of the golden mean: too little courage would make us excessively fearful, but too much would place us in extreme danger. The virtue of courage would be the midpoint between those two extremes. Virtues that may be useful for health care providers to embrace include compassion, benevolence, respect, honesty, and kindness. Beauchamp and Childress (2001) suggest that virtue ethics can serve as a useful adjunct to other theories and principles of ethics that enable individual perspectives on both the right action and the right motive.

Critical Thinking

Virtue Ethics and Respect for Clients

Virtue ethics suggests that respectfulness is a worthwhile virtue to be embraced by nurses. How would acting on the virtue of respectfulness make a difference in the way you treat clients and their partners during the perinatal period? Would you listen to client concerns or suggestions differently? What special considerations might be needed for clients with different cultural backgrounds?

Nursing Ethics

As bioethics has developed, nursing has begun to question whether there is a unique set of ethics for nursing and how those ethics might be embodied. Based on the work of Noddings (1984), who helped to link caring to ethics; Benner and Wrubel (1989), who linked caring and nursing in a very practical sense; and others, an ethics of caring that is applicable to nursing practice has emerged. The **ethic of care** is a perspective that recognizes the personal concerns and vulnerabilities of clients in health and illness. Nurses, operating under the tenets of an ethic of care, would be willing to provide care to achieve therapeutic goals without expectation of reciprocity, because of a desire to be a caring individual.

Gadow (1988) suggests that nurses have a covenant to care by alleviating another's vulnerability. Wicker (1988) indicates caring may help bring clients' lives into balance, even if curing cannot occur. Benner and Wrubel (1989) propose that caring creates possibility because it focuses on others and identifies personal concerns. To be considered moral, caring must be an overriding value to guide action and apply to all persons in similar circumstances. Additionally, caring considers the welfare of others and incorporates empathy, support, and compassion (Fry, 1988). An ethic of care enables nurses to respond to others as worthy, with no expectation of reciprocity (Benner, Tanner, & Chesla, 1996). Bishop and Scudder (2001) propose that rather than merely applying principles, the moral sense of nursing is articulated through the "caring presence of nurses that achieves the therapeutic intent of nursing practice" (p. xi).

According to Noddings (1984), the ethical self exists in relationship with others. Caring relationships are grounded in an ideal vision, in which we hold our best selves. Caring involves reciprocity; our desire to care is rooted in previous relationships, where others have cared for us and we have cared for others. Moral behavior arises from a natural impulse to care, preserving the fundamental goodness of these experiences. Ethical caring occurs because of the desire to be a caring person. Caring relationships permit the caregiver to view the world from the perspective of the recipient of care. From that perspective, the one caring is able to set aside personal agendas and place herself or himself at the disposal of the recipient.

Benner et al. (1996) perceive that the ethical and clinical knowledge of the nurse are inseparable and are learned experientially. Through experience, nurses develop an ethical comportment that encompasses a practical "know-how" of relating to clients in a respectful and supportive way. The ethical comportment aids in protecting those who are vulnerable, promoting growth and health, or fostering a peaceful death. These skills can be developed within a socially based practice, through the

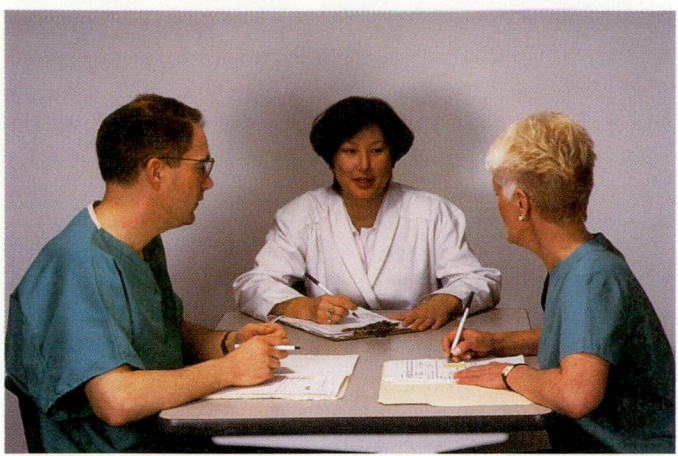

Figure 4-2   Consultation with health care team members is an important part of maintaining an autonomous practice. Good communication promotes safe care and facilitates discussion of ethical issues.

stories of others, and through other experiences, permitting nurses to move from the status of a novice to that of a skilled practitioner (Figure 4-2).

Nursing ethics are therapeutic in the sense that they promote the well-being of clients. "Nursing ethics should evoke thinking about concrete practice in ways that help nurses individually and collectively to fulfill the moral sense of nursing" (Bishop & Scudder, 2001). Nurses, working from a framework of caring, should consider the individual needs of clients and attempt to respond in a caring, personalized manner. Advocacy on behalf of clients should be an example of engaging in a therapeutic ethic of nursing. Treating clients holistically—not simply as a body in need of repair—is another way of engaging in ethical nursing practice. Recognizing that nursing is practiced in a context with many players, including administrators, physicians, and other care providers, nurses should feel a particular sense of commitment to clients and their families and be an advocate on their behalf.

Critical Thinking

Caring and Personal Agendas

According to the tenets of an ethic of care, nurses should be able to set aside their personal agendas when caring for clients. This may be difficult to achieve. Is it possible to put aside personal agendas and focus on the needs of the client? How might you go about leaving your personal agenda behind when giving care? What are the risks of setting aside a personal agenda? What are the potential rewards?

Ethics and Holism

Holistic ethics is a philosophical perspective that merges the concept of unity and wholeness of all people and nature (Keegan, 1995). Acts are performed by people who have a desire to do good and to contribute to the unity of the self and the universe. Correct acts are ones that reflect the enlightened consciousness of the individual and are judged by the effects that the act has on the nature of the individual and the larger self. From this perspective, holistic ethics encompasses elements of both utilitarian and deontological thinking. Outcomes are important, but there is also a concern for the intrinsic nature of the act.

The *Code of Ethics for Holistic Nurses* provides guidance for action and identifies responsibilities for self and others (American Holistic Nurses Association, 1995). The code expresses that nurses have fundamental responsibilities for health promotion, facilitation of healing, and alleviation of suffering. It suggests that nurses have an obligation to self, demonstrated by modeling health behaviors and achieving harmony in life. Nurses have a primary responsibility to clients that reflects an awareness of the holistic nature of human beings. Nurses are responsible for cooperating with co-workers and maintaining competence. Nurses practicing within a holistic framework should work to meet the health-related and social needs of the public and facilitate healing by manipulating the environment to promote peace, harmony, and nurturance.

Ethical Principles

Four major principles guide ethical thinking in nursing practice. These include respect for autonomy, nonmaleficence; beneficence, and justice. These principles may be used in conjunction with the theoretical perspectives discussed as guidelines to help resolve ethical dilemmas. Other principles such as veracity and fidelity will also influence decision making. Each of these ethical principles is equally important in the consideration of ethical dilemmas, although some dilemmas may cause us to focus more emphasis on one principle than another.

Respect for Autonomy

Autonomy refers to individual independence in holding a particular view, making choices, and taking action based on values and beliefs (Beauchamp & Childress, 2001). Respect for autonomy requires that others be treated in a way, such as noninterference in decision making or actions, that enables autonomous action. The concept of respect for autonomy recognizes the inherent worth of the individual and that a competent human being is qualified to make decisions in his or her own best interests (Miller, 1981). For autonomous choice to occur, individuals must

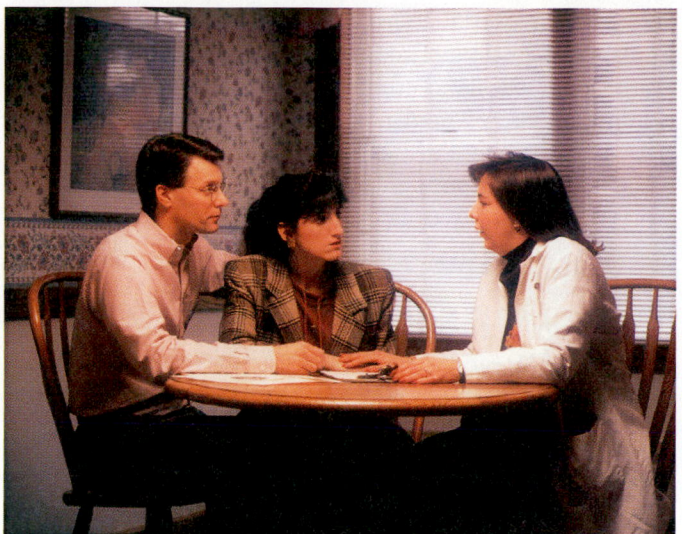

Figure 4-3   Providing information plays a significant role in promoting the autonomy of pregnant women and their families. (Photo courtesy of Bellevue, The Women's Hospital, Niskayuna, NY)

be aware of the alternatives and consequences. The concept of informed consent is firmly rooted in the principle of respect for autonomy and is discussed later.

Although respect for autonomy implies that individuals have the right to make choices, it also focuses on the relationship of individuals to the communities in which they live (Figure 4-3). For example, while individuals can anticipate that community members will respect their autonomy, they also must respect the autonomy of others. We are not given license to perform any act simply because we have autonomous choice. In fact, there are some specific instances where autonomy may be limited. Autonomy of children is routinely restricted because parents believe a child's welfare is promoted by making decisions on behalf of the child. An individual may not be competent to make decisions. For example, clients who are confused or lack the mental capacity to make decisions may have limited autonomy. Another reason for limiting autonomy is when an action could generate harm or when benefit would be derived from restricting autonomy (Mappes & DeGrazia, 1996).

Nonmaleficence

Nonmaleficence refers to the concept of preventing harm to others and is an important principle for nurses. **Harm** is the interference with the mental or physical well-being of others (Beauchamp & Childress, 2001). Many basic rules are nonmaleficent, including not killing, not causing pain, not disabling, and not depriving of freedom. Nonmaleficence encompasses both harm and the risk of harm. The harm may be either intentional or unintentional. As nurses, we have the obligation to exercise due care in professional practice so that unintentional harms do not occur. **Due care** is a legal and ethical standard of performance by which professionals abide. As professionals, nurses must possess sufficient knowledge and skills and render care that is cautious, diligent, and thoughtful.

Beneficence

Beneficence means doing good and may include: prevention of harm, removal of evil, and promotion of good (Frankena, 1973). As nurses our goal is to promote the welfare of clients in our care, so beneficence is a key to our actions. Because the goods and services we have to offer are sometimes limited by our resources, unlimited beneficence is not always possible. In these instances, combining the principle of beneficence and the principle of justice may be helpful.

An issue related to beneficence is what happens when the health care provider's desire to promote client welfare clashes with the client's autonomous decisions. **Paternalism** is the interference with the liberty of another in which the interference is justified by promoting the well-being of that individual (Beauchamp & Childress, 2001). One example of paternalism would be a situation in which a person coerces another to do something that is perceived to be beneficial. This situation frequently causes conflict in health care. For example, maternal-child nurses possess knowledge and expertise about care during and after pregnancy. Education and experience allow these nurses to make suggestions to clients about behavioral modification that should be made to promote a healthy pregnancy. These might include recommendations regarding diet, exercise, smoking, and alcohol intake. How should nurses respond when clients fail to make the changes suggested, even when clients know the potential consequences of failing to modify behavior? The principle of autonomy would suggest that nurses support the client's choices, whereas the principle of beneficence would suggest that nurses override the mother's autonomy to ensure that suggested changes are made. The second choice could be considered paternalistic in nature.

Critical Thinking

Autonomy

Sometimes competent clients make decisions that may be potentially harmful. When this situation occurs:

- Can health providers ever overrule the client's decision? If so, under what circumstances?

- How would you work to promote this client's autonomy?

Justice

Justice refers to how we divide benefits and burdens in our society (Beauchamp & Childress, 2001). For example, health care is a benefit that promotes the health and well-being of individuals in our society. However, paying for health care is a burden. Because our health care resources are not unlimited, we must decide on the fairest system for allocation of both the benefit and resources of health care and the burden of paying for care. A basic principle of justice is that, in distribution of resources, equals should be treated equally and nonequals treated unequally. In health care, pregnant women need access to prenatal care. So all pregnant women should be treated equally in terms of access to care. However, some pregnant women experience greater complications during their pregnancy, causing them to need more sophisticated care. According to this rule, these women would receive additional care not given to women who do not need it (i.e., nonequals are treated unequally).

Depending on the benefit or burden to be divided, the material principles of justice may be invoked to decide how to distribute society's goods. The **material principles of justice** provide a set of guidelines that can be used to justify the distribution of benefits. They offer the following concepts to defend distribution decisions:

- Equality, in which everyone receives an equal share
- Need, for which those who need more receive more
- Contribution, in which goods are received in proportion to productive labor
- Effort, in which the amount of work is rewarded
- Merit, for which rewards are given according to achievement
- Free market exchange, in which wealth and income would be derived from a natural distribution of talent and abilities (Beauchamp & Childress, 2001)

Veracity and Fidelity

Other principles or rules that affect ethical decision making and conflict resolution include veracity and fidelity, both important concepts for nurses. **Veracity** is truthfulness: nurses are truthful with clients in their care. **Fidelity** is keeping promises: if nurses make promises to clients, they keep them. Both these rules reflect respect for others and are essential for establishing trust in relationships.

Code for Nurses

Another guide for nurses in making ethical decisions is the *Code for Nurses with Interpretative Statements* published by the American Nurses Association (1985). **Codes** represent people's acceptance of the obligations and responsibilities entrusted to them by society. The purpose of codes is to provide guidance for action, although codes are not necessarily binding. The *Code for Nurses* has evolved over the past 40 years and currently includes 11 principles for nursing practice: The American Nurses Association Code (Box 4-1) clearly identifies that the fundamental principle of respect for persons is central to nursing practice. Ac-

---

Box 4-1

American Nurses Association Code for Nurses

1. The nurse provides services with respect for human dignity and the uniqueness of the client, unrestricted by considerations of social or economic status, personal attributes, or the nature of health problems.

2. The nurse safeguards the client's right to privacy by judiciously protecting information of a confidential nature.

3. The nurse acts to safeguard the client and the public when health care and safety are affected by the incompetent, unethical, or illegal practice of any person.

4. The nurse assumes responsibility and accountability for individual nursing judgments and actions.

5. The nurse maintains competence in nursing.

6. The nurse exercises informed judgment and uses individual competence and qualifications as criteria in seeking consultation, accepting responsibilities, and delegating nursing activities to others.

7. The nurse participates in activities that contribute to the ongoing development of the profession's body of knowledge.

8. The nurse participates in the profession's efforts to implement and improve standards of nursing.

9. The nurse participates in the profession's efforts to establish and maintain conditions of employment conducive to high-quality nursing care.

10. The nurse participates in the profession's effort to protect the public from misinformation and misrepresentation and to maintain the integrity of nursing.

11. The nurse collaborates with members of the health professions and other citizens in promoting community and national efforts to meet the health care needs of the public.

Note. From *Code for Nurses with Interpretive Statements* (p. 1), by American Nurses Foundation/American Nurses Association, 1985, Washington, DC: Author. Reprinted with permission.

cording to the code, nurses are to support human dignity and to safeguard the client's welfare.

Ethical Decision-Making Model

Many ethics texts or articles suggest a series of steps that can be used to resolve an ethical dilemma (Davis et al., 1997: Thompson & Thompson, 1990; Silva, 1990; Waithe, Duckett, Schmitz, Crisham, & Ryden, 1989). These steps encourage individuals to focus on the situation, gather information, apply ethical theories and principles to guide reasoning, and propose actions for dilemma resolution. By engaging in critical thinking, guided by the model, dilemma resolution can occur. Although the number and sequence of steps may vary, similarities exist among models. A composite framework incorporating common aspects of decision-making models can be found in Box 4-2. One of the things that the framework requires is ascertaining which ethical theories and principles are to be applied for dilemma resolution. Additionally, the decision maker must determine how to weight the theories and principles, that is, which theory or principle should be the most influential in deciding the correct action? This process is necessary because theoretical perspectives or ethical principles may be in conflict with one another.

To apply the model to a dilemma, nurses should review the case with which they are dealing by responding to the suggested questions. Sometimes nurses feel impatient with having to stop and answer questions, particularly when they are in a situation that may be emotional or frustrating. However, efforts will be rewarded because issues will be clarified, and reasoning based on ethical principles and theories offers perspectives to approach the problem and helps provide a rationale for action. Unfortunately, nurses sometimes find themselves engaged in dilemmas that require resolution over short periods—from seconds to minutes. For this reason, it is helpful to discuss case scenarios with others and practice using the ethical decision-making framework to increase awareness of issues and potential

---

Nursing Tip — *Getting Support When an Ethical Dilemma Occurs*

Sometimes you may find yourself dealing with an ethical dilemma. In addition to using the dilemma resolution format suggested in this chapter, you may feel that you need some additional support. Support may come from several places.

- There may be administrative support on your nursing unit or clinic.
- Some institutions have a nursing ethics committee for the purpose of providing a forum for nurses to discuss ethical dilemmas they encounter.
- Many institutions have more generalized ethics committees, which are multidisciplinary bodies that discuss and make recommendations about actions that would be appropriate to resolve a dilemma.

Find out what resources your institution has and how nurses can use them.

Box 4-2

Ethical Decision-Making Framework

Context
- Who is involved and how are they involved?
- What is the setting of the situation?
- What other information is needed for dilemma resolution?
- What personal beliefs of the nurse may have an impact on this situation?

Clarification of Issues
- What are the ethical issues involved?
- Who should decide the issue?

Identification of Alternatives and Potential Outcomes
- What are the possible alternatives and the potential outcomes of each?

Ethical Reasoning
- What ethical theories and principles have bearing on this situation? How?
- Should some principles or theories be given greater weight in the decision-making process? Why?
- What legal or social constraints are factors in this decision?
- What special obligations might be present in my role as a nurse?

Resolution
- Based on the reasoning above, what is the best action in this situation?
- What would be the best strategy for carrying out this action?

Evaluation
- What were the outcomes of the action?
- Should the same action be chosen when a similar dilemma arises in the future? Why or why not?

Client Education

Advance Directives

Ordinarily, nurses specializing in women's health care do not think about teaching clients about advance directives. However, completion of these documents helps clients ensure that their wishes are carried out in circumstances in which they are no longer considered competent. Knowledge of advance directives helps both providers and clients to consider the encompassing totality of the life cycle from birth to death. Consider the following teaching points:

- A Living Will, or a Directive to Physicians and Family or Surrogates—as it is known in some states—permits individuals to indicate their wishes about the medical care that they want to receive in the event of a terminal illness or irreversible condition.
- A medical power of attorney (sometimes known as a durable power of attorney for health care) permits individuals to appoint someone to make decisions regarding medical care when they are no longer able to do so.
- Each state has specific laws regarding completion of advance directives. Information regarding specific regulations regarding advance directives can be obtained from health care institutions or from organizations, such as Choice in Dying.
- Copies of a living will or medical power of attorney should be given by the client to the person designated as the decision maker and to health care providers.
- Having these documents in place helps to ensure that wishes are followed, even if the client is no longer competent.

Client Education

Working with Clients Considering an Abortion

- Provide relevant information about the pregnancy when it becomes available.
- Remember that religious beliefs and effects on other family members may influence abortion decisions.
- Allow clients time to make the decision. A single clinic or office visit is usually not sufficient time for most clients.
- Identify potential sources of client support and assess the adequacy of these sources.
- If clients choose to have an abortion, help them recognize that it is normal to feel a sense of loss after the procedure.

resolutions. A case study applying the decision-making framework is provided later in this chapter.

Selected Dilemmas in Maternal-Child Practice

Several dilemmas and controversial issues relating to maternal-child practice are now discussed.

Abortion

Elective abortion, the willful or purposeful termination of a pregnancy, usually within the first trimester, is a controversial issue. The ethics of abortion have been debated, especially considering the question: "up to what point of fetal development and under what circumstances is abortion morally acceptable, if ever?" Individuals with a conservative view toward abortion would propose that abortion is always wrong. A more liberal perspective suggests that abortion should be available to those who desire to terminate their pregnancies, while a moderate view would advocate abortion in selected instances.

Since the 1973 U.S. Supreme Court decision in the case of *Roe v. Wade*, the right of women to choose abortion has been available in the United States, and the debate over the ethical implications has continued. The *Roe v. Wade* decision permitted women to choose abortion within the first trimester, but permitted states the option to regulate abortion to protect the life of the mother during the second trimester. States were also permitted to regulate or prohibit abortion after 28 weeks of pregnancy—the age of fetal viability. Subsequent Supreme Court decisions (*Beal v. Doe* and *Maber v. Roe*) suggested that states were not required to spend federal funds to pay for elective abortions, thereby restricting access to abortion for women who do not have money.

Despite persistent efforts to limit abortion through denial of Medicaid funding for abortions and through gag rules prohibiting care providers who are working in clinics that receive federal funding from offering abortion as an option to pregnant women, abortion remains a legal option for women in this country. However, proposed legislation to limit late-term abortions is underway. Although the U.S. Supreme Court recognized personal privacy derived from constitutional amendments as a legal basis for permitting women and physicians to elect pregnancy termination, ethical debate continues to be divisive. Some opponents of abortion feel that life begins at conception, and, therefore, it deserves protection similar to that extended to other humans. Opponents feel abortion is killing and deprives the victim (fetus) of the basic right to life, including the experiences, activities, and enjoyment constituting an individual's future (Marquis, 1996). Those who support the right to choose abortion argue that the fetus does not necessarily have the right to use a woman's body during pregnancy (Thompson, 1996). Another argument supporting the right to choose abortion suggests that there are two senses of being human—a biologic one derived from genetics and a moral one that is contingent on being a full-fledged member of the moral community. If one uses the moral sense of being human, a fetus would never qualify for equal protection of life (Warren, 1996).

Consider some of the following situations: Mary G., an unmarried 16-year-old, discovers she is pregnant; after amniocentesis disclosed the presence of Down syndrome, Shirley B., a 38-year-old woman, is considering terminating her pregnancy; although she did not report it, Fay C. was raped 3 months ago and is now pregnant. Each of these is a scenario in which a woman might want to consider an abortion. However, decision making in this process can be complex and lonely to navigate. Maternal-child nurses often find themselves in a position of providing support for women who are making decisions about whether to terminate a pregnancy. The client education box suggests interventions for nurses working with clients who are considering abortion.

Maternal-Fetal Conflict

The following situations are examples of maternal-fetal conflict:

- Annie Z., a pregnant client in your care, continues to use cocaine in spite of education about the harmful effects on the fetus and referrals to a drug abuse program.
- Bess Y. is still smoking during her pregnancy even though she is aware the habit can adversely affect her pregnancy.
- As a result of extended labor, Betty O. has been scheduled for a cesarean section; however, Betty wishes to continue with the labor process and have a vaginal delivery.
- During her second trimester, Nancy D. has been told that she needs to have intrauterine fetal surgery. She considers the procedure risky and wants to refuse.

In each of these instances, pregnant women are being asked to modify behavior or to submit to treatment to benefit their developing fetus. Although most pregnant women would say they want a healthy baby, modifying

Critical Thinking

Late-Term Elective Abortions

Reflect on how you feel about clients who want an abortion during the second trimester when they discover a major defect in the developing fetus? How would you support this woman and her family? How would you manage this situation if the client's decision was different from the decision you would make?

behaviors or submitting to unwanted intervention during pregnancy is not easy. Maternal-fetal conflict occurs when the interests of a pregnant woman are divergent from the interests of the fetus. For example, a client who smokes may have difficulty stopping a habit that she knows is unhealthy for her fetus. One role of health care providers is to make recommendations that in their opinion are beneficial to the pregnancy. When the pregnant woman disagrees, conflict is inevitable. One way of describing this situation is that there is a conflict between the ethical principles of respect for autonomy (the pregnant mother's decision) and beneficence (what health care providers perceive as beneficial to the fetus). Maternal-fetal conflict has become a more prominent problem with the advent of technology that enables fetal diagnosis and management. The ethical question becomes whether a pregnant woman and her fetus represent one client, and the pregnant woman serves as the decision maker, or the mother and fetus are really two clients, each with rights and privileges that may compete with one another. In a two-client model, decision-making control could be removed from a pregnant woman and given to another individual who would be responsible for making decisions on behalf of the fetus.

Consider the situation in which a physician has told a woman that she must have a cesarean section and she refuses the intervention. In such a time-limited and potentially risky situation, attempts to use the legal system for problem resolution have ensued. In fact, court-ordered cesarean sections have occurred (Lindgren, 1996). Unfortunately, such court-ordered treatments are coercive and create a conflict between the perceived interests of the woman and the fetus (Lindgren, 1996).

Three competing values may be present in maternal-fetal conflicts: autonomy of the pregnant woman, protection of the fetus, and protection of the common good (Andrews & Patterson, 1995). Ordinarily, the right of the person to make autonomous decisions is the most highly valued. The principles of nonmaleficence and beneficence are used to justify mandating intervention for protection of the fetus. Another argument supporting fetal intervention is that if a woman has chosen to continue a pregnancy, then she has a responsibility to make her

Reflections from Families

It was like a nightmare. I found out that my pregnancy might not be normal and then had to have an ultrasound. Waiting to find out the results was really hard . . . I couldn't sleep. Once I knew for sure there was a problem, I had to decide what to do—whether to keep the pregnancy—and that was even harder than waiting. I wanted to do the right thing, but making the decision to terminate the pregnancy was hard, even though I always have thought of myself as pro-choice.

pregnancy and therefore her fetus as healthy as possible. A woman's failure to do so may leave her open to more coercive tactics. An argument to support the mother's autonomy is that the fetus maintains its life though the woman's body and as such is inseparable from it. Therefore, a pregnant woman should have sufficient autonomy to make decisions on her own behalf and on behalf of the fetus. Pregnant women do have a responsibility to protect their fetuses, but it does not follow that coercive public policies should force them to do so. Chervenak and McCullough (1992) suggest that a combined approach, based on the viability of the fetus, be a guide in consideration of maternal-fetal conflict. Viable fetuses that could survive outside the uterus should be treated under a beneficence-based obligation to promote fetal welfare. However, if the fetus was pre-viable because of gesta-

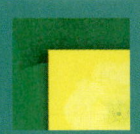

CASE STUDY/CARE PLAN
APPLICATION OF AN ETHICAL DECISION-MAKING FRAMEWORK

Marcella G. is a 26-year-old woman who is 5 months pregnant. She has been coming to your clinic for prenatal care since her third month of pregnancy. On her initial visit, another nurse identified that Marcella has a history of active cocaine use. At that time, counseling was given regarding the destructive effects that cocaine could have on the fetus and mother, and a referral to a drug treatment program was made. Now, 2 months later, you discover that the referral appointment has not been kept and that Marcella continues to use cocaine.

Context

Marcella, the client, and the nurse are the primary players. The fetus may be considered a player, if the two-client model, consisting of the fetus and the mother, is used, rather than the one-client model, in which the mother is responsible for decisions on behalf of both herself and the fetus. There may be other health care providers, such as a nurse practitioner, physician, or social worker, who would also be concerned about the continued drug use. The setting is a prenatal clinic. Your personal beliefs are also important: you may feel that maintaining the autonomy of pregnant clients is important or that protection of the fetus has priority.

Clarification of Issues

You must decide your action based on the information that drug use continues. You feel that expectant mothers should make autonomous decisions, but you also recognize that the fetus is at physiologic risk if drug use continues. While the client is a participant in the dilemma, the nurse should decide what her (own) next actions should be.

Identification of Alternatives and Potential Outcomes

1. The nurse could do nothing and let the clinic visits continue, with Marcella using drugs throughout her pregnancy. The potential outcome is that Marcella would continue her prenatal care but the fetus would suffer harm because of the drug use. Also, Marcella would not receive help for her addiction, and the nurse violates legal mandate to report use of illegal substance.

2. The nurse can try to persuade Marcella to enter a drug treatment program for the remainder of her pregnancy. This action would support Marcella's autonomy and promote a better pregnancy outcome. Trust for the nurse-client relationship would be maintained.

(continues)

tional age or not viable because of the severity of a defect, then the mother's autonomy should prevail in decision making.

Whether nurses support the one-client or two-client model of the pregnant woman and fetus, they should work to maximize the client's understanding of behaviors that support good fetal outcomes. They should continue to work to get substance abusers into treatment programs. If a woman is refusing a cesarean section, care providers should seek to find out why. A better understanding may facilitate a resolution that is agreeable to both mother and care provider. Mishkin and Povar (1993) suggest that health care decision making is a joint enterprise between caregivers and their clients, in which client autonomy and professional standards of care are complementary. In the instance of refusal of fetal surgery,

procedures are not routine and involve risk. Thus, the maternal considerations should be thoroughly addressed. Care providers should seek to provide accurate information and support the mother's autonomous decision.

Critical Thinking

Maternal-Fetal Rights: One-Client or Two-Client Model

Do you perceive pregnant women to fit the one-client or the two-client model? Why?

---

3. The nurse could report Marcella's continued drug use and see if she could force Marcella to enroll in a treatment program. Coercive behaviors would negate Marcella's right to privacy and autonomy. Trust in the nurse-client relationship would be eroded. However, the fetus would benefit from a drug-free environment.

Ethical Reasoning

If a two-client model—in which the mother and fetus have an equivalent moral status—is assumed, arguments would center around the obligation the mother has to the fetus. If you approached this problem from a utilitarian perspective, you would try to examine the action that would produce the best possible outcome for all concerned, but with a real concern that the mother meet her fetal obligations. Using a one-client model, the autonomy of Marcella in promoting the welfare of the fetus would be important. The nurse favoring a fetal-rights stance would believe that if Marcella wanted to procreate, then she has a special obligation to the fetus. Reporting Marcella and forcing drug program enrollment would probably improve fetal outcome. However, the outcome would be better for all three parties—mother, fetus, and nurse—if the nurse could convince Marcella to enroll in the program on her own volition. The principle of respect for autonomy would help to focus on the unity of the mother and fetus and their mutual welfare. The body of the mother is integral to maintaining fetal safety. Doing nothing to intervene in the process would be the worst option because both the welfare of the mother and the fetus are negated. From a deontologic perspective, the nurse would have to decide the correct action that promotes the autonomy and welfare of pregnant women who use drugs. If the virtue of integrity is considered paramount for practice, the nurse must intervene. The second option of voluntary entry into a drug program would preserve professional integrity of the nurse as well as support maternal autonomy and promote maternal and fetal welfare. Using an ethic of care, the nurse would feel an obligation to promote client well-being and advocate on behalf of the client. This action would be further supported by the *Code for Nurses*, because the nurse would act on behalf of the client to promote the welfare of mother and fetus in the context of respecting client choices. Coercion would be difficult under these circumstances. One legal consideration would be Marcella's parental status if she has positive results on a drug screen at the time of delivery. Potentially, the child could be placed in custody until drug rehabilitation is successfully completed. In this circumstance, if Marcella does not remain drug-free, she could permanently lose custody of her baby.

Resolution

The second option of voluntary entry into the drug program is the best option of the three. To try and coercively modify behavior would be counterproductive. Efforts to maintain the nurse-client relationship should continue. Blaming and hostility on the part of the nurse discourages further efforts to seek help.

Evaluation

Ideally, the outcome would be that Marcella entered the treatment program. Even if Marcella did not initially agree to enroll, the nurse should continue to monitor her pregnancy and continue to encourage help-seeking behaviors. Care should include education, treatment referral, complication prevention, and promotion of optimal parenting.

Genetic Mapping

As mapping of the human genome continues, rapid advances are being made in the nature and amount of information that is available to health care consumers. Genetic mapping identifies individual genes, their function, and DNA sequences. The human genome has been mapped and the genome project was completed ahead of schedule. Many benefits can potentially be derived from this newfound knowledge. Preventive treatments may be available in more instances, and cures for lethal diseases may be found. For example, parents at risk for Huntington's disease—a progressive neurologic disorder—could elect to have preimplantation genetic testing. In this testing, an embryo developed through in vitro fertilization would have a genetic analysis completed on one or two cells before cell differentiation. Only embryos without the gene for Huntington's disease would be implanted.

However, genetic information could also be used to great detriment. Insurance agencies or employers may discriminate against individuals or groups who carry particular genes. A central ethical issue in genetics is how to balance the need for genetic information with an individual's right to privacy, particularly when the health care system is moving toward a client-based longitudinal electronic health record (Gostin, 1995). A longitudinal health record would be an electronic database containing all data relevant to an individual's health status over a lifetime. Such a database would be available to a wide variety of individuals or institutions, permitting a loss of confidentiality regarding personal health information. Potentially, an individual could lose health benefits or employment or face stigmatization if sensitive genetic information were disclosed.

In addition to privacy, there are other issues related to genetic testing. If testing resources are inadequate—which is often the case with a new technology—it may be difficult to determine who should have priority for testing. Should testing be done for genetic disorders that are currently untreatable? Or should testing be done for parents who wish to choose the gender of their child? Prenatal testing can also create agonizing choices, such as when parents face the choice of whether to terminate a pregnancy because genetic screening indicates the presence of a defect (Penticuff, 1996).

Although many of these questions are difficult to answer, some suggestions about how to approach genetic screening are offered (Penticuff, 1996). Before screening, consideration should be given to the benefits that will be derived and the therapeutic capabilities of treating identified disorders. Laboratory facilities must be adequate and tests should be reliable. Counseling should be available before and after testing so that the need and appropriateness for testing can be explained and the explanation of the findings and their implications can be given. Genetic screening should be voluntary, done with the informed consent of the individual. Findings should remain confidential, disclosed only with the consent of the person tested. However, to ensure confidentiality of information, rigorous safeguards must be legislated; otherwise, insurance providers could secure information and deny coverage (Penticuff, 1996; Gostin, 1995).

Reproductive Technology

The availability of reproductive technologies has produced a new set of ethical dilemmas. These technologies encompass a broad range of techniques, including in vitro fertilization, gamete intrafallopian transfer, zygote intrafallopian transfer, ovum transfer, embryo adoption, embryo hosting, and surrogate parenting. Questions about the use of reproductive technologies have produced a number of court cases because ethical resolution of issues is lacking. The Roman Catholic Church has rejected many of these techniques because of the belief that procreation is the function of marriage and because multiple zygotes must be developed to secure a viable one (Tschudin, 2003). An alternate perspective supporting the use of technology in insemination is that sexual intimacy and procreation are separate activities (Bandman & Bandman, 1995).

Surrogate motherhood, in which one woman contracts to carry a pregnancy to term for another woman, also poses many problems. Cases have ended in court proceedings, with the surrogate mother not wanting to give up the newborn to the biologic father and his wife. In another instance, none of the contracting parties wanted to keep a newborn with multiple disabilities. Who should be responsible for the emotional welfare and cost of care for this child? At issue is the surrogate mother's right to make an agreement to bear a child and whether that agreement can be broken. Beneficence is a useful ethical principle when considering the welfare of the child born into a surrogate situation.

Unanswered questions surrounding reproductive technologies include:

■ To whom should reproductive technologies be available—all who request them or only to married individuals or to those with adequate financial resources?

Critical Thinking

Pregnancy Termination for Genetic Defects

Reflect on what you believe about genetic defects. Are there defects that should always be terminated? Are there other genetic defects that never should be terminated?

■ Who has ownership of the remaining frozen embryos—the father, the mother, or the potential infant who would be represented through state protection? Lawsuits have occurred during divorces to prevent one spouse from obtaining ownership of frozen embryos.

■ Should donors remain anonymous and can they be compensated?

HIV Status Determination

During pregnancy, women infected with untreated human immunodeficiency virus (HIV) have a 25% to 35% chance of transmitting the infection to their unborn child. Transmission can potentially occur via the placenta, during delivery, or through breastfeeding. While many states have instituted anonymous testing of all newborns to establish the prevalence of HIV infection, prenatal testing is not mandated. Prenatal testing has become a more urgent issue since treatment with the antiviral drug zidovudine (AZT or ZDV) has decreased perinatal transmission of HIV (Downes, 1995).

The ethical conflict of HIV screening is related to the client's right to privacy and autonomy to make decisions regarding care versus the benefit that might potentially be derived from accurate knowledge regarding HIV status of the population. Advantages to knowing HIV status include knowing that infected mothers could be at greater personal risk because the pregnancy may alter cell-mediated immunity. Knowledge of HIV status during pregnancy could promote correct diagnosis and treatment, which would decrease complications and the risk of perinatal transmission. However, diagnosis of HIV infection has special social and financial considerations. In addition to the emotional impact of such a diagnosis, employment and insurance may be lost once the diagnosis is disclosed. Also, fear of being tested may prevent some women from seeking prenatal care. Although it may be medically beneficial to establish the diagnosis, policies mandating HIV testing may deter women from receiving care. Insisting that testing be done would undermine the client's autonomy, her right to privacy, and restrict her liberty to control her body.

Nurses need to maintain an open mind when counseling HIV-infected pregnant women. The risk of HIV transmission must be considered in light of the significance of the pregnancy to this woman and the availability of treatment. Women should be informed about the risks of HIV and counseled accordingly. Nurses must be careful to listen to client concerns about testing and treatment options. Treating clients with respect and developing trusting relationships may facilitate testing and treatment (Downes, 1995; Schmeltzer & Whipple, 1991).

Female Circumcision

As more women from other countries immigrate to North America, nurses are seeing a greater incidence of female circumcision, which is also sometimes termed "female genital mutilation" (Gibeau, 1998). Female circumcision is a cultural practice that can involve removal of the prepuce and clitoris or may extend to excision of the labia minora, excision of the labia majora, and closure of the vagina, leaving a small opening (infibulation). Sometimes considered a rite of passage or a mechanism for socialization into the role of a woman, the practice has persisted, particularly in Northern Africa. Female circumcision is considered by some to be a sign of purity and is essential to maintain family honor and to be a desirable mate for marriage (Lane & Rubinstein, 1996; Lightfoot-Klein & Shaw, 1991). Opposition to female circumcision has occurred because it is perceived as subjugation of women.

Female circumcision has also come under criticism because of significant short- and long-term health implications. Short-term complications include hemorrhage, shock, infection, and damage to urethra, vagina, and anus. Long-term complications include recurrent vaginitis and urinary tract infections, keloid scar formation, persistent infection, cysts, vulvar abscesses, dysmenorrhea, painful intercourse, and increased morbidity and mortality related to childbirth (Gibeau, 1998; Lightfoot-Klein & Shaw, 1991). During childbirth, the infibulation must be cut and then resutured following delivery.

National and international groups (including the World Health Organization and UNICEF) have opposed female genital circumcision on the basis of it being a health risk and a human rights violation (Gibeau, 1998). In 1997, federal laws became effective that prohibit female genital surgeries from being performed in the United States on girls under age 18. Yet, the dilemma remains: how can nurses be sensitive to cultural beliefs and also promote practices that enhance the well-being of clients? Nurses may encounter clients who request to be reinfibulated following delivery or may have clients who request female circumcision for their daughters.

Critical Thinking

HIV Testing for Pregnant Clients

The issue of HIV testing for all pregnant women is controversial. One issue surrounding mandatory testing is what would be done for women who are found to be HIV-infected. Treatment with AZT has been found to reduce the incidence of perinatal transmission. Should pregnant women who are infected be required to submit to treatment to reduce the possibility of HIV transmission to the fetus? What consideration should be given to the wishes of the pregnant woman regarding treatment preferences?

The cultural significance of practices must be recognized, even when they differ from the nurse's cultural norms. Women who practice female circumcision come from cultures in which the practice is considered to be normal. While Western concerns make ending female genital surgeries a priority, in the context of other cultures, other priorities, such as ending physical abuse, promoting education, or stabilizing economics, may prevail (Lane & Rubinstein, 1996). Nurses should recognize that practices exist in Western culture that could be considered equally destructive. For example, breast augmentation to meet a Western cultural standard that large breasts are desirable may be considered abnormal. Often, the principle of autonomy guides the care that nurses provide. However, when cultural practices are physically harmful, such practices are difficult to support. One strategy to resolve the ethical dilemmas of this issue is to express respect for cultural practices but also work to shed new light on the negative health outcomes of female genital surgeries (Lane & Rubinstein, 1996).

Alternative or Complementary Therapies

Alternative or complementary therapies are health-related techniques and practices that are meant to promote healing and, in some instances, complement mainstream medical practices. The focus of these therapies is to treat the person holistically, recognizing that the mind, body, and spirit interact with the environment as a whole. Examples of complementary therapies can include, but are not limited to, healing touch, acupuncture, massage therapy, use of guided imagery, nutrition, yoga, dance, aromatherapy, and folk remedies. The use of complementary and alternative therapies is increasing in health care, and some nurses now incorporate these care modalities into their practices (Simon, 1999). Although client use of alternative therapies is increasing, clients do not necessarily inform their care providers that they are undergoing these therapies, because these practices have been devalued in the past (Nash, 1999). Nurses must be sensitive to client needs with respect to alternative therapies. The principle of respect for autonomy indicates that clients have a need to be informed about potentially useful therapies and make decisions regarding their use. The principle of beneficence indicates that positive acts to improve the welfare of clients should be supported; the principle of nonmaleficence indicates that care should be taken so that harm is not done to clients through either the provision of or withholding of potentially therapeutic opportunities (Nash, 1999). Nurses need to investigate client use of alternative therapies and explore how these practices may be beneficial.

LEGAL ISSUES

As professionals, nurses are both ethically and legally accountable for their practices. Care of pregnant women and newborns requires specialized knowledge, communication, and teamwork among health care providers. Accurate assessment, reporting, and documentation are essential to safe and effective nursing care. When pregnancy and childbirth are involved, most people anticipate normal deliveries and healthy babies. However, adverse events resulting from poor nursing care in the labor room accounted for 128 (17.4%) of a total of 747 malpractice cases in a study conducted by Beckmann (1996). In these cases, poor nursing assessment and medication errors contributed to maternal injuries and death. The purpose of this section is to examine basic aspects of the laws and standards that govern nursing practice, including suggestions for promoting quality care throughout pregnancy.

Basic Legal Concepts

We live according to laws that set minimum standards for behavior. Laws are derived from federal, state, or local sources and provide a necessary order for individuals living within a society. Laws also extend to professional nursing practice that have developed along with laws governing medical practice.

There are two major divisions of law: criminal and civil. **Criminal law** addresses public concerns and punishes the wrongs that threaten a group or society; **civil law** is concerned with and punishes wrongs against the individual (Hall, 1996). Laws are derived from three major sources: statutory law, or those laws passed through legislative process; regulations, which are established by the executive branch (such as president or governor); and case law, sometimes referred to as common law, which is derived from judicial decisions on specific cases. Some laws from each of these sources concern nurses. Statutory laws, through nurse practice acts, define what constitutes the scope and practice of nursing and determine educational qualifications and titling for registered nurses. The Board of Nurse Examiners for each state helps to establish regulations governing nursing practice and can make decisions regarding issuing or suspending licenses for practice (Figure 4-4). Case law may identify a minimum standard to which a health care provider is expected to adhere. For example, the need for institutions to identify an effective chain of command for dealing with emergencies has been set through case law (Mahlmeister, 1996).

A **tort** is a civil wrong that may be caused either intentionally or unintentionally. **Negligence** occurs when there is an unintentional wrong caused by the failure to act as a reasonable person would under similar circum-

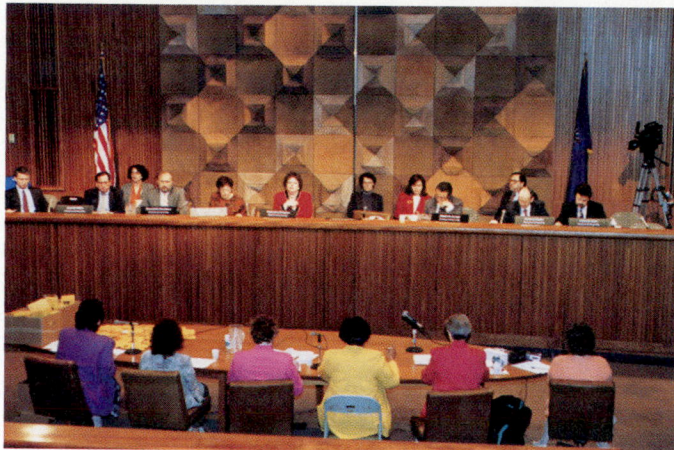

Figure 4-4 Nurses must be involved in legislative activities that are a means of regulating nursing practice.

(Photo courtesy of the New York State Nurses Association)

stances (Mahlmeister, 1996). **Malpractice** is a type of negligence involving the actions of professionals who failed to perform as other competent professionals would in the same set of circumstances. Four components must be present to demonstrate malpractice, including duty, breach of duty, client injury, and proximate cause (Mahlmeister, 1996). In a case of malpractice, the defendant must have a duty toward the injured person. For example, a nurse has a duty to provide safe care for a client. That duty must have been breached. In other words, the professional must have failed to act in such a way that the standards of practice were upheld. A common question asked in cases of a breach of duty is: Did the nurse act in a way that a reasonable, prudent nurse would act in a similar situation? Next, an injury must have occurred. The potential for injury is not adequate for establishing malpractice, there must have been an actual injury. Last, the resulting injury must be directly caused by the negligence that occurred. Consider the example of a postpartum client, who had an epidural block, and, while under the influence of the drug, fell and sustained a head injury, because the nurse left the bed rails down and had not instructed the client to seek assistance in walking. The nurse would be considered negligent for not providing safeguards that a reasonable and prudent nurse would have provided under similar circumstances.

Another way of looking at causation is through proving the injury would not have occurred except that the nurse failed to act in a reasonable and prudent manner. As professionals, nurses are expected to possess specialized knowledge and are liable for their actions. The concept of **liability** means that each person is accountable for his or her acts that fail to meet the standards of the profession (Mahlmeister, 1996).

Standards of Care

In addition to laws, standards of care also guide nursing practice. **Standards of care** are documents developed by professional groups to establish a level of practice agreed upon by members of the profession. In many instances, these standards reflect the minimum expectations required of professionals for a safe practice. Because standards are based on current knowledge, they are dynamic and may be subject to change as new information becomes available. Standards of care are sometimes used in legal situations as a yardstick for determining if negligence occurred. Nurses should be knowledgeable about professional standards of practice in their specialty and practice within those guidelines. This professional accountability serves nurses well when issues of liability arise (Mahlmeister, 1996).

A standard used in women's health is published by the Association of Women's Health, Obstetric, and Neonatal Nurses (AWHONN, 1998). These standards are divided into standards for care and professional performance; guidelines for women's, perinatal, and newborn health; acute care; community and home care; and administration. The standards of care section uses the nursing process format and addresses assessment, diagnosis, outcome identification, planning, implementation, and evaluation. The section on professional performance addresses quality of care, performance appraisal, education, collegiality, ethics, collaboration, research, resource utilization, practice environment, and accountability (AWHONN, 1998). The guidelines suggest actions appropriate to nursing practice in specific areas of maternal-child nursing.

Additional sources of standards are the scope and standards for nursing practice developed by each state's Board of Nurse Examiners, and standards developed by individual institutions and found in policy and procedure manuals. Sometimes it is difficult for nurses to assess whether they are practicing within the scope and standards of nursing. Suggested questions that nurses may ask to determine the acceptability of their practices or any given activity include (Flores, 1997, pp. 6–7):

- Is the activity consistent with the state's Nurse Practice Act and rules and regulations of the Board of Nurse Examiners?

- Is the activity in accordance with established policies and procedures of the institution?

- Is the activity supported by research or in the scope and standards of practice statements?

- Does the nurse possess the required knowledge and demonstrated competency in performing the activity?

- Would a reasonable and prudent nurse perform the activity in this setting?
- Is the nurse prepared to assume accountability for the provision of safe care and the outcomes rendered?

If nurses are knowledgeable and able to respond affirmatively to each of these questions, then the activity in question should be within the scope and standards of practice. Flores suggests that referring to a decision-making model such as this one becomes more automatic with routine use, ensuring more critical thinking about practice issues and empowering nurses to be proactive.

Practicing Safely in Perinatal Settings

A holistic, interpersonal approach to care and adequate documentation are essential components of safe nursing practice and serve to reduce the risks of liability. Competent care requires a team approach, with nurses playing a key role in assessment and communication (Fiesta, 1995). McMullen and Philipsen (1995) offer suggestions to decrease litigation and to improve care throughout a client's pregnancy. Believing that interpersonal care and communication are important factors in reducing liability, they suggest that nurses establish good rapport with clients and their families. Nurses should encourage input from clients and families, allowing sufficient time for questions and dialogue. These measures enhance communication, health teaching, and interpersonal relationships. Good rapport with clients helps them to feel respected and well cared for during pregnancy (Philipsen & McMullen, 1994b). These measures also improve continuity of client care and reduce potential liability.

Policies and procedures are also an important factor in safe nursing practice. Policies and procedures should be updated regularly and should be realistic within the framework of practice (McMullen & Philipsen, 1995). When new practices become accepted, institutions should revise existing policies to reflect correct practice guidelines so that nurses are not left in the position of trying to implement updated practices that are not in the hospital procedure manual. Nurses also should be able to perform the outlined procedures within the context of the work setting. Otherwise, the policy should be examined and a safe, but more feasible, policy substituted. Nurses should be aware of what constitutes safe practice and know how policies are changed in their institution.

As institutions cut costs, the skill mix of the nursing staff may change, leading to greater use of unlicensed assistive personnel (UAPs) for providing client care. To efficiently practice, registered nurses are responsible for delegating selected care tasks to UAPs. The function of UAPs is to complement performance of nursing functions rather than to substitute for the registered nurse. To promote safe practice, nurses should be familiar with state regulations governing delegation, so that appropriate tasks are delegated for UAPs to carry out. The *Standards and Guidelines for Professional Nursing Practice in the Care of Women and Newborns* (AWHONN, 1998) suggest that task delegation should be based on client needs and the knowledge and skill of the provider designated to perform the task.

During pregnancy, the prenatal care offered should meet nationally established standards and be documented accordingly. An area of particular concern during the first trimester of pregnancy is giving adequate information to the client regarding the availability of prenatal tests, such as chorionic villus sampling, amniocentesis, triple screen of alpha-fetoproteins, and screens for some teratogenic communicable diseases (Philipsen & McMullen, 1994a).

Later in pregnancy, testing remains a significant issue. Once again, nurses should be careful to inform clients about the availability of specific testing, including the potential risks and benefits, and record the expectant mother's response (Philipsen & McMullen, 1994b). Even routine test results, such as those from urinalysis, blood cell counts, and blood pressure measurement, should be documented.

Another legal issue centers around antepartum clients being discharged from labor and delivery because they are not yet ready to deliver. Before discharge, there should be documentation of at least two assessments, noting any change in client condition and a baseline fetal monitor strip from 20 to 30 minutes of observation. Assessment should include vital signs and examination of the cervix. The physician or nurse-midwife must be notified of the client's presenting condition and reassessment before discharge (Rommal, 1996). If clients are discharged before delivery, written discharge instructions should be reviewed, signed by the mother, and a copy given to the mother (McMullen & Philipsen, 1995). This opportunity presents an excellent chance to answer any questions a mother may have.

Critical Thinking

Unrealistic Hospital Policy

You are a nurse working in labor and delivery. One of the policies of your institution is that all women in the first stage of labor be monitored every 15 minutes and a charted entry regarding their status be made. Checks may include vital signs, assessment of fetal heart rate, and vaginal examination. While you feel that frequent checks are important, the staffing of your unit does not allow nurses sufficient time to meet this policy. Consequently, nurses do not follow this policy. How would you respond to this situation?

Nurses must be knowledgeable about the expected practices of physicians and question the appropriateness of physician orders when deviations from standards occur. In the process of reporting emergencies, nurses must be familiar with the established chain of command in the institution. Nurses should know when to activate the chain of command and when it is appropriate to move up the chain of command (Mahlmeister, 1996). When seeking help, nurses should remember that prompt reporting facilitates problem resolution and that persistence can help ensure that clients receive appropriate care. Following these guidelines should promote safe client care and reduce opportunities for negligence to occur.

Legal Issues in Maternal-Child Practice

Two issues that nurses often encounter in maternal-child practice are informed consent and the right to privacy.

Informed Consent

Based on a client's right to self-determination, **informed consent** demands that information regarding treatment procedures be given to clients and their consent secured. To obtain a valid consent, clients must be presented with information regarding the course of treatment; methods by which the treatment is carried out; any alternative forms of treatment available, including the inherent risks and benefits of each option; and risks of nontreatment. If any of these areas is not included, then the consent process is incomplete.

Physicians are responsible for determining the competency of clients and providing information to clients for consent. If permissible by hospital policy, nurses can witness consent documents, but should witness the physician obtaining the signature on the form (Figure 4-5). If nurses feel that a valid consent is lacking, then the nursing supervisor or physician should be notified (Fiesta, 1994).

Closely related to informed consent is the right of competent individuals to refuse treatment. In maternal-child nursing, treatment refusal carries particular significance because the well-being of the fetus may be affected by maternal decisions. The issue of viewing pregnant women by a one-client or two-client model affects the right of refusal. Every effort should be made to ensure that pregnant women are well-informed of their options and that treatment decisions are not coercive.

Right to Privacy

In recognition of care providers having access to sensitive information about clients, certain legal, professional, and ethical standards have been developed to help ensure a client's right to privacy. A client's right to privacy means that nurses should not unnecessarily expose a client's body or disclose information to unauthorized parties. During labor and delivery, many personnel may be in and

> ### Reflections from Nurses
>
> In the United States, fathers are encouraged to play an active role during pregnancy and the birth process. However, in other cultures men do not participate in the event of birthing. As a nurse, I find it challenging to manage family dynamics when caring for a family whose values differ from mine. To provide sensitive care, I make an effort to ask the pregnant woman if she will have a partner or coach during the labor and delivery process. Her answer helps me better understand her expectations of support during the childbirth experience.

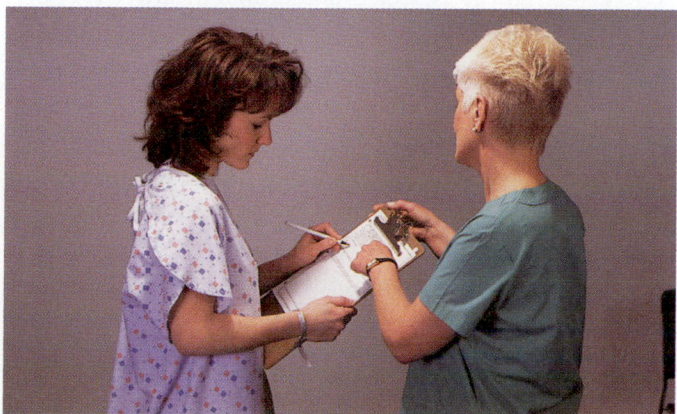

Figure 4-5   Nurses can play an important role in a client's informed consent.

> ### Nursing Tip   Building Knowledge and Experience
>
> Knowledge and experience are powerful tools in practice. Be knowledgeable about maternal-child nursing and about the standards of care and policies that govern practice. Make critical analysis of client care part of a daily routine. Find expert practitioners who integrate ethical practice and promote high standards of care. These tasks strengthen the quality of your practice and provide a mechanism for you to become an experienced nurse.

WEB ACTIVITIES

••• Explore the Internet Encyclopedia of Philosophy: http://www.utm.edu. Many of the selections here reflect a more theoretical aspect of ethics. Review the portion of this chapter that discusses ethical theories and principles. What more can you discover about these areas on this Web site?

••• Visit and explore the Web site for advance directives: http://www.partnershipforcaring.org. How might this information be useful to you personally as well as to you in your role as a nurse working in women's health?

••• Visit the American Nurses Association Web site: http://www.ana.org. Click on the ethics site. What kind of position statements do you find there that are related to the topic of ethics and women's health? Think about women's health from a broad perspective and remember to include issues such as childbearing, violence against women, genetics, HIV, and eldercare.

••• Explore a consumer information website regarding HIPAA privacy regulations: http://www.nc/net.org/healthprivacy

out of the client's room. To protect privacy, only those responsible for care should have room access. Measures, such as drawing a curtain or closing doors during examinations, should be taken to afford privacy. Casual conversation in the hall or elevators about clients under care should be avoided. Health care providers should access information only for clients in their care. It is often tempting to review a chart of a friend or colleague receiving care. However, a client's right to privacy would prohibit securing this information.

The Health Insurance Portability and Accountability Act (HIPAA) was passed in 1996. This law includes protections for coverage for workers who change health insurance plans. One of the important aspects of this law is that health care organizations that accept insurance (covered entities) must be in compliance with the rules governing privacy and confidentiality of health care information. The federal government mandated that all employees of a health care agency had to have completed HIPAA training by April 2003 to ensure that the agency was compliant with maintaining privacy and confidentiality. This confidentiality also pertains to any researcher who wants to access client records.

Key Concepts

■ Ethics provides rules and principles that can be used for resolving ethical dilemmas. Ethical decisions tend to be reflective and may be influenced by values, beliefs, and personal interpretations.

■ Laws are rules that represent the minimum standard of morality and govern the behavior of individuals. Laws are written to promote the welfare of society.

■ Standards of care are developed by professional groups to establish a level of practice agreed upon by members of the profession.

■ Utilitarianism is an ethical theory that focuses on the consequences of action. Actions bringing about good consequences are considered the best.

■ Deontology is an ethical theory that is concerned with doing the right action rather than with the consequences of the action. Actions selected should be ones that could be followed in other similar situations.

■ Virtue ethics focus on developing desirable personal attributes and acting in a manner that is congruent with those attributes.

■ An ethic of care is a nursing perspective that recognizes the personal concerns and vulnerabilities of clients in health and illness. Nurses, operating under the tenets of an ethic of care, would be willing to provide care to achieve therapeutic goals without expectation of reciprocity.

■ In holistic ethics there is a concern both for the outcome of a decision and the intrinsic nature of the act itself. Acts are selected based on a desire to do good and to contribute to the unity of the self and universe.

■ Respect for autonomy recognizes the right of competent individuals to make informed choices on their own behalf.

■ Nonmaleficence suggests that health care providers must exercise due care to prevent client harm.

■ Beneficence is an ethical principle focusing on promoting the welfare of others.

■ Justice provides a mechanism for making decisions about dividing benefits and burdens within society.

■ The American Nurses Association *Code for Nurses* supports the concept of respect for persons and safeguarding a client's welfare. The code offers guidance for nursing actions.

■ Ethical decision making is best when conducted in a systematic manner that carefully examines characteristics of the situation and uses ethical theories and principles as tools.

■ Malpractice occurs when professionals are negligent and fail to perform as other professionals would in a similar set of circumstances. Malpractice consists of a breach of duty, resulting in client injury that is directly related to the negligence.

■ Interpersonal care and good communication are key factors in reducing the risks of liability.

■ Nurses should be proactive in their care approach, that is, be knowledgeable about perinatal nursing practice, legal issues, and standards of care. Adequate client assessment, communication with other care providers, and documentation are essential to safe practice.

Review Questions and Activities

1. The ethical perspective focusing on a sense of commitment to clients and advocacy on their behalf is:
   a. Virtue ethics
   b. Deontology
   c. Ethic of caring
   d. Utilitarianism

   The correct answer is c.

2. The ethical principle concerned with distributing benefits and burdens is:
   a. Respect for autonomy
   b. Justice
   c. Nonmaleficence
   d. Beneficence

   The correct answer is b.

3. Due care is both an ethical and legal concept that indicates that care providers should:
   a. Encourage client decision making
   b. Promote client autonomy
   c. Divide benefits carefully
   d. Exercise caution to prevent unintentional harms

   The correct answer is d.

4. A health care provider interferes with the decisions of a competent person for the purpose of promoting the competent person's welfare. This statement is an example of:
   a. Paternalism
   b. Beneficence

   c. Autonomy
   d. Due care

   The correct answer is a.

5. Discuss informed consent with your classmates. Have one group describe the kinds of information that might be disclosed about a cesarean section when using the reasonable person standard. Another group can describe the information that might be given when using the community standard. The third group should describe information to be given when using the individual client standard. Share your information with the other groups and compare the nature of the information divulged. What ethical principles support the concept of informed consent?

6. Review the case study. What other arguments or viewpoints might be considered for trying to persuade Marcella to enter the drug rehabilitation program or for coercing her into the program? In this situation, what type of actions would the one-client model support? What actions would a two-client model permit? Which would be the best model to use in your ethical thinking? Why?

7. While a client was in labor, health care providers failed to note early signs of fetal distress, although a later review of fetal-monitor readouts clearly indicated that distress occurred. Following delivery, the baby appears to be healthy and has Apgar scores that are within normal limits. As a nurse, you are being pressured to omit those sample monitor strips from the labor and delivery record. What legal and ethical obligations should you consider as you respond to this situation? How will these obligations influence your response? Are there ever circumstances where modifying the medical record would be appropriate? Why or why not?

References

American Holistic Nurses Association. (1995). *Code of ethics for holistic nurses.* Raleigh, NC: Author.

American Nurses Association. (1985). *Code for nurses with interpretative statements.* Washington, DC: Author.

Andrews, A., & Patterson, E. (1995). Searching for solutions to alcohol and other drug abuse during pregnancy: Ethics, values, and constitutional principles. *Social Work, 40*(1), 55–64.

Association for Women's Health: Obstetric, and Neonatal Nurses. (1998). *Standards and guidelines for professional nursing practice in the care of women and newborns* (5th ed.). Washington, DC: Author.

Bandman, E., & Bandman, B. (1999). *Nursing ethics throughout the lifespan* (4th ed.). Norwalk, CT: Appleton & Lange.

Beauchamp T., & Childress, J. (2001). *Principles of biomedical ethics* (5th ed.). New York: Oxford University Press.

Beckmann, J. (1996). *Nursing negligence: Analyzing malpractice in the hospital setting*. Thousand Oaks, CA: Sage.

Benner, P., & Wrubel, J. (1989). *The primacy of caring: Stress and coping in health and illness*. Menlo Park, CA: Addison.

Benner, P., Tanner, C., & Chesla, C. (1996). *Expertise in nursing practice: Caring, clinical judgment and ethics*. New York: Springer.

Bishop, A., & Scudder, J. (2001). *Nursing ethics: Holistic caring practice (2nd ed.)*. Boston: Jones & Bartlett.

Chervenak, F., & McCullough, L. (1992). Fetus as patient: An ethical concept. *Contemporary OB/GYN, 37*(10), 11–16, 22.

Davis, A., Aroskar, M., Liaschenko, J., & Drought, T. (1997). *Ethical dilemmas in nursing practice* (4th ed.). Stamford, CT: Appleton & Lange.

Downes, J. (1995). The ethical dilemmas of mandatory prenatal and newborn HIV testing. *Nursing Connections, 8*(4), 43–50.

Fiesta, J. (1994). *Twenty legal pitfalls for nurses to avoid*. Clifton Park, NY: Thomson Delmar Learning.

Fiesta, J. (1995). Assessment and communication. *Nursing Management, 26*(6), 22, 24.

Flores, K. (1997). Scope of practice, Part III: The decision-making model, *RN Update, 28*(4), 6–7.

Frankena, W. (1973). *Ethics* (2nd ed.). Englewood Cliffs, NJ: Prentice Hall.

Fry, S. (1988). The ethic of caring: Can it survive in nursing? *Nursing Outlook, 36*(1), 48.

Gadow, S. (1988). Covenant without cure: Letting go and holding on in chronic illness. In J. Watson & M. Ray (Eds.), *The ethics of care and the ethics of cure: Synthesis in chronicity*. New York: National League for Nursing.

Gibeau, A. (1998). Female genital mutilation: When a cultural practice generates clinical and ethical dilemmas. *Journal of Obstetric, Gynecologic, and Neonatal Nursing, 27*(1), 85–91.

Gostin, L. (1995). Genetic privacy. *Journal of Law, Medicine, & Ethics, 23*, 320–330.

Hall, J. K. (1996). *Nursing ethics and law*. Philadelphia: W. B. Saunders.

Jones, S. (1996). Genetics: Changing health care in the 21st century. *Journal of Obstetric, Gynecologic, and Neonatal Nursing, 25*(9), 777–783.

Kant, I. (1981). *Grounding for the metaphysics of morals* (J. Ellington, Trans.). Indianapolis, IN: Hackett. (Original work published 1785)

Keegan, L. (1995). Holistic ethics. In B. Dossey, L. Keegan, C. Guzzeta, & L. Krolkmeier, (Eds.), *Holistic nursing: A handbook for practice* (pp. 137–151). Gaithersberg. MD: Aspen.

Lane, S., & Rubinstein, R. (1996). Judging the other: Responding to traditional female genital surgeries. *Hastings Center Report, 26*(3), 31–40.

Lightfoot-Klein, H., & Shaw, E. (1991). Special needs of ritually circumcised women patients. *Journal of Obstetric, Gynecologic, and Neonatal Nursing, 20*(2), 102–107.

Lindgren, K. (1996). Maternal-fetal conflict: Court-ordered cesarean section. *Journal of Obstetric, Gynecologic, and Neonatal Nursing, 25*(8), 653–656.

Mahlmeister, L. (1996). The perinatal nurse's role in obstetric emergencies: Legal issues and practice issues in the era of health care redesign. *Journal of Perinatal and Neonatal Nursing, 10*(3), 32–46.

Mappes, T., & DeGrazia, D. (1996). *Biomedical ethics* (4th ed.). New York: McGraw-Hill.

Marquis, D. (1996). Why abortion is immoral. In T. Mappes & D. DeGrazia (Eds.), *Biomedical ethics* (4th ed., pp. 441–444). New York: McGraw-Hill.

McMullen, P., & Philipsen, N. (1995). Fetal well being III: Strategies to diminish liability and improve client care in all trimesters. *Nursing Connections, 8*(1), 50–53.

Miller, B. (1981). Autonomy and the refusal of lifesaving treatment. *Hastings Center Report, 11*(4), 22–28.

Mishkin, D., & Povar, G. (1993). Decision making with pregnant patients: A policy born of experience. *Journal on Quality Improvement, 19*(8), 291–302.

Nash, R. (1999). The biomedical ethics of alternative, complementary, and integrative medicine. *Alternative Therapies, 5*(5), 92–95.

Noddings, N. (1984). *Caring: A feminine approach to ethics and moral education*. Los Angeles: University of California Press.

Penticuff, J. (1996). Ethical dimensions of genetic screening: A look into the future. *Journal of Obstetric, Gynecologic, and Neonatal Nursing, 25*(9), 785–789.

Philipsen, N., & McMullen, P. (1994a). Fetal well being I: The health care provider's responsibility in the first trimester. *Nursing Connections, 7*(2), 32–33.

Philipsen, N., & McMullen, P. (1994b). Fetal well being II: Health care providers' responsibility in late pregnancy. *Nursing Connections, 7*(3), 52–54.

Rommal, C. (1996). Risk management issues in the perinatal setting. *Journal of Perinatal and Neonatal Nursing, 10*(3), 1–31.

Ross, W. D. (1994). The personal character of duty. In P. Singer (Ed.), *Ethics* (pp. 332–337). New York: Oxford University Press.

Scanlon, C. (1994). Ethics survey looks at nurses' experiences. *The American Nurse, 26*, 1, 22.

Schmeltzer, S., & Whipple, B. (1991). Women and HIV infection. *Image, 23*(4), 249–255.

Silva, M. (1990). *Ethical decision making in nursing administration*. Norwalk, CT: Appleton & Lange.

Simon, J. (1999). The explosion of complementary and alternative therapies. *Nursing Diagnosis, 10*(3), 91.

Singer, P. (Ed.). (1994). *Ethics* (pp. 185–188). New York: Oxford University Press.

Thompson, J. (1996). A defense of abortion. In T. Mappes & D. DeGrazia (Eds.), *Biomedical ethics* (4th ed., pp. 445–452). New York: McGraw-Hill.

Thompson, J., & Thompson, H. (1990). Ethical decision making: Process and models. *Neonatal Network, 9*(1), 69–70.

Tschudin, V. (2003). *Ethics in nursing (3rd ed.)*. Philadelphia: W. B. Saunders.

Waithe, M., Duckett, L., Schmitz, K., Crisham, P., & Ryden, M. (1989). Developing case situations for ethics education in nursing. *Journal of Nursing Education, 28*(4), 175–180.

Warren, M. A. (1996). On the moral and legal status of abortion. In T. Mappes & D. DeGrazia (Eds.), *Biomedical ethics* (4th ed., pp. 434–440). New York: McGraw-Hill.

Wicker, P. (1988). Discussion group summary: When caring doesn't mean curing. In J. Watson & M. Ray (Eds.), *The ethics of care of the ethics of cure: Synthesis in chronicity*. New York: National League for Nursing.

Suggested Readings

Dossey, B., Keegan, L., Guzzeta, C., & L. Krolkmeier, C. (1995). *Holistic nursing: A handbook for practice*. Gaithersberg, MD: Aspen.

Resources

American Nurses Association, 600 Maryland Avenue, SW, Suite 100 West, Washington, DC 20024-2571, 800-274-4262, http://www.ana.org

The Association of Women's Health, Obstetric, and Neonatal Nurses (AWHONN), 2000 L Street, NW, Suite 740, Washington, DC 20036, 800-673-8499, http://www.awhonn.org

Internet Encyclopedia of Philosophy, http://www.iep.utm.edu

Partnership for Caring, 1620 Eye Street NW, Suite 202, Washington, DC 20006, 202-296-8071, http://www.partnershipforcaring.org

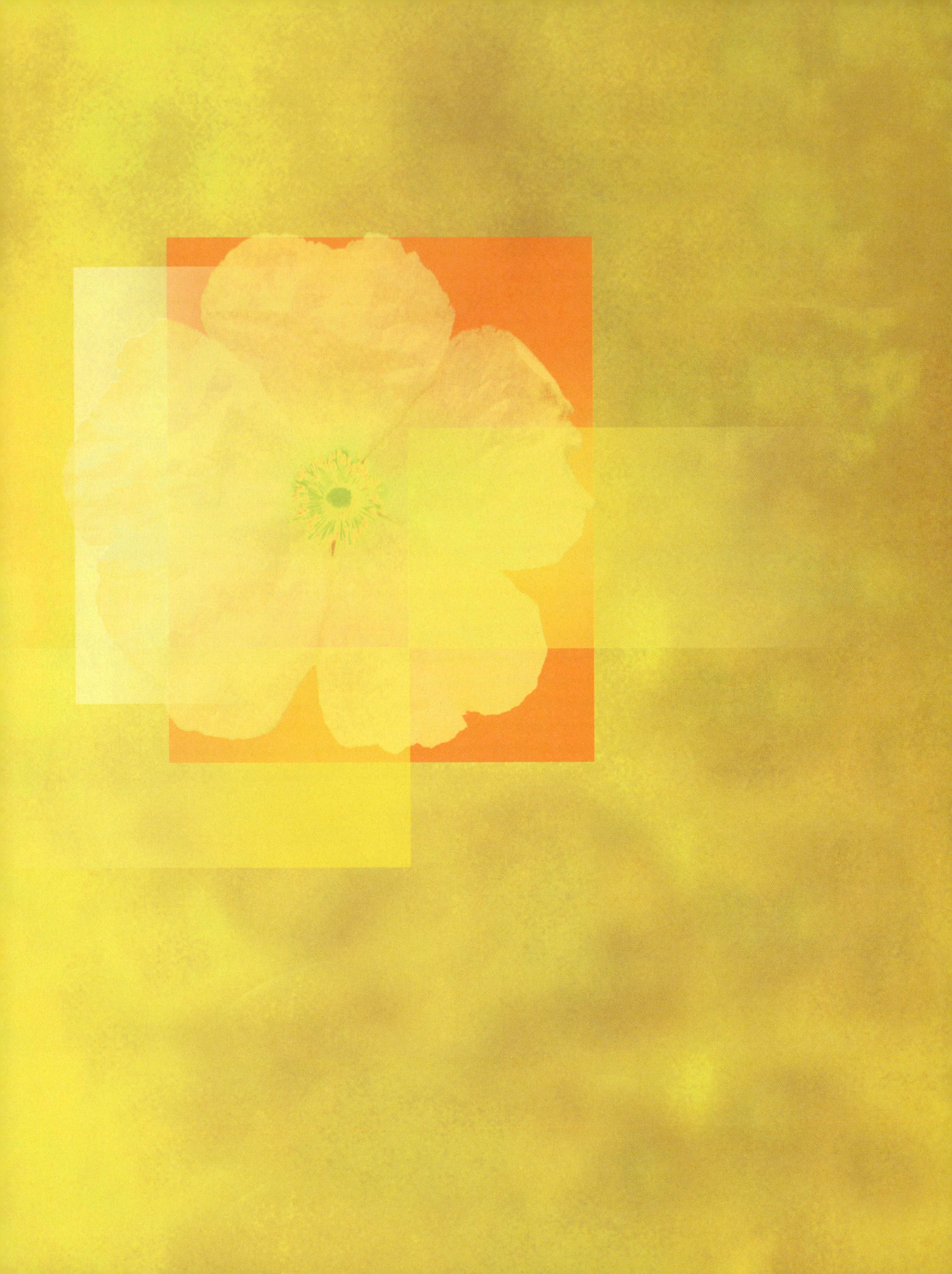

UNIT 2

Health Care of Women across the Life Span

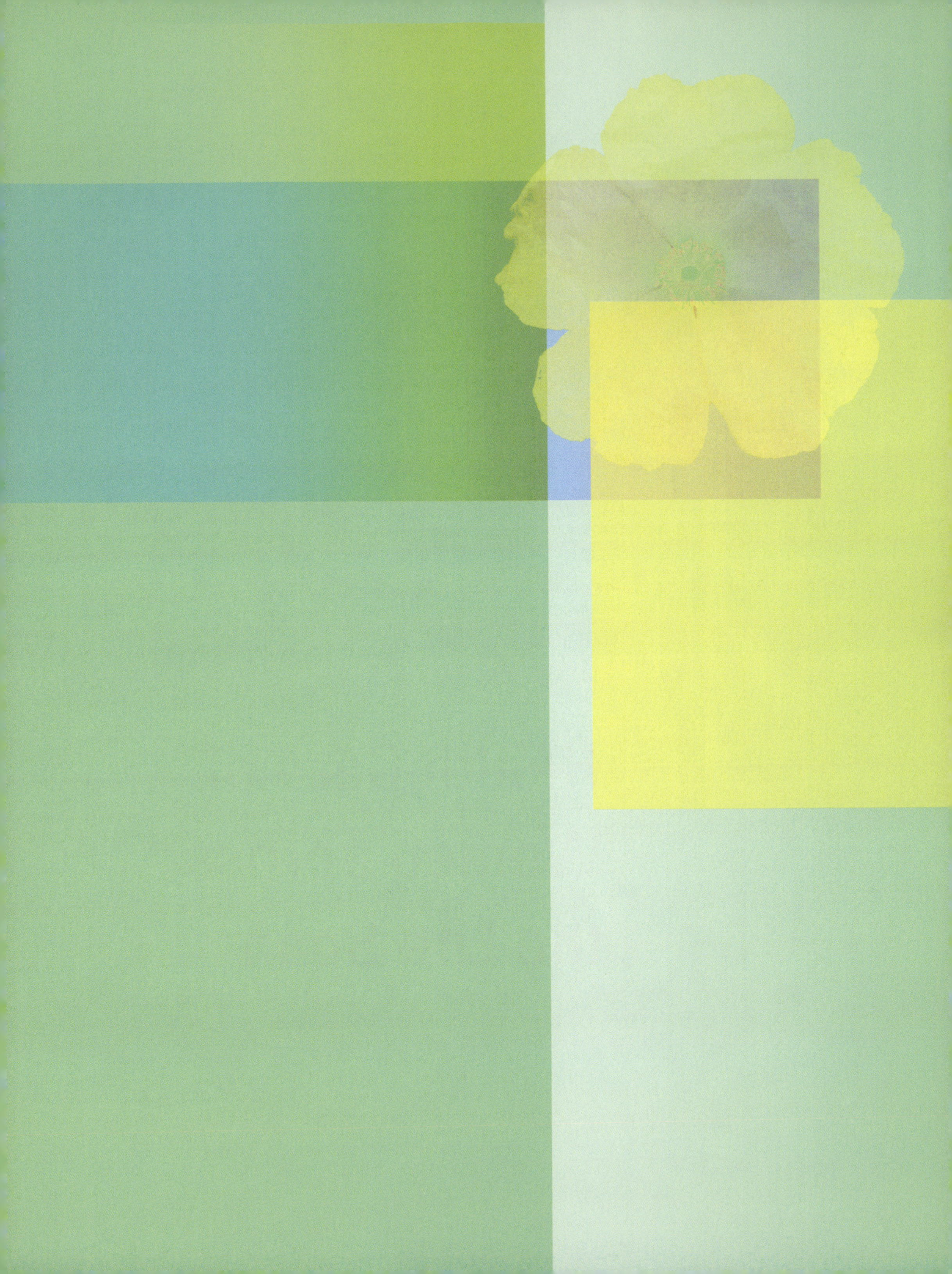

CHAPTER 5

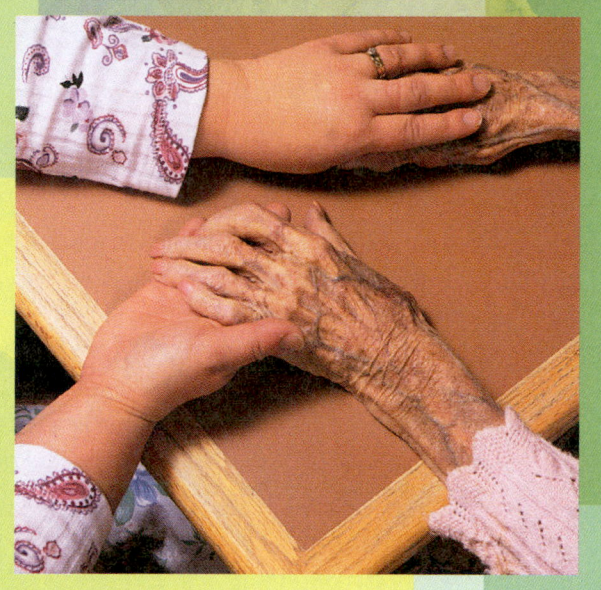

PROMOTING WOMEN'S HEALTH

Women have unique health needs across the life span. Physiologic differences between men and women are present before birth and continue throughout life. Psychosocial and cultural contexts differ for men and women as well. One important role for nurses is to promote women's health in any health care setting. Nurses can best fulfill this role by being aware of the developmental issues and nutritional needs of women as well as any concerns specific to women. Women are most frequently the victims of violence and assault. Nurses have opportunities to support women's self-care efforts in health promotion over the life span. The following questions are designed to help nurses clarify their personal feelings and increase their awareness of these health-related issues for women.

- How do women develop differently from men?
- What social behaviors are expected of women that are different from those of men?
- What can a woman do to promote her health at different points in her development?
- What can younger women do to promote healthy aging?
- How do nutritional needs change for women of different ages?
- How does a family make common meals that meet the nutritional needs of all members?
- What are my feelings about women who repeatedly are abused by a partner?
- What are my feelings about men who abuse women?

Key Terms

Acquaintance rape
Adolescence
Anencephaly
Anorexia nervosa
Anovulatory cycle
Assault
Basal metabolism
Binge eating
Body mass index (BMI)
Bulimia nervosa
Calorie
Corpus luteum
Daily Reference Values
    (DRVs)
Date rape
Dietary Guidelines for
    Americans
Encephalocele
Femicide
Food Guide Pyramid
Gonadotropin-releasing
    hormone (Gn-RH)
Heme iron
Hypochromic anemia
Hypothalamic-pituitary-
    ovarian axis
Insoluble fiber

Menarche
Menopause
Microcytic anemia
Nonheme iron
Nutrition Facts Food
    Label
Obesity
Osteoporosis
Ovulation
Perimenopause
Perpetrator
Pseudomenstruation
Puberty
Rape
Recommended Dietary
    Allowances (RDA)
Reference Daily Intakes
    (RDIs)
Soluble fiber
Spina bifida
Stranger rape
Stress incontinence
Tanner Stages
Thelarche
Wife rape

Competencies

Upon completion of this chapter, the reader should be able to:

1. Determine physiologic development using the Tanner Stages.
2. Describe the three phases of the menstrual cycle.
3. Discuss the physiologic changes of the peri- and postmenopausal stages.
4. Discuss self-care methods across the life span.
5. Describe the common nutritional guidelines used to advise normal, healthy women on recommended eating practices to provide optimum nutrition.
6. Identify key nutrients of importance in a woman's dietary intake pattern.
7. Classify a woman's body size based on her BMI.
8. Identify factors that may support a system in which abuse occurs.
9. Identify risk factors for abuse or neglect.
10. Describe the legal responsibilities of the nurse involved with mandatory reporting and documentation of abuse.

Thisisection focuses on health care of women across the life span. Included in this chapter are concepts related to female physical and psychosocial development, issues in female nutrition, and issues related to violence against women.

WOMEN'S DEVELOPMENT ACROSS THE LIFE SPAN

As women age, their health care choices may be influenced by many factors. Resources may be limited by fixed incomes, chronic illness, and loss of family and life partners. There are more women in the U.S. population than there are men, and a woman's life expectancy is 79 years compared with 72 years for men (Commonwealth Fund, 1997). As a result, additional health resources are used by women. By understanding the physiologic and psychosocial needs of women who are aging, nurses can better direct clients to the most appropriate resources available.

The discussion begins with the cellular changes that differentiate the female from the male reproductive system and continues to the hormonal effects at birth. The female adolescent's physical, emotional, and cultural development are examined. The discussion proceeds to the young adult, the woman during midlife, and the mature woman. Included are specific self-care and cultural cues to assist the nurse in providing culturally appropriate health care to women throughout their lives.

Prenatal through Early Adolescent Years

Initial differentiation between genders begins at fertilization at the time in which the genetic sex is determined by chromosomes XX (female) or XY (male). After the female genetic sex is determined, development of the reproductive system occurs in three phases: ovarian development, duct development, and the development of the external genitalia. By 10 weeks' gestation, the ovaries can be identified. By approximately 16 weeks' gestation, the cells that will later make up the ovarian follicles can be identified (Blackburn & Loper, 2003).

The development of the external genitalia is complete before that of the internal reproductive organs. Differentiation of male from female external genitalia occurs in the absence of androgens. The clitoris develops. The urethra and vaginal orifice open into the vestibule. The labia majora and labia minora develop from the surrounding connective tissue. The development of the external genitalia is complete at approximately 12 weeks' gestation (Blackburn & Loper, 2003).

During the newborn assessment shortly after birth, both female and male infants may exhibit signs of circulating maternal estrogens. The newborn's breasts may seem slightly swollen and enlarged, with nipple size ranging from 1.0 to 1.5 cm. The swelling will resolve in time and rarely lasts beyond the first month of life. Assessing the development of the newborn's breast tissue also aids in determining gestation.

Not only is the breast tissue affected by maternal hormones, the female genitalia of the newborn also are affected by maternal estrogens. The labia minora and labia majora appear engorged, and the labia minora may be more prominent than is the labia majora. A pinkish-white mucoid vaginal discharge also may be noted in the diaper. This is termed **pseudomenstruation** and is a sign of maternal transfer of estrogen. On resolution of the maternal hormonal effects, the childhood hormonal values are maintained at a static level until just before the onset of puberty.

Adolescence

Adolescence can be defined as the passage from childhood to maturity. Adolescence begins with the appearance of secondary sex characteristics and ends with cessation of growth and lasts from approximately ages 11 to 18 years. **Puberty** is the onset of the process of physical maturity. At puberty the secondary sex characteristics begin to develop and the capability of sexual reproduction is attained. The events leading to puberty occur in a timed sequence that is initiated with the secretion of the gonadal hormones and the development of the secondary sexual characteristics (Stedman, 2000). As girls move through

adolescence, they become concerned with appearance, beauty, and their changing bodies. As adolescent females begin to mature physically, they look to their peers for recognition and validation. They begin to make choices based on the interaction of the social group and peer relationships rather than on family recommendations. Emotional maturity is related to life experiences and the ability to make appropriate life choices and therefore often occurs many years after physical maturity. The cultural influences of the family and peer group in turn influence the life choices of the adolescent.

The age of pubertal growth ranges from 8 to 14 years. Any visible sign of pubertal development before age 8 years in girls is considered precocious and needs further medical investigation (Thiedke & Rosenfeld, 2001). The age of puberty may be determined by health status, genetics, and nutrition. Theories suggest that a minimum body weight of 48 kg and a minimum percent of body fat, 17%, are necessary for **menarche**, the onset of menstruation, to occur (Speroff, Glass, & Kase, 1999).

Physiologic Changes

The onset of puberty and menarche occur as a physiologic response to hormonal pulses associated during the sleep cycle. The pulses are cues of the **hypothalamic-pituitary-ovarian axis**, which is the transport mechanism of a hormone from the hypothalamus that stimulates the release of gonadotropins that, in turn, stimulates the ovaries to release estrogen and progesterone. The pulses begin between the ages of 6 and 8 years with the nighttime release of **gonadotropin-releasing hormone (Gn-RH)** from the hypothalamus. Gn-RH flows to the anterior pituitary gland, causing the release of the gonadotropins, or luteinizing hormone (LH) and follicle-stimulating hormone (FSH). LH and FSH stimulate the ovary to release estrogens, progestins, and androgens. Early hormonal stimulation precipitates the developing changes in the female reproductive organs: the breasts, labia, vagina, and uterus. Changes in the reproductive organs typically occur 2 years before the onset of menstruation (Blackburn & Loper, 2003). Hormonal stimulation also leads to rapid growth of the axial skeleton, resulting in the so-called growth spurt frequently experienced before the onset of menses.

External Development

The **Tanner Stages** are the five stages of female and male physical development outlined by Tanner (1981) and recognized today as the standard in adolescent physical development (Tables 5-1 and 5-2). Stage 1 is the state of preadolescence, in which there are no signs of physical maturity. Stage 5 represents full maturity of the breast and pubic hair development. The initial visible sign of puberty in the female is **thelarche**, or the prominence of glandular tissue in the breast behind the nipple, also called the

Table 5-1	Sexual Maturity Rating for Female Breast Development
DEVELOPMENTAL STAGE	**DESCRIPTION**
	1. Preadolescent stage (before age 10) Nipple is small, slightly raised.
	2. Breast bud stage (after age 10) Nipple and breast form a small mound. Areola enlarges. Height spurt begins.
	3. Adolescent stage (10–14 years) Nipple is flush with breast shape. Breast and areola enlarge. Menses begins. Height spurt peaks.
	4. Late adolescent stage (14–17 years) Nipple and areola form a secondary mound over the breast. Height spurt ends.
	5. Adult stage. Nipple protrudes; areola is flush with the breast shape

Table 5-2	Sexual Maturity Rating for Female Genitalia
DEVELOPMENTAL STAGE	**DESCRIPTION**
Stage 1 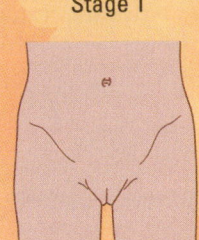	No pubic hair, only body hair (vellus hair)
Stage 2 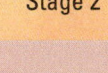	Sparse growth of long, slightly dark, fine pubic hair, slightly curly and located along the labia (ages 11 to 12)
Stage 3 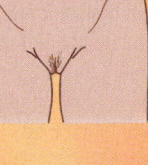	Pubic hair becomes darker, curlier, and spreads over the symphysis (ages 12 to 13)
Stage 4 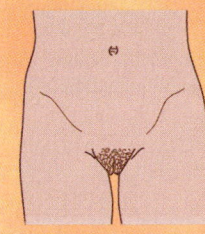	Texture and curl of pubic hair is similar to that of an adult but not spread to thighs (ages 13 to 15)
Stage 5 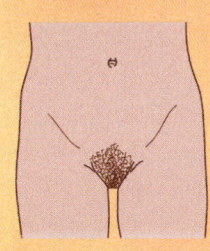 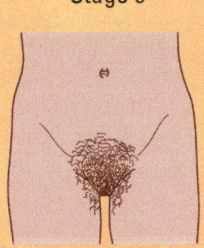	Adult appearance in quality and quantity of pubic hair; growth is spread to inner aspect of thighs and abdomen

breast bud. Simultaneously, or shortly thereafter, the first sign of pubic hair development is noted sparsely on the labia majora and mons pubis. This is indicative of Tanner Stage 2. Stage 3 reveals further enlargement of the breast mound (the areola and breast as one unit). A slight darkening of the areola pigment may be noted. Sparse, dark, curly hair is noted over the mons pubis. In Stage 4, separation of the areola-nipple unit above the breast occurs. The pubic hair appears adultlike but is limited to the mons pubis and labia. The final stage, Stage 5, reveals further nipple-areola development, with increased pigmentation and the enhancement of Montgomery's tubercles and ducts on the areola. The pubic hair is adultlike, with

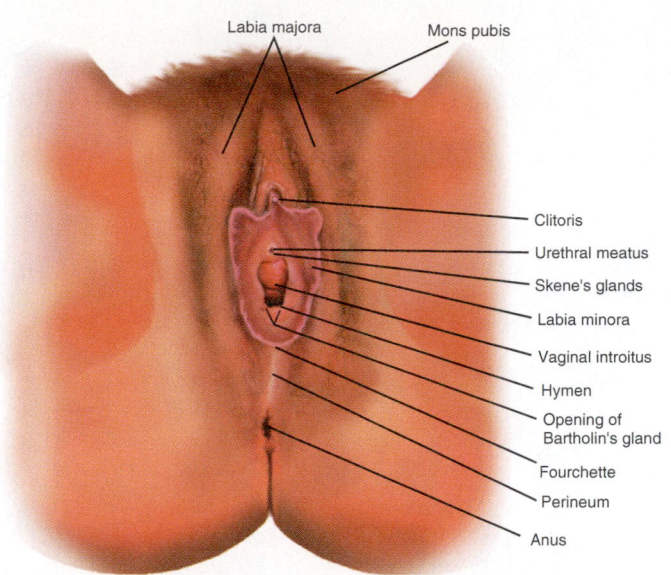

Figure 5-1 External structures of the female genitalia.

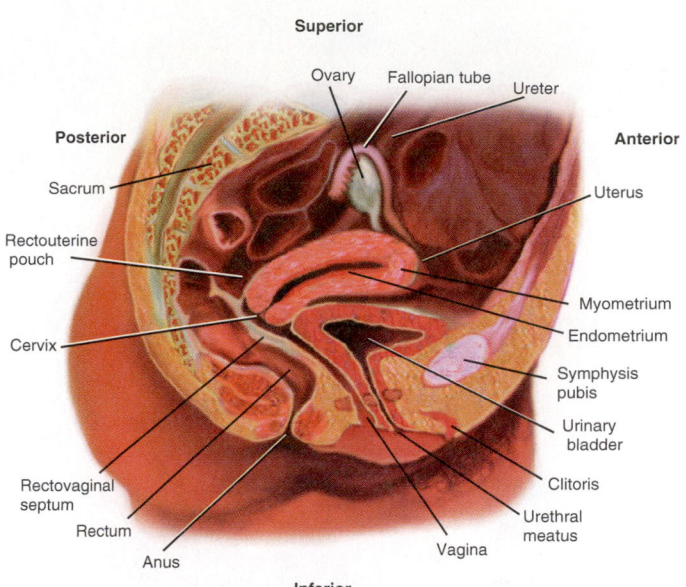

Figure 5-2 Female internal pelvic organs.

extension to the inner thighs. By Tanner Stage 5, the labia majora increases to twice the size of the labia minora. The vaginal orifice becomes more prominent, and the urethral orifice becomes less prominent (Blackburn & Loper, 2003). The external structures of the female genitalia are shown in Figure 5-1. The Tanner Stages are of great assistance in educating adolescents about the chronologic stages of their physical development.

Internal Development

As the external physiologic characteristics change, the internal structures of the female organs also develop. The vagina lengthens and increases in size. The pH of the vaginal secretions decreases to an acidic pH (pH of 5), and the amount of the vaginal secretions increases. The acidic pH and increase in secretions support conception. The uterus also increases in size and length to prepare for fertility. The ovaries increase in size but at a slower rate than does the uterus. The internal structures of the female pelvis are illustrated in Figure 5-2.

As estrogen is released, the ovary develops a complex vasculature network in preparation for ovulation. Once the vascular compartments are fully developed, and a sufficient amount of estrogen is released, the estrogen stimulates the anterior pituitary to release LH that, in turn, causes ovulation to occur.

Breast Development

Breast development is the first visible sign of puberty. The breast is made up of 15 to 20 lobes of glandular tissue supported by fibrous connective and adipose tissues. Within each lobe of glandular tissue there are 20 to 40 lobules lined with epithelial cells called acini cells, which

produce milk in lactating women. The lobules are connected by lactiferous ducts that empty into a lactiferous sinus near the nipple. Montgomery's tubercles are located on the lateral edges of the areola and provide natural secretions for the lactating breast. The fibrous tissue provides support to the glandular tissue of the breasts, as do the suspensory ligaments known as Cooper's suspensory ligaments. Figure 5-3 depicts the internal anatomic structures of the breast. Usually the breasts develop simultaneously; however, the breasts may develop in an asynchronous manner, with one breast developing faster than the other. As the breasts develop to Tanner Stage 5, it is not unusual for a woman to have one breast that is slightly larger in caliber than the other.

Menarche

Menarche is the beginning of the menstrual function, or the onset of the first menstrual period as a result of the hypothalamic-pituitary-ovarian axis. The mean age of menarche is approximately 12 years. The age range varies from 9 to 17 years (Speroff, Glass, & Case, 1999). Menarche may be delayed in adolescents who are lean. Conversely, girls who are obese, that is, whose body weight is 20% to 30% more than their ideal weight may begin menses early (Williams, Larsen, Kronenberg, Melmed, & Polonsky, 2003). Initially, menstruation is irregular and sporadic. The duration of the menstrual cycle ranges from 21 to 45 days, with an average of 28 days. The bleeding may vary from very light to very heavy and last from 2 to 7 days. Menstrual bleeding that lasts longer that 10 days is considered abnormal or dysfunctional. Anovulatory cycles account for 90% to 95% of all dysfunctional bleeding that occurs. An **anovulatory cycle** is a menstrual cycle that

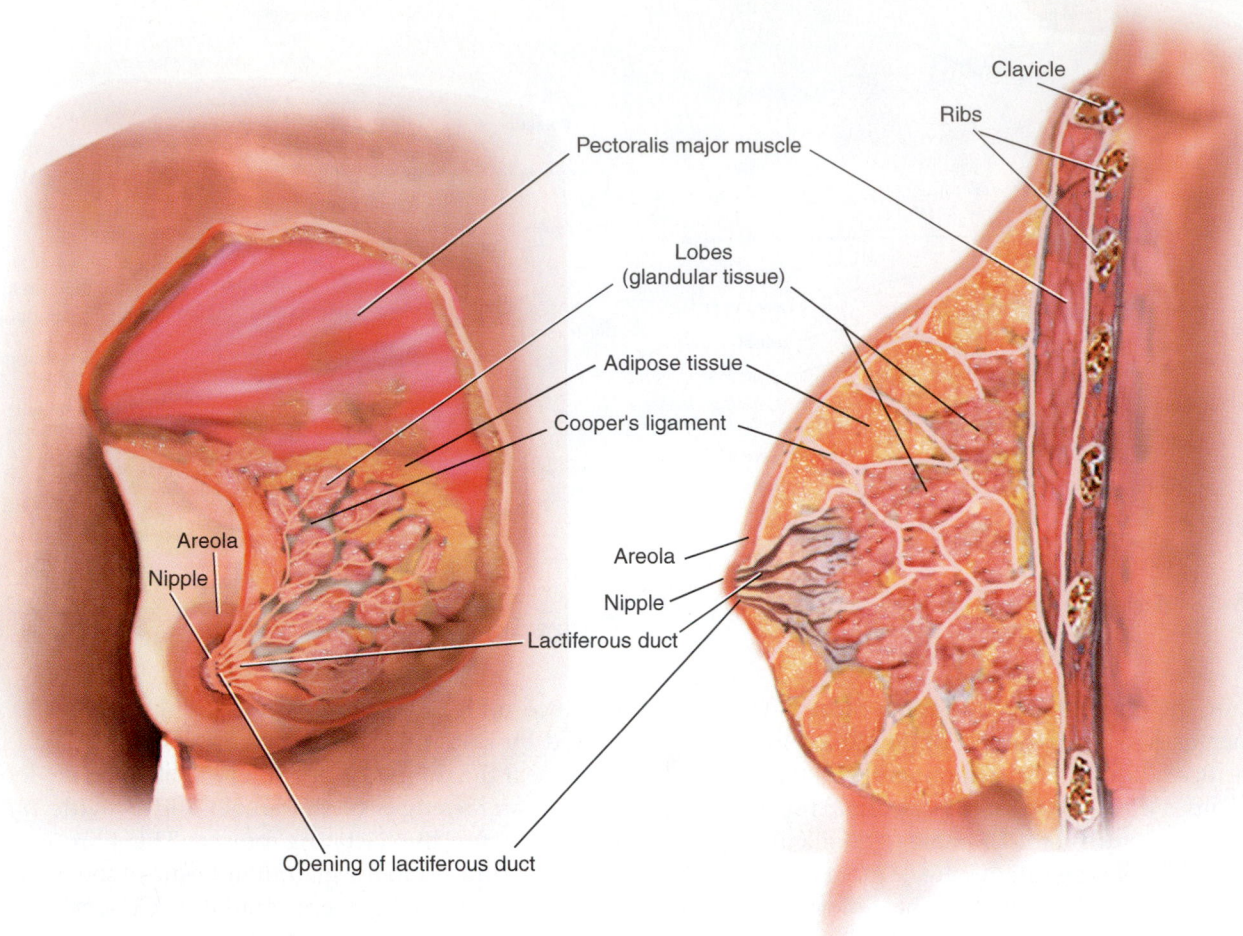

Figure 5-3   Anatomical structures of the female breast.

occurs in the absence of ovulation. An adolescent may have anovulatory cycles for the first several years of menstruation. The cause of anovulatory cycles in the adolescent usually is an immature hypothalamic-pituitary-ovarian axis; however, in some cases, a pathological cause may be established (Dealy, 1998).

The Menstrual Cycle

There are three phases of the menstrual cycle. The phases occur as a result of the effects of hormonal influence on the ovaries and uterus (Figure 5-4). As menarche approaches, the Gn-RH pulses increase in frequency and intensity. The first day of the menstrual bleeding is considered day 1 of the cycle and is considered the menstrual phase, or phase one. At this time, levels of estrogen, progestin, LH, and FSH are relatively low. Gn-RH continues to stimulate the anterior pituitary to release FSH, which acts as a stimulus on the ovary to release estrogen in preparation for the developing follicles and provides thickening of the uterine lining.

By day 5 to 7, a single follicle has assumed dominance (Hatcher et al., 2000). This is phase two, also termed the proliferative-follicular phase. Estrogen levels in the blood begin to increase, sending a message to the anterior pituitary gland to decrease the circulating levels of FSH. As the woman approaches day 14, or midcycle, the continued increase in estrogen stimulates the release of LH from the anterior pituitary. The LH surge is responsible for **ovulation**, or the release of the dominant follicle in preparation for conception, which occurs within the next 10 to 12 hours after the levels of LH have peaked.

Phase three, or the secretory-luteal phase, begins after ovulation. Once the dominant follicle is released the remnant cyst of the follicle releases estrogens, progesterone, and androgens. The remnant cyst of the dominant follicle left behind in the ovary is termed the **corpus luteum**. The corpus luteum is a yellow mass in the ovary formed by an ovarian follicle that has matured and discharged its ovum. The estrogen levels begin to decrease after the surge in LH, and progesterone levels begin to increase. There is a second increase in estrogen levels that coincides with the release of progesterone from the corpus luteum. The endometrial lining changes in substance to provide a glycogen-rich environment to foster implantation. FSH and LH levels decrease as a result of the increasing estrogen and progesterone levels. If implantation, fertilization,

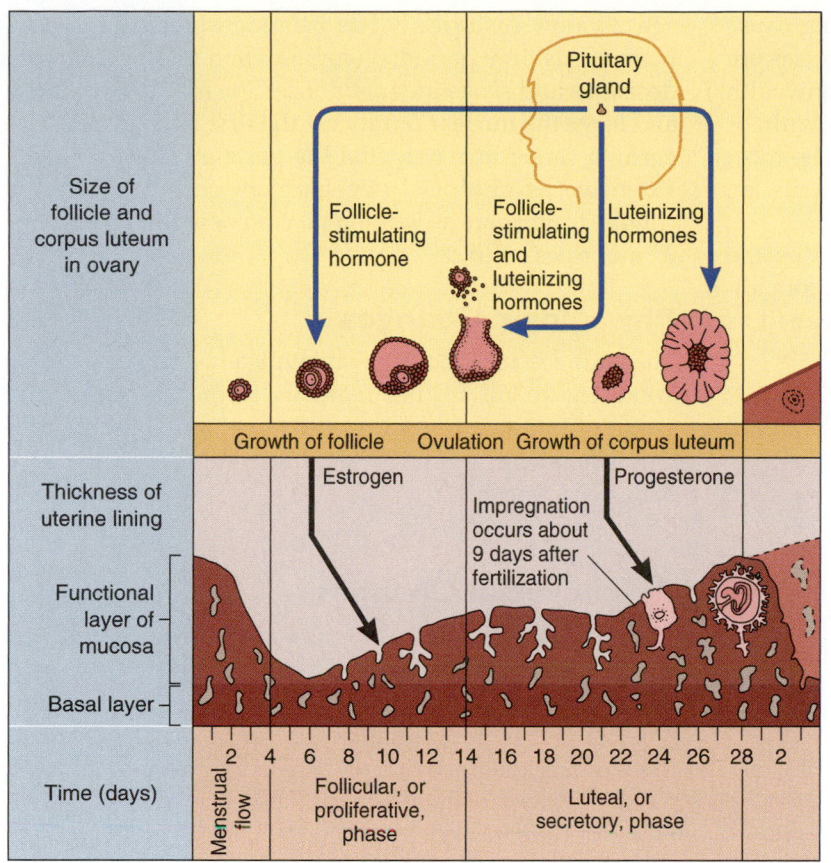

Size of follicle and corpus luteum in ovary	
Thickness of uterine lining	
Functional layer of mucosa	
Basal layer	
Time (days)	

Figure 5-4   Events of the menstrual cycle.

or pregnancy does not occur, the corpus luteum regresses and the estrogen and progesterone levels decrease, which results in menstruation, returning to day 1 of the cycle (Hatcher et al., 2000). If pregnancy (implantation) occurs, the corpus luteum continues to produce estrogen and progesterone, thus prohibiting menstruation.

Psychosocial Changes

A young woman approaches normal physical development over a span of years. Her emotional development also occurs as a lengthy process. Changes in body image, function, the onset of menses, and relationships play a role in the perception of what is normal in her eyes. Girls are socialized in the context of their environment and relationships. Erikson (1950) identified the adolescent developmental task as "identity versus role confusion" in his developmental theory. This developmental phase supports the premise that emotional maturity is based on separation and independence, meaning that the adolescent must detach herself from current relationships to be able to grow and develop a new, productive adult identity.

Peer acceptance is extremely important. Behaviors related to dress, activities, and habits follow individual peer norms. Weight is also a factor in development of self-concept. An average weight is valued most by teens. Second is thinness, and least valued is being overweight

(Fogel & Woods, 1995). As the peer group becomes more powerful, girls emphasize their own self-worth in the context of their relationships, further enhancing self-esteem.

Cultural Influences

The adolescent's sense of self also is dependent on the cultural context in which she lives. Based on data from the Centers for Disease Control and Prevention (as cited in Rosenfeld et al., 1997), adolescent girls' self-esteem varied based on ethnicity. Black girls cited higher levels of self-esteem than did Hispanic or Caucasian girls. Hispanic girls had the greatest decrease in self-esteem and were most likely to report emotional distress. The decrease in self-esteem may be due to discrimination; inadequacy of the education received; and the influence of additional factors, such as poverty and gang involvement.

Self-Care Considerations

The opportunity to provide self-care knowledge to adolescents is tremendous. Through anticipatory guidance and trusting relationships, health information and education can be provided to the adolescent. Because adolescents generally are healthy, the focus should be on primary and secondary preventive practices. Primary preventive practices target those diseases and maladies that can be prevented. Primary prevention consists of practices such as wearing seat belts, receiving immunizations, and following instructions for safe sex. Secondary prevention includes screening for diseases, breast self-examination, and Pap smear screening.

As the adolescent matures psychologically, she will begin making independent choices and pursue a degree of autonomy establishing her identity. Risk-taking behavior is most prevalent during adolescence, as teens may be unable to utilize abstract thinking and view themselves as immune to danger. Some degree of risk taking during adolescence signifies autonomy and independence. Serious forms of risk taking, however, can lead to disaster.

Critical Thinking

Teenage Sexual Behavior

Nearly half of all teenaged girls admit to being sexually active. Many teens have anal or oral sex so they won't get pregnant. How accurate do you think these figures are? Given this high percentage, should adolescents have access to contraception without parental consent?

Accidental and unintentional injury is the leading cause of death in adolescents. The second and third causes are homicide and suicide, respectively (Commonwealth Fund, 1997). Risk-taking behavior may occur with or without knowledge of the potential aftermath. The most serious forms of risk-taking behavior in adolescents are substance abuse and sexual activity.

Adolescents report binge drinking as early as the eighth grade (14%), with 23% of high-school seniors admitting to binge drinking. Binge drinking is defined as four to five or more drinks once in a 2-week period of time (Commonwealth Fund, 1997). Alcohol use in adolescents also is related to poor academic performance, early sexual activity, and troubled social environments (Rosenfeld et al., 1997). Cigarette smoking is on the rise in young women compared with young men. One in four women admit to smoking. This year, more women will be smoking than men (Centers for Disease Control and Prevention [CDC], 1995). Teens underestimate the power of nicotine addiction and find quitting difficult. In providing anticipatory guidance to adolescents, nurses should focus on the benefits of abstaining from tobacco products such as fresh breath, whiter teeth, and increased exercise and performance ability (Wallis, Kasper, Reader, & Brown, 1998).

Engaging in early sexual activity is another form of risk-taking behavior in adolescents. In young women, early sexual activity can lead to pregnancy, sexually transmitted diseases, and pelvic inflammatory disease. Nearly 50% of all high-school students report engaging in sexual activity, which is a decrease from 70% in 1995 (CDC, 1999). On average, 48% of high-school girls admit to "ever having" sexual intercourse and 52% of high-school boys admit to "ever having" sexual intercourse (CDC, 1999). Although the rate at which U.S. teenagers engage in sexual intercourse is on the decline, as is teen pregnancy, the United States continues to have the highest teen pregnancy rates of the developed nations. Teen pregnancy continues to be a major health care issue for adolescents.

Adolescence is a time of discovery. In finding a sense of self, the young woman also will find a sense of responsibility. With the support of their environment, adolescents prepare for a productive adulthood through positive choices, accepting responsibility, and ultimately psychological maturity through their relationships. If they are unable to achieve their identity, adolescents will have difficulty making decisions and playing a productive role in society.

Young Adulthood to Perimenopausal Years

This period spans roughly the years between 15 and 44, although the childbearing years are typically considered to be from ages 18 to 39 years. Pregnancy outside of this age window historically has been considered high risk. During this time period, a woman often makes major life decisions and seeks independence. She may go to college and leave the nuclear family for the first time. Choices regarding career and potential life partners also are made. Extensive psychosocial development occurs during the childbearing years as women take on new roles and leave former roles behind.

Physiologic Changes

The young adulthood years are typically characterized by good health and further maturity of the body. Nursing care and interventions are geared toward promoting optional health through healthy diet, exercise, and good habits. The specific physiologic changes of pregnancy are outlined in detail in Chapter 10.

Psychosocial Changes

The psychosocial changes that occur during pregnancy should be considered from the point of view that pregnancy is a cycle of change in women's lives. Even as partners plan for their pregnancies, ambivalence is present as the woman imagines the new challenges as a mother. As women anticipate their labor and delivery, they ask themselves questions. "Will I be a good parent?" "Will I be able to provide an adequate home?" During the first trimester, a woman must adjust to being pregnant. Some of the physiologic and psychosocial effects of early pregnancy, include nausea, vomiting, and emotional lability.

In the second trimester of pregnancy, the expectant mother focuses on fetal growth and her altered body image. In the third trimester, the pregnant woman often focuses on preparation for the delivery. She may begin to prepare space in the home for the infant. She may also

---

Reflections from Families

I knew that I wanted to be pregnant, but at times I had overwhelming anxiety and fear of the unknown. It was the right time in our lives to have a baby. I thought we were prepared, but I wasn't sure. Initially, I was nauseated and felt bad all of the time. I thought it was some kind of sign that the pregnancy was in trouble. My health care provider explained to me that what I was going through both physically and emotionally was normal. I never realized that pregnancy could be such a time of great joy and anxiety at the same time.

begin to focus on the event of labor and delivery. When her due date approaches, she becomes eager for birth to occur yet may be apprehensive about labor and delivery.

Throughout the pregnancy, during the birth process, and immediately postpartum, the mother will further develop the capacity to give and care for her infant. The pregnant woman may feel more comfortable asking questions of the nurse. It is important to assess for any emotional discomfort or anxiety that the woman or her partner may be feeling. Development of a birth plan may provide a feeling of control and decision making for the client.

Cultural Influences

The cultural patterns and behaviors the woman had assimilated during earlier years will continue in this period. She may prefer to spend time with friends who share her cultural practices or may seek out those with different ideas as a means of expanding her own viewpoint. In providing care for clients in the childbearing years, nurses have the opportunity to provide support when they understand clients in the context of their own cultures.

Self-Care Considerations

Self-care considerations for women in young adulthood center on achieving and maintaining health. Good health is promoted through practices such as a healthy diet, stress management, exercise, reduced caffeine and alcohol intake, monthly breast self-examination, and yearly Pap tests.

Perimenopausal to Mature Years

The middle years, generally considered to be from 45 to 64 years, may be the most challenging and productive years of a woman's life. She may have completed her childbearing and is now focusing on a career, or she may have initially focused on her career and is now considering childbearing. If her children are young, their demands on her time may need to be balanced with the demands of her career. Her parents may be aging and may require more care and assistance. The woman's physiologic and hormonal changes demand attention. Some women may no longer feel the need to regularly see a care provider. Women may struggle with self-image and physical appearance related to aging. This time also is one in which women are accessing health care for physical changes and perimenopausal symptoms. There is an abundance of health information available to women on the Internet and in other media sources. The nurse should assist and support women in their quest for valid knowledge.

Physiologic Changes

The physiologic and hormonal changes that occur during midlife are known as perimenopause. Perimenopause is the time before cessation of menses or menopause. A woman may be considered to be in perimenopause for 5 to 10 years, or until cessation of menses for 1 year. During this time period, the woman may have normal menses, spotting, or absence of a monthly menstrual cycle. A woman who has not had a menstrual period for 1 year is considered to be in menopause. As a woman approaches her 40s, she begins to have fewer ovulatory cycles. The ovary may only have several thousand follicles remaining at this time and may be less sensitive to gonadotropin stimulation (Speroff et al., 1999). In turn, the follicles, by way of the feedback system, produce less estrogen. The decrease in estrogen does not provide for maturation of the endometrial lining, and, therefore, menses may not occur. Eventually, estrogen production decreases sufficiently to affect estrogen-dependent tissues, such as the breasts, bone, mucous membranes, heart, neuroendocrine system, and reproductive organs.

The glandular tissue of the breasts atrophies with the loss of circulating estrogen. The glands and lobules are replaced with fat. The skin becomes less elastic, and the breasts become soft and pendulous.

Women lose calcium from bone as a normal process of aging. With the loss of estrogen during the peri- and postmenopause periods, the bone loss is dramatic. Decreased levels of calcium intake and high levels of physical activity that results in less than 10% body fat also contribute to bone loss before the midlife years. A woman may lose 1% of her bone density per year for 5 to 10 years after menopause. The bone loss may result in back pain and compression. Fractures also may occur with bone stress. When women lose bone, they are diagnosed with **osteoporosis**. Osteoporosis is bone loss owing to a decrease in calcium absorption or the loss of estrogen. Osteoporosis can be a devastating disease, leading to fractures, loss of independence, and potentially death (Society for Women's Health Research, 1999). It is important to continue to provide education to women about their risk for osteoporosis and to develop a plan for prevention (Figure 5-5). An osteoporosis prevention plan would include high calcium intake (approximately 1,000 mg for premenopausal women and 1,500 mg for postmenopausal women) and weight-bearing exercise 3 to 4 times a week. Hormone replacement therapy also may be an option for women experiencing menopause.

Heart disease is the leading cause of death in women and is responsible for more deaths than breast, ovarian, and uterine cancers combined (Society for Women's Health Research, 1999). As a woman approaches menopause, her risk for heart disease becomes equal to that of a man's. Additional risk factors for heart disease must be considered when providing nursing care to the woman in midlife.

Diminished estrogen levels are responsible for atrophy of the skin and mucous membranes of the mouth,

Nursing Alert

Risk Factors for Heart Disease

- Age over 60 years
- Obesity
- Cigarette smoking
- Hypertension
- Diabetes mellitus
- Sedentary lifestyle
- Family history

Note. From *2000 Heart and Stroke Statistical Update*, by the American Heart Association, 1999, Dallas, TX: Author.

urethra, vagina, and bladder. The skin becomes less elastic and taut. It may appear dry and loose, which may lead to increased wrinkling. There is also drying and thinning of the mucous membranes around the mouth and within the urogenital system.

The effects of estrogen loss on the urinary system can be quite disturbing for women. Decreasing circulating levels of estrogen cause a loss of elasticity of the urethra, resulting in frequency and urgency of urination. An overall loss of muscular support within the pelvis may add to the woman's urinary tract symptoms. Complaints of stress incontinence and urge incontinence may occur in this phase of life. Stress incontinence is the most common type of incontinence in women under 60 years of age.

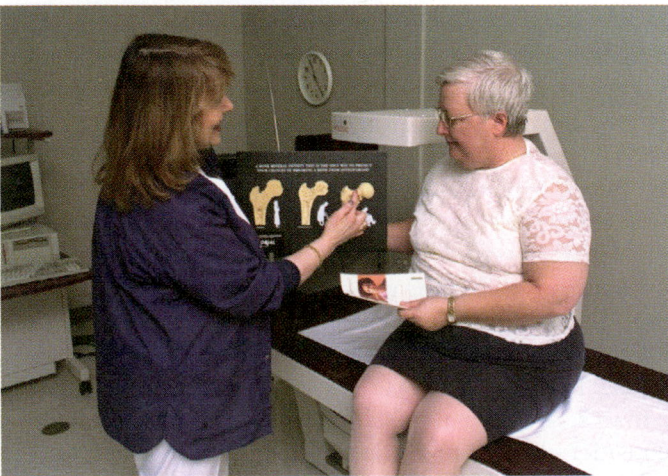

Figure 5-5   As women approach menopause, osteoporosis prevention education is critical in promoting optimal health.

Stress incontinence is an involuntary discharge of urine with a cough, sneeze, or laughter owing to the loss of muscular support at the neck of the urethra. Urge incontinence is less common than is stress incontinence. Although nonsurgical and surgical interventions are available, many women may be uncomfortable initiating a discussion about incontinence. The nurse-client relationship provides a non-threatening mechanism to bring that information forward through the educational process.

The reproductive organs also are affected by the loss of circulating estrogen. The vagina decreases in depth and the uterus decreases in size. The ovaries shrink. The vaginal skin thins, and the rugae diminish. There is an increase in vaginal pH from an acidic state to a neutral or alkaline state. Sexual intercourse may be uncomfortable, and trauma may occur as a result of thinning vaginal epithelium. Water-soluble lubricants may provide comfort during sexual intercourse.

Changing estrogen levels also result in vasomotor instability, causing hot flashes or flushing. Sympathetic activity increases, resulting in a rapid heart rate. Skin temperature also increases, resulting in a flash or sensation of warmth. Night sweats may occur, and nighttime wakening as a result of night sweats may cause sleep deprivation. Hot flashes and sleep disturbance are the most common symptoms of menopause.

Until recently, hormonal replacement therapy (HRT) estrogen with progestin, was recommended for menopausal women who had not had a hysterectomy. This recommendation was based on earlier research findings that associated less cardiovascular problems and reduction of unpleasant menopausal symptoms with use of HRT. In July 2002, the Women's Health Initiative, a large multisite, controlled clinical trial, terminated the Prempro (progestin plus estrogen) arm of the study owing to an increase in the global risk index (Writing Group for the Women's Health Initiative Investigators, 2002). The primary risks related to breast cancer and cardiovascular problems. Current recommendations are for more individualized decisions based on a careful assessment of risks and benefits. Prempro is not recommended as a preventive measure for cardiovascular health and should be used in low dosages for only short periods of time for symptom relief. The estrogen-only arm of the study for women without a uterus is still continuing at the time of this writing.

Psychosocial Changes

Women's perceptions of the midlife period have changed over the past 20 years. In the past, many women identified their sense of self with the child rearing or spousal role. More recent studies have revealed an understanding of stressful life events, such as physical changes, physical limitations, empty nest concerns, and changes in interpersonal relationships; however, the women are positive

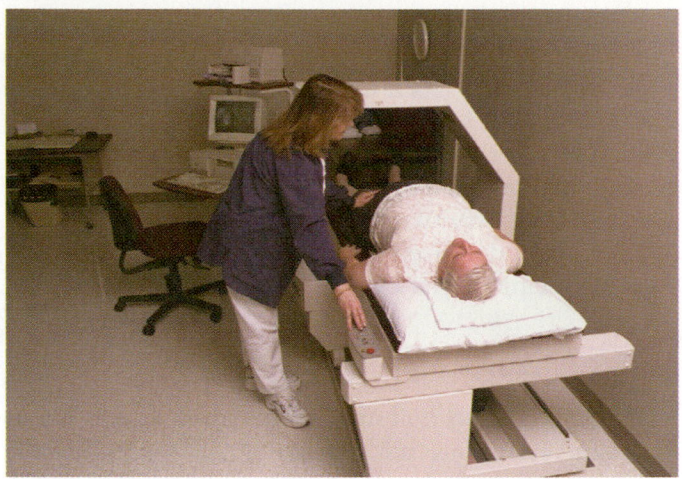

A.

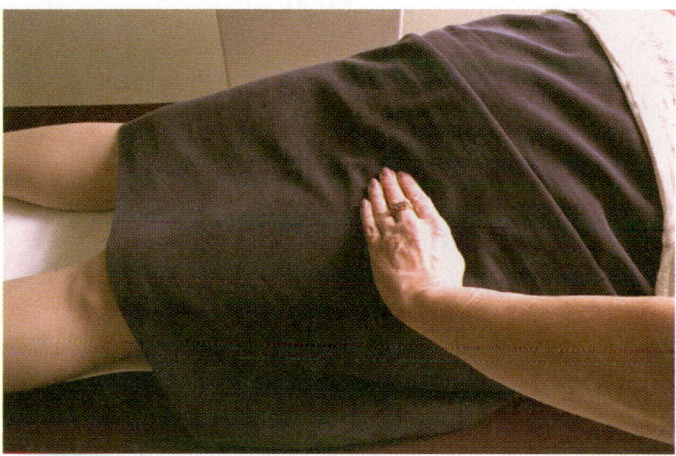

B.

Critical Thinking

Menopause

A 45-year-old woman is beginning to notice changes in her menstrual cycle. Her cycles are increasingly longer (approximately 45 days), with a shortening duration. She is concerned about how these changes may affect her lifestyle and her health. Some of her friends at work have told her that they felt their health was negatively impacted when they went through menopause. As the nurse involved with this client's primary care:

- How would you initiate anticipatory guidance?
- In what key areas would you provide health education?
- How would you address the "concerns of friends?"

in their overall outlook (Woods & Mitchell, 1997). Women's psychosocial issues related to midlife are attributed to managing the busy demands of daily life (Woods & Mitchell, 1997).

Cultural Influences

Cultural perceptions of midlife are not clearly understood. Women's lifestyles and social interactions influence health. In some cultures, as a woman ages her social status may increase and she may be valued as a life expert. In other cultures, a woman's social status may decrease and she may be devalued. As her ability to reproduce declines nurses must be sensitive to woman's roles in different cultural groups.

Self-Care Considerations

Nurses are ideal candidates to educate clients regarding the self-care measures that can be taken during midlife. As physiologic symptoms begin to occur, the nurse may have the first contact with the client. Clients experiencing hot flashes should be educated on symptom management.

In an effort to maintain bone density, all clients should be advised to perform weight-bearing exercises and maintain a calcium intake of 1,000 mg/d of elemental calcium. Bone density testing may be advised to determine a baseline bone density, as well as to determine the client's risk for fracture (Figure 5-6).

Be advised that women may have difficulty in expressing sexual difficulties. Because nurses are excellent counselors and educators and because communication is a core component of nursing curriculum, nurses should develop communication strategies in working with women at midlife.

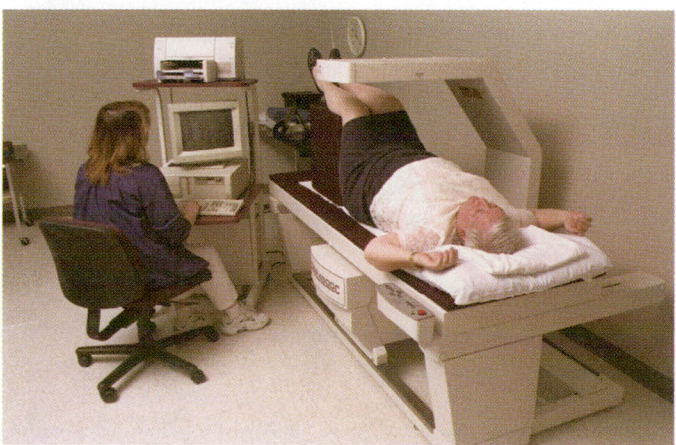

C.

Figure 5-6   A bone density scan should be done to determine a baseline as well as to determine a client's fracture risk. A. Positioning the client. B. Aligning the scanner. C. Reading the results.

Women should also be reminded to perform monthly breast self-examinations and have annual mammograms after the age of 50. As a woman ages, her risk for breast cancer increases, with the majority of breast cancers being diagnosed after age 50 (American Cancer Society, 1999). Educational information regarding hormone replacement therapy or alternatives should be provided at this time. Women should feel comfortable and confident in performing their own self-examinations.

Mature Years

The perceptions of mature women (aged 65 and older) regarding health are not determined by the number of chronic illnesses they might have but by how the women feel. Perry and Woods (1995) asked a group of women ranging in age from 70 to 91 years. "What does being healthy mean to you?" The research of these authors led them to write the following quote about health and women of advanced age: "Health involves the appreciation of life, experiencing joy and happiness. To be free from sickness does not guarantee health. Likewise, health can be experienced despite chronic illness and disability, because being healthy is a philosophy or way of living" (p. 55).

Physiologic Changes

Physiologic concerns of the aging woman are multifocal and affect all body systems (Figure 5-7). Some changes in the integumentary system, for example, wrinkles, spots on the skin, and graying hair, may have a different social and psychological effect on women than on men related to the expectations and values that our culture has placed on youth and beauty in women.

As estrogen declines, further changes in the reproductive organs occur. The ovaries and uterus decrease in size. The vagina shortens and secretions decrease and become more alkaline, which can increase the risk of atrophic vaginitis. The supportive musculature of the reproductive organs weakens, increasing risk of uterine prolapse. Breast tissue diminishes and breast cancer risk increases with age. Libido and need for intimacy remain unchanged, and positive relationships with others become even more important in avoiding loneliness and depression.

Psychosocial Changes

The physiologic processes that occur as a result of aging directly affect the psychological health and social interactions of women who are aging. The woman must make adjustments in her own life owing to changes in functional status; in many cases, the woman also must provide care for an aging partner. Considerations are made for retirement that may cause lifestyle changes for the woman living on a fixed income. The aging woman may choose to either identify with a social group or isolate herself. Independent living may not be an option for some women, yet alternatives may be unsatisfactory.

Depression is more common in women than in men. The lifetime risk for major depression in women is 20% to 25%; at any point in time, 5% to 10% of women are suffering from a depressive disorder (Speroff & Darney, 2001). Depression is related not only to physiology but to the

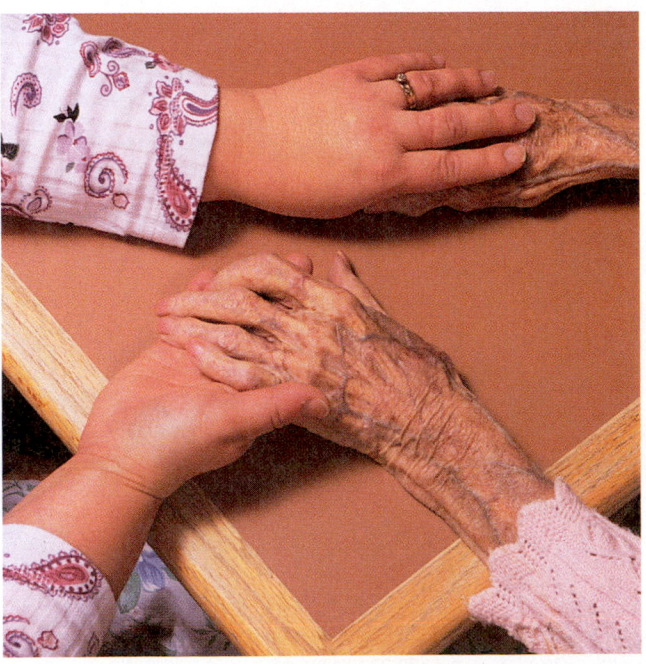
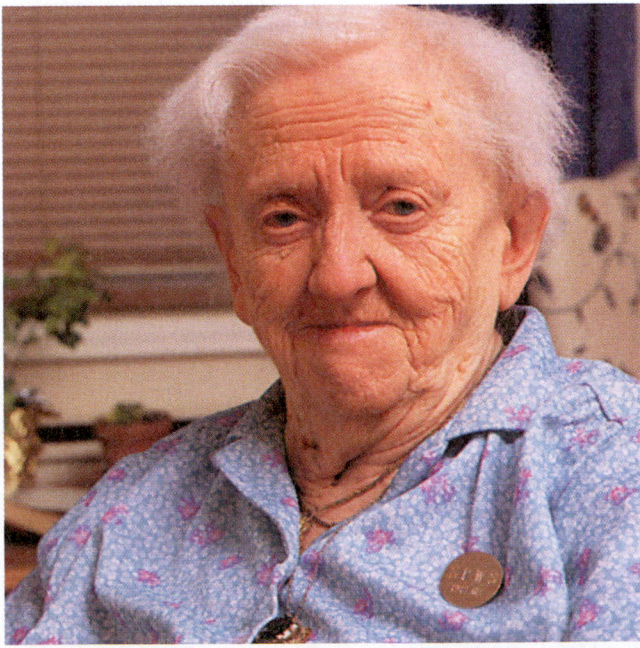

Figure 5-7   Changes in the skin and hair are some of the more visible effects of aging.

social and economic factors unique to women. Because of decreased physical abilities related to aging, social isolation, and economic problems, older women should be screened for depression.

Thiedke and Rosenfeld (2001) outlined some of the sociologic tasks of older women, including the following:

- Adjusting to declining physical strength and health
- Adjusting to retirement and its reduced income
- Adjusting to changes in the health of one's spouse
- Establishing an explicit affiliation with one's age group
- Adopting and adapting to social roles in a flexible way
- Establishing satisfactory physical living arrangements

Cultural Influences

Although aging in American society often has been devalued, in some cultures women gain social status after childbearing and as they age. In the case of women who are aging, instructions and health education must be delivered in a trusting, personal manner. When provided respectfully, the information is more likely to be valued and the advice followed. Health information and education relayed in a kind, caring, and respectful way can be successful in breaking down cultural barriers, and in encouraging trust in the care provider.

Self-Care Considerations

Safety is a major self-care focus for mature women. Nurses providing care for the aging population must become proficient in assessing functional and cognitive status. Initial assessments of the aging woman can be done from the waiting room as she walks to the exam room, noting gait, comfort, posture, and balance.

During the interview/health history for an office visit or admission to the hospital, a medication history should be taken. Because of the nature of many chronic illnesses, multiple medications may be prescribed. Self-care education should be provided in an easy to understand format using printed materials with a large font. The instructions must extend beyond prescription medication to include over-the-counter medications and herbal preparations as well. The client can be encouraged to use a single pharmacy with computerized records to reduce the risk of adverse drug interactions.

Nursing Implications

There are many gender-related issues in the development of women. These are physiologic, psychological, and social in nature. A number of health-related issues surround reproduction, and nurses should be sensitive to the multifaceted processes by which women become mothers. The hormonal changes in women from menarche through menopause have manifestations beyond the reproductive organs. Nurses are in a position to educate women about these developmental changes and to provide counseling and support. Many times women may be more comfortable discussing these issues with a nurse than with other health care providers. Nurses can apply their understanding about women's developmental issues to female clients in whatever arena they encounter clients. It does not need to be restricted to maternity care. Nurses can provide information and support about these issues for individual clients or to groups of clients. Many times nurses are asked to speak to community groups about women's issues. This is an excellent opportunity to give sound health information about women's development.

WOMEN'S NUTRITION ACROSS THE LIFE SPAN

Nutrition is a vital aspect of the health of women at all ages, and is particularly important during the childbearing years. Nutrition has also been identified as an area of lifestyle that can be modified to reduce risks for chronic diseases. Nurses have long been engaged in nutritional counseling interventions, and a good nutritional assessment and appropriate interventions should be a part of every nursing plan. Nurses who are providing care to women should be especially concerned about nutrition, because women generally procure and prepare food for the entire family. Nutrition during pregnancy has implications for both the mother and the fetus. The mother's nutrition before pregnancy is also important for the health of the fetus.

This section focuses on the nutritional concerns of women throughout their life cycle, with a major focus on needs during pregnancy. Emphasis is placed on the factors contributing to healthy lifestyles during the stages of a woman's life. Nutrients of special concern to women and nutritional needs during select times of a woman's life are highlighted. Prevention of major illnesses is the

---

Nursing Tip   *Health Care versus Family Care*

It is important to consider culture and familial influence when carrying out nursing interventions. Individuals are more likely to adhere to nursing care instructions and health education when their family members also are instructed and believe in the process.

focus. Finally, there is a brief discussion of the major nutritional concerns related to the primary causes of morbidity and mortality in women.

Nutritional Guidelines

Nutritional guidelines can come in different forms. The Dietary Guidelines for Americans, the Food Guide Pyramid, culturally adapted food guides, and Nutrition Facts food labeling will be discussed.

Dietary Guidelines

Dietary Guidelines for Americans was the first joint publication effort of the Department of Health and Human Services and the Department of Agriculture. They are mandated by public law to be revised every 5 years (USDA, 2000). *Dietary Guidelines for Americans* provides guidance on diet and health to the general population with practical recommendations that meet nutritional requirements, promote health, support an active lifestyle, and reduce the risk of chronic disease.

The guidelines for 2000 include the following 10 recommendations:

- Aim for a healthy weight.
- Let the food pyramid guide your food choices.
- Eat a variety of grains daily, especially whole grains.
- Eat a variety of fruits and vegetables daily.
- Keep food safe to eat.
- Choose a diet low in saturated fat that is also low in cholesterol and moderately low in total fat.
- Choose beverages and foods that limit intake of sugar.
- Choose and prepare foods with less salt.
- Drink alcoholic beverages in moderation.
- Be physically active each day.

Food Guide Pyramid

The Food Guide Pyramid was first introduced in 1992, published by the Department of Agriculture and Department of Health and Human Services (USDA & DHHS, 1992). The Food Guide Pyramid translates the dietary guidelines for Americans into practical eating portions that meet the dietary guidelines and, if foods are chosen carefully, they also meet the recommended daily allowances (RDA) and Dietary Reference Intakes (DRI).

The Food Guide Pyramid was designed to graphically illustrate the dietary guidelines for Americans, emphasizing balance, moderation, and variety. The Food Guide Pyramid can be modified to fit the cultural preferences of clients by using foods customary to their culture and to fit differing age groups by modifying the types of foods and the serving sizes. Depending on cultural food preferences, food groupings may be modified to adequately adjust for a client's nutrient requirements. Figure 5-8 presents the traditional Food Guide Pyramid.

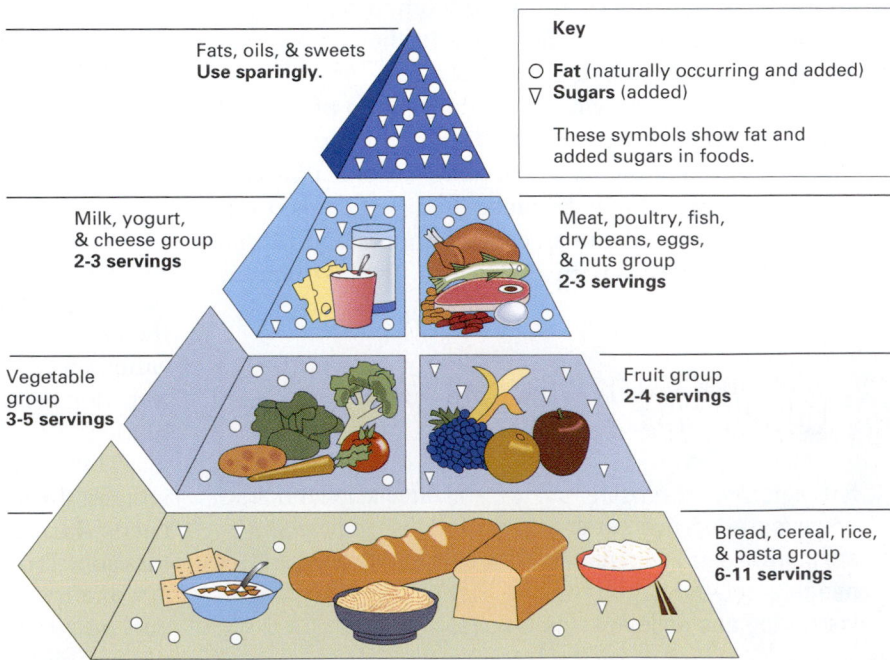

Figure 5-8 Food Guide Pyramid.

Courtesy of United States Departments of Agriculture and Health and Human Services (1992). The food guide pyramid: A guide to daily food choices. Washington, DC, (leaflet no. 572)

Culturally Adapted Food Guides

While the basic nutritional requirements and guidelines generally apply to all people, nutritionists and nurses have long been aware of cultural differences in eating patterns and food preferences. Translating nutritional requirements into cultural food practices has sometimes been challenging. The Food Guide Pyramid can be adapted to be used with clients from various cultures or with specific dietary practices, such as those common to Asian, Mediterranean, and Latin American diets (Townsend & Roth, 2003).

All of the food pyramids limit saturated fats to protect against heart disease. The Asian, Mediterranean, and Latin American plans give greater daily predominance to heart-healthy monounsaturated fats. As *Dietary Guidelines for Americans* (USDA, 2000) suggests, the fat content of the diet should be kept low: total fat, saturated fat, and cholesterol. The total daily fat intake should be no more than 30% of the total calories, and saturated fats should comprise no more than 10% of total calories.

Nutrition Facts Food Label

Another tool designed to aid people in selecting a healthy diet is the **Nutrition Facts food label**, which was introduced in 1993 (FDA, 1993). Nutrition labeling on processed packaged foods includes credible health and nutrient content claims and standardized serving sizes (FDA, 1999). The items, with amounts per serving, that must be included on the food label are illustrated in Figure 5-9.

The food manufacturer can voluntarily include additional information on food products. The percent daily values (DV) are based on a 2,000-calorie diet. Clients must adjust their intake of nutrients based on their estimated caloric consumption each day and on the serving size they consume. The DVs are based on two sets of standards. One is based on the **Daily Reference Values (DRVs)**, which are the standards for daily intake of total fat, saturated fat, cholesterol, total carbohydrate, dietary fiber, and protein. The total fat DRV is based on diets that provide 30% of total calories as fat; saturated fat is set at 10% of total calories. The DRV for total carbohydrates is based on 60% of the total calories, and for protein, on 10%.

The other standard used to calculate percent daily values on nutrition labels is the **Reference Daily Intakes (RDIs)** (Nutrient Data Laboratory, 2001). This standard addresses the vitamin and mineral content of foods. It provides legal standards set by the U.S. Food and Drug Administration (FDA) for labeling foods and supplements uniformly. The RDIs generally represent the highest values of vitamins and minerals in the 1968 **Recommended Dietary Allowances (RDA)** (Food & Nutrition Board, 1989) tables for nutrients in any age group over age 4, excluding pregnant and breast-feeding women. The

RDA lists the average daily nutrient intake levels recommend for healthy Americans. The Nutrition Facts labels make it possible for consumers to compare products easily, based on the product's contribution of fat, cholesterol, sodium, and other major nutrients.

Nutritional Needs across the Life Span

Adolescence

For women, adolescence is a special time of growth and development. In this discussion, adolescence covers ages 11 to 18.

Nutrition Facts

Serving Size 1/2 cup (114g)
Servings Per Container 4

Amount Per Serving

Calories 90	Calories from Fat 30

% Daily Value

Total Fat 3g	**5%**
Saturated Fat 0g	**0%**
Cholesterol 0mg	**0%**
Sodium 300mg	**13%**
Total Carbohydrate 13g	**4%**
Dietary Fiber 3g	**12%**
Sugars 3g	
Protein 3g	

Vitamin A	80%	•	Vitamin C	60%
Calcium	4%	•	Iron	4%

• Percent Daily Values are based on a 2,000 calorie diet. Your daily values may be higher or lower depending on your calorie needs:

	Calories	2,000	2,500
Total Fat	Less than	65g	80g
Sat Fat	Less than	20g	25g
Cholesterol	Less than	300mg	300mg
Sodium	Less than	2,400mg	2,400mg
Total Carbohydrate		300g	375g
Fiber		25g	30g

Calories per gram:
Fat 9   •   Carbohydrate 4   •   Protein 4

Figure 5-9   Sample nutrition facts food label.

Nutritional Needs

Nutrient requirements increase greatly during this time as a result of rapid growth, the onset of puberty, and an increase in body mass. Sufficient dietary calories must be provided so that protein is available for growth. Adequate calcium intake is another main concern for the adolescent because 45% of the skeletal mass is formed during this period; calcium is also important in the prevention of future osteoporosis. The new Daily Reference Intake (DRI) Adequate Intake (AI) for calcium is 1,300 mg/day for girls aged 9 to 18 (Food & Nutrition Board, 1997). This is equal to at least four and one-half servings of calcium-rich foods each day. If teens are also pregnant, they have additional nutritional needs.

The typical food habits of adolescents are characterized by an increased tendency toward skipping meals, snacking, inappropriate consumption of fast foods, dieting, and fad diets (Table 5-3). Adolescence is a time when peer influence is often greater than parental influence. The teen's search for independence, challenge of existing values, concern about body image, search for self-identity, and coping with the pressures of a quickly changing world influence dietary behavior.

Nutritional Concerns

Eating disorders frequently begin during adolescence in girls. When dealing with the rapid physiologic and psychologic changes experienced in this stage of life, adolescent females tend to alter their eating behavior to gain control over this aspect of their life (Giannini, Newman, & Gold, 1990). The groups affected by eating disorders have expanded from the traditional young, Caucasian, affluent girl or woman, whose illness is a reflection of disturbed family relationships, to include women and men of all ethnic backgrounds. The national chapters of Anorexia Nervosa and Related Eating Disorders, Inc. (ANRED) and Anorexia Nervosa and Associated Disorders (ANAD) estimate that 20% of the population between ages 12 and 30 is experiencing a major eating disorder. Today's society promotes the ideal physique for males and females as being thin with a high lean body mass ratio. Western society's media images and high fashion industry perpetuate and reinforce these often unattainable body images, which stereotype slim and obese people.

Anorexia Nervosa.   Anorexia nervosa is self-starvation motivated by excessive concern with weight and an irrational fear of becoming fat; it was first reported as early as 1868 (Frisch & Frisch, 2002). People with anorexia excessively control and restrict their caloric intake and have an unrealistic view of their body fat stores and body shape. They are often perfectionists in their daily lives. The medical complications of anorexia nervosa are similar to those seen in starvation: slow resting heart rate, low blood pressure, amenorrhea (disruption of the menstrual cycle), and hypothermia (complaints of being cold). The skin is often cool and there may be a loss of scalp hair. Soft lanugo (fine, soft, blonde) hair may appear on the face and trunk area. The normal amount of body fat for females (20% to 25%) decreases to an extremely low level (7% to 13%).

The most serious medical complications of anorexia nervosa are damage to the cardiovascular system and sudden death (Kaplan & Sadock, 2003). Irregular heart rhythms may occur, especially with deficiencies in potassium, magnesium, or phosphorus. Treatment for anorexia nervosa is successful in about 50% of cases. The focus of treatment is on gradually restoring body weight, improving self-esteem and attitudes about weight and body shape, and normalizing eating and exercise patterns and behavior. Antidepressant medications and family therapy are often used.

Bulimia Nervosa.   Bulimia nervosa is characterized by behaviors that are the opposite of those seen in anorexic clients. Binge eating, which is excessive consumption of calories over a short period of time; purging by self-induced vomiting; use of laxatives or diuretics, or both; excessive exercise; and periods of severe caloric restriction are the typical patterns of the bulimic client. The client with bulimia often hides food, eats in secret, is depressed, and may be a substance abuser. In contrast to the close-knit, orderly, often rigid family of clients with anorexia nervosa, instability and conflict characterize the families of clients with bulimia nervosa. Clients with bulimia appear impulsive and out of control and usually have a normal body weight or are slightly overweight. Bulimia is more common in athletes and ballet dancers than in other groups. The medical complications related to the anatomic and physiologic changes characteristic of bulimia are often severe. The body is constantly adjusting to the feast or famine cycle. As a consequence of self-induced vomiting, severe erosion of the dental enamel, loss of teeth, esophagitis, hiatal hernia, esophageal tear or rupture, hypochloremic alkalosis, hypokalemia, shock, and other symptoms may occur. If ipecac is used to induce vomiting, myocardial ipecac toxicity may develop, causing fatal dysrhythmias and potentially fatal myocarditis. Laxative abuse may result in chronic hypokalemia, along with renal tubular damage. Binge eating may also create marked gastric dilation, gastric rupture, or post-binge pancreatitis. Enlargement of the parotid glands may occur and can become disfiguring. Treatment for bulimia consists of nutritional counseling to replace the disordered eating patterns with regular meals and snacks, and psychologic counseling to improve self-image and attitudes toward body weight. Antidepressants are often useful in the treatment plan.

Table 5-3   Nutrient and Calorie Content of Some Fast Foods Compared with Recommended Daily Allowances (RDA) for 16-Year-Old Girl

	WEIGHT (oz)	CALORIES	PROTEIN (g)	FAT (g)	CALCIUM (mg)	IRON (mg)	SODIUM (mg)	VITAMIN A (RE)	THIAMIN (mg)	RIBOFLAVIN (mg)	NIACIN (mg)	VITAMIN C (mg)
Hamburger	3½	250	12	11	56	2.2	463	14	0.23	0.24	3.8	1
French fries	2	160	2	8	10	0.4	108	0	0.09	0.01	1.6	5
Chocolate milk shake	10	335	9	8	374	0.9	314	59	0.13	0.63	0.4	0
Pizza	4	300	15	9	220	1.6	700	106	0.34	0.29	4.2	2
Soda	12	160	0	0	11	0.2	18	0	0	0	0	0
Doughnut	2	210	3	12	22	1.0	192	5	0.12	0.12	1.1	0
Potato chips	2	315	3	21	15	0.6	300	0	0.09	0	2.4	24
Chocolate bar with peanuts	1½	225	6	16	75	0.6	30	12	1.0	1.0	2.1	0
RDAs for 16-year-old girl		2,200	44	73	1,200	15	500	800	1.1	1.3	15	60

Binge Eating. **Binge eating** is a disorder of periodic binge eating that is not normally followed by vomiting, the use of laxatives, or excessive exercise. Several thousand calories are consumed within a short period of time. Binge eating twice a week for 6 months is usually required for diagnosis. Stress, depression, anger, anxiety, and other negative emotions usually prompt the binge-eating episodes. Nutrition and psychologic counseling help focus on the disordered eating pattern and the underlying feeling or circumstances surrounding the event. Antidepressants may again be part of the treatment plan.

Eating disorders are often seen in fashion models, wrestlers, figure skaters, gymnasts, dancers, drill teams, competitive athletes, flight attendants, actors, and persons training to be dietitians, all of whose careers may depend on their ability to maintain a particular body weight. Close attention should be given to the degree of body-size conformity placed on adolescents by their coaches, agents, peers, or parents. The evaluation and treatment of clients with eating disorders often requires an interdisciplinary team approach that includes professionals in psychiatry, psychology, general medicine, nutrition, nursing, and social work. The family must be involved in the treatment and care of the client over an extended period.

Obesity. **Obesity** is defined as a body weight that is 20% over the ideal. Obesity is increasing in the United States at an alarming rate. Many common health conditions are increasing along with overweight and obesity. Recent studies show that 50% of adults in the United States are overweight or obese: this reflects a 25% increase over the past 30 years (Mokdad et al., 1999).

Excess weight has been seen in conjunction with increased rates of cardiovascular disease, type 2 diabetes mellitus, hypertension, stroke, hyperlipidemia, osteoarthritis, and some cancers. Concerted initiatives need to be undertaken to prevent and treat overweight children and adolescents, or the health care system will be more and more overwhelmed with adults seeking treatment for obesity-related health conditions. The physical, social, environmental, and psychologic factors contributing to this malady must be assessed and addressed by a multidisciplinary health care team of physician, nurse, psychologist, dietitian, social worker, and others.

Adulthood

The nutritional needs of women in the reproductive phase of their life are set forth in the Recommended Dietary Allowances and the Dietary Reference Intakes (Food & Nutrition Board, 1997, 1998, 2000). Updates to the nutrient needs of all individuals are continually being reviewed and periodically published. The key nutrients of concern to women are addressed in the following section, with specific nutritional concerns for pregnancy, lactation, and

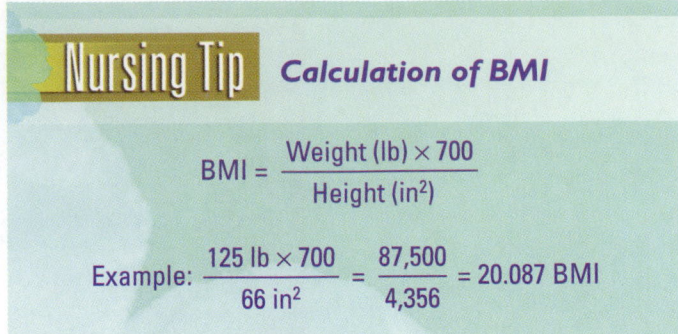

Nursing Tip · *Calculation of BMI*

$$BMI = \frac{Weight\ (lb) \times 700}{Height\ (in^2)}$$

$$Example: \frac{125\ lb \times 700}{66\ in^2} = \frac{87,500}{4,356} = 20.087\ BMI$$

old age. Periodic review of the nutritional literature is essential to keep practice and guidance current.

The body weight of a client reflects her past history of nutritional habits. The current recommendations are to determine a client's ideal body weight based on the **body mass index (BMI)**. The BMI represents a ratio of the relationship between height and weight.

The interpretation of the BMI calculation is as follows: less than 18, severe underweight; 18 to 20, low body weight; 20 to 25, normal body weight; 25 to 30, overweight; 30 to 40, obese; and more than 40, gross obesity. Tables are available for a quick calculation.

Nutritional Needs

Nutritional need vary across the life span. Necessary vitamins, minerals, and elements are discussed in the following section.

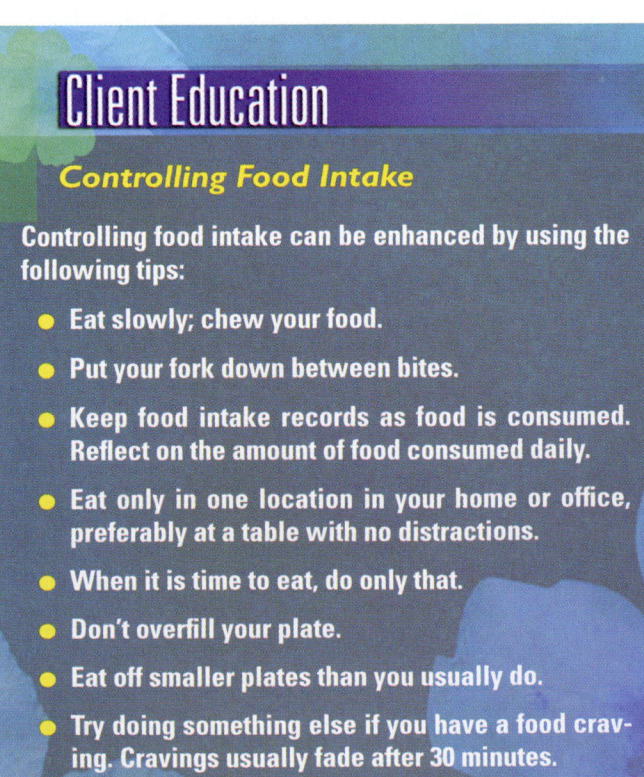

Client Education

Controlling Food Intake

Controlling food intake can be enhanced by using the following tips:

- Eat slowly; chew your food.
- Put your fork down between bites.
- Keep food intake records as food is consumed. Reflect on the amount of food consumed daily.
- Eat only in one location in your home or office, preferably at a table with no distractions.
- When it is time to eat, do only that.
- Don't overfill your plate.
- Eat off smaller plates than you usually do.
- Try doing something else if you have a food craving. Cravings usually fade after 30 minutes.

Calories or Energy Needs. The amount of energy provided to the body by food is measured in **calories**. The body uses the energy from foods for growth, tissue repair, and maintenance; to fuel muscular activity; to process nutrients; and to maintain body temperature. **Basal metabolism** is the energy used to support the body functions while the body is at rest. To calculate the basal metabolic rate (BMR) for females, multiply body weight by 10.

The final category of energy needs of the body is dietary thermogenesis, also called specific dynamic action (SDA) of foods, diet-induced thermogenesis, and thermic effect of foods. This is the heat or energy expended during digestion of food and the absorption and use of nutrients. Dietary thermogenesis requires approximately 10% of the body's total energy needs. By adding these three categories of energy needs by the body, a good estimate of caloric needs can be determined.

The composition of energy nutrients found in foods determines their caloric content. Each gram of carbohydrate or protein contains four calories. Each gram of fat contains nine calories. Alcohol contains seven calories per gram. The information in Nutrition Facts food labels assists consumers in determining the number of calories per serving of food.

Critical Thinking

Determining Caloric Needs

The following formula may be used to determine caloric needs:

130 lb woman × 10 = 1,300 calories for BMR

+ 1,300 calories × 30% (average activity level) = 390 calories for activity

+ 1,690 calories × 10% (SDA) = 169 calories

Total caloric needs/day = 1,859 calories

Therefore, approximately 1,859 calories per day would be necessary for this woman to maintain her body weight. Since each pound of body weight equals 3,500 calories, to lose 1 pound a week, this woman would need to consume 500 fewer calories per day or to consume 250 fewer calories per day and increase her activity expenditure by 250 calories per day. If this woman desired to gain 1 pound of weight per week, she would need to increase her caloric intake by 500 calories per day. What are the caloric needs for a woman weighing 145 lb?

Protein. The protein requirement for adult women is 0.8 kg body weight. The need for increased protein for the pregnant woman is 30% greater than when nonpregnant. This translates into an increase of 10 to 14 additional grams of protein per day during the last half of pregnancy. The increased need should be expected as a result of the increase in both maternal and fetal tissue formation. Adequate calories must be consumed so that protein can be used for the body's building and synthetic processes.

Calcium. Calcium is a mineral needed for strong bones and teeth, neural transmission, and muscle contractions; it also plays a role in cells and cell membranes, blood clotting, and other functions. Nearly 99% of the body's calcium is in the bones and teeth. Calcium is in a dynamic state in the body, always being moved from the bloodstream to the bones, according to the body's needs. The remaining 1% of calcium is found in body fluids. Calcium is required to maintain normal blood pressure and for the absorption of vitamin B_{12}. In 1997, the Food and Nutrition Board, recommended 1,300 mg/day of calcium for ages 9 through 18 and 1,000 mg/day for ages 19 to 50, for both males and females. The benefit of calcium intake on weight-bearing sites, such as the hip, is enhanced in women with high levels of physical activity.

If a woman does not regularly consume dairy products or other foods high in calcium each day, a calcium supplement of at least 600 mg/day is recommended. Calcium in the form of calcium carbonate, calcium citrate, or calcium phosphate, in supplements that carry the United States Pharmacopoeia (USP) symbol, have been shown to be highly absorbable. Clients should discuss possible interactions among calcium supplements and prescription or over-the-counter medications with their physician or pharmacist. Table 5-4 offers an overview of calcium sources.

Vitamin D. Vitamin D plays an important role in calcium absorption and bone mineralization. Vitamin D allows calcium to leave the intestines and enter the bloodstream to be absorbed and allows the bones to release more calcium and the kidneys to retain more calcium in the body. Because it is a fat-soluble vitamin, it is stored in the liver. Vitamin D intake is recommended at 5μg (200 IU) per day for adults over age 19, even during pregnancy and lactation. For adults between ages 51 and 70, the DRI is 10 μg (400 IU) per day, increasing to 15 μg (600 IU) per day for individuals over age 70.

Sources of vitamin D include vitamin D-fortified cow's milk or margarine, eggs, and butter. Adequate exposure of the skin to sunshine, that is, about 30 minutes of direct sunlight on the hands and face without sunscreen two to three times weekly, may be enough for the body to produce an adequate amount of vitamin D. Synthesis of

Table 5-4   Overview of Selected Vitamins and Minerals

NUTRIENT	FUNCTION	SOURCES	DEFICIENCY	TOXIC EFFECTS
Calcium (Ca)	• Aids in bone and teeth formation • Promotes muscle contraction and relaxation • Aids blood clotting • Aids in nerve transmission • Promotes normal heart rhythm • Needs vitamin D for absorption	• Milk • Cheese • Sardines • Salmon • Green leafy vegetables • Whole grains	• Rickets • Osteoporosis • Tetany • Poor tooth formation	• Kidney stones • Deposits in joints and soft tissue • May inhibit iron and zinc absorption
Vitamin D	• Stimulates absorption of calcium and phosphorus for good bone mineralization	• Yeast • Fish liver oils • Fortified milk and cereals	• Rickets • Malformed teeth • Bone deformities	• Hypercalcemia • Kidney stones • Cardiovascular damage
Folate (folic acid)	• Is necessary for synthesis of RNA and DNA • Promotes amino acid metabolism, red and white blood cell formation	• Green leafy vegetables • Meat • Eggs • Yeast	• Glossitis • Diarrhea • Macrocytic anemia	• None known
Vitamin B_{12} (cobalamin)	• Promotes normal function of all cells, especially of the nervous system • Promotes blood formation • Promotes carbohydrate, protein, and fat metabolism • Aids in synthesis of RNA and DNA • Is necessary for folate metabolism	• Fresh shrimp, oysters, meats, milk, eggs, and cheese	• Pernicious anemia • Anorexia • Indigestion • Paresthesia of hands and feet • Poor coordination • Depression	• None known
Iron	• Aids in formation of hemoglobin • Whole grains • Aids in antibody formation	• Meat • Egg yolk • Legumes • Prunes • Raisins • Apricots	• Iron deficiency anemia	• Hemochromatosis • GI cramping • Vomiting • Nausea • Shock • Convulsions • Coma

vitamin D may be reduced in winter months, in darker-pigmented individuals, and in those living with high concentrations of atmospheric ozone. For women in northern climates or those with little exposure to sunlight, such as office workers, nursing home residents, and house-bound persons, supplementation should be considered if the diet is inadequate. The recommended intake of vitamin D for individuals with osteoporosis may be increased by the physician to 10 µg (400 IU) per day. Rich sources of vitamin D include fortified milk (400 IU per quart), high-fat fish (250 to 800 IU per serving), canned fish (200 to 500 IU per serving), and cod liver oil (400 IU per teaspoon). Table 5-4 provides an overview of vitamin D.

Folate.   Folate, sometimes referred to as folacin or folic acid, is a B vitamin found in many vegetables, beans, fruits, whole grains, and fortified breads and cereal products. Routine supplementation with folate should occur at least 1 month before conception through the first trimester of pregnancy. All women in the reproductive years should consume at least 400 µg of folic acid per day from fortified foods, vitamin supplements, or a combination of the two, in addition to a varied, healthful diet. Because more than 30% of pregnancies are unplanned, the March of Dimes recommends that women consume 1 mg of folic acid per day during their childbearing years. The folic acid fortification of widely consumed cereal and grain products should have a remarkable effect in reducing the number of pregnancies affected by neural tube defects (NTD), when these products are consumed with synthetic supplements of folic acid (Lewis, Crane, Wilson, & Yetley, 1999).

Dietary sources of folate include meat, fish, poultry, eggs, fortified whole-grain breads, fortified cereals, peanuts, leafy green vegetables, and yeast extract. Liver is an excellent source, with 3.5 ounces of chicken livers containing 700 µg of folic acid and 3.5 ounces of beef liver containing 217 µg of folic acid.

Sufficient body supplies of folic acid before and during conception and for up to 13 weeks after conception help guard against birth defects of the brain and spine (NTDs) that occur when the neural tube does not close completely, as in **spina bifida** (in which the spinal canal does not close and protrudes out of the back), **encephalocele** (in which the brain protrudes through a defect in the skull), and **anencephaly** (a fatal condition in which a baby is born with a severely underdeveloped brain and skull and dies shortly after birth). In the United States, more than 3,000 infants per year are born with NTDs, about 4 of every 1,000 births. Babies with the other NTDs live longer,

Reflections from a Young Adult

My grandmother recently fell and broke her hip for the second time. All her life she's been a heavy smoker and coffee drinker and not very big on dairy products, especially milk. I guess I never really appreciated the link among good dietary habits, a healthy lifestyle, and overall physical health and well-being. Most of my life I've done what I've wanted and been very healthy, but seeing my grandmother's troubles really motivates me to watch my habits and consider their impact on my long-term health.

with paralysis, neurologic damage, and possibly bowel and bladder incontinence. Women who have had one infant with an NTD are considered to be at high risk for having another infant with an NTD. Four mg of folate per day, compared to 400 µg for all other women of childbearing age, is recommended for these women, beginning at least 1 month before pregnancy and throughout the first trimester of pregnancy. This treatment has been shown to reduce the risk of the mother having another NTD-affected child by about 70%.

Women aged 19 and older need 400 µg of dietary folate equivalent (DFE) per day. One DFE = 1 µg food folate = 0.6 µg folic acid (from fortified food or supplement) consumed with food = 0.5 µg of synthetic (supplemental) folic acid taken on an empty stomach. Refer to Table 5-4.

Vitamin B$_{12}$.   Vitamin B$_{12}$ is needed to build red blood cells and to keep the nervous system healthy. It is also essential for the normal use of folate and helps protect against the risk factors characteristic of heart disease and atherosclerosis. This vitamin is only found in animal food sources. The best sources of this vitamin are meats, fish, poultry, shellfish, eggs, milk, and milk products. Some brands of soymilk products are fortified with vitamin B$_{12}$. Vegetarians consuming no animal products (vegans) need 2.4 µg per day of vitamin B$_{12}$. Care should be taken to get adequate amounts of this vitamin, either through the diet or a multi-vitamin and mineral supplement. Impaired absorption of this vitamin accounts for more than 95% of the cases of vitamin B$_{12}$ deficiency in the United States.

Deficiency of vitamin B$_{12}$ can mean the development of pernicious anemia. The name was given to this deficiency disease in 1822 when pernicious meant "to lead to death." This deficiency causes macrocytic, megaloblastic anemia, in which red blood cells have delayed and abnormal nuclear maturation. See Table 5-4.

The RDA is 2.4 µg per day for vitamin B$_{12}$ for both adolescents and adults. In pregnancy, the recommendation increases to 2.6 µg, and in lactation to 2.8 µg/day.

Iron.   Iron is a trace mineral that functions to transport oxygen to the cells as a component of hemoglobin and myoglobin. Iron is also required by several enzyme systems and helps convert energy for normal cell activities. Iron is stored intracellularly as ferritin and hemosiderin, primarily in the liver, spleen, bone marrow, and other organs. In general, for menstruating females, the iron recommendation is 15 mg/day. The recommendation decreases past the age of 51 to 10 mg/day. For pregnancy, the recommended level doubles to 30 mg/day, and during lactation, the recommended level returns to the menstruating female level of 15 mg/day. Refer to Table 5-4.

If dietary intake is inadequate, the stored iron is used to meet the body's need for iron. Only after depletion of iron stores do hematocrit levels begin to fall. Signs of iron deficiency are the depletion of the iron stores, **microcytic** (small cell size) **anemia**, and **hypochromic** (lacking in color) **anemia**. Iron deficiency anemia is the most common nutritional deficiency in the United States. The incidence in high-risk populations ranges from 10% to 50%: in menstruating women, 5% to 14%; in males in early adolescence, 4% to 12%; in children ages 1 to 2, 9%. There is currently an interagency group, consisting of the Micronutrient Initiative and the University of Toronto, presenting the technology to fortify salt with iron, in addition to iodine, to address the severe levels of iron deficiency anemia existing worldwide.

Iron in the diet consists of two forms. **Heme iron** (iron from animal sources) constitutes about half of the iron in the diet. **Nonheme iron** (dietary iron sources other than from meats, in which the iron is not bound to hemoglobin) comprises the remaining half of the iron found in animal sources and all of the iron found in plant sources, including grains and cereals. There is greater absorption of nonheme iron when it is taken with a good dietary source of ascorbic acid, like orange juice or oranges. Nonheme iron is less absorbable when taken with tea (tannic acid), dairy products (calcium phosphate), many cereals (phytates), bran, oxalates, and antacids. Heme iron is absorbed four to five times better than nonheme iron. Nonheme iron accounts for a larger percentage of total human iron intake. On the average, about 10% of iron consumed is absorbed. The rate of absorption varies with need and the form of the iron consumed.

Administration of the iron supplement between meals or at bedtime increases absorption rates. If a client has iron-deficiency anemia and therapeutic levels of iron (more than 30 mg/day) are given to treat the anemia, the client should also be given 15 mg of zinc and 2 mg of copper because of the interference of iron with the absorption and use of these trace minerals.

Fiber. Dietary fiber is a complex carbohydrate, mainly composed of the indigestible parts of plant cell walls. Dietary fiber is connected to better colon health, a reduced incidence of type 2 diabetes mellitus, lower blood pressure and cholesterol levels, and less risk of cardiovascular disease. Individuals who eat a lot of whole grain cereals and bread products and fruits and vegetables with the skins seem to have less constipation and diverticulitis. Dietary fiber (20 to 35 g/day) from a wide variety of food sources, such as fruits, vegetables, legumes, and whole grains is recommended. When fiber intake is increased, it should be done gradually. In addition, 1 to 2 quarts of additional fluid should be consumed with the additional fiber. This helps with possible constipation problems. Participating in regular physical exercise is recommended to manage constipation.

There are two types of fiber: insoluble and soluble. **Insoluble fiber** resists absorption into the body. It moves quickly through the digestive tract, absorbing water and making the stools softer and bulkier. The rapid passage of food through the intestines is believed to reduce the potential for carcinogens to interact with the intestinal surface. However, this hypothesis is under study. Insoluble fiber is found primarily in whole grains, nuts, seeds, vegetables, cooked dried beans, and dried peas or legumes.

Soluble fiber reduces blood cholesterol levels. It can bind bile acids or coat the intestines, thus inhibiting the absorption of cholesterol. Soluble fiber includes pectins, gums, and mucilages that dissolve in water. Some key sources of soluble fiber are oat bran, barley, apples, fruits, seaweed, and cooked dried beans and peas (legumes).

Water. Water is an essential, vital nutrient, often overlooked in recommendations. It is an essential nutrient because it is required in amounts that exceed the body's ability to produce it. It is necessary for the transport of nutrients in the body and for body temperature maintenance and serves as a solvent for minerals, vitamins, amino acids, and glucose. Water provides a means for the elimination of waste materials and toxins from the body in urine. Approximately 60% of the adult's body is composed of water with two-thirds of this water distributed intracellularly and one-third extracellularly. Water accounts for 50% to 80% of body weight, depending on the level of lean body mass. Usual recommendations for adults are to drink 8 to 10 cups (1 cup = 8 oz = 237 mL) of water per day, or 30 mL/kg of body weight, with a minimum of 6 cups (1500 mL) for small individuals. More daily fluid is required: (1) in hot, dry climates or high altitudes; (2) with a high-fiber diet; (3) with a diet high in al-

Nursing Tip — *Fluid Requirements for Adolescents and Adults*

More daily fluid is required in:

1. Hot climates
2. High-fiber diets
3. Diets high in alcohol, caffeine, or both
4. Increased activity
5. Pregnancy and lactation

Early signs of dehydration include headache, fatigue, loss of appetite, flushed skin, heat intolerance, lightheadedness, dry mouth, stomach burning, and dark urine with a strong odor. Dehydration may also be associated with premature labor. Additional fluid is needed during pregnancy and lactation.

cohol or caffeine; and (4) with increased activity. Early symptoms of dehydration include headache, fatigue, loss of appetite, flushed skin, heat intolerance, lightheadedness, dry mouth and eyes, a burning sensation in the stomach, and dark urine with a strong odor.

Mature Years

The age group that is most rapidly gaining members in the United States is that of elderly persons (over 65); those over age 85 are in the fastest-growing subgroup. In 1995, there were 3.6 million persons over age 85. By 2040, over 12 million people may be over age 85; and by 2050, two thirds of all Americans over age 85 may be women (Administration on Aging, 2000).

As aging occurs, the nutrients needed to maintain optimal nutritional status stay relatively high, but the caloric needs decrease because of lower levels of activity and decreased rates of metabolism. The diet of aging individuals should be nutrient-dense to obtain essential nutrients in a limited number of calories. Emphasis should be placed on consuming a diet high in fruit and vegetables, low-fat meats, fortified dairy products, and enriched and fortified high-fiber breads and cereals. Limited consumption of fats, sweets, and alcohol is advised, because these foods are high in calories but low in other essential nutrients. The older adult usually needs about 1,600 calories daily. The daily calcium intake should increase to 1,200 mg/day and vitamin D, to 10 μg/day for women age 50 and older.

Women should determine their nutritional health by watching for signs of poor nutrition. Anyone with three or more risk factors should consult a physician, registered dietitian, or other health care professional.

Nursing Alert

Dietary Risk Factors for the Aging Woman

- **D**isease
- **E**ats poorly
- **T**ooth loss or mouth pain
- **E**conomic hardship
- **R**educed social contact
- **M**any medicines
- **I**nvoluntary weight loss or gain
- **N**eeds assistance in self-care
- **E**lderly, over age 80

COLLABORATIVE CARE

Teams for Women's Healthcare

Nurses working with women in any setting may be collaborating or referring women to other professionals and resources. These may include some of the following:

- Physicians: pediatricians, obstetricians, gynecologists, family practice, internists, and other specialists
- Advanced practice nurses: Certified Nurse Midwives, nurse practitioners (women's health, family, neonatal, pediatric, and other specialties)
- Social workers
- Nutritionists
- Psychologists and psychiatrists
- Health educators
- Community health workers

Nursing Implications

Many times the nurse has the best opportunity to discuss nutritional issues with clients. To effectively counsel clients about nutritional changes, the nurse must be aware of nutritional needs and be able to assess for nutritional risks of deficiency or excess. In nutritional counseling, the entire family must be considered, as most meals are prepared for the entire family rather than for individual members. Women are crucial in nutritional counseling because they generally make all the food choices as they shop, plan menus, cook, and serve the family's food. Eating patterns are infused with cultural beliefs and practices, and these practices are passed on from generation to generation. Eating patterns are also heavily influenced by social networks and activities. For example, teenagers are likely to adopt eating patterns of their peers rather than their family. However, as adults they will revert back to family eating patterns. The availability of food and economic resources are also important in a family's dietary decision making. All of these factors illustrate the difficulty of making dietary changes.

Nurses can follow the nursing process, beginning with an assessment that includes a 24-hour recall of dietary intake, validation of whether this is a typical eating pattern, and assessment of resources for getting and preparing foods. Cultural beliefs and eating patterns should also be assessed. These data should be analyzed for nutritional adequacy. Interventions may consist of connecting the family with available resources for acquisition of food or nutritional services. Providing the family

Client Education

Resources for Food Programs

If clients have difficulty managing their food budget to meet food costs, refer them to a registered dietitian or social worker who can assist them. There are several federal nutrition programs designed to improve the nutritional status of pregnant and lactating women, their infants, and children up to age 5. The Special Supplemental Food Program for Women, Infants, and Children (WIC) certifies individuals meeting the current federal guidelines to be at nutritional risk and living on a household income of 185% or less of the federal poverty level income. Other supplemental nutrition programs may also be available for the client, such as food stamps and the Cooperative Extension—Expanded Food and Nutrition Education Program (EFNEP). These are for lower-income individuals who need to enhance their access to adequate nutrition and receive sound nutrition education.

with information about healthier eating behaviors is an important intervention. However, interventions to alter a family's dietary choices and methods of food preparation involve more than providing information. Evaluation of interventions is necessary and should be undertaken for referrals to community agencies and educational interventions and should be incorporated into an ongoing engagement with the family.

VIOLENCE AND ABUSE AGAINST WOMEN

Violence against women in the United States is a serious threat to their health and welfare (Paluzzi & Houde-Quimby, 1996). Abuse can be verbal, financial, emotional, and physical. This section focuses on interpersonal violence and abuse against women of all ages and their children.

Intimate Partner Violence

Intimate partner violence is sometimes referred to as *intimate partner abuse, domestic violence, domestic abuse, spouse abuse,* or *wife battering,* all of which describe intentional violent or controlling behavior by a current or former intimate partner. In 1996, some 840,000 women experienced aggravated **assault** (the intentional act of inflicting physical injury on another person), rape, and assaultive victimization by their current or former spouses, boyfriends, or girlfriends (Greenfield et al., 1998). On average, each year from 1992 to 1996, 8 of every 1,000 women received nonfatal injuries from willful or intentional abusive acts by their intimate partners. In addition, women are eight times more likely than are men to be assaulted by intimate partners (Greenfield et al., 1998). Each abusive interaction has the potential to be deadly. From 1976 through 1996, 29.7% of women victims of murder were killed by husbands, ex-husbands, and nonmarital partners compared with 5.9% of male victims (Greenfield et al., 1998). Among murder victims for every age group, females are much more likely than are males to have been murdered by intimate partners (Cooper & Eaves, 1996). Thousands of deaths occur as a result of repeated assaults over many years (Hodges, 1993). Coercive behaviors of the **perpetrator** (the person accused of a criminal offense), such as belittlement, physical assaults, and stalking, can escalate to **femicide** (murder of a female). Of murders attributed to intimate partners, 75% were female victims. Femicide is the major cause of death for Black women aged 15 to 34 years and the seventh leading cause of premature death for all women in the United States (Hambleton, Clark, Symaya, Weissman, & Horner, 1997). According to the Federal Bureau of Investigation, in 1996, 30% of all women victims of murder were slain by husbands or boyfriends (Uniform Crime Reports for the United States, 1996).

Sexual Assault

Rape is defined as sexual penetration of another by force or threat of force, without consent. Abuse by an intimate partner accounts for half of all rapes of women over 30 years old (Jones, 1994). In one study, Murdoch and Nicholand (1993) found that one in four women in the military under the age of 50 had been physically abused within the past year. Of enlisted women, 31% had been forced to have nonconsensual sex.

Two major categories of rape exist: acquaintance rape and stranger rape. **Acquaintance rape** occurs when a perpetrator with whom the victim has had a previous nonviolent relationship uses deceit and coercion to obtain sex. Two types of acquaintance rape are wife rape and date rape. **Wife rape** is a forced sexual experience with a common-law or legally married spouse; **date rape** is rape that occurs between a dating couple without consent of one of the participants. **Stranger rape** is a nonconsensual sexual experience between a victim and an assailant who are strangers. Stranger rape is sudden and is more likely to involve violence, with or without the use of a weapon (Marx, Wie, & Gross, 1996). By 1993, all 50 states had passed laws making marital rape a crime. Studies have estimated that 14% to 25% of wives are forced by their spouses to have sexual intercourse against their will at some time during the course of their marital relationship

Critical Thinking

Risks of Being Raped

- What would you say to a woman who asks if it is possible to contract AIDS or gonorrhea as an outcome of being raped?
- What are her options for sexually transmitted disease testing?
- What are her options for preventing conception?

Nursing Tip   *Helping Survivors of Rape*

What you can say to a survivor of intimate partner violence or rape:

- I am afraid for the safety of you and your children.
- Violence only gets worse over time.
- You know when it would be safest to leave, and we are here for you when you are ready.
- You do not deserve to be hit.
- It is not your fault.
- Let me help you figure out a safety plan for you and your children.

(Resnick, Kilpatrick, Walsh, & Vernonen, 1991; Russell, 1990). Many rapes are unreported, particularly by teenage victims.

To assess and provide care to a person who experiences rape, nurses must first understand the psychological effect of rape trauma syndrome. This syndrome is characterized as a response to the extreme stress and profound fear of death, which most survivors experience (Figure 5-10). Rape trauma syndrome begins with an acute or immediate phase of disorganization followed by a long-term process of reorganization that occurs as a result of attempted or forcible sexual assault. The majority of women report symptoms of avoidance and denial, which may prevent them from seeking help and participating in legal prosecution (Kramer & Green, 1991). Nurses may use information on the prevalence of symptoms of post-traumatic stress disorder (PTSD) to help in identification and provision of anticipatory guidance to survivors of sexual assault. Many cities have rape crisis centers and nurses can receive special education to become sexual assault nurse examiners (SANE).

Cultural Influences

No ethnic or socioeconomic group of women is immune to domestic violence. The National Victims Survey found no significant difference in the rates of severe abuse among Caucasian, Black, or Hispanic American women (Campbell, Masaki, & Torres, 1997). Unfortunately, women belonging to minority groups often face racism and anti-immigrant

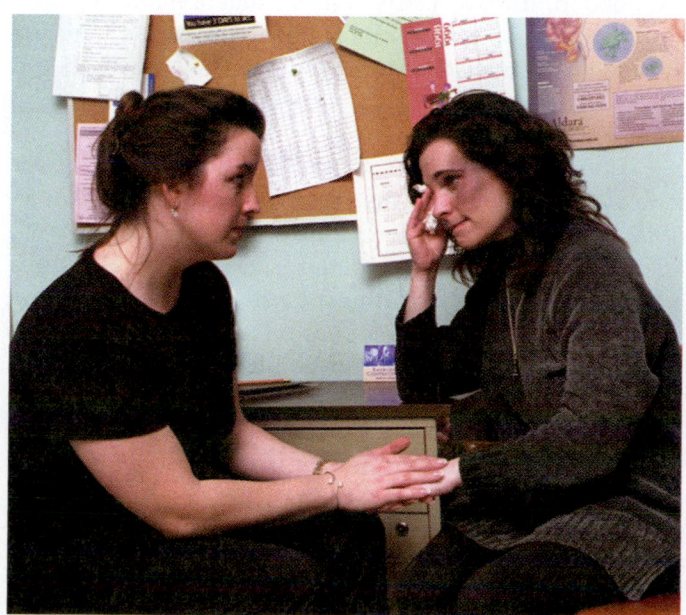 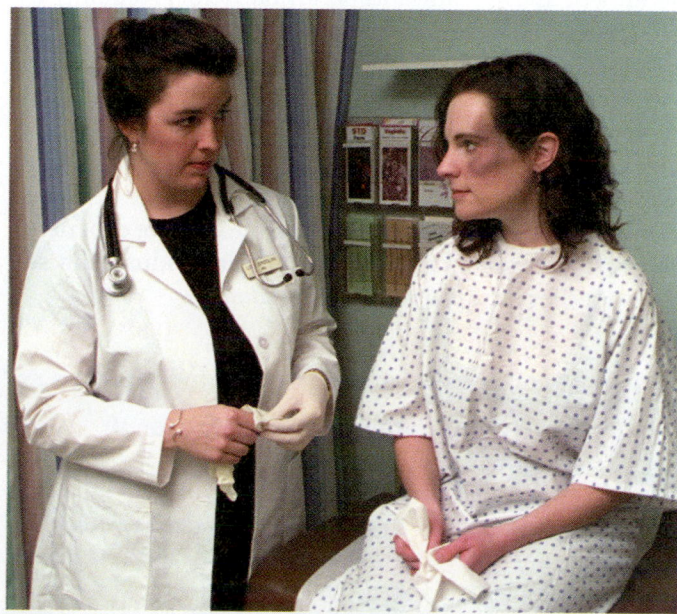

Figure 5-10   Caring for a woman who has survived an assault requires compassion and sensitivity during both the interview and physical examination.

Client Education

Culturally Appropriate Solutions

For clients experiencing violence, refer to the following:

- Bilingual and bicultural programs within the community

- Support groups that meet in predominantly local areas (e.g., shelters and churches), which provide shared experiences for persons of the same race

- National African American Women's Health Project, which uses model community-based self-help programs, community-based health centers, films, and publications

- Immigrant and Refugee Women, Immigrant Assistance Line: English and Spanish, 415-554-2444; Cantonese, Mandarin, and Vietnamese, 415-554-2454

- Native Americans, Women of Nations: 612-222-5830

- Additional sources, which can be found by looking in the blue or white pages of your local telephone directory under Domestic Abuse Information and Treatment Centers, Social Service Organizations, Human Service Organizations, Shelters, Women's Organizations, or Family Services

sentiment that create additional barriers to ending the abuse. Male batterers may use culture and immigration status to control their partners (e.g., claiming that battering is an acceptable cultural practice or threatening to report the woman for deportation if she does not do as told). Fewer services and less information are available to battered women of color, primarily because of economic restraints. Awareness of cultural influences on the abusive experience can assist nurses in approaching and individualizing services for the client in a more caring manner.

Nursing Tip Overcoming Cultural Biases

Culturally astute nurses are aware of their own biases and how they may affect their perceptions and relationships with clients from other cultures. You should seek information about other cultures through interactions with clients and community experts and through reading.

Research studies suggest that Black women are more likely than are Caucasian women to report abuse and other violent crimes to the police (Bachman & Coker, 1995; Hutchison, Hirschel, & Pesackis, 1994).

Portrait of an Abuser

Chronic alcohol use and illicit drug use are among the most prevalent risk factors for being an abuser (Fagan, Barnett, & Patton, 1988; Greenfield et al., 1998; Hotaling & Sugarman, 1986: Kantor & Straus, 1989; Ptacek, 1998). Roberts (1988) found that at the time of the assault, 70% of perpetrators were under the influence of drugs, alcohol, or both. Even higher rates of drug and alcohol use were seen in a study by Brookoff (1997): 92% of perpetrators used illicit drugs or alcohol on the day of the assault. Coleman and Strauss (1983) reported rates of violence almost 15 times higher for husbands who were "often" versus "never" drunk in the past year. Abuser's drinking patterns, especially binge drinking, are associated with marital violence across all ethnic groups and social classes (Kantor, 1993).

Battering is more than an isolated case of the person "blowing up." It is a process of deliberate intimidation intended to coerce the person being abused (i.e., girlfriend or boyfriend, spouse, significant other, child, or older person) into doing the will of the abuser. It is behavior that shows an established set of control behavior. In reality the man who abuses his wife and children is not "out of control," rather, he is very much "in control." The perpetrator enforces control in a way that compares to brainwashing. Coercive techniques are used to set up a regulating situation for domestic violence. These techniques include isolation, monopolization of perception, induced debility and exhaustion, threats, occasional indulgences, demonstration of the abuser's omnipotence, degradation, and enforcement of trivial demands (Jones, 1994; Willson, 1998).

The Cycle of Violence

The cycle of violence was first described by Walker in 1962 (Paluzzi & Houde-Quimby, 1996). Walker (1984) identified family violence patterns as consisting of three phases: the tension-building phase, the acute battering phase, and the honeymoon phase. The cyclic behavior begins with a time of tension-building arguments, progresses to violence, and settles into a making-up or calm period. The time between the acute battering and honeymoon phases was identified by Curnow (1997) as the open-window phase, when the battered victim is most receptive to receiving help. With time, this cycle of violence increases in frequency and severity as it is repeated over and over again.

The traditional view of a woman who is battered is that of a dependent victim, one psychologically unable to take steps to stop the abuse (Campbell & Fishwick, 1993;

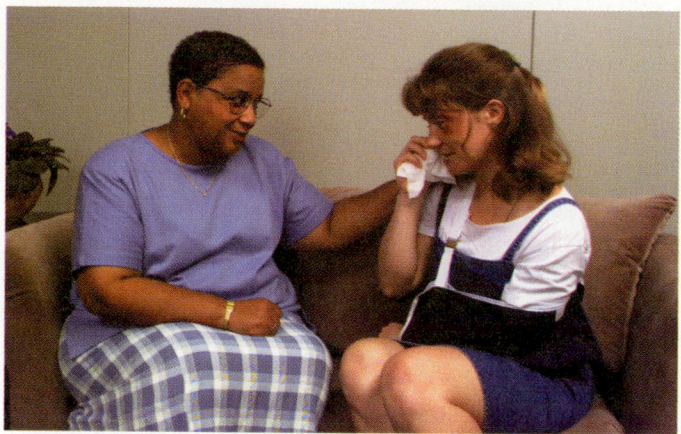

Figure 5-11   Nurses need to be skilled in recognizing when a client who is battered is most receptive to help and most likely to accept the reality of the abusive situation.

Gondolf, 1998; Gondolf & Fisher, 1988). This traditional perspective fails to see the potential present in these women that enables them to survive. These women will seek help; and it is important for nurses to understand when that will occur, learn effective interventions, and provide empirical information as to the impact of those interventions (Figure 5-11).

Understanding Walker's cycle of violence can assist nurses in identifying the process and timing of interventions for women who are stalked and abused.

Nursing Implications

Minimum components of a safety plan include preparatory steps for ensuring safety during violent episodes, or details about how the woman who is being abused will leave the relationship. Community resources (e.g., women's shelters, the police, the district attorney's office, women's centers, and hotline phone numbers) are reviewed, and referrals are offered or made at the time of

Critical Thinking

Evaluating the Risks and Benefits of Leaving an Abusive Spouse Because of the Children

- Is it better for a woman to leave an abusive spouse and rear the children in a single-parent home?
- What if the single parent has financial difficulties?
- What are the benefits and risks of keeping the family together "for the children's sake"?

Nursing Alert

Abuse Assessment Screening

Questions that help you screen for abuse:

- Has anyone ever hit, slapped, restrained, or hurt you physically or emotionally?
- Are you afraid of your partner* at times? Of your previous partner?**
- Have you ever felt unsafe in your home situation?**
- Does your partner like to boss you around?
- If your partner does not get his own way, how does he act?
- Have you been forced to have sexual relations or engage in sexual activities that you are uncomfortable doing?
- When arguing with your partner, does he threaten to hurt you or the children?
- Has your partner ever stopped you from leaving home, visiting family or friends, or going to work or school?
- Do you have a say in how to spend money?
- Are any of these things occurring now?

Note. Interview the woman alone, not with her partner.
*Partner, spouse, boyfriend, ex-husband, or ex-boyfriend.
**Quick screening questions.

the visit. The nurse should assess the client's risk of danger privately, maintaining confidentiality, and must maintain a nonjudgmental demeanor. Each encounter with a client can foster disclosure of the extent of intimate partner violence and empower the client to develop strategies that increase her safety. The nurse should discuss methods of limiting the danger, such as removing guns from the house and attempting to avoid arguments in high-risk rooms, such as the kitchen, garage, or any room with objects that are potential weapons. The nurse should help the client prepare a decisive escape plan. First, the client should consider how she will exit the house, for example, by which door or window. Second, the client needs to plan what to take with her when leaving: purse, car keys, cash, and important papers. The client should know to keep these items nearby. She should gather together important documents and be sure they are secure and easy to access. Personal documents she will need include birth certificates, social security cards, and her driver's license;

Nursing Alert

Safety Planning

Help a client plan for safety or escape by considering the following:

- Is it safe for the woman and her children to go home?

- Are there weapons in the home?

- Has there been an increase in the frequency or severity of the violence?

- Has the woman been hospitalized in the past as a result of the intimate partner violence?

- Has the abuser threatened to kill the woman or himself?

- Has the woman thought of committing or tried to commit suicide?

- Does the abuser hurt the children?

- Has the woman attempted or is she planning to leave the relationship?

Nursing Tip   Sequelae of Abuse

Abuse of women is likely to be the precursor of chronic disease, substance abuse, and mental health problems, which affect women of all ethnic backgrounds and socioeconomic classes (Grisso & Ness, 1996). All those who experience or witness abuse suffer psychological consequences.

medical documents include health insurance identification cards and policies; and financial information includes bank account numbers.

A safety plan includes seeking out supportive family members or friends who will assist the woman in leaving the relationship, provide shelter, and call the police when violence is suspected. Integral to all safety planning is referral to community agencies that assist women who are abused. It is important to discuss the woman's concerns about using community agency resources. Fear of physical retaliation after reporting the abuse to the police is a common concern. Does filing assault charges against one's partner stop the abusive behaviors or just make them worse? Some research findings indicate that police intervention is associated with decreased levels of abuse. Research-based clinical practice can assist the nurse in helping the abused woman overcome her fears by building on knowledge and dispelling myths.

Threats of abuse, physical assaults, and the increased risk of homicide experienced by women who are abused affect their health and carry a tremendous amount of morbidity. Campbell and Lewandowski (1997) identified multiple violence-associated illnesses that ranged from minor difficulty with mental concentration and headaches to irritable bowel syndrome and post-traumatic stress disorder.

Women who are abused seek health care interventions at emergency departments; prenatal clinics; general medi-

cine practices; and social support agencies, such as women's shelters (Klein, Campbell, Soler, & Ghez, 1997). When the abusive relationship becomes violent, women most often seek help and protection from legal enforcement agencies (McFarlane, Soeken, Reel, Parker, & Silva, 1997). In large urban police departments, specialty units provide services for domestic violence victims (Berry, 1998).

Violence against women creates a public health problem that mandates nurses to implement preventive strategies. Nurse clinicians are called on to assess the dangerousness of abusive relationships for their clients in a variety of settings and to offer care, resources and referrals as appropriate (Figure 5-12). These assessments frequently are based on a history of abuse, the nurse clinician's intuition, and the clinician's knowledge of risk factors for homicide (Campbell, 1995; Gondolf, 1998). Nurse clinicians refer or are mandated to report women who are abused to the criminal justice system, that is, the police or the district attorney's office.

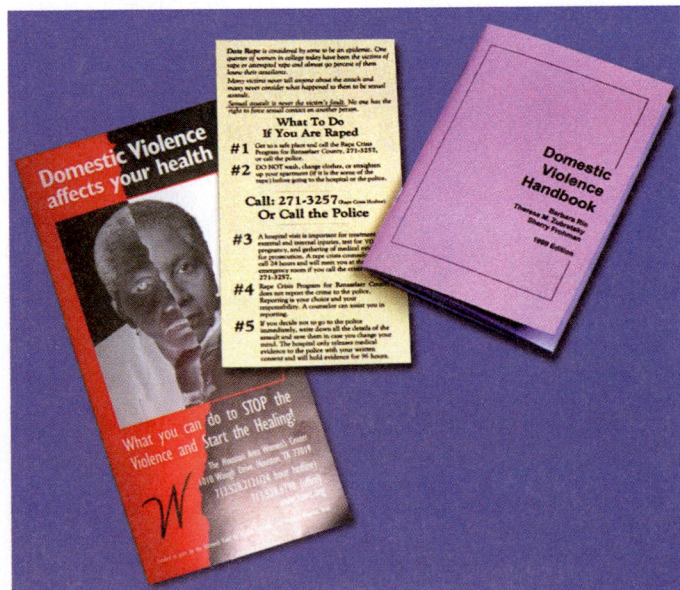

Figure 5-12   In addition to physical and emotional support, nurses can share literature and make referrals for clients who have experienced violence.

WEB | ACTIVITIES

••• Where would you find information specific to the risk for osteoporosis on the internet in an effort to better educate your midlife clients on their risks?

••• Visit the U.S. Department of Agriculture Web site. Use it to plan a daily menu for a 15-year-old girl; a pregnant 31-year-old woman; and a 65-year-old woman.

••• Visit the National Dairy Council home page. Do they outline calcium needs for pregnancy and lactation? What foods do they recommend as the best sources for calcium?

••• Search the Web for sites addressing abuse, violence, and rape. Do these sites offer information on the different types of assault (e.g., acquaintance rape versus date rape)? Are there resources for families as well as health care providers?

••• Check the sites of some of the major nursing and health care organizations, such as NANDA, the National League for Nursing and American Psychiatric Association. Do these sites include information on abuse, violence, and rape?

••• Search government Web sites for support groups for survivors of violence and self-help programs for abusers. Are research studies available online?

Key Concepts

■ Physiologic gender differentiation occurs at fertilization at the time in which the genetic sex is determined by chromosomes XX or XY.

■ The maternal transfer of estrogen causes changes in the newborn's breast tissue and genitalia that resolve shortly after birth.

■ Physical maturity and emotional maturity do not occur simultaneously, which frequently leads to adolescent conflicts.

■ Individual cultural beliefs may impact the care of the woman throughout the life span.

■ Hormonal changes during the midlife years bring on additional physiologic changes.

■ Health education and self-care measures are key in providing positive support to women during the midlife years.

■ Physiologic and psychosocial issues continue to affect women as they age. Functional assessment is key in providing self-care and maintaining a safe environment for the client.

■ A woman's overall health throughout the life span is greatly affected by her nutrition and lifestyle choices.

■ Adolescents need to strive for a balanced diet while keeping consumption of junk foods to a minimum.

■ Eating disorders are most prevalent in the adolescent years and stem from an unhealthy, distorted body image.

■ Women of all ages should work toward a target weight for their height and body type.

■ As a woman ages, the nutrient needs to maintain optimal nutritional status stay relatively high but the caloric needs decrease as a result of lower activity level and decreased metabolic rates.

■ Domestic violence is a public health problem with great consequences, including the physical, mental, and emotional pain of the victim.

■ The economic cost of violence and abuse is felt by the health care industry, the legal system, and business communities.

■ The nurse is an essential provider of domestic violence prevention, screening, and referral to community resources.

■ Minimum components of a safety plan include a private interview, preparatory steps for ensuring safety or for leaving the relationship, and a listing of community resources.

■ Subsequent client encounters are opportunities for nurses to re-question the client about abuse and her safety.

Review Questions and Activities

1. What causes dysfunctional uterine bleeding during adolescence?
   a. Abnormal periods
   b. Anovulatory cycles
   c. Poor diet
   d. Poor grades

   The correct answer is b.

2. What is the most visible sign of puberty?
   a. Social withdrawal
   b. Weight gain
   c. Enlargement of the breast bud
   d. Anger

   The correct answer is c.

3. How can the Tanner Stages be defined?
   a. Emotional changes of the aging woman
   b. Thelarche
   c. Stages of adolescent physical development
   d. Menarche

   The correct answer is c.

4. What is the second phase of the normal menstrual cycle?
   a. Ovulation
   b. Secretory-luteal phase
   c. Menstruation
   d. Proliferative-follicular phase

   The correct answer is d.

5. The corpus luteum regresses with decreases in estrogen and progestin, resulting in menstruation, when what does not occur?
   a. Ovulation
   b. Cysts
   c. Menarche
   d. Implantation

   The correct answer is d.

6. Record all the food that you eat for 24 hours.
   a. Analyze your list and compare it to the recommended daily intakes for your age group.
   b. Calculate your body mass index (BMI).
   c. Make nutritional recommendations for yourself based on the above data.

7. On your next trip to the grocery store, check labels and identify 15 popular foods that have over 10 grams of fat per serving. Note the serving size on the label.

8. Outline appropriate nursing care for a rape survivor.

9. Suggest approaches to ensure that psychosocial support of a woman who has experienced rape is provided.

10. Develop an escape plan for a wife who is battered and has two school-age children.

References

Administration on Aging. (2001). *Aging into the 21st century*. Washington, DC: U.S. Bureau of Census.

American Cancer Society. (1999). *Breast cancer facts and figures 1999/2000*. Atlanta, GA: American Cancer Society.

American Heart Association. (1999). *2000 heart and stroke statistical update*. Dallas, TX: American Heart Association.

Bachman, R., & Coker, A. L. (1995). Police involvement in domestic violence: The interactive effects of victim injury, offender's history of violence, and race. *Violence and Victims, 10*, 91–106.

Berry, D. B. (1998). *The domestic violence sourcebook: Everything you need to know*. Los Angeles: Lowell House.

Blackburn, S., & Loper, D. (2003). *Maternal, fetal, and neonatal physiology: A clinical perspective* (2nd ed.). Philadelphia: W. B. Saunders.

Brookoff, D. (1997). *Drugs, alcohol, and domestic violence in Memphis*. [NIJ Research Preview.] Washington, DC: National Institute of Justice.

Campbell, J. C. (1995). Prediction of homicide of and by battered women. In J. Campbell (Ed.), *Assessing dangerousness: Violence by sexual offenders, batterers, and child abusers* (pp. 96–113). Thousand Oaks, CA: Sage.

Campbell, J. C. & Fishwick, N. (1993). Abuse of female partners. In J. C. Campbell & J. Humphreys (Eds.), *Nursing care of survivors of family violence* (pp. 68–104). St. Louis, MO: Mosby.

Campbell, J. C., & Lewandowski, L. A. (1997). Mental and physical health effects of intimate partner violence on women and children. *Psychiatric Clinics of North America, 20*, 353–374.

Campbell, D. W., Masaki, B., & Torres, S. (1997). In E. Klein, J. Campbell, E. Soler, & M. Ghez (Eds.), *Ending domestic violence: Changing public perceptions/halting the epidemic* (pp. 64–87). Thousand Oaks, CA: Sage.

Centers for Disease Control and Prevention (CDC). (1995). Tobacco use and usual source of cigarettes among high school students. United States. *Morbidity and Mortality Weekly Report, 45*, 413–418.

Centers for Disease Control and Prevention. (1999). Youth behavioral risk surveillance. *Morbidity and Mortality Weekly Report, 49*(SS05), 1–96.

Coleman, D. H., & Straus, M. (1983). Alcohol abuse and family violence. In E. Gottheil, K. A. Druley, T. E. Skoloda, & H. S. Waxman (Eds.), *Alcohol, drug abuse, and aggression* (pp. 104–124). Springfield, IL.: Charles Thomas.

Commonwealth Fund. (1997). *Selected facts on U.S. women's health*. New York: Columbia University Press.

Cooper, M., & Eaves, D. (1996). Suicide following homicide in the family. *Violence and Victims, 11*(2), 99–112.

Curnow, S. A. M. (1997). The open window phase: Helpseeking and reality behaviors by battered women. *Applied Nursing Research, 10*(3), 130.

Dealy, M. (1998). Dysfunctional uterine bleeding in adolescents. *Nurse Practitioner: The American Journal of Primary Health Care, 23*(5), 12–23.

Erikson, E. (1950). *Childhood and society*. New York: W. W. Norton.

Fagan, R. W., Barnett, O. W., & Patton J. B. (1988). Reasons for alcohol use in maritally violent men. *American Journal of Drug and Alcohol Abuse, 14*, 371–392.

Fogel, C., & Woods, N. (1995). *Women's health care: A comprehensive handbook*. London: Sage Publications.

Food and Drug Administration. (1993). *FDA Consumer* Special Issue. FDA (1999). The Food Label FDA Background, May 1999.

Food and Nutrition Board, National Academy of Sciences. Institute of Medicine. (1997). *Dietary reference intakes, 1997*. Washington, DC: National Academy Press.

Food and Nutrition Board, National Academy of Sciences, Institute of Medicine. (1997). *Dietary reference intake for calcium, phosphorous, magnesium, vitamin D, and fluoride.* The Standing Committee on the Scientific Evaluation of Dietary Reference Intakes. Washington, DC: National Academy Press.

Food and Nutrition Board, National Academy of Sciences, Institute of Medicine. (2000) *Dietary reference intakes for vitamin C, vitamin E, selenium, and carotenoids.* Washington, DC: National Academy Press

Food and Nutrition Board, National Academy of Sciences, Institute of Medicine. (1998). *Dietary reference intakes: thiamin, riboflavin, niacin, vitamin B6, folate, vitamin B12, pantothenic acid, biotin, and choline.* Washington, DC: National Academy Press.

Food and Nutrition Board, National Academy of Sciences, National Research Council. (1989) *Recommended dietary allowances, revised 1989* (10th ed.). Washington, DC: National Academy Press.

Frisch N. C., & Frisch L. E. (2002). *Psychiatric mental health nursing* (2nd ed.). Clifton Park, NY: Thomson Delmar Learning.

Giannini, J. A., Newman, J., & Gold, M. (1990). Anorexia and bulimia. *American Family Physician, 41,* 169–176.

Gondolf, E. W. (1998). *Assessing woman battering in mental health services.* Thousand Oaks, CA: Sage.

Gondolf, E. W., & Fisher, E. R. (1988). *Battered women as survivors: An alternative to treating learned helplessness.* Lexington, MA: Lexington.

Greenfield, L. A., Rand, M. R., Craven, D., Klaus, P. A., Perkins, C. A., Ringel, C., et al., (1998). *Violence by intimates: Analysis of data on crimes by current or former spouses, boyfriends, and girlfriends* (NCJ-167237). Washington, DC: U.S. Department of Justice, Bureau of Justice Statistics.

Grisso, J. A., & Ness, R. B. (1996). Update in women's health. *Annals of Internal Medicine, 125,* 213–214.

Hambleton, B. B., Clark, G., Symaya, D. V., Weissman, G., & Horner, J. (1997). HRSA's strategies to combat family violence. *Academic Medicine, 72*(1), S19–S24.

Hatcher, R., Trussel, J., Stewart, F., Cates, W., Stewart, G., Guest, F., et al. (2000). *Contraceptive technology.* New York: Ardent Media.

Haynes, M. (1996). Geriatric gynecologic care of minorities. *Clinical Obstetrics and Gynecology, 39*(4), 946–958.

Hodges, K. (1993). Domestic violence: A health crisis. *North Carolina Medical Journal, 54,* 213–216.

Hotaling, G. T., & Sugarman, D. B. (1986). An analysis of risk markers in husband to wife violence: The current state of knowledge. *Violence & Victims, 1,* 101–124.

Hutchinson, I. W., Hirschel, J. D., & Pesackis, C. E. (1994). Family violence and police utilization. *Violence and Victims, 9,* 299–313.

Jones, A. (1994). *Next time she'll be dead: Battering and how to stop it.* Boston: Beacon.

Kantor, G. K. (1993). Refining the brushstrokes in portraits of alcohol and wife assaults. In S. E. Martin (Ed.). *Alcohol and interpersonal violence: Fostering multidisciplinary perspectives* (NIH Publication 93-3496, NIH Monograph 24; pp. 281–290). Washington, DC: National Institutes of Health.

Kantor, G. K., & Straus, M. A. (1989). Substance abuse as a precipitant of wife abuse victimizations. *American Journal of Drug and Alcohol Abuse, 15,* 173–189.

Kaplan H. L., & Sadock B. J. (2003). *Kaplan & Sadock's synopsis of psychiatry* (9th ed.). Baltimore: Williams & Wilkins.

Klein, E., Campbell, J., Soler, E., & Ghez, M. (1997). *Ending domestic violence: Changing public perceptions/halting the epidemic.* Thousand Oaks, CA: Sage.

Kramer, T., & Green, B. (1991). Posttraumatic stress disorder as an early response to sexual assault. *Journal of Interpersonal Violence, 6*(2), 160–173.

Lewis, C. J., Crane, N. T., Wilson, D. B., & Yetley, E. A. (1999). Estimated folate intakes: Data updated to reflect food fortification, increased bioavailability, and dietary supplement use. *American Journal of Clinical Nutrition, 70,* 198–207.

Marx, B. P., Wie, V. V., & Gross, A. M. (1996). Date rape risk factors: A review and methodological critique of the literature. *Aggression and Violent Behavior, A Review Journal, 1*(1), 27–45.

McFarlane, J., Soeken, K., Reel, S., Parker, B., & Silva, C. (1997). Resource use by abused women following an intervention program: Associated severity of abuse and reports of abuse and reports of abuse ending. *Public Health Nursing, 14,* 244–250.

Mokdad, A. H., Serdula, M. K., Dietz, W. H., Bowman, B. A., Marks, J. S., & Koplan, J. P. (1999). The spread of the obesity epidemic in the U.S., 1991–1998. *Journal of the American Medical Association, 282,* 1519–1522.

Murdoch, M., & Nicholand, K. L. (1993). *Women veterans' experiences with domestic violence and with sexual harassment while in the military.* Retrieved from http://www.fvpf.org/fund/thefacts/veteran.html

Nutrient Data Laboratory (2001). *Recommended dietary intakes* Retrieved March 16, 2004 from http://www.nal.usda.gov/fnig

Paluzzi, P. A., & Houde-Quimby, C. (1996). Domestic violence: Implications for the American college of nurse-midwives and its members. *Journal of Nurse Midwifery, 41,* 430–435.

Perry, J., & Woods, N. (1995). Older women and their images of health: A replication study. *Advanced Nursing Science, 18*(1), 51–61. Alley, N., Acheson, Admire, J. (eds.).

Ptacek, J. (1998). Why do men batter their wives? In R. K. Bergen (Ed.), *Issues in intimate violence* (pp. 181–195). Thousand Oaks, CA: Sage.

Resnick, H., Kilpatrick, D., Walsh, C., & Vernonen, L. (1991). Marital rape. In R. Ammerman & M. Herson (Eds.), *Case studies in family violence.* New York: Plenum.

Roberts, A. (1988). Substance abuse among men who batter their mates: The dangerous mix. *Substance Abuse Treatment, 5,* 83–87.

Russell, D. E. H. (1990). *Rape in marriage.* New York: MacMillan.

Society for Women's Health Research, (1999). *What do women suffer from?* Washington, DC: Author.

Speroff, L., Glass, R., & Kase, N. (1999). *Clinical gynecologic endocrinology and infertility* (6th ed.). New York: Lippincott, Williams & Wilkins.

Speroff, L. & Darney, P. (2001). *A clinical guide for contraception* (3rd ed.). Baltimore: Williams & Wilkins.

Stedman, T. (2000). *Stedman's medical dictionary* (27th ed.). New York: Lippincott, Williams & Wilkins.

Tanner, J. (1981). Growth and maturation during adolescence. *Nutrition Reviews, 39*(2), 43–55.

Thiedke, C. C., & Rosenfeld, J., (2001). *Women's health* (AAFP). Baltimore: Williams & Wilkins.

Townsend, C. E., & Roth, R. A. (2003). *National and diet therapy* (8th ed.). Clifton Park, NY: Thomson Delmar Learning.

Uniform Crime Reports for the United States. (1996). *Who are the victims* Retrieved from http://www.ojp.usdoj.gov/vawo/manual/who.htm

United States Department of Agriculture. (2000). *2000 Guidelines for Americans* (5th ed.). Washington, DC: National Academy Press.

U.S. Departments of Agriculture & Department of Health and Human Services. (1992). *The food guide pyramid*. Home and Garden Bulletin No. 252.

Walker, L. E. (1984). *The battered woman syndrome*. New York: Springer.

Wallis, L., Kasper, A., Reader, G., & Brown, W. (1998). *Textbook of women's health*. New York: Lippincott, Williams & Wilkins.

Williams, R., Larsen, P., Kronenberg, H., Melmed, S., & Polonsky, K. (2003). *Williams textbook of endocrinology* (10th ed.). Philadelphia: W.B. Saunders.

Willson, P. (1998, 5 April). Domestic violence: Are nurses hiding the facts? *The Internet Journal of Advanced Nursing Practice, 2*(1). Retrieved October 31, 2003, from http://www.ispub.com/journals/ijanp.htm

Woods, N., & Mitchell, E. (1997). Women's images of midlife: Observations from the Seattle midlife women's health study. *Health Care for Women International, 18,* 439–453.

Writing Group for the Women's Health Initiative Investigators. (2002, July 17). Risks and benefits of estrogen plus progestin in healthy postmenopausal women: Principal results from the Women's Health Initiative randomized controlled trial. *Journal of the American Medical Association Express, 288*(3), 321–333.

Suggested Readings

Allen, K. M., & Phillips, J. M. (1997). *Women's health across the life span: A comprehensive perspective*. Philadelphia: Lippincott-Raven.

American Medical Association. (1999). Patient page: Benefits and dangers of alcohol. *Journal of the American Medical Association, 281*(1), 104.

Anliker, J., Damron, D., Ballesteros, M., Langenberg, P., Havas, S., Mettger, W., et al. (1999). Using the stages of change model in a 5-a-day guidebook for WIC. *Journal of Nutrition Education, 31,* 175A–176A.

Bailey, L. B. (1998). Dietary reference intakes for folate: The debut of dietary folate equivalents. *Nutrition Reviews, 56,* 294–299.

Callister, L. (1995). Cultural meanings of childbirth. *Journal of Obstetric, Gynecologic, are Neonatal Nursing, 24*(4), 327–331.

Campbell, J. C. (1995). Making the health care system an empowerment zone for battered women: Health consequences, policy recommendations, introduction, and overview. In J. C. Campbell (Ed.), *Assessing dangerousness: Violence by sexual offenders, batterers, and child abusers* (pp. 3–22). Thousand Oaks, CA: Sage.

Campbell, J. C., & Campbell, D. W. (1996). Cultural competence in the care of abused women. *Journal of Nurse Midwifery, 41,* 457–462.

De Sevo, M. (1997). Keeping the faith: Jewish traditions in pregnancy and childbirth. *Lifelines, 1*(4), 46–49.

Gilligan, C. (1993). *In a different voice: Psychological theory and women's development*. Cambridge, MA: Harvard University Press.

Greene, G. W., Rossi, S. R., Rossi, J. S., Velicer, W. F., Fava, I. L., & Prochaska, J. O. (1999). Dietary applications of the stages of change model. *Journal of the American Dietetic Association, 99,* 673–678.

Hagen, P. T. (1997). *Mayo health quest: Guide to self-care*. Rochester, MN: Mayo Clinic.

Jacobson, M. S., Rees, J. M., Golden, N. H., & Irwin, E. (Eds.). (1997). Adolescent nutritional disorders: Prevention and treatment. *Annals of the New York Academy of Sciences, 817.*

Kleiner, S. M. (1999). Water: An essential but overlooked nutrient. *Journal of the American Dietetic Association, 99,* 200–206.

Kristal, A. R., Glanz, K., Curry, S. J., & Patterson, R. E. (1999). How can stages of change be best used in dietary interventions? *Journal of the American Dietetic Association, 99,* 679–684.

Locksmith, G. J., & Duff, P. (1998). Preventing neural tube defects: the importance of periconceptional folic acid supplements. *Obstetrics & Gynecology, 91,* 1027–1034.

McMann, M. C. (1999). *Taking control: Women and health. A primer on women's health*. Houston, TX: Women's Fund for Health Education and Research.

Nichols, F. & Humenick, S. (2000). *Childbirth education: Practice, research and theory* (2nd ed.). Philadelphia: W. B. Saunders.

Obermeyer, C. (2000). Menopause across cultures: A review of the evidence. *Menopause: Journal of the North American Menopause Society, 7*(3), 184–192.

Pennington, J. A. T. (1998). *Bowes and Church's food values of portions commonly used* (17th ed.). Philadelphia: Lippincott.

Position of the American Dietetic Association and Dieticians of Canada: Woman's health and nutrition. (1999). *Journal of the American Dietetic Association, 99,* 738–751.

Rorie, J-A. L., & Barger, M. K. (1996). Primary care for women: Cultural competence in primary care services. *Journal of Nurse Midwifery, 41*(2), 92–100.

Wallace, H. (1999). *Family violence: Legal, medical, and social perspectives* (2nd ed.). Boston, MA: Allyn & Bacon.

Wildman, R. E. C., & Medeiros, D. M. (2000). *Advanced human nutrition*. Boca Raton, FL: CRC Press.

Resources

Abuse During Pregnancy: A Protocol for Prevention and Intervention Continuing Education Credits Available from the March of Dimes, 800-367-6630, http://www.modimes.org

American Cancer Society, 1599 Clifton Road, Atlanta, GA 30329, 800-ACS-2345, http://www.cancer.org

American Diabetes Association. Everything you need to know, from nutrition to exercise to who's at risk for diabetes. http://www.diabetes.org

American Dietetic Association—Your Link to Nutrition and Health! Offers food tips and dietitian services, http://www.eatright.org

American Heart Association, 7272 Greenville Avenue, Dallas, TX 75231. For Women's health information call 1-888-MY-HEART, http://www.americanheart.org

Association of Women's Health, Obstetric, and Neonatal Nurses (AWHONN), 2000 L Street, NW, Suite 740, Washington, DC 20036, 800-673-8499, http://www.awhonn.org

Centers for Disease Control and Prevention (CDC). CDC serves as the national focus for developing and applying disease prevention and control, environmental health, and health promotion and education activities designed to improve the health of the people of the United States, http://www.cdc.gov

Commission on Dietary Supplement Labels—established by Congress in the Dietary Supplement Health and Education Act of 1994 and appointed by Former President Clinton, http://www.health.gov/dietsupp

Department of Health and Human Services, National Heart, Lung, and Blood Institute. Offers basic health information as well as clinical guidelines, http://www.nhlbi.nih.gov

Family Violence: A Self-Study Guide for Health Care Professionals in Primary Care. The Family Peace Project, Medical College of Wisconsin, 414-548-6903

Family Violence Prevention Fund, 383 Rhode Island Street, Suite 304, San Francisco, CA 94103–5133. http://www.endabuse.org, 415-252-8900

Food, Nutrition, and Consumer Services (FNCS) ensures access to nutritious, healthful diets for all Americans. Through food assistance and nutrition education for consumers, FNCS encourages consumers to make healthful food choices, http://www.fns.usda.gov

Food and Nutrition Information Center. Food and nutrition topics listed alphabetically. Great Web site for clients, http://www.nal.usda.gov/fnic

Harvard Eating Disorders Center conducts research, mentors developing scientists, and expands knowledge about eating disorders, their detection, treatment, and prevention, http://www.hedc.org

Healthfinder. Useful Web site for clients to conduct searches for specific health conditions, health news, and useful health resources. Also available in Spanish, http://www.healthfinder.gov

How to Identify and Document Genital and Non-Genital Injuries, Health Education Alliance, Monterey, CA, 800-404-3258.

Improving the Health Care Response to Domestic Violence: A Resource Manual for Health Care Provider, Family Violence Prevention Fund, San Francisco, CA, 415-252-8900

International Food Information Council Foundation (IFIC). IFIC's purpose is to bridge the gap between science and communications by collecting and disseminating scientific information on food safety, nutrition and health, http://www.ific.org

Medscape offers daily news and updates concerning health and medicine. Easy search option beneficial to clients, http://www.medscape.com

National Association of Anorexia Nervosa and Associated Disorders (ANAD) is the oldest national nonprofit organization helping eating disorder victims and their families. In addition to its free hotline counseling, ANAD operates an international network of support groups for sufferers and families, and offers referrals to health care professionals who treat eating disorders, across the United States and in 15 other countries, http://www.anad.org

National Coalition Against Domestic Violence (NCADV), P.O. Box 18749, Denver, CO 80218–0749, 303-839-1852, http://www.ncadv.org

National Coalition for Women with Heart Disease, 818 18th St., NW, Suite 730, Washington, DC 20036, 202-728-7234, http://www.womenheart.org

National Domestic Violence Hotline, 1-800-799-SAFE

National Nutritional Foods Association's (NNFA) principal voice on issues of research, technology and quality in the health foods industry, the Science and Quality Assurance Department also serves as an information resource on scientific issues, http://www.nnfa.org

National Osteoporosis Foundation, 1232 22nd Street, NW, Washington, DC 20037–1292, 202-223-2226, http://www.nof.org

SAMHSA's National Clearinghouse for Alcohol and Drug Information. SAMHSA is the federal agency charged with improving the quality and availability of prevention, treatment, and rehabilitative services in order to reduce illness, death, disability, and cost to society resulting from substance abuse and mental illnesses, http://www.health.org

Silent Witness National Initiative, 7 Sheridan Avenue South, Minneapolis, MN 55405, 612-377-6629, Fax: 612/374-3956, E-mail: info@silentwitness.net, http://www.silentwitness.net/

U.S. Department of Health and Human Services, Food and Drug Administration (FDA). News, drug updates, and search options, http://www.fda.gov

U.S. Department of Justice office of Justice Programs Office of the General Counsel, Attention: FOIA staff, 810 7th St. NW, Room 5400, Washington, DC 20531, 202-307-0790

U.S. Department of Labor, Women's Bureau, http://www.dol.gov/wb

U.S. Food & Drug Administration, Center for Food Safety & Applied Nutrition provides voluntary dietary supplement adverse event reporting, and product information, such as labeling, claims, package inserts, and accompanying literature. http://www.cfsan.gov

Violence Against Women Office, U.S. Department of Justice, 202-616-8894, http://www.ojp.usdoj.gov/vawo

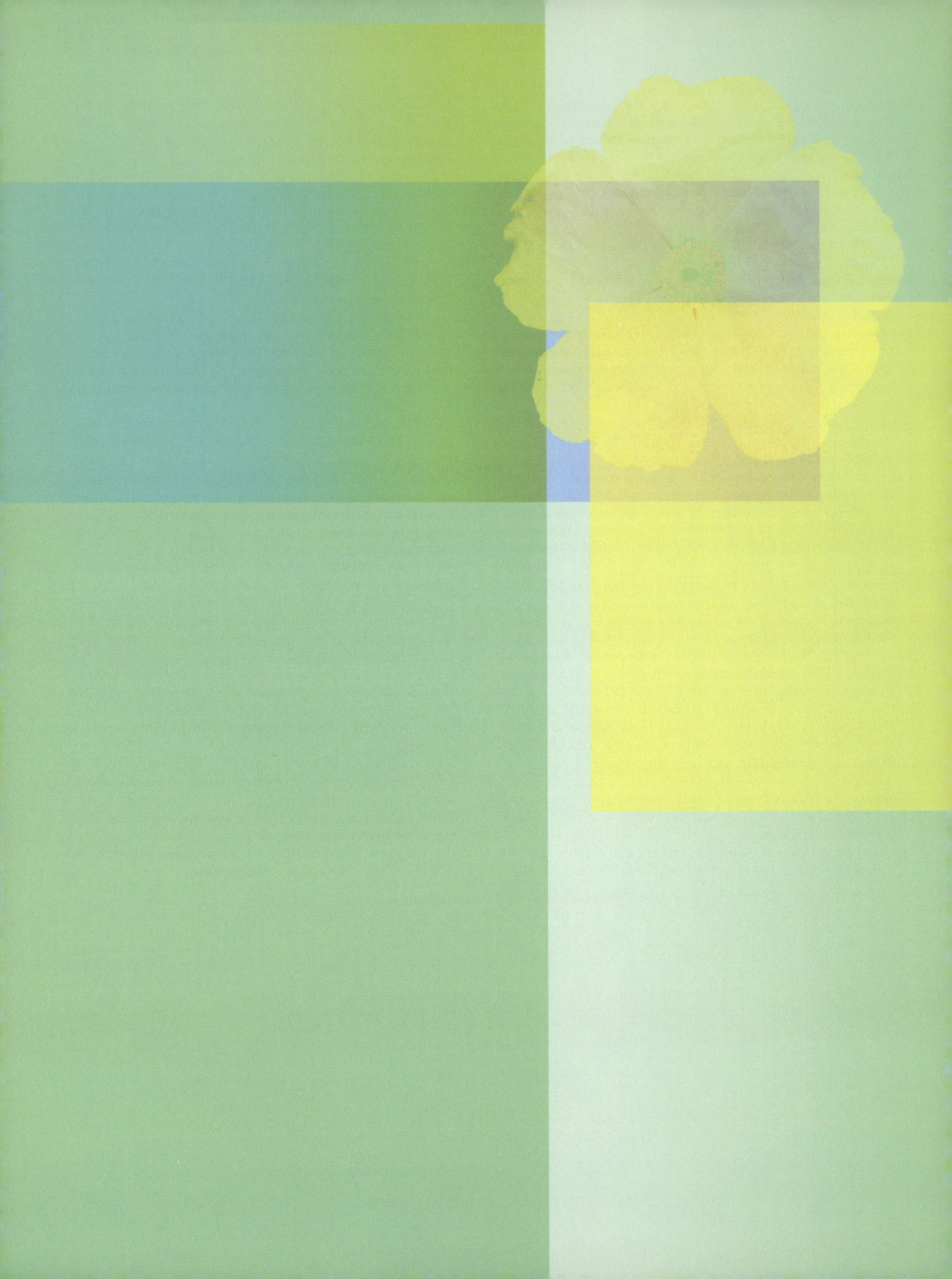

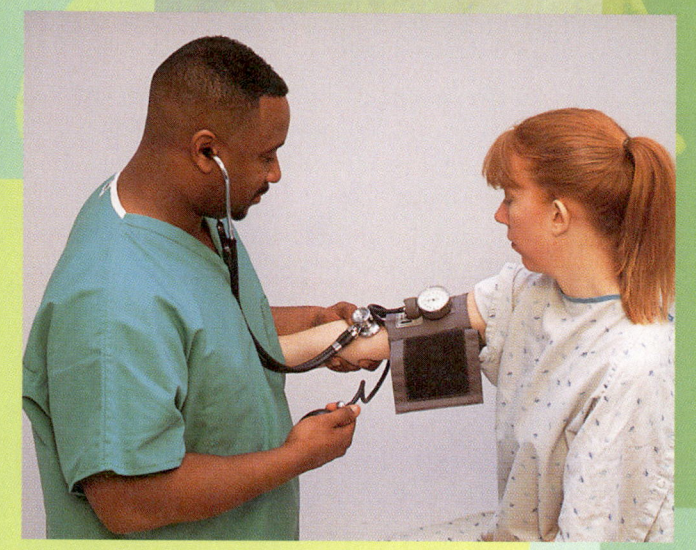

CHAPTER 6

HEALTH CARE ISSUES AND REPRODUCTIVE CONCERNS

A more comprehensive view of women's health has recently emerged, which includes not only reproductive health conditions but also other health conditions that affect women over the life span. These health conditions include those that affect both men and women, such as cardiovascular disease, although these diseases may affect women differently than men. Use the following questions to examine your personal feelings.

- Are women my age likely to live longer than men?
- Are women likely to be healthier in later years than men?
- Is there anything wrong with women taking drugs for which efficacy was based on research that included only male subjects?
- Are more women apt to die from breast cancer or heart disease?
- Am I doing all I can to help women reduce their risk of breast cancer, lung cancer, heart disease, and HIV infection?

Key Terms

Amenorrhea
Birth rate
Cancer
Carcinoma in situ
Cervical infection
Dysfunctional uterine
bleeding (DUB)
Dysmenorrhea
Endometriosis
Estrogen deficiency
vulvovaginitis
False discharge
Fertility rate
Fibroadenoma
Fibrocystic changes
Fibroid tumor
Health promotion
Health protection
Invasive breast cancer
Invasive cancer
Lactation discharge
Life expectancy
Localized breast cancer
Mastectomy

Menopause
Metastatic breast cancer
Morbidity rate
Mortality rate
Nipple discharge
Osteoporosis
Pap smear
Pathologic discharge
Pelvic inflammatory
disease (PID)
Pelvic relaxation
Physiologic discharge
Polycystic ovary
syndrome
Premenstrual syndrome
(PMS)
Primary amenorrhea
Primary dysmenorrhea
Screening
Secondary amenorrhea
Secondary
dysmenorrhea
Vaginal infection

Competencies

Upon completion of this chapter, the reader should be able to:

1. Discuss the historical perspective of women's health in the United States.
2. Describe the leading causes of death (mortality) and disease (morbidity) in women from childhood to old age.
3. Discuss the factors that put women at an increased risk of death and disease over the life span and describe methods of health promotion, disease prevention, and screening.
4. Describe subjective and objective data, laboratory test results, and procedure result data for women's reproductive health conditions.
5. Discuss usual therapeutic interventions for women's reproductive health conditions.
6. Identify risk factors for woman's reproductive health conditions.
7. Discuss the nursing process steps appropriate for each woman's reproductive health condition.

Women's health care has become a priority in the United States in the last two decades. This is evidenced by consumer activism and major commitment by governmental agencies, research institutions, and service delivery systems to redefine women's health care, expand the research focus on women's health issues, and implement expanded prevention and intervention programs. Women with different ethnic, cultural, and religious backgrounds have unique health beliefs and behaviors that affect their overall health status.

HISTORICAL PERSPECTIVE OF WOMEN'S HEALTH

Until recently, there was no such entity as women's health care. Women received care as adults who happened to have additional health conditions relating to childbearing and diseases of the reproductive system. This care relied primarily on a disease model in which diagnosis and treatment of reproductive health problems were the focus. Little attention was given to prevention, health promotion, risk factors, and nonreproductive health conditions of women across the life span, including the years before or after the reproductive years.

History of Reproductive Health Care in the United States

Historically, women's health care revolved around reproduction. Women's gynecologic health care was focused on women of reproductive and postmenopausal age, involving primarily birth control, pregnancy, delivery, infertility, and conditions of the reproductive system.

Over the centuries, midwives provided most reproductive care. Women, through experience and handed-down knowledge, cared for women in their community during pregnancy and childbirth. In the United States, midwifery was a respected profession until the mid-1800s. At about that time, the profession of medicine became better organized, and care of pregnant women became the province of physicians, most of whom were men. Physicians considered midwives ignorant and unskilled because they received no formal education. In the late 1800s and early 1900s, the medical community, in many states, convinced public health authorities that midwifery should be abandoned. The medical profession blamed immigrant midwives for the high maternal and infant mortality rate of the immigrant population. The medical profession's rejection of midwifery denied poor women access to reproductive health care.

Women did not enter the profession of medicine in any great numbers until the late 1970s. It was not until the 1990s that women entered medical school in about the same proportion as men. Concurrent with the increase in enrollment of women in medical schools was the demand for an expanded concept of women's health, a resurgence of the profession of midwifery, expansion of the role of nursing, and support for advanced practice nurses to provide primary health care. In addition, many individuals, groups, and organizations were effective in increasing the focus of the scientific community on women's health. Some of these included the National Women's Health Network, the Society for the Advancement of Women's Health Research, and the Boston Women's Health Book Collective.

Today, women's health care is provided by a broad array of health disciplines, including nursing, medicine, public health, social work, and midwifery. While preventive health care has been viewed as important to the overall health and welfare of society for the past 30 years, little focus has been on women's preventive health care issues until the present.

Current View of Women's Health Care

A newer view of women's health covers the life span. The foundation for the physical and emotional health of adult women begins in childhood. Gender differences in diet, exercise, values, and roles have an impact on the biologic and psychological development of women. Diet and exercise affect bone density, growth, and body image in later life. Values and roles affect health-seeking behaviors, economic status, prevention behaviors, nutrition and exercise habits, and fertility rates. **Fertility rate** is defined as the number of births per 1,000 women, ages 15 to 44. Educational level affects socioeconomic status, self-esteem, and access to care. Given a normal life expectancy, one-third of a woman's life is lived after menopause. **Life expectancy** is defined as the average number of years for which a group of individuals of the same age is expected to live. Health

status after menopause is affected not only by the previous biologic factors but also by psychological development, sociocultural environment, and economic status. Many reproductive and gynecologic issues are intrinsically related to biologic factors. Social roles, economic level, race, culture, psychological development, and religious beliefs also affect biologic factors.

Sensitivity to gender issues, racial and cultural backgrounds, sexual orientations, personality types, marital status, economic status, patterns of risk-taking behaviors, genetic and environmental risk factors, and age are now considered essential to providing comprehensive health care to women. A newer approach to women's health includes health promotion and health protection throughout the life span (Foster, 1994). **Health promotion** includes consideration of adequate nutrition intake, development and maintenance of physical fitness, development and use of stress management skills, attainment and maintenance of optimal bone density, and avoidance of hazardous substances, including tobacco, alcohol, and drugs (Figure 6-1). **Health protection** includes provision of safe childbearing through adequate prenatal and postnatal care, safe delivery, and effective family planning for child spacing and desired family size; it also includes prevention, early diagnosis, and appropriate treatment for infections, cancer, cardiovascular and respiratory disease, diabetes, and other chronic illnesses (Foster, 1994).

Women's health encompasses conditions that are not specific to the reproduction system, including those found in both men and women, but which may be expressed differently in women. Some diseases, such as osteoporosis, occur more frequently in women than in men. Some

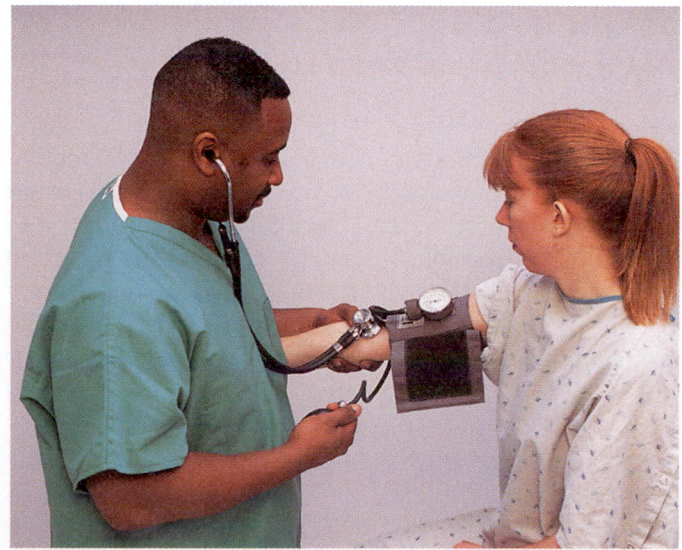

Figure 6-1   Health promotion for women of all ages includes regular physical exams.

diseases, such as HIV infection, historically occurred more frequently in men, but manifest differently in women; some diseases, such as heart disease, occur commonly in both genders but manifest differently in women (Cohen, 1997).

Sociocultural Influences

Women's health concerns reflect the diversity of women's cultural, economic, and physical environments, which affect the duration and quality of life. Unfortunately, women continue to experience serious threats to their physical and mental well-being. Despite living an average of 6 years longer than men, women have poorer health and greater disability from disease than men (U.S. Census Bureau, 1999). Women who live in poverty and are poorly educated have shorter life spans, higher rates of illness and death, and more limited access to health care services. The majority of single heads of households in the United States are women, putting them at a greater risk for poverty. Women, in general, have greater problems obtaining access to primary health care, and have a poorer quality of life with more acute symptoms, chronic conditions, and disabilities from health problems than do men (Wentz, 1994).

A positive factor influencing women's health care is the growing number of women who are developing political power and consumer interest in changing national policy regarding women's health. Women have become more involved in promoting reproductive choices, which give them control over their bodies and life choices. The availability of the birth control pill in the 1960s gave women the power to make their own choices about when to have children. Today, more women are demanding participation in health care decisions on an individual level and in health care policy at local, state, and national levels.

National Response to Women's Health Issues

In the last 20 years, a variety of federal agencies responded to the national concern that women's health issues were not being adequately addressed. In 1986, the National Institutes of Health (NIH) established a policy to encourage inclusion of women in clinical trials. The major reason women were previously excluded was the potential risk to the fetus if the woman became pregnant while participating in a study, or unknown risks for subsequent pregnancies.

In 1990, NIH created the Office of Research on Women's Health (ORWH) in response to public demand. The ORWH was established to strengthen and enhance the prevention, diagnosis, and treatment of illness in women and to enhance research related to diseases and conditions that affect women.

In 1992, the NIH undertook the Women's Health Initiative, which is a 15-year study of major diseases and conditions, including heart disease, stroke, breast cancer, colon and rectal cancer, depression, and osteoporosis, in a sample of 160,000 postmenopausal women at 45 centers across the country. This is the largest clinical study ever undertaken in the United States, with $625 million appropriated for the initiative. The Women's Health Initiative includes three major types of study:

1. Surveillance study to identify specific risk factors for disease

2. Clinical trial, involving 45,000 individuals, to study the role of diet modification and hormone replacement therapy in the prevention of cardiovascular diseases, cancer, and osteoporosis

3. Prevention study, carried out in 60 communities, to determine effective methods for incorporation of health-promoting behaviors

The Women's Health Initiative provided recognition that women have many nonreproductive years of life, during which they are at great risk for cardiovascular disease, cancer, osteoporosis, and depression. This is the first major study that recognized that heart disease is the leading cause of death for women and that heart disease develops later in life in women than in men. The study's premise is that understanding the role of risk factors for cancer, osteoporosis, and cardiovascular disease will provide future treatment recommendations for the care of women who are postmenopausal (National Institutes of Health, 1994).

Nursing Tip

The Mission and Mandate of the Office of Research on Women's Health

- Increase research into diseases, disorders, and conditions that affect women.

- Establish a research agenda for NIH for the future directions in women's health research

- Ensure that women are included in NIH-supported research.

- Support the advancement of women in biomedical careers.

Note. Adapted from the Office of Research on Women's Health. *ORWH's Mandate.* Retrieved July 16, 2003, from http://www4.od.nih.gov/orwh/overview.html

DEMOGRAPHIC DATA FOR AMERICAN WOMEN

The overall health of both men and women has improved in the 20th century. Life expectancy has increased for both genders, with life expectancy of women exceeding that of men. A century ago, many women died during their reproductive years from complications of childbearing and infections. Advancements in maternity care, immunizations, antibiotic therapy, public sanitation, and biomedicine have been major factors in increasing the life expectancy of women. It is estimated that, in the 21st century, the life expectancy for both genders will continue to increase (Table 6-1). Longevity will result from technological advances and more effective prevention and treatment of acute and chronic disease. Research on the biology of aging, including the study of the cellular aging process, may increase life expectancy in the future. As women live longer, chronic conditions that affect older women will be more prevalent. Health care providers and delivery systems must be prepared for the increased numbers of women needing preventive and restorative care in the future. See Table 6-2 for a breakdown by race and gender.

Population Shift

As the baby boom generation (persons born between 1946 and 1964) reaches age 65, there will be major economic and sociologic changes, resulting in increased demands for health care, fewer workers to support the Medicare program, a large aging population, and an increased interest in healthy living. A major proportion of this generation will be made up of women, who will live longer than men but not necessarily healthier. Women significantly outnumber men in the over-age-65 group because premature deaths are almost twice as high for men in earlier decades

Table 6-1	Projections of Life Expectancy for People Born 2000–2010					
	CAUCASIAN (YRS)		AFRICAN AMERICAN (YRS)		ALL OTHER RACES (YRS)	
YEAR	FEMALE	MALE	FEMALE	MALE	FEMALE	MALE
2000	80.5	74.2	74.7	64.6	77.5	68.3
2005	81.0	74.7	75.0	64.5	78.1	69.1
2010	81.6	75.5	75.5	65.1	78.7	69.9

Note. Adapted from Table No. 118, Statistical Abstract of the United States, 1996.

Table 6-2	Life Expectancy: in Years, by Race, Sex, and Age, 1998					
	ALL RACES		CAUCASIAN		AFRICAN AMERICAN	
AGE	FEMALE	MALE	FEMALE	MALE	FEMALE	MALE
At Birth	79.5	73.8	80.0	74.5	74.8	67.6
10	70.2	64.6	70.6	65.2	66.6	59.0
20	60.3	55.0	60.8	55.5	56.2	49.5
30	50.6	45.7	51.0	46.1	46.7	40.6
40	41.1	36.4	41.4	36.8	37.5	31.9
50	31.8	27.6	32.0	27.9	28.8	23.9
60	23.2	19.6	23.3	19.7	21.0	17.1
70	15.5	12.8	15.6	12.8	14.1	11.5
80	9.2	7.5	9.1	7.5	8.7	7.1
85 & over	6.7	5.5	6.6	5.4	6.6	5.5

Note. Adapted from Table No. 5, *National Vital Statistics Report*, Vol. 48, No. 11, July 24, 2000.

than for women. Men die in earlier years as a result of motor vehicle accidents, homicides, suicides, heart attacks, and AIDS (CDC, 2000). This results in a higher age-adjusted mortality rate for males than females. This trend has been observed throughout the 20th century and results in approximately 70% of persons over age 85 being women (U.S. Census Bureau, 1999). The major shift in the population is the increasing number of elderly women.

Race and Ethnicity

Ethnic and racial diversity has varied over time in the United States. In the early 1990s, approximately 84% of the women living in the United States were Caucasian, 13% were Black, 8% were Hispanic, and 3% were of other races. Projections indicate a continuing change in racial diversity over time, with increases in Black and Hispanic populations. The National Center for Health Statistics (NCHS, 1992) reported that the number of babies born to Hispanic women reached record highs; births to Hispanic women comprised 18% of the total births across the nation in 1995. This increase in births is the result of high fertility rates among Hispanics, particularly recent immigrants. The increased Hispanic birth rate contrasts with birth rates of other groups that have been stable or have declined (NCHS, 1998). **Birth rate** is defined as the number of births per 1,000 population.

Employment

Historically, there have always been more men than women in the labor force. However, in the last several decades, more women are participating in the labor force than ever before in the history of the United States. In 1976, 31% of women with infants under age 1 were in the labor force. In 1998, 59% of women with infants under 1 one year were working outside the home (U.S. Census Bureau, 2000).

Men earn more than women, even when men and women work in the same occupations. Women earn between 60% and 80% of what men in comparable positions earn, regardless of race and ethnicity, although this gap appears to be closing in some areas. The same disparity exists at all levels of education for women. Black and Hispanic women earn less than Caucasian, Black, and Hispanic men.

Education

The more education, the better the health status, for both men and women. Education has an important influence on socioeconomic status. The overall trend in the United States reflects a more educated population, with the younger population being more educated than the older population (USCB, 1999). The percentages of high school completion vary by race. Among Caucasians, 87.7% had earned high school degrees or higher; among Blacks, 77.4% among non-Hispanic Asian and Pacific Islanders, 84.7%, and among Hispanics, 56.1% (U.S. Census Bureau, 1999).

Since 1970, there has been a steady increase in the number of women who have completed college. In 1970, 8.1% of women completed college compared to 19.3% in 1993. However, there is great variation among racial groups. In 1993, Asian women were most likely to be college-educated, 27% of whom had college educations in comparison to 12.4% Black women and 8.5% Hispanic women.

Since education is positively associated with health status, persons who have not completed at least high school are at higher risk for poor health. Lower levels of education are seen in conjunction with poorer nutrition, decreased access to health care, and increased likelihood of risk behaviors, such as smoking.

Marital Status

Both men and women are marrying later in life. The median for first marriages is rising to 24.8 for women and 27.1 for men (U.S. Census Bureau, 2003). In 1950, the marriage rate was 11.1 per 1,000 population as compared to 9.9 in 1999 (USDHHS, 2000b). As the marriage rate has decreased, the divorce rate has increased from 2.6 per 1,000 in 1950 to 4.1 in 1999 (USDHHS, 2000b). This leaves many women in the position of being a single parent.

Fertility and Birth Rates

The fertility rates of women in the United States have declined from 87.9 per 1,000 women in 1970 to 65.9 per 1,000 in 1999 (National Vital Statistics Report, 2000). The overall birth rate has decreased from 24.1 in 1950 to 14.5 in 1999 (USDHHS, 2000b).

Trends in childbearing differ among women of various ages and are reflected in age-specific birth rates. Women are having children later in life than before. There has been

Nursing Tip   *Current Reasons Women Delay Childbirth*

- Ability to control the timing of childbirth through the use of contraception
- Establishing careers before having children
- Marrying later in life
- Availability of modern technology to enhance fertility

an increase in the birth rate for women aged 30 to 34 (U.S. Census Bureau, 1999). Clearly there has been a trend toward more women giving birth later, when they are in their 30s and 40s.

Birth Rates for Adolescent Mothers

Birth rates for adolescent mothers rose from 1980 to a high in 1992 and have dropped steadily since then. The Centers for Disease Control and Prevention (CDC, 2002) reported that in 1997 there had been a decrease in sexual intercourse by teenagers from 1990 to 1995. About 50% of teenagers ages 15 to 19 reported that they had never had sexual intercourse in 1995 compared with 55% in 1990. This is consistent with the downward trend in the birth rate for teen mothers between 1990 and 1999.

Birth Rates for Unmarried Women

Births to unmarried women in the United States have dramatically increased, from a total of 399,000 in 1970 to 1,260,000 in 1996 (U.S. Census Bureau, 1999). Births to unmarried adolescents ages 15 to 19 have also increased although the rate declined from 14.1 per 1,000 in 2001 to 13.9 in 2002 (CDC, 2003). There has been a dramatic increase in the number of births to women age 20 and older. This is because of the increase in the proportion of women in the population over age 20.

Unmarried mothers and their children are of concern. Statistically, they are at greater risk for poverty, limited education, poor health, and social problems, such as dropping out of school, behavior problems, and delinquency. Unmarried women under age 25 are at greater risk than their married counterparts as a result of living below the poverty line, not completing high school, having poorer health, and having less access to care.

MORTALITY AND MORBIDITY

One way to measure the health of the nation or subgroups within the population is to examine mortality and morbidity data. **Mortality rate** refers to the total number of deaths in a population over a specific period of time. **Morbidity rate** refers to the total number of persons in a population who currently have a specific disease or condition.

Leading Causes of Death

The leading causes of death for both men and women in the United States according to the U.S. Census Bureau (1999) are illustrated in Table 6-3.

More men than women die from cancer, COPD, accidents, suicide, and chronic liver disease. More women die from cerebrovascular disease, pneumonia, diabetes, and nephritis (U.S. Census Bureau, 1999).

Table 6-3   Leading Causes of Deaths for Females and Males, 1998

CAUSE OF DEATH	DEATHS PER 100,000 POPULATION		
	BOTH SEXES	FEMALE	MALE
All causes	864.7	853.5	876.4
Heart disease	268.2	268.3	268.0
Cancer	200.3	189.7	213.6
Stroke	58.6	70.4	46.3
COPD	41.7	40.2	43.2
Accidents	36.2	25.2	47.7
Pneumonia	34.0	36.8	31.0
Diabetes	24.0	25.4	22.4
Suicide	11.3	(NA)	18.6
Nephritis	9.7	9.9	(NA)
Chronic liver disease	9.3	(NA)	12.4

Note. Adapted from Table No. 8, N*ational Vital Statistics Report*, Vol. No. 11, July 24, 2000.

Cardiovascular Disease

Cardiovascular disease is the leading cause of death for both men and women in the United States. Approximately one of every two female deaths in the United States results from cardiovascular diseases. Forty-nine percent of women die within 1 year of a heart attack compared with 31% of men. This may be because cardiovascular disease presents differently in women than in men and is not recognized by health care providers when an emergency situation occurs. Even though there has been a major reduction in the number of deaths from heart disease in the United States, heart disease remains the major overall health problem facing women today.

Even though cardiovascular disease is the leading cause of death for both sexes, there has been a decrease in deaths from cardiovascular disease in the past three decades. There are more than three times more deaths from heart disease than from breast and lung cancer combined (National Vital Statistics Report, 2000).

The prevalence of heart disease increases as women age. The increased risk for cardiovascular disease in women may be the result of the decrease in estrogen at menopause. The prevalence increases to one in three at age 65 and older. Cardiovascular disease typically develops in women 10 to 15 years later than in men. The risk of coronary artery disease for younger women is less than for men the same age, but as women age, mortality from heart disease increases. By age 75, the incidence of heart disease is essentially the same in both sexes. The prevalence of

Nursing Tip
Preventing Cardiovascular Disease

- Quit smoking
- Follow a low-fat, low-cholesterol diet
- Exercise at least three times per week
- Maintain a normal body weight
- Have periodic blood pressure checks

heart disease varies by race and ethnicity. For both men and women, Blacks have a higher death rate from cardiovascular disease than Caucasians (USDHHS 2000a).

There has been pervasive inattention by both health care providers and women themselves to the importance of cardiovascular disease in women. Women tend to fear having a heart attack less than having breast cancer. Women who have heart attacks are twice as likely as men to die because they lack access to appropriate medical care, are less aware of symptoms that could be related to

cardiovascular disease, and are not provided with appropriate medical interventions.

Stroke is the third leading cause of death for women. It kills more than twice as many women annually as breast cancer. Stroke and heart disease cause almost twice as many deaths in women than all types of cancer combined (USDHHS, 2000a).

Cancer

Cancer is uncontrolled growth or spread of abnormal cells resulting from malfunction of genes that control cell growth and cell division (American Cancer Society [ACS], 2000). The majority of cancerous diseases result from gene mutation; heredity accounts for only 5% to 10% of cancers (ACS, 2000). Cancer is the second leading cause of death for both men and women living in the United States; one of every four deaths results from cancer. However, when specific age groups are considered, cancer is the leading cause of death in women ages 25 to 64 but not in men. Mortality and morbidity rates vary according to gender (Figure 6-2).

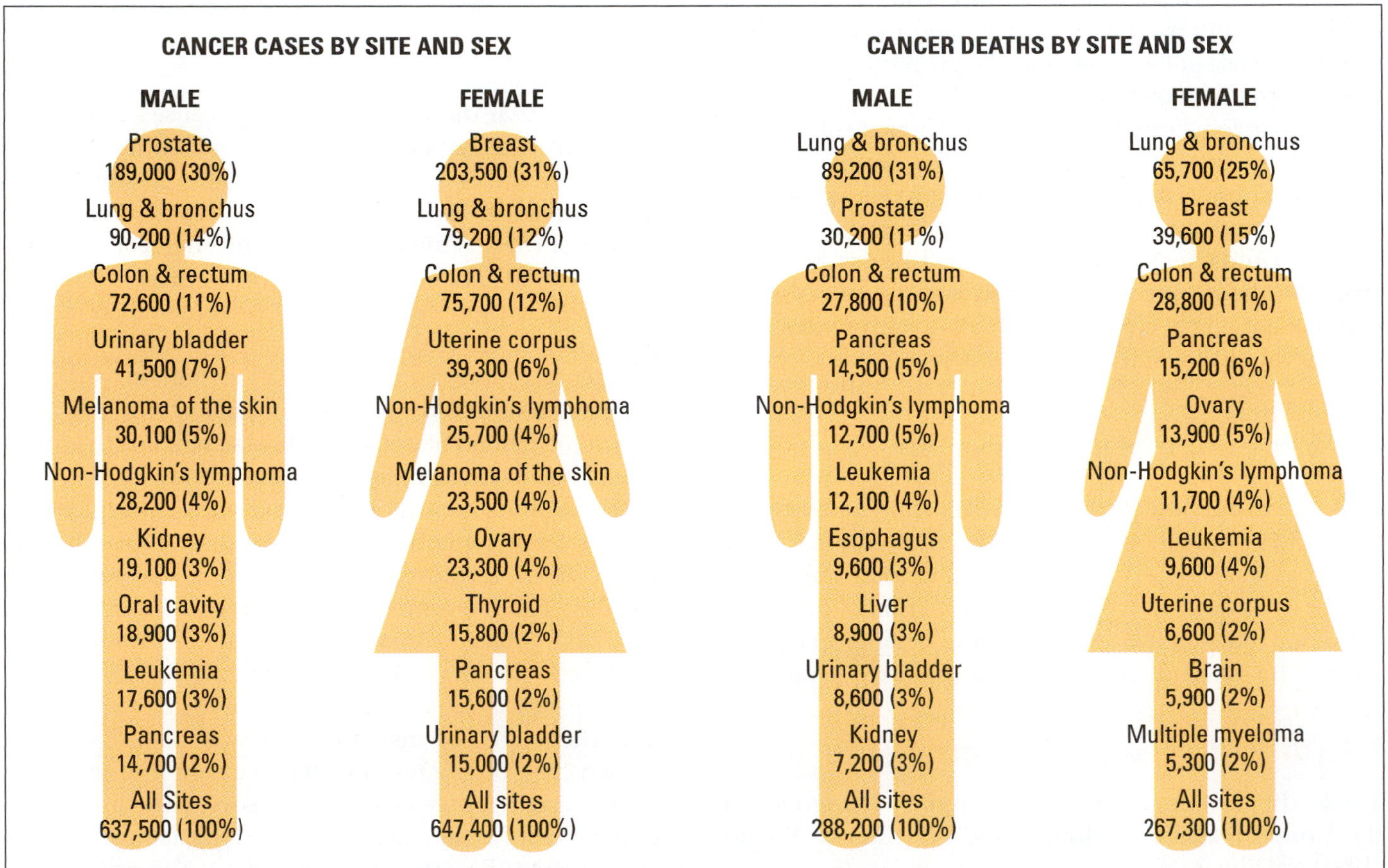

CANCER CASES BY SITE AND SEX

MALE	FEMALE
Prostate 189,000 (30%)	Breast 203,500 (31%)
Lung & bronchus 90,200 (14%)	Lung & bronchus 79,200 (12%)
Colon & rectum 72,600 (11%)	Colon & rectum 75,700 (12%)
Urinary bladder 41,500 (7%)	Uterine corpus 39,300 (6%)
Melanoma of the skin 30,100 (5%)	Non-Hodgkin's lymphoma 25,700 (4%)
Non-Hodgkin's lymphoma 28,200 (4%)	Melanoma of the skin 23,500 (4%)
Kidney 19,100 (3%)	Ovary 23,300 (4%)
Oral cavity 18,900 (3%)	Thyroid 15,800 (2%)
Leukemia 17,600 (3%)	Pancreas 15,600 (2%)
Pancreas 14,700 (2%)	Urinary bladder 15,000 (2%)
All Sites 637,500 (100%)	All sites 647,400 (100%)

CANCER DEATHS BY SITE AND SEX

MALE	FEMALE
Lung & bronchus 89,200 (31%)	Lung & bronchus 65,700 (25%)
Prostate 30,200 (11%)	Breast 39,600 (15%)
Colon & rectum 27,800 (10%)	Colon & rectum 28,800 (11%)
Pancreas 14,500 (5%)	Pancreas 15,200 (6%)
Non-Hodgkin's lymphoma 12,700 (5%)	Ovary 13,900 (5%)
Leukemia 12,100 (4%)	Non-Hodgkin's lymphoma 11,700 (4%)
Esophagus 9,600 (3%)	Leukemia 9,600 (4%)
Liver 8,900 (3%)	Uterine corpus 6,600 (2%)
Urinary bladder 8,600 (3%)	Brain 5,900 (2%)
Kidney 7,200 (3%)	Multiple myeloma 5,300 (2%)
All sites 288,200 (100%)	All sites 267,300 (100%)

*Excludes basal and sqamous cell skin cancers and in situ carcinoma except urinary bladder.
Percentages may not total 100% due to rounding

©2002, American Cancer Society, Inc., Surveillance Research

Figure 6-2 Leading sites of new cancer cases and deaths—2002 estimates. (Reprinted from *American Cancer Society Cancer Facts and Figures, 2002*)

Client Education

Recommendations for Early Cancer Detection

● Tell clients that persons ages 20 to 40 should have a cancer-related checkup every 3 years, and clients over age 40 should be seen yearly. Examination should include counseling as well as examinations of the thyroid, lymph nodes, and skin.

● Encourage women age 40 and older to have a mammogram and a clinical breast examination each year. Women ages 20 to 39 should have a clinical breast examination every 3 years.

● Teach clients how to perform a breast self-examination.

● Provide breast self-examination information (appropriate for age, language, and culture of client).

● Teach your client the appropriate time of month for breast self-examination.

● Explain to the client that people age 50 and older should be screened for colorectal cancer every 5 to 10 years (depending on the recommendation of their physician).

● Inform all sexually active women and women age 18 and older of the importance of having an annual pelvic examination and Pap smear.

● Explain to your client what to expect during a pelvic examination, particularly before your client's first pelvic examination.

● Encourage your client to schedule routine office visits for screening.

● Schedule an appointment with your client to reinforce the discussion of the importance of follow-up for early cancer detection and breast self-examination (ACS, 2000).

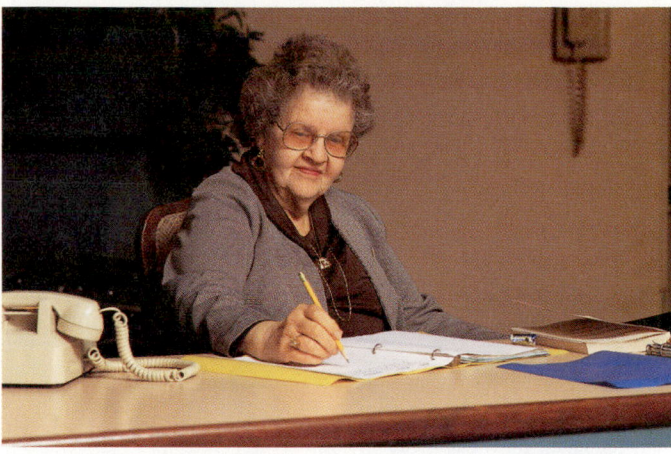

Figure 6-3 Nearly 4/5 of all cancer cases occur in adults over the age of 55.

because of the decrease in male lung cancer rates. As people get older, their cancer risk increases. Americans aged 55 and older receive nearly 80% of all cancer diagnoses (ACS, 2000) (Figure 6-3). Some inroads in prevention and health promotion have been made, which reduces mortality rates. Some of these include reduction in tobacco use, diet modification, cancer screening procedures, and progress in treatment based on research (Wingo et al., 1998).

Lung Cancer

Since 1985, lung cancer has been the leading cause of cancer death among women in the United States. Over the past 30 years, the lung cancer death rate among American women has increased nearly 400%, almost exclusively from cigarette smoking. From 1992 to 1996, mortality rates from lung cancer decreased significantly in men (down 1.7% per year), but rates for women increased (up 0.9% per year) (ACS, 2000). The dramatic increase in smoking among women has caused lung cancer to surpass breast cancer as a cause of death in women. Since 1987, more women have died from lung cancer than breast cancer, which was the major cancer killer of women for more than 40 years (ACS, 2000).

The death rate for lung cancer has risen despite medical advances and early diagnosis, which may be related to women lagging behind men in quitting smoking. Lung cancer symptoms of persistent cough, chest pain, bronchitis, sputum with bloody streaks, and recurring pneumonia usually do not appear until the advanced stages of the disease (Figure 6-4). An additional concern is the increasing use of tobacco among youth. Teenage girls' smoking rates have increased from 27% to 37% between 1991 and 1997 (USDHHS, 2000b). Lung cancer from smoking is the most preventable cause of death today (ACS, 2000). Tobacco use in the United States causes the death of nearly one in every five Americans.

Breast cancer rates increased significantly from 1973 to 1990 but were level from 1990 to 1995. Death rates for the four major cancers (lung, breast, prostate, and colorectal) decreased significantly from 1990 to 1995 (Wingo, Ries, Rosenberg, Miller, & Edwards, 1998). The decline in mortality rates was greater in men than women, largely

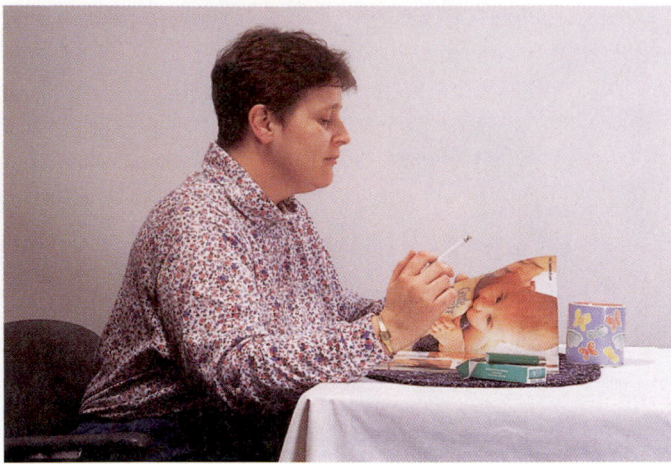

Figure 6-4   Lung cancer is the leading cause of cancer death in women.

The following facts can be used to educate clients:

■ People who cease to smoke, regardless of age, live longer than people who continue to smoke.

■ Smokers who cease to smoke before age 50 have half the risk of dying within the next 15 years compared with those who continue to smoke.

■ Smoking cessation substantially decreases the risk of lung, laryngeal, esophageal, oral, pancreatic, bladder, and cervical cancers.

■ Smoking cessation lowers the risk for other major diseases, such as coronary heart disease and cardiovascular disease.

Nurses and other health care providers have both the opportunity and the means to help clients modify smoking behavior.

Breast Cancer

Breast cancer is the second most prevalent cancer in women. The American Cancer Society estimates that one of every eight women in the United States will develop breast cancer during her lifetime (American Cancer Society, 2000). This method of computing risk assumes that every woman has an equal chance for breast cancer and

Client Education

Smoking Cessation

● Obtain smoking history from every client regardless of the reason for health care.

● Encourage every client who smokes to stop smoking.

● Identify benefits of smoking cessation.

● Identify risks of smoking.

● Help the client set a specific date to stop smoking.

● Schedule follow-up visits with the client to reinforce cessation.

● Provide smoking cessation literature that is appropriate for age, language, and culture.

● Develop appropriate collection of literature for client population served and knowledge of community smoking cessation programs.

● Reinforce advice to the client by arranging for other health care providers to also counsel the client.

● Chart smoking history and counseling given at each client visit.

● Provide access to nicotine patch or other products to reduce nicotine addiction.

Nursing Alert

The American Cancer Society's Recommendations for Early Detection of Breast Cancer

● Women over age 40 should have a breast screening mammogram every year.

● Between the ages of 20 and 39, women should have a breast examination by a health provider every 3 years and every year after age 40.

● Women age 20 and older should perform breast self-examinations every month.

● If any changes in breast tissue are noted (lumps, swelling, dimpling, skin changes, redness, or nipple discharge), a health provider should be contacted immediately.

● Discuss any new changes in breast tissue with a health provider.

Note. From *Cancer Facts and Figures—2000*, by the American Cancer Society, 2000, Atlanta, GA: Author.

that every woman will live to be 110 years old; therefore, the risk cited can be misleading. The chance of developing breast cancer for an average 40-year-old woman is 1 in 1,000. The risk increases as women get older. In 1998 it was projected there would be 178,700 new cases of invasive breast cancer and 43,500 deaths from breast cancer (ACS, 1998). Incidence of new cases of breast cancer increased by about 4% per year during the 1980s but has leveled off in recent years. The increase in new cases was attributed in part to the earlier detection of breast cancer through increased use of breast self-examination (Figure 6-5), clinical breast examination, and diagnostic screenings, including mammography (NCHS, 1992).

The incidence of breast cancer is highest in Caucasian women (113.2 per 100,000) and lowest among Native American women (11.6 per 100,000).

Mortality rates continue to decline with the largest decrease occurring in younger women. These decreases have occurred in both Caucasian and Black women. These decreases are likely due to earlier detection and improved treatment (ACS, 2000). Mammography is the best method for early detection of breast cancer and has attributed to

Client Education

Breast Self-Examination (Recommendations of the American Cancer Society)

By regularly examining her own breasts, a woman is likely to notice any changes that occur. The best time for breast self-examination (BSE) is about a week after your period ends, when your breasts are not tender or swollen. If you are not having regular periods, do BSE on the same day every month. Women who are pregnant, breast-feeding, or have breast implants also need to do regular BSE.

Lying Down

- Lie down with a pillow under your right shoulder and place your right arm behind your head (Figure 6-5 A).
- Use the finger pads of the three middle fingers on your left hand to feel for lumps in the right breast.
- Press firmly enough to know how your breast feels. A firm ridge in the lower curve of each breast is normal. If you're not sure how hard to press, talk with your doctor or nurse.
- Move around the breast in a circular, up-and-down line or wedge pattern (Figure 6-5B). Be sure to do it the same way every time, check the entire breast area, and remember how your breast feels from month to month.
- Repeat the examination on your left breast, using the finger pads of the right hand. (Move the pillow to under your left shoulder.)

Standing Before a Mirror

- Repeat the examination of both breasts while standing, with your one arm behind your head (Figure 6-5C). The upright position makes it easier to check the upper and outer part of the breasts (toward your armpit). This is where about half of breast cancers are found. You may want to do the standing part of the BSE while you are in the shower. Some breast changes can be felt more easily when your skin is wet and soapy.
- Gently squeeze the nipple to check for discharge (Figure 6-5D).
- Repeat the examination on the alternate side.
- For added safety, you can check your breasts for any dimpling of the skin, changes in the nipple, redness, or swelling while standing in front of a mirror right after your BSE each month (Figure 6-5E).
- Raise your arms over your head to visualize the breast contour and the lower quadrants (Figure 6-5F).
- Place your hands on your hips and press inward to flex the pectoral muscles, which may enhance skin dimpling or puckering (Figure 6-5G).
- If you find any changes, see your health care provider right away.

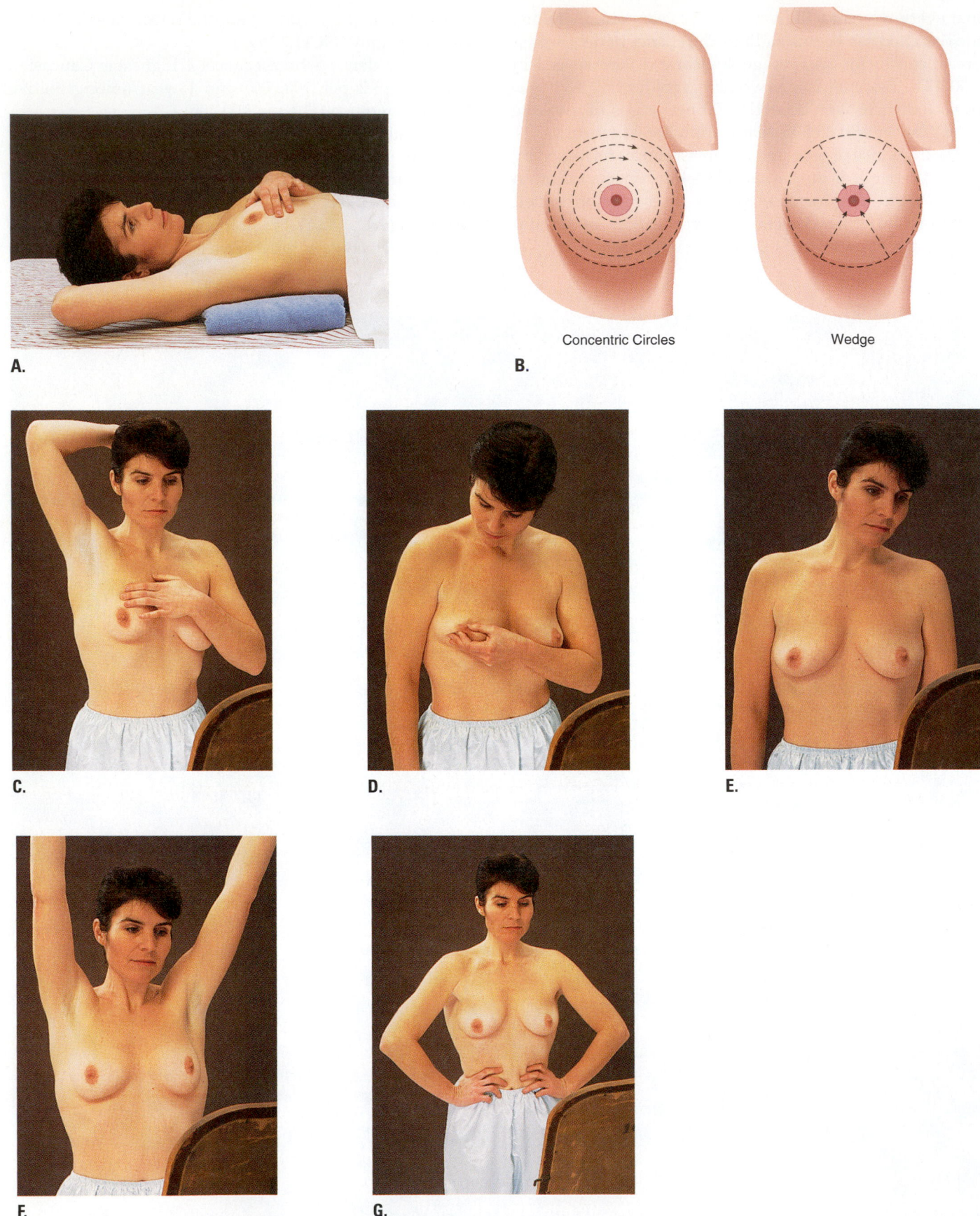

Concentric Circles   Wedge

A.

B.

C.

D.

E.

F.

G.

Figure 6-5   Breast Self-Examination.

Nursing Alert

Breast Cancer Risk Factors

- Family history of breast cancer (first-degree relative, i.e., mother, sister, daughter)

- Biopsy-confirmed atypical hyperplasia

- Early menarche (before age 12)

- Late menopause (after age 55)

- Recent use of oral contraceptives or post-menopausal estrogen therapy

- Never having children or having the first child after age 30

- High socioeconomic status and high level of education

- Alcohol consumption of more than 2 to 5 drinks per day

- Presence of *BRCA*-1 or *BRCA*-2 gene

Nursing Alert

Examining Nipple Discharge

If a client is found to have abnormal nipple discharge:

1. Wear gloves before proceeding with the assessment.
2. Note the following: color, consistency, amount of discharge, unilateral or bilateral, spontaneous, or provoked.
3. With a sterile, cotton-tipped swab, obtain a sample of the discharge so that a culture and sensitivity testing and Gram stain may be done.
4. Follow your institution's guidelines for sample preparation.

the decrease in breast cancer deaths due to early detection (Figure 6-6).

Breast self-examination is important for detecting physical signs and symptoms of breast cancer. Women can examine their own breasts to detect a breast lump,

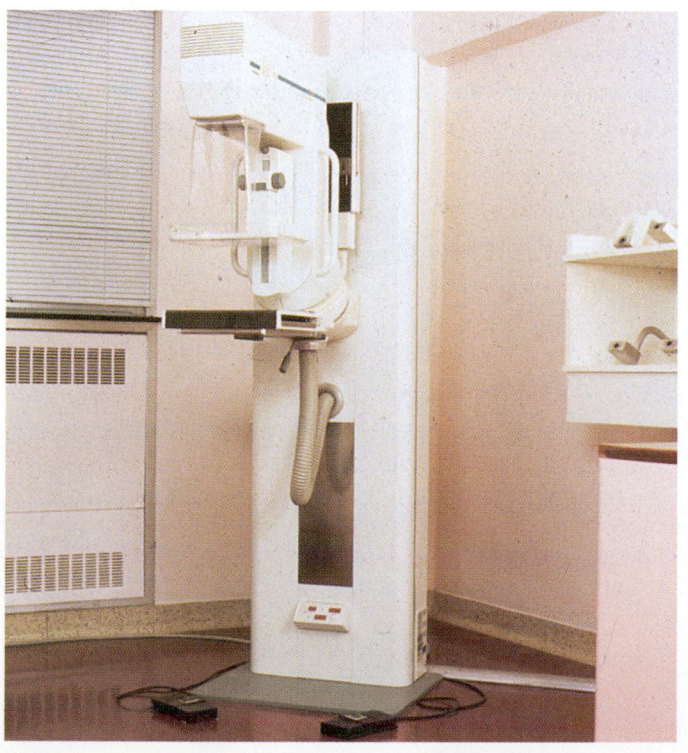

A.

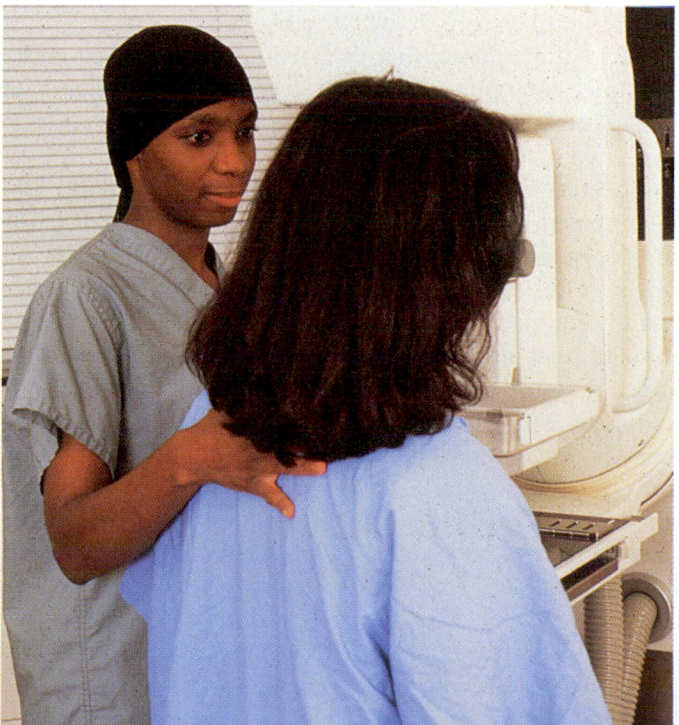

B.

Figure 6-6   A. Mammography unit. B. Client positioning for mammogram.

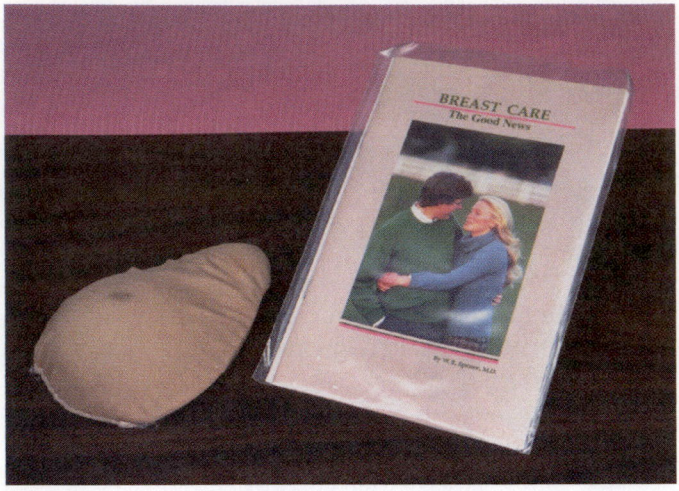

A.

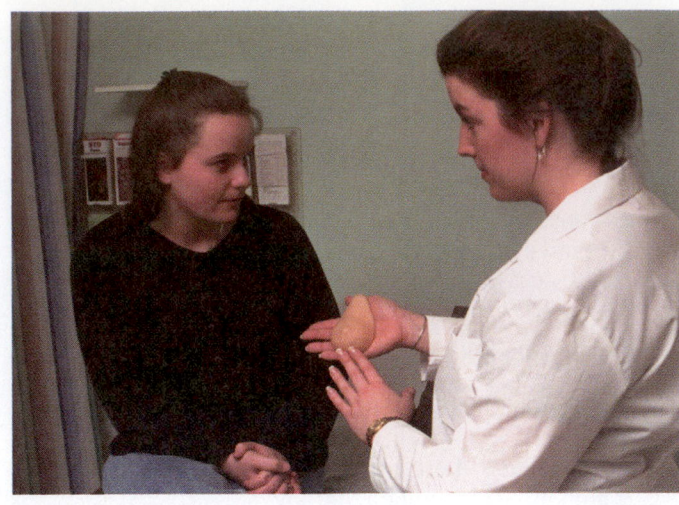

B.

Figure 6-7 A. Breast exam educational materials. B. Nurse teaching client breast exam techniques with a model.

swelling, distortion, dimpling, nipple pain, scaliness, or retraction (see Figure 6-7) (ACS, 2000). Many women experience breast pain or tenderness, which is often seen in conjunction with benign conditions of the breast. Breast pain is not normally the first symptom of breast cancer. The American Cancer Society recommends that women ages 20 to 39 have a clinical breast examination every 3 years and a monthly self-examination.

The risk of breast cancer rises as women age, most notably after age 40. Breast cancer occurs more frequently in Caucasian women over age 35 than in Black women of comparable age. Risk factors for breast cancer include personal or family history of breast cancer, biopsy-confirmed atypical hyperplasia, early menarche, late menopause, recent use of oral contraceptives or post-menopausal estrogens, never having children or having the first live birth at a late age, and a higher level of education and socioeconomic status (ACS, 1998). Other factors implicated in increased risk of breast cancer are alcohol use, high-fat diets, and exposure to chemical carcinogens. Some of the possible risk factors for breast cancer are amenable to lifestyle changes, such as poor diet, lack of exercise, and alcohol use. Because most of the established risk factors are not amenable to change through lifestyle or prevention strategies, the major focus has been on early detection and early treatment. A small percentage of breast cancers (1% to 5%) are associated with a genetic predisposition (genes *BRCA*-1, *BRCA*-2 and possibly other as yet unidentified genes).

Malignant Breast Conditions

Malignant breast conditions are life-threatening and life-altering, both emotionally and physically. In 2000, Johnson predicted, "An estimated 175,000 new cases of breast cancer among women will be diagnosed (in 2000), and 43,000 women will die of this disease." The primary risks for development of breast cancer are female gender and increasing age (Thomas & Greifzu, 2000).

Localized Breast Cancer

Localized breast cancer has not metastasized (spread), is usually less than 2 centimeters in size, is considered non-

Critical Thinking

Oral Contraceptives and Cancer Risk

There have been recent studies indicating a correlation between estrogen-based oral contraceptive use and breast cancer, with a two- to fourfold increased risk noted for some populations. During the breast assessment, the client asks you about the association between oral contraceptives and increased breast cancer risk because she is considering switching from oral contraceptives to another method of birth control. How would you respond?

invasive beyond the breast, and has potential for the best client outcome. The lower the stage of breast cancer at diagnosis, the better the outcome. According to the tumor, nodal involvement, and metastasis (TNM) method of staging cancer, localized ductal or lobar breast cancer meets the criteria for TNM stage 0 or stage 1. Stage 0 criteria include cancer in situ (localized), confined to the milk duct or the lobe, and with no occurrence of metastases. Stage 1 criteria include size less than 2 centimeters, infiltration to surrounding breast tissue, and no lymph node involvement (Thomas & Greifzu, 2000).

Management of localized breast cancer, in which the cancer is confined to one area, can include lumpectomy (to remove the tumor and a small amount of surrounding tissue) and radiation therapy. Adjacent lymph nodes may be removed. The woman is not a candidate for lumpectomy if she has more than one tumor, tumors in more than one quadrant of the breast, or diffuse calcifications; has had previous radiation therapy to the area; has large breasts; has a tumor located under the nipple; or has small breasts with a large tumor mass-to-breast mass ratio (Thomas & Greifzu, 2000).

Invasive Breast Cancer

Invasive breast cancer has extended beyond the local epithelium and has the potential to spread from the breast to other parts of the body. Invasive breast cancer meets TNM criteria for stages 2 and 3. TNM stage 2 criteria are size between 2 and 5 centimeters and tumor cells that have spread to adjacent axillary lymph nodes; stage 3A criteria include size less than 5 centimeters and fixed (attached to each other or to surrounding tissue) to adjacent axillary lymph nodes; and stage 3B criteria include tumor of any size; spread to the skin, chest wall, or mammary lymph nodes; and no metastases to distant organs (Thomas & Greifzu, 2000).

Management depends on the size of the tumor, involvement of lymph nodes, and type of tumor cells (positive or negative estrogen receptors). The usual treatment includes mastectomy, radiation, chemotherapy, or a combination of these. Adjuvant hormone therapy may be added to the treatment plan.

Metastatic Breast Cancer

Metastatic breast cancer is breast cancer that has spread to other parts of the body. It meets the criterion for TNM stage 4, which is metastasized tumors of any size (Thomas & Greifzu, 2000). Once metastases occur, there is no cure and life expectancy is short. Thus, therapeutic intervention is primarily supportive in nature.

Nursing Implications

Nursing assessment for breast conditions involves careful medical and gynecologic history taking, with special emphasis on breast history, including results and frequency of BSE, breast trauma, breast stimulation, and assessment for

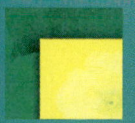

CASE STUDY/CARE PLAN
CLIENT WITH BREAST CANCER

A 51-year-old, single, woman visits a community women's health clinic with a chief complaint of a lump in her left breast. Client states, "I am afraid of cancer. I am afraid I will die." The woman wrings her hands, eyes dart back and forth and she looks toward her sister as if for help.

Physical examination reveals a 3 cm solid mass with an irregular, dimpled surface in the inner quadrant of the left breast in the 10 o'clock position. Mammography indicates a potentially malignant mass, and she is referred for biopsy. Biopsy reveals the mass is malignant, and a mastectomy is scheduled.

Assessment

- Nulliparity, sporadic practice of BSE, and sporadic use of the health care system.
- Mammography results indicate malignant breast cancer.
- Biopsy results document diagnosis of malignant breast neoplasm.

(continues)

Nursing Diagnosis

Fear related to breast cancer diagnosis.

Expected Outcomes   Client will:

1. Identify emotional feelings related to diagnosis of breast cancer.

2. Relate understanding of usual medical and surgical treatments for breast cancer.

3. Discuss perception of effect of mastectomy, radiotherapy, and chemotherapy on her life.

4. List coping strategies for incisional pain, radiation discomfort, and chemotherapy side effects.

Planning   The nurse must ensure that all information is presented at the client's level of understanding, with involvement of family and support persons as needed or appropriate.

NOC   Anxiety control

NIC   Anxiety reduction

Nursing Interventions	Rationales
1. Discuss client's emotional feelings regarding breast cancer diagnosis. Facilitate client's use of support system. Refer client to local breast cancer support group.	1. Acknowledging client's feelings is supportive of her emotional response and demonstrates caring and a concerned attitude. Diagnosis of breast cancer is a shock, and she will need a support system to help her cope. The local breast cancer support group has volunteers who have experienced breast cancer and support clients through all stages of the grieving, treatment, and recovery phases.
2. Explain the anticipated level of discomfort, physical sensations, anticipatory grieving, procedures, and outcome for mastectomy (loss of breast, removal of lymph nodes), radiotherapy (fatigue, itching or peeling skin).	2. Information facilitates understanding and acceptance of condition; anticipatory guidance reduces fear.
3. Discuss client's perception of the effect of mastectomy, radiotherapy, and chemotherapy on her life (e.g., job, family, friends).	3. Women's perception affects planning and compliance.
4. Describe potential coping strategies for incisional pain (pain medication, relaxation techniques), radiation effects (sunscreen, protective cotton clothing to decrease additional skin irritation), and chemotherapy effects (antiemetic medication, cap to decrease hair loss, balanced nutrition to decrease fatigue). Provide client with choices for coping strategies.	4. Anticipatory guidance decreases fear and increases compliance. Providing woman with choices increases sense of control and enhances self-esteem.

Evaluation

- Client states that she can expect to have her breast and lymph nodes under her arm removed.
- Client states that she will need to come for radiation treatments after surgery each day for 5 to 6 weeks.
- Client states that she may have skin irritation and will have chemotherapy, possibly for 3 to 8 months, depending on the schedule chosen by her oncologist.
- Client states that she may have some nausea, vomiting, fatigue, and hair loss, and she will be given medication to control her nausea.
- Client states that she will not be able to work as a dishwasher at the cafe while she is recovering and undergoing radiation and chemotherapy.
- Client states that she will move in with her sister while she is recovering and taking radiation and chemotherapy treatments.
- Client states that she can take medication for pain and nausea.

symptoms of specifically suspected breast conditions. Physical assessment focuses on the collection of data regarding the suspected breast condition, including necessary laboratory tests and collection of biopsy specimens.

Nursing diagnoses may include the following:

■ Pain related to screening, diagnostic procedures, surgical procedures

■ Fear related to medical condition and selected therapeutic intervention

■ Grief related to body image change or prognosis

■ Deficient knowledge related to specific breast condition, screening, diagnosis, or intervention procedures

Nursing plans include specific actions that the client completes to achieve the highest level of wellness possible or to achieve peace regarding prognosis. Sample goals include the following:

■ Consume food portions according to the daily recommendations in the food pyramid or as required on the basis of medical diagnosis from 24-hour diet recall; intention to consume suggested foods and intention to modify detrimental food intake.

■ Complete daily exercise (walking 30 minutes per day, any prescribed exercise required for restoration of function after surgery).

■ Understand instructions regarding prescriptive medications.

■ Return to the health care facility for scheduled follow-up visits.

■ Call the health care provider regarding adverse effects of prescriptive medications as instructed.

■ Call health care provider regarding any adverse symptoms of breast condition as instructed.

■ Have all questions answered to her satisfaction.

■ Understand health promotion counseling.

Nursing interventions involve educating the woman regarding the diagnosis, consequences, interventions, specific procedures; her choices; counseling regarding expected outcomes; emotional support; reduction of fears,

---

Nursing Tip   *The Client After Mastectomy*

There are four types of **mastectomy** (excision of the breast). In a simple mastectomy, only the breast is removed. In a modified radical procedure, the breast and lymph nodes from the axilla are removed (Figure 6-8). In a radical mastectomy, the breast, lymph nodes from the axilla, and pectoral muscles are removed (Figure 6-9). This procedure is rarely performed. In a subcutaneous mastectomy, the skin and nipple are left intact, but the underlying breast tissue and lymph nodes are removed. The client who has undergone a simple, modified radical, or radical mastectomy has had the breast amputated from the chest wall.

Reconstruction techniques include synthetic implants, tissue expansion techniques (in which a temporary device is placed in a subpectoralis-subserratus position between the anterior chest wall and skin and is then inflated with saline over a period of weeks), and latissimus dorsi myocutaneous flap breast reconstruction. A myocutaneous flap reconstruction involves transferring skin from the back or the abdomen to the anterior chest wall.

Assessment of the client who has had a mastectomy is guided by the type of mastectomy and the presence or absence of reconstructive surgery. Follow the standard assessment procedures and modify your technique to suit the amount of breast tissue and the presence, if any, of a nipple. Always begin the assessment on the unaffected breast. Mastectomy clients should continue to perform monthly breast self-examinations to determine if masses have returned to the excised area. Annual clinical evaluations and mammograms are also recommended.

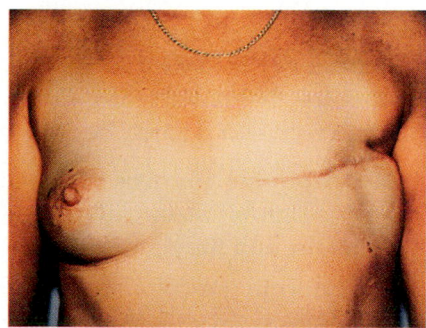

Figure 6-8   Modified Radical Mastectomy. (Courtesy of Steven M. Lynch, MD)

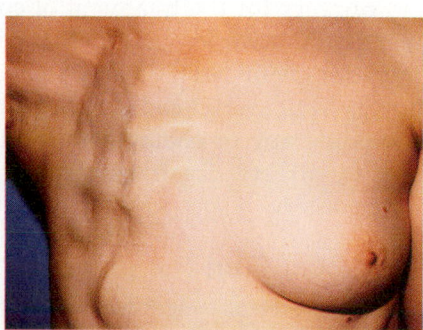

Figure 6-9   Radical Mastectomy. (Courtesy of Steven M. Lynch, MD)

anxiety, stresses, and concerns; advocacy; and relief of current or future pain.

Women who seek care for breast conditions are demonstrating concern and are usually ready to learn about protecting the health of their breasts. Breast and general health promotion and disease prevention strategies include recommendations for regular exercise and for diet from the food pyramid to maintain normal BMI; avoiding or stopping smoking; performing self-assessments; and scheduling provider assessments and screenings as necessary.

Colorectal Cancer

Colorectal cancer ranks third as a cause of cancer deaths in women and is three times more prevalent than uterine cancer. Invasive colorectal cancer is the most preventable visceral cancer. Most cases arise from adenomatous polyps that take approximately 10 years to progress to an invasive stage.

Colon cancer was estimated to be responsible for 11% of all cancer deaths in the year 2000. Risk factors include family history, ulcerative colitis, first-degree family history of adenomas or colorectal cancer, and a personal history of adenomas or of ovarian, endometrial, or breast cancer. Possible additional risk factors include inactivity, high-fat diets, low-fiber diets, and inadequate intake of fruit and vegetables (ACS, 2000).

If detected at an early stage, colorectal cancer can be successfully treated with surgery (U.S. Preventive Services Task Force, 1996). Recommendations for early detection for both men and women, beginning at age 50, include:

- Performing a fecal occult blood test (FOBT) and flexible sigmoidoscopy; if normal, repeat the FOBT annually and the sigmoidoscopy every 5 years, or
- Performing a colonoscopy; if normal, repeat every 10 years, or
- Performing a double-contrast barium enema; if normal, repeat every 5 to 10 years, and
- Performing a digital rectal examination in addition to the above diagnostic tests

Surgery for the treatment of colorectal cancer is frequently curative for cancers that have not spread. Treatment for clients whose cancer has deeply perforated the bowel wall or spread to the lymph nodes includes chemotherapy or chemotherapy plus radiation in addition to surgery. Treatment can be performed before or after surgery.

Cervical Cancer

Rates of cervical cancer have decreased steadily over the past several decades. Rates for Blacks decreased more rapidly than for Caucasians; however from 1992 to 1996,

the mortality rate for Black women continued to be more than twice that for Caucasian women (ACS, 2000). This decrease results largely from early detection through the use of the Pap smear. The **Pap smear** is a screening device for cervical cancer. Endocervical cells are obtained by use of a cervical brush and then examined for abnormal cells by electron microscopy. Hispanic and Native American women have a higher incidence and higher death rates than Caucasian women. Rates for carcinoma in situ reach a peak for both Black and Caucasian women between ages 20 and 30. **Carcinoma in situ** is defined as cancer that involves only the cells in the organ in which it

Nursing Alert

Risk Factors for Cancer of the Female Genitalia

Evaluate each client for risk factors, and counsel the client regarding diminishing risk factors that are behavior dependent. Suspected carcinoma of the female genitalia requires an immediate referral.

Cervical Cancer

- Early age at first intercourse
- Multiple sex partners
- Prior history of human papillomavirus
- Tobacco use
- Family history

Endometrial Cancer

- Early or late menarche (before age 11 or after age 16)
- History of infertility
- Failure to ovulate
- Unopposed estrogen therapy
- Use of tamoxifen
- Obesity
- Family history

Ovarian Cancer

- Advancing age
- Nulliparity
- History of breast cancer
- Family history of ovarian cancer

Vaginal Cancer

- Daughters of women who ingested diethylstilbestrol during pregnancy

Note. From *Health Assessment & Physical Examination* (2nd ed.), by M. E. Z. Estes, 2002, Clifton Park, NY: Delmar Learning.

Nursing Alert

Risk Factors for Cervical Cancer

- Early age at first intercourse
- Multiple sexual partners
- Sex with partners who have had multiple sexual partners
- Smoking
- History of human papillomavirus (HPV) infection
- Low socioeconomic status

began and that has not spread to any other tissue. **Invasive cancer** is defined as cancer that has spread or infiltrated beyond the original site or organ. Over 25% of invasive cervical cancers occur in women older than age 65, and 40% to 50% of all women who die from cervical cancer are over age 65 (ACS, 1998). Invasive cervical cancer is defined as cancer that has spread from the surface of the cervix to the deeper tissues of the cervix.

Signs and symptoms for cervical cancer include abnormal vaginal bleeding or spotting and abnormal vaginal discharge. Pain is known as a late symptom for cervical cancer.

Risk factors for cervical cancer include early age at first intercourse, multiple sexual partners or partners who have had multiple sexual partners, smoking, and low socioeconomic status (ACS, 2000). Cervical cancer risk is closely linked to sexual behavior and sexually transmitted human papillomavirus (HPV) infection. Early detection and treatment has caused a marked decrease in mortality from cervical cancer. Early detection through Pap smear testing is recommended because 8 to 9 years is generally required for precancerous changes to progress to invasive carcinoma, also known as infiltrating cancer. Almost all early-stage cancers can be effectively treated. Pap smears can detect precancerous changes years before invasive cancer sets in.

Medical management for abnormal cervical cell development or cervical cancer includes local excision, cryotherapy, electrocoagulation, or carbon dioxide laser therapy to destroy the abnormal cells (Bristow & Montz, 2000). Surgery, radiotherapy, or radiotherapy and chemotherapy combined are the usual therapeutic interventions when cervical conditions have progressed to invasive cervical cancer (Moore, 1997).

Cervical cancer is very treatable, with high survival rates. Most cervical cancers are treated with surgery, radiation therapy, or both. In situ cancers may be treated with cryotherapy, which destroys cells with extreme cold, or electrocoagulation, which destroys cells with intense heat that is generated by an electric current (ACS, 2000).

It is recommended that all women who are or have been sexually active or have reached age 18 should have annual Pap smears (Figure 6-10). This recommendation has been adopted by the major organizations (U.S. Preventive Services Task Force, 1996). The recommendation permits Pap testing

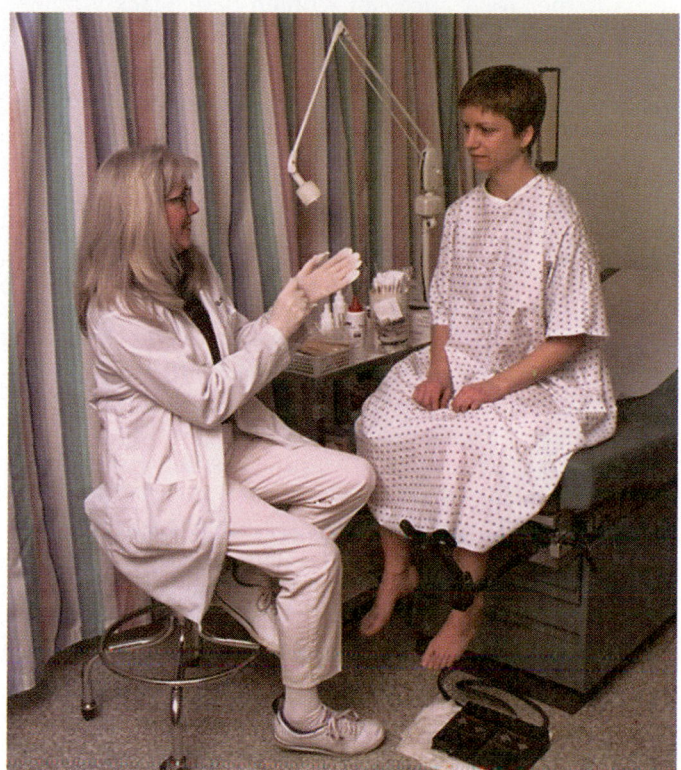

A.

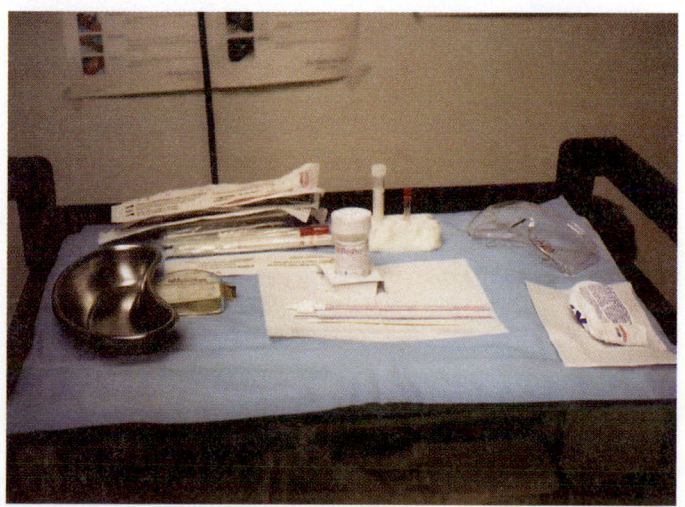

B.

Figure 6-10   A. The nurse and client prepare for a pelvic exam. B. Materials needed for a gynecologic exam.

less frequently after three or more normal annual test results, at the discretion of the health care provider and client.

Endometrial Cancer

An estimated 36,100 cases of cancer of the body of the uterus, usually of the endometrium, were diagnosed in 2000 (ACS, 2000). Mortality rates are also relatively constant (ACS, 1998). Although incidence of endometrial cancer is higher for Caucasian women than Black women, Black women have higher mortality rates (ACS, 2000).

Endometrial cancer is rarely seen in women under age 50, but the risk rises sharply in women in their late 40s to mid-60s. The incidence of endometrial cancer increased rapidly during the years when unopposed estrogen was commonly used to treat menopausal women. Estrogen replacement therapy (ERT) was more common among Caucasian women, resulting in higher rates of endometrial cancer. Unopposed estrogen therapy for menopause is no longer recommended because of the increased risk of endometrial cancer.

Signs and symptoms for endometrial cancer are similar to that of cervical cancer: abnormal uterine bleeding or spotting. Late manifestations of the disease include pain and systemic symptoms (ACS, 2000).

Risk factors for uterine cancer include those factors that expose the endometrium to estrogen, including (ACS, 1998):

- Unopposed estrogen therapy
- Therapy with tamoxifen
- Early menarche (before age 12)
- Never having children
- Late menopause (after age 55)
- History of failure to ovulate
- Infertility
- Diabetes
- Gallbladder disease
- Hypertension
- Obesity

There is preliminary evidence suggesting that a high-fat diet increases the risk of developing uterine cancer. Factors associated with a lower risk of endometrial cancer are having multiple children, use of oral contraceptives that combine both estrogen and progestin, and use during menopause of ERT combined with progesterone therapy. Endometrial cancer is treated by surgery, radiation therapy, hormonal therapy, chemotherapy, or a combination of these treatments, depending on the stage of the cancer (ACS, 2000).

Survival rates women with for uterine cancer are good when the disease is treated early; the 5-year survival rate for early-stage endometrial cancer is 95% (American Cancer Society, 2000).

Ovarian Cancer

One in 70 women develop ovarian cancer. Approximately 23,100 new cases of ovarian cancer occurred in 2000, with an estimated 14,500 deaths (ACS, 2000). The average age at diagnosis is 63. Approximately 90% of cases occur in Caucasian women. Risk factors for ovarian cancer include a family history of ovarian cancer (in first-degree relatives, such as mother, sister, daughter), nulliparity, older age at the time of first pregnancy or live birth, fewer pregnancies, use of fertility drugs, high-fat diet, and a personal history of breast, endometrial, or colorectal cancer. Women who have had breast cancer or have a family history of breast or ovarian cancer are at increased risk. Alteration in BRCA-1 or BRCA-2 genes has been noted in women with ovarian cancer, and pregnancy and the use of oral contraceptives appear to reduce the risk of ovarian cancer (ACS, 2000).

Ovarian cancer usually shows no signs or symptoms until late in development. Enlargement of the abdomen from accumulation of fluid is the most common sign (ACS, 2000). Usually ovarian tumors are of considerable size by the time they are detectable by pelvic examination. Women over age 40 who present with persistent symptoms of vague digestive disturbances (stomach discomfort, distention) that cannot be explained by any other cause may need an ovarian cancer evaluation, including a thorough pelvic examination (ACS, 2000).

As of 2000, screening tests available for ovarian cancer include an annual pelvic examination, which includes bimanual palpation of the ovaries, and pelvic ultrasonography. Improvements in diagnostic methods continue, including identification of the breast and ovarian cancer gene on chromosome 17.

Only 25% of ovarian cancers are diagnosed early in the localized stage, with the survival rate at this stage being 95% for 5 years (ACS, 2000). For women with regional ovarian cancer, the survival rate is 79%; the survival rate for progressive disease is 28% (ACS, 2000).

Chronic Conditions

Women live longer than men, but they are not necessarily living better. This is particularly true during later life, when they are more likely to have chronic disease. Chronic diseases that women are more likely to be affected by and which are discussed following include osteoporosis, Alzheimer's disease, immune disorders, urinary incontinence, mental illness, and substance abuse (USDHHS, 2000b). In every age group, more women than men experience and seek care for illness and disability.

Nursing Alert

Risk Factors for Osteoporosis

- Caucasian women
- Premature menopause
- Sedentary lifestyle
- Excessive caffeine intake
- Regular alcohol use
- Excess salt intake
- Postmenopause
- Insufficient dietary calcium
- Smoking
- Family history of osteoporosis

Osteoporosis

Osteoporosis is a disorder characterized by excessive loss of bone density. Osteoporosis affects over 25 million Americans; more than 80% of them are women. This disease affects one-third to one-half of postmenopausal women. The rates for osteoporosis increase dramatically for women as they age (Davidson & DeSimone, 2002). Hip fractures are the most serious consequence of osteoporosis, with more than 250,000 people hospitalized with hip fractures annually. About one-third of these become totally dependent, and one-half never walk again.

Prevention of osteoporosis should span the entire lifetime. Approximately 60% of a woman's bone mass develops by age 18, and peak bone density is achieved by the late 20s. To build and maintain bone density, women should eat calcium-rich foods, get regular exercise, and avoid tobacco and excessive consumption of alcohol or caffeine. Treatment includes calcium and vitamin D supplementation and medications to strengthen bone structure.

Alzheimer's Disease

Alzheimer's disease occurs more frequently in women than in men and increases with age—dramatically so after age 85. In 1998, there were 22,725 deaths from Alzheimer's disease, with most deaths occurring after age 75 (USDHHS, 2000a). The disease usually begins after age 65, and the risk goes up with age. Younger people may have Alzheimer's disease, but it is less common. About 3% of the population aged 65 to 74 have Alzheimer's disease. Alzheimer's disease is not a normal function of aging, although about 50% of the population over age 85 years may have the disease.

Immune Disorders

Immunologic diseases occur more frequently in females than males. Autoimmune thyroid disease occurs 15 times more frequently in women than men. Rheumatoid arthritis occurs three times more frequently in women than men, and leads to disability and decreased life expectancy. Systemic lupus erythemathosus (SLE) occurs nine times more frequently in women than men and is three times more prevalent in Black women than in Caucasian women. Systemic sclerosis affects women four times as frequently as men. Diabetes mellitus and multiple sclerosis occur more frequently in women (USDHHS, 2000b).

Urinary Incontinence

Eleven million older women in the United States have urinary incontinence. Women are more frequently affected than men; approximately 2 million men experience the condition. Approximately 50% of persons residing in nursing homes are incontinent. Urinary incontinence is the 10th leading cause of hospitalization. More diapers are sold in the United States to women over age 65 than are used for babies. Although half of all elderly people experience episodes of incontinence, it is a problem of younger women also. Ten to thirty percent of women in the 15–65 age group develop incontinence as a result of weakened pelvic muscles or pelvic trauma (Shimp & Peggs, 2000).

Mental Illness

Mental health is crucial to a woman's well-being. Some of the most common mental disorders, including depression and anxiety, occur in approximately twice as many women as men. It is estimated that there are currently 7 million women in the United States with clinical depression. An estimated 12% of women experience a major form of depression at some time in their lives, compared with 7% of men. Women are twice as likely as men to suffer from clinical depression. Suicide was the fourth leading cause of death among women aged 25 to 44 in 1998 (USDHHS 2000a). Women are more likely than men to attempt suicide but are far less likely to die as a result, primarily because men are more likely to use a firearm. Of women who have depression, about 75% are untreated. Most drugs to treat depression have been studied in clinical trials on men. The effects of hormones on depression and their interaction with psychotropic drugs have not been well studied and are therefore largely unknown. Women who have had a history of substance abuse or physical or sexual abuse are particularly at risk for depression, eating disorders, and anxiety disorders.

Substance Abuse

The abuse of alcohol and other legal and illicit drugs is a serious and growing problem among U.S. women. There are approximately 10 million alcoholics in the United States, of which 30% to 50% are women. Women are less likely to use or abuse alcohol than men but have a 50% to 100% higher death rate from alcoholism than men. Alcohol use during pregnancy poses a serious threat to the developing fetus. Heavy drinking during pregnancy has been clearly implicated in severe birth defects, including mental retardation, abnormal face and neck features, nervous system disorders, and delayed growth. Use of alcohol during pregnancy occurs more frequently in single women, smokers, teenagers, and those with little education. In 1998, approximately 4.5 million women aged 15 to 44 were currently illicit drug users, of which one-third were raising children. Women tend to be more easily addicted to tranquilizers than men.

Smoking in women has increased parallel to the tobacco industry's aggressive marketing to women, particularly to teenage girls. Smoking contributes substantially to deaths and disability from cancer, lung disease, heart disease, and stroke. Smoking is the leading cause of premature births and increases the risk of miscarriage, mental retardation, and low birth weight. Exposing children to secondhand smoke increases the risk of sudden infant death syndrome (SIDS), recurrent otitis media, and severe respiratory illness. Smoking cessation programs have been more successful in males than in females. By age 25, one in three women is a smoker. The number of women who are heavy smokers has also increased in the last two decades.

AGE-SPECIFIC ISSUES

Certain health alterations are more prevalent in certain age groups, and are grouped accordingly in the following discussion.

Infancy to Young Adulthood

Less than 1% of all deaths of females occur in girls aged 1 to 4. Accidents are the leading cause of death in this age group, followed by other causes (USDHHS, 2000a) (Table 6-4).

Between ages 5 and 14, the death rate for female children drops by 50%. Accidents continue to be the leading cause of death, followed by other causes (Table 6-5). In this age group, boys have almost twice the death rate from accidents that girls do (National Vital Statistics Report, 2000).

The major cause of death and illness among all children is injury, both intentional and unintentional. Injury accounts for over half of all deaths in this age group (Figure 6-11).

Girls are prone to autoimmune diseases, including systemic lupus erythematosus (SLE), juvenile rheumatoid arthritis, and thyroid disease.

Table 6-4	Leading Causes of Deaths by Age and Sex for Ages 1–4: 1998		
CAUSE OF DEATH	**DEATHS PER 100,000 POPULATION**		
	BOTH SEXES	**FEMALE**	**MALE**
All causes	34.6	31.4	37.6
Accidents	12.7	10.5	14.9
Congenital anomalies	3.7	3.7	3.7
Cancer	2.4	2.4	2.4
Homicide	2.6	2.4	2.9
Heart disease	1.4	1.3	1.5
Pneumonia and influenza	1.0	1.0	0.9
Septicemia	0.6	0.5	0.7
Perinatal-related	0.5	0.5	0.5
Stroke	0.4	0.4	(NA)
Benign neoplasms	0.3	0.3	(NA)

Note. Adapted from Table No. 8, *National Vital Statistics Report*, Vol. No. 11, July 24, 2000.

Table 6-5	Leading Causes of Deaths by Age and Sex for Ages 5–14: 1998		
CAUSE OF DEATH	**DEATHS PER 100,000 POPULATION**		
	BOTH SEXES	**FEMALE**	**MALE**
All causes	19.9	16.2	23.4
Accidents	8.3	6.1	10.4
Cancer	2.6	2.3	2.9
Homicide	1.2	1.1	1.3
Congenital anomalies	0.9	0.9	1.0
Heart disease	0.8	0.7	1.0
Suicide	0.8	0.4	1.2
COPD	0.4	0.4	0.4
Pneumonia and influenza	0.3	0.3	0.3
Benign neoplasms	0.2	0.2	0.2
Stroke	0.2	0.2	0.2

Note. Adapted from Table No. 8., *National Vital Statistics Report*, Vol. No. 11, July 24, 2000.

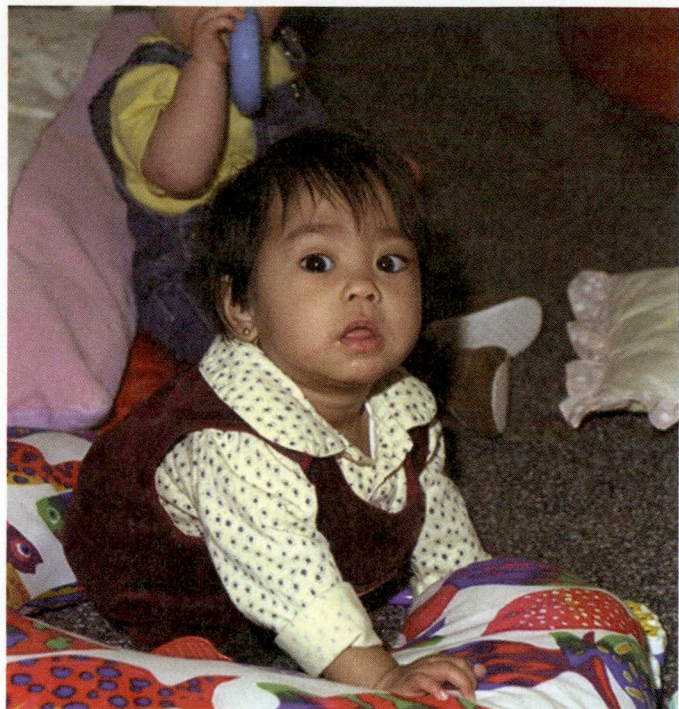

Figure 6-11   Injury is the major cause of morbidity and mortality in young children.

Young Adulthood to Perimenopausal Years

As girls, ages 15 to 24, become adolescents and young adults, the leading cause of death continues to be accidents. The leading causes of death for this age range are listed in Table 6-6. During this period, males have almost three times the risk of dying as females, with most deaths attributable to accidents, homicide, and suicide (U.S. Census Bureau, 1999).

Nursing Alert

Common Risk-taking Behaviors among Adolescents

- Accidental and unintentional injuries
- Homicide
- Suicide
- Alcohol and other drug use
- Cigarette smoking
- Sexual activity
- Body piercing and tattooing

Table 6-6	Leading Causes of Deaths by Age and Sex for Ages 15–24: 1998		
CAUSE OF DEATH	**DEATHS PER 100,000 POPULATION**		
	BOTH SEXES	**FEMALE**	**MALE**
All causes	82.3	43.5	119.3
Accidents	35.9	19.1	51.9
Homicide	14.8	3.0	24.8
Suicide	11.1	3.3	18.5
Cancer	4.6	3.7	5.4
Heart disease	2.8	2.1	3.5
Congenital anomalies	2.8	1.1	1.3
COPD	0.6	0.5	0.8
Pneumonia and influenza	0.6	0.6	0.6
AIDS	0.5	0.6	0.6
Stroke	0.5	(N/A)	0.6

Note. Adapted from Table No. 8, *National Vital Statistics Report*, Vol. No. 11, July 24, 2000.

For adult women between ages 25 and 44, the risk of dying is more than double that of the previous age range, with cancer being the leading cause of death (Table 6-7).

From ages 15 to 44, accidents, cancer, heart disease, suicide, and AIDS are the most frequent causes of death in both genders (Figure 6-12). The most frequent causes of ill

Table 6-7	Leading Causes of Deaths by Age and Sex for Ages 25–44: 1998		
CAUSE OF DEATH	**DEATHS PER 100,000 POPULATION**		
	BOTH SEXES	**FEMALE**	**MALE**
All causes	157.7	107.4	208.8
Accidents	32.6	16.5	48.9
Cancer	25.7	28.0	23.4
Heart disease	20.2	11.9	29.0
Suicide	14.6	6.0	23.5
AIDS	10.4	5.1	15.7
Homicide	9.8	4.6	15.0
Chronic liver disease	4.7	2.9	6.5
Stroke	4.0	3.9	4.1
Diabetes	3.0	2.4	3.6
Pneumonia and influenza	2.3	1.9	2.7

Note. Adapted from Table No. 8, *National Vital Statistics Report*, Vol. No. 11, July 24, 2000.

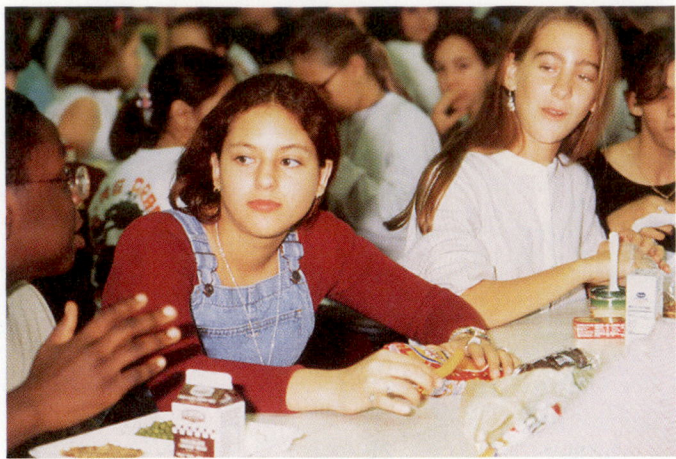

Figure 6-12 Adolescents are most at risk for mortality from accidents, cancer, heart disease, suicide, and AIDS.

Table 6-8	Leading Causes of Deaths by Age and Sex for Ages 45–54: 1998		
CAUSE OF DEATH	**DEATHS PER 100,000 POPULATION**		
	BOTH SEXES	**FEMALE**	**MALE**
All causes	664.0	501.9	836.9
Cancer	231.9	209.9	255.3
Heart disease	174.9	101.5	253.2
Accidents	31.9	18.0	46.8
Stroke	26.8	23.3	30.6
Diabetes	22.9	21.1	25.8
COPD	22.7	21.2	24.3
Chronic liver disease	19.3	10.1	29.0
Suicide	14.1	6.4	22.4
Pneumonia and influenza	10.5	8.2	13.0
AIDS	7.2	(NA)	12.1

Note. Adapted from Table No. 8, *National Vital Statistics Report*, Vol. No. 11, July 24, 2000.

health among women are eating disorders, autoimmune diseases, depression, alcohol and tobacco use, sexually transmitted diseases (STDs), reproductive problems, homicide, and sexual abuse. Intervention strategies that can reduce or prevent serious illness or death in this age group address women at risk and risky behaviors associated with the diseases and illnesses. Alcohol is often a causative factor in motor vehicle accidents and violence that ends in homicide and suicide. Risky sexual behavior puts women at risk for STDs, HIV infection, cervical cancer, unwanted or unplanned pregnancies, pelvic inflammatory disease (PID), atopic pregnancy, and infertility. Smoking puts women at risk for lung and other cancer, heart disease, and COPD.

Perimenopausal to Mature Years

For mature women, ages 45 to 64, the risk of dying is more than five times that of women aged 25 to 44. Approximately 14% of all female deaths occur in this age range. The leading causes of death for men and women are summarized in Table 6-8.

Women in the menopausal to mature years are a fast-growing segment of the population because of the aging of the baby boom generation. These years are important because of menopause and the fact that many chronic conditions first appear. The rates of some chronic conditions increase markedly in the population between the ages of 45 and 64. During these years, one out of seven women has heart disease. Approximately 3% of women in this age group have a major depressive episode. Major reasons for hospitalization of women in this age range include heart disease, cancer, gallbladder disease, benign tumors, psychosis, and diabetes.

The three major risk factors for the diseases that relate to morbidity and mortality during this period are smoking, obesity, and a sedentary lifestyle. The drop in estrogen lev-

els at menopause is a factor in the increased incidence of heart disease and osteoporosis. The Women's Health Initiative is conducting the largest and most expensive clinical trial ever conducted to determine whether women should begin hormone replacement therapy at menopause, how long it should be continued, and whether it will reduce the incidence of heart disease and osteoporosis.

Mature Years

While many women aged 65 and over lead full and productive lives, statistics show that women in this age group die at a rate that is almost seven times higher than women 45 to 64 years of age. Death of women aged 65 and over accounts for 8 of 10 female deaths annually. Heart disease is the major killer of both men and women (Table 6-9).

Older women experience a significant number of chronic illnesses. Frequently, older women have multiple health problems that can be compounded by social and psychological problems, including loneliness, isolation, and loss of independence (Figure 6-13).

HEALTH PROMOTION AND DISEASE PREVENTION

In recent years, health promotion has become a major goal for the United States and many other countries of the world. The World Health Organization defines health promotion as a process, action, program, or endeavor to

Table 6-9	Leading Causes of Deaths by Age and Sex for Ages 64 and Over: 1998		
CAUSE OF DEATH	**DEATHS PER 100,000 POPULATION**		
	BOTH SEXES	**FEMALE**	**MALE**
All causes	5096.4	4754.9	5582.4
Heart disease	1760.6	1658.4	1906.1
Cancer	1116.8	912.7	1407.2
Stroke	404.5	438.2	356.5
COPD	284.6	240.2	347.8
Pneumonia and influenza	241.2	233.6	252.1
Diabetes	142.4	139.1	146.9
Accidents	95.9	83.2	113.9
Nephritis	65.8	59.9	74.2
Alzheimer's disease	65.2	76.7	48.7
Septicemia	55.3	56.1	54.1

Note. Adapted from Table No. 8, *National Vital Statistics Report*, Vol. No. 11, July 24, 2000.

obtain the goal of complete physical, mental, and social well-being. Other definitions have included concepts of self-care, health-promoting behaviors, empowerment, development of healthy lifestyles, maintenance or enhancement of well-being, and healthy environments.

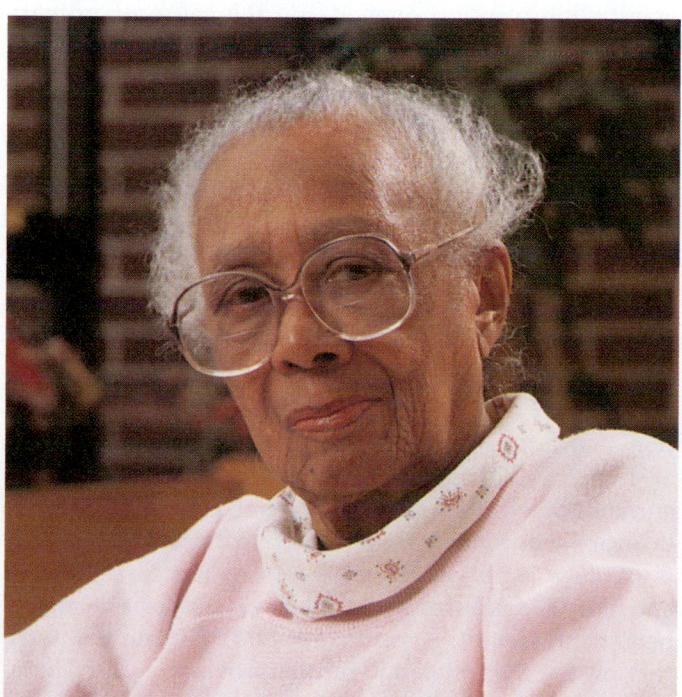

Figure 6-13   Despite health alterations, older adults often embody grace and dignity.

Not only are there many definitions of health promotion and disease prevention, there are differing sets of preventive services recommended by government agencies, professional organizations, voluntary associations, and academic experts. However, in spite of this, there seems to be basic agreement among authorities on recommendations for the major types of preventive care. The U.S. Preventive Services Task Force (1996) published its report in the *Guide to Clinical Services*, which is widely regarded as the premiere reference source on the effectiveness of clinical preventive services, including screening tests for early detection of disease, immunizations to prevent infections, and counseling for risk reduction.

Types of Preventive Services

The three major types of preventive services include screening, immunization, and counseling.

Screening

Screening is the process of completing a test or examination to detect the most characteristic sign or signs of a disorder or disease that may require further investigation. Screening sensitivity and specificity and positive predictive value must be considered when evaluating and selecting screening tests. There is little value in performing screening tests without close tracking of results and the necessary follow-up testing. Analysis of screening tests must adhere to national standards for accuracy in testing and reporting of results. Clients should be clearly informed of the potential cost and side effects of necessary follow-up testing and treatment as appropriate.

Immunizations

Immunizations can prevent or postpone serious disorders. The National Vaccine Advisory Committee has set standards for childhood immunization practices, and the National Coalition for Adult Immunization has developed standards for adult immunization practices.

Counseling

The third method to implement preventive care is counseling. The U.S. Preventive Services Task Force (1996) described 10 principles for client education and counseling with which all health care professionals should be familiar. These principles include:

1. Develop a therapeutic alliance.
2. Counsel all clients.
3. Ensure that clients understand the relationship between behavior and health.
4. Work with clients to assess barriers to behavioral change.

5. Gain commitment from clients to change.

6. Involve clients in selecting risk factors to change.

7. Use a combination of strategies.

8. Design a behavior modification plan.

9. Monitor progress through follow-up contact.

10. Involve office staff.

Preventive services should be provided at a level of comprehension consistent with the age and learning skills of the client.

The following are recommendations for development of preventive services.

- Preventive services must become an integral part of all health services, including nursing.
- Protocols for prevention must continue to be developed.
- Screening must be useful, that is, have the ability to detect conditions that are treatable, and be completed at the right time.
- Screening must be acceptable to the client.
- Prevalence of a condition must be sufficient to justify the cost of the screening.
- Immunizations can prevent or postpone serious disorders.
- Counseling is an integral component of prevention.
- Nurses must continue to strive for excellence and sensitivity in providing prevention education, counseling, and screening.
- Counseling must be culturally appropriate.

WOMEN'S HEALTH CONDITIONS

Women are living longer now than ever before. Thus, a woman can expect to experience a variety of health conditions resulting from the aging process, as well as the normal physiologic "wear and tear" that occurs on a daily basis. Women can realistically expect to live into their 80s, and they want to have a high quality of life throughout their life span. Nurses can facilitate the achievement of women's goals for quality of life by assessing their clients' health conditions and developing an individualized plan to reduce the adverse effects of disease. Conditions addressed in this section include menstrual, breast, pelvic, and menopausal conditions.

Menstrual Cycle Abnormalities

In general, abnormal conditions of the menstrual cycle are deviations from what is normal for an individual woman. The condition may occur in the frequency or length of the cycle, volume or length of menstrual flow, or the total number of years of menstruation.

Menstrual cycle conditions are a readily noticeable concern. Common conditions may be classified as amenorrhea, dysfunctional or abnormal uterine bleeding, dysmenorrhea, endometriosis, or premenstrual syndrome. Refer to Table 6-10 for a list of menstrual cycle conditions and to Table 6-11 for therapeutic interventions for menstrual cycle conditions. Box 6-1 lists additional alterations in menstrual cycle function.

Amenorrhea

Amenorrhea is the absence or lack of menses during the reproductive years. Normal causes of amenorrhea include pregnancy, lactation, and menopause. Other causes can be pathologic and may include stress, excessive exercise, eating disorders, weight loss, a low body mass index (BMI), or other potentially life-threatening disorders. Amenorrhea can be classified as primary or secondary.

Primary Amenorrhea

Primary amenorrhea is the absence of menarche until age 16 or the absence of the development of secondary sex characteristics and menarche until age 14 (Keene, 1999). Causes of primary amenorrhea may involve hypothalamic, pituitary, enzymatic, or chromosomal abnormalities; genitourinary tract abnormalities; or drug therapy. The primary symptom is failure to experience menarche when there has been development of secondary sex characteristics or without such development as in Turner syndrome. Therapeutic intervention depends on the cause of primary amenorrhea and usually includes estrogen replacement therapy (ERT) to prevent osteoporosis or to stimulate development of secondary sexual characteristics.

Secondary Amenorrhea

Secondary amenorrhea is the absence of menses for at least 6 months or for three cycles after menarche (Keene, 1999; McGee, 1997). Secondary amenorrhea is more common than primary amenorrhea and is often caused by physiologic responses to pregnancy, lactation, or anovulation (Keene, 1999). In addition to absence of menses, the woman may have diseases related to endocrine dysfunction that are causing the secondary amenorrhea, such as hypothyroidism, hyperthyroidism, adrenal disease, chronic hepatic disease, chronic renal disease, or polycystic ovary syndrome. Women athletes who train vigorously or women with anorexia often experience secondary amenorrhea because of the effects of the relationship of height and weight, percentage of body fat, and malnutrition on the hypothalamic-pituitary-ovarian axis. Therapeutic intervention for secondary amenorrhea includes cyclic progesterone, when the cause is anovulation; oral contraceptives, for the woman who desires contraception;

Table 6-10   Menstrual Cycle Conditions

CONDITION	DATA SUBJECTIVE	OBJECTIVE	LABORATORY OR PROCEDURE
Amenorrhea			
Primary amenorrhea	No menarche	Secondary sex characteristics	Thyroid function tests
			Blood glucose level
		Reproductive tract anomalies	Karyotype (Turner syndrome)
			Laparoscopy (ovarian pathology)
Secondary amenorrhea	3 or more missed menstrual periods	Previous gynecologic procedures or problems	Decreased thyroid function tests
	Menstrual pattern	Weight gain or loss	Increased blood glucose level
		Major life events	Increased serum prolactin level
		Exercise level	Laparoscopy to detect polycystic ovary syndrome
		Thyroid size	Ultrasound to detect ovarian cysts
		Exophthalmia	
		Moon facies	
		Hirsutism	
		Delayed deep tendon reflexes	
		Breast atrophy	
		Thinning hair	
		Temporal baldness	
Abnormal or Dysfunctional Uterine Bleeding			
Bleeding between menstrual periods	Possible uterine abnormality	Anemia	Low thyroid function, pituitary function (FSH or LH)
	Irregular bleeding	Pregnancy test	hCG studies (for anovulation)
	Heavy bleeding	CBC (complete blood count) for anemia or infection	Increased prolactin level
	Prolonged bleeding	Ultrasound	
	Light bleeding	Endometrial biopsy to rule out endometrial cancer	
	Short or long cycles		
Dysmenorrhea			
Primary dysmenorrhea	Mild to severe cramping, lasting 2–4 days before menses to third day of menses	Nulliparity	Ultrasound
		Age (adolescence to early 20s)	
	GI symptoms: bloating, nausea, vomiting	Normal results on physical examination	
	Back, thigh, and headache pain		
	Family history		
Secondary dysmenorrhea	Increasingly painful menses	Third or fourth decade of life	Elevated WBC count if STD or PID is present
	Dyspareunia	Endometriosis	Cultures for gonorrhea and chlamydia
	Painful defecation	PID, STD	Ultrasound
	Rectal pressure	Increased uterine size	Laparoscopy (endometriosis)
	Heavy or irregular bleeding	Endometritis	
		Salpingitis	
		Leiomyomata	

(continues)

Table 6-10   Menstrual Cycle Conditions *(continued)*

CONDITION	SUBJECTIVE	OBJECTIVE	LABORATORY OR PROCEDURE
Endometriosis			
Dysmenorrhea	Infertility Cyclic dyspareunia Dyschezia GI symptoms Pelvic heaviness Chronic pelvic pain (may radiate to thighs) Abnormal bleeding	Uterus may be fixed Possible adnexal mass(es) Pelvic tenderness	Ultrasound monitoring of implants Laparoscopy
Premenstrual syndrome			
Cluster of symptoms at luteal phase	Depressed mood Mood swings Irritability Difficulty in concentration or coping Fatigue Edema Breast tenderness Headache (premenstrual) Sleep disturbances Abdominal bloating Increased appetite Weight gain Food cravings Acne Heart palpitations Anxiety Hostility	Signs of stress Emotional lability	None

bromocriptine, when the woman is experiencing hyper-prolactinemia; gonadotropin-releasing hormone (GnRH), when the cause is hypothalamic failure; and thyroid hormone replacement therapy, when the cause is hypothyroidism. In addition, the woman who is hypoestrogenic is given calcium and ERT to prevent development of osteoporosis.

Dysfunctional Uterine Bleeding

Dysfunctional uterine bleeding (DUB) is "any significant deviation from the usual menstrual pattern" (Keene, 1999, p. 75). DUB occurs more often in adolescents and perimenopausal women. An estimated 20% of women seek therapeutic intervention at some point in their lives for DUB (Smith, 1998). The differences from the usual bleeding pattern may include hypermenorrhea and menorrhagia, intermenstrual bleeding and metrorrhagia, menometrorrhagia, oligomenorrhea, polymenorrhea, or

hypomenorrhea; refer to Box 6-1 for an explanation of these terms.

Causes of DUB include hormonal abnormalities, such as anovulation (no egg release); pregnancy-associated events; pelvic inflammatory disease (PID); trauma; neoplasm; endometriosis; and anatomic or systemic disease.

A woman may report characteristics of oligomenorrhea when she experiences a scant amount of menstrual bleeding or cycles more than 35 days apart. Therapeutic interventions include:

- Oral contraceptives for menstrual cycle control
- Administration of high doses of estrogen and progesterone to produce therapy withdrawal bleeding (pharmaceutical dilation and curettage, removal of uterine contents)
- Cyclic progesterone therapy for chronic anovulatory bleeding (bleeding when no egg is released)

Table 6-11   Management of Menstrual Conditions

CONDITION	USUAL THERAPEUTIC INTERVENTIONS
Amenorrhea	
Primary amenorrhea	Hymenectomy for imperforate hymen Nutritional correction of low BMI Hormone replacement for endocrine dysfunctions
Secondary amenorrhea	Nutritional correction for high/low BMI Estrogen and/or progesterone replacement therapy Thyroid hormone replacement therapy
Dysfunctional or abnormal uterine bleeding	
	Hormone replacement therapy (oral contraceptive pill use, combined estrogen and progestin therapy, progestin therapy alone) Iron supplements for anemia Possible ablation of endometrium
Dysmenorrhea	
Primary dysmenorrhea	NSAIDs or prostaglandin synthetase inhibitors OCPs
Secondary dysmenorrhea	Antibiotics for infection Treatment specific to underlying cause
Endometriosis	
	NSAIDs Surgical removal or ablation of endometrial implants GnRH agonists Medroxyprogesterone (Provera) Continuous OCP therapy
Premenstrual syndrome	
	Education regarding syndrome Stress reduction techniques Regular exercise and sleep habits Smoking cessation Support groups Regular, balanced meals with low intake of sodium and caffeine Diuretic agent at time of symptoms NSAIDs Prostaglandin synthetase inhibitors Selective serotonin reuptake inhibitors (SSRIs) OCPs GnRH agonist (extremely severe symptoms)

Box 6-1

Menstrual Cycle Alterations

- **Hypermenorrhea or menorrhagia:** Excessive menstrual bleeding, either in duration or amount, during regularly occurring menstrual cycles.
- **Hypomenorrhea:** Decreased menstrual bleeding, either in duration or amount, occurring at regular intervals.
- **Intermenstrual bleeding:** Irregular vaginal bleeding, usually not caused by menses and not excessive in amounts, occurring between regular menstrual cycles.
- **Menometrorrhagia:** A combination of menorrhagia and metrorrhagia. Irregular, frequent, possibly excessive, or prolonged vaginal bleeding, which may or may not be menstrual.
- **Metrorrhagia or intermenstrual bleeding:** Bleeding of normal amount but occurring at irregular intervals.
- **Oligomenorrhea:** Light menstrual bleeding or infrequent menses, which occur in cycles at least 35 days apart.
- **Polymenorrhea:** Frequent menses that occur in cycles no more than 21 days apart.

■ Nonsteroidal anti-inflammatory drugs (NSAIDs) to reduce the amount of menstrual bleeding

■ Endometrial ablation (separation) to decrease or eliminate menstrual bleeding by eliminating the tissue sloughing

■ Hysterectomy (removal of uterus), when abnormal uterine bleeding cannot be corrected by more conservative methods

Dysmenorrhea

Dysmenorrhea is painful menses or cramping during menstruation. Typically dysmenorrhea begins up to 48 hours before onset of menses and resolves within 2 to 4 days of onset or by the end of the menstrual period (Ugarriza, Klinger, & O'Brien, 1998). Dysmenorrhea can be classified as primary or secondary.

Primary Dysmenorrhea

Primary dysmenorrhea is painful menses with a uterine cause, but without pelvic pathology, and usually occurs within 1 to 3 years of menarche (Ugarriza et al., 1998). Painful uterine contractions stimulated by prostaglandin produced by the endometrium during menses are most often identified as the cause for primary dysmenorrhea. Symptoms of primary dysmenorrhea may include sharp, intermittent suprapubic pain radiating to the back or thighs; headache; fatigue; backache; flushing; dizziness; and syncope. Typically, adolescents do not experience dysmenorrhea until menstrual cycles become ovulatory. Women often experience reduction in dysmenorrhea after pregnancy. Therapeutic interventions for primary dysmenorrhea are directed toward reduction of symptoms and include NSAIDs started 1 to 3 days before the onset of menstrual flow (to decrease prostaglandin production) and oral contraceptives, to decrease endometrial proliferation and, therefore, the amount of prostaglandin produced by the endometrium.

Secondary Dysmenorrhea

Secondary dysmenorrhea is painful menses resulting from a pathologic process, such as pressure from outside the uterus, tissue ischemia, cervical stenosis, congenital abnormality (imperforate hymen), endometriosis, ovarian cysts, PID, or uterine fibroid tumors (Ugarriza et al., 1998). Symptoms may begin earlier in the cycle and last longer than the symptoms of primary dysmenorrhea,

with specific symptoms other than pain. These symptoms can include breast tenderness and a change in bowel habits. Therapeutic intervention usually involves correction of the cause.

Endometriosis

Endometriosis is a chronic disorder resulting from the implantation of endometrial tissue outside the uterus. Pelvic sites of endometrial tissue implantation include the cervix, cul-de-sac, ovaries, fallopian tubes, pelvic peritoneum, uterine broad ligaments, and bowel (Figure 6-14) (Corwin, 1997). Distant sites of endometrial tissue implantation occur less commonly and can include the abdominal wall, kidneys, spleen, gallbladder, diaphragm, lung, stomach, or breasts. Each of these sites will bleed during the menstrual cycle. The disorder affects nearly one in seven women of childbearing age. Endometrial tissue, regardless of location, responds to cyclic ovarian hormone fluctuations. However, there is no place for the endometrial tissue to be sloughed off; blood shed from the endometrial tissue implants accumulates locally dur-

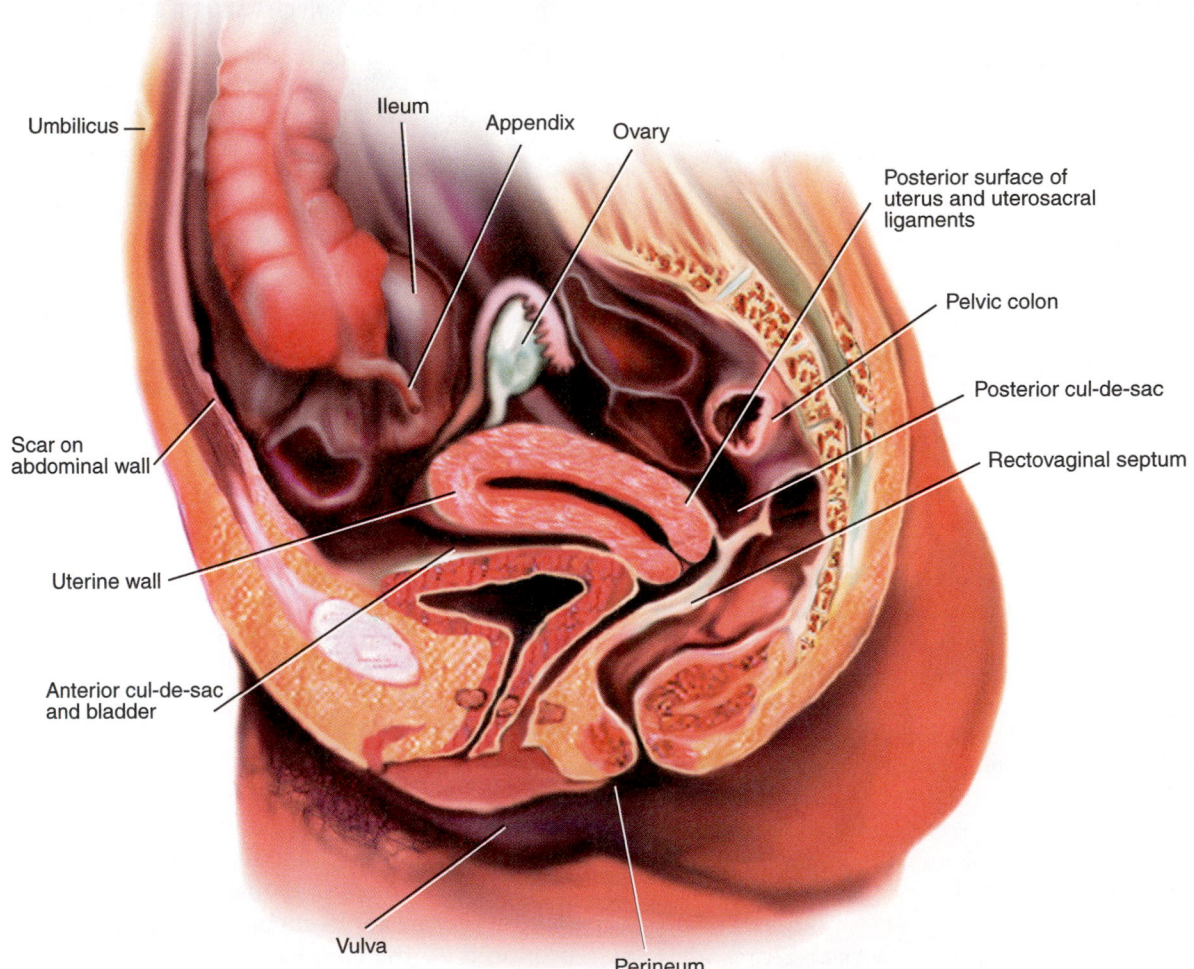

Figure 6-14   Common sites of endometriosis.

ing menses. Often, women experience short menstrual cycles (less than 28 days), increased duration of bleeding (7 days or more), excessive bleeding (for at least 5 days), and significant cramping (Corwin, 1997). The woman experiences symptoms of pain, inflammation, or pelvic heaviness, depending on the duration of the disorder, location of endometrial tissue implants, and the phases of the menstrual cycle. The intensity and duration of symptoms seem to be greater in women with more advanced disease. Such women may experience chronic pelvic pain, frequent low back pain and heaviness, dyspareunia, cyclic painful defecation or rectal bleeding, cyclic diarrhea, cyclic flank pain, or cyclic hematuria or dysuria.

Therapeutic intervention is focused on stopping the progressive destruction of pelvic organs caused by the progression of endometrial implants and preserving fertility options for the woman. Endometrial implants are removed surgically or ablated with laser or electrocautery to preserve childbearing capability. NSAIDs aid in pain control by reducing prostaglandin production by the endometrial implants during menses. In addition, temporary relief can be achieved by continuous administration of gonadotropin-releasing hormone (GnRH) to prevent release of luteinizing hormone (LH), thus causing temporary cessation of menstruation. If suppression of menstrual cycles lasts longer than 6 months, low-dose ERT or estrogen and progesterone replacement therapy is usually begun to prevent bone loss and alleviate symptoms of menopause.

Premenstrual Syndrome

Premenstrual syndrome (PMS) is a cyclic cluster of behavioral, emotional, and physical symptoms that occurs during the luteal phase of the menstrual cycle. The symptoms must be sufficiently severe to interrupt normal activity before the diagnosis can be made (Ugarriza et al., 1998). The cause is unknown but is thought to be related to hormonal changes. Since 1987, PMS has been recognized as a mental disorder (Ugarriza et al., 1998). For most women with PMS, symptoms are noticed from 2 to 12 days before the onset of menses and resolve within 24 hours of the onset of menses and vary in severity. An estimated 30% to 40% of women of childbearing age are believed to experience PMS to some degree (Ugarriza et al., 1998).

Women may experience one or more of the recognized symptoms, which can be classified as affective, cognitive, autonomic, behavioral, neurologic, dermatologic, a result of fluid or electrolyte imbalances, neurovegetative, or algetic (painful). Affective symptoms include sadness, anxiety, anger, irritability, and mood swings. Cognitive symptoms manifest as decreased concentration, indecision, paranoia, rejection sensitivity, and suicidal ideation. Autonomic symptoms include nausea, diarrhea, palpitations, and perspiration. Behavioral symptoms are demonstrated by decreased motivation, poor impulse control,

decreased efficiency, and social isolation. Clumsiness, seizures, dizziness, paresthesias (numbness or tingling), and tremors are the neurologic symptoms. Dermatologic symptoms are acne or greasy or dry hair. Fluid or electrolyte imbalances may cause bloating, weight gain, oliguria (decreased urine), or edema (swelling). Neurovegetative symptoms include insomnia, hypersomnia, anorexia, fatigue, lethargy, agitation, and libido (sex drive) change. Pain experienced by women with PMS can manifest as headaches, breast tenderness, and joint and muscle pain.

Therapeutic interventions for PMS are designed to achieve alleviation of symptoms, since PMS is not a disease. No single treatment has been effective. Women are taught to modify diet, increase exercise, alleviate stress, and change activities of daily living to reduce the intensity of symptoms, reduce fatigue, enhance the ability to sleep, and reduce stress.

Nursing Implications

Nursing assessment for menstrual conditions involves careful medical and gynecologic history taking, assessment of symptoms, and assessment for specific suspected conditions. The interview should begin with a discussion of medical and gynecologic history and lifestyle behaviors, which permits establishment of rapport, before asking more personal questions specific to characteristics of the menstrual cycle. The physical assessment focuses on collection of data regarding the suspected menstrual cycle abnormality, including collection of laboratory test samples and specimens.

The nursing diagnosis can be formulated once the condition is identified. Nursing diagnoses are individualized for the client and her condition. Applicable nursing diagnoses may include:

- Pain related to a specific menstrual condition
- Fear related to the medical diagnosis
- Anxiety related to unknown outcomes
- Deficient knowledge related to limited experience (or information) regarding (specific menstrual cycle condition)

Planning includes specific actions the woman should complete to achieve the highest level of wellness. There is a greater guarantee of compliance when plans are designed in collaboration with the client. Sample planning goals may include:

- Consume correct proportions of foods recommended in the food pyramid, as evidenced by a 24-hour diet recall.
- Exercise by walking 30 minutes each day.
- Take any prescriptive medications as written.

Client Education

Women's Health Problems

For the client to successfully achieve her outcome goals, she must know the following:

1. **Expected, unexpected, and adverse effects of her medication**

2. **Correct scheduling of medication according to her daily schedule**

3. **Convenient reminders for taking medication (i.e., when she brushes her teeth or some other routine activity)**

4. **Rationale for change in lifestyle behaviors as they affect her treatment regimen**

5. **Effects, outcomes, and physical sensations for all assessment procedures and treatment procedures**

6. **Rationale and recommended schedule for follow-up assessments**

7. **Reinforcement that all medication must be taken, leftover medication must be discarded, primary provider must be informed when medication is discontinued before scheduled end of therapy, and medication must not be shared among family members or friends**

- Understand instructions regarding prescriptive medications.
- Return to the health care facility as scheduled for follow-up visits.
- Call the health care provider if adverse effects of prescriptive medications occur.
- Call the health care provider if symptoms do not improve.
- Have questions answered to satisfy need for information.
- Understand health promotion counseling.

Breast Conditions

Women's breast conditions are intimately connected with personal and social images of women. Thus, breast conditions have the potential to generate significant emotional and physiologic effects. Breast conditions can be categorized as benign or malignant. Table 6-12 lists data related to breast conditions and Table 6-13 lists therapeutic interventions. Malignant (cancerous) breast conditions were discussed earlier in the chapter.

Benign Breast Conditions

Benign breast conditions are noncancerous changes in the breast and account for the majority of breast conditions. For the most part, benign breast conditions are related to physiologic changes and include fibrocystic changes, fibroadenoma, and nipple discharge. Evaluation and characteristics of breast masses are outlined in Tables 6-14 and 6-15 and in Figures 6-16–6-18.

Fibrocystic Changes

Fibrocystic changes are age-related changes most commonly involving cyst formation and thickening of breast tissue: the result is "lumpy" breasts. The "lumps" may be tender or painful. The tenderness may be present throughout the cycle or episodic. Women who report fibrocystic changes often experience cyclic, bilateral nodularity, usually in the upper outer quadrant of the breast or in the axillia, and increased tenderness or pain before the onset of menses (Baron & Walsh, 1995). The nodularity feels like fibrous thickening or lumpiness without a clear outline and may disappear after the menstrual period. The changes are thought to be caused by estrogen and progestin changes, imbalances, or fluctuations and occur in premenopausal women or chronically in women aged 35 to 50. When the changes result from atypical hyperplasia, the woman's risk for development of breast cancer increases (White, Griffith, Nenstiel, & Dyess, 1996). There does not seem to be an association between fibrocystic nodularity and increased risk of breast cancer. Therapeutic interventions are limited to differentiating between fibrocystic changes and breast cancer. Screening interventions include clinical breast examination, mammography, and ultrasonography. Contents of fluid-filled cysts are aspirated and evaluated to determine if neoplastic cells are present. Aspiration of the cyst often eliminates the cyst, but the cyst may reform.

Fibroadenoma

Fibroadenoma is a painless solid breast mass or tumor, which has well-defined borders, is mobile, often feels oval-shaped, frequently feels "rubbery," tends to reach a size of 1 of 3 centimeters, and does not change in response to cycling hormone levels (Brucker & Scharbo-DeHaan, 1991). The woman may report a discrete, mobile, seed-sized, or marble-sized "lump" (with no nipple discharge) in one or both breasts. The cause of fibroadenoma is an overgrowth of breast tissue, which occurs most often between the ages of 20 and 40; however, it may not be discovered until the perimenopausal or postmenopausal period (Brucker & Scharbo-DeHaan, 1991). Therapeutic interventions are focused on establishing the benign diagnosis. Screening techniques include mammogram and ultrasound. The mass may be evaluated using fine-needle aspiration biopsy or excision (removal) biopsy.

Table 6-12 Common Conditions of the Breast

CONDITION	DATA SUBJECTIVE	OBJECTIVE	LABORATORY OR PROCEDURE
Benign Conditions			
Fibrocystic changes	Lump(s) Pain Tenderness Bilateral	Palpable, movable, rubbery, firm, smooth, distinct mass(es) Bilateral	Mammogram Ultrasound examination Fine-needle aspiration for biopsy Possibly excisional biopsy
Fibroadenoma	Lump(s) Nontender	Firm, smooth, discrete mass(es) Often bilateral	Mammogram Ultrasound examination Possibly excisional biopsy
Nipple discharge	Unilateral or bilateral discharge Pain (duct ectasia)	Multicolored or gray, thin-to-thick discharge (must be expressed) Nipple fixation Discharge from multiple ducts	Cytologic examination of discharge Hemostix (blood detection strip)
	Spontaneous discharge most often from one nipple only (intraductal) Papilloma (if multiple papillomas, discharge can be bilateral)	Serosanguinous discharge Usually one duct (unless multiple papillomas)	Cytologic examination of discharge Hemostix Surgical biopsy
	Bilateral milky discharge (galactorrhea)	Milky color From multiple ducts Possibly signs of hypothyroidism or pituitary enlargement	Visual field testing Pituitary MRI Hemostix
Malignant Conditions			
Localized cancer	Lump(s) Possibly unilateral nipple discharge	Palpable, nondiscrete, movable or fixed mass(es) Abnormal results on mammogram Nipple discharge that is bloody, serous, serosanguinous, or watery	Mammogram Ultrasound examination Biopsy Hemostix Cytologic examination of discharge
Invasive cancer	Lump(s) Possible nipple discharge	Hard, nondiscrete, fixed mass(es) Dimpling Nipple flattening or deviation (unilateral)	Mammogram Ultrasound examination Biopsy with cytologic examination Hemostix and cytology (for any discharge)
	May also include: nipple skin change, such as itching, burning, "weeping," bleeding ulceration (Paget's disease)	Nipple discharge Peau d'orange (Figure 6-15) appearance Nipple skin changes Venous prominence (unilateral) Swelling (unilateral)	Mammogram Ultrasound examination Biopsy Cytologic examination of discharge Hemostix Biopsy
Metastatic cancer	Lump(s) Skin changes Arthralgia Bone pain Shortness of breath Possible spontaneous nipple discharge	Masses of varying size Hard, fixed lymph nodes Dimpling the skin Skin erythema Bloody, serous, serosangiunous, or watery discharge from single duct	Bone scan Chest X-ray film Hemostix Cytologic studies

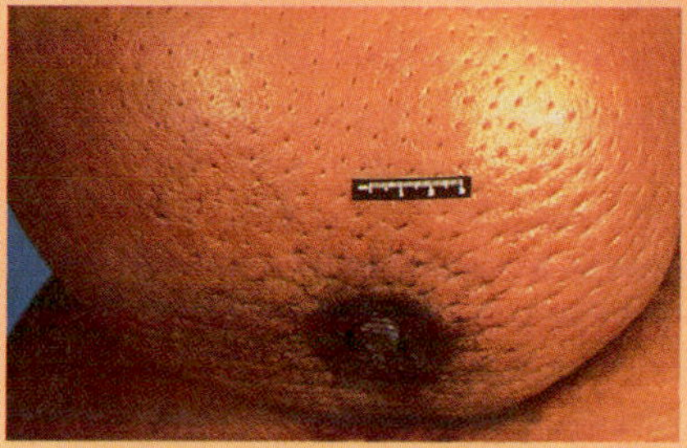

Figure 6-15 Peau d'orange. (Courtesy of Dr. S. Eva Singletary, University of Texas, M.D. Anderson Cancer Center)

Table 6-13 Management of Conditions of the Breast	
CONDITION	USUAL THERAPEUTIC INTERVENTIONS
Benign Conditions	
Fibrocystic changes	Consider avoiding methylxanthine (caffeine) Avoid tobacco Wear well-fitting bra Diuretic agent for premenstrual symptoms Clinical breast examination annually (every 6 months if there is a familial risk for breast cancer) Baseline mammogram at age 35, every 1 to 2 years from age 40 to age 50, annually after age 50
Fibroadenoma	Excisional biopsy for solid lumps not clearly identified as benign by other methods Follow-up clinical breast examinations and mammograms (see fibrocystic changes)
Nipple discharge	Evaluation for possible malignancy Follow-up clinical breast examinations and mammograms (see fibrocystic changes) Bromocriptine (Parlodel) for galactorrhea Surgery (depending on cause)
Malignant Conditions	
Localized cancer	Radiation Lumpectomy (breast-conserving surgery)
Invasive cancer	Surgery Combination therapy: chemotherapy, hormone therapy, radiotherapy
Metastatic cancer	Combination therapy: chemotherapy, hormone therapy, radiotherapy Possibly autologous marrow transplant Consider thoracentesis and paracentesis, if shortness of breath is a symptom

Nipple Discharge

Nipple discharge is fluid produced by and accumulating within a secretory unit of the breast and exiting through the nipple (Arnold & Neiheisel, 1997). The woman may notice nipple discharge on her bra or night clothing. Nipple discharge can be categorized as lactation, physiologic, pathologic, or false discharge.

Lactation Discharge. **Lactation discharge** is any secretory discharge occurring as a physiologic response to the normal hormonal stimulation of pregnancy, postpartum, or the period following weaning of the infant (Arnold & Neiheisel, 1997). The discharge is usually thin and white and discharged from both breasts. With continued stimulation, the woman may continue to experience lactation discharge for several weeks to years after weaning the infant. The lactation discharge is not harmful. Therapeutic interventions involve education regarding the cause of the discharge and the recommendation to limit or avoid stimulation of the breasts.

Physiologic Discharge. **Physiologic discharge** is the result of physiologic conditions affecting all breast tissue equally (i.e., bilaterally), involving secretory tissue in each breast, and resulting in milky-white or multicolored (yellow, green, or gray) fluid. Usually milky, nonlactation nipple discharge is referred to as galactorrhea. Occurrences or practices that are characteristic of galactorrhea include hyperprolactinemia (an elevated serum prolactin level); menarche or menopause; intake of exogenous estrogens or progestins, dopamine antagonist medications, or opiates; sexual or mechanical nipple stimulation; and traumatic anterior thoracic nerve stimulation. Thus, the discharge is not part of a disease process. Therapeutic interventions include reassurance and counseling.

Pathologic Discharge. **Pathologic discharge** is the result of pathologic conditions affecting the hypothalamic-pituitary axis, prolactin levels, or breast diseases, and, thus, may affect both breasts (Arnold & Neiheisel, 1997). Pathologic conditions that cause hyperprolactinemia include tumor of the pituitary gland, Addison's disease, and hypothyroidism. The nipple discharge associated with such conditions is thin and milky. Some causes of pathologic galactorrhea are benign and include intraductal papilloma (benign epithelial neoplasm), duct ectasia (inflammatory response to stagnation of breast duct secretions), and breast infections. Nipple discharge caused by intraductal papillomas tends to be serous or bloody and may be secreted from only one breast, unless one or more intraductal papillomas are present in each breast. The color of the nipple discharge caused by ductal ectasia can

Table 6-14   Evaluation of Breast Mass Characteristics

If a breast mass is noted during palpation, the following information should be obtained regarding the mass. Always note if one or both breasts are involved.

Location	Identify the quadrant involved or visualize the breast with the face of a clock superimposed on it. The nipple represents the center of the clock. Note where the mass lies in relation to the nipple, e.g., 3 cm from the nipple in the 3 o'clock position.
Size	Determine size in centimeters in all three planes (height, width, and depth).
Shape	Qualify the mass as round, ovoid, matted, or irregular.
Number	Note if lesions are singular or multiple. Note if one or both breasts are involved.
Consistency	Qualify the mass as firm, hard, soft, fluid, or cystic.
Definition	Note if the mass borders are discrete or irregular.
Mobility	Determine if the mass is fixed or freely mobile in relation to the chest wall.
Tenderness	Note if palpation elicits pain.
Erythema	Note any redness over involved area (Figure 6-16).
Dimpling or retraction	Observe for dimpling (Figure 6-17) or retraction (Figure 6-18) as the client raises arms overhead and presses her hands into her hips.

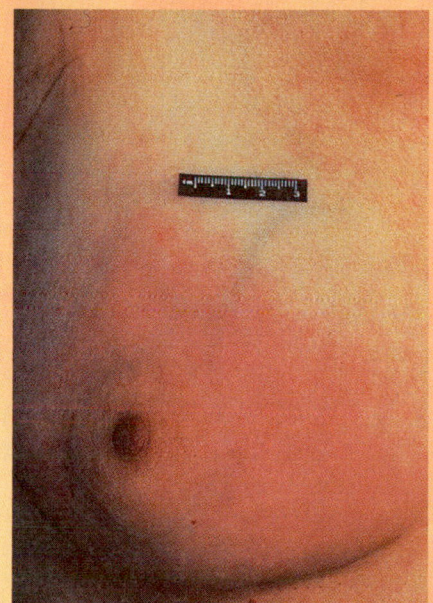

Figure 6-16   Erythema with Abnormal Vascular Pattern Secondary to Inflammatory Breast Cancer. (Courtesy of Dr. S. Eva Singletary, University of Texas, M.D. Anderson Cancer Center)

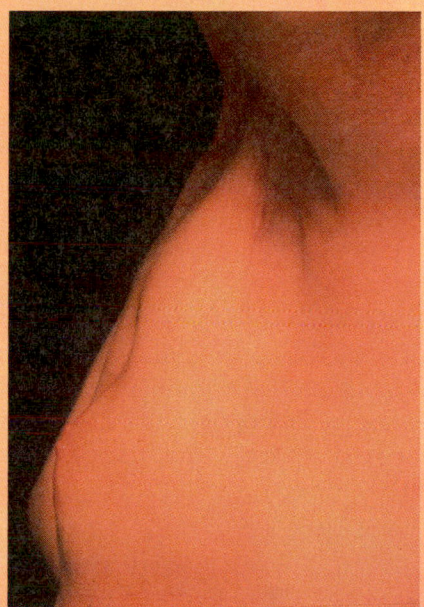

Figure 6-17   Dimpling of Left Breast Tissue. (Courtesy of Dr. S. Eva Singletary, University of Texas, M.D. Anderson Cancer Center)

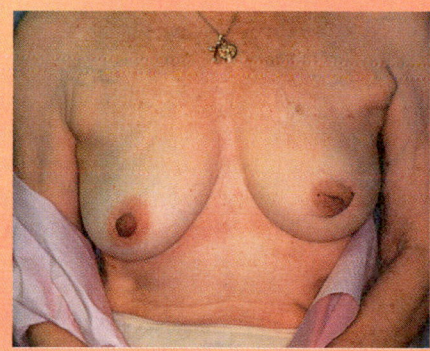

Figure 6-18   Nipple Retraction on Left Breast. (Courtesy of Steven M. Lynch, M.D.)

be bloody, brown, cream-colored, gray, green, purulent, or white and can vary from thin to extremely thick. Breast infections usually result in purulent nipple discharge. Therapeutic interventions involve individualization of treatment to the cause of the discharge. Lactogenic medications can be eliminated or the dose reduced, antibiotics are administered for infectious processes, exercise habits causing the discharge can be altered, and referral for

biopsy for suspected malignant discharge establishes the cause of the discharge (Arnold & Neiheisel, 1997).

Of greatest concern is diagnosis of the pathologic discharge accompanying breast cancer. Fortunately, the majority of pathologic nipple discharges are caused by benign pathologic processes, but occasionally, pathologic nipple discharge is caused by breast cancer (Arnold & Neiheisel, 1997). In such cases, the discharge is most often

Table 6-15   Characteristics of Common Breast Masses

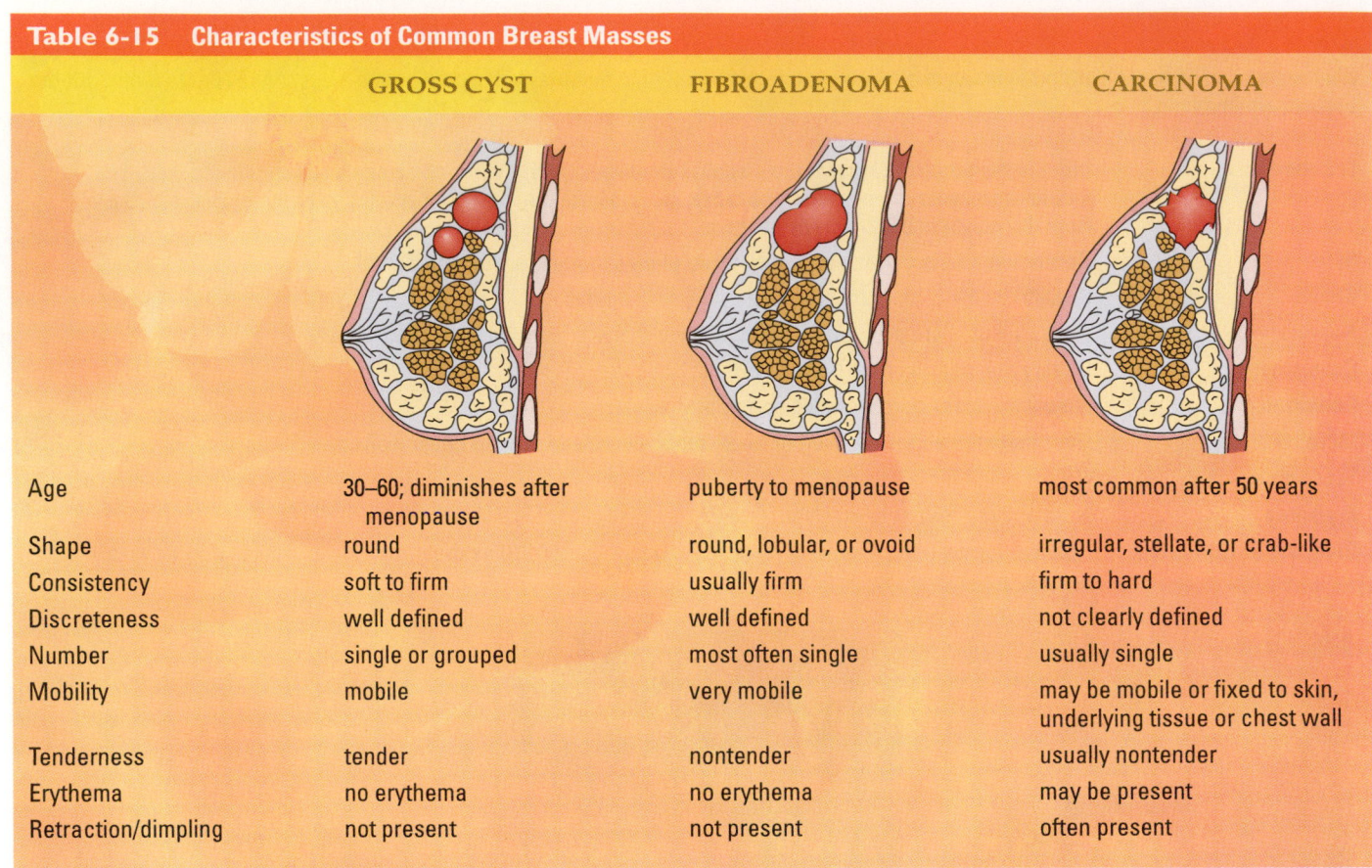

	GROSS CYST	FIBROADENOMA	CARCINOMA
Age	30–60; diminishes after menopause	puberty to menopause	most common after 50 years
Shape	round	round, lobular, or ovoid	irregular, stellate, or crab-like
Consistency	soft to firm	usually firm	firm to hard
Discreteness	well defined	well defined	not clearly defined
Number	single or grouped	most often single	usually single
Mobility	mobile	very mobile	may be mobile or fixed to skin, underlying tissue or chest wall
Tenderness	tender	nontender	usually nontender
Erythema	no erythema	no erythema	may be present
Retraction/dimpling	not present	not present	often present

spontaneous, associated with a breast mass, and a "classically unilateral, single-duct discharge" (Arnold & Neitheisel, 1997, p. 109). Usually, the discharge associated with breast cancer is bloody, serous, and watery: the bloody discharge ranges from bright red to black and the serous discharge is thin, sticky, and yellow to light orange (Arnold & Neiheisel, 1997).

False Discharge.   **False discharge** refers to fluid appearing on the nipple or areolar surface that is not secreted by breast tissue (Arnold & Neiheisel, 1997). Conditions associated with false nipple discharge include any dermatologic disease (eczema, bacterial or viral dermatitis), nipple trauma, or Paget's disease (inflammatory, malignant neoplasm). The fluid appearing on the nipple or areola may be bloody, clear, colored, purulent, serous, or viscous. Management includes treatment of the disease causing the discharge (e.g., antibiotics, topical dermatologic medication).

Pelvic Conditions

Pelvic conditions can be categorized as infectious, benign, or malignant conditions. Infectious conditions include vaginal, cervical, and pelvic inflammatory infections

(PID). Benign conditions may affect the cervix, uterus, and ovaries. Malignant conditions, discussed previously, can be cervical, uterine, or ovarian. Table 6-16 lists criteria for pelvic conditions, and Table 6-17 lists usual therapeutic interventions for pelvic conditions.

Infectious Conditions

Infectious conditions of the pelvis include vaginal infections, cervical infections, and PID. Infections may be caused by bacterial, viral, fungal, or protozoal organisms.

Vaginal and Cervical Infection

A **vaginal infection** is inflammation of the vagina, and a **cervical infection** is inflammation of the cervix. Many of the infectious organisms are sexually transmitted (chlamydia, gonorrhea, trichomoniasis, herpes simplex infection, human papilloma virus infection), while others are overgrowth of organisms normally or frequently found in the vagina (yeast, Döderlein's bacillus, beta-hemolytic streptococci). Postmenopausal women who are not receiving ERT or hormonal replacement therapy may experience atrophic vaginitis caused by the response of the vaginal environment to decreased estrogen levels. Bacterial vaginosis (inflammation caused by an overgrowth of

Table 6-16   Pelvic Conditions

	DATA		
CONDITION	**SUBJECTIVE**	**OBJECTIVE**	**LABORATORY OR PROCEDURE**
Infections			
Cervicitis	Spotting (especially after sexual intercourse) Increase in vaginal discharge May be asymptomatic	Yellowish-white discharge Red, edematous, friable cervix Cervical motion Tenderness Grayish-green discharge, with cervix having strawberry-like appearance (trichomoniasis)	Wet mount for WBCs count, trichomonads Cultures for *C. trachomatis, N. gonorrhoeae* HSV Numerous white blood cells
Bacterial vulvovaginosis	Increased vaginal discharge Odor after sexual intercourse	Homogenous gray-white discharge Musty or fishy odor on "whiff" test	pH of discharge using pH sensitive strips Wet mount (clue cells) Positive amine test
Monilial vulvovaginitis	Itching, burning Discharge Dyspareunia	Thick, curd-like vaginal discharge Vulvar or vaginal erythema Edematous cervix Possibly friable cervix	Wet mount (budding hyphae, leukocytes)
Atrophic vulvovaginitis	Vaginal dryness Vaginal irritation and burning Itching Postcoital spotting	Vulvar and vaginal atrophy Pale, thin, friable vaginal mucosa Sparse pubic hair	No lab test is reliable. A maturation index can be done with the Pap smear to provide some data
Pelvic inflammatory disease	Lower abdominal pain or tenderness Chills and fever Nausea and vomiting Increased vaginal discharge Irregular bleeding Malaise Dysmenorrhea Dyspareunia Postcoital spotting Dysuria	Lower abdominal rebound tenderness Cervical motion tenderness Hypoactive bowel sounds Adnexal fullness, tenderness Mucopurulent cervical discharge Cervical friability Body temperature of over 100.4°F	C-reactive protein Erythrocyte sedimentation rate Positive gonorrhea and chlamydia cultures Ultrasound for fluid in cul-de-sac or pelvic mass or abscess Wet mount
Benign Conditions			
Pelvic relaxation			
Uterine prolapse	Backache Pelvic pressure or heaviness	Cervix descended into vagina or through introitus	Bimanual pelvic exam
Cystocele	Urinary frequency, urgency, incontinence Dyspareunia Vaginal pressure Urinary tract infections Incomplete bladder emptying	Bulging of anterior vaginal wall	Postvoid urinary retention Postvoid analysis of urinary retention determines the severity of the condition
Rectocele	Difficult defecation Vaginal pressure Rectal fullness	Bulging of posterior vaginal wall	Rectal exam reveals the severity of rectocele
Enterocele	Vaginal pressure Abdominal pain Loose stools	Bulging of cul-de-sac or posterior vaginal wall	

(continues)

Table 6-16   Pelvic Conditions (continued)

CONDITION	DATA		
	SUBJECTIVE	OBJECTIVE	LABORATORY OR PROCEDURE
Functional Conditions			
Polycystic ovary syndrome	Often asymptomatic Amenorrhea or oligomenorrhea Dysfunctional uterine bleeding Infertility Irregular menstrual cycles	Obesity Hirsutism Acne Enlarged ovaries Enlarged clitoris Voice changes Alopecia	Elevated LH Level Ultrasound examination of ovarian size and follicles Endometrial biopsy for hyperplasia Hyperinsulinemia Serum glucose Serum prolactin level
Premature ovarian failure	Amenorrhea Hot flashes Night sweats Vaginal dryness Dyspareunia	Vaginal atrophy Vulvar atrophy Uterine atrophy	Testosterone level ↑FSH and LH levels ↓Thyroid function tests ↑Prolactin level
Structural Conditions			
Fibroid tumors	Most are asymptomatic Possible pressure discomfort Possible hypermenorrhea Pain if tumor is twisted Pelvic pressure Deep pelvic pain Dyspareunia	Abnormal results on pelvic examination Anemia from hypermenorrhea Palpation of painless, mobile, smooth uterine mass or nodule	Ultrasound examination Pelvic magnetic resonance imaging (MRI) These tests identify the location and size of fibroids
Malignant Conditions			
Cervical cancer	Blood-tinged, watery vaginal discharge Abnormal vaginal bleeding Postcoital spotting or bleeding Dyspareunia Abdominal, back, or flank pain	Enlarged cervix Foul-smelling discharge Anemia Leg edema	Pap smear Colposcopy, cervical, and endo-cervical sampling for cytology
Endometrial cancer	Metrorrhagia (premenopausal) Pelvic pain or bloating (advanced disease) Postmenopausal bleeding	Uterus may be abnormal on palpation	Endometrial biopsy for cytology
Ovarian cancer	Changes in bowel or bladder function Abdominal fullness, discomfort Dyspareunia Irregular bleeding Fatigue Back pain Shortness of breath Pelvic pressure	Ascites Possible pelvic mass Weight loss	Blood level of CA-125 Vaginal ultrasound Barium enema MRI or CT scan with contrast Laparotomy

anaerobic bacteria) accounts for 40% to 50% of vaginitis, vulvovaginal candidiasis (yeast infection) accounts for 20% to 25%, and vaginal trichomoniasis (a sexually transmitted protozoal infection) accounts for 15% to 20% (Cullins, Dominguez, Guberski, Secor, & Wysocki, 1999).

Women who come for treatment of vaginal infection typically relate symptoms of vaginal discharge; pruritus; local irritation; dysuria (painful urination); and dyspareunia (painful intercourse). If the woman has bacterial vaginosis, she often complains of a "fishy" odor of the vaginal discharge, especially after sexual intercourse. If the vaginitis is

Table 6-17   Management of Pelvic Conditions

CONDITION	USUAL THERAPEUTIC INTERVENTIONS	CONDITION	USUAL THERAPEUTIC INTERVENTIONS
Structural Conditions		**Infection**	
Fibroid Tumors	Iron and progestins (small tumors and minimal symptoms)	Cervicitis Vaginitis	Medication specific to the causative organism (metronidazole for tricho-moniasis, acyclovir for herpes simplex virus, ceftriaxone for gonorrhea, doxycycline for chlamydia)
	Surgery (myomectomy, hysterectomy) GnRH agonists (short-term therapy only) Annual pelvic ultrasound to monitor size of tumors		
		Bacterial vulvovaginosis	Metronidazole, clindamycin
Pelvic Relaxation		Monilial vulvovaginitis	Terconazole
Uterine prolapse	Kegel exercises, ERT, vaginal pessaries (mild prolapse) Hysterectomy	Trichomoniasis	Metronidazole
		Pelvic inflamma-tory disease	Cefoxitin or cefotetan and doxycycline; or clindamycin and ofloxin; or clindamycin and gentamicin
Cystocele	Kegel exercises, vaginal pessaries for uterine prolapse, ERT Surgical repair		ERT or hormone replacement therapy Vaginal lubricant (K-Y Jelly, Replens) Atrophic vaginitis
Enterocele	Weight reduction Vaginal pessary Surgical repair	**Malignant Conditions**	
Rectocele	High-fiber diet Regular bowel habits Increased fluid intake Stool softeners Vaginal pessary Surgical repair	Endometrial cancer	Surgery: total abdominal hysterectomy and bilateral salpingo-oophorectomy (TAH-BSO) or TAH-BSO followed by radiotherapy or intrauterine radiation followed by TAH-BSO (depends on stage of cancer) Chemotherapy and/or progestin therapy for distant metastases
Functional Conditions		Cervical cancer	Cryosurgery, loop electrosurgical excision procedure (LEEP), cone biopsy, laser surgery, or hysterectomy for pre-invasive dysplasia Total vaginal hysterectomy TAH, radical hysterectomy with lymph node dissection (depending on size of lesion) Radiation (advanced disease)
Polycystic ovary syndrome	Diet modification (obesity) Weight reduction Stress management (decrease excess androgen) Hair removal (hirsutism) Medroxyprogesterone for cyclic withdrawal bleeding Clomiphene for ovulation induction ERT or oral contraceptives (for hyperandrogenism) Possible ovarian wedge resection	Ovarian cancer	Surgery (from unilateral oopherectomy to TAH-BSO) and/or node excision (depends on stage of cancer) Radiotherapy Chemotherapy
Premature ovarian failure	Hormone replacement therapy		

caused by *Candida*, pruritus, dysuria, and vulvovaginal irritation tend to be the primary complaints. The woman who has trichomoniasis usually complains of copious yellowish or greenish discharge with a foul odor, pruritus, vulvovaginal irritation, and dysuria. Table 6-18 contains a description of vaginal discharges. Women should be taught how to perform a self-inspection of the external genitalia (Figure 6-19).

Based on the Centers for Disease Control and Prevention (CDC) recommendations, therapeutic intervention for bacterial vaginosis is intravaginal metronidazole or clindamycin cream (Cullins et al., 1999). CDC recommendations for vulvovaginal candidiasis are intravaginal terconazole cream or suppositories. Oral metronidazole is the CDC recommendation for treatment of trichomoniasis (Cullins et al., 1999) Since trichomoniasis is considered a sexually transmitted disease (STD), the woman's partner must be treated simultaneously and she must avoid sexual intercourse until the disease is cured.

Table 6-18 Description of Vaginal Discharges

CHARACTERISTIC	NORMAL	NONSPECIFIC VAGINITIS	TRICHOMONAL	CANDIDAL	GONOCOCCAL
Color	White	Gray	Grayish yellow	White	Greenish yellow
Odor	Absent	Fishy	Fishy	Absent	Absent
Consistency	Nonhomogenous	Homogenous	Purulent, often with bubbles	Cottage cheese-like	Mucopurulent
Location	Dependent	Adherent to walls	Often pooled in fornix	Adherent to walls	Adherent to walls
Anatomic Appearance					
Vulva	Normal	Normal	Edematous	Erythematous	Erythematous
Vaginal mucosa	Normal	Normal	Usually normal	Erythematous	Normal
Cervix	Normal	Normal	May show red spots	Patches of discharge	Pus in os

Note. From *Health Assessment & Physical Examination* (2nd ed.), by M. E. Z. Estes, 2002, Clifton Park, NY: Delmar Learning.

Pelvic Inflammatory Disease

Pelvic inflammatory disease (PID) is inflammation of the uterus, fallopian tubes, or ovaries, or a combination, caused by ascent of vaginal flora or bacteria. At least 1 million women, 70% of whom are younger than age 25, are estimated to have PID annually (Mott, 1998). The ma-

Nursing Alert

Criteria for Diagnosis of Pelvic Inflammatory Disease

- Uterine/adnexal tenderness **or**
- Cervical motion tenderness **and** any of the following:

Oral temperature >101°F (>38.3°C)

Abnormal cervical or vaginal mucopurulent discharge

Presence of white blood cells (WBCs) on saline microscopy of vaginal secretions

Elevated erythrocyte sedimentation rate

Elevated C-reactive protein

Laboratory documentation of cervical infection with *N. gonorrhoeae* or *C. trachomatis*

Note. From "Sexually Transmitted Diseases Treatment Guidelines," by the Centers for Disease Control and Prevention, 2002, *Morbidity and Mortality Weekly Report, 51* (RR-6), pp. 1–75.

Nursing Tip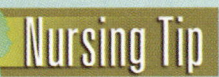

Treatment Guidelines for Pelvic Inflammatory Disease

Parenteral and Oral Regimen for Hospitalized Clients

Cefotetan 2 g IV every 12 hours

OR

Cefoxitin 2 g IV every 6 hours

PLUS

Doxycycline 100 mg orally or IV every 12 hours

for 24 hours after clinical improvement **THEN**

Clindamycin 450 mg orally four times/day for 14 days

Oral Regimen for Outpatient Treatment

Ofloxacin 400 mg orally twice/day for 14 days

OR

Levofloxacin 500 mg orally once/daily for 14 days

WITH OR WITHOUT

Metronidazole 500 mg orally twice/day for 14 days

Note. From "Sexually Transmitted Diseases Treatment Guidelines," by the Centers for Disease Control and Prevention, 2002, *Morbidity and Mortality Weekly Report, 51* (RR-6), pp. 1–75.

Women should be encouraged to examine their external genitalia once a month, following these steps:

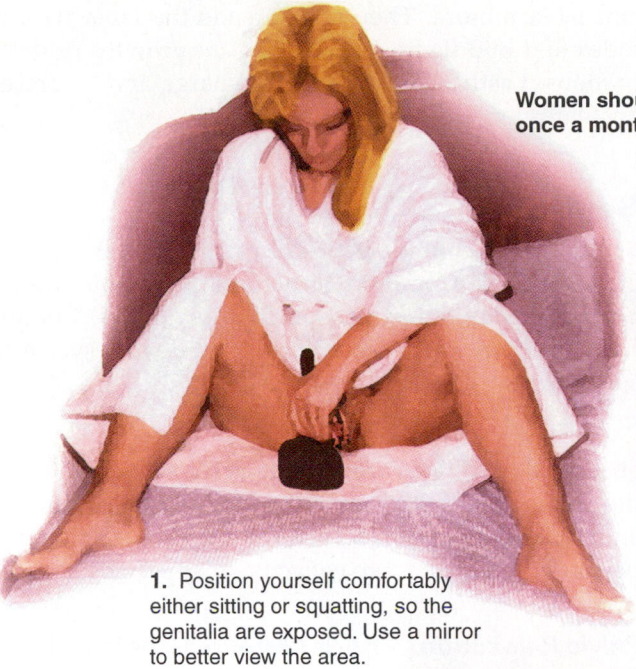

1. Position yourself comfortably either sitting or squatting, so the genitalia are exposed. Use a mirror to better view the area.

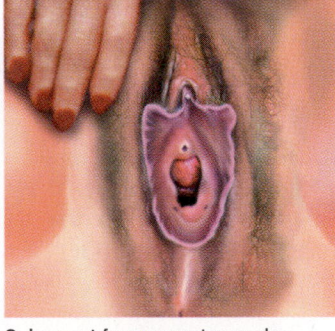

2. Inspect for symmetry, moles, growth, changes in skin color, inflammation, irritated areas, and infestations.

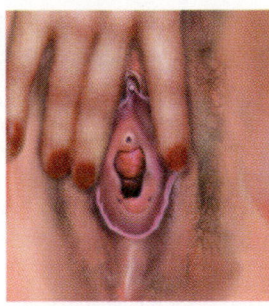

3. Using the index and middle fingers, gently spread the labia to inspect the clitoris and inner sides of the labia.

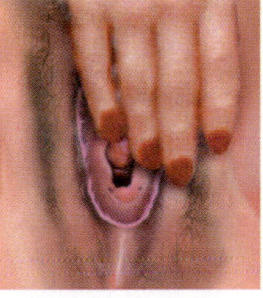

4. Using the finger pads, gently palpate the vulvar region, noting any lumps, nodules, irregularities, or tenderness.

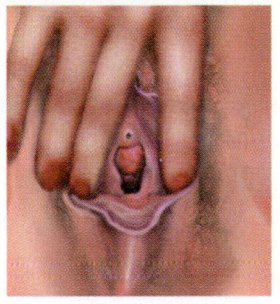

5. Using the index and middle fingers, spread the vaginal opening slightly and palpate the tissue for moistness, elasticity, lumps, nodules, irregularities, or tenderness.

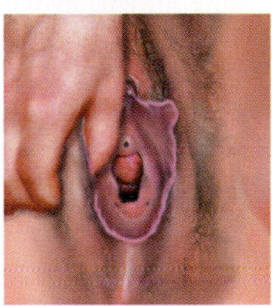

6. Insert the thumb inside the labia and gently compress the tissue between the thumb and index finger, noting any lumps, lesions, or tenderness.

Figure 6-19   Steps to follow to perform vulvar self-examination.

jority of PID infections are caused by chlamydia and gonorrhea, ascending from the vagina. High-risk women are those who are age 25 or younger, have multiple sex partners, do not use barrier protection, douche, and use intrauterine devices. PID is often undiagnosed and the treatment is delayed, which increases the risk for infertility, ectopic pregnancy, and chronic pelvic pain.

Nursing Implications

Nursing assessment for infections includes assessment for risk, symptoms, medical history, gynecologic history, and lifestyle behaviors. Physical assessment focuses on data and specimen collection to aid diagnosis of the specific infection (see Table 6-16).

Nursing diagnoses are formulated after diagnosis of infection. Applicable nursing diagnosis may include the following:

- Pain related to infection
- Fear related to the diagnosis
- Deficient knowledge related to limited experience regarding the disorder

Nursing plans include specific actions the client completes to achieve the highest level of wellness possible. Sample goals may include the following:

- Take prescriptive medication as written.
- Understand instructions regarding prescriptive medication(s).

■ Return to health care provider as scheduled for follow-up assessment of infection status.

■ Notify health care provider of adverse effects of prescribed medication(s).

■ Notify health care provider of failure of symptoms to improve as expected.

■ Adopt recommended change in lifestyle behavior to prevent recurrence of infection.

■ Have questions answered to her satisfaction.

■ Understand health promotion counseling.

Nursing interventions involve teaching, counseling for prevention, and explaining prescribed medications. Women with multiple sexual partners should be counseled about:

■ The risks for infection

■ Recommendations for annual screening for chlamydial and gonorrheal infections

■ Testing for chlamydial and gonorrheal infections 3 to 6 months after starting a relationship with a new sexual partner

■ The need for sexual partners to be treated each time chlamydial and gonorrheal infections occur

■ Eliminating douching, because such practices destroy the lactobacilli residing in the vagina and may force bacteria from the vagina into the uterus

■ Distinguishing between normal vaginal discharge and discharge characteristic of vaginal infection

Educational nursing intervention includes explaining the dangers of self-diagnosis of vaginal infection and use of over-the-counter or herbal therapies instead of seeking early diagnosis and therapeutic intervention at the first sign of a vaginal infection. Nurses should provide emotional support and therapeutic communication to overcome a client's embarrassment regarding vaginal infections and to help clients understand that the delicate balance of the vaginal ecosystem can be disturbed by a variety of factors (Cullins et al., 1999).

When a woman presents with a pelvic infection, the nurse can use such a moment to explain the vulvar self-examination to her. The woman can be encouraged to perform the vulvar examination at the same time of the month as she performs BSE. To perform the vulvar examination, she lies down, spreads and flexes her knees, and prepares to palpate the inguinal area and vulva with the flat surface of her hand to detect enlarged lymph nodes. Then, using a mirror, she inspects the entire vulvar surface (the area between her legs from the top of her pubic hair to the rectum), looking for any growths or discolorations. She inspects surfaces of both the labia majora and labia minora. Then she spreads the labia with her index and middle fingers, looking for growths or discolorations. Lastly, she looks for discharge and, if present, evaluates for odor, amount, and color.

Benign Pelvic Conditions

Benign pelvic conditions can be categorized as structural or functional. Common structural conditions include pelvic relaxation and uterine fibroid tumors. Common functional conditions include polycystic ovary syndrome.

Structural Conditions

Structural conditions are changes in the size or position of the pelvic organs, including the bladder, uterus, ovaries, and rectum. Common structural changes involving the pelvic organs are known collectively as pelvic relaxation.

Pelvic Relaxation. **Pelvic relaxation** is the loss of pelvic muscle support of the pelvic organs, which may result in development of a cystocele (bulging of the posterior wall of the bladder into the anterior vaginal wall), enterocele (bulging of the bowel into the posterior cul-de-sac and vaginal wall), rectocele (bulging of the anterior wall of the rectum into the posterior vaginal wall), or uterine prolapse (protrusion of the uterus into the vaginal canal). The causes of pelvic relaxation include permanent damage to connective tissue or muscular structure during the stretching and trauma of vaginal birth, chronically increased intraabdominal pressure (from heavy lifting, obesity, straining with constipation, ascites, coughing with obstructive respiratory disease), aging-related muscle atrophy (estrogen deficiency), and congenitally weak connective-tissue strength (elasticity). The woman may experience urinary incontinence, urgency, or frequency; constipation or difficult defecation; pelvic pressure; dyspareunia; walking or sitting discomfort; or protrusion of an organ through the introitus (Lucas, 1999).

Therapeutic interventions for pelvic relaxation depend on the stage of relaxation. First-degree prolapse consists of descent of the cervix into the lower third of the vagina; second-degree is descent of the cervix to the introitus or less than 1 centimeter through the introitus; third-degree is descent of the cervix 1 centimeter beyond the introitus; and fourth-degree is descent or prolapse of the uterus and cervix through the introitus (Lucas, 1999). Women with first- or second-degree stages may increase muscle support for the pelvic organs by performing Kegel exercises several times per day or using a vaginal pessary to provide support for the pelvic organs. For the woman with a third- or fourth-degree prolapse, weakness of the pelvic musculature is irreversible and hysterectomy is usually the treatment of choice (Lucas, 1999).

Fibroid Tumors. **Fibroid tumors** (leiomyomas) are benign tumors arising in the myometrium, which can protrude into the uterine cavity (submucous leiomyomas), bulge through the outer uterine layer (subserous leiomyomas), or grow within the myometrium (intramural leiomyomas). The cause is proliferation of smooth-muscle cells. The tumors usually do not grow more than 1 to 2 centimeters per year; thus, the tumor growth can be watched until the uterus reaches a 4- to 5-month gestation size as a result of tumor growth (Lucas, 1999). By the time the uterus reaches this size, the woman may be experiencing excessive urination, backache, pelvic pressure, abdominal discomfort, hypermenorrhea, anemia, or pressure on the ureters (Lucas, 1999). The tumors are dependent on estrogen for growth and, thus, grow more rapidly during pregnancy. The tumors are found more often during the fourth or fifth decades of life, affect 1 out of 5 Caucasian women, affect 1 of 3 Black women, and occur more often in nulliparous, nonsmoking women who take oral contraceptive pills (Grabo, Fahs, Nataupsky, & Reich, 1999). Anovulatory menstrual cycles (unopposed estrogen) are thought to be the cause of fibroid tumor growth during the perimenopausal period (Grabo et al., 1999). The resulting distortion of uterine shape and size contributes to interference with conception, pregnancy maintenance, and fetal growth and development (Grabo et al., 1999).

Therapeutic intervention depends on the woman's desire for future childbearing. If she does not desire future pregnancies and the tumors are large (at least 4-months' gestation size), she may choose to have a hysterectomy (Lucas, 1999). If she desires future childbearing, she may have a myomectomy to remove submucosal tumors before conception. Hormone therapy may be used for short-term intervention to decrease the size of the fibroid tumors. However, the woman will experience menopausal symptoms and is at risk for osteoporosis if the intervention is continued for more then 6 months.

Functional Conditions

Functional conditions include changes in function of the pelvic organs, such as polycystic ovary syndrome.

Polycystic Ovary Syndrome. **Polycystic ovary syndrome** (PCOS) is a complex endocrine disorder associated with long-term anovulation and an excess of androgens circulating in the blood. The syndrome is characterized by formation of cysts in the ovaries. PCOS is the leading cause of amenorrhea in premenopausal women. It is the cause for amenorrhea in 30% of all women, oligomenorrhea in 75% of women, and hirsutism (excess body hair) in 87% of women. Causes of PCOS are the results of anovulation, such as ovarian failure, hypothalamic or pituitary suppression, and adrenal enzyme dysfunction. The syndrome begins with an imbalance of leutinizing hormone (LH) and follicle-stimulating hormone (FSH), with LH levels elevated and FSH levels low to normal. The result of the hormone imbalance is continued follicular development, elevated estrogen levels, anovulation, and formation of multiple ovarian cysts. Endocrine involvement results in hyperestrogenemia, adrenal androgen excess, ovarian abnormalities, hyperprolactinemia, and hyperinsulinemia. Women typically seek health care for amenorrhea or irregular menstrual cycles, infertility, hirsutism, acne, or obesity.

Medical management for PCOS is targeted to the woman's primary concern (e.g., amenorrhea, hirsutism, infertility, obesity). Combination oral contraceptives or GnRH agonists can be used for hyperandrogenic effects (e.g., male-pattern hair growth and acne). Amenorrhea and anovulation associated with PCOS place the woman at increased risk for endometrial cancer at a young age and for postmenopausal breast cancer. Medroxyprogesterone (Provera) can be used for treatment of the PCOS amenorrhea.

Nursing Implications

Nursing assessment for pelvic conditions involves assessing risk factors, current symptoms, and medical and gynecologic history. Physical assessment focuses on the collection of data to rule out or confirm pelvic condition and identification of the need to collect specimens for laboratory tests and for additional diagnostic procedures (see Table 6-16).

Nursing diagnoses are formulated after the pelvic condition is identified. The diagnoses are individualized for the client and based on the identified pelvic condition. Applicable nursing diagnoses may include the following:

- Pain related to pelvic conditions
- Fear related to procedures and treatment
- Anxiety related to effects of condition or treatment on future childbearing
- Deficient knowledge regarding (specific pelvic condition)

Nursing plans include specific actions that the client will complete to achieve the highest level of wellness possible. Sample goals may include the following:

- Develop strategies for coping with pain.
- Consume recommended foods, based on the food pyramid, daily.
- Reduce stress and promote wellness by exercising at least 30 minutes daily (e.g., walking, swimming, biking).
- Take prescriptive medication as written.

Reflections from a Newlywed

I was vacationing at the beach with my new husband. The first day, we went for a long walk on the beach and I developed a little pain and stiffness in my lower back, which I attributed to the car ride, sleeping on a thin mattress, and walking in soft sand. About 3 AM the next morning, I was awakened by cramping and non-specific pain in my lower pelvis. Thinking it was gas, I got up to go to the bathroom and could barely stand upright. After another half hour, the pain was no better—even a little worse. I was sweating and then was chilled and had a loose bowel movement. We called the ambulance, having no idea where the nearest hospital was. On the way, I vomited, my pulse was erratic, and I was generally miserable. When we arrived at the hospital, they drew blood, took a urine sample, and gave me a CAT scan. After considering everything from gas to kidney stones to appendicitis, they discovered through ultrasound that I had an ovarian cyst that had swollen and caused the ovary to twist around. Laparoscopic surgery proved that ovarian torsion was present, causing the cessation of blood flow that basically killed the ovary. I also had a cyst on the other ovary, but the doctor was pretty sure that was a "functional" cyst, which is pretty normal. During the surgery they removed the cyst, the ovary, and the fallopian tube.

I was 33, newly married, and had just stopped taking oral contraceptives and was looking forward to starting a family. I had always had an annual pelvic examination and Pap smear and had never before experienced any irregularity or cysts. We were very concerned about how having only one ovary would affect our ability to conceive, but we've been reassured it should be no problem.

■ Understand instructions regarding prescriptive medication(s).

■ Return to health care provider for follow-up visits as scheduled.

■ Notify health care provider of adverse effects of medications.

■ Notify health care provider of failure of symptoms to improve.

■ Answer questions to her satisfaction.

■ Become informed about choices for medical management.

■ Understand expected outcomes of therapy.

■ Understand health promotion activities.

Nursing intervention involves education, consequences and prevention of the condition (if possible), specific procedures in and the outcomes of the therapeutic intervention plan, prescription medications, consequences of "doing nothing," assisting the woman with informed decision making and serving as client advocate. Nurses must provide emotional support for each woman, especially the woman who is embarrassed.

Menopause

Menopause is the result of the decline in ovarian function (estrogen production). **Menopause** refers to the end of menses, just as menarche refers to the beginning of menses. Menopause is determined when the woman experiences no menstrual periods for 12 months.

Every woman will experience menopause at some point in her life, most often at about ages 49 to 51, and thus, experience the physiologic effects of estrogen deficiency in tissues containing estrogen receptors. Even though the severity of symptoms varies from woman to woman, most women experience menopausal symptoms. Typical menopausal symptoms are related to vasomotor instability, urogenital atrophy, and psychological discomforts.

Vasomotor Instability

Vasomotor instability is commonly known as "hot flashes" or "hot flushes." The hot flash is uncontrollable, unpredictable, uncomfortable, and embarrassing and prompts many women to seek relief. Women experience the hot flash as an intense heat sensation, beginning in the upper chest or neck, progressing to the head, and demonstrated by a reddening of the skin. It occurs either occasionally (one or two a day) or frequently (several in an hour) (LeBoeuf & Carter, 1996). For many women, hot flashes are more severe at night, resulting in night sweats and contributing to insomnia. The cause of hot flashes is

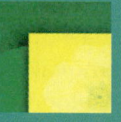

CASE STUDY CARE PLAN
CLIENT WITH BACTERIAL VULVOVAGINOSIS

A 19-year-old with a complaint of "another vaginal infection" is being examined in the nurse practitioner clinic at the city health department. Client states, "I've got another infection. There's lots of discharge on my pants and it smells bad when I have sex." Her latest Pap smear (after a period of 2 years of failure to keep her scheduled appointments) reveals an abnormal result, suggestive of HPV infection. Her history indicates that she is single, never married; gravida 4, para 4 (each child has a different father); has had multiple sex partners; delivered her first baby at age 14; has been treated numerous times in the STD clinic; and has smoked 1 to 2 packs of cigarettes daily since age 10. On examination, copious, homogenous, gray, malodorous discharge is observed. A wet-mount examination of the discharge shows clue cells and the "whiff" test is positive for amine odor. The diagnosis is bacterial vulvovaginosis.

Assessment

- Positive results on "whiff" test.
- Wet-mount examination reveals copious clue cells (epithelial cells covered with bacteria), no lactobacilli present, and WBCs too numerous to count.

Nursing Diagnosis

Ineffective health maintenance related to risk-taking behaviors, as evidenced by chief complaint and subjective, objective, and laboratory data.

NOC	Knowledge: Health behaviors
NIC	Health education
Expected Outcomes	Client will:
	1. Describe risk factors for cervical cancer.
	2. Identify cervical cancer risk factors specific to herself.
	3. Relate strategies she is willing to use to reduce her personal cervical cancer risk.
Planning	The nurse should take into account the client's developmental maturity and target education and materials to a level the client understands.

Nursing Interventions

1. Discuss cervical cancer risk factors (cigarette smoking, early age at first sexual intercourse, first childbirth before age 20, history of STDs (especially HPV infection), multiple sexual partners.
2. Assist client in relating risk factors to herself.
3. Discuss potential strategies to decrease risk for cervical cancer (i.e., stop smoking, "safe sex"). Facilitate implementation of cervical cancer reduction strategies.

Rationales

1. Teaching is more effective when it builds on a woman's existing knowledge base. Official list of risk factors may help late adolescent accept reality of vulnerability to cancer.
2. Awareness of the reality of risk increases the likelihood that the woman will change lifestyle behaviors.
3. Information permits informed decision making. Verification of woman's understanding permits correction of misinformation. Her involvement in planning increases compliance.

Evaluation

- Client is able to state cervical cancer risk factors in her own words.
- Client identifies cigarette smoking, young age at first sexual intercourse and first childbirth, multiple sexual partners, frequent STDs and HPV infection, abnormal Pap smear results.

Client Education

Kegel Exercises

Every woman should be taught to use Kegel exercises every day to prevent or improve urinary incontinence. Kegel exercises contract the pubococcygeus muscle (the muscle supporting the pelvic organs) by alternately contracting and relaxing the muscle controlling the rectum. The client is instructed to first relax the muscle as she would for defecation. She may visualize the process better if she conceptualizes her pelvic floor muscle as an elevator. When the elevator is in the basement, the muscle is relaxed. She contracts (or squeezes) the muscle enough to raise the elevator to the first floor, then contracts the muscle a little more to raise the elevator to the second floor, and contracts the muscle a little more to raise the elevator to the third floor, where she holds it for 3 seconds at first and gradually increases the time each week by 2 to 3 seconds, until she sustains the contraction for 10 seconds. She then relaxes the muscle by descending the elevator to the second, then first, and finally the basement floor. She maintains relaxation for 3 seconds (increasing the relaxation time as she increases the contraction time) and repeats the process 10 times. She is instructed to complete 6 to 8 sets of 10 repetitions per day. She can use a variety of triggers to remind her to complete a set of Kegel exercises. Some events used as triggers include a stop at a red light or stop sign while driving, the ringing of the telephone, or a commercial while watching television.

unknown and the response of the brain to surges of LH levels is not well understood.

Intervention for vasomotor instability responses may include hormone replacement therapy (HRT). An additional nonprescription intervention may include vitamin E therapy (DeMasters, 2000). Nursing interventions frequently include recommendations to wear nonsynthetic

Nursing Tip   *Managing Menopause*

Women should discuss management of menopausal symptoms and use of HRT thoroughly with their healthcare provider to determine the risks and benefits.

fabrics (cotton or silk) and loose clothing, dress in layers for easy removal of clothing during a hot flash, place two sets of cotton sheets on the bed for easy removal of damp sheets during the night, maintain normal blood glucose levels (small, frequent, nutritious meals), drink at least 6 to 8 glasses of water per day to maintain fluid balance, and avoid intake of substances associated with hot flashes (such as spicy foods, alcohol, and caffeine).

Urogenital Atrophy

Urogenital atrophy is the response of the estrogen receptor tissues to loss of estrogen. Such responses typically include a thinning and decreased elasticity of the vaginal epithelium and walls; change in color of vaginal epithelium to pale, almost whitish-pink; vaginal narrowing and shortening; progressive decrease in vaginal rugae and vaginal secretions; increased vaginal pH; vaginal dryness and itching; dyspareunia; and lower urinary tract symptoms (LeBoeuf & Carter, 1996). With loss of estrogen, the genitourinary tract epithelium loses peripheral blood flow, resulting in loss of tone and development of urinary incontinence and a shortened urethra. This loss of tone may result in development of cystocele and rectocele (Crandall, 1997). In addition, cystocele increases urinary incontinence and rectocele increases constipation. Vaginal dryness results in dyspareunia, a risk for tearing the vagina during sexual intercourse, and development of atrophic vulvovaginitis (inflammation of the vulva or vaginal epithelium).

HRT as a therapeutic intervention successfully reverses the physiologic responses of the urogenital tissues to loss of estrogen (DeMasters, 2000). Since oral or transdermal HRT can take several weeks to reverse urogenital atrophy, some providers prescribe topical estrogen for the woman to apply for a short time, along with oral or transdermal HRT. Studies are not complete on risk factors associated with estrogen use.

Nonprescriptive nursing interventions often include recommendations to increase vaginal moisture by using a lubricant (K-Y Jelly, Replens), continue sexual activity to increase blood flow to the genitourinary tissues, spend more time in foreplay to increase vaginal lubrication, and try to find a position during sexual intercourse that decreases the discomfort of dyspareunia (Crandall, 1997). Performing six to eight sets of 10 repetitions of Kegel exercises daily can reduce episodes of urinary incontinence and increase structural support to pelvic organs. In addition, eliminating substances known to cause frequent urination and bladder irritation, such as caffeine, artificial sweeteners, and even some fruit juices, may decrease episodes of urinary incontinence. Increasing water and fresh vegetable intake and walking for exercise can decrease constipation.

Psychological Conditions

Psychological disturbances of menopause include the mood swings, irritability, and changes in short-term memory thought to be related to declining estrogen levels. Decreases in circulating estrogen directly affect neurotransmitters responsible for regulating mood, appetite, sleep, and pain perception (Wasaha & Angelopoulos, 1996; Crandall, 1997). The changes in mood are responses similar to the psychological and emotional responses of premenstrual syndrome and postpartum blues, conditions related to the decrease in hormone levels. In addition, the menopausal woman is usually experiencing the role and lifestyle changes (retirement, widowhood, caring for sick parents, caring for grandchildren, beginning a career or second career) characteristic of the aging process, along with the accompanying insomnia. Thus, the combination of such changes and the decline in circulating estrogen can intensify psychological and emotional responses to both processes.

Alzheimer's disease is a chronic, progressive disease of mental deterioration and disability, the incidence of which increases from 5% of women over age 65 to 25% to 50% of women over age 85 (Cotter, 1997); this condition may be present as menopause begins.

Nursing Implications

Nursing assessment for menopausal conditions involves careful personal and family history taking, and assessment for personal and familial risk factors, symptoms, and how the client has been coping with the symptoms. Physical assessment is focused on data collection for a diagnosis of the menopausal condition. Identification of necessary laboratory tests and diagnostic procedures also must be done.

Nursing diagnoses are individualized to each woman and her specific menopausal condition. Applicable diagnoses may include the following:

- Pain (mild or moderate) related to (specific menopausal condition)
- Grief related to mid to late life losses
- Deficient knowledge related to limited experience (or information) regarding (specific menopausal condition)
- Ineffective coping related to lack of acceptance of prognosis for (specific menopausal condition)

Nursing plans include specific actions the woman and her family will complete to achieve the highest possible level of wellness. Sample goals may include the following:

- Consume recommended foods based on the food pyramid in serving sizes to meet body requirements, including intake of calcium from foods or supplements.

- Exercise 30 minutes per day at least 3 to 4 times per week.
- Take prescriptive medication(s) as written.
- Understand instructions regarding prescriptive medication(s).
- Understand therapeutic intervention plan.
- Notify health care provider of adverse effects of medication(s).
- Notify health care provider of failure of symptoms to improve.
- Return to health care provider for scheduled follow-up visits.
- Have questions answered to her satisfaction.
- Understand health promotion counseling.

Nursing interventions for menopausal conditions include education regarding reduction of risk factors for each woman, emphasizing prevention strategies, and explaining therapeutic interventions to ensure successful compliance. Nursing interventions for each menopausal condition described must be explained, encouraged, and evaluated. In addition, education should focus on health-promoting nutrition, maintenance of appropriate weight for height (BMI), and exercise.

WEB ACTIVITIES

- • • • Visit the American Cancer Society's Web site. What are the 5-, 10-, and 20-, year survival rates for the cancers discussed in this chapter?

- • • • Visit some of the Web sites listed in the Resources section, such as the American Cancer Society and the American Heart Association. Using the health promotion guidelines that they post, develop a teaching plan for a woman at risk for cervical cancer and cardiovascular disease.

- • • • Search the CDC's Web site for statistics on various conditions discussed in this chapter. Is geographic information also included?

- • • • Search for information on some of the disorders in this chapter, such as endometriosis. Are there Web sites available? Do they offer "healthy-living" guidelines? Can you volunteer to be part of a clinical trial if you have some of these conditions?

Many women are often frightened and confused regarding taking HRT because of conflicting news reports of research findings. Nurses can help women discuss with their provider the research studies and benefits of HRT in comparison to the adverse potential of each woman's risk for each menopausal condition. Nurses can also help educate women on the short duration of administration of HRT recommended to help alleviate perimenopausal symptoms.

Research has shown the risk for endometrial cancer is almost eliminated by adding progestin to estrogen use (DeMasters, 2000). Some research findings indicate women who use HRT may have a lower endometrial cancer risk than women who do not. Other research findings seem to indicate that HRT is protective against colorectal cancer. The large study (Women's Health Initiative) on use of estrogen/progesterone HRT for perimenapausal women was stopped due to slightly higher risks for breast cancer and cardiovascular problems in women on HRT. The estrogen-only arm of the study continues, and may help prevent osteoporosis. Additional reports from the Woman's Health Initiative, will be completed in the next few years and may provide answers to many of the questions and concerns of women and, most likely, create new questions.

Key Concepts

■ Historically, little attention has been given to health issues or conditions that affect women.

■ Because of technologic advances and more effective prophylactic treatment for acute and chronic diseases, both women and men are expected to live longer.

■ The leading cause for mortality in women is heart disease, followed by cancer and stroke, which account for two-thirds of all deaths among women.

■ Factors that put women at increased risk of mortality and morbidity are smoking, obesity, and sedentary lifestyle. Prevention strategies to minimize these factors are essential.

■ Risk factors for breast cancer include age over 50, female gender, history of ovarian or endometrial cancer, and history of first-degree relatives with breast cancer.

■ Menstrual cycle alterations relate to frequency and length of cycle, amount of flow, and number of years cycles are experienced.

■ Endometriosis is a chronic disorder caused by implantation of endometrial tissue outside the uterus; it affects 1 in 7 women of childbearing age.

■ Premenstrual syndrome affects 30% to 40% of women of childbearing age and is characterized by behavioral, emotional, and physical symptoms.

■ Common benign breast conditions include fibrocystic changes, fibroadenoma, and nipple discharge.

■ Infections in the pelvic area include vaginal, cervical, and pelvic inflammatory diseases, which may be caused by bacteria, viruses, fungi, or protozoa.

■ Menopause may be accompanied by hot flashes, urogenital atrophy, mood swings, irritability, and estrogen loss, which may increase the risk of cardiovascular disease and osteoporosis.

Review Questions and Activities

1. The Office of Research and Women's Health has as its mission all of the following except:
   a. Promotion of healthy behavior in women
   b. Improvement of health of minority women
   c. Recruitment of women for legislative positions
   d. Provision of greater access to health services for women

   The correct answer is c.

2. The Women's Health Initiative is a:
   a. 10-year study of breast cancer
   b. Clinical trial to study cardiovascular drugs in women
   c. Longitudinal study of nurses
   d. 15-year study of major diseases and conditions of postmenopausal women

   The correct answer is d.

3. Life expectancy in the United States is:
   a. Decreasing faster in the last 10 years than ever before
   b. Longer for men than women
   c. Longer for women than men
   d. Higher for Black women than Caucasian women

   The correct answer is c.

4. The highest birth rates are occurring in:
   a. Blacks
   b. Caucasians
   c. Hispanics
   d. Asians

   The correct answer is c.

5. The two leading causes of death for both sexes are:
   a. Heart disease and stroke
   b. Cancer and stroke
   c. Heart disease and cancer
   d. Heart disease and accidents

   The correct answer is c.

6. Heart disease in women:
   a. Occurs more frequently than in men at all ages
   b. Decreases slightly after age 65

c. Increases after menopause, with an incidence similar to that in men by age 75

d. Occurs more frequently in Caucasian women than in Black women

The correct answer is c.

7. Accidents are the leading cause of death in women in all of these age groups except:
a. 5 to 14 years
b. 15 to 24 years
c. 25 to 44 years
d. 45 to 64 years

The correct answer is d.

8. Cancer deaths in the United States are:
a. Increasing in men and decreasing in women
b. Decreasing in men and increasing in women
c. Increasing in both men and women
d. Decreasing in both men and women

The correct answer is d.

9. The leading cause of cancer deaths in women is:
a. Lung
b. Cervical
c. Ovarian
d. Breast

The correct answer is a.

10. Lung cancer in women is:
a. Decreasing because of a decrease in smoking habits of women
b. Increasing because of an increase in smoking habits of women
c. Difficult to treat, but easy to detect
d. Less important as a cause of death in women than breast cancer

The correct answer is b.

11. Risk factors for breast cancer include:
a. Family history
b. History of HPV infection
c. Early menopause
d. Low-fat diet

The correct answer is a.

12. Ovarian cancer is:
a. Common among young Black women
b. Easy to detect with the Pap smear
c. Likely to carry a good prognosis once it is detected
d. Frequently detected late in its course

The correct answer is d.

13. Cancer prevention programs for women include all of the following except:
a. Smoking cessation
b. Periodic screening
c. Bone density index measurement

d. Elimination of unopposed estrogen use for menopause

The correct answer is c.

14. The following statements are true regarding osteoporosis *except*:
a. It affects one-third to one-half of postmenopausal women
b. It increases as women age
c. It puts women at high risk for hip fractures
d. It occurs as a result of arthritis

The correct answer is d.

15. Depression in women:
a. Occurs less frequently than in men
b. Tends to be treated in only about 75% of women with the condition
c. Is twice as likely to occur in women than in men
d. Is easy to treat with psychotropic drugs developed in research on women

The correct answer is c.

16. You are counseling a perimenopausal client regarding prevention of osteoporosis. You recommend that she increase her dietary intake of which of the following?
a. Milk and iron
b. Calcium and vitamin D
c. Magnesium and vitamin C
d. Magnesium and phosphorus

The correct answer is b.

17. You are explaining the intervention strategies for PMS to a 28-year-old client. You recommend that during the latter part of her cycle she limit which of the following?
a. Exercise
b. Fluid intake
c. Fruits and vegetables
d. Salt and caffeine intake

The correct answer is d.

18. You are completing the chief complaint interview for a 17-year-old with dysmenorrhea. You will assess for which of the following symptoms?
a. Food cravings
b. Heart palpitations
c. Abnormal bleeding
d. Duration of her pain

The correct answer is d.

19. You are counseling a 40-year-old who has come to the clinic because she found a "lump" in her breast last night. She is frantic because she believes she has cancer. The clinical breast examination reveals firm, smooth, discrete masses in both breasts. You reinforce the physician's impression that what she is

feeling is most likely a noncancerous "lump" and that she should have which of the following evaluation procedures first?

a. Lumpectomy
b. Mammogram
c. Excisional biosy
d. Stereotactic biopsy

The correct answer is b.

20. You are collecting data from a 37-year-old client who you suspect may have fibroid tumors. You expect her subjective data to include which of the following symptoms?

a. Urinary urgency
b. Difficult defecation
c. Cyclic migraine headaches
d. Deep pelvic pain dyspareunia

The correct answer is d.

21. You are completing the chief complaint interview with a client who states that she has a continuous blood-tinged, watery discharge; postcoital bleeding; and dyspareunia. Based on her subjective data, you suspect which of the following medical diagnoses?

a. Cervical cancer
b. Hypermenorrhea
c. Pelvic relaxation
d. Polycystic ovary disease

The correct answer is a.

22. The chief complaint interview on a client reveals vaginal discharge with itching and burning. The client also reveals she experiences dyspareunia. If her diagnosis is monilial vulvovaginitis, you would expect the wet mount slide to contain which of the following?

a. Bacteria
b. Clue cells
c. Trichomonads
d. Budding hyphae

The correct answer is d.

References

American Cancer Society. (1998). *Cancer facts and figures—1998.* Atlanta, GA: Author.

American Cancer Society. (2000). *Cancer facts and figures—2000.* Atlanta, GA: Author.

American Cancer Society. (2002). *Cancer facts and figures—2002.* Atlanta, GA: Author.

Arnold, G. C., & Neiheisel, M. B. (1997). A comprehensive approach to evaluating nipple discharge. *Nurse Practitioner, 22*(7) 96, 98-102, 105-111.

Baron, R. H., & Walsh, A. (1995). Nine facts everyone should know about breast cancer. *American Journal of Nursing, 95*(7), 29-33.

Bristow, R., & Montz, F. (2000). Cervical cancer. In S. B. Ranson (Ed.), *Practical strategies in obstetrics & gynecology,* Philadelphia: PA, W. B. Saunders.

Brucker, M. C., & Scharbo-DeHaan, M. (1991). Breast disease: The role of the nurse midwife. *Journal of Nurse-Midwifery, 36*(1), 63-73.

Centers for Disease Control and Prevention (CDC). (2003). Retrieved July 16, 2003, from http://www.cdc.gov/nchs

Centers for Disease Control and Prevention. (2002). Sexually transmitted diseases treatment guidelines. *Morbidity and Mortality Weekly Report, 51*(RR-6), 1–75.

Centers for Disease Control and Prevention. (2000, July 2). *National Vital Statistics, (48,* 11).

Cohen, M. (1997). Natural history of HIV infection in women. *Obstetrics and Gynecology Clinics of North America, 24*(8), 743–758.

Corwin, E. J. (1997). Endometriosis: Pathophysiology, diagnosis, and treatment. *American Journal of Primary Health Care, 22*(10), 35-36, 38-42, 45-46, 48-51, 55.

Cotter, V. T. (1997). Hormonic convergence: Finding balance through hormone replacement therapy. *Association for Women's Health, Obstetrics, and Neonatal Nurses Lifelines, 1*(1), 37-42.

Crandall, S. G. (1997). Menopause made easier. *RN, 60*(7), 46-50.

Cullins, V. A., Dominguez, L., Guberski, T., Secor, R. M., & Wysocki, S. J. (1999). Treating vaginitis. *Nurse Practitioner, 24*(10), 46-63.

Davidson, M., & DeSimone, M. (2002). Osteoporosis update. *Clinician Reviews, 12*(4), 76–82.

DeMasters, J. (2000). A clinician's guide to understanding the dilemma. *Association for Women's Health, Obstetrics, and Neonatal Nurses Lifelines, 4*(2), 26-35.

Estes, M. E. Z. (2002). *Health assessment & physical examination* (2nd ed.). Clifton Park, NY: Delmar Learning.

Foster, J. C. (1994). A woman's health agenda. *Holistic Nurse Practice, 8,* 74–88.

Grabo, T. N., Fahs, P. S., Nataupsky, L. G., & Reich, H. (1999). Uterine myomas: Treatment options. *Journal of Obstetric, Gynecologic, and Neonatal Nurses, 28*(1), 23-31.

Johnson, C. L. (2000). Update on breast and cervical cancers, *Association for Women's Health, Obstetrics, and Neonatal Nurses Lifelines, 4*(1), 20–21.

Keene, G. F. (1999). Office gynecology: Common reproductive tract disorders. *Clinician Reviews, 9*(1), 58–80.

LeBoeuf, F. J., & Carter, S. G. (1996). Discomforts of perimenopause. *Journal of Obstetric, Gynecologic, and Neonatal Nursing, 25*(2), 173–180.

Lucas, B. D. (1999). Five reasons to consider a hysterectomy. *Patient Care for the Nurse Practitioner, 2*(9), 28–50.

McGee, C. (1997). Secondary amenorrhea leading to osteoporosis. *Nurse Practitioner, 22*(5), 38–64.

Moore, G. J. (ed.). (1997). *Women and cancer.* Boston: Jones and Bartlett.

Mott, A. M. (1998). Prevention and management of pelvic inflammatory disease by primary care providers. *American Journal for Nurse Practitioners, 2*(6), 7–15.

National Center for Health Statistics. (1992). *Health, United States, 1990* (DHHS Publication No. (PHS) 91-1232). Hyattsville, MD: Public Health Service.

National Center for Health Statistics. (1998). *Births of Hispanic origin, 1989–1995.* Washington, DC: Author.

National Center for Health Statistics. (2000). [No title]. Retrieved November 12, 2003, from http://www.cdc.gov/nchs.

National Institutes of Health. (1994). *Women's health initiative*. Bethesda, MD: Author.

Office of Research on Women's Health. (2003). *ORWH's mandate*. Retrieved July 16, 2003, from http://www4.od.nih.gov/orwh/overview.html.

Shimp, L. A., & Peggs, J. F. (2000). Urinary incontinence. In M. A. Smith & L. A. Shimp, (Eds.), *Women's health care*. New York: McGraw Hill.

Smith, C. B. (1998). Pinpointing the cause of abnormal uterine bleeding. *Women's Health Primary Care 1*(10), 835–844.

Thomas, S., & Greifzu, S. P. (2000). Oncology today: Breast cancer, *RN, 63*(4), 41–45.

Ugarriza, D. N. Klinger, S., & O'Brien, S. (1998). Premenstrual syndrome: Diagnosis and prevention. *Nurse Practitioner, 23*(9), 40–58.

U.S. Census Bureau. (1999). *Statistical abstract of the United States: 1999* (119th ed.). Washington, DC: Author.

U.S. Census Bureau. (2003). *Census 2000 gateway*. Retrieved December 16, 2003, from http://www.census.gov/main/www/cen2000.html.

U.S. Department of Health and Human Services, Center for Disease Control and Prevention, National Center for Health Statistics. (2000a). *Deaths: Final data for 1998* (Vol. 48, No. 11). Washington, DC: Author.

U.S. Department of Health and Human Services. Office on Women's Health. (2000b). *Women's health issues: An overview*, Washington, DC: Author.

U.S. Preventive Services Task Force. (1996). *Guide to clinical preventive services* (2nd ed.). Baltimore: Williams & Wilkins.

Wasaha, S., & Angelopoulos, F. M. (1996). What every woman should know about menopause. *American Journal of Nursing, 96*(1), 24–33.

Wentz, A. C. (1994). Women's health issues. In *Advances in internal medicine* (Vol. 40, pp. 1–28). St. Louis, MO: Mosby Year Book.

White, G. L., Griffith, C. J., Nenstiel, R. O., & Dyess, D. L. (1996). Breast cancer: Reducing mortality through early detection. *Clinician Reviews, 6*(9), 77–102.

Wingo, P. A., Ries, L. A., Rosenberg, H. M., Miller, D. S., & Edwards, B. K. (1998). Cancer incidence and mortality, 1973–1995. *Cancer, 82*, 1197–1207.

Women's Health Report of the Public Health Task Force on Women's Health Issues. (1985). *Public Health Report, 1*, 74–106.

Suggested Readings

Baker, S. (1998). Menstruation and related problems and concerns. In Youngkin, E. Q., & Davis, M. S. (Eds.), *Women's health: A primary care clinical guide* (pp. 139–160). Stamford, CT: Appleton & Lange.

Igoe, B. A. (1997). Symptoms attributed to ovarian cancer by women with the disease. *Nurse Practitioner, 22*(7), 122–143.

Mosca, L., Manson, J. E., Southerland, S. E., Lange, R., Manolio, T., & Barret-Conner, E. (1997). American Heart Association Medical/Scientific Statement. *Cardiovascular disease in women: A statement for healthcare professionals from the American Heart Association. Circulation, 96*(7), 2468–2482.

National Institutes of Health, (2002). *Osteoporosis and related bone disorders*. National Resource Center (NIHORBD-NRC).

Poma, P. A. (1997). A simple strategy for managing perimenopausal bleeding. *Contemporary Nurse Practitioner, 2*(3), 21–26.

Siris, E. S., & Schussheim, D. H. (1998). Osteoporosis: Assessing your patient's risk. *Women's Health in Primary Care, 1*(1), 99–106.

Wong, C., Froelicher, E., Bacchetti, F., Barron, H., Gee, L., Selby, J., et al. (1997). Influence of gender on cardiovascular mortality in acute myocardial infarction patients with high indications for coronary angiopathy. *Circulation, 96* (Suppl. 9), 51II–57II.

Resources

Agency for Health Care Research and Quality, 540 Gaither Road, Rockville, MD 20850, 301-427-1364.

American Cancer Society (ACS), 1599 Clifton Road, NE., Atlanta, GA 30329-4251, 404-320-333, 1-800-227-2345, http://www.cancer.org

American Heart Association 1615 Stemmons Freeway, Dallas, TX 75207, 748-7212, http://www.American heart.org.

Cansearch: A Guide to Cancer Resources, http://www.canceradvocacy.org

Centers for Disease Control and Prevention 1-800-311-3435, http://www.cdc.gov

Food and Drug Administration (FDA), HFI-40, Rockville, MD 20857, 1-888-463-6332, http://www.fda.gov

Health and Human Services, 200 Independence Avenue, S.W., Washington, DC 20201, 202-619-0257, 1-877-696-6775, http://www.hhs.gov

Journal of the National Cancer Institute, Oxford University Press, Journals Subscription Department, Great Clarendon Street, Oxford OX2 6DP, U.K. +44 (0) 1 865353907, http://jnci.oupjournals.org

Medical/Health Sciences Libraries, Hardin Library for the Health Sciences, 600 Newton Rd., University of Iowa, Iowa City, IA 52242-1098, 319-335-9871, http://www.lib.uiowa.edu

Medline Plus: http://www.nln.nih.gov/medlineplus

Morbidity and Mortality Weekly Report, John W. Ward, M.D., Editor Epidemiology Program Office MS C-08, Centers for Disease Control and Prevention, 1600 Clifton Rd., Atlanta, GA 30333, Fax: 404-639-4198, http://www.cdc.gov/mmwr

National Alliance of Breast Cancer Organizations, 9 East 37th Street, 10th Floor, New York, NY 10016, http://www.nabco.org

National Breast Cancer Coalition, 1707 L Street NW, Suite 1060 Washington DC. 20036, 1800-622-2838, 202-296-7477 http://www.stopbreastcancer.org

National Cancer Institute (NCI) CancerNet, Public Inquiries Office, Building, 31, Room IOA03, 31 Center Drive, MSC 2580, Bethesda, MD 20892-2580, 301-435-3848, 1-800-4-Cancer, http://www.cancer.gov

National Center for Health Statistics, National Center for Health Statistics, Division of Data Services, 3311 Toledo Road, Hyattsville, MD 20782, 301-458-4636, http://www.cdc.gov/nchs

National Institutes of Health, 9000 Rockville Pike, Bethesda, MD 20814, 301-496-4000, http://www.nih.gov

National Library of Medicine, 8600 Rockville Pike, Bethesda, MD 20894, 888-346-3556, http://www.nlm.nih.gov

Occupational Safety and Health Administration, Office of Public and Consumer Affairs, U.S. Department of Labor, Room N3637, 200 Constitution Ave NW, Washington, DC 20210, 1-800-321-OSHA, http://www.osha.gov

Susan G. Komen Breast Cancer Foundation, 800-I'M AWARE 462-9273.

Y-ME National Breast Cancer Organization, 800-221-2141 (9 AM to 5 PM CST), 312-986-8228 (24 hours), http://www.y-me.org

UNIT 3

Human
Reproduction

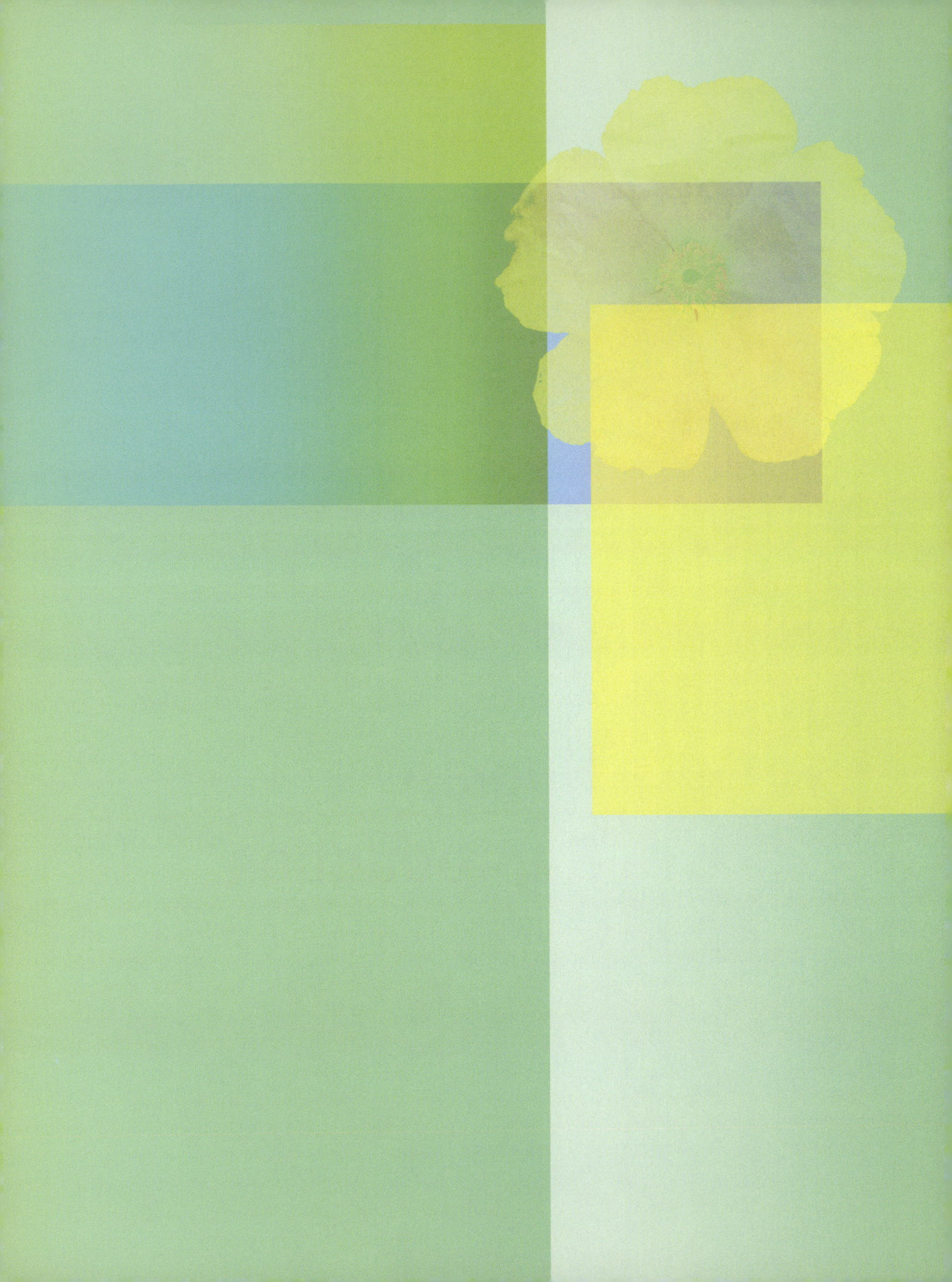

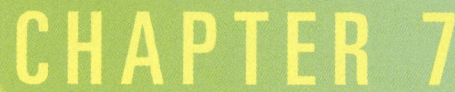

CHAPTER 7

REPRODUCTION, SEXUALITY, INFERTILITY, AND FAMILY PLANNING

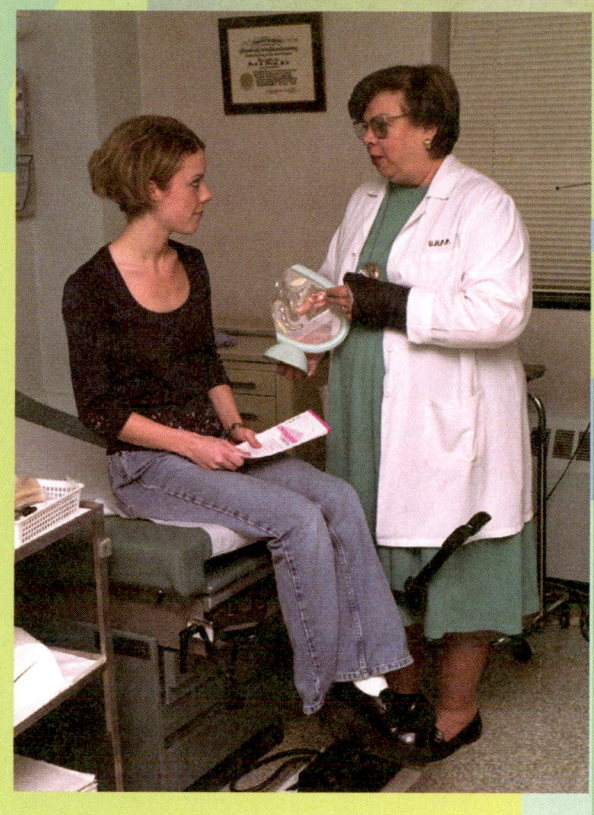

Terms dealing with menstruation and sexuality often are value-laden. The following questions can be used to explore personal knowledge, values, and beliefs that may affect your ability to care for women and their partners:

- Do I understand the interrelationship of menstruation and ovarian function? Can I explain the relationship clearly to clients of various ages and educational levels?
- What do I think about men or women whose choices, such as drug use or sexual activity, may have affected their fertility?
- How do I feel about pregnancy, the decision to have children, and the decision not to have children?
- Which terms do I use to describe menses, sexuality, and body parts? Are these terms value-laden? Are they appropriate to the client's level of education and understanding? Which issues affect the use of certain terms?
- Do my attitudes toward sexuality influence my delivery of health care?
- What is my attitude toward couples who fail to effectively use contraceptives?

Key Terms

Abortion
Anovulatory
Cervical cap
Coitus interruptus
Contraception
Corpus luteum
Desire phase
Diaphragm
Emergency
  contraception
Endometriosis
Endometrium
Estrogen
Excitement phase
Family planning
Follicular phase
Follicle-stimulating
  hormone (FSH)
Galactorrhea
Germ cells
Gonadal
Gonadotropin-releasing
  hormone (Gn-RH)
Graafian follicle
Human chorionic
  gonadotropin (hCG)
Hydrocele
Hypothalamic-pituitary-
  gonadal axis
Implantable contraception
Infertility
Injectable contraceptive
Leydig cells
Libido
Luteal phase

Luteinizing hormone
Menarche
Menopause
Menses
Menstrual phase
Mittelschmerz
Neurohormonal
Orgasmic phase
Ovulation
Ovulation prediction
Perimenopause
Plateau phase
Precocious
Progesterone
Proliferative phase
Prostaglandins
Puberty
Refractory period
Resolution phase
Secretory phase
Seminiferous tubules
Serial monogamy
Sexual dysfunction
Spermatogenesis
Spermatozoa
Sperm capacitation
Spermicide
Spinnbarkeit
Sterilization
Testosterone
Tubal ligation
Vaginal ring
Varicocele
Vasectomy

Competencies

Upon completion of this chapter, the reader should be able to:

1. Explain the menstrual cycle in terms of the ovarian, endometrial, and neurohormonal components.
2. Identify the normal ages of onset and cessation of menses and factors related to normal variations.
3. Describe normal menstruation in terms of length of cycle, flow, and quantity of blood loss.
4. Describe spermatogenesis.
5. Discuss factors related to male and female infertility.
6. List key components of an infertility examination and a rationale for their inclusion.
7. Discuss the emotional impact of infertility.
8. Describe regimens to treat infertility, including assisted reproductive technology.
9. Discuss the currently available methods of contraception.
10. Identify the risks and benefits of each form of contraceptive device.
11. Discuss the mechanism of action of each form of contraception.
12. Describe the steps in successful reproductive decision-making.
13. Describe some of the implications of an uplanned and unwanted pregnancy.
14. Use the nursing process to assist the client in determining the need for contraception.

C onsidering the coordination of the complex body systems required for reproductive functioning, it is amazing that conception and birth occur. Yet within that complexity, finely ordered events produce cyclic changes that can be predicted. In women the most evident result of this neurohormonal interplay, the menstrual cycle, provides a basis for understanding the physiology of reproduc-

tion. (The term **neurohormonal** pertains to hormones formed by secretory cells and liberated by nerve impulses.) To grasp the usually predictable events which are driven by the functioning of the ovary, it is helpful to start at the beginning of human sexual development. In men the physiology is not quite as complex; however, a number of organs and systems are involved with reproduction.

This chapter describes the physiology of the female and male reproductive systems. Normal parameters for functioning are provided as guidelines for assessment. Sexuality, sexual dysfunction, and infertility are discussed. Their emotional impact and clinical guidelines for assessment and treatment are presented. Finally, family planning methods are discussed in some detail. The emotional impact and clinical guidelines for assessment and treatment are presented.

NORMAL SEXUAL DIFFERENTIATION

In human embryos, sexual development is a product of genetic and hormonal influences, which determine the differentiation of the internal systems and formation of external genitalia. **Gonadal** (referring to the ovaries in the female and the testes in the male) development begins at 5 to 6 weeks' gestation, with testicular differentiation at 7 weeks' gestation. At this time the production of **testosterone**, a potent, naturally occurring androgen (male) hormone, begins. Testosterone regulates the development of the penis, testes, scrotum, seminal vesicles, prostate gland, and genital duct system.

Without the activity of the Y chromosome, ovarian development occurs 2 weeks later. In the female ovary, 5 to 7 million **germ cells**, the precursors of ova, are evident by 20 weeks' gestation. By birth, this number has already decreased to 1 to 2 million cells. By puberty, the number of germ cells is approximately 300,000. This decrease continues until menopause when only thousands are left. The ovaries provide varying amounts of **estrogen** (female sex hormone) and **progesterone** (antiestrogenic hormone) needed for the production of eggs (oocytes) from these germ cells. The ovaries coordinate the development and sloughing of the **endometrium** (lining of the uterus), resulting in the menstrual cycle. Thus, these two events, the ovarian and the endometrial cycles, occur at the same

COLLABORATIVE CARE

Caring for the Client with Sexual Problems, Infertility, and Family Planning

The nurse's role in caring for the client with sexual problems, infertility, or family planning is primarily that of providing education and support. To fulfill this function, the nurse may need to collaborate with physicians, geneticists, social workers, and case managers.

Client Education

Adolescence and Puberty

Puberty, the development of secondary sex characteristics and the ability to reproduce, can be a tumultuous time for parents and teens. It is quite common for the mother of an adolescent girl to have questions about when certain developmental events can be expected in her daughter's life. The nurse may be the person who is first approached to provide this information. The following is a synopsis of the range of normal events:

- The average age of menarche in the United States is 12.8 years.

- Menarche usually is a mid to late event in puberty and usually occurs after the development of pubic and axillary hair, breast buds, and genital changes.

- A young girl who has not developed secondary sex characteristics by the age of 14 years should be evaluated by a physician.

- A young girl who develops secondary sex characteristics but does not begin menses within two years also should be evaluated by a physician.

time and produce **ovulation** (release of a mature ovum) and **menses** (monthly bleeding from the lining of the uterus).

Female Reproductive Function

The onset of menstrual bleeding, or **menarche**, usually occurs between 9 and 16 years of age (Speroff, Glass, & Kase, 1999). Several factors may affect the age of onset of menses, including family history, geographic location, general health, and nutrition. Current information supports the importance of body weight in determining the time of menarche (Speroff, Glass, & Kase, 1999). Moderately overweight girls begin menstruation earlier than do those of normal weight. Girls with very low body fat, such as those having anorexia and girls who participate in strenuous athletics, may have delayed menarche.

For 12 to 18 months after menarche, menses may be irregular, cycles are often **anovulatory** (without release of an egg), and the menstrual flow may be very heavy or very light. It is important to be aware that pregnancy can

Nursing Tip — *Iron and Menstruation*

Blood loss from menstruation results in approximately 0.5 mg of iron being lost with each milliliter of blood, explaining why women tend to have lower hemoglobin levels than do men, especially women with heavy menses. These iron deficits can be overcome through dietary means by eating liver and other foods rich in iron or by taking a multivitamin with iron.

Nursing Tip — *Menopause*

It is important to realize that the diagnosis of menopause, and the end of reproductive functioning, is not made until 1 year after the last menses. Thus, it is wise to counsel women to continue contraception throughout the perimenopausal years.

Note. From *Clinical Gynecological Endocrinology and Infertility* (6th ed.), by L. Speroff, R. H. Glass, and N. G. Kase, 1999, Phildelphia: Lippincott.

result during this time, and appropriate education should be provided. Parents may seek evaluation with concerns that their daughter may be experiencing early (**precocious**) puberty (Smith & Hornberger, 1997), irregular or heavy menses, or delayed menses. Often, explaining the wide range of what is considered to be normal is all that is required. Conversely, the child under 8 years of age who has pubertal changes, such as menarche, requires further evaluation because there may exist important growth implications or another underlying disease. Likewise, with delayed menses, a girl over the age of 17 years could have a genetic, hormonal, or hypothalamic-pituitary disorder. Anatomic defects of the uterus and vagina also must be ruled out.

A menstrual cycle refers to the time that passes from the first day of one menstrual period to the first day of the next menstrual period. The normal cycle length can range from 21 to 36 days, although 95% of women have cycles between 25 and 32 days. A working number used to describe a so-called normal cycle is 28 days. Timing of the cycle begins on the first day of bleeding, or day 1 of the cycle. Bleeding usually continues for 3 to 5 days, with 1 to 8 days considered to be within normal limits. The amount of blood lost averages 30 mL (1 oz) per cycle but ranges from 20 to 80 mL (0.67 to 2.67 oz). Blood loss usually is greater during the first 3 days of the cycle because the precise hormonal events leading to menses affect the entire endometrium (cellular lining of the uterus that is shed monthly at the time of menses) at the same time, resulting in generalized sloughing of the endometrial tissue.

Normally, menstruation continues until **menopause** (cessation of menses), which occurs between the ages of 35 and 60 years (Byyny & Speroff, 1996). Menopause is determined to be present when a woman has completed 1 year without menses. For as many as 15 years before the cessation of menses, women may experience changes in their cycle, such as heavier or lighter bleeding and changes in the length or duration of menses. This time is described as the **perimenopause** and is a result of changes in ovarian

function. In the United States, 51 years of age is the average time of menopause (Speroff et al., 1999).

Endometrial Activity

The activity of the endometrium during the menstrual cycle can be described as the menstrual, proliferative, and secretory phases. The endometrium is prepared for implantation of a fertilized ovum by the ovarian hormones. When implantation does not occur the tissue sloughs and new tissue begins to build for the next cycle. This cycle of growth and regression occurs approximately 300 to 400 times in the adult human female. Specific changes in the endometrium occur in the various phases of the menstrual cycle.

The **menstrual phase** is the time during which the woman experiences vaginal bleeding. It begins with day 1 of the menses and continues for about 5 days, during which time almost two thirds of the endometrial tissue is lost. The lost tissue has been described as having evidence of necrosis and white cell infiltration as well as fragmentation of vessels and glands.

The **proliferative phase** describes the endometrium from the end of menses through ovulation, which occurs on or about day 14 of the normal 28-day cycle. The growth of the glands of the endometrium is associated with increased estrogen levels produced by the ovary. The tissue of the endometrium has changed and grown from being dense and approximately 0.5 mm thick to being spongy and 3.5 to 5.0 mm thick, an increase of 7 to 10 times in size.

The **secretory phase** continues from the time of ovulation (days 14 to 28) under the combined effects of estrogen and progesterone. The endometrium stops growing but increases in vascularity and the glycogen-producing glands occur. With the increased blood and glycogen, the tissue is ready for implantation. Without fertilization and implantation, estrogen and progesterone levels decrease, leading to decreased blood supply to the tissue. As blood vessels constrict and relax, leading to separation of the prepared endometrial layer, necrosis of the tissue results in menstruation. Even during menses, increasing estrogen levels produced by the ovary begin the healing process, and the endometrium begins to regenerate and prepare for the next cycle.

Ovarian Regulation

In the reproductive aspect of a woman's life there are baselines of all sex hormones. Fluctuations also occur that establish the menstrual cycle. The main organs of regulation are the hypothalamus and pituitary in the brain and the ovaries in the pelvis (Speroff et al., 1999). These structures are termed the hypothalamic-pituitary-gonadal axis and form a feedback loop that controls hormone production. Although a delicate interplay and regulation between the brain and ovaries exist, the ovaries actually drive the process of ovulation. Two phases can be used to describe the functioning of the ovary as it regulates the menstrual cycle and the development of an egg, the follicular and the luteal phases.

The **follicular phase** refers to maturation of the follicle, leading to the production of an egg and ovulation. The **luteal phase** refers to the secretion of hormones from the corpus luteum, which is formed from the follicle that produced the egg. The corpus luteum continues to secrete estrogen and progesterone. These hormones prepare and maintain the endometrium for implantation of the fertilized ovum. Again, it is important to remember that the menstrual cycle is driven or regulated by these ovarian hormones. Thus, the visible evidence of the hormone fluctuations and ovarian functioning is menses. When a woman's cycle is regular and predictable, without the aid of hormone therapy, she probably is ovulating.

As well as producing the steroid hormones estradiol and progesterone and small amounts of testosterone, the ovaries produce oocytes or eggs. At 4 to 6 days before menses, ovarian follicles begin to grow independent of hormonal stimulation. For most follicles, growth is limited, and they never reach maturity. Under the influence of hormones, a single follicle is chosen to reach maturity by day 5 to 7 in the cycle. Termed the *preantral* or *primary follicle*, the selected follicle continues to enlarge. It is surrounded by a membrane, the zona pellucida. The size and number of layers of the cells increase under the influence of estrogen, and follicular fluid begins to increase. The maturing follicle or **graafian follicle** continues growing until ovulation occurs. Typically, in a 28-day cycle, ovulation would be on day 14; however, the day of ovulation varies according to the number of days needed for maturation of the follicle. The follicular phase may vary in length from 7 to 22 days and determines the length of the cycle. That is, the follicular phase may vary in length but the luteal phase is consistently 14 days. Thus, menses will begin 14 days after ovulation.

Ovulation

Although not always considered a phase of the ovarian cycle, multiple important events occur at the time of ovulation that warrant special note. Physical and hormonal events take place to enhance the possibility of fertilization (Speroff et al., 1999). The increased estrogen levels at this time have prepared the endometrium for implantation but also change the characteristics of the cervical mucus. The role of cervical mucus is to facilitate sperm transport into the uterus. Before ovulation, cervical mucus threads are 1 to 2 cm long, increasing to 12 to 24 cm and becoming thin, clear, and copious when ovulation occurs. The increased elasticity is called **spinnbarkeit** and facilitates sperm transport into the uterus (Figure 7-1). The cervix becomes softer and the os opens. Some women can determine the time of ovulation because they experience pain in the lower abdomen called **mittelschmerz**.

Hormonal events include an increase in androgen levels. Androgens are hormones derived from testosterone that increase libido and prepare the follicle for ovulation. **Prostaglandins** are chemicals produced by many bodily systems, including those of the female reproductive system. Prostaglandins increase and, although the exact action is not known, may act to thin the follicle wall and contract smooth muscle in the cell wall to facilitate release of the oocyte.

The luteal phase begins with ovulation as the cells of the ovary that produced the egg increase in size and accumulate lutein. Lutein is a yellow pigment that gives the name to the **corpus luteum**, or *yellow body*. The corpus luteum continues to produce estrogen and progesterone. Progesterone levels increase rapidly for nearly 8 days as this hormone suppresses the growth of new follicles. The corpus luteum begins to degenerate on days 9 to 11 when not sustained by the hormone of early pregnancy, **human chorionic gonadotropin (hCG)**. When pregnancy occurs, hCG prevents regression of the corpus luteum, which continues to produce hormones until 9 or 10 weeks' gestation. By this time the placenta has assumed production of the needed steroidal hormones estrogen and progesterone.

When pregnancy does not occur, the corpus luteum begins to degenerate and the levels of estrogen and progesterone decrease, stimulating the start of a new cycle. This continuing cycle of events, although controlled by the follicle, which will ovulate, are under the direction of

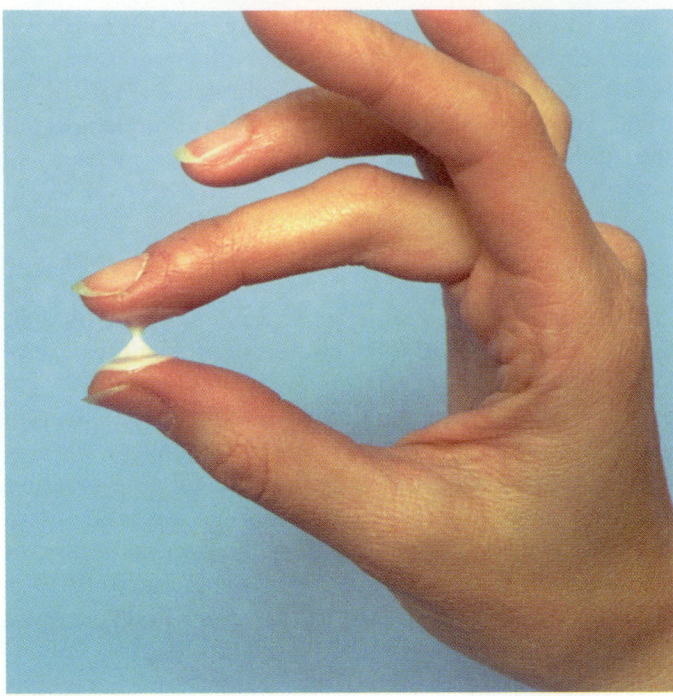

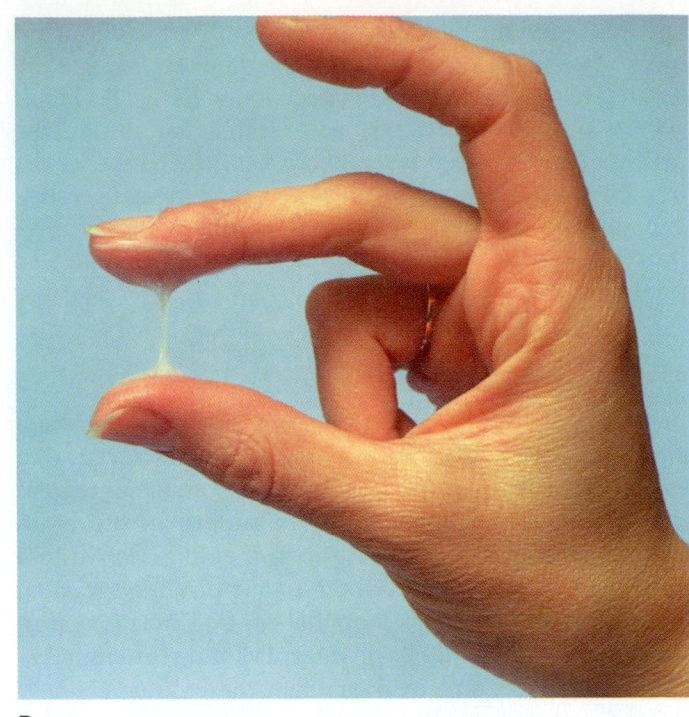

A.

B.

Figure 7-1   Spinnbarkeit test. A. Before ovulation, cervical mucus is thick, preventing transport of sperm. B. At ovulation, secretions become thinner and elastic, facilitating sperm transport.

the anterior pituitary and hypothalamus. The **hypothalamic-pituitary-gonadal axis** is a triad of the hypothalamus, pituitary, and ovaries that regulates the hormones of reproduction and that must function in synchrony for conception to occur.

Hormonal Regulation

The hypothalamus functions similarly to a thermostat, sensing hormone levels in the blood (Speroff et al., 1999). Depending on the set levels, the hypothalamus sends a message to the anterior pituitary to either increase or decrease the amounts of the specific hormone needed. As well as regulating the ovaries, the hypothalamus also plays a regulatory function in growth hormone, thyroid-stimulating hormone (TSH), and the adrenal hormones.

The hypothalamic hormone that controls the gonadotropins is called **gonadotropin-releasing hormone (Gn-RH)**. When the hypothalamus senses a decrease in the level of hormones produced by the ovary, Gn-RH is released into the blood. The hypophyseal portal system provides a mechanism by which the hypothalamus and anterior pituitary communicate. The anterior pituitary receives the message that more or fewer hormones are needed and either stimulates or suppresses the release of hormones.

The hormones produced by the pituitary are **follicle-stimulating hormone (FSH)**, which stimulates the ovary to

prepare a mature ovum for release, and **luteinizing hormone (LH)**, which is responsible for the release of the ovum. The anterior pituitary also produces the hormone prolactin, which regulates milk production. With the release of FSH and LH, events in the ovary are regulated to produce the hormones needed to support the development of the oocyte and for ovulation. As the ovary is preparing an egg for ovulation, the endometrium is being prepared to support the implantation and growth of the fertilized egg. Preparation of the endometrium is primarily under the influence of estrogen. Estrogen is the hormone responsible for the secondary sex characteristics of the female.

During the second phase of the cycle the corpus luteum produces progesterone, which stimulates the secretory phase and supports the continued growth of the endometrium. When fertilization does not occur 8 to 10 days after ovulation, the corpus luteum degenerates and progesterone levels rapidly decrease. This rapid decrease results in progesterone levels below those needed to sustain the endometrium, and menstruation begins. With the decrease in progesterone levels the hypothalamus is stimulated to increase secretion of Gn-RH, and the cycle begins again (Speroff et al., 1999).

An understanding of the complexity and interrelatedness of the hypothalamic-pituitary-gonadal axis provides a basis for understanding and treating many of the problems related to the reproductive system. The diagnosis of problems such as dysfunctional uterine bleeding, amenorrhea, and infertility and the appropriate treatment can be determined based on this knowledge.

Male Reproductive Function

The genetic sex of the fetus is determined at conception. The male and female reproductive systems, however, are similar until differentiation begins at 5 to 6 weeks' gestation, and testicular development occurs by 7 weeks' gestation. In utero, the fetal gonads are active and secrete either estrogen or testosterone. As noted previously, in the male, the hormone testosterone regulates development of the penis, testes, scrotum, seminal vesicles, prostate gland, and genital duct system. During childhood, hormones are inhibited. During puberty, however, the hypothalamus begins to produce increased levels of Gn-RH, which stimulate the anterior pituitary to produce FSH and LH. Hormones produced in the hypothalamus, pituitary, and testes are responsible for **spermatogenesis**, or development of sperm cells. This system is analogous to the hypothalamic-pituitary-ovarian axis in the female, which produces an ovum.

Follicle-stimulating hormone stimulates the production of primary spermatocytes in the **seminiferous tubules**, which are the tubes that carry semen from the testes. Concurrently, LH stimulates the **Leydig cells** in the testes to produce testosterone. Testosterone encourages maturation of the **spermatozoa**, or sperm.

Testosterone is essential for spermatogenesis and also stimulates the production of seminal fluid. Testosterone is responsible for secondary sexual characteristics such as the distribution of body hair, increased muscle mass, and enlargement of the vocal cords. The sexual drive is thought to be controlled by testosterone. The action of testosterone continues throughout life, including the development of sperm. Levels of this hormone decrease as men age, however, resulting in decreased hair distribution, reduced body mass, and decreased sexual activity. This decrease in testosterone has led to the suggestion that men have a series of physical and emotional changes comparable with those that occur during menopause in women.

Development of sperm in the testes takes approximately 70 days. After leaving the testes the sperm remains in the epididymis for 12 to 26 days, during which time they mature. The semen, which forms the ejaculate, contains sperm and secretions from the prostate, vas deferens, and seminal vesicles. Being a complex system, it is apparent that many factors can affect male fertility, even events that occurred days to months before the sperm is developed. Some of the factors that affect male fertility can be as simple as wearing tight-fitting underwear, excessive use of hot tubs, or use of marijuana. A combination of events also may affect male fertility, including infection, a varicocele, and injury.

Once ejaculated, sperm can live from 2 to 3 days in the female genital tract but with decreasing activity after 24 hours, whereas an ovum is fertile for only 24 hours. The relative long life of sperm enhances the capacity for fertilization of an ovum.

In addition to the purely physiologic processes in men and women that regulate fertility, there are behaviors involved in procreation that society has termed *sexuality*.

SEXUALITY

Sex, sexual behavior, and *sexuality* are terms that often are used synonymously. In reality, they are different but related concepts. Sex is one of four primary drives, including thirst, hunger, and avoidance of pain. Sexual behavior refers to those practices involving sexual intercourse and other behaviors involving stimulation of the genitalia and other erogenous zones for the purpose of procreation or gratification. Sexuality is a complex concept that deals with the quality of being sexual, sexual activity, sexual orientation, and sexual receptivity or interest. Sexuality encompasses issues related to human sexual response; sexual orientation; and beliefs, attitudes, and social and cultural patterns related to sexual matters. The expression of sexuality is influenced by ethical, spiritual, cultural, and moral factors.

Sexuality and sexual function are important to a woman's health and well-being. The nurse plays a significant role in assisting women and men to understand their sexual health, sexual development, and sexuality (Figure 7-2). In fact, the holistic framework requires that the nurse be able to assist clients with concerns related to sexuality. Nurses, like other health care providers, can be uncomfortable discussing such personal topics with their clients. This unease may stem from vulnerability related to inadequate experience in dealing with clients with sexual difficulty, lack of information, or misinformation on the part of the nurse. Sexual awareness is required on the part of the client; however, cultural influences may inhibit conversation about such matters.

Many women have questions about their sexuality or sexual function. In fact, it has been estimated that as many as 60% of women have questions related to their sexuality (Baram, 2002). Many times women are hesitant to discuss these personal problems with anyone. Women may be most uncomfortable asking questions related to sexuality when cared for by someone of the opposite sex. Because of the awkwardness of discussing personal issues with providers, there is a tendency to seek information from other women or from the lay press. Occasionally, this practice leads to myth and misinformation. The tendency to obtain partial information and misinformation makes it very important for the nurse to assess the client's perception of her situation before institution of a plan of care.

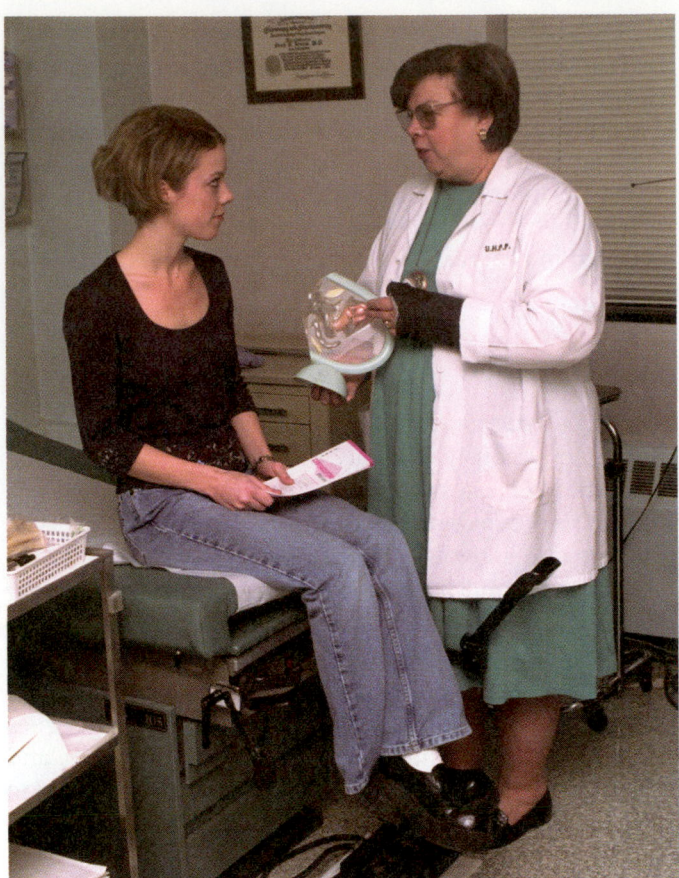

Figure 7-2 Nurses play an important role in helping clients understand their sexual health and development.

Sexual dysfunction can produce multifaceted and severe alterations in a woman's physical and mental health. Even if the question is one of health promotion, the nurse is in an excellent position to help women voice their questions and to dispel myths. Before these things can happen, the nurse must have an adequate understanding of the complexity of sexuality and the interaction of its components. Typically, this information is not high priority in educational programs and may not be discussed. In fact, it has been the practice at some institutions to relegate the study of sexuality to prenursing courses. The resulting

Nursing Tip *Being Nonjudgmental*

In the United States, body piercing and tattooing currently are trends. It is common to see piercing of navels, nipples, tongues, and the clitoris. These practices have roots in sexuality and sexual mores. You have the duty to accept the client's practices even when they differ from your own values.

general lack of information decreases the likelihood that the nurse will feel comfortable with this subject matter. Providing information about sexuality requires that the nurses have a nonjudgmental accepting attitude to allow women who have been enculturated never to discuss sex to do so in a public setting. Some women may not even have the vocabulary to voice their questions and concerns. The nurse may have to teach some women the names of body parts and their functions before being able to assist in answering questions or solving problems. Assistance may take many forms. A woman who has been sexually abused, for example, may have great difficulty tolerating a simple vaginal examination. A woman who is a lesbian may not participate in routine gynecologic care because she does not want her health care providers to know about her lifestyle. The young adolescent may not understand how to insert a tampon and may be very uncomfortable about seeking such information.

The nurse is required to closely examine personal values through self-reflection and rely on cultural competence to assist women with their sexual concerns (Figure 7-3). It is important that the nurse does not inject personal biases and other factors into the nurse-client interaction that will produce negative outcomes.

Human Sexual Response

Masters and Johnson (1966) are renowned for their study of human sexual response. They conceptualized the human sexual response consisting of four phases: excitement, plateau, orgasmic, and resolution. These phases occur in men and women and are associated with a number of physiologic changes. Contemporary sources include a fifth phase, which has been identified as the desire phase.

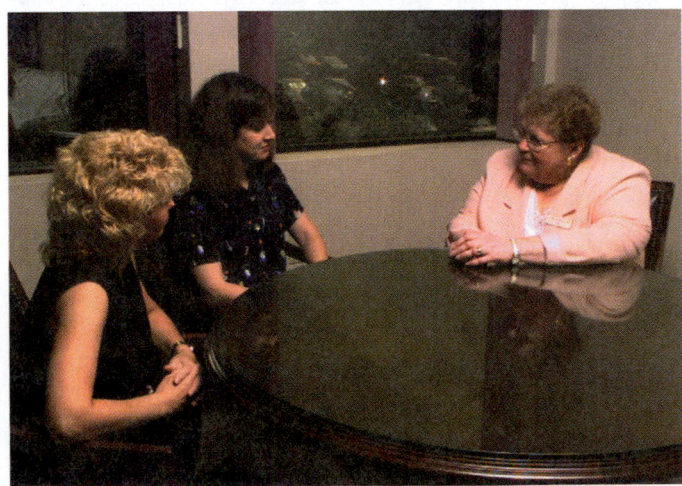

Figure 7-3 During the health history and interview, the nurse must remain nonjudgmental when discussing clients' practices and lifestyle choices.

The **desire phase** is conceptualized as being present before the other four phases. The desire phase has been described as the motivation or inclination to be sexual. Baram (2002) indicates that internal cues, such as fantasies, or external cues, such as an interested partner, may trigger sexual desire. Baram further states that desire also depends on proper neuroendocrine function. Other influences include sexual orientation, sexual preferences, mind-set, and the environment. All of these factors affect an individual's **libido**, their conscious or unconscious sexual desire.

The **excitement phase** occurs as a result of internal or external cues. During this phase the woman experiences increased vaginal lubrication, engorgement of the blood vessels of the breast and pelvis, and a sense of muscular tension. She also experiences increased heart rate, respiratory rate, and blood pressure. Besides the increase in muscular tension, many women experience flushing of the skin over the chest, neck, and face known as *sexual flushing*. These skin changes are the result of surface vasodilation, which produces congestion of the vessels with blood. The woman's nipples also become erect. Because of pelvic vasocongestion, the clitoris and labia become swollen. The vagina becomes distended and elongated, and the vaginal opening constricts, forming what is called an orgasmic platform (Kohn & Kaplan, 2000).

The man's response during the excitement phase includes changes in the scrotum, penis, and breasts. The scrotal sac becomes thickened and is elevated against the body owing to shortening of the spermatic cord. The penis becomes engorged with blood, which increases its circumference and length. This penile state is called an erection. As in the woman, the man's nipples become erect and he may experience the same sexual flushing of the chest, neck, and face.

The **plateau phase** of sexual response follows the excitement phase. During the plateau phase, women experience the most heightened sense of sexual tension. The labia become congested with blood to the extent that they may have a bluish hue. The change in color may be more difficult to recognize in dark skin types. There is full vaginal expansion as well as elevation of the uterus out of the pelvis in preparation for entry of the penis. By this phase, 75% of women experience sexual flushing. Tachycardia and hyperventilation occur as does a modest increase in blood pressure of 20 to 60 mmHg (Cohen, Kenner, & Hollingsworth, 1991).

The man's response during the plateau phase includes an increase in coronal circumference of the penis with continued erection. The testicles increase in size and are elevated against the body. As in the woman, there is generalized muscular tension that increases in intensity as orgasm approaches. The man also experiences tachycardia, hyperventilation, and increased blood pressure. The

systolic pressure increases by 20 to 80 mmHg, and the diastolic pressure increases by 20 to 40 mmHg (Cohen et al., 1991).

In the **orgasmic phase** the woman experiences elongation of the vaginal canal. There is an intense desire for sexual release as a result of blood vessel congestion. This sensation builds until the woman reaches orgasm. During this time the woman experiences an increase in blood pressure, tachycardia, and hyperventilation.

As the man enters the orgasmic phase, he experiences muscular contractions of the accessory reproductive organs, including the vas deferens, seminal vesicles, and ejaculatory duct. The sphincters of the bladder relax, and contractions of the urethra and perirectal muscles occur. Ejaculation occurs as the man achieves orgasm. As in the woman, the man experiences further tachycardia, hyperventilation, and blood pressure elevation.

During the **resolution phase** release of muscular tension occurs. The woman experiences a feeling of warmth and relaxation. Physiologic changes that took place in the previous phases of the response are reversed within 5 to 10 minutes (Baram, 2002). Resolution is slower when orgasm has not been achieved. Findings by Masters and Johnson suggest that women actually may experience a very short **refractory period**, that is, time before they are interested in experiencing intercourse again. Women are capable of multiple orgasms.

The man experiences a longer resolution phase. Immediate decrease in penile erection occurs after ejaculation, with partial decrease in vasocongestion. Within a few minutes after ejaculation, complete remission of erection occurs. There is a refractory period in which the man cannot achieve another erection. The time of the refractory period is somewhat variable; however, it is unusual for men to achieve multiple orgasms as do women.

Saks (1999) indicated that there is a physiologic difference in the brains of men and women after orgasm. There is a hippocampal neurologic discharge in the brain that makes men sleepy. In women, there is no such discharge. Women may experience a spurt of energy after orgasm.

American Sexual Practices

The public image of sex in America bears very little resemblance to what occurs in reality. Television portrays men and women as sexual beings who must be thin, beautiful, and young. The results of these myths are false expectations, deficits in self-esteem, broken relationships, and perhaps even a decline in physical health. When one tries to untangle the reality of sexuality, however, it becomes apparent that a realistic picture is almost impossible to ascertain. Masters and Johnson spent their entire careers scientifically analyzing the human sexual response, and many questions still remain unanswered.

In the late 1960s and 1970s, federal agencies studied sexuality, sexual practices, and homosexuality in an attempt to uncover the truth about sexuality in America (Michael, Gagnon, Laumann, & Jolata, 1994). Many of these studies were flawed and biased, and therefore, myths sometimes were perpetuated.

In 1994, Michael et al. undertook a survey to study sexuality that was designed to eliminate some of the flaws in previous research. The survey consisted of a sample of 3,432 Americans. Responses of the participants were compared with U.S. census data on the variables of gender, age, education, marital status, and race and ethnicity. The study group was found to represent 97.1% of American adults from 18 to 49 years of age. The following is a description of findings from the survey and may assist the nurse in making decisions about so-called normal sexuality.

When asked how many sexual partners they had had in the past 12 months, participants responded as follows: 11.1% of men and 13.7% of women denied having sexual partners, 67.6% and 75.5% had one partner, 9.6% and 6.3% had two partners, and 11% and 4.5% had three or more partners, respectively. These data support the notion that most American men and women participate in monogamous relationships. These data, however, do not address the concept of serial monogamy as a sexual practice. **Serial monogamy** is a term used to describe the practice of having one sexual partner at a time but several partners during a lifetime. There has been speculation that a factor in the exceedingly high divorce rate in the United States is the great value Americans have placed on monogamy (Michael et al., 1994). It is speculated that when a person become sexually dissatisfied with a relationship with a spouse, divorce enables that person to leave the relationship and still maintain the value of monogamy. This is a characteristic of serial monogamy. In reality, divorce is a much more complex phenomenon.

Sexual Preferences

The next question addressed by the survey (Michael et al., 1994) related to gender preference. The question was "Have your sex partners in the past 12 months been exclusively male, male and female, or exclusively female?" In answer to this question, 98.3% of women and 96.3% of men reported heterosexual (opposite gender) relationships; 1.0% of men and 0.5% of women reported bisexual relationships; and 2.6% of men and 1.2% of women reported homosexual (same gender) relationships.

Frequency of intercourse is a factor that is commonly discussed among couples concerning what is normal and was addressed in the survey. Frequency of intercourse was analyzed based on gender, age, marital status, education, religion, and race and ethnicity. The norm for frequency of intercourse was several times monthly: 37% of men and 36% of women reported having intercourse several times monthly; 26% of men and 30% of women reported having intercourse two to three times weekly; and only 8% of men and 7% of women reported engaging in intercourse four or more times weekly. These findings suggest there is a wide range of what is considered normal behavior concerning frequency of intercourse. Frequency of intercourse becomes a problem for couples when expectations are different between the two members of the sexual dyad.

Age is a factor in frequency of participation in intercourse. Men under the age of 30 years reported engaging in intercourse more frequently (two to three times per week). Men over 40 years of age more commonly (43%) reported engaging in intercourse several times per month. Women in all age categories most commonly reported intercourse several times per month. Similar findings were obtained concerning marital status, education, religion, and race and ethnicity. This group of variables can have immeasurable influence on one's sexuality and sexual behavior.

This study also examined sexual practices and preferences. Vaginal intercourse had the widest appeal for men and women. The least preferred sexual practice was forcing a partner to have sex or being forced to have sex of any type.

Masturbation (self-stimulation) was another sexual practice studied. Findings suggested that masturbation is not rare. It is a practice preferred by men more than women but common in both genders. In this study, fewer than 6 out of 10 (60%) of men in the 18- to 24-year-old age group and 7 out of 10 (70%) of all men reported masturbating in the past year. Fewer than 4 out of 10 (40%) of women in the 18- to 24-year-old age group and 3 out of 10 (30%) of women over 54 years of age masturbated. Nearly half of women in their 30s reported masturbating. It has been speculated that masturbation is not as common as once thought among young men because it is perceived by them to be an activity indicating immaturity. It also has been suggested that masturbation is controlled by social factors and cultural influences (Michael et al., 1994).

Among the group of most sexually active persons, approximately 85% of men and 45% of women living with a sexual partner reported masturbating in the past year. Married persons were more likely to masturbate than were those living alone. These findings led the researchers to conclude that masturbation is not a substitute for other sexual practices but is an activity that stimulates and is stimulated by other sexual activity.

A change has occurred in American culture involving the meaning and place of sexuality (D'Emilio & Freedman, 1997). The view that sex is a family-centered process with the aim of reproduction, as was conceptualized in the colonial era, has changed to the view that sex is for personal pleasure. In the 19th century, sexuality was focused more on intimacy and romance. In contemporary times the attitude exists that sexuality is linked to personal identity, individual desire, and personal fulfillment.

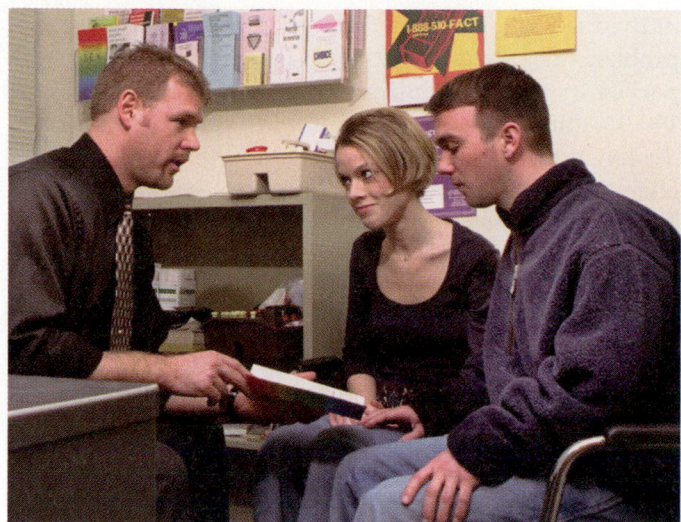

Figure 7-4   An important element in sex education and counseling is sharing information on contraceptive options.

The focus is away from procreation and continually is being reshaped by the nature of the economy, the family, and politics. For example, the availability of abortion for the woman with limited means may change depending on politics because funding for abortion may be decreased by the federal government in an administration having antiabortion sentiment.

One of the factors that has contributed greatly to the contemporary view of sexuality is contraception, or prevention of pregnancy (Figure 7-4). In the 1920s and 1930s there was much resistance to the idea of contraception. When oral contraceptives became available in the 1960s, the social and sexual cultures had changed to the extent that contraceptive practices became acceptable. Sexual abstinence was less likely as marriage and childbearing were more likely to occur later in life after completion of education. It was considered more socially acceptable for couples to live together; however, childbearing was more likely to be delayed until marriage. Unintended pregnancy is sometimes the precipitating event that leads to marriage in cohabiting couples. In sexual relationships, contraception and conception may be the key to the relationship, especially when partners do not agree about sexual matters. In fact, some believe that women do not control their destiny until they control their fertility (D'Emilio & Freedman, 1997).

Media and advertising have contributed greatly to how women view their sexuality. For example, advertisements offer suggestions about clothing and a vast array of personal grooming products to make women feel more attractive sexually. The media has greatly influenced our sexuality, and increasingly so in the past few decades.

As sexuality has changed, so have attitudes about sexual preference. During the era of World War II, homosexuality was considered a psychiatric problem. In the decades since then, homosexuality has been viewed as sexual deviance and most recently as an alternative lifestyle. Even though homosexuality is not the predominant sexual preference in the United States, evidence exists that it is becoming more widely accepted culturally. Evidence of this acceptance can be seen in the laws that have changed to enable marriage and adoption of children by couples of the same gender. Even the rigid structure of the military is exhibiting some flexibility by no longer questioning service people about their sexual preference.

Pregnancy and Sexuality

Pregnancy is a time when sexual issues may come to the forefront. Couples may express concerns about maintaining a sexual relationship throughout their pregnancy. Certain changes may take place in normal sexual response that are related to the physiologic changes of pregnancy (Alteneder & Hartzell, 1997). In fact, there may be changes in each trimester. In the first trimester, the woman may be less interested in sex because of fatigue, nausea, or adaptation to pregnancy. In the second trimester, her interest may increase. As she nears term, however, she may experience some discomfort unless there are position changes to allow for the increase in her abdominal size. Education and support may assist the couple in maintaining a positive sexual relationship.

Women who are sexually abused in childhood may develop gender and sexual identities that emphasize self-worth based on sexuality (American College of Obstetricians and Gynecologists, 2000). These women are likely to have particular problems with sexual issues during pregnancy.

Sexuality and Aging

There is not an abundance of evidence related to sexuality and aging. There are physiologic changes that occur with aging, as well as attitudinal factors, physical illnesses, and social factors that can affect sexuality as a woman ages. Two physiologic changes in women are likely to affect a woman's sexuality as she grows older. Decreases in the rate of production and volume of vaginal lubrication can lead to vaginal dryness and a sense of tightness, irritation, or burning after intercourse (Byyny & Speroff, 1996). Some loss of elasticity of the vaginal muscles also occurs that limits the woman's ability to tolerate deep or prolonged thrusting. These changes can result in postcoital spotting and soreness. These atropic symptoms can be relieved or eliminated by the use of lubricants, a change in coital position, or hormone replacement therapy.

Even after menopause women have sexual desire. Women in their 60s and 70s may continue to be sexually active depending on their health and social circumstances (Figure 7-5). Many times older women have outlived their

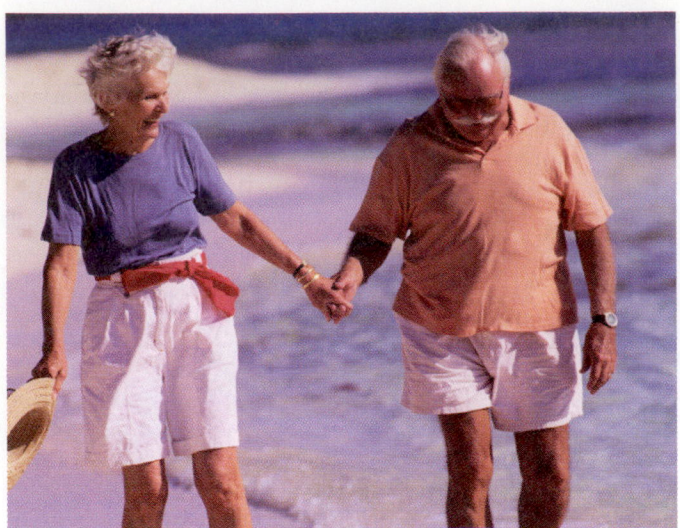

Figure 7-5   Sexual expression and intimacy are elements of partnerships throughout the life cycle.

husbands and thus their opportunity for sexual expression is limited.

Byyny & Speroff (1996) suggest that younger people and health care providers underrate the interest older people have in sex. These authors submit that the two most important factors influencing interest in sex are strength of the relationship and health of both partners. They further suggest that sexual activity among the aging is more influenced by culture and attitude than by nature and physiology.

SEXUAL DYSFUNCTION

Sexual dysfunction is the disturbance of one or more of the phases of human sexual response. The diagnosis is based on clinical judgment and must be evaluated in the biopsychosocial context in which it occurs (Vermillion & Holmes, 1997). In other words, sexual dysfunction may be biologic, psychologic, or social in nature or the result of a combination of any of these variables. Because the disturbance is so complex, a thorough assessment must be undertaken to determine the cause.

Epidemiologic data concerning sexual dysfunction are sparse and reflect the hesitancy to discuss such matters by clients and some health care providers. Sexual dysfunction can affect males and females; however, it is unclear statistically which gender is more greatly affected.

Evaluation of Sexual Dysfunction

The nurse can make a major contribution to the care of couples with sexual dysfunction by providing an atmosphere that allows discussion of personal, highly emotional topics. The nurse often is the person with whom individuals share their feelings. Evaluation of sexual problems begins with taking a sexual history from both parties in the relationship (Van Sickle & Rosenstrock, 1999). Although it is not the nurse's role to treat sexual dysfunction, the practitioner should have enough knowledge to discuss normal compared with dysfunctional behavior and make appropriate referrals.

The PLISSIT model has been identified as a useful one in general care settings for discussing sexual concerns (Katz, 2000). PLISSIT is an acronym for permission, limited information, specific suggestions, and intensive therapy. The PLISSIT model also has been used successfully to address sexual concerns during pregnancy (Alteneder & Hartzell, 1997).

Permission

When taking a sexual history, the nurse should ask open-ended, nonjudgmental questions that identify what the woman considers to be her normal sexual activity. This approach gives the woman permission to express concerns and ask questions.

Limited Information

The nurse should be familiar with sexual terms, sexual anatomy and physiology, and sexual norms and should be able to determine which limited information is needed to assist the woman with her problem. Many times information is all that is necessary to resolve the problem.

Specific Suggestions

The nurse should have enough knowledge to make suggestions for alleviation of client concerns. In pregnancy, for example, women may have dreams that they find unacceptable. It may be sufficient to let them know that many pregnant women experience emotionally charged dreams. If this information is not sufficient, however, the nurse can make a suggestion for referral to another health care provider who has expertise in dealing with such problems.

Intensive Therapy

The nurse should know her limitations concerning time and expertise and should make referrals for complex or time-consuming cases. In making the referral, it is wise for the nurse to suggest that the client needs someone with more skill rather than insinuate there is something abnormal about the client's problem.

Normal sexual function is sometimes an unknown factor and often a taboo subject for many individuals. Open communication and a supportive attitude from caregivers can increase sexual knowledge and discredit myths.

INFERTILITY

As noted previously, when one considers the complex physical and hormonal sequence of events required for conception and pregnancy, it is amazing that normal births ever occur. For pregnancy to occur the female ovary must produce a mature egg, capable of being fertilized, which must be transported through the fallopian tube into the uterus where the hormonally prepared endometrium supports implantation. The male testes must produce an adequate quantity of mature, motile sperm, capable of surviving the arduous trip through his reproductive system, into the vagina, through the cervical mucus, uterus, and fallopian tube to join with the ovum. With each normal ovulatory cycle, there is about a 25% chance of pregnancy resulting. For most couples, pregnancy may not occur for 6 months to 1 year with unprotected intercourse.

Clearly, many factors affect fertility. The ability to have children, however, is considered a normal expectation of adult life. **Infertility** is defined as the inability to conceive after 1 year with appropriately timed coitus without the use of contraception. The inability to carry a fetus to viability is also an important infertility factor. Infertility affects almost 15% of couples (Silverberg, 2000), with the risk increasing for women after 35 years of age. After this age, nearly one third of women desiring a child are unable to conceive (Wallach, Garcia, Rosenwak, & Seifer, 1998). For those who have difficulty or are unable to conceive, infertility can be devastating.

It is estimated that there were 4.5 million women who reported infertility in 1982 (Stephen & Chandra, 1998) as compared with 4.8 million in 1988 and 6.2 million in 1995. This increase is thought to be multifactorial. Proposed factors include delayed childbearing by a number of baby-boomers in society, the decreased popularity of permanent sterilization as a means of contraception, and an advance in age limits beyond 35 years as a criterion to qualify for infertility treatment. More couples are seeking fertility assistance because it is an acceptable and treatable condition. Also, the waiting list for adoption is typically 2 to 10 years. The result has been that many couples wait until later in life to attempt a first pregnancy.

The financial and psychological costs of infertility can be immense (Jerka, Schuett, & Foxhall, 1996). Estimates of the financial costs of infertility treatment vary according to the technology used. However, Van Voorhis (1998) noted that "In 1992, the overall cost per delivery was $30,252." Psychologic sequelae described include depression, guilt, stress, loss, grief, disturbances of self-esteem, relationship problems, and even divorce. Estimates of financial costs often are inexact but include direct medical costs, such as drugs, ovulation prediction kits, physician fees, laboratory tests, hospitalizations, and radiologic examinations. Indirect costs may include expenses related to food and transportation when seeking care, lost wages, and extended care of children while the parents are undergoing testing. Other elusive costs may be incurred related to pain and grief or psychologic counseling.

Factors Affecting Fertility

Because of the complexity of determining the cause of infertility and its expense, it is important that both partners be involved in the process from the beginning. A thorough assessment, which can be time-consuming, expensive, and emotionally burdensome, may be required to produce a live birth. For the infertile couple the evaluation and treatment may be positive experiences because they offer hope.

Female Factors

Approximately 40% of the time female factors are the cause of infertility. Within this group of women, for 40% the major reason is failure to ovulate (Rosenthal, 1997). Another 40% have either tubal or pelvic problems. The remaining 20% have unusual problems or unexplained infertility.

Perhaps the single most important factor in female infertility is aging (Sauer, 1998). Although the causes of infertility are many, the decision to delay childbearing may result in difficulty in achieving a pregnancy. The decline in fertility with age has several components. With increasing age, there is higher risk of spontaneous abortion. The incidence of pelvic or tubal problems increases. Finally, the endocrine changes that begin 10 to 15 years before menopause lead to decreased fertility.

Problems of Ovulation

For most women (95% to 98%) the presence of monthly menstrual cycles with premenstrual symptoms indicates an ovulatory cycle. Although its value has become more controversial with more sophisticated test measures (Illions & Thompson, 1997), taking the basal body temperature (BBT) can be a helpful and inexpensive indicator of ovulation for the woman experiencing monthly menses. The BBT should be evaluated after two menstrual cycles. A biphasic temperature pattern suggests ovulation.

The woman who is having irregular or infrequent menses or who is not having menses should be evaluated for ovulatory dysfunction (Kaplan, 1996). Common signs of problems of ovulation other than alterations in menses are **galactorrhea** (nipple discharge); signs of androgen excess, such as facial hair or male pattern hair growth; alterations in thyroid or adrenal functioning; and weight changes.

Ovarian Abnormalities. Anovulation may be a result of ovarian abnormalities such as hypogonadism (Turner's syndrome), a genetic disorder, or external causes such as radiation or chemotherapy (Seaman, Telich-Vidal, & Sable, 1997). A cause that occasionally is overlooked is the use of oral contraceptives, which were initially prescribed to regulate menses or for the treatment of acne. Ovarian tumors or polycystic ovaries may prevent ovulation owing to changes in the feedback mechanism regulating ovarian function.

Hormonal Abnormalities. Abnormalities of hormonal functioning or ovarian failure may result in anovulation (Prior, 1997; Anasti, 1998). Irregularities in any of the sectors of the hypothalamic-pituitary-ovarian axis may alter the hormonal balance needed for ovulation. Appropriate levels of the adrenal, thyroid, and pituitary hormones also are needed. General poor health, inadequate nutrition, stress, and excessive exercise affect ovarian function.

Tubal Structural Problems
Fertilization usually occurs in the outer portion of the fallopian tube, which also provides transport for the embryo into the uterus for implantation. Obstruction or narrowing of the tube can lead to the inability to conceive or tubal pregnancies. Blockages may be a result of congenital defects, infections, or endometriosis (Spielvogel, Shwayden, & Coddington, 2000). Infection is the most common cause of scarring, however, and can result from organisms such as *Neisseria gonorrhoeae*, *Chlamydia trachomatis*, *Mycoplasma*, and *Mycobacterium tuberculosis*. Seemingly minor surgery such as appendectomy or laparoscopy also may cause infection or adhesions, with resultant infertility.

Structural Problems of the Uterus
Infertility related to uterine problems is often structural in origin. Although fibroid tumors (leiomyomata) themselves usually are not a cause of infertility, they may obstruct the fallopian tubes or interfere with implantation. Although somewhat rare, congenital malformations may interfere with implantation or the ability to carry a fetus to term. An inadequate endometrium also may impede fertility because implantation may not be successful. An inadequate endometrium can result from Asherman's syndrome, a thinning of the uterine lining after surgical procedures, or inadequate hormonal production.

Endometriosis has gained the reputation for being the cause of many cases of infertility (Berube, Marcoux, Langenum, & Maheux, 1998). **Endometriosis** is the implantation of uterine endometrium outside the uterus. The exact mechanism is not known but a reflux through the tubes at the time of menses is thought to explain the unusual implantation sites. Although the most common sites for endometriosis are in the lower pelvis and bowel, it has been seen on the diaphragm, lungs, and brain. Again, it is difficult to correlate the severity of the endometriosis with

infertility because a woman with very few visible implants may be unable to conceive, whereas a woman with a severe case may have no problem conceiving. The exact reason for the resultant infertility also is not known. The infertility may be merely from obstructing implantation or adhesions, or it may be a result of a much more complex problem involving the body's response to foreign tissue (Seltzer & Pearse, 1995). Abnormal uterine division, such as bicorunate, unicornuate, or septal uterus, may also result in infertility.

Structural Problems of the Vagina and Cervix
As the vagina and cervix are developing, a variety of congenital structural abnormalities may occur that could interfere with the transport, implantation, or growth of the embryo. There may be two vaginal vaults, two cervixes, imperforate hymen, irregularly shaped uterus or tubes, or the cavities within either may be misshapen. Although these structural problems may be determined by physical examination, other diagnostic tests such as ultrasonography may be needed.

In addition, infections may change the cervical mucus and vaginal secretions that aid sperm motility and viability. Historically, cervical mucus and vaginal secretions were of greater concern. The use of intrauterine insemination, however, has lowered the incidence of these problems.

Male Factors
Male factors account for 35% to 40% of infertility. The incidence of male reasons for infertility is summarized in Box 7-1.

A semen analysis, a simple noninvasive screening test, should be an early, if not first, step in assessing a couple experiencing infertility. It is important that the specimen be collected and analyzed properly. After at least 48 hours of abstinence, a specimen obtained by masturbation should be collected in a clean container. The specimen should remain at body temperature and be delivered

---

Box 7-1

Male Factors Associated with Infertility

- Idiopathic, 70%–75%
- Testicular disorders (surgery, trauma), 10%–13%
- Genital tract obstructions, 8%–10%
- Sperm autoimmunity, 4%–6%
- Hormonal disorders, 1%
- Ejaculation, sexual dysfunction, 1%

to the laboratory in 30 to 45 minutes. Because of the variability between specimens, it is suggested that the test be repeated in 2 to 4 weeks. Findings in a normal semen analysis are provided in Table 7-1.

Even the parameters in Table 7-1 are not necessarily predictive of fertility because there are many possibilities for error, including laboratory error, error in the way in which the specimen was collected, or events that occurred 3 months before the test that may have affected spermatogenesis, such as an illness or injury.

Many factors should be considered when the cause of a low sperm count seems to be idiopathic (Bigelow, Jarrell, Young, Keefe, & Love, 1998). Increased scrotal heat owing to activities, such as frequent hot tub or sauna use, chronic infections causing increased body temperature, and sitting at a desk or in a car or bike riding for long periods, can cause a decreased sperm count. Sons of mothers who took diethylstilbestrol (DES) while pregnant have been shown to have reduced sperm counts. Trauma to the testes and surgery also can affect sperm production or cause adhesions, resulting in obstructions (Silber, 2000). The use of drugs or alcohol is a factor that may cause low sperm count. Environmental factors such as exposure to toxic drugs, chemicals, and anesthetic gases also have been implicated in low sperm counts.

Testicular disorders account for approximately 10% to 13% of male infertility (Illions & Thompson, 1997). These disorders include cryptorchidism (undescended testes) and other congenital abnormalities or malformations. Obstructions of the genital tract (8% to 10%) can result from congenital abnormalities, trauma or surgery, and genital infections. Abnormalities in hormonal functioning, including the thyroid, pancreas, and pituitary, can impair fertility. Ejaculation or sexual dysfunction, which may be physical or psychologic, also may result in an inability to reproduce. Even when sperm count and mobility seem adequate, an immune response to the sperm in the male or female may decrease fertility.

Unexplained Infertility

For approximately 10% of infertile couples no specific causative problem can be identified. Possibly, each partner has minor problems that alone cannot explain the infertility but in combination prevent fertility (Guzick, 2000). For couples such as these, assisted reproductive technology may be of benefit. Often, however, these couples will require support and encouragement to seek other alternatives, such as adoption.

Assessment of the Infertile Couple

When a couple presents with concerns about infertility, it is important to understand that men and women are very concerned and possibly emotionally fragile. Many couples have read and tried many of the common folklore remedies to achieve pregnancy. Depending on their own values, or those of their culture, the ability to bear children can be very important. Entering a medical setting for evaluation is in itself, for some, an admission of failure. In addition, much concern can center on which partner is at fault. Before even beginning the medical aspects of care, it is important to understand and assist the couple to understand their motivation for pregnancy and be prepared to offer support. The couple should understand that the evaluation and treatment for infertility will be stressful and will involve both partners throughout the process. It is important to meet with the couple together. Some time also should be spent alone with each individual because there may be issues the person would prefer not to discuss in the presence of his or her partner.

The first and perhaps most valuable step in the evaluation for infertility is taking a detailed medical and fertility history from each partner. An outline for this history is shown in Box 7-2.

Table 7-1	Normal Semen Analysis
ELEMENT	**QUANTITY OR QUALITY**
Volume	2.0 mL or more
Sperm concentration	20 million/mL or more
Motility	50% or more with forward progression, or 25% or more with rapid progression within 60 min of ejaculation
Morphology	30% or more normal forms
Leukocytes	Fewer than 1 million/mL
Immunobead test	Fewer than 20% with adherent particles
SpermMar test	Fewer than 10% with adherent particles

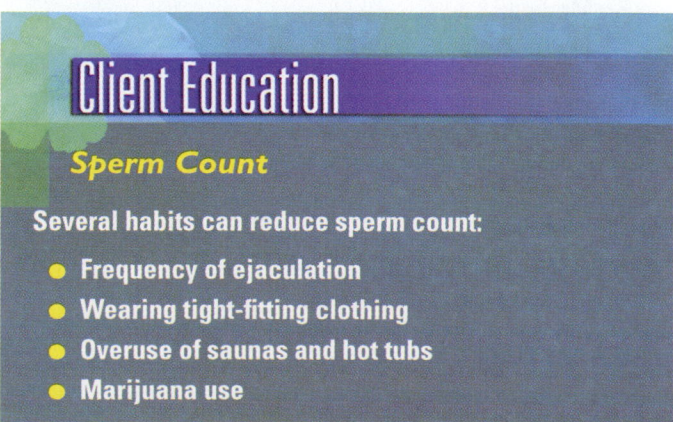

Client Education

Sperm Count

Several habits can reduce sperm count:

- **Frequency of ejaculation**
- **Wearing tight-fitting clothing**
- **Overuse of saunas and hot tubs**
- **Marijuana use**

Box 7-2

Evaluation of Infertility

Female History

1. Age

2. Fertility history
   How long the pregnancy has been sought
   Prior pregnancies: age at conception, outcome of
      each pregnancy
   Prior contraception: method, complications,
      length of time without contraception
   Use of an intrauterine device
   Abortions: number, type

3. Menstrual history
   Date of last menstrual cycle
   Age of menarche
   Characteristics of menses: interval, duration,
      regularity, predictability (breast tenderness,
      bloating), dysmenorrhea
   Awareness of ovulation, change in cervical mucus,
      mittelschmerz (midcycle pelvic pain), midcycle
      spotting
   Polycystic ovaries, ovarian cysts

4. Medical history
   Major diseases: diabetes, tuberculosis, tumors
   Treatments for disease, including medications
      and chemotherapy
   Sexually transmitted infections: gonorrhea, syphilis,
      chlamydia, herpes
   Hormonal irregularities: adrenal, thyroid, pituitary
      (hyperprolactinemia)

5. Surgical history
   Laparoscopy or other reproductive surgery
   Appendectomy
   Endometriosis
   Any abdominal surgery
   Dilation and curettage

6. Medications
   In utero exposure to DES
   Hormones, including oral contraceptives
   Antibiotics
   Tretinoin (Retin-A)

7. Occupation
   Exposure to radiation, toxic drugs, chemicals,
      anesthetic gases

8. Personal and sexual habits
   Alcohol or drug use (cocaine, marijuana, inhalants,
      and so on)

Smoking
Extremes of weight gain or loss
Douching
Frequency of intercourse; use of lubricants
Timing of intercourse for optimum conception
Pregnancy with other partners
Number of other partners (risk of sexually trans-
   mitted infections and antibody reaction to sperm)

Male History

1. Fertility history
   Age
   Previous children
   Frequency of intercourse; difficulties associated
      with function, including erection and ejaculation

2. Medical history
   Major diseases: diabetes; tuberculosis; renal,
      thyroid, or adrenal diseases; other hormonal
      imbalances
   Mumps after childhood
   Abnormality or disease of the genital tract, tumors,
      epididymitis, prostatitis
   Acute illness in past 3 months
   Sexually transmitted infections and treatment

3. Surgical history
   Genital surgery, including hernia repair,
      retroperitoneal surgery, and prostate surgery

4. Medications
   List all drugs being taken, both prescription and
      over the counter (some may affect
      spermatogenesis, others function)

5. Occupation (sitting for long periods affects
      spermatogenesis)
   Exposure to radiation, toxic drugs, chemicals,
      anesthetic gases

6. Personal and sexual habits
   Alcohol or street drug use (cocaine, marijuana,
      inhalants, and so on)
   Smoking
   Wearing of tight underwear or biking shorts
      (elevates temperature)
   Use of hot tubs (temperature)
   Use of personal lubricants; condom use
   Frequency of intercourse (very frequent
      ejaculation can reduce sperm count)

Physical Assessment and Diagnostic Tools

In many infertility practices the medical history is completed by the nurse. Often the physician or nurse practitioner will complete the physical examination, with the nurse providing assistance and much of the education. An overview of tools commonly used in infertility assessment is given in Table 7-2. Typically, the woman's examination is done in the office of the infertility practice; however, the man may be referred to a urologist for evaluation. In the man's examination, the presence of secondary sexual characteristics and genital abnormalities should be noted. Key evaluations include undescended testes and absence of the vas deferens. Attention should be paid to the presence of a varicocele, or abnormal blood vessels in the scrotum. A varicocele and the presence of a hydrocele, fluid in the scrotum, may be related to infertility.

In the woman, attention is paid to secondary sexual characteristics, such as breast development, pattern of facial and genital hair distribution, and the presence of acne. These characteristics are indicators of sexual maturity and, therefore, the ability to conceive. The thyroid should be palpated carefully for enlargement or nodules. The breasts should be evaluated for normal development and the presence of discharge. Surgical scars may indicate abdominal surgery, with resultant adhesions affecting reproductive function. A complete pelvic examination, including inspection of the external genitalia, should be performed to rule out anatomic abnormalities and infection. With the pelvic examination, cultures should be taken and a Pap smear performed. The first visit is an ideal time to offer preconceptual counseling, including testing for blood type, Rh antibodies, and immunity to measles. Vaccines should be discussed and possibly administered when indicated for measles, hepatitis B, and other immunizations as recommended. Teaching should include the need to use contraception until the immunizations have been completed. This recommendation is not likely to be received positively by the couple who so desperately want to conceive a pregnancy.

Before any further evaluation is done, a semen analysis should be obtained. This is the easiest and least invasive test that can be performed and often is overlooked.

Nursing Tip *Understanding the Menstrual Cycle*

Many couples do not understand when the fertile time of the menstrual cycle occurs. Before considering an infertility workup, it is important to explore basic knowledge about sexuality, reproduction, and timing of intercourse. Helping the woman to be more aware of how her body functions, when ovulation occurs, and midcycle changes in the cervical mucus can assist couples in achieving conception.

Table 7-2 Tools Used to Assess Infertility

TEST	INSTRUCTIONS	FINDINGS
Basal body temperature (BBT)	Used to confirm ovulation and time intercourse. Temperature can be taken orally, rectally, or vaginally with a regular thermometer, but special BBT thermometers or newer digital ones may be easier to read. Temperature must be taken on awakening, before any activity. The chart should be started on day 1 of the cycle. All events, such as intercourse, variations in normal activity, and illness, should be recorded.	Typically, the temperature decreases slightly (0.2°F) 24–36 h before ovulation and increases (0.4–0.8°F) 24–72 h after. Temperature stays elevated for 11–16 d. This biphasic pattern indicates ovulation. The most fertile time is 3–4 d before ovulation and 1–2 d after. Coitus every other day during this time is suggested.
Endometrial biopsy	A sample of the endometrial tissue lining the uterus to determine the uterine response to hormonal stimulation. Performed 2–3 d before an expected menstrual period. Danger of pregnancy loss exists, and a pregnancy test should be performed before this biopsy. Usually done in the physician's office with the use of a pipelle, a thin catheter inserted into the uterine cavity. Taking ibuprofen decreases possible cramping and discomfort. Helpful in diagnosing a luteal phase defect.	The pathology report will describe the influence of hormones on the uterus.

(continues)

Table 7-2   (continued)

TEST	INSTRUCTIONS	FINDINGS
Hysterosalpingogram	An X-ray study to determine if the uterine cavity and fallopian tubes are open and healthy. Performed 2–5 d after the end of menses. Special evaluation and possible alternative treatment should be considered if a history of pelvic inflammatory disease, pelvic mass, or sensitivity to iodine exists.	Abnormalities of the structure of the uterus or tubes may be identified. Narrowing or occlusion of the tubes can be seen.
Laboratory evaluations	Based on medical history and physical examination, additional blood or urine tests may be ordered to evaluate the function of ovaries, pituitary, adrenal, hypothalamus, thyroid, and other glands to determine the cause of infertility.	Test parameters vary and are determined by the laboratory. Abnormalities may require further testing or treatment.
Laparoscopy	Procedure using an endoscope to view the pelvin organs. May be abdominal or vaginal. Treatments may be performed as problems are identified. Uterine abnormalities such as fibroids, adhesions, and endometriosis may be identified and removed. Used to retrieve eggs for reproductive technology. Usually suggested when no other cause of infertility is found.	Depending on the findings, treatment usually is performed at the same time to correct abnormalities. Findings might include fibroids, endometriosis, adhesions, ovarian cysts, and tubal blockages.
Ovulation predictor kit	A urine test used to predict ovulation based on luteinizing hormone (LH) measured in the urine. Available over the counter, the kits cost $30–$40/mo and include 5–10 tests. LH triggers ovulation, which occurs 20–48 h after the LH surge. LH can be detected in the urine 8–12 h after its peak levels. Urine should be tested at the same time each day. Some tests require first morning voiding. Be sure to read instructions in the kit.	False-positive results can be obtained owing to menopause, pregnancy, and polycystic ovaries. Instructions in the kit will describe the findings.
Postcoital test	Evaluates cervical mucus to determine adequacy of mucus and the ability of sperm to travel within it. Intercourse should occur after 48 hours of abstinence within 24–48 h of ovulation. Cervical mucus is examined by obtaining a sample during pelvic examination 2–8 h after coitus.	The mucus should be described in terms of quantity, clarity, viscosity, pH, spinnbarkeit, and sperm characteristics of number, motility, and forms. Normal findings are described as 5–10 morphologically normal sperm with linear motility in thin, clear, copious, acellular mucus with spinnbarkeit >8 cm.
Semen analysis	Semen should be collected by masturbation after 2–3 days' without ejaculation. Collect in a clean, dry container. Be sure to collect entire ejaculate; do not use withdrawal or condoms for collection. Special sheaths can be used, if required. Specimen should be kept warm and delivered to the laboratory in 30–60 min. Two or three specimens may be required over several months because spermatogenesis takes 2.5 months.	Normal values: Volume, 2–6 mL Viscosity, liquid within 30 min pH, 7–8 Count, more than 20 million/mL Motility, more than 40% moving Morphology, more than 50% mature and normal
Ultrasonography	Sound waves used to evaluate the structure of the pelvic organs and monitor ovulation by identification of follicles and release of the ova. Also used to evaluate the fetus during pregnancy. Identifies ectopic pregnancies, endometriosis, and submucosal fibroids. May be performed abdominally or vaginally.	Structural abnormalities can be identified. Size, development, and maturation of ovarian follicles can be monitored, and status for egg retrieval provided.

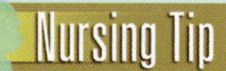

Nursing Tip   *Basal Body Temperature*

The basal body temperature (BBT) test has become less popular since the advent of the ovulation prediction kits because the BBT is less accurate.

The ordering of further diagnostic tests will depend on the findings of the medical history and physical examination.

After the first examination, couples who have not previously kept a BBT chart may be asked to keep this record for 1 or 2 months. With newer technology such as the ovulation predictor kit and hormonal assays, however, the BBT may not be required.

Reflections from an Infertile Couple

We wanted to have a child very badly, but after 3 years of marriage and unprotected regular intercourse we had no pregnancy. After a long discussion with my husband, we decided to seek medical advice. We decided the best way to proceed was for me to visit my gynecologist.

We had no idea how impersonal and cold the whole process would be. You are asked to distance yourself from the emotional aspects of sexuality and focus on the mechanics of conception. My husband remembers the semen analysis as being the most challenging. He was given a sterile container, shown to a room, and told to produce a semen specimen. No further instructions were given. My most embarrassing time was when we had a postcoital test scheduled. The physician wanted me to be seen in his office within 2 hours after intercourse to examine my vaginal secretions under the microscope. On a bad traffic day, it can take 2 hours to travel from our home to his office. We had to rent a motel room near my husband's workplace and have intercourse during his lunch hour because we both had missed so much work. I'm not sure health care providers understand how stressful some of these tests can be.

Management of Infertility

After the findings of the history, physical examinations, laboratory tests, and other diagnostic tests are reviewed, a therapeutic regimen to treat the underlying cause of the infertility is decided on with the couple. It is very important that the couple understand each treatment considered for their situation. In planning their care the health care provider also must take into consideration influences such as the ages of the partners, how long they have been trying to conceive, health care insurance coverage or financial resources, and any cultural or religious concerns. Generally, less invasive and less complex treatments are tried first, moving progressively to more involved procedures or combinations of therapies (Angard, 1999). Treatment decisions will depend on the couple's desires. Because of the expense of infertility treatment, both financial and emotional, communication about the proposed treatments, possible side effects, and potential effectiveness is very important.

Laparoscopy

Laparoscopy is one of the most important diagnostic and therapeutic tools used in infertility. It allows direct visualization of peritoneal structures and definitive diagnosis of endometriosis, adhesions, and abnormalities in structure or function of the pelvic organs. During the procedure, treatment of adhesions, ablation of endometriosis, and restoration of patency of the fallopian tubes may be accomplished. Occasionally, a myoma or fibroid may

Nursing Tip   *Cancer and Fertility*

As cure rates for cancer have improved, both men and women who have or have had cancer are considering the effects of the cancer and cancer treatments on their fertility. Although the cancer itself may affect the ability to conceive, treatment with surgery, chemotherapy, or radiation may damage reproductive capability. With increased awareness, more emphasis is being put on preserving reproductive function. Cryopreservation (freezing) of sperm, decreased toxicity of chemotherapy, and the use of shielding during radiation have been used. Hormonal suppression of gonadal activity has been suggested as a means of preserving gonadal function.

It is important to be aware of the implications of cancer on fertility and that couples may desire pregnancy after cancer therapy. Education, information, and emotional support can assist these clients in making treatment decisions.

interfere with fertility and may be removed during laparoscopy. A general anesthetic typically is used and carbon dioxide gas is used to distend the abdomen for better visualization. It is important to inform the woman that there may be some discomfort, such as cramping from manipulation of the pelvic organs and shoulder pain as a result of the gas used.

Artificial Insemination

Artificial insemination, with either the partner's or donor's sperm, allows for semen to be placed in the vagina near the cervical os. This is most appropriate when infertility is a result of problems with sperm production or ejaculation. Intrauterine insemination provides a means to bypass cervical mucus problems when the tubes appear to be open, allowing for fertilization in the tubes. For this procedure, a washed sperm specimen is prepared and inserted high into the uterus at the appropriate time in the cycle.

The use of donor sperm presents health and ethical issues that should be discussed clearly with the person seeking insemination. Standards for testing, preparation, and storage of sperm have been established and reduce the possibility of infection with the human immunodeficiency and hepatitis viruses. The couple also has the option to describe criteria used for donor matching, such as ethnic and physical characteristics.

Hormonal Therapy

A disturbance in ovulation usually is treated with one or more hormones, depending on the cause of the problem. Many times medications are available to assist in the management of infertility (Table 7-3). Bromocriptine, clomiphene, human menopausal gonadotropins, Gn-RH, and purified FSH are used to induce ovulation. hCG stimulates ovulation. Progestins may be used to support the luteal phase of the cycle. Before these drugs are used, thyroid, pituitary, and adrenal disorder must be diagnosed and treated.

Assisted Reproductive Technology

Although many advances in the diagnosis and treatment of infertility have improved the chances of pregnancy, for some couples pregnancy would be impossible without the use of advanced technology. Assisted reproductive

Table 7-3	Medications for Treatment of Ovarian Disorders	
DRUG	**PURPOSE**	**ADMINISTRATION**
Bromocriptine (Parlodel)	Inhibits prolactin secretion by the pituitary, which interferes with the secretion of gonadotropin-releasing hormone (Gn-RH) Used in the presence of galactorrhea or elevated prolactin levels	2.5 mg, orally, twice daily (because of side effects, may start with 2.5 mg at bedtime increasing to twice daily)
Clomiphene (Clomid, Serophene)	Induce ovulation. May produce multiple gestation. Incidence of twins may be slightly higher (Wolf, 2000).	50 mg, orally, starting day 5 of the cycle for 5 days. If no ovulation, increase dosage by 50 mg/mo up to 200–250 mg. If no pregnancy by 3–4 mos, reevaluate.
Gn-RH Leuprolide (Lupron)	Reduces endometriosis of fibroids and suppresses LH surge	May be given intravenously, intranasally, or subcutaneously; dose will vary according to method
hCG (APL, Pregnyl, Profasi, Novarel)	Stimulates LH surge, and triggers ovulation Used in conjunction with clomiphene, hMG, and FSH.	10,000 IU given IM
Human menopausal gonadotropin or menotropins (Pergonal, Humegon, Repronex)	Stimulate follicle growth in the ovaries, often with multiple eggs. For women who fail to respond to clomiphene. Watch for hyperstimulation syndrome.	Made from equal amounts of follicle-stimulating hormone (FSH) and luteinizing hormone (LH). 75 or 150 IU injected intramuscularly daily starting day 3–5 for 7–14 d based on estrogen blood levels and ultrasound monitoring of follicles.
Progesterone (Provera)	For luteal phase defects	Given as vaginal or rectal suppository
Purified FSH (Metrodin, if available)	Induces ovulation in clomiphene-resistant women with higher levels of LH than FSH	Daily intramuscular (IM) injections starting early in the cycle

Note. The data in column 2, item 2, are from "Ovulation Induction," by L. J. Wolf, 2000, *Clinical Obstetrics and Gynecology, 43*(4), pp. 902–915.

Clomiphene (Clomid)

Pharmacologic Class	Avoid in pregnancy (Pregnancy Category X)
Therapeutic Class	Ovarian stimulant
How Supplied	50 mg tablets
Indications for Use	Ovulation induction to treat infertility resulting from ovarian failure
Chemical Effect	Stimulates the hypothalamus and pituitary to increase secretion of LH and FSH
Therapeutic Effect	Through negative feedback, the hypothalamus and pituitary are stimulated to secrete LH and FSH to promote ovulation; one of the most common methods of ovulation induction
Dosage	50 mg/day for 5 days beginning on the first day of the cycle; may be increased to 100 mg/day for 5 days
Side Effects and Adverse Reactions	Ovarian hyperstimulation is possible, resulting in multiple pregnancy. Ovarian cysts are possible as are abdominal bloating and blurred vision.
Contraindications	Pregnancy, liver disease or history of liver disease, ovarian cysts, polycystic ovarian disease
Nursing Considerations	Avoid if possibly pregnant (give after menstrual period). Note history of hepatic dysfunctions (contraindicated with liver disease).
Client Teaching	Take at same time of day. Stop if pelvic pain, abdominal distention, or blurred vision occurs or if pregnancy is suspected.
Laboratory Finding	May cause dizziness or lightheadedness.

technology (ART) involves the use of in vitro fertilization (IVF), gamete intrafallopian transfer (GIFT), and embryo transfer (ET). Typically, ovulation is induced with the use of fertility drugs to produce several mature follicles from which eggs can be retrieved. In IVF and ET, the eggs are aspirated from the ovarian follicles and fertilized outside the woman's body. IVF is most appropriate when the tubes are absent or blocked. In this process the eggs are fertilized and, after 48 hours, the embryo is inserted into the uterus for implantation. In GIFT and ET, at least one tube must be open. In ET, the eggs are fertilized outside the body but placed in the tube and enter the uterus for implantation. In GIFT, the retrieved egg and prepared sperm are drawn into a catheter separately and injected into the tube so that fertilization can take place in the tube. These methods have been in use for almost 20 years and have been successful in many cases.

New technology has provided the means for retrieving sperm from the testes when ejaculation is not possible, injecting sperm into the ova (intracytoplasmic sperm injection, or ICSI), cryopreservation of embryos for future pregnancies, and surrogate pregnancies. Future advances may include cloning, chromosome manipulation, the transfer of cell components from one cell to another, and biochemically assisted hatching of the egg to improve the chances of fertilization (American Society for Reproductive Medicine, 1998).

As technology has expanded, ethical and legal issues have emerged. The ethical issues that have arisen include the use of technology for sex selection, pregnancies in much older women, and the use of donor eggs and embryos.

Legal issues defining parenthood, the use of embryos and sperm after death or divorce of the spouse, and the disposal of embryos cause concern. Nurses need to be aware of these issues and help clients address them as possible outcomes.

The use of technology is not without cost. ART can be very expensive, and pregnancy is not guaranteed (Angard, 1999). Many couples have undergone numerous cycles without success. Insurance companies have varying policies as to what will be covered, and often very little is included in the policy. Clearly, the financial and emotional impact can be immense, and nurses may be in the position to help couples deal with giving up the hope of having a biologic child. Support groups such as Resolve are also helpful for couples dealing with infertility.

Nursing Implications

All nurses should be familiar with the terminology and substance of information concerning sexuality, reproductive function, sexual dysfunction, fertility, and infertility. This information is essential in dealing with clients in any clinical setting. The nurse is viewed by the public as someone who has this knowledge and is very capable of taking very technical material and relaying it in terms that almost anyone can understand. Every nurse should be equipped with information to take an accurate and adequate sexual and reproductive medical history. Every nurse should be aware of the PLISSIT model and be familiar with its use in screening for sexual dysfunction, and be able to identify resources that couples could refer to if they are having problems with sexuality or fertility.

Some nurses choose to work in the field of sexual counseling or infertility. These nurses need more extensive education and training to develop expertise. Sometimes these nurses participate in teams who undertake the infertility workup or in surgery where the ART is pursued.

FAMILY PLANNING

Family planning involves cognitive decisions and behavioral practices that enable a woman to conceive a wanted pregnancy and avoid an unwanted or a badly timed pregnancy. Family planning decisions are complex and may be made by the woman, her partner, or the couple together. These decisions are made in a number of ways.

Each year in the United States, 49% of pregnancies are unintended (Dailard, 2000). The unintended pregnancy rate is approximately 3.5 million pregnancies per year in the United States (La Valleur, 2000). A pregnancy may occur at a time in a woman's life that she recognizes is inappropriate for having a child. Many of these unplanned and badly timed pregnancies involve women under the age of 20 years. This section prepares the nurse to assist women of childbearing age in many different settings to adapt and identify their health care needs regarding how many children they will have and the timing of having children.

Reproductive decision-making is discussed as are currently available methods of contraception and nursing care to meet the health care needs of women of childbearing age. For the nurse, an understanding of reproductive decision-making is important because many times women do not recognize or have knowledge of choices they have. Understanding there is a choice is necessary before the woman can determine if she wants a method of contraception and which method is best for her.

Reproductive Decision-Making

In nearly every situation in life, one has choices about the actions one takes. Many of the choices have such obvious negative consequences that they are quickly eliminated and thus it may appear as if there are no choices. For example, every student has a choice to refuse to turn in required course work, take examinations, or attend classes. Most students do not consider these options viable choices because the consequences generally are undesirable.

In reproductive decision-making, **contraception**, or prevention of pregnancy, often is the topic for which couples will seek information. Interestingly, despite the fact that choosing a contraception method often is a decision made jointly by couples, little is known about how men and women differ in this regard. Grady, Klepinger, and Nelson-Wally (1999) found that women ranked pregnancy prevention as the most important factor and ranked the health risks associated with the method and protection

from sexually transmitted diseases (STDs) second. By contrast, men considered protection from STDs as the most important factor. It is likely that women make most decisions regarding reproduction because the direct consequences of pregnancy have the greatest impact on women.

Ideally, reproductive decision-making is a rational process based on the premise that human beings are agents with free will. Nurses need to honor the choices of their clients and become aware of their personal values. This awareness is helpful so that the nurse does not impose personal values on clients. Rational decision-making is a logical process based on accurate information. A rational approach allows for an active rather than a passive approach to decision-making. An active approach involves projective planning in which individuals assess the situation; consider available options; and examine the risks, benefits, and consequences of various options (Figure 7-6). Box 7-3 identifies the steps in this process.

Factors Affecting Reproductive Choices

Although the rational process appears straightforward, in reality, decision-making is complex. In a study of 800 women, 75% changed contraceptive methods at least once and reported 1,889 method choices and gave 1,036 reasons for changing (Matteson & Hawkins, 1997). In another study that examined prenatal contraceptive decision-making with postpartum behavior, only 54% of women planning to use oral contraceptives actually used them and 31% of women planning to use condoms used them (Miller, Laken, Ager, & Essenmacher, 2000). Psychological factors, sociocultural factors, and spiritual and religious beliefs and values influence choices. Many women find themselves with unintended pregnancies because they were passive and made no decision. Reproductive decision-making can be life altering and is an area in

---

Box 7-3

Steps in Rational Decision-Making

- Recognize that there is a decision to be made and identify the problem.
- Seek information about options for problem resolution.
- Evaluate the options based on risks, benefits, and feasibility.
- Select the most acceptable option.
- Develop a realistic plan to implement the option.
- Implement the option.
- Evaluate the plan and make revisions or adaptations to resolve obstacles.

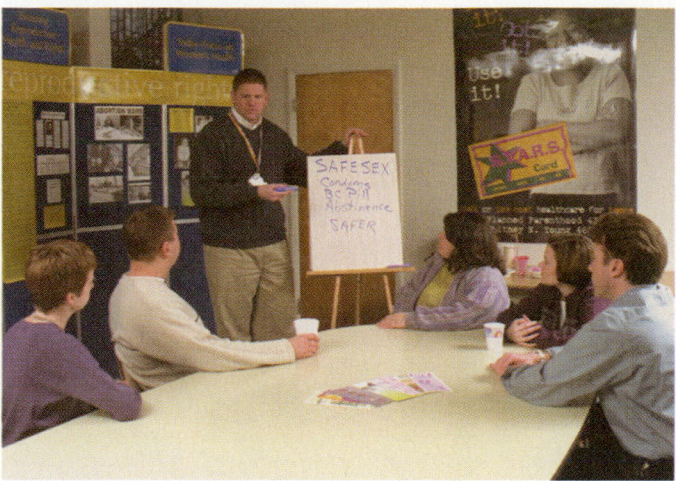

Figure 7-6   Rational decision-making in family planning is based on having accurate information about various options and their associated risks and benefits.

which nurses often are engaged with clients in helping to make these decisions.

Psychological Influences

Reproductive decisions often are influenced by feelings about one's self. For example, a young man may feel his self-concept is enhanced by performance in sexual activity. A young woman may feel that achieving pregnancy enhances her self-esteem. Sometimes women may agree to sexual activity to satisfy a sense of belonging, to feel needed, or to feel important. The accompanying emotional issues involving sexuality and relationships may cloud a logical process.

In their study of female psychology, Gilligan, Ward, and Taylor (1988) found that females make decisions based on relationships rather than by using an objective, purely rational process. The importance of the role of attachment and connection in a young woman's decision-making is reiterated over multiple studies, which may help to understand the gender differences in reproductive decision-making. Ironically, the use of contraception is lower in couples who have just met than in couples with an established relationship. In a study of sexually active females under 18 years of age, 52% who had just met their sexual partner used no method compared with 24% who were going steady (Manning, Longmore, & Giordano, 2000). Adolescent females who first had sex with a man 6 or more years older than they had an even greater decreased rate of practicing contraception.

Pender's (1996) Health Promotion model specifies personal and experiential factors as strong predictors for health-promoting behaviors. Pender also identifies a client's perceptions about the benefits and barriers to a health-related behavior as core areas of intervention. A sense of *self-efficacy*, or judgment about personal capability to execute actions, is another psychological aspect of health behaviors.

Sociocultural Influences

The immediate social situation or social group greatly influences reproductive decision-making. Decisions often reflect the patterns of one's immediate social group. Pender (1996) identified family, peers, providers, norms, support and models, and the situational influences as important contributors to client behavior. Cultural values regarding sexuality and gender roles, the power dimensions of adolescent's lives, and economic disadvantage exert powerful influences on decision-making (Gage, 1998). Adolescents, in particular, are influenced by peer pressure and may subject themselves to unprotected intercourse through the belief that everyone does it. The peer group also may influence the adolescent female if the group regards the use of contraception as a label of sexual activity, thus dissuading the use of planned contraception. With these pressures, she may not consider the consequences, weigh the options, or consider her own needs and aspirations. Oddens (1997) found that contraceptive use was principally determined by social influences, attitudes, and self-efficacy.

Social circumstances are significant in making decisions regarding reproductive actions. For example, a woman with little money may not be able to afford to purchase contraceptives. A homeless woman may not use contraceptives because it is inconvenient and she has nowhere to keep them to have available when needed. A woman also may agree to sexual intercourse through the influence of romantic surroundings and a persuasive partner.

Cultural beliefs, values, and customs structure gender roles and reproductive behavior. It is important for nurses to understand the client's cultural beliefs about the acceptable age of childbearing, marriage requirements, how the father is chosen, spacing of pregnancies, and health behaviors during pregnancy. The general culture influences behavior through movies, music, and other media. Exposure of young children to explicit sexual activity has resulted in increasingly younger children acting and dressing as adults. Some have speculated that this exposure contributes to early sexual activity in adolescents.

Spiritual and Religious Influences

Spiritual and religious beliefs impact reproductive decision-making. Many belief systems condone sexual activity only within marriage, and some view sexual activity only for the express purpose of procreation. In other systems, sexual intimacy between a couple may be viewed as being sacred. The Roman Catholic Church, for example, does not condone the use of most contraceptives or abortion. The only acceptable method is natural family planning. For Muslims, and southern Baptists, although contraception is acceptable, there may be religious objections to abortion.

Readiness for Decision-Making

Honoring the client's need to make the best decision for herself, while providing the best information and facilitating the rational decision-making process, is best achieved through a process of shared decision-making (Figure 7-7). This process is increasingly advocated as the ideal model for the medical encounter and has the following characteristics: client and provider are (1) both involved, (2) share information, (3) build consensus regarding the plan, and (4) reach an agreement on implementation (Charles, Gafini, & Whelan, 1997).

Freedom to Make Choices

Rational decision-making is based on the premise that clients are agents with free will to make choices; however, in reality, not all clients are free to make choices. Women who are victims of rape or sexual violence have had their freedom compromised. In some states, minors are not free to obtain contraceptive methods or abortion without parental consent. In other states, minors seeking medical care, including contraceptive information, methods, and, in some cases, abortions, are considered emancipated minors. Thus, health care providers can legally provide services without parental notification, approval, or consent. Nurses need to be aware of institutional policies and state practice regulations.

Many health care providers assume that the woman is free to make reproductive decisions independently; however, in many cultures this is not the case. The decisions regarding children and contraception reside with the husband, are shared between husband and wife, or involve the entire extended family.

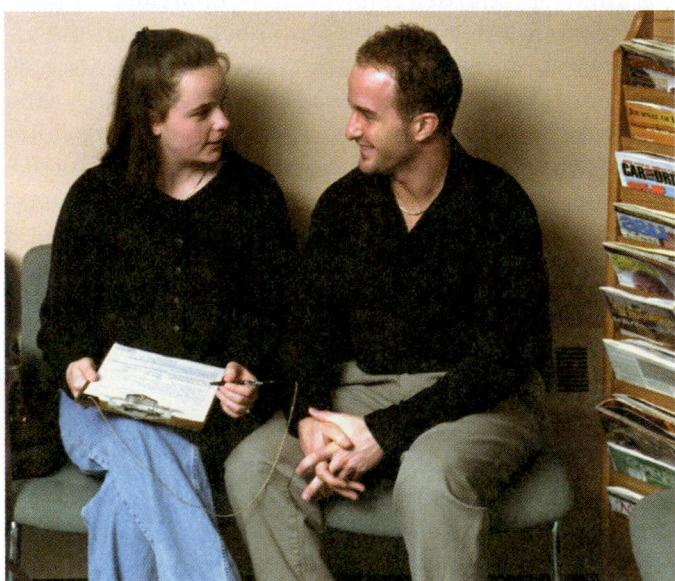

Figure 7-7   Rational decision-making is based on the premise that clients are agents with free will to make choices.

Nursing Tip

Clinical Assessment of Reproductive Decision-Making

- Is the client free to make a choice?
- Is the client competent to make a choice?
- Does the client recognize situations in which she has a choice?
- Does the client have adequate knowledge to make an informed choice?
- Can the client reasonably implement the choice? What are the barriers or obstacles to using this contraceptive method?

Competence to Make Choices

Cognitive skills of abstract thinking are necessary to contemplate the risks, benefits, and consequences of various options. Persons without these skills need special consideration, and the health care provider may need to take more responsibility in the decision-making process to find a responsible party to make decisions. Young adolescents may not have developed abstract thinking and the ability to project into the future to process the potential consequences of sexual intimacy. In these cases, nursing interventions may need to facilitate the development of these skills and the processing of projecting the consequences of choices.

Recognition of Decision Points

Decisions are more likely to be reactive or passive and, therefore, not reasoned when the client is unaware that she is at a decision point or that options are possible. One nursing intervention may be simply to make the client aware that she has an opportunity for choices. For example, an adolescent female may not recognize that she can refuse to have intercourse unless her boyfriend uses a condom. Closely related to the recognition of choice is being aware of options. For example, a woman cannot make a decision to use an emergency method of contraception after intercourse if she is unaware of that option.

Three decision points are relevant to contraceptive use: (1) sexual activity, (2) preventive contraception, and (3) emergency contraception. Differentiating these decision points may be useful in recognizing opportunities for choices.

Sexual Activity.   Some women make generalized decisions about sexual activity. For example, a woman may decide to be abstinent until after marriage, or after finishing school, or until she gets a job. Another may feel that if she has a sexual encounter with a particular individual, then she has made a decision related to that relationship and no longer has choices as to whether she will have sexual relations with that person in the future.

Choices about sexual activity often are not made proactively. Many women think that proactive decisions inhibit spontaneity. Women should recognize that they have choices regarding if, with whom, when, and where intercourse should occur. Each opportunity for intercourse is a decision point.

Preventive Contraception. Most contraceptive decisions are made to avoid or postpone pregnancy. In contrast, making a decision to have a baby is the most proactive approach. Some women do not use contraceptives because they feel they are not vulnerable to pregnancy because they are too old or too young, or it is not the fertile period in their menstrual cycle. Many women fail to use contraception when they have sporadic sexual encounters or are not in a stable relationship. This is not a good rational decision because pregnancy can result from one sexual encounter and the chances for partner support are decreased.

Emergency Contraception. Postcoital contraception, also known as **emergency contraception**, is now more readily available and includes pregnancy termination, morning-after contraception, and RU 486. Many women, however, are not aware of these options. Because a postcoital method may be inconsistent with some belief systems, preventive contraception may be more appropriate.

Knowledge Level

Informed reproductive decision-making involves more than awareness of options; it requires accurate information regarding the risks, benefits, and consequences of each option. Informed reproductive decision-making includes weighing the risks, benefits, and consequences of not using contraception. This process allows the client to make a choice regarding the risk-benefit ratio with which she is comfortable. Knowledge of how to effectively use the contraceptive method also is important and needs to be considered (Figure 7-8). A survey by Fuchs, Prinz, and Koch (1996) found that most women are poorly informed about oral contraceptive use and are largely unaware of the important long-term noncontraceptive benefits.

Implementation of the Choice

The nurse also must be aware of contraindications and obstacles to use. In this process of information sharing, the nurse might share her knowledge of medical contraindications. For example, a woman with a history of thromboembolism should not take certain oral contraceptives. The client also might share her knowledge of potential obstacles to use. For example, an adolescent may be uncomfortable touching herself and thus would be a poor candidate for the female condom or many of the barrier methods.

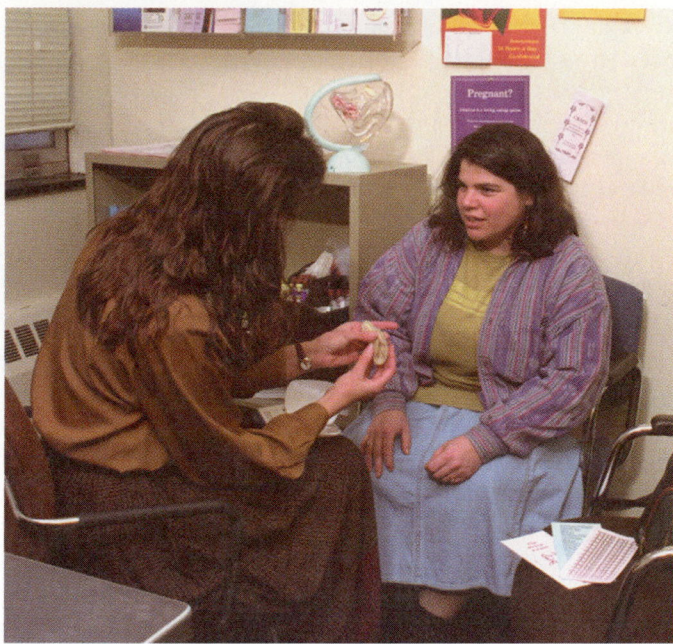

Figure 7-8 Clients must understand and return-demonstrate proper use of contraceptive devices to ensure their effectiveness.

Possible barriers and obstacles should be explored: Which actions on the part of the client are necessary to effectively use the chosen method? An adolescent without transportation may not be able to come to the clinic to get an injection every 3 months. When a teenager is living at home and believes her parents will not approve of contraception, a method that provides evidence for her parents to detect is not a good choice. A woman may choose condoms as her preferred method; however, if her partner refuses to use them, she needs to have an alternative plan. A woman may choose oral contraceptives but, in reality, cannot remember to take them regularly.

By assessing the decision-making process and the client's knowledge, the nurse can be more effective in facilitating satisfactory use of contraceptives. This interactive approach involving the client and family members as appropriate may promote greater effectiveness of contraceptive strategies.

Contraceptive Methods

Contraceptive methods currently available are either reversible or permanent (Figure 7-9). Reversible methods vary in the time required for reproductive capacity to return on discontinuance, and they vary in the frequency of administration necessary to prevent unwanted pregnancy. Permanent methods vary in regard to when the method becomes permanent. For example, oral contraceptives must be taken daily, whereas injectible methods may require administration every 3 months. An excellent

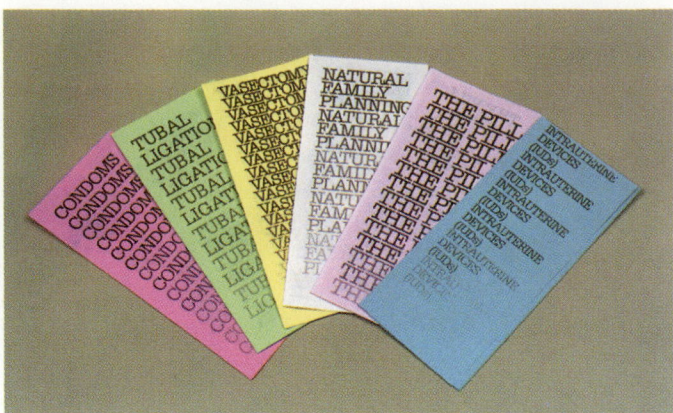

Figure 7-9 In addition to face-to-face teaching, clients should be offered printed information on family planning choices.

example with regard to permanent methods is that the vasectomy is not considered permanent until follow-up sperm counts show that the count has approached or reached zero.

Reversible Methods

The numbers and kinds of reversible contraceptive methods is ever expanding. Each year several new products are marketed that are designed to refine those products already available or meet the needs of women who experience side effects.

Oral Methods

Oral methods of contraception include combined oral contraceptives and progestin-only contraceptives.

Combined Oral Contraceptives. Combined oral contraceptives have been available to women since the 1960s. The Food and Drug Administration approved this type of contraception in 1960 (Speroff & Darney, 2001). Approximately 60 million women worldwide have used combined oral contraceptives as a method of choice (Speroff & Darney, 2001).

There are three basic types of combined oral contraceptives (COC): monophasic, biphasic, and multiphasic pills. Monophasic COCs contain estrogen and progestin in the same dosage for 21 days of the menstrual cycle. If 28 pills are in the package, the remaining 7 pills may be inert or iron pills. Biphasic pills may have a stable dose of estrogen throughout the cycle and an increase in progesterone in the second half of the cycle, or the dosage of both hormones may change in the second half of the cycle. This type of COC was designed to alleviate problems some women have with breakthrough bleeding. Multiphasic COCs have three different dosages of estrogen and progesterone during the monthly cycle. This type of COC also was designed to alleviate the side effects and break-

through bleeding some women experience with monophasic or biphasic COCs.

Pharmacology

Combined oral contraceptives are composed of steroids of the hormones estrogen and progesterone. Two types of estrogens have been used in the formulation of COCs. Mestranol was used in the pills having a higher dose when COCs initially were developed. It was determined, however, that mestranol was broken down to ethinyl estradiol before its use. In contemporary COCs, ethinyl estradiol is the only estrogen available in these preparations.

The net effect is that estrogen prevents breakthrough bleeding by potentiating the action of progestin and enabling lower doses of progestin to be used for the same effect.

By contrast, progestin diminishes the release of leuteinizing hormone (LH) by the anterior pituitary gland. LH ordinarily is released in pulses, with a sharp increase in pulsatile action immediately before ovulation. In fact, a surge of LH is responsible for release of the mature ovum at the time of ovulation. Progestins make cervical mucus less receptive, making it impervious to sperm passage. Progestins make the endometrium less receptive to implantation. Progestins also influence secretions and peristalsis of the fallopian tubes, impeding mobility of the sperm and ovum.

Types of Combined Oral Contraceptives

Numerous preparations of COCs are sold by various pharmaceutical companies (Figure 7-10). Each year there are additional kinds of preparations added to the list. The wide variety of preparations meets individual needs and reduces undesired side effects or management problems. Table 7-4 contains some of the currently available preparations.

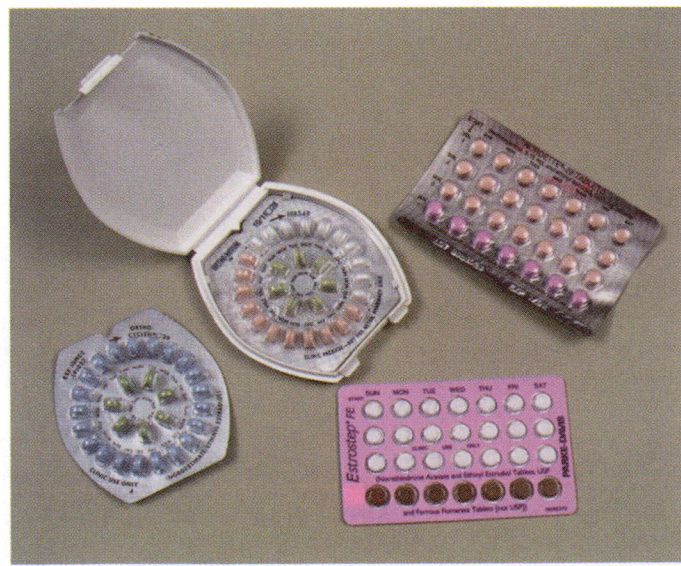

Figure 7-10 Birth control pills.

Table 7-4 Currently Available Combined Oral Contraceptives

MONOPHASIC PREPARATIONS		BIPHASIC PREPARATIONS	MULTIPHASIC PREPARATIONS
Alesse	Norethin 1/35E	Gracial	Estrostep
Brevicon	Norethin 1/50M	Jenest	Jenest
Demulen	Norinyl 1 + 35	Mircette	Ortho-Novum 7/7/7
Demulen 1/35	Norinyl 1 + 50	Ortho-Novum 10/11	Ortho Tri-Cyclen
Desogen	Norlestrin 1/50		Tri-Cyclen
Genora 1/35	Ortho-Cept		Tri-Levlen
Genora 1/50	Ortho-Cyclen		Tri-Norinyl
Levlen	Ortho-Novum 1/35		Triphasil
Loestrin Fe 1.5/30	Ortho-Novum 1/50		
Loestrin Fe 1/20	Ovcon-35		
Lo/Ovral	Ovcon-50		
Modicon	Ovral		
Nelova 1/35E			
Nelova 0.5/35			
Nordette			

Efficacy

The combined oral contraceptive is the most effective reversible method available to women today. When used correctly, the failure rate is less than 1% (Jensen & Speroff, 2000).

Benefits and Risks

Combined oral contraceptives offer contraceptive benefits and noncontraceptive benefits. Both kinds of benefit make it to a woman's advantage to choose oral contraception. COCs are relatively inexpensive, safe, effective, and easy to use. Return to fertility usually occurs within three months on discontinuance of this method.

Contraceptive Benefits

Over the past 30 years, no drug has been as well studied as has the COC. Most women who use COCs do so for contraception. COCs are highly reliable. When used appropriately, COCs are more than 99% effective (Jensen & Speroff, 2000). Successful use of COCs is highly related to the woman's understanding about how the preparation works and compliance with certain practices. These practices are summarized in the Client Education box.

Noncontraceptive Benefits

Combined oral contraceptives offer several important noncontraceptive benefits that reduce morbidity and mortality in women. The number of these recognized benefits has increased with data gathered from many women who have used COCs over many years (Burkman, 2001).

■ *Protection against Ovarian Cancer* Ovarian cancer is the fourth leading cause of cancer death in American women and has the highest mortality rate of any gynecologic cancer. Its onset is insidious. By the time of detection, ovarian cancer has metastasized in 60% of cases. There is a survival rate of 40% at 5 years for women treated for ovarian cancer.

When a woman has ever used them, COCs offer a 40% to 80% reduction in the risk for ovarian cancer (Burkman, 2001). The degree of protection increases with the length of use. A minimally protective effect is present with 3 to 6 months of use. The protective effects of COCs last at least 15 years after discontinuance. This reduction in risk is present in all four subtypes of ovarian cancer.

■ *Protection against Endometrial Cancer* The incidence of endometrial cancer is reduced by the use of COCs. Overall, studies suggest that there is a reduction in risk of 50% beginning approximately 1 year after initiation of use (Burkman, 2001). The reduction is apparent in all histologic subtypes of endometrial cancer. Protection lasts up to 15 years after discontinuance of the medication.

Nursing Tip *Understanding COCs*

Clients who are considering the use of combined oral contraceptives should have the benefit of information about mechanism of actions, benefits, risks, adverse effects, and contraindications to assist them in making their decision.

■ *Reduction in Incidence of Salpingitis* Salpingitis has been reduced with the use of COCs. The mechanism of action is thought to be a chemical reaction in the woman's body that changes the cervical mucous and impedes ascent of infectious organisms. It has been estimated that a 50% reduction in hospital admissions for salpingitis can be attributed to COCs (Burkman, 2001).

■ *Reduction in Incidence of Ectopic Pregnancy* Combined oral contraceptives have been given credit for reducing the rate of ectopic pregnancy (implantation of fertilized egg outside of the uterus) by approximately 90% (Burkman, 2001). The mechanism of action is thought to be through inhibition of ovulation. This is a secondary benefit to preventing salpingitis.

■ *Prevention and Treatment of Functional Ovarian Cysts* The relatively new low-dose COCs reduce the incidence of functional ovarian cysts by preventing ovulation. Preparations containing 50 µg of ethinyl estradiol have been associated with reducing cyst formation. If a woman

Client Education

Oral Contraceptives

Women who are going to use combined oral contraceptives (COCs) should understand several important points about their successful use.

1. COCs, especially low-dose preparations, are more likely to be effective when taken the same time every day.

2. COCs may be begun on the Sunday after the first day of the woman's menses. If she begins the pill immediately it should be effective in 7 to 10 days. If she wants to be really safe, she may want to consider using a backup method with the pill for the first month.

3. The woman should know that COCs do not offer protection against exposure to the human immunodeficiency virus (HIV). She or her partner should use a condom in combination with the pill for this type of protection.

4. The woman needs to know that there are various types and dosages of COCs, and they are not necessarily interchangeable.

5. When a woman forgets to take one pill, it should be taken when she remembers; the next pill should be taken at the regularly scheduled time.

6. When a woman misses more than one pill, there is the possibility of escape ovulation. She should use a backup method along with the pill for 7 days or refrain from intercourse for the remainder of the cycle (Hatcher et al., 1998).

7. When starting a new preparation, the woman should know it might take 3 months for hormone levels to stabilize. Breakthrough bleeding may diminish after the third cycle is completed (Lynch, 2000).

8. The woman should be aware of signs and symptoms that should warn her to discontinue the pill immediately, including the following ACHES:

   Abdominal pain (severe) or yellowing of skin

   Chest pain (severe), cough, shortness of breath

   Headaches (severe), dizziness, weakness, numbness

   Eye problems (vision loss or blurring), speech problems

   Severe leg pain (calf or thigh)

   If any of these signs or symptoms occurs, the woman should stop taking her pills immediately and contact a health care provider.

9. The woman should know about less serious conditions that may occur and do not require immediate discontinuance of the pill but do require evaluation by a health care provider. Many of these symptoms and conditions can be easily alleviated or treated so that the woman may continue to use combined oral contraceptives. The use of COCs in the presence of relative contraindications requires clinical judgment on the part of the health care provider (Speroff & Darney, 2001). Relative contraindications include migraine headaches, hypertension, uterine fibroids, gestational diabetes, elective surgery, epilepsy, sickle cell disease, diabetes, and gallbladder disease.

has recurrent functional cysts, use of COCs may eliminate recurrence (Hatcher et al., 1998).

■ *Menstrual Cycle Benefits* Women who have heavy menses and those with painful menses benefit from the use of COCs. The resulting increase in progestin is likely to decrease flow and reduce or eliminate cramping some women experience during menstruation.

■ *Reduction in Incidence of Benign Breast Disease* The reduction of benign breast disease is thought to be due to inhibition of ovulation. When a woman ovulates, certain proliferative breast changes occur. When ovulation ceases, these changes typically do not occur. The decrease in benign breast changes occurs even at the lowest dose of oral contraceptive.

■ *Reduction in Acne* Acne can vary from person to person and can be worse at certain times in the same person. Certain COCs can be very effective in reducing or eliminating the incidence of acne. In the very young woman who has acne the benefits increase if she also has menstrual cramping or functional ovarian cysts.

■ *Improvement in Bone Mineral Density* Bone mineral density peaks in women between the ages of 20 and 25 years, stays constant for approximately 10 years, and progressively decreases during the later reproductive years (Burkman, 2001). Estrogens act on bone by increasing absorption of calcium and directly decreasing reabsorption of calcium through inhibition of osteoclasts. One case control study indicates that there is a 25% reduction in hip fracture risk among women who use COCs.

■ *Reduction in Risk for Colorectal Cancer* There is growing epidemiologic evidence that oral contraceptives protect women against colorectal cancer. Although the exact mechanism of action for this protection is unknown, it has been hypothesized that reduction in bile acid concentration may explain the protective effect (Burkman, 2001). The reduction in risk may be from 40% to 50%.

■ *Reduction in Risk for Uterine Fibroids* Uterine fibroids are benign uterine tumors that increase in size and cause heavy menses. Research has shown a 70% reduction in risk for developing fibroids among women using oral contraceptives (Jensen & Speroff, 2000).

Indications

Combined oral contraceptives are used specifically for family planning but also may be used to treat certain gynecologic conditions. Young women often have problems with cycle control. These women may benefit from the use of COCs to regulate irregular cycles, reduce flow, and control dysmenorrhea. Women with polycystic ovarian syndrome may benefit from COCs because they reduce circulating androgens. Premenstrual symptoms may be

improved with the use of COCs. Older women often experience anovulatory cycles with heavy bleeding owing to unopposed estrogen and also can benefit from COCs. This type of bleeding often is associated with perimenopause. COCs also can help alleviate other perimenopausal symptoms as well in women who do not have contraindications up to age 50 (Long, 1998).

Contraindications

Absolute and relative contraindications have been described related to oral contraceptives. If the woman has an absolute contraindication to the pill, she should not be given oral contraceptives under any circumstances. If she has a relative contraindication to the pill, she may take the pill under certain circumstances with direct supervision of her physician. Box 7-4 describes the absolute contraindications to oral contraception, and Box 7-5 describes the relative contraindications.

Box 7-4

Absolute Contraindications to the Use of Combined Oral Contraceptives

- Presence or a history of deep venous thrombosis or pulmonary embolism
- Cerebrovascular accident or a history
- Coronary artery or ischemic heart disease, or a history of either
- Structural heart disease complicated by pulmonary hypertension, atrial fibrillation, or subacute bacterial endocarditis, or a history of any of these conditions
- Diabetes with nephropathy, retinopathy, or neuropathy, or other vascular disease
- Diabetes of over 20 years duration
- Breast cancer
- Pregnancy
- Lactation
- Liver problems
- Headaches
- Major surgery
- Cigarette smoker over the age of 35 years
- Blood pressure levels over 160/100

Note. Data adapted from *Contraceptive Technology* (17th ed.), by R. A. Hatcher, J. Trussell, F. Stewart, W. Cates, G. Stewart, F. Guest, et al., 1998, New York: Arden Media.

Box 7-5

Relative Contraindications to the Use of Combined Oral Contraceptives

- Absence of menses
- Spotting or breakthrough bleeding
- Right upper quadrant pain
- Midepigastric pain
- Migraine headaches
- Severe, nonvascular headaches
- Galactorrhea
- Jaundice and pruritis
- Depression

Note. Data adapted from *Contraceptive Technology* (17th ed.), by R. A. Hatcher, J. Trussell, F. Stewart, W. Cates, G. Stewart, F. Guest, et al., 1998, New York: Arden Media.

Nursing Alert

COC Contraindications

Be sure to tell your clients that certain drugs interact with COCs to reduce their efficacy, including:

- carbamazepine (Tegretol)
- griseofulvin (Fulvicin)
- phenobarbital
- phenytoin (Dilantin)
- rifabutin (Mycobutin)
- rifampin (Rifadin)
- topiramate (Topamax)

Note. Data adapted from *Contraceptive Technology* (17th ed.), by R. A. Hatcher, J. Trussell, F. Stewart, W. Cates, G. Stewart, F. Guest, et al., 1998, New York: Arden Media.

Side Effects

Most women experience relatively few side effects of the pill. Many times, side effects may be eliminated by changing pill formulation or dosage. Some side effects that have been reported are weight gain, breast tenderness, breakthrough bleeding, depression, decreased libido, and nausea. Table 7-5 describes the side effects and their relationship to hormones in the pills.

Another common concern is the effect of COCs on the lipid profile (Long, 1998). The concern was that the pill had adverse effects on the lipid profile by causing elevated triglycerides, which have been associated with cardiovascular disease and stroke. It appears that low-dose pills and the new progestins have moderated this risk for users.

Progestin-Only Contraceptives. A progestin-only contraceptive also is referred to as a minipill. This type of preparation is especially attractive for women who want oral contraception and cannot take COCs. This would include women who cannot take or do not tolerate estrogen, lactating women, and women with chronic medical conditions.

Three brands of progestin-only pills currently are available in the United States. The trade names are Nor-Q.D., Micronor, and Ovrette. Nor-Q.D. and Micronor contain norethindrone, 0.35 mg; Ovrette contains norgestrel, 0.075 mg.

Pharmacology

Unlike the COC, the minipill does not act by preventing ovulation. Instead, its mechanism of action is that the progestin acts to make the endometrium hostile to implantation and the cervical mucus becomes thick and impermeable (Speroff & Darney, 2001). Approximately 40% of women will ovulate while taking the minipill.

Efficacy

The minipill is considered to be more than 99% effective when used properly. It must be taken at the same time each day because there is a higher potential for ovulation and pregnancy than with the COC when a dose is late or missed. There is no significant metabolic effect, and fertility returns to normal almost immediately after discontinuance (Speroff & Darney, 2001).

Benefits and Risks

Minipills are of benefit to women who are unable to take COCs. In lactating women and women over the age of 40 years, the protection approaches 100% with proper use (Speroff & Darney, 2001). This high rate of efficacy in these groups may be due to the decreased fertility in this client population. The World Health Organization states that progestin-only pills have no adverse effects on lactation and can be started as early as 6 weeks postpartum (Adams, 2000). The minipill also is useful for women who

Table 7-5 Side Effects of Combined Oral Contraceptive Related to Hormones and Dosage

General Side Effects

Estrogen Excess	*Estrogen Deficiency*	*Progestin Excess*	*Androgen Excess*
Chloasma	Nervousness	Appetite increase	Acne
Chronic nasopharyngitis	Vasomotor symptoms	Depression	Cholestatic jaundice
Gastric influenza		Fatigue	Hirsutism
Hay fever and allergic rhinitis		Hypoglycemia	Increased libido
Urinary tract infection		Decreased libido	Oily skin and scalp
		Neurodermatitis	Rash and pruritis
		Weight gain	Edema

Reproductive Side Effects

Estrogen Excess	*Estrogen Deficiency*	*Progestin Excess*	*Progestin Deficiency*
Breast changes	Absence of withdrawal bleeding	Cervicitis	Breakthrough bleeding
Cervical extrophy	Continuous bleeding	Decreased flow	Delayed withdrawal bleeding
Dysmenorrhea	Hypomenorrhea	Moniliasis	Dysmenorrhea
Hypermenorrhea	Pelvic relaxation		Heavy flow with clots
Menorrhagia	Atropic vaginitis		
Clotting with menses			
Increased breast size			
Mucorrhea (mucus discharge)			
Uterine enlargement			
Uterine fibroid growth			

Cardiovascular Side Effects

Estrogen Excess	*Progestin Excess*
Capillary fragility	Hypertension
Cerebrovascular accident	Leg vein dilation
Deep vein thrombosis	
Telangiectasis	
Thromboembolic disease	

Premenstrual Side Effects

Estrogen Excess or Progestin Deficiency
Bloating
Dizziness
Edema
Headache
Irritability
Leg cramps
Nausea and vomiting
Visual changes
Weight gain

Note. Data adapted from *Managing Contraceptive Pill Patients*, by R. P. Dickey, 2001, Durant, OK: Essential Medical Information Systems.

experience decreased libido with COCs. The minipill offers many of the same noncontraceptive benefits as do COCs; however, these benefits may be at a reduced level. Because it is thought that the minipill produces no metabolic effect, it should be safe for use in women who have diabetes and those over the age of 35 years. Return to fertility is almost immediate on discontinuance.

In the first year of use, there typically is a 5% failure rate among the general population. This rate is slightly higher than that of COCs but better than use of no contraceptive, which has a pregnancy rate of 80% within 1 year of unprotected intercourse.

Women who use the minipill will develop more functional ovarian cysts, which usually will resolve without treatment. The major problem with use of the minipill is that of breakthrough bleeding.

Indications

As is the combined oral contraceptive, the minipill is designed to be used as a contraceptive. It also may be used to decrease bleeding related to unopposed estrogen. Some minipills can be used for emergency contraception, which is discussed later in this chapter.

Contraindications

Minipills should not be used in the presence of pregnancy. Progestin is considered a teratogen to the unborn fetus. The minipill also is contraindicated in women who have breast cancer, women taking certain medications, and women who have liver disease.

Side Effects

The major side effect of the minipill is irregular bleeding. Women who use this method may not have regular menses for the duration of its use. They may have irregular periods of spotting. Because the bleeding is light, however, this side effect is not bothersome for some women.

Dermatologic Methods

The United States Food and Drug Administration has approved the first contraceptive patch (Figure 7-11). It is a prescription device available for the first time in 2002. Marketed by the Ortho McNeil Pharmaceutical Company, it is a patch replaced weekly for 3 weeks each month. The fourth week, no patch is worn. This device is thought to be 99% effective when used correctly; evidence indicates that a higher dose may be necessary for women weighing over 250 pounds. Hormones contained in the patch are similar to those found in combined oral contraceptive, and, therefore, some women should not use the patch. Further information can be obtained from the Ortho Evra Web site (http://www.orthoevra.com).

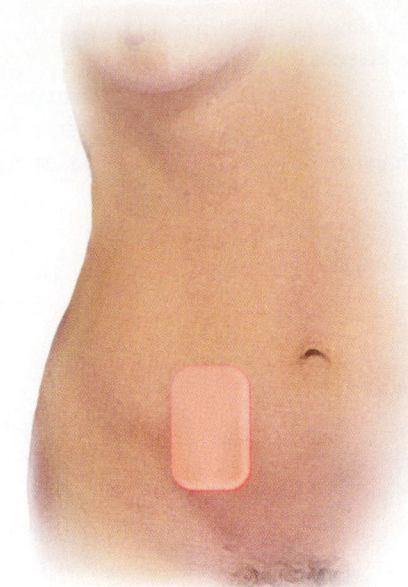

Figure 7-11 The contraceptive patch is a newly released method of contraception.

Intrauterine Methods

The intrauterine device has been available in the United States for more than 70 years, although it has only been accepted widely as a contraceptive device for the past 40 years (Figure 7-12). Present perceptions of this method are strongly influenced by some problems that arose with one particular IUD in the 1970s. That IUD was called the Dalkon Shield. Some women using Dalkon Shields developed pelvic inflammatory disease (PID). At the time, there was much discussion about safety, resulting in all but one type of IUD being removed from the market. Today, there is some discussion that the major contributing factors to removal from the market were ignorance of the facts, fear of medical liability, inadequate medical training in insertion, and confusion about the mechanism of action. As a result, physicians stopped recommending this method (Department of Health and Human Services [DHHS] & the National Institute of Child Health and Human Development [NICHHD], 1996). The IUD has been re-released for use but is not as widely used as it was before removal from the market.

Two types of IUD are currently available in the United States: the copper device Paragard T 380A and devices that utilize the hormone progesterone, such as Progestasert and Mirena. Mirena is the newest device in which the hormone levonorgestyl is utilized.

Composition. The Paragard has a 380 mm^2 exposed surface of copper on its arms and stem. The Progestasert con-

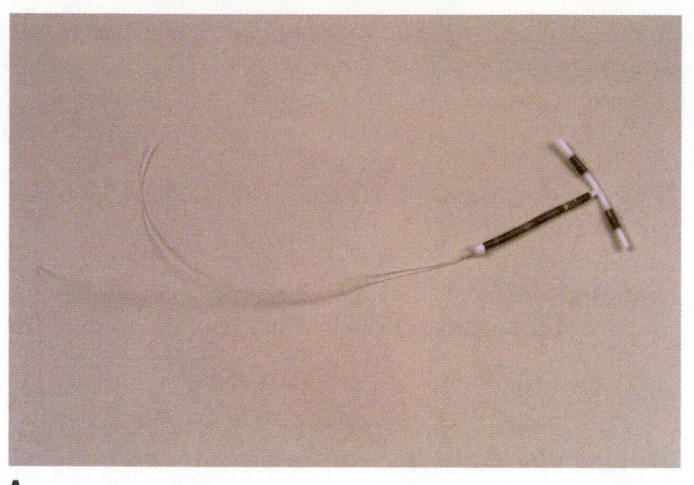

A.

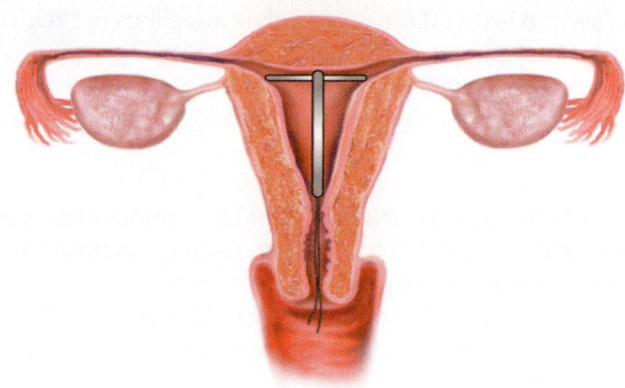

B.

Figure 7-12   A. Intrauterine device (IUD). B. Proper insertion of an IUD.

tains a reservoir of 38 mg of progesterone that is released at a rate of 65 µg/d (Nelson, 2000). Some other types of IUD from previous years with an unlimited life span may remain in use even though they are not available on the market today.

Mechanism of Action.   It is thought that the IUD works by interfering with sperm transport from the cervix to the fallopian tubes. This interference makes viable sperm scarce in the fallopian tube. It is also thought that the IUD inhibits sperm capacitation and survival. **Sperm capacitation** is the process by which the sperm becomes hypermobile and there is a breakdown of the plasma membrane and merging with the acrosomal membrane, which allows the sperm to bind with the zona pellucida of the ovum (Speroff et al., 1999). It is thought to inhibit implantation. It also is thought that the IUD alters the biochemical or cellular composition of uterine fluid, or both, causing impairment of the viability of gametes (DHHS & NICHHD, 1996).

The copper IUD is a functional spermicide. The copper ions released from the device interfere with sperm motility and create a reaction to the foreign body that results in a spermicidal endometrium (Nelson, 2000). Progestasert is believed to act through thickening the cervical mucus and rendering it impermeable to sperm.

Efficacy.   The copper IUD has a first-year failure rate of 0.7% with typical use. The copper T has a 10-year failure rate of 2.1% to 2.7% (Nelson, 2000). Progestasert has a first year failure rate of 2% with typical use. The median time from removal of the IUD to planned pregnancy is 3 months (Nelson, 2000).

Benefits and Risks.   In properly selected women, the IUD can offer a method of contraception for those who cannot or do not want to take oral contraceptives. The woman should be in a mutually monogamous relationship with her partner. The IUD is ideally suited to women who have chronic medical problems that restrict their use of hormones (Kjos, 1997). Unlike pills that must be taken daily, the IUD provides prolonged protection. Paragard is approved for 10 years of use before replacement; Progestasert is approved for 1 year of use before replacement (Stewart, 1998).

The IUD requires little maintenance. The woman should check the length of the tail string in her vagina after each menses. If the string is not found, she should notify her health care provider immediately.

Insertion issues are related to IUDs. The two most serious problems are vasovagal response and uterine perforation. A vasovagal response involves rapid decrease in blood pressure on insertion of a probe or IUD into the uterus. It occurs in approximately 1% of women on manipulation of the cervix. This response usually is mild and transient; however, occasionally, the woman will require resuscitation. Therefore, resuscitation equipment should be immediately available.

Perforation of the uterus occurs in approximately 1 in 770 to 1,600 insertions (Nelson, 2000). Most perforations occur when the uterine sound is inserted to determine the depth of the intrauterine cavity. Using current techniques that do not require the use of uterine sound has reduced this risk.

Indications.   Client selection is an important consideration when using the IUD. The woman should have had a previous pregnancy, must not have a history of PID, and must be in a monogamous relationship. The woman who has never been pregnant has a smaller uterine cavity and thus is at risk for expulsion.

Mishell (1996) indicated four misconceptions that prevent more women from choosing IUDs. The first reason is the fallacy that IUDs work as an abortifacient, resulting in failure of implantation of a fertilized egg. The second is that IUDs cause pelvic infections or PID. The third fallacy is that IUDs cause ectopic pregnancies. The fourth reason is the belief that the problems encountered in the past with the Dalkon Shield are common to all IUDs.

Contraindications. Nelson (2000) enumerates contraindications for IUD insertion. General contraindications include pregnancy, acute cervicitis, a distorted uterine cavity, uterine or cervical carcinoma, unexplained vaginal bleeding, severe immunocompromise, and multiple sexual partners.

Specific contraindications for IUD insertion include issues specific to copper or progesterone (Nelson, 2000). Contraindications to copper devices include uterine cavity size of less than 6 or greater than 9 cm, copper allergy, Wilson's disease, severe anemia, heavy menses, and severe dysmenorrhea. Contraindications for the progesterone device are uterine cavity size of less than 6 or greater than 9 cm, a history of ectopic pregnancy, and diabetes.

Side Effects. Bleeding and cramping are the two most common side effects encountered after insertion of the IUD. These symptoms usually are minimal and temporary; however, occasionally, they occur to the extreme, necessitating removal of the device.

Other adverse effects include infection, accidental pregnancy, and expulsion of the device (Nelson, 1995). Infection is related to insertion and STD. These side effects make client selection a very important factor.

Intravaginal Methods

The **vaginal ring** (which delivers steroids through the vaginal mucosa) is a contraceptive device that had its beginnings in the 1970s (Ballagh, 2001). It became apparent that drug absorption could occur in the vaginal mucosa. Duncan at Upjohn first patented vaginal delivery of sex steroids through a polysiloxane tube or disk in 1970. Since that time, more than a dozen patents for contraceptive rings have been filed.

Various ring designs have been used. Modifications have been made to ensure sustained, even steroid release over a period of time. The result has been a highly effective product.

Composition. Vaginal rings are available that contain progestins alone or a combination of estrogen and progestin.

Mechanism of Action. The steroids are absorbed through the upper vaginal mucosa. In the combination form of the intravaginal ring, ethinyl estradiol is released

at 20 mg/d and norethindrone at 1 mg/d. These dosages are equivalent to those in oral contraceptives. The mechanism of action is through prevention of ovulation, increased viscosity of cervical mucus, and endometrial atrophy.

Types of Intravaginal Devices. Ballagh (2001) described various types of vaginal rings. The progestin-only rings may include progesterone, etonogestrel, levonorgestrel-norgestrel, megestrol, nestorone, or norgestrienone. Combined estrogen-progestin devices can contain the previously mentioned progestins in combination with ethinyl estradiol.

Benefits and Risks. One of the benefits of the vaginal ring is that it does not require the rigor necessary to use oral contraceptives. The vaginal ring allows a sustained release of steroids over a 3-week period. The method is reversible by the woman. The only requirement for discontinuance is nonreplacement of the device at the end of the use-free week. Acceptance of the ring is high among women, except those who find placing a foreign object in their vagina unacceptable (Grow & Almed, 2000).

Indications. The vaginal ring is designed for women who do not want to use a method that must be administered daily, for example, women who travel or who do not have a permanent place to store pills. The woman who uses the vaginal ring must be comfortable inserting and removing an object from her vagina. Vaginal rings also are useful in relieving menopausal symptoms. Nuvaring is a brand of vaginal ring available in the United States.

Contraindications. Because the steroids from the ring are absorbed directly from the vaginal mucosa into the bloodstream, use of the vaginal ring is contraindicated in women who cannot use oral estrogen or progestins.

Adverse Effects. Occasionally, the vaginal ring can be expelled when straining to have a bowel movement or on tampon removal. Some women experience discomfort with intercourse when the vaginal ring is in place. Some women have an odor that they attribute to the ring. Some women also complain of vaginal discharge they attribute to the vaginal ring.

Nursing Tip　*Vaginal Ring*

The vaginal ring is designed to be left in the vagina for 3 weeks and removed for 1 week to allow menses. The ring may be removed or remain in place during intercourse.

Nursing Tip   *Condom Use*

Care must be taken to leave space at the end of the male condom when it is applied. If this space is not allowed, there is a tendency for the condom to break. The condom must be removed before the penis becomes flaccid. The condom also must be secured at the base of the penis as it is removed to avoid having the condom remain in the vagina when the penis is withdrawn.

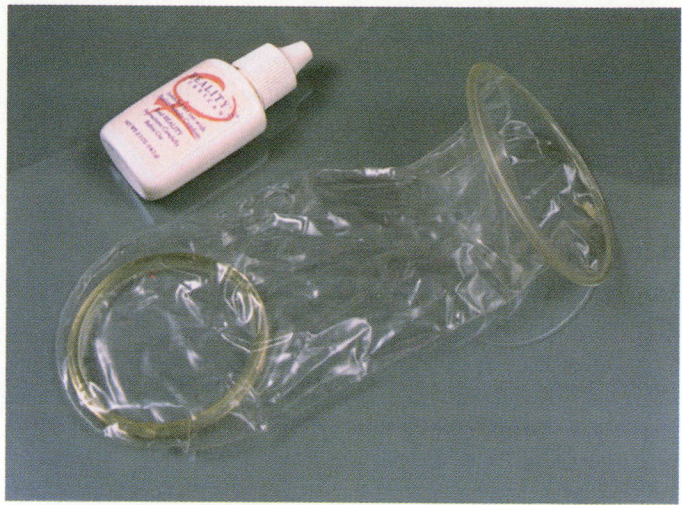

A.

Barrier Methods

Barrier methods of contraception include condoms, diaphragms, and cervical caps. Spermicide is a chemical barrier method.

Condoms.   Condoms are available for men and women. Condoms are the most frequently used barrier method of contraception. Six billion condoms were sold worldwide in 1990 (Speroff & Darney, 2001). They are sold without a prescription at most drug stores and in other public places. Condoms are available in various colors and textures and with a lubricant inside that contains a spermicide (Figure 7-13). Condoms have a typical effectiveness rate of 88% and a theoretical effectiveness rate of 98%. The difference in the two rates has to do with improper use, lack of use, and breakage.

The female condom has been available since the 1990s (Figure 7-14). It is inserted into the vagina and covers the perineum. It is a polyurethane sheath 7.8 cm in diameter and 17 cm long. It contains two polyurethane rings. One ring is at the closed end of the sheath and is designed to

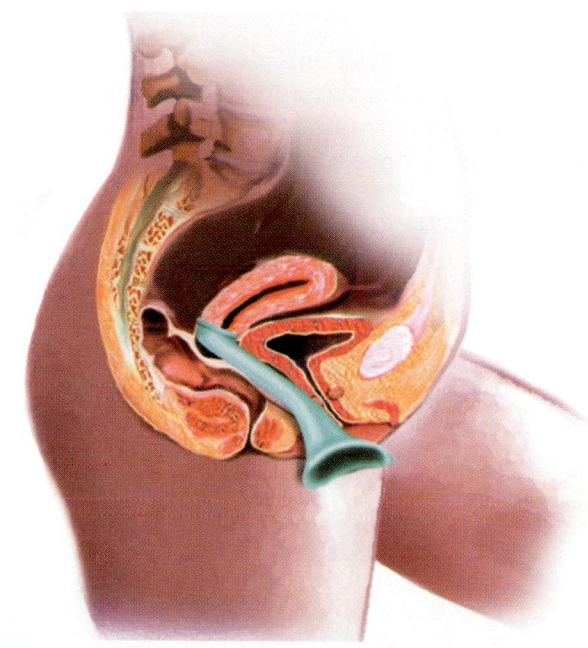

B.

Figure 7-14   A. Female condom. B. Proper insertion of a female condom.

be placed into the vagina. The ring at the open end remains outside the vagina after insertion. The outside portion of the female condom provides some protection for the external genitalia of the woman and the base of the penis of the man during intercourse. Unlike the lubricant in the male condom, the female condom does not contain spermicide.

Male condoms have been available for centuries and have been made of sheepskin and other materials. Currently, the most prevalent material is latex. Latex condoms have pores small enough to protect against the HIV virus and herpes simplex viruses.

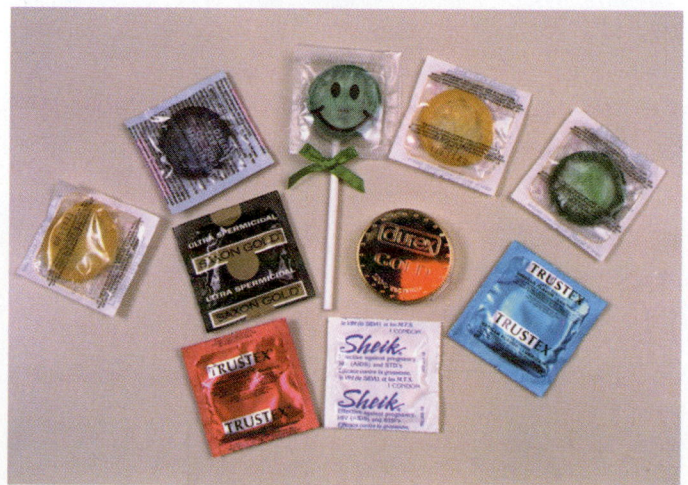

Figure 7-13   Male condoms.

Mechanism of Action

The condom acts as a barrier to prevent sperm from entering the vagina during intercourse. Both types of condom are designed for single use. Because the mechanism of action is as a barrier, a worn or torn condom negates its action.

Benefits and Risks

Condoms are inexpensive, readily available, require no contact with the health care system, and when used properly are quite effective as a method of contraception. When applied properly, condoms are almost as reliable as the oral contraceptive. The major risks of contraceptive failure with the condom involve use failure caused by breakage, accidental removal, or partner dissatisfaction with its use.

Indications

Both male and female condoms are indicated for use as a contraceptive device and as a method to prevent STDs. There are a number of reasons a couple may decide to use the condom as the primary form of contraception.

Contraindications

Condoms should not be used by the person with an allergy to latex.

Side Effects

If a person is sensitive to latex or spermicide, hypersensitivity reactions to the male condom may develop. Hyper-

Nursing Alert

Extra Precaution

Cautious women should use a spermicide as a secondary means of contraception in case of failure of the primary mode.

sensitivity is less likely to develop with use of the female condom because it is not made of latex.

Diaphragm. The **diaphragm** is a latex device available by prescription from a health care provider. The woman must be measured for adequate fit. Diaphragms are measured in millimeters and come in several sizes and styles to meet the needs of nulliparous and multiparous women. Measurement is so important to effectiveness that a woman must be refitted if she delivers a child or has a substantial weight change (Figure 7-15).

Mechanism of Action

The diaphragm is designed to be a receptacle for the spermicide. The diaphragm is fitted snuggly behind the symphysis pubis anteriorly. The sides of the diaphragm should extend laterally to encompass the entire cervix and rest in the lateral fornices. In the posterior dimension, when fitted properly, the cervix rests inside the diaphragm.

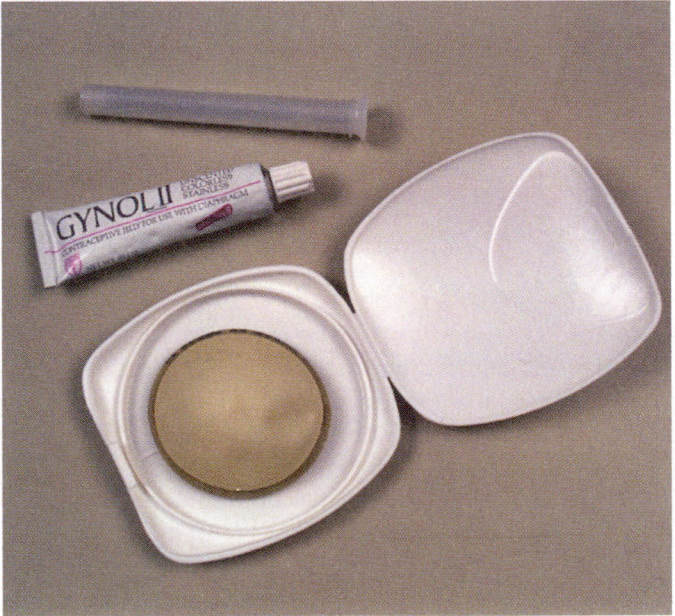

A.

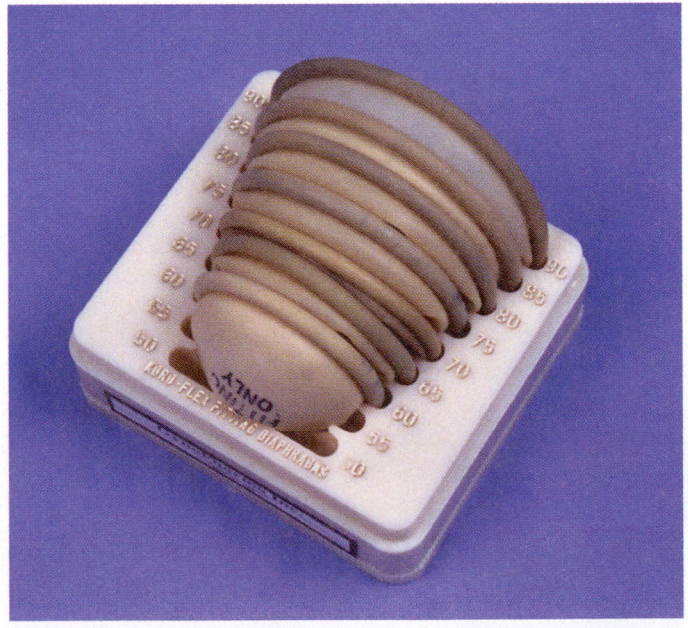

B.

Figure 7-15 A. Diaphragm with contraceptive jelly. B. Various sizes of diaphragms to be fitted by the health care provider.

Client Education

Diaphragm Care

When cleaning the diaphragm for storage, cornstarch or powder should not be used on the diaphragm. These substances can affect the integrity of the latex. When vaginal lubricants are used for intercourse, they should be water-based. Petroleum-based products increase the risk of disintegration of the latex.

The diaphragm must be positioned properly on insertion to avoid exposure of the cervix by the erect penis. This requires that the woman feel comfortable enough with checking the placement of the diaphragm with her fingers after insertion for proper placement.

The diaphragm requires care and proper storage. When these precautions are not taken, there is risk of use failure. The result may be an accidental pregnancy. When intercourse is repeated without additional application of spermicide there is risk for acquiring STDs and unintended pregnancy.

A spermicidal gel is placed inside the dome of the diaphragm and around the rim to ensure that sperm do not enter. It is important to emphasize that the diaphragm is not effective without a spermicide, as sperm can travel around the diaphragm and reach the os. If intercourse is undertaken more than once, additional spermicide should be applied into the vagina. The diaphragm should remain in place for 6 hours after intercourse. On removal, care should be taken to wash the diaphragm with a mild soap and water solution and allow it to dry before it is returned to its case for storage.

Benefits and Risks

The diaphragm is a long-established contraceptive device that requires little upkeep. Its theoretical failure rate is 6%, giving it the potential as an excellent method of contraception. The failure rate in typical use is somewhat higher (18%) because of the need to insert the diaphragm before intercourse. It must be left in place for 6 hours after intercourse and may remain in place up to 24 hours (Speroff & Darney, 2002). When properly cared for, the diaphragm can be used for 2 years without replacement. However, it must be inspected frequently for holes or deterioration of the latex.

Contraindications

There are no contraindications for the use of a barrier device. However, women who have allergies to latex or

spermicide would probably not want to use this method. Hatcher et al. (1998) suggest that women at high risk for failure use another method. Women at risk are those who have intercourse three or more times per week; who are under age 30 years; whose personal style or sexual patterns make consistent use difficult; who have had previous contraceptive failures; who have ambivalent feelings about the desirability of a pregnancy; and who intend to delay and not prevent pregnancy. These women are least likely to have success with this method.

Cervical Cap. The **cervical cap** is a rubber or latex barrier device designed to be applied to the cervix (Figure 7-16). It must be fitted to the woman by the health care provider to conform to the cervix. When properly fitted, the cervical cap is a few millimeters in diameter larger than is the cervix. The device is folded for insertion and fits against the cervix with suction. Once inserted, the device must be checked to ensure it is applied to the cervix and that suction is applied. Spermicide is placed in the dome of the cup and remains in place until the cervical cap is removed.

Benefits and Risks

The cervical cap is similar to but has an advantage over the diaphragm. Additional spermicide does not need to be applied with each act of intercourse. The cervical cap can be left in place for 36 to 48 hours after intercourse but should not remain inserted for prolonged periods of time. After a few days women may complain of a foul-smelling discharge.

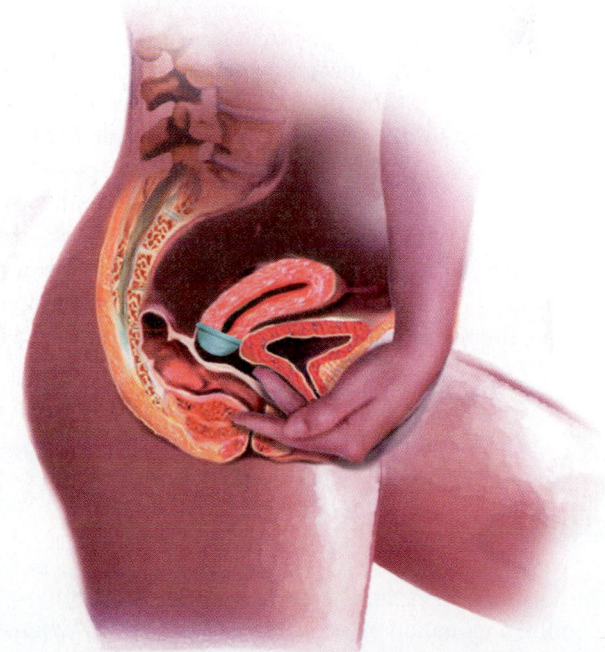

Figure 7-16 Proper insertion of a cervical cap.

Some women cannot wear the cervical cap because of irregularity of the cervical contour or other reasons. The cap must be left in place for 6 hours after intercourse because there may still be motile sperm in the vagina. Because the efficacy of the device depends on maintaining suction of the cap against the cervix and there may be dislodgment of the device during intercourse, the possibility of an accidental pregnancy exists.

Side Effects

When a cervical cap is left in place too long the potential for infection and cervical erosion exist. Antibiotics to treat the infection and another method of contraception may be required until the infection is healed. Cervical erosion may affect the outcome of the woman's Pap smear and also may necessitate removal of the device and use of another method.

Spermicide. **Spermicide** is a chemical method of contraception based on varying formulations of the chemical nonoxynol. The delivery system for this chemical can be foam, sponge, gel, cream, suppository, or film (Figure 7-17). This type of contraceptive has a failure rate of about 20% when used alone. When used in combination with another barrier method, its rate of effectiveness increases. Hatcher et al. (1998) suggest that the combination of spermicide and a barrier method is one of the safest contraceptive options. Each spermicidal device must remain in the vagina for a period of time after intercourse that is sufficient to kill the sperm. This means the woman should not bathe or douche for 6 hours after intercourse.

Types of Spermicide

Contraceptive gel, foam, or cream are designed to be used in combination with diaphragms and cervical caps. Spermicides, however, can be used alone. Spermicides come with applicators, and, therefore, a measured dose of the product will be used with each application. Suppositories can be used alone or with a condom. The woman must allow 15 to 30 minutes before intercourse for dispersion of the medication. Contraceptive film can be used alone or in combination with a diaphragm or cervical cap. When used alone, the film should be placed high in the vagina in

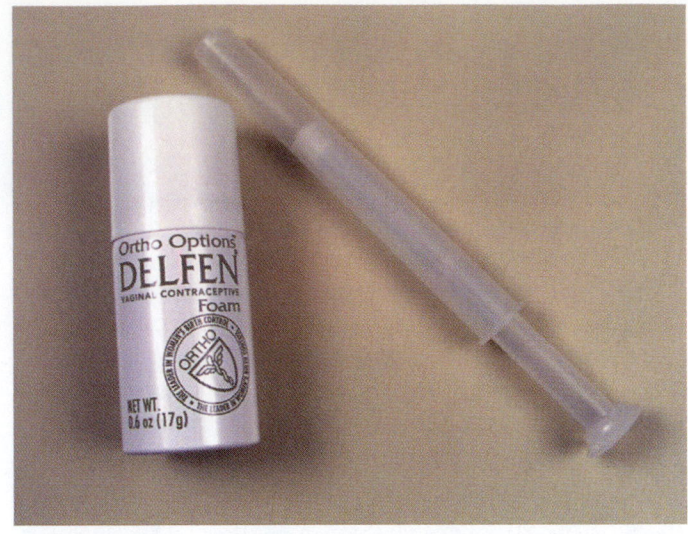

A.

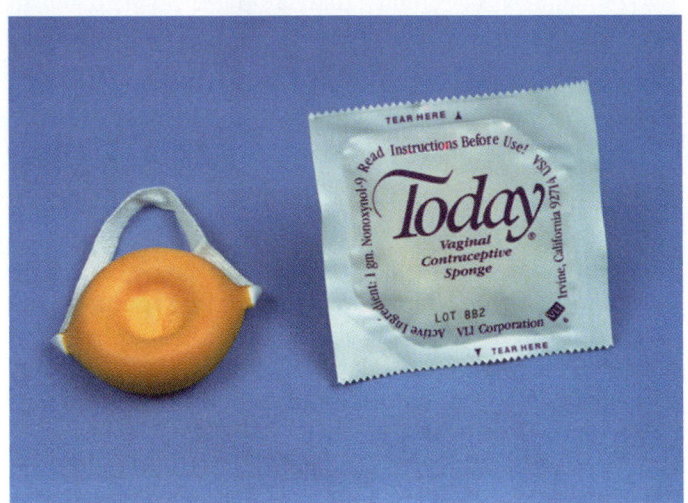

B.

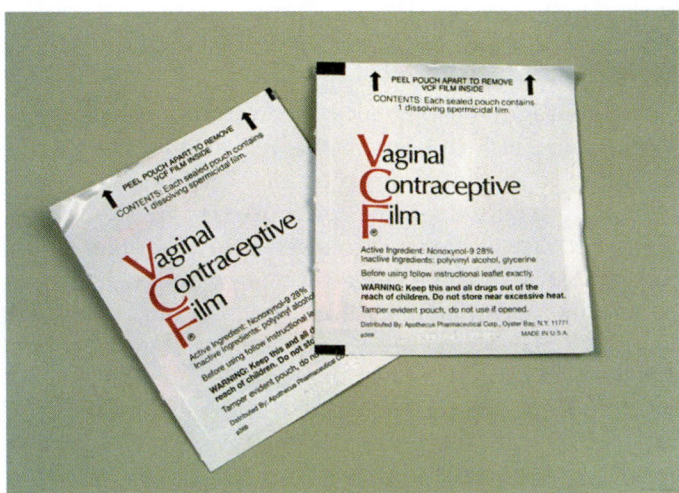

C.

Figure 7-17   Spermicides. A. Foam. B. Sponge. C. Film.

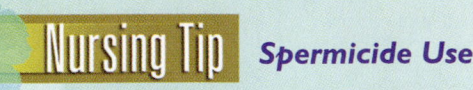

Nursing Tip   *Spermicide Use*

When using one of the spermicides for contraception, a second application of the product is necessary when intercourse is repeated.

contact with or near the cervix. When used with the diaphragm, the film should be used inside the diaphragm near the cervix. Fifteen minutes is required for the insert to dissolve so that the spermicide is available for use.

Mechanism of Action

Nonoxynol 9, the spermicide available in the United States, is a surfactant that destroys the sperm cell membrane. Other spermicides are used in other parts of the world.

Benefits and Risks

Spermicide may lower the risk of becoming infected with an STD by as much as 25% (Hatcher et al., 1998). Spermicides are stored easily for those who have intercourse infrequently. Another benefit may be that the male partner does not have to be involved with this type of method. It is an excellent backup method in case a woman runs out of pills or expels her IUD.

One of the disadvantages of this type of product is allergy or sensitivity to the ingredients. This sensitivity will result in skin irritation. Frequent use results in a greater likelihood of irritation. Some of the products effervesce and some women dislike this feeling. Use of the sponge or diaphragm may result in frequent yeast infections.

Implantable Methods

When **implantable contraception** (contraceptive device surgically implanted) is discussed, Norplant comes to mind (Figure 7-18). This device had been available in the United States for approximately 13 years prior to being removed from the market. Several other types of implantable devices are available. Over 6 million women worldwide have used levonorgestrel (Norplant) (Meckstroth & Darney, 2000). In 2003, Norplant was removed from the market due to manufacturing problems.

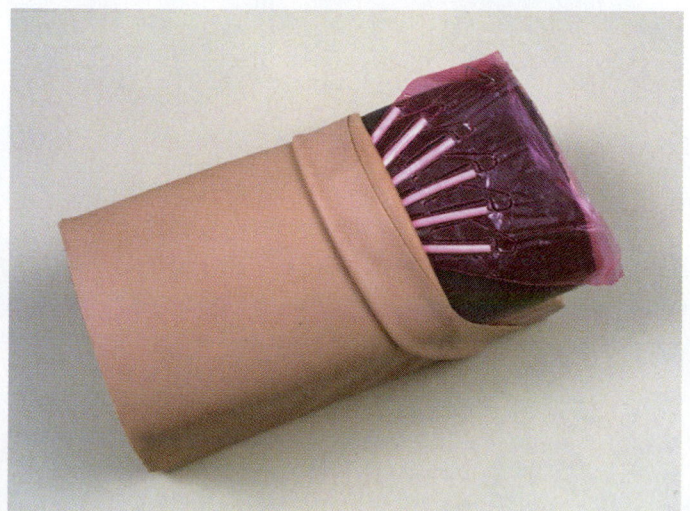

Figure 7-18   Implantable contraceptive.

Meckstroth & Darney (2000) discussed the new types of implantable devices that are becoming available. Norplant is still available in the standard six-capsule form; a new device, which is called Jadelle, that contains two rods of levonorgestrel is available. A second type of implant called Implanon is available in a single rod for implantation. Uniplant is a silastic capsule containing nomegestrol acetate that can be implanted as a single silastic capsule. Biodegradable implants include Capronor and Anuelle, which are under investigation. Capronor is a single biodegradable capsule, and Anuelle is marketed in the form of biodegradable pellets.

Composition.   Each of these implantable devices contains a progestin. Norplant contains six levonorgestrel capsules. Jadelle contains two levonorgestrel capsules. Implanon contains a single rod of the progestin etonogestrel, which is a metabolite of desogestrel. Uniplant contains nomegestrol acetate, which is a 19-nor-progesterone derivative. Nestorone is a potent progestin. Capronor contains levonorgestrel and Anuelle contains norethindrone (Meckstroth & Darney, 2000).

Mechanism of Action.   Pregnancy is prevented in several ways. Inhibition of ovulation is one mechanism of action but not the primary one. Some women continue to ovulate infrequently. Changes in the cervical mucus and endometrium are the primary mechanism of action.

Efficacy.   Several factors that affect the efficacy of this method include progestin concentration, the woman's weight, and her age. Another factor in effectiveness is the period of time that has passed since insertion. Implantable devices are thought to be more effective initially when inserted in the first 5 to 7 days of the menstrual cycle. A backup method is used for 1 week after insertion.

Benefits and Risks.   A benefit of this type of contraceptive method is that once implanted, the woman has long-term contraception. Norplant is effective for 5 to 7 years' use, although it has been approved for 5 years' use. Norplant II/Jadelle has been approved for 3 to 5 years' use before replacement is required. Implanon has been approved for 3 years' use before replacement is required. Uniplant has been approved for 1 year of use; Nestorone has been approved for 2 years' use; Capronor is approved for 1 year of use; and Anuelle is approved for 2 years' use.

Implants require a minor surgical procedure for insertion and removal. Removal sometimes can be complicated by broken or deeply placed implants or bleeding. Scar tissue around the implants may also contribute to difficulty in removal.

Indications. Implantable devices are designed to be used only for contraception.

Contraindications. Absolute contraindications for this type of product include active thrombophlebitis or thromboembolic disease, undiagnosed genital bleeding, acute liver disease, benign or malignant liver tumors, and known or suspected breast cancer. Refer to Box 7-6 for additional contraindications.

Side Effects. These implants are thought to have little metabolic effect. Menstrual changes occur in about 75% of users (Meckstroth & Darney, 2000). Alterations in the pattern of menstrual bleeding may occur. In the first 3 months of use, menses are likely to be prolonged, with spotting between menses. Other side effects that occur less frequently include headaches, weight change, acne, ovarian cysts, and mood changes.

Some women have a local foreign body reaction producing inflammation and occasionally infection of the insertion site. There are no data suggesting the products used in implants can potentiate autoimmune disease (Meckstroth & Darney, 2000).

Box 7-6

Relative Contraindications to the Use of Implantable Contraceptives

- Heavy cigarette smoking in women over 35 years of age (15 or more cigarettes daily)
- History of ectopic pregnancy
- Diabetes mellitus
- Hypercholesterolemia
- Severe acne
- Hypertension
- History of cardiovascular disease
- Gallbladder disease
- Severe vascular or migraine headaches
- Severe depression
- Chronic disease that affects the immune system
- Concomitant use of certain medications such as phenobarbital, phenytoin, carbamazepine, and rifampin

Note. Adapted from *A Clinical Guide to Contraception*, by L. Speroff and P. D. Darney, 2001, Baltimore: Williams & Wilkins.

Injectable Methods

Depo-Provera (depot medroxyprogesterone acetate, or DMPA) is a progestin-only **injectable contraceptive** administered intramuscularly (IM) every 3 months (Figure 7-19). Lunelle is a combination of medroxyprogesterone and estradiol cypionate (MPA/E2C), designed to be given IM monthly. Lunelle has been voluntarily taken off the market by the pharmaceutical company due to a manufacturing problem, though it is still available on the Internet.

Mechanism of Action. Depot medroxyprogesterone acts by inhibiting ovulation. The 150 mg dose inhibits ovulation for 3 months. The mechanism of action for Lunelle also is through inhibition of ovulation, and a dose of 0.5 mL provides contraception for 1 month.

Benefits and Risks. Depot medroxyprogesterone allows for 3 months' contraception without any effort on the part of the woman. DMPA is effective and well tolerated by most women and is safe for use by women who are lactating.

If subsequent DMPA injections do not occur within 14 weeks, there is real potential for method failure and an unplanned pregnancy. Clients should be instructed to come in for reinjection immediately at 12 weeks to avoid an unplanned pregnancy.

Lunelle has a very high efficacy. Its failure rate is estimated at 0.1 per 100 women-years (Kaunitz, 2001). Return to fertility is rapid after discontinuance of the injection.

In contrast with DMPA, Lunelle must be administered monthly. This regimen requires more frequent reproductive decision-making. The safety and adverse event profile are similar to that of combined oral contraceptives.

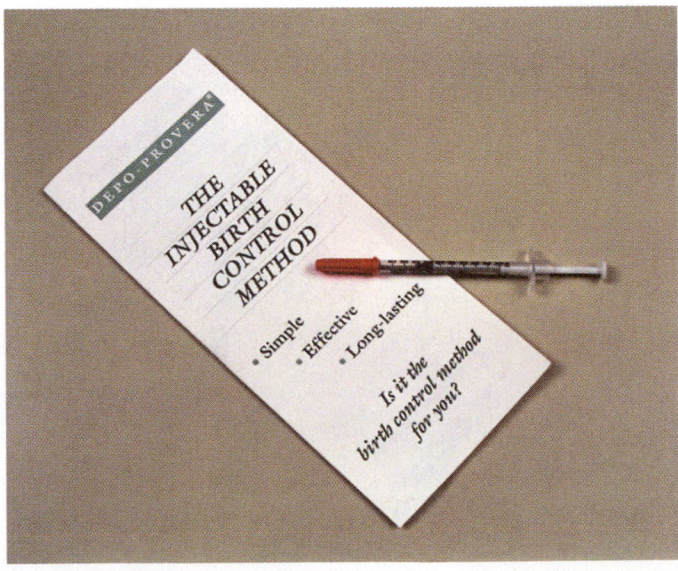

Figure 7-19 Injectable contraceptive.

> ### Nursing Tip   *Timing of Injectable Contraception*
>
> It is best to administer either injectable product, DMPA or Lunelle, within the first 5 days of the menstrual cycle to ensure that the woman is not pregnant and allow time to prevent ovulation.

Indications. Depot medroxyprogesterone and Lunelle are used only for contraception.

Contraindications. Contraindications for DMPA include known or suspected pregnancy, undiagnosed vaginal bleeding, active thrombophlebitis, history of thromboembolic disorder, current or past history of cerebrovascular accident, liver dysfunction, known or suspected malignancy of the breast, and known hypersensitivity to DMPA.

Contraindications for Lunelle include known or suspected pregnancy, undiagnosed vaginal bleeding, thrombophlebitis or a history of thrombophlebitis or thromboembolic disease, cerebrovascular disease, coronary artery disease, cholestatic jaundice, and carcinoma of the endometrium. Known hypersensitivity to the medication also is an absolute contraindication.

Side Effects. The side effects of DMPA can include menstrual, weight, and mood changes. Menstrual changes are very common in women who use DMPA. In the first 3 months of use, heavy and irregular bleeding is most common. After 3 months, amenorrhea becomes more common. Menstrual disturbances are likely to be the reason women discontinue this form of contraception.

Weight gain is a problem encountered by many women and is a factor involved in discontinuance of contraception. Some women who use DMPA complain of weight gain. This weight gain, however, has not been validated by controlled studies.

The overall incidence of depression in women who use DMPA is low but does exist. Women who use Lunelle are less likely to experience menstrual changes. They may experience weight gain similar to that with DMPA. There are no reports of mood change with Lunelle. There have been reports of decreased libido with both products.

Natural Family Planning Methods

Two methods are available as natural family planning devices. Coitus interruptus is primarily controlled by the man, and ovulation prediction is primarily controlled by the woman.

Composition. Coitus interruptus involves removal of the male penis from the vagina before ejaculation. It is probably one of the least effective methods of contraception, with a failure rate of 19% (Hatcher et al., 1998). This method, however, is much preferable to using no contraceptive method with a failure rate of 85%.

Ovulation prediction, also known as the rhythm method, is the female natural family planning method. The woman predicts her fertile period through the use of basal body temperature charts, cervical mucus changes, or both. She abstains from intercourse for the period of time during which she is fertile. When timing intercourse, the woman must determine the day on which she ovulates and take into account that the male sperm is active for 48 hours and the ovum is susceptible to fertilization for 24 hours.

Mechanism of Action. Both of these methods, in fact, are barrier devices because they place time or distance between the sperm and ovum to prevent conception.

Benefits and Risks. These methods are inexpensive and, when used properly, can be effective. Caution must be used with coitus interruptus because seminal fluid may escape before ejaculation and before removal of the penis from the vagina. The result can be an unwanted pregnancy.

With ovulation prediction methods, it is not safe to assume that because ovulation occurred on day 14 of one cycle that it will do so each month. Ovulation at another time can result in an unplanned pregnancy.

Indications. Natural family planning methods are for those persons who do not believe in or cannot use other methods. These methods are vastly more reliable than is intercourse without the use of any method.

Contraindications. There are no known contraindications to natural family planning.

Emergency Contraception

Emergency contraception, also known as the "morning-after" pill, is available to prevent unintended pregnancy. This type of contraception has been available in the United States for approximately 20 years but it is not widely used or known by women. In the United Kingdom, however, the method has been used over 4 million times with few reported side effects (Grow & Almed, 2000).

Several types of postcoital contraception are available. Hormonal methods include administration of the COC, progestins, gonadotropin-releasing hormone (Gn-RH) agonists, antiprogestins, and high-dose estrogen Gn-RH agonists. The copper IUD also may be used for these purposes. Surgical abortion is also an option.

Combined Oral Contraceptives. In 1974, Yuzpe published the first results of successfully using 100 µg of ethinyl estradiol and 1 mg/dL norgestrel in combination as a single dose for emergency contraception. The current standard is to give the equivalent of 100 µg of ethinyl estradiol and 1 mg of levonorgestrel in combination for this purpose (Hatcher et al., 1998). The medication must be initiated within 72 hours of unprotected intercourse, and a second dose of the medication is given 12 hours after the initial dose. Table 7-6 summarizes some of the protocols used in contemporary health care.

Mechanism of Action

If COCs are administered before ovulation, ovulation may be delayed or suppressed for that menstrual cycle. The suppression is through action on the anterior pituitary. If administered after ovulation, the action is thought to be through suppression of endometrial hormone receptors, possibly leading to inadequate maturation of the endometrium and thus preventing implantation (La Valleur, 2000).

Efficacy

After treatment, the pregnancy rate ranges from 0.5% to 2.5%. The variation has to do with when in the menstrual cycle the woman had unprotected sex, how soon she received treatment, and whether the woman develops side effects such as vomiting.

Table 7-6	Emergency Contraception with Combined Oral Contraceptives
TRADE NAME	DOSAGE
Alesse	five pink pills immediately and five pink pills in 4 hours
Levlen	four orange pills immediately and four orange pills in 12 hours
Lo/Ovral	four pills immediately and four pills in 12 hours
Nordette	four orange pills immediately and four orange pills in 12 hours
Ovral	two pills immediately and two pills in 12 hours
Prevens	two pills immediately and two pills in 12 hours
Tri-Levlen	four yellow pills immediately and four yellow pills in 4 hours
Triphasil	four yellow pills immediately and four yellow pills in 4 hours

Note. Adapted from *Contraceptive Technology* (17th ed.), by R. A. Hatcher, J. Trussell, F. Stewart, W. Cates, G. Stewart, F. Guest, et al., 1998, New York: Ardent Media.

Benefits and Risks

Emergency contraception with COCs offers women a chance to prevent an unwanted pregnancy for a number of reasons. There are no noncontraceptive benefits to be had because of the short-term nature of this regimen.

Risks with this method include failure of the method to prevent pregnancy. Failure will result in the woman having to decide whether to seek pregnancy termination or continue the pregnancy.

Indications

Postcoital contraception is designed as a secondary method of contraception, not as a first choice. Women who repeatedly find themselves in need of this type of contraception are not being proactive in their reproductive decision-making and require counseling.

Contraindications

The only absolute contraindication to emergency contraception with COCs is pregnancy. Use of progestin-only emergency contraception may be best for the woman with a history of thromboembolism.

Side Effects

The major side effects of emergency contraception using COCs are nausea and vomiting. Providing an antinauseant medication before taking the COCs can reduce this side effect. There may be an increased incidence of ectopic pregnancy if conception does occur. There may be menstrual disturbance even in the absence of pregnancy because of the high doses of hormones involved in emergency contraception regimens. Other side effects can include headache, fatigue, and mood swings (La Valleur, 2000).

Progestin-Only Pills. Levonorgestrel has been used in Europe and China for emergency contraception. It is given in a dose of 0.75 mg within 72 hours of unprotected intercourse, and the dose is repeated in 12 hours (La Valleur, 2000). Hatcher et al. (1998) determined that this dose could be obtained by taking 20 yellow tablets of Ovrette immediately and 20 additional tablets in 12 hours. Currently, one 0.75 mg formulation is available that is marketed solely for emergency contraception. The trade name is Plan B. Each of these packets contains two levonorgestrel tablets. One tablet is for immediate use, and the other is for use in 12 hours. This medication must be used within 72 hours of unprotected intercourse (Speroff, 2000).

Antiprogestins. Mifepristone (RU 486) is a synthetic steroid that prevents progesterone from binding to its receptors. Mifepristone has been used extensively in Europe as an abortifacient and as an emergency contraceptive method (Thomas, 2001).

Benefits and Risks

A benefit of this type of emergency contraception is that it is a medical rather than a surgical approach to pregnancy termination. This method is less invasive and has fewer complications than does surgery. Pills are easier to obtain than is a surgical procedure and are very effective. Despite the many benefits, this drug has been very controversial in this country because of questions about when life begins.

Indications

Mifepristone has been investigated for use as an abortifacient and as an emergency contraceptive method. Mifepristone is more effective the earlier in the pregnancy it is used (Cates & Ellertson, 1998).

Contraindications

Contraindications to administering this drug are known or suspected pregnancy unless there is commitment to pregnancy termination. Mifepristone also is not used with known or suspected ectopic pregnancy or if there is an undiagnosed adnexal mass. Mifepristone should not be used in clients who have adrenal failure and clients who use long-term steroid therapy. It should not be used in clients who have hemorrhagic disorders or who are using anticoagulants. Clients who have an allergy to the product should not use it.

Side Effects

The major side effects are cramping and vaginal bleeding. Cramping usually can be managed with acetaminophen (Tylenol) with codeine. ASA (aspirin) and ibuprofen (Aleve, Motrin) are avoided because they are antiprostaglandins

and would tend to negate the actions of mifepristone. Bleeding usually is mild but occasionally can be heavy, depending on the age of gestation. When heavy bleeding is a problem, dilatation and curettage may be required.

Intrauterine Devices. Intrauterine devices can be used for emergency contraception. The device should be inserted within 5 to 10 days after unprotected intercourse. In addition to the usual mechanism of action, an IUD inserted for emergency contraception acts as a toxin to the blastocyst (La Valleur, 2000). The IUD is extremely effective as an emergency contraceptive in selected clients.

Surgical Methods. Abortion can be a medical or a surgical procedure. The purpose of abortion is to terminate a pregnancy. It is not designed to be used as a primary method of contraception but is more appropriate as a backup method in case of failure of the primary method (Table 7-7).

Although this surgical procedure has been legally available in the United States since 1973, abortion is still very controversial. Many Americans do not approve of pregnancy termination in any form. The result of this division of thought has been observable in numerous attempts to reverse legalization of abortion. Zealots have tried to prevent women from entering clinics where abortions are performed, picketed clinics, and even have bombed abortion clinics.

Several methods are used for abortion. The choice of methods depends on factors such as the gestational age of the pregnancy. Vacuum extraction can be used only early in the pregnancy. Dilation and evacuation have been

Table 7-7	Types of Abortions	
TYPE OF ABORTION	**PROCEDURE**	**NURSING CARE**
D&C (dilation and curettage)	Cervical os is dilated and then a suction curette is used to empty the contents of the uterus.	• Ensure that equipment is available and ready to use. • Assist the physician and provide emotional support for the client.
D&E (dilation and evacuation)	Cervix is dilated, a curette is used to scrape the uterus and then suction is used.	• Ensure that equipment is available and ready to use. • Assist the physician and provide emotional support for the client.
Saline	Injection of hypertonic solution into the uterus, followed by Cytotec (misoporstal) and/or Pitocin (oxytocin) to induce labor.	• Ensure that equipment is available and ready to use. • Assist the physician and provide emotional support for the client.
Methotrexate Sodium (Amethopterin MTX)	Used for early first trimester ectopic pregnancies.	• This is off-label use of this drug without FDA approval. • It has been used to terminate ectopic pregnancies. • Advise the client that the products can be aborted immediately after prostaglandin or up to 6 weeks.
RU 486	Used in the first trimester only and usually followed by Cytotec p.o. to complete the process.	• Heavy bleeding may occur—if severe, contact the physician. • Assist in management of pain, nausea, vomiting, diarrhea, or headache.

used to abort pregnancies that have progressed beyond the time at which vacuum extraction or aspiration is possible.

Permanent Methods

Sterilization refers to the use of a surgical procedure to produce permanent loss of reproductive capability. Surgical sterilization has become very common for married couples who have decided to permanently limit the size of their family. More women have surgical sterilization than do men.

Female Methods

Worldwide more than 190 million couples use sterilization as their contraceptive method (Pati & Cullins, 2000). Sterilization is the most prevalent method used by married couples in the United States and is used by 39% of couples. Female tubal sterilization, also called **tubal ligation**, accounts for 72% of the sterilization procedures performed in the United States. Female sterilization can be done by tubal ligation or hysterectomy or bilateral oophorectomy. Hysterectomy usually is used when a gynecologic problem exists at the same time the woman wants permanent sterilization. When a woman has no gynecologic problem, tubal ligation can be performed immediately after delivery by minilaparotomy. A small abdominal incision is made through which the fallopian tubes are grasped and a segment of each is removed. Tubal ligation at any other time usually is a laparoscopic procedure in which a small periumbilical incision and a small lower quadrant incision are made. The tubes may be cauterized, or a clip may be placed on the tube to allow for later removal (Figure 7-20). The woman considering tubal ligation should know that it is a permanent sterilization method. Reversal of this procedure has been done; however, such attempts are not always successful and can be expensive.

Some health care providers believe that the appropriate time for a woman to have a tubal ligation is early in the menstrual cycle so there is no possibility for pregnancy. Many times the woman is using birth control pills as a method of contraception, which lessens the importance of when the procedure is done because the woman is not ovulating. If the woman is taking birth control pills, the remainder of the cycle of pills should be taken after the procedure to prevent hormonal problems associated with stopping the pills before the cycle is completed.

Benefits and Risks. Tubal ligation is effective immediately and is considered permanent. These are two very great benefits for women and couples who have finished childbearing. There are no devices to use or details to remember. Laparoscopic tubal ligation can be performed easily on an outpatient basis. It is quite common for a woman to have the surgery on Friday and return to work on Monday.

Although the tubal procedure is considered permanent, there is a small failure rate. Occasionally, the tube will reopen. When this occurs, an unwanted pregnancy may result. In this case, some women have had the procedure a second time. Others decide they want their partner to undergo the next procedure.

Indications. Permanent female sterilization should be reserved for those women who have completed their family. A common discussion with these women includes directions by the health care provider for the woman to consider what her thoughts would be if something would happen to her existing family. If the woman thinks she might want to have more children under those circumstances, she may be encouraged to use a different method of birth control.

Contraindications. Contraindications for this method include women whose health condition is not good enough to withstand the procedure. This contraindication is uncommon.

Side Effects. Tubal ligation is a common procedure but is not without complications. The woman has a risk of death from anesthesia or infection. The mortality rate of tubal ligation has been reported to be 1 to 2 deaths per 100,000 procedures. This mortality rate compares favorably with that of hysterectomy, which is 5 to 25 deaths per 100,000 procedures, and childbirth, which is 8 deaths per 100,000 live births in the United States (Pati & Cullins, 2000). Other potential injuries include hemorrhage and damage to the bladder or bowel. Another long-term potential side effect is that the woman may regret having had the procedure;

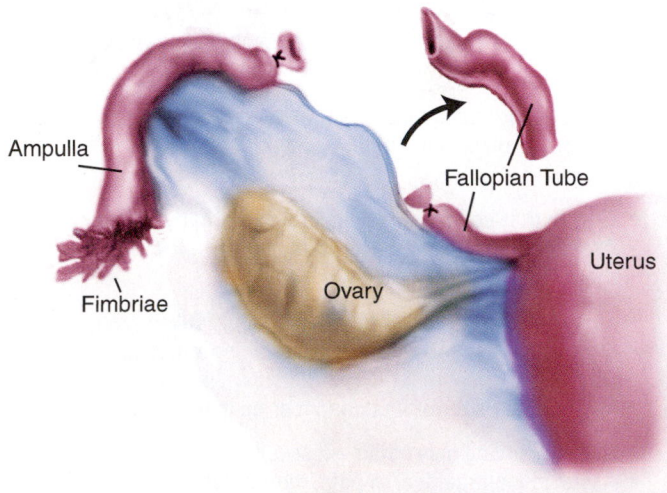

Figure 7-20   Tubal ligation.

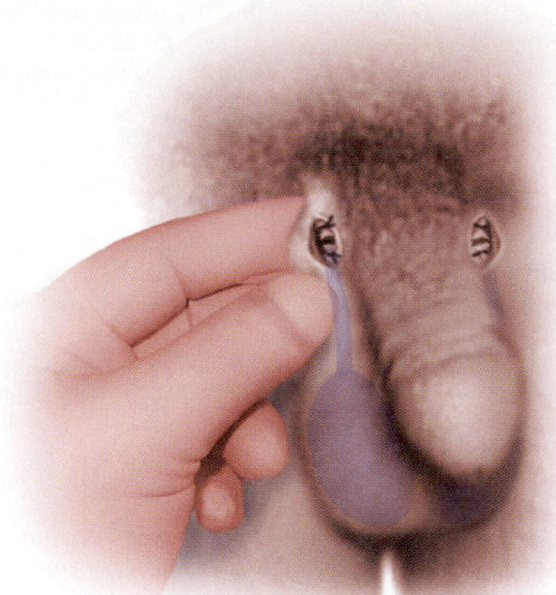

Figure 7-21   Vasectomy.

WEB ACTIVITIES

••• What support groups, chat rooms, or resources can you locate for infertile couples?

••• Search the Internet under the key words "fertility," "infertility," and "artificial insemination." What links can you find?

••• Visit the Web site of a pharmaceutical company such as Glaxo or Mead Johnson. Do they offer information on their infertility drugs?

••• Go to http://www.aasect.org, the Web site for the American Association of Sex Educators, Counselors, and Therapists. What three major sexual concerns can you identify that are of importance to women using its on-line journal?

••• Go to the NARAL homepage at http://www.naral.org. What are the issues of interest to this group?

••• Go to http://nrlc.org. What is the agenda for this group?

reversal of a tubal ligation is typically only about 25% successful. The final side effect would be failure of the procedure to provide contraception.

Male Methods

The male sterilization procedure is called vasectomy. The vas deferens transport sperm from the epididymis to the seminal vesicle for mixture with other seminal fluids before ejaculation. **Vasectomy** ligates the vas deferens, thus interrupting sperm transport (Figure 7-21). The procedure can be done in an outpatient setting under local anesthesia.

As is sterilization in women, vasectomy is considered permanent. Reversal of the procedure has been done but is not always successful. About 90% of vasectomy reversals are effective, but only 50% return to a fertile sperm count and are able to father a child. Postoperative follow-up is important in vasectomy because the sperm count does not immediately decrease to zero. Vasectomy is not considered effective until the man has had two negative sperm counts.

Nursing Implications

Nurses often are in a position to provide information about contraception to women who are undecided about the method of contraception they want to use. The nurse must stay informed about the new technologies that are being developed because many times these methods may be preferable for the woman for a number of reasons.

Advanced practice nurses in many settings are able to prescribe and/or insert contraceptive devices. These practitioners should remain current in the contraceptive devices and methods available.

Key Concepts

■ Couples experiencing infertility or sexual dysfunction undergo a highly emotionally charged situation that also may be technically difficult.

■ Many times a couple's problems with infertility or sexuality are multifactorial and may require prolonged interaction with the health care system for diagnosis and treatment.

■ To some couples, conception is more important than most other things in their lives.

■ With new advances in technology, conception is occurring in couples in whom it would not have been possible in the recent past.

■ The new assisted reproductive technologies carry ethical considerations with which society must deal.

■ To use a contraceptive effectively requires the use of a rational decision-making process.

■ To use the least effective contraceptive method will prevent unwanted pregnancy significantly better than will unprotected intercourse.

■ Complex factors influence a couple's choice and use of contraception.

■ To assist couples in family planning, the nurse must realize the couple may have a very different value system from that of the nurse. The nurse will need to understand the client's perspective to be helpful.

Review Questions and Activities

1. What is the most common male factor in infertility?

2. What is the most common female factor in infertility?

3. Why is infertility sometimes difficult to diagnose and treat?

4. Which cultural practices do humans have related to fertility and sexuality?

5. Which components relate to the experience of sexual dysfunction?

6. What is serial monogamy, and how is it an important concept in American culture?

7. What are your ethical beliefs about freezing and storing fertilized ova?

8. With new information forthcoming, what reproductive technologies may be available in the coming century?

9. Which factors are involved in the reproductive decision-making process?

10. What is the difference in the mechanism of action between combined oral contraceptives and the minipill?

11. What are the absolute and relative contraindications of COCs?

12. What is the difference between monophasic, biphasic, and triphasic birth control pills?

13. What time limitations are involved with emergency contraception?

14. What are the reasons the IUD is not used more widely?

References

Adams, D. M. (2000). Breastfeeding and oral contraceptives: Exploring opinions and options. *Lifelines, 4*(3), 45–47.

Alteneder, R., & Hartzell, D. (1997). Addressing couples' sexual concerns during the childbearing period: Use of the PLISSIT model. *Journal of Obstetric, Gynecologic, and Neonatal Nursing, 26*(6), 651–658.

American College of Obstetricians and Gynecologists (ACOG). (2000). *Adult manifestations of childhood sexual abuse.* ACOG Educational Bulletin. Washington, DC: Author.

American Society for Reproductive Medicine. (1998). *Induction of ovarian follicle development and ovulation with exogenous gonadotropins.* Washington, DC: Author.

Anasti, J. N. (1998). Premature ovarian failure: An update. *Fertility & Sterility, 70*(1), 1–14.

Angard, N. T. (1999). Diagnosis infertility: These treatments can help couples achieve pregnancy. *Lifelines, 3*(3), 22–29.

Ballagh, S. A. (2001). Vaginal ring hormone delivery systems in contraception and menopause. *Clinical Obstetrics and Gynecology, 44*(1), 106–113.

Baram, D. A. (2002). Sexuality and sexual function. In J. S. Berele (Ed.), *Novak's gynecology* (13th ed.). Baltimore: Williams & Wilkins.

Berube, S., Marcoux, S., Langenum, M., & Maheux, R. (1998). Fecundity of infertile women with minimal or mild endometriosis and women with unexplained infertility. *Fertility & Sterility, 69*(6), 1034–1049.

Bigelow, P. L., Jarrell, J., Young, M. R., Keefe, T. J., & Love, E. J. (1998). Association of semen quality and occupational factors: Comparison of case control analysis and analysis of continuous variables. *Fertility & Sterility, 69*(1), 11–18.

Burkman, R. T. (2001). Oral contraceptive: Current status. *Clinical Obstetrics and Gynecology, 44*(1), 62–72.

Byyny, R. L., & Speroff, L. (1996). *A clinical guide for the care of older women: Primary and preventive care* (2nd ed.). Baltimore: Williams & Wilkins.

Cates, W., & Ellertson, C. (1998). Abortion. In R. Hatcher (Ed.), *Contraceptive technology* (17th ed.). New York: Ardent Media.

Charles, C., Gafini, A., & Whelan, T. (1997). Shared decision-making in the medical encounter: What does it mean? (Or it takes at least two to tango). *Social Science and Medicine, 44*(5) 681–692.

Cohen, S., Kenner, C., & Hollingsworth, A. (1991). *Maternal, neonatal, and women's health nursing.* Springhouse, PA: Springhouse.

Dailard, C. (2000). *Issues in brief: Abortion in context in the United States: Alan Guttmacher Institute.* (Retrieved March 3, 2001, from http://www.agi-usa.org.)

D'Emilio, J., & Freedman, E. B. (1997). *Intimate matters: A history of sexuality in America* (2nd ed.). Chicago: University of Chicago Press.

Department of Health and Human Services (DHHS) & The National Institute of Child Health and Human Development (NICHHD). (1996). IUD's: State-of-the-art conference. *Clinical Courier, 14*(12), 1–7.

Dickey, R. P. (2001). *Managing contraceptive pill patients.* Durant, OK: Essential Medical Information Systems.

Fuchs, N., Prinz, H., & Koch, U. (1996). Attitudes to current oral contraceptive use and future developments: The women's perspective. *European Journal of Contraceptive and Reproductive Health Care, 1*(3) 275–284.

Gage, A. J. (1998). Sexual activity and contraceptive use: The components of the decision making process. *Studies in Family Planning, 29*(2) 154–166.

Gilligan, C., Ward, V., & Taylor, J. (1988). *Mapping the moral domain.* Cambridge, MA: Harvard University Press.

Grady, W. R., Klepinger, D. H., & Nelson-Wally, A. (1999). Contraceptive characteristics: The perceptions and priorities of men and women. *Family Planning Perspectives, 31*(4), 168–175.

Grow, D. R., & Almed, S. (2000). New contraceptive methods. *Obstetrics and Gynecology Clinics of North America, 27*(4), 901–916.

Guzick, D. S. (2000). When infertility can't be explained. *Contemporary Ob/Gyn, 45*(9), 102–111.

Hatcher, R. A., Trussell, J., Stewart, F., Cates, W., Stewart, G., Guest, F., et al. (1998). *Contraceptive technology* (17th ed.). New York: Ardent Media.

Illions, E. H., & Thompson, R. J. (1997). Office evaluation of the infertile couple. In V. L. Seltzer & W. H. Pearse (Eds.), *Women's primary health care*. New York: McGraw-Hill.

Jensen, J. T., & Speroff, L. (2000). Health benefits of oral contraceptives. *Obstetrics and Gynecology Clinics of North America, 27*(4), 705–721.

Jerka, J., Schuett, S., & Foxhall, M. J. (1996). Loneliness and social support in infertile couples. *Journal of Obstetric, Gynecologic, and Neonatal Nursing, 25*(1), 55–60.

Kaplan, C. R. (1996). Work-up of infertility: Diagnosis and treatment of anovulation. *The Female Patient, 21*(3), 35–42.

Katz, A. (2000). Birds do it, bees do it, let's talk about it: The nurse's role in sexual counseling. *Lifelines, 4*(5), 40–41.

Kaunitz, A. M. (2001). Injectible long-acting contraceptives. *Clinical Obstetrics and Gynecology, 44*(1), 73–91.

Kjos, S. L. (1997). Contraception for women at risk: A case for the intrauterine device. *Contemporary Ob/Gyn, 42*(11), 105–121.

Kohn, I. I., & Kaplan, S. A. (2000). Female sexual dysfunction: What is known and what can be done. *Contemporary Ob/Gyn, 45*(2), 25–46.

La Valleur, J. (2000). Emergency contraception. *Obstetrics and Gynecology Clinics of North America, 27*(4), 817–839.

Long, V. E. (1998). Between childbearing and menopause: Contraceptive options for women over 40. *Advance for Nurse Practitioners, 6*(12), 52–58.

Lynch, C. M. (2000). Breakthrough bleeding with ocs: Practical management considerations. *Contemporary Ob/Gyn, 12* (Suppl.), 3–19.

Manning, W. D., Longmore, M. A., & Giordano, P. C. (2000). The relationship context of contraceptive use at first intercourse. *Family Planning Perspectives, 32*(3), 104–110.

Masters, W. H., & Johnson, V. E. (1996). *Human sexual response*. Boston: Little Brown.

Matteson, P. S., & Hawkins, J. W. (1997). Women's patterns of contraceptive use. *Health Care of Women International, 18*(5), 455–466.

Meckstroth, K. R., & Darney, P. D. (2000). Implantable contraception. *Obstetrics and Gynecology Clinics of North America, 27*(4), 781–815.

Michael, R. T., Gagnon, J. H., Laumann, E. O., & Jolata, G. (1994). *Sex in America: A definitive survey*. Boston: Little Brown.

Miller, V. L., Laken, M. A., Ager, J., & Essenmacher, L. (2000). Contraceptive decision making among Medicaid-eligible women. *Journal of Community Health, 25*(6), 473–480.

Mishell, D. R. (1996). IUDs: Historical perspective and mechanisms of action. In D Mishell (Ed.), *Intrauterine Contraception in the U.S.: A current perspective*. Little Falls, NJ: Health Learning Systems.

Nelson, A. (1995). Patient selection is the key to IUD success. *Contemporary Ob/Gyn, 40*(10), 49–62.

Nelson, A. L. (2000). The intrauterine contraceptive device. *Obstetrics & Gynecology Clinics of North America, 27*(4), 723–740.

Oddens, B. J. (1997). Determinants of contraceptive use among women of reproductive age in Great Britain and Germany. II: Psychological factors. *Journal of Biosocial Science, 29*(4), 437–470.

Pati, S., & Cullins, V. (2000). Female sterilization: Evidence. *Obstetrics and Gynecology Clinics of North America, 27*(4), 859–899.

Pender, N. (1996). Health promotion in nursing practice. Stamford, CT: Appleton & Lange.

Prior, J. (1997). Ovulatory disturbances and amenorrhea: A physiologic approach to diagnosis and therapy. In J. A. Rosenfeld (Ed.), *Women's health in primary care*. Philadelphia: Williams & Wilkins.

Rosenthal, M. R. (1997). Ovulatory disturbances and amenorrhea: A physiologic approach to diagnosis and therapy. In J. A. Rosenfeld (Ed.), *Women's primary health care*. Baltimore: William & Wilkins.

Saks, B. (1999). Sexual dysfunction: Sex, drugs, and women's issues. *Primary Care Update for Ob Gyns, 6*(2), 61–65.

Sauer, M. V. (1998). Motherhood at any age? Egg donation not intended for everyone. *Fertility & Sterility, 69*(3), 187–188.

Seaman, E. K., Telich-Vidal, M., & Sable, D. (1997). Effects of cancer treatment on fertility. *Contemporary Ob/Gyn, 42*(5), 31–52.

Seltzer, V. L., & Pearse, W. H. (1995). *Women in primary health care: Office practice and procedures*. New York: McGraw-Hill.

Silber, S. J. (2000). Evaluation and treatment of male infertility. *Clinical Obstetrics and Gynecology, 43*(4), 854–888.

Silverberg, K. M. (2000). Evaluation of the couple with infertility in a managed care environment. *Clinical Obstetrics & Gynecology, 43*(4), 844–853.

Smith, K., & Hornberger, L. (1997). Rewards of caring for and the health promotion of women adolescents. In J. A. Rosenfeld (Ed.), *Women's health in primary care*. Baltimore: Williams & Wilkins.

Speroff, L. (2000). Oral contraceptives and carbohydrate metabolism. *Dialogues in Contraception, 6*(4), 18.

Speroff, L., & Darney, P. D. (2001). *A Clinical Guide for Contraception* (3rd ed.). Baltimore: Williams & Wilkins.

Speroff, L., Glass, R. H., & Kase, N. G. (1999). *Clinical gynecological endocrinology and infertility* (6th ed.). Philadelphia: Lippincott.

Spielvogel, K., Shwayden, J., & Coddington, C. C. (2000). Surgical management of adhesions, endometriosis, and tubal pathology in women with infertility. *Clinical Obstetrics and Gynecology, 43*(4), 916–928.

Stephen, E. H., & Chandra, A. (1998). Updated projections of infertility. *Fertility and Sterility, 70*(1), 30–34.

Stewart, G. K. (1998). Intrauterine devices. In R. Hatcher (Ed.), *Contraceptive technology* (17th ed.). New York: Ardent Media.

Thomas, M. A. (2001). Postcoital contraception. *Clinical Obstetrics and Gynecology, 44*(1), 101–105.

Van Sickle, M., & Rosenstrock, H. (1999). Taking a sexual history: Which questions to ask. *The Female Patient, 24*(3), 33–40.

Van Voorhis, B. J. (1998). Infertility treatment: What is a cost-effective approach? *Drug Benefits Trends, 10*(2), 22–29.

Vermillion, S. T., & Holmes, M. M. (1997). Sexual dysfunction in women. *Primary Care Update for Ob-Gyns, 4*(6), 234–240.

Wallach, E. E., Garcia, J., Rosenwak, Z., & Seifer, D. K. (1998). Fertility over 35: Improving the odds. *Contemporary Ob/Gyn, 43*(5), 106–118.

Wolf, L. J. (2000). Ovulation induction. *Clinical Obstetrics and Gynecology, 43*(4), 902–915.

Suggested Readings

Bachman, G. A., Coleman, E., Driscoll, C. E., & Renshaw, D. (1999). Patients with sexual dysfunction: Your guidance makes a difference. *Patient Care for the Nurse Practitioner, 2*(4), 14–25.

Berman, J. R., Berman, L. A., & Goldstein, I. (1998). Sexual dysfunction: Past, present, and future. *The Female Patient 23*(12), 45–51.

Heiman, J. R., & Meston, C. M. (1997). Evaluating sexual dysfunction in women. *Clinical Obstetrics and Gynecology, 40*(3), 616–629.

Holland, K. L., & Finger, W. W. (1999). Chronic pelvic pain and sexual trauma in women. *The Female Patient, 24*(1), 13–18.

Leiblum, S. R. (2000). Redefining female sexual response. *Contemporary Ob/Gyn, 45*(11), 120–126.

Meana, M., Binik, Y. M., Khalife, S., & Cohen, D. R. (1998). Biopsychosocial profile of women with dyspareunia. *Obstetrics and Gynecology, 90*(4, P.1), 583–589.

O'Donahue, W., Dopke, C. A., & Swingen, D. N. (1997). Psychotherapy for female sexual dysfunction: A review. *Clinical Psychology Review, 17*(5), 537–566.

Rammer, E., & Friedrich, F. (1998). The effectiveness of intrauterine insemination in couples with sterility due to male infertility with and without a woman's hormone factor. *Fertility and Sterility, 69*(1), 31–36.

Reichart, G. A. (1998). Female circumcision: What you need to know about genital mutilation. *Lifelines, 2*(3), 31–34.

Renshaw, D. (1994). Unconsummated marriage: A neglected aspect of sexual dysfunction. *The Female Patient, 19*(5), 55–60.

Rhodes, J. C., Kjerulff, K. H., Lagenberg, P. W., & Guzinski, G. M. (1999). Hysterectomy and sexual functioning. *Journal of the American Medical Association, 282*(20), 1934–1941.

Ringel, M. (1999). Patients with sexual dysfunction: Your guidance makes a difference. *Patient Care for the Nurse Practitioner, 2*(4), 14–24.

Sarwer, D. B., & Durlak, J. A. (1996). Childhood sexual abuse as a predictor of adult female sexual dysfunction: A study of couples seeking sex therapy. *Child Abuse and Neglect, 20*(10), 963–972.

Taneepanichskul, S., Reinprayoon, D, & Jaisamrarm, U. (1999). Effects of DMPA on weight and blood pressure in long-term acceptors. *Contraception, 59*(3), 301–303.

Ullman, S. R. (1997). *Sex seen: The emergence of modern sexuality in America.* Berkeley, CA: University of California Press.

Resources

Infertility

American Society for Reproductive Medicine, 1209 Montgomery Highway, Birmingham, AL 35216, Office: 205-978-5000, http://www.asrm.com

Hannah's Prayer, a Christian network, P.O. Box 5016, Auburn, CA 95604-5016

International Council on Infertility Information Dissemination (INCIID), P.O. Box 6836, Arlington, VA 22206, Voice: 520-544-9548, Fax: 703-379-1593, INCIIDinfo@inciid.org, www.inciid.org

Resolve, 1310 Broadway, Somerville, MA 02144, Business office: 617-623-1156, Helpline: 617-623-0744, http://www.resolve.org

Family Planning

Alan Guttmacher Institute, http://www.agi-usa.com. This organization provides a broad range of information about family planning.

Family Planning Network, http://www.familyplanning.net

Planned Parenthood Federation, http://www.plannedparenthood.org

Sexual Dysfunction

American Association of Sex Educators, Counselors and Therapists (AASECT), P.O. Box 5488, Richmond, VA 23220, http://www.aasect.org

American Psychiatric Association, 1400 K Street, N.W., Washington, DC 20005, http://www.psych.org

American Psychological Association, 750 First Street, N.E., Washington, DC 20002, http://www.apa.org

Society for Human Sexuality, 1122 E. Pike St., Seattle WA 98122, http://www.sexuality.org

CHAPTER 8

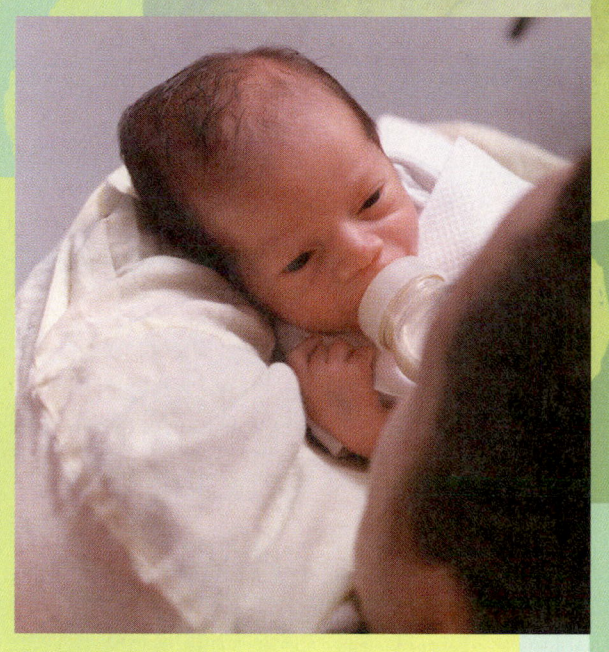

GENETICS AND GENETIC COUNSELING

Genetic counseling has been defined as a specialized type of family counseling related to genetic risks. A great portion of nursing education is dedicated to the teaching and application of mental health methodology. Even if you are not a practicing psychiatric-mental health nurse, you have been exposed to these techniques and approaches during your education. They are extremely helpful in a genetic counseling situation and, as a member of a genetic counseling team, you are contributing invaluable expertise and experience to this process. However, the nurse in a genetic counseling team is often faced with ethical issues that may bring to mind past personal and professional experiences. They require some preparation on the part of the practitioner, and you may want to review, before the occasion, some of your personal and ethical value systems. For example:

- How would you respond to the often-heard questions: "Tell me what you would do in my place" and "Help me make this decision."
- Could you maintain a strictly nondirective approach to counseling? Is it even desirable to be nondirective?
- Are you able to support the decision of a client (for example, not to have amniocentesis in a high-risk genetic situation) that goes against your moral values?
- How do you feel about giving a client referral information that may lead him or her to an outcome contrary to your beliefs?

Key Terms

Allele
Alpha-fetoprotein (AFP)
Amniocentesis
Aneuploidy
Autosome
Chromosome
Clastogen
Cytogenetics
Deletion
Diploid
Dominant
Euploid
Gamete
Gametogenesis
Gene
Genetic counseling
Genotype
Haploid
Hemizygous

Heterozygote
Homologous
Homozygous
Karyotype
Meiosis
Mitosis
Monosomy
Mosaicism
Multifactorial
Mutation
Nondisjunction
Pedigree (Genogram)
Phenotype
Polygenic
Proband
Recessive
Translocation
Trisomy

Competencies

Upon completion of this chapter, the reader should be able to:

1. Discuss the genetic etiology of human disease, emphasizing the difference between gene alterations and chromosomal abnormalities.
2. Discuss the numerical and structural features of chromosomes.
3. Compare and contrast the stages of gamete formation in oogenesis and spermatogenesis.
4. Define and characterize meiotic and mitotic chromosome nondisjunction.
5. Differentiate between euploidy and aneuploidy, and discuss mechanisms that lead to aneuploidies.
6. Discuss the normal function of structural genes and analyze their derangements in Tay-Sachs disease, phenylketonuria, and Lesch-Nyhan syndrome.
7. Differentiate between transmission of alleles in dominant and recessive patterns.
8. Compare characteristics of single-gene and multifactorial inheritance.
9. Describe the major clinical manifestations of selected autosomal and X-linked disorders. Analyze their significance in prenatal testing.
10. Describe the major features of selected disorders that result from numerical and structural chromosomal abnormalities and discuss their effects on women's health care.
11. Analyze the consequences of screening for genetic diseases.
12. Discuss the various elements of genetic counseling and their effect on the family.
13. Compare and contrast various procedures and methods used in prenatal diagnosis.

Medical genetics is a relatively new branch of an old science. Familial occurrences of specific traits have been cited in the literature for centuries. With discoveries in genetic disorders, the focus of genetic research was turned to identifying the protein (enzyme) products of specific genes and to relating them to disease process (Cox & Sinclair, 1997).

The field of cytogenetics, or the study of chromosomes with a special focus on chromosome abnormalities, was launched by the first discovery of a human chromosomal abnormality, trisomy 21, which is the causative event in Down syndrome. Many other chromosomal disorders were subsequently defined, and cytogenetics was the standard working tool of geneticists for many years.

In the early 1960s, the technique of prenatal diagnosis was to be totally revolutionized by the development of genetic amniocentesis. In this technique, a sample of amniotic fluid is removed, and cells that were sloughed off by a developing fetus are studied. This allows geneticists to identify both biochemical defects and chromosome anomalies. The process of genetic counseling, which up to this point was based, at best, on statistical predictions and fixed-risk figures, now could be done on a personal level, as geneticists began to provide genetic information about a specific pregnancy. In the early 1970s, Sarah Lawrence University in New York began to offer the first master's degree program in genetic counseling, with a curriculum based on a strong foundation of genetics and psychology. The addition of gene cloning to the armamentarium of medical genetics set the pace for genetic engineering and potential gene correction of hereditary diseases.

The purpose of this chapter is to provide the reader with baseline essentials of genetics and to awaken an interest in further reading.

CHROMOSOMAL BASIS OF INHERITANCE

A **gene** is a segment of nucleic acid that contains genetic information necessary to control a certain function, such as the synthesis of a polypeptide. A **chromosome** is a filament-like nuclear structure consisting of chromatin that stores genetic information as base sequences in DNA, and whose number is constant in each species. When attempting to generate a list of human genetic disorders, one soon discovers that some are classified under gene alterations (e.g., sickle cell disease, galactosemia, cystic fibrosis), while others represent chromosomal abnormalities (e.g., Turner syndrome; Down syndrome; cri du chat, or cat's cry syndrome). Although such numerical or structural chromosomal aberrations automatically affect large groups of genes, a small gene alteration does not alter chromosome structure and number. Alterations in single genes (single-gene disorders) or even in large groups of genes (polygenic disorders) may be a lesion too small to cause an alteration in chromosomal structure and cannot be identified by karyotype analysis. A **karyotype** is the chromosomal constitution of an individual, which is represented by a laboratory-made display, in which chromosomes are arranged by size and centromere position. This concept is easily understood when one considers that human somatic cells (nucleated cells, with the exception of ova and spermatozoa) contain approximately 100,000 genes, distributed in the form of tightly coiled DNA molecules along 46 chromosomes. If all chromosomes were the same size, each would carry approximately 2,300 genes. However, since human chromosomes vary in size, the larger the chromosome, the greater the number of genes carried. Therefore, the clinical manifestations of numerical chromosome alterations increase in severity in proportion to the increasing size of the involved chromosome. For example, a **trisomy** (a condition caused by the presence of an extra chromosome that is added to a given chromosome pair and results in a total number of 47 chromosomes per cell) in which the extra chromosome is one of the smallest size, group G (Down syndrome, or trisomy 21), produces malformations that are much more compatible with life than a trisomy involving a larger chromosome, group D (Patau syndrome, or trisomy 13).

Chromosome Number and Structure

When grouped in a karyotype (Figure 8-1) for cytogenetic analysis, somatic cell chromosomes, usually derived from small lymphocytes collected from circulating blood, are arranged according to size (groups A through G, in

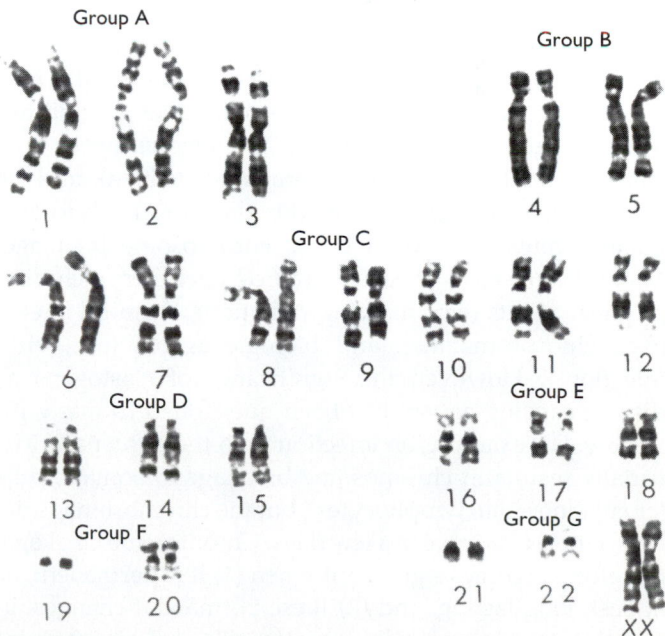

Figure 8-1 Karyotype of a human female cell. Chromosomes obtained from a peripheral blood lymphocyte culture. (Courtesy of Dr. David Ledbetter, Department of Human Genetics, University of Chicago)

> ### Nursing Tip *Genetic Counseling*
>
> Nurses need additional preparation to act as genetic counselors. All nurses, however, should be alert for women or families who might benefit from genetic counseling. Additionally, nurses should assess family reactions to genetic disorders and consider engaging other members of the health care team.

decreasing size) and position of the centromere (metacentric, submetacentric, and acrocentric chromosomes). Group A chromosomes consist of pairs 1 through 3, group B include pairs 4 and 5, and group C include pairs 6 through 12; groups D (pairs 13 to 15) and G (pairs 21 and 22) are the large and small acrocentric chromosomes, respectively; group E contain pairs 16 to 18; and group F include pairs 19 and 20. The X chromosome approximates the size and shape of a group C pair, and the Y chromosome is similar to a group G chromosome. Short chromosome arms are designated as *p* (for *petit*, or small in French), long arms as *q*. This nomenclature allows for quick recognition of chromosomal structural features or abnormalities. For example, the designation 46, XX, B(5)p⁻ indicates a deletion (⁻) of a portion of the small arm (p) of chromosome pair number 5 of the B group, occurring in a female (XX) with a normal chromosome number (46). This is the typical chromosome pattern found in the cri du chat (cat's cry) syndrome. When stained with special techniques, each homologous chromosome pair displays a different, constant pattern of banding (e.g., Giemsa stain banding as depicted in Figure 8-1). Banding techniques, developed in the early 1970s, allow the exact classification of chromosomes in groups and the identification of alterations in chromosome structure, such as deletions and translocations. The term **deletion** refers to the loss of chromosomal material, and **translocation** is the misplacement of genetic material from one chromosome to another.

Patterns of Chromosome Anomalies

The normal structure of chromosomes is subject to alterations that result from breakage and rearrangement. Chromosome breakage has long been recognized as a significant source of genetic abnormalities. The term **clastogen** (i.e., chromosome-breaking agent, from *clastos*, to break, and the suffix, *gen*, an agent) was coined in the early 1970s to designate agents that could cause chromosome breakage. Many clastogens have been identified since then, including physical agents (e.g., ionizing radiation), chemical agents (e.g., chlorpromazine), and biologic agents (e.g., viral infections). However, the significance of clastogens as disease-causing agents has been questioned in many instances. For example, an infection with the influenza virus usually results in chromosome breakage in somatic cells (circulating small lymphocytes), but the chromosome structures return to normal in a few days. Chromosome breakage, therefore, becomes significant when (1) it is permanent, or at best, long-lasting; and (2) these permanent changes, in addition to appearing in somatic cells, are also present in germ cells and thus have the potential of being transmitted to the offspring. Figure 8-2 depicts some of the possible consequences of chromosome breakage.

Chromosome breakage resulting in loss of the broken fragment is termed "chromosome deletion," which may have significant clinical consequences, such as cri du chat syndrome. In addition, chromosome breakage may also result in unstable end points ("sticky ends"), which predisposes chromosomes to a variety of rearrangements of the resulting fragments. One such rearrangement is a translocation, by which a chromosomal fragment reunites with another nonhomologous chromosome. Two types of translocations have clinical significance: reciprocal and robertsonian. In a reciprocal translocation, breaks occur in two different chromosomes and the fragments are mutually exchanged, resulting in derivative chromosomes. Robertsonian translocations occur when the short arms of two acrocentric chromosomes (pairs 13 to 15 of group D, and pairs 21 and 22 of group G) are lost, and the remaining long arms fuse at the centromere, forming a "single

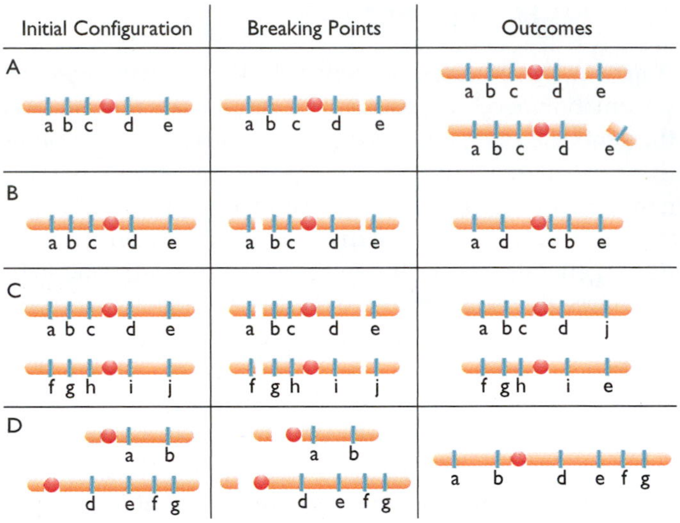

Figure 8-2   Examples of structural rearrangements after chromosomal breakage. Initial chromosome constitution, breaking points, and consequences of the breaks and rearrangements are shown. In panel A, a break occurs between markers *d* and *e*. Three consequences are: the resulting chromosomes, bearing markers *a* through *d* have undergone a deletion. The severed fragment may stay aligned with the rest (top example), the space being narrower than the length of the fragment: chromosome gap. Or it may be lost (bottom example): chromosome break. In panel B, the initial chromosome suffers two breaks (between markers *a* and *b* and between *d* and *e*). The center portion undergoes a pericentric inversion, resulting in a newly arranged chromosome, in which the markers are sequenced *a*, *d*, *c*, *b*, and *e*. Panel C depicts an exchange of genetic material between chromosomes bearing markers *a* through *e* and *f* through *j*. Since no genetic material was lost, only rearranged, this is termed a balanced translocation. Panel D represents a robertsonian translocation between two acrocentric chromosomes (one from group G, the small chromosome, the other from group D, the large chromosome). Loss of the short arms and fusion at the centromere results in a translocated chromosome. If no significant genetic material is lost, this is also a balanced translocation, causing no clinical manifestations.

chromosome." Both types result in individuals who have the same amount of genetic information, although "rearranged," and therefore no clinical manifestations are expected. These persons are termed "balanced translocation carriers." However, if this person reproduces, there is a chance that the translocated chromosome will be present in the gamete that undergoes fertilization by a normal gamete. The resulting zygote will have a gene imbalance caused by the extra chromosomal (genetic) material, and the child will be at risk for physical and mental abnormalities.

Distribution of Chromosomes during Cell Division

Human somatic cells are **diploid** (a cell which contains two copies of each chromosome). Such a diploid chromosome number is represented by the notation 2n=46. A **haploid** chromosome constitution (n=23) is found in germ cells, the male and female **gametes** (spermatozoa and ova). Somatic cell chromosomes are represented by 44 **autosomes** (the 22 pairs of chromosomes, which do not greatly influence sex determination at conception) and two sex chromosomes, XX in females and XY in males. As somatic cells multiply by **mitosis**, each daughter cell receives the same chromosome number as the initial cell. This equitable chromosome sharing results from a phenomenon termed "disjunction." During anaphase, chromatids of each chromosome separate and migrate to opposite poles of the cell, guided by microtubules of the mitotic spindle

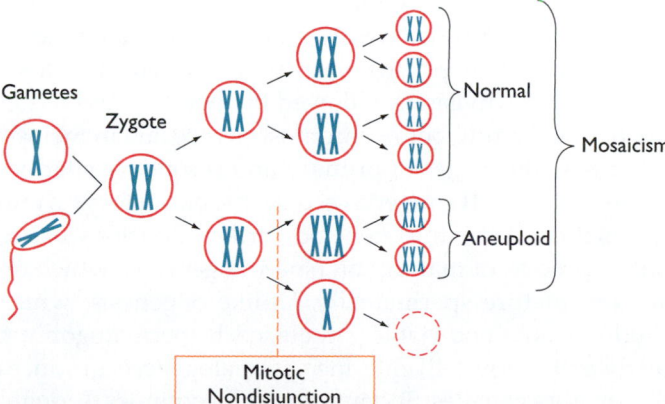

Figure 8-3   Consequences of chromosome nondisjunction occurring during mitosis, after a normal zygote was formed by fertilization of two normal gametes. (Only one chromosome pair is represented.) Following the first mitosis, the upper cell originates a normal line of cells with the correct chromosome number. The bottom cell undergoes nondisjunction, resulting in a line of cells with one extra chromosome. (The monosomic cell is not viable and there are no further divisions.) The outcome is a mosaic individual with two cell lines, one containing the normal chromosome number, the other aneuploid.

(Figure 8-3). Disruption of this orderly chromosome distribution occurs in **nondisjunction**. Through failure of homologous chromosomes or chromatids to separate properly during meiotic (meiosis I or II) or mitotic anaphase, daughter cells will have different chromosome numbers (e.g., 45 and 47, instead of 46 and 46). Cells that are **monosomic** (the aneuploid condition of having a chromosome represented by a single copy in a somatic cell) tend to degenerate and die, but those with the extra chromosome (trisomic) continue to divide and generate a complete line of trisomic cells.

Mitotic Nondisjunction and Mosaicism

When mitotic nondisjunction occurs during embryonic development, the trisomic cell line multiplies rapidly with the normal cell line, and an individual with **mosaicism** for that particular chromosome results. Mosaicism, therefore, results in an individual (mosaic) with two or more genetically different cell populations. The chromosomal notation for a male with a mosaic type of Down syndrome, for example, is 46, XY/47, XY, G(21)$^+$. The slash (/) indicates a dual cell population, in which one has the normal chromosomal constitution (46, XY), while the other carries the extra G(21) chromosome ($^+$) and has a total number of 47 chromosomes.

Oogenesis and Spermatogenesis

The halving of chromosome number that occurs in **gametogenesis** (a series of mitotic and meiotic divisions occurring in the gonads that leads to the production of gametes) takes place during the first division (meiosis I) of meiosis. **Meiosis** is a reductional type of cell division, in which the chromosome number is halved. The second division (meiosis II) is an equational, mitosis-like cell division. As somatic chromosomes are shared by the products of the first meiotic division, each daughter cell receives one member of each autosomal pair and one of the sex chromosomes (either the X or the Y). As a result, women can form only X-bearing ova, but men can produce X-bearing and Y-bearing spermatozoa.

Oogenesis

The process of oogenesis (Figure 8-4) begins during prenatal development and comprises three main phases: cell proliferation by mitosis, reduction of chromosome number and genetic recombination through meiosis, and maturation of oocytes. During fetal development, early germ cells divide by mitosis until the stages of oogonia and primary oocytes are reached. These cells still have a diploid chromosome number (2n=26). Primary oocytes then enter meiosis I and, at birth, they are found at an arrested stage, termed "dictyotene," which persists until puberty. Starting at menarche, shortly before each ovulation, the primary

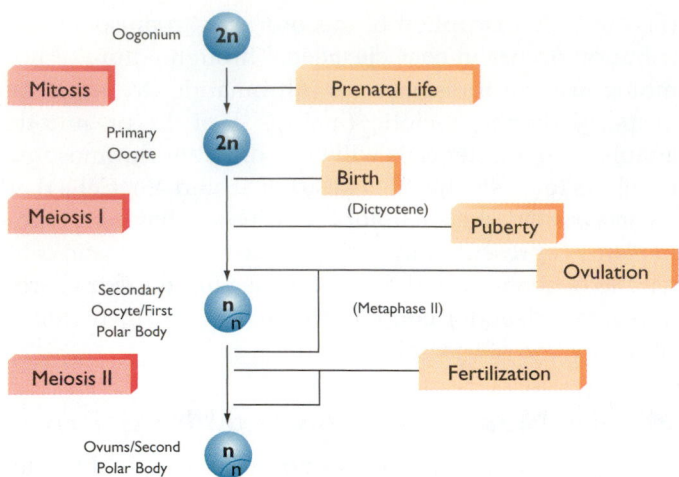

Figure 8-4   Oogenesis. Depicted here are the various types of cell division, the resulting cell types, and the time elapsed from primordial oogonium to mature ovum. First ovum is released at menarche, the last one immediately before menopause. Permanence of the latter in the ovary, approximately 52 years.

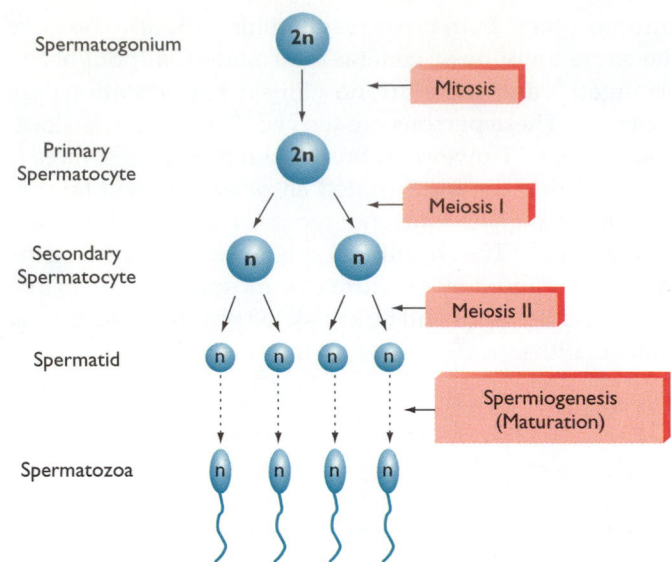

Figure 8-5   Spermatogenesis. Different cell divisions and resulting cells. Approximate time elapsed from spermatogonia to mature spermatozoa is 75 days, followed by a further 10 to 12 days of maturation in the epididymis.

oocyte resumes cell division and completes meiosis I, now with the number of chromosomes reduced to the haploid number (n=23). The outcome of meiosis I is one secondary oocyte and one first polar body. At ovulation, the nucleus of the secondary oocyte initiates meiosis II (the first polar body degenerates). At this point, if fertilization does not occur, the secondary oocyte degenerates and dies without completing meiosis II. However, if fertilization occurs, the nucleus of the secondary oocyte resumes and completes meiosis II as the male pronucleus approaches it. The product of meiosis II is one ovum and one secondary polar body (which later degenerates). The female pronucleus contained in the ovum now fuses with the (haploid) male pronucleus and forms a diploid zygote, which evolves into the embryo, fetus, and newborn infant.

Of the approximately 2 million oocytes present at birth, only about 300,000 are present at puberty. Of these, only approximately 400 reach full maturity, which ends in monthly ovulation during reproductive years. The remaining follicular units undergo progressive atresia, by apoptosis, a physiologic phenomenon that persists throughout those years. From a genetic perspective, the long duration of the first meiotic division, while the oocyte continues its metabolic functions, may be responsible, at least in part, for the occurrence of meiotic errors, such as nondisjunction. From a teratogenic viewpoint, an ovum fertilized at an advanced age has remained in the ovaries since birth and therefore has been exposed to a variety of environmental (internal and external) influences. This long-term exposure may account for the linear relationship between maternal age and birth defects discussed later.

Spermatogenesis

Unlike oogenesis, in which oocytes are produced prenatally, the process of sperm production only begins at puberty (Figure 8-5). As in oogenesis, three sequential steps can be identified in spermatogenesis: intense cell proliferation by mitosis, the recombination and reduction events of meiosis, and spermiogenesis (maturation of spermatozoa). At puberty, testicular endocrine cells, called Leydig cells or interstitial cells, increase in number and begin to produce testosterone, which initiates spermatogenesis. The process of spermatogenesis is characterized by a series of mitotic divisions, followed by meiosis I and II. Reduction in the number of chromosomes occurs in meiosis I, between the stages of primary and secondary spermatocytes. Meiosis II converts secondary spermatocytes into spermatids. After this step, no further divisions occur, only a process of maturation (spermiogenesis), which results in mature spermatozoa. Unlike oogenesis, which produces only one viable gamete, each spermatogonium (early male germ cell) entering spermatogenesis produces four mature gametes. Spermatogenesis continues throughout a lifetime, but declines with age.

Meiotic Nondisjunction and Aneuploidy

Meiotic nondisjunction is a major cause of **aneuploidy**, an abnormal chromosome pattern in which the total number of chromosomes is not a multiple of the haploid number, n = 23. Nondisjunction can occur during meiosis I and II, during both oogenesis and spermatogenesis, resulting in gametes with an aneuploid chromosome number (for ex-

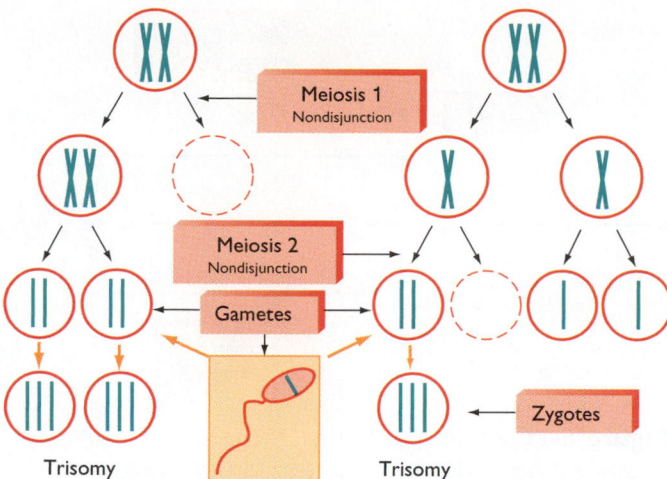

Figure 8-6   Outcomes of meiotic chromosome nondisjunction occurring during meiosis 1 (left) and meiosis 2 (right). (Only one chromosome pair is represented.) Nondisjunction at meiosis 1 results in one aneuploid and one monosomic cell (which does not survive). Meiosis 2 produces two aneuploid gametes, which, on fertilization by normal, euploid gametes, will produce trisomic zygotes. Likewise, nondisjunction at meiosis 2 also results in aneuploid gametes, and subsequently in trisomic zygotes.

ample, 22 and 24, instead of 23 and 23) (Figure 8-6). As in the case of somatic cells, gametes lacking a chromosome are not likely to survive. The gametes with an extra chromosome are more viable, and on fertilization, a normal gamete will produce an aneuploid zygote. The most common aneuploidies in humans are trisomies. For example, as a result of meiotic nondisjunction, a spermatozoon carrying an extra G(21) chromosome, that is, 24, X or Y, G(21)$^+$ may fertilize an ovum with a normal chromosomal constitution, 23, X. The result will be a zygote with 47 chromosomes, including the extra G(21), which will develop into an infant with Down syndrome, or G(21) trisomy. The chromosome notation for a female with free trisomy-type Down syndrome, for example, is 47, XX, G(21)$^+$. Unlike the mosaic case described, all somatic cells in this person contain the extra G(21) chromosome. The addition of one chromosome to one of the pairs (trisomy) creates a relatively small aneuploid alteration in the total chromosome number (46 to 47), which is usually quite compatible with life. However, the addition of one or more chromosomes to each pair (increments of the haploid number, 23) results in triploid cells with 69 chromosomes (46+23) or tetraploid cells with 92 chromosomes (46+23+23). The product of this uniform addition of chromosomes to all of the original pairs is termed euploidy. A **euploid** cell is one whose chromosome number is a multiple of 23. But even in the case of triploid individuals (3n=69) the genetic imbalance is of such magnitude that the few infants who are carried to term have severe mul-

tiple abnormalities that limit their life span to a few hours or days.

GENE STRUCTURE AND FUNCTION

Genes are sequences of DNA that determine a certain biologic function. Many are structural genes and carry the necessary information to promote the synthesis of proteins (polypeptides). Others are regulatory and control the function of other genes or groups of genes. A **mutation** (alteration) of a structural gene may result in the synthesis of an abnormal protein (e.g., enzyme) with potential clinical consequences. The following four figures illustrate some mechanisms of gene-protein interaction. Figure 8-7 represents the normal metabolic conversion of a substance A into an end-product K, via by-products B, C, D, and so on. Enzymes b and c, whose synthesis is controlled by genes β and δ, catalyze steps B $\Rightarrow$ C, and C $\Rightarrow$ D, respectively. A feedback loop ensures physiologic levels of K.

In Figure 8-8, a mutation has occurred in gene β, preventing normal (quantitative or qualitative) synthesis of enzyme b, and the consequent interruption of the pathway between B and C. Continuous uptake of A will

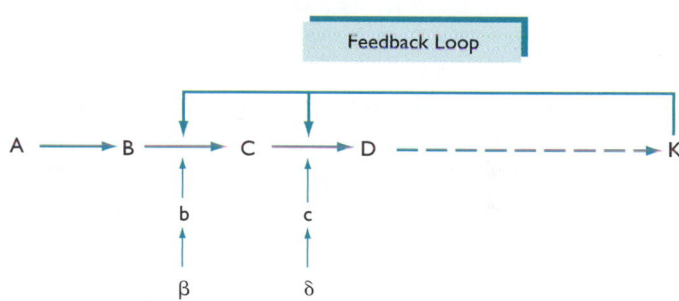

Figure 8-7   Normal sequence of events in the metabolic conversion of product *A* into end product *K*, mediated by enzymes *b* and *c*, which are encoded by genes β and δ, respectively.

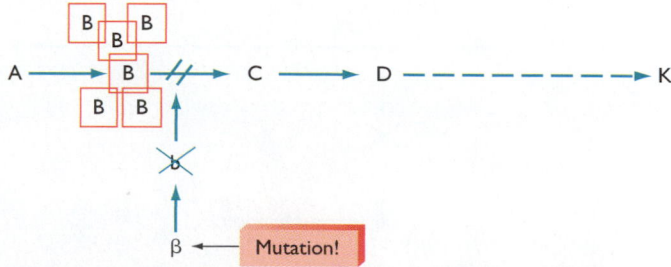

Figure 8-8   Consequences of a mutation in gene β resulting in lack of enzyme *b*, interruption of the metabolic pathway, and accumulation of by-product *B*. Prototype gene dysfunction in Tay-Sachs disease.

produce two results: accumulation of B, and depletion of all products beyond the block. An example of this situation is Tay-Sachs disease (a GM_2 gangliosidosis): mutation of the Tay-Sachs gene (β) causes the lack of the enzyme hexosaminidase A (HexA), represented by (b), and whose absence results in accumulation of ganglioside GM_2 (B) in nerve cells, producing all the clinical manifestations of this progressive neurologic disorder.

Figure 8-9 depicts a mutation in gene δ, blocking the synthesis of enzyme c, and interrupting the metabolic conversion of C into D. In this instance, an alternative pathway $C \Rightarrow E \Rightarrow F$ is opened. This event may have two outcomes: product F may eventually be converted into K, with no significant clinical consequences, or F may represent the end point to the alternative pathway and begin to accumulate until it reaches toxic levels. The example here is phenylketonuria (PKU), an inborn error of metabolism that creates an intolerance to the amino acid phenylalanine. The missing enzyme here (c), which results from mutation in the PKU gene (δ), is phenylalanine hydroxylase. The alternative pathway leads to the formation and accumulation of phenylketones (F), which, in combination with phenylalanine deficiency, prevents the postnatal completion of myelination of nerves and results in profound mental retardation.

Figure 8-10 represents a genetic alteration of the enzyme d, which mediates the feedback loop controlling ideal concentrations of K. As a result, K may accumulate to toxic levels. The prototype genetic disease here is Lesch-Nyhan syndrome, in which d is the enzyme hypoxanthine-guanine phosphoribosyl transferase (HGPRT) and K is uric acid. Accumulation of uric acid to extremely high levels, plus HGPRT deficiency, results in mental retardation and a tendency for self-mutilation in affected persons.

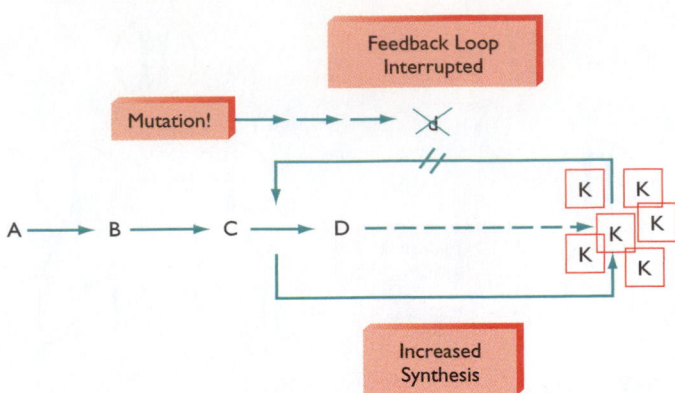

Figure 8-10   Consequences of a mutation in the gene encoding for enzyme *d*, which is involved in the feedback control loop for end-product *K*. As a result, increased synthesis of *K* is observed, eventually reaching toxic levels. Prototype gene dysfunction in Lesch-Nyhan syndrome.

SINGLE-GENE (MENDELIAN) INHERITANCE

The concept of gene, by definition, does not determine the expression of that gene. A gene is defined as a segment of nucleic acid that contains genetic information necessary to control a certain function, such as the synthesis of a polypeptide. For example, the gene for Tay-Sachs disease is a site on a chromosome that controls the synthesis of the enzyme HexA. The possible expressions of this gene would be HexA$^+$, indicating the command for synthesis of HexA, or HexA$^-$, indicating the lack of such command, resulting in the absence of the enzyme. Such alternate forms of gene expression are termed **alleles** of the gene HexA. The genetic constitution of an individual at any given locus is called **genotype**, whereas the expression of that gene's function in terms of measurable or observable features of the individual is termed **phenotype**. Whether or not a gene is expressed in the phenotype depends on the arrangement of its alleles and on the concepts of dominance and recessivity. A mutation in the original, or "wild-type" allele, in this case HexA$^+$, may result in a different allele, such as HexA$^-$.

Dominant Gene Inheritance Pattern

Consider a gene with two alleles, the normal ("wild-type") represented by (+), and the mutant allele represented by (−). Figure 8-11 illustrates the three possible arrangements for the alleles in persons carrying that gene. Represented here are pairs of somatic **homologous** chromosomes (chromosomes with matching genes) where that gene is located. The model may also be used to illustrate

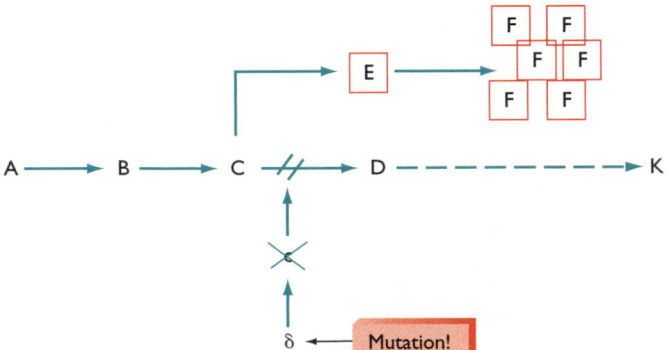

Figure 8-9   Consequences of a mutation in gene δ, resulting in lack of enzyme *c*, interruption of the metabolic pathway, and opening of an alternate pathway. The outcome is accumulation of by-product *F*. Prototype gene dysfunction in phenylketonuria (PKU).

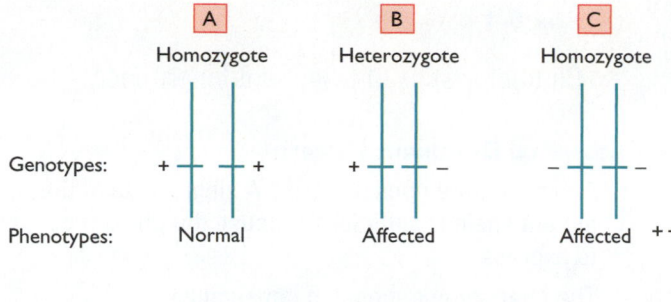

Figure 8-11   Dominant inheritance pattern. Schematic of the three possible allelic arrangements of a dominant gene: genotypes and possible phenotypes. Note absence of carrier state.

the X chromosome pair in women. The first individual (A) received from each parent a copy of the normal allele (+/+). The second person (B) received from one parent one copy of the normal allele and from the other, one copy of the mutated allele (+/–). The third person (C) received from each parent a copy of the mutated allele (–/–). These are the only possible mathematical combinations, given one gene with two alleles. Persons (A) and (C) are **homozygous** for either allele (+/+) or (–/–). A homozygous person, or homozygote, is an individual possessing a pair of identical alleles of a given gene. Person (B) is termed a **heterozygote**, that is, an individual who has two different alleles at a given locus (+/–).

Now, imagine determining by physical examination the phenotypes of these three individuals. Person (A) carries normal alleles and displays a normal phenotype. Person (C) has only mutant alleles and exhibits an affected phenotype. Person (B), the heterozygote, also displays an affected phenotype, but the clinical manifestations in person (C), the homozygote for the mutant alleles, are more severe. When this type of correlation between genotypes and observed phenotypes is obtained, the mode of inheritance is termed **dominant**. This term implies that in the heterozygote (person B) the expression of the mutant allele dominates over the expression of the normal allele. In other words, in the case of dominant genes, the presence of one copy of the mutant allele is sufficient to express the phenotype. And by extension, two copies of the mutant allele bring about a more accentuated expression of that characteristic. In summary, a dominant allele is one that is phenotypically expressed in single copy (heterozygote) and in double copy (homozygote).

In addition to the patterns of phenotypic expression described above, conditions exist that may cause a variation of expression. These include incomplete penetrance and variable expressivity.

A gene is said to have reduced or incomplete penetrance in a population when a proportion of persons who possess that gene do not express the phenotype. Usually, those who do express the affected phenotype have a complete expression of the phenotype, with all features of the syndrome present. A gene is said to have variable expressivity when individuals possessing that gene display the features of the syndrome in various degrees of expression, from mild to severe.

Vertical Transmission of Dominant Genes

A clear understanding of transmission patterns requires a few general guidelines. First of all, most genetic diseases are rare. The probability that two affected persons will produce offspring is very low for most diseases (exceptions to this rule are discussed later). Second, depending on the disease, if one parent is affected, he or she is much more likely to be heterozygous (+/–) than homozygous (–/–) for the mutant allele. Usually, an individual homozygous for the mutant allele experiences physical or mental abnormalities at a much more severe level. Those assumptions being accepted, two questions remain:

1. What are the chances for transmitting the mutant allele to the offspring?
2. What are the risks for the offspring being affected?

The outcomes of these matings are best expressed by the use of Punnett squares (Figure 8-12).

An individual who is homozygous for the mutant allele of a dominant gene (–/–) may contribute that allele (–) to all of his or her offspring. Since a single copy of the

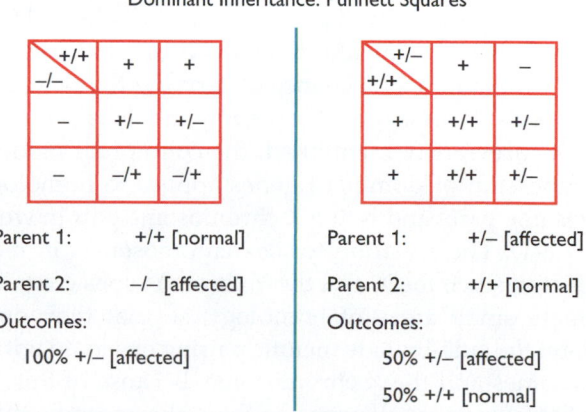

Figure 8-12   Punnett squares depicting transmission of a dominant gene and resulting offspring's genotypes and phenotypes. Genotypes of the parents (top left cell), the possible gametes produced by each parent (single symbols), and the result of their random combination at fertilization. Possible outcomes in each pregnancy.

mutant allele is sufficient for the expression of the phenotype, all children will be affected, regardless of the genotype of the other parent. Panel 1 of Figure 8-12 illustrates the mating of such an affected homozygote with an unaffected partner. However, because of the often severe physical and mental signs found in an affected homozygote, the mating represented in panel 2 is more often encountered. Here, an affected heterozygote (+/−) will have equal chances of contributing the mutant allele (−) or the normal allele (+) to the offspring. (Random chromosome segregation during meiosis results in half of all gametes carrying the mutant allele and half carrying the normal allele.) Any time the mutant allele (−) of a dominant gene is transmitted to the offspring, the phenotype is expressed, regardless of the genotype of the other partner. Since most genetic disorders are rare, the mating illustrated in panel 2 of Figure 8-12, in which the other parent is unaffected (+/+), is representative of the majority of cases. In such mating, each pregnancy carries a 50% chance of being affected (+/+) and a 50% chance of being unaffected (−/−). These probability figures are fixed for each time conception occurs in the same set of parents, because each pregnancy is a statistically independent event.

However rare dominant diseases may be, in some circumstances, the symptoms brought about by the condition, serve to bring affected individuals together and increase their social interaction. One such example is achondroplasia. Because of their short stature, achondroplastic dwarfs tend to associate with persons who have the same syndrome. Here again the homozygote for the mutant allele (−/−) is often not carried to term or is born with severe malformations (e.g., hydrocephaly). Therefore, even in the absence of genotype determination, it is more likely that two socially adept achondroplastic dwarfs are both heterozygotes (+/−). In such cases, each pregnancy produced by this couple has a 25% chance of being genotypically and phenotypically unaffected (+/+), a 50% chance of being affected with dwarfism like the parents (+/−), and a 25% chance of carrying the severe stigmata of the homozygote for the mutant allele (−/−).

As previously mentioned, the conceptual model for transmission of dominant genes applies to homologous autosome pairs and to the X chromosome pair in women (Box 8-1). The situation for sex chromosomes in men is different, since the X and the Y chromosomes contain extremely small areas of homology, so that they do not exhibit the side-by-side meiotic pairing observed with the autosomes and the X chromosome. Because of this, men are **hemizygous** for all genes on the X chromosome that do not have a homologous site on the Y, and their alleles are represented as single copies. Therefore, in the inheritance of an X-linked dominant gene, the single-copy presence of its normal or mutant allele results in the expression of the normal or mutant phenotype, respectively.

Box 8-1

Characteristics of Dominant Inheritance

Autosomal Dominant Pattern*

1. A carrier state does not exist. A single dose of the mutant allele is sufficient to cause the phenotype to express.
2. The phenotype appears in consecutive generations. Affected persons tend to have an affected parent.
3. Children of an affected parent have a 50% chance of inheriting the mutant allele and being affected.
4. Phenotypically normal persons in a family pedigree are free of the mutant allele and do not transmit the phenotype to their offspring.
5. Both males and females are equally likely to be affected.
6. Homozygotes for the mutant allele are likely to be more severely affected.

X-Linked Dominant Pattern*

1. Both males and females can be affected, but women are usually less severely affected than men.
2. Affected males do not transmit the mutant allele to their sons.
3. All daughters of an affected male are affected and have a 50% chance of passing the mutant allele to their sons and daughters.

Unless otherwise specified, affected persons' partners are unaffected.

Recessive Gene Inheritance Pattern

The term **recessive** suggests the idea of "hidden" or "occult." In a genetic connotation, it reflects the behavior (expression) of the mutant allele in the heterozygote. A recessive allele is one whose phenotypic expression occurs in a homozygous or hemizygous condition; in the heterozygote, a recessive allele is masked by its dominant homologous counterpart. For example, Figure 8-13 illustrates the relationships between genotypic and phenotypic expression of a recessive gene with two alleles, (+) representing the normal or "wild-type" allele and (−) representing the mutated allele. Here again, the concepts apply to autosome pairs and the X chromosome pair in females. In the expression of a recessive gene, individuals (A) and (B) display both a normal (unaffected) phenotype, and only (C), who inherited two mutant alleles from both parents, is affected. This means that a recessive disease can

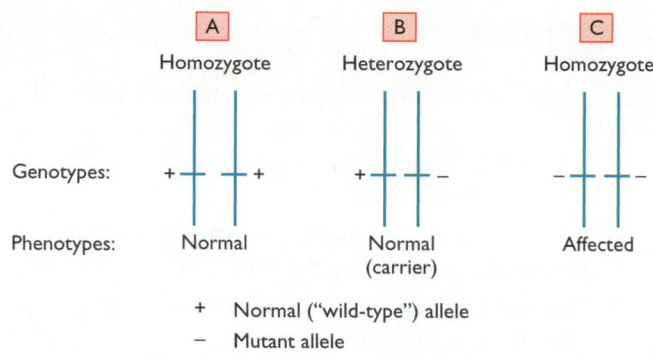

Figure 8-13   Recessive Inheritance Pattern. Schematic of the three possible allelic arrangements of a recessive gene. Genotypes and possible phenotypes. Note the introduction of a heterozygous carrier (B).

only be phenotypically expressed when two copies of the mutant allele are present, and, therefore, both parents must equally contribute to this outcome. In other words, in the heterozygote, the mutant allele is recessive (hidden), and the effect of the normal allele predominates (dominates), causing a normal phenotype to express. The difference between (A) and (B), however, is significant; whereas (A) can produce only gametes (ova or spermatozoa) with normal alleles, (B) carries the mutant allele and thus 50% of the gametes produced transmit this allele. This situation illustrates the concept of carriers for a genetic disease, that is, individuals who are clinically normal (or nearly normal), but who are potential transmitters of the disease.

Identification of such carriers is of paramount importance for genetic counseling. In the case of an unaffected couple who produce a child with a recessive disease, identification is easy. Because they each must contribute a mutant allele, they must be considered obligate carriers, even in the absence of specific carrier testing for that gene. Specific tests to detect heterozygous carriers of a variety of genetic diseases are available, but it would be impractical and certainly not cost-effective to screen all prospective parents without specific risk factors with all available tests. Genetic screening for carriers is usually limited to populations at risk, either because they belong to a high-risk group for a certain disorder (e.g., Ashkenazi Jews and Tay-Sachs disease) or because of a family history. Carriers for certain specific disorders can be identified by tests before conception (e.g., sickle cell disease), by means of routine screening, or after conception by means of prenatal diagnosis (e.g., Tay-Sachs disease).

Vertical Transmission of Recessive Genes

One of the most common situations in clinical practice is that of an asymptomatic couple who produce a child with a recessive disorder. Most people who seek genetic counseling fall into this category. The surprise element of this scenario is understandable if the following factors are considered:

1. Genetic disorders are rare, and, therefore, the chances that both parents will be heterozygous for the same gene are remote.

2. Many people remain childless for years, or they may have produced healthy children before the one affected and are unaware that they carry a harmful gene.

3. Even when both parents are carriers, the transmission by each parent of the mutant allele (which results in an affected child) does not always occur.

Box 8-2 summarizes characteristics of recessive inheritance.

Box 8-2

Characteristics of Recessive Inheritance

Autosomal Recessive Pattern*

1. A carrier state exists; both males and females can be carriers.

2. Both males and females are equally likely to be affected.

3. The disease appears to "skip a generation." Members of that generation who have affected children are asymptomatic carriers.

4. Carrier parents have a 25% chance to produce an affected child in each pregnancy.

5. Parent consanguinity (mating between blood relatives) may be a factor when a child is affected with a *rare* recessive disease.

X-Linked Recessive Pattern*

1. Most affected persons are male; affected females are extremely rare.

2. Male-to-male transmission of the X-linked mutant allele does not occur. Males transmit their X chromosomes to their daughters.

3. All daughters of an affected male are (heterozygous) **carriers**, none are **affected** (homozygotes).

4. Sons of carrier females have a 50% chance of inheriting the mutant allele and being **affected** (hemizygotes). Daughters have a 50% risk of inheriting the mutant allele and being (heterozygous) **carriers**.

Unless otherwise specified, all affected or carrier persons' partners are normal.

Recessive Inheritance: Punnett Squares

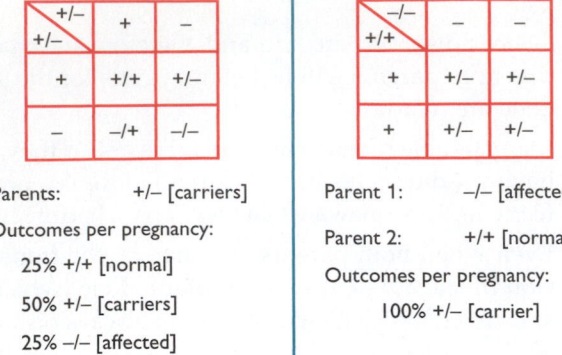

Parents: +/− [carriers]

Outcomes per pregnancy:

   25% +/+ [normal]

   50% +/− [carriers]

   25% −/− [affected]

Parent 1:   −/− [affected]

Parent 2:   +/+ [normal]

Outcomes per pregnancy:

   100% +/− [carrier]

Figure 8-14   Punnett squares depicting transmission of a recessive gene and resulting offspring's genotypes and phenotypes. The genotypes of the parents (top left cell), the possible gametes produced by each parent (single symbols), and the result of their random combination at fertilization. Results are possible outcomes in each pregnancy.

As with dominant inheritance, the best visualization of transmission of recessive genes is obtained through Punnett squares. Panel 1 of Figure 8-14 illustrates the example described previously. Both parents are asymptomatic heterozygous carriers (+/−) for a recessive gene. On forming gametes, each parent has a 50% chance of passing on the mutant allele (−). Random combination of these alleles during conception results, in each pregnancy, in a 25% chance of producing a child with a normal phenotype (+/+), a 50% chance of producing an asymptomatic carrier like themselves (+/−), and only a 25% chance of producing an affected child (−/−). Panel 2 of Figure 8-14 demonstrates that even when one of the parents is affected (−/−), the other parent's genotypically normal (+/+) contribution ensures that they cannot produce an affected child (−/−). All their children will be carriers (+/−). However, in very common diseases, such as sickle cell disease among Blacks, it is possible that an affected person (−/−) and a heterozygous carrier (+/−) will produce an affected child (−/−). The risk for this event in every pregnancy is 50%, with another 50% probability of producing a carrier (+/−) that is, 50% carrier/50% affected.

POLYGENIC AND MULTIFACTORIAL INHERITANCE

Risk calculation with single-gene disorders follows strict Mendelian rules and is fairly straightforward. However, very few phenotypes are completely controlled by the action of a single gene. The majority of traits in the human body are controlled by several genes working together to produce the final effect; these are **polygenic** traits. When environmental factors also contribute to the expression of

Box 8-3

Characteristics of Multifactorial Inheritance

1. No clearly defined pattern of inheritance exists within a single family.
2. The recurrence risk increases when more than one family member has the trait.
3. The recurrence risk increases with increasing severity of the malformation.
4. The recurrence risk increases with consanguinous parents (mating between blood relatives).

the phenotype, these are **multifactorial** traits. One of the primary characteristics of polygenic and multifactorial inheritance is the existence of a *continuous variation* in the trait, as opposed to an all-or-nothing distribution: for example, distribution of height or the distribution of various body shapes. Box 8-3 summarizes characteristics of multifactorial inheritance.

Included in the many pathologic conditions that are polygenic and multifactorial in nature are coronary artery disease, diabetes mellitus, hypertension, obesity, and common psychiatric illnesses, such as schizophrenia and bipolar disorder. Even though an undeniable genetic predisposition to these conditions exists, they are heavily influenced by environmental factors, such as lifestyle, dietary habits, and stressful events.

Risk determination in polygenic and multifactorial inheritance is made on the basis of *empirical observation* of a large number of cases, followed by a specific statistical analysis for each trait. For several disorders, risk prediction and determination tables exist that take into consideration family history, number of cases in the family, and extent or severity of the malformations. By consulting these tables, the nurse and other clinicians can help clients understand the likelihood of genetic disorders occurring in future pregnancies.

SINGLE-GENE DISORDERS

By comparison with multifactorial inheritance, single-gene disorders are in the minority. However, precise molecular information has been developed using monogenic disorders as a framework. The work of Ingram (1956) on sickle cell disease is a clear example. McKusick's latest (2000) online cataloguing of *Online Mendelian Inheritance in Man* (OMIM) lists 11,807 single-gene disorders, of which 11,072 are autosomal, 637 are X-linked, 38 are Y-linked, and the remaining 60 result from mitochondrial gene action (see Resources). Table 8-1 lists some examples of monogenic disorders, their mode of inheritance, and frequency of occurrence.

Autosomal Dominant Disorders

Selected autosomal dominant disorders are discussed in this section, including achondroplasia, Ehlers-Danlos syndrome, familial hypercholesterolemia. Marfan syndrome, neurofibromatosis (type 1), osteogenesis imperfecta, and polycystic kidney disease.

Achondroplasia

The most common form of dwarfism (adult stature, 48 to 52 inches) is achondroplasia, characterized by shortened limbs, especially proximally (rhizomelia), and a normal length torso. Common features include lordosis, prominent forehead with flattened nasal bridge, and short hands with stubby fingers. Life span and IQ are within normal limits among heterozygotes. One of the common complaints is backaches and there is an increased risk of

spinal cord compression. Gynecologic problems include premature menarche, enlarged breasts, and premature menopause. Pregnancy often results in increased mechanical and locomotive burden. Skeletal malformations also affect the normal progress of pregnancy and delivery: because of a small chest cavity, harmful cardiorespiratory conditions may develop, and because of a contracted pelvis, delivery by cesarean section is often recommended. Increased paternal age may be a factor in producing a child with achondroplasia.

Ehlers-Danlos Syndrome

This genetic disease is an umbrella term for a group (with nine subtypes) of disorders of connective tissue that result in hyperelasticity of skin, hyperflexible joints, vascular fragility, and poor wound healing. Common complications include a tendency, for bruising, hernias, and varicose veins, all of which increase during pregnancy. Poor wound healing and a predisposition to hemorrhaging are risk factors during and after delivery (e.g., an episiotomy may be complicated by these factors). The life span may

Table 8-1 Selected Single-Gene Disorders		
DISORDER	**CLASSIFICATION**	**FREQUENCY**
Achondroplasia	Autosomal dominant	1:26,000
Albinism (occulocutaneous)	Autosomal recessive	1:10,000 to 1:12,000
Cystic fibrosis	Autosomal recessive	1:2,000 to 1:2,500 (all persons) 1:17,000 (Blacks)
Cystinuria	Autosomal recessive	1:10,000
Duchenne muscular dystrophy	X-linked recessive	1:3,000–5,000 (males)
Ehlers-Danlos syndrome	Autosomal dominant	1:150,000
Familial hypercholesterolemia	Autosomal dominant	1:200 to 1:500
G6PD deficiency	X-linked recessive	1:10 (Black males) 1:50 (Black females)
Hemophilia A (classic)	X-linked recessive	1:2,500 to 1:5,000 males
Hemophilia B (Christmas)	X-linked recessive	1:30,000 males
Huntington disease	Autosomal dominant	1:18,000 to 1:25,000 (U.S. and U.K.) 1:333,000 (Japan)
Hypophosphatemic vitamin D–resistant rickets	X-linked dominant	1:20,000
Marfan syndrome	Autosomal dominant	1:10,000 to 1:20,000
Mucopolysaccharidoses	Autosomal recessive	1:20,000 (type III most common)
Neurofibromatosis type I	Autosomal dominant	1:4,000 to 1:5,000
Osteogenesis imperfecta	Autosomal dominant	1:20,000 (all types combined)
Phenylketonuria	Autosomal recessive	1:15,000
Polycystic kidney disease	Autosomal dominant	1:200 to 1:1,250
Sickle cell disease	Autosomal recessive	1:400 to 1:600 (Blacks)
Tay-Sachs disease	Autosomal recessive	1:3,600 (Ashkenazi Jews) 1:360,000 (all other groups)

be limited by vascular events, such as aneurysms and rupture of large vessels. Even though the three most common variants are inherited as autosomal dominant traits, autosomal recessive and X-linked inheritance patterns have been reported. Prenatal diagnosis is possible in type V, since enzyme (lysyl oxidase) activity is present in normal amniotic cells.

Familial Hypercholesterolemia

Also called hyperlipoproteinemia IIa, this is one of various disorders of lipoproteins, along with abetalipoproteinemia and familial combined lipoproteinemia. Familial hypercholesterolemia (FH) is one of the most common single-gene disorders, in which the manifestations are sensitive to environmental (dietary) variations, to the point of being classified at times as a multifactorial disorder. However, individuals who are homozygous for this gene tend to develop severe and life-threatening conditions, such as early onset of atherosclerotic disease that affects the coronary, cerebral, and peripheral circulation. Postmortem examination of young children (ages 3 and 4) and young adults has revealed early arterial changes with lipid deposition and some plaque formation. Variants of the FH gene have been described, increasing the genetic complexity of this disease. Prenatal diagnosis has been accomplished by measurement of the hydroxymethylglutaryl coenzyme A (HMG CoA) reductase.

Marfan Syndrome

Marfan syndrome is another disorder of connective tissue, involving a triad of ocular, skeletal, and cardiovascular alterations. The most common ocular abnormality is a partial dislocation of the lens. Common skeletal findings include tall stature, arachnodactylic ("spider-like") hands and feet, and scoliosis. Severe scoliosis may compromise respiratory function in pregnant women with Marfan syndrome. The major life-threatening risk, however, is the frequent occurrence of aortic fusiform or dissecting aneurysms. Fifty percent of aortic aneurysms in affected women under age 40 occur during pregnancy, with rupture most likely to occur in the third trimester (Godfrey, 1993). Aortic valve abnormalities found in Marfan syndrome also contribute to an increased mortality rate during pregnancy. As a point of curiosity, historians have suggested that President Abraham Lincoln had Marfan syndrome and may have died from a dissecting aneurysm if he had not been felled by the assassin's bullet. Average life span with Marfan syndrome is 40 to 50 years.

Neurofibromatosis

The hallmark of type I multiple neurofibromatosis (MNF I), or von Recklinghausen disease, is the development of multiple soft tumors of peripheral nerves, or neurofibromas, and an abnormal skin pigmentation. In early childhood, the disease presents with multiple brown (or café-au-lait) spots, usually on the torso, and then progresses, from adolescence onwards, in the form of neurofibromas. This progression has also been reported in association with pregnancy, with the possibility of some regression after delivery. An important finding is that apparently, affected infants born to affected mothers have a worse prognosis than those who had affected fathers and those without a family history (fresh mutations) (Simpson & Golbus, 1992). This fact emphasizes the importance of genetic and reproductive counseling for clients with MNF I. As many as 75% of clients with MNF I go through life without developing some of the complications of this disease: scoliosis, moderate to severe mental retardation, learning difficulties, hypertension, seizures, spinal cord or root compression, optic gliomas, pheochromocytomas, and malignant changes in the neurofibromas (Seashore & Wappner, 1996).

Osteogenesis Imperfecta Type I

All four types of osteogenesis imperfecta (OI) involve osteoporosis and recurrent fractures of long bones with minimal trauma. Type I disease is also characterized by blue sclera, conductive deafness (secondary to otosclerosis), and discolored teeth resulting from dentinogenesis defects. (Type II results in perinatal lethality with multiple fractures during gestation and birth.) Life span of type I OI is usually normal in spite of the multiple fractures throughout life. Pregnancy in women with OI type I is complicated by respiratory difficulties among those with kyphoscoliosis and by cephalopelvic disproportions among those with previous pelvic fractures. Special precautions during delivery must also be observed for the safeguard of both mother and child (who may also have OI). In some cases, OI has been identified prenatally via sulfate incorporation test.

Polycystic Kidney Disease

This is a fairly common disorder that causes cysts in the kidneys, liver, pancreas, and spleen. Renal cysts may remain asymptomatic until the third or fourth decade of life, when the onset of renal failure or hypertension prompts a diagnosis of polycystic disease. Occasionally, an enlarged kidney is detected on X-ray studies before the onset of other symptoms, such as hematuria and proteinuria. Polycystic renal disease accounts for approximately 10% of all adult cases of chronic renal failure (Gabow, 1993). Since asymptomatic women have no related complications during pregnancy and the risk for a harmful outcome increases with progressing renal disease, it is important that reproductive counseling be provided to women with a family history of polycystic renal disease who want to have children. Prenatal diagnosis has been accomplished through linked polymorphism genetic tests.

Autosomal Recessive Disorders

The most common autosomal recessive disorders include cystic fibrosis, mucopolysaccharidoses, phenylketonuria, sickle cell disease, and Tay-Sachs disease.

Cystic Fibrosis

Cystic fibrosis (CF) is the most common lethal genetic disease affecting Caucasians. Clinical manifestations include abnormal exocrine gland function with pancreatic insufficiency and malabsorption, chronic pulmonary disease, and excessive salt in sweat (sodium in excess of 60 mmol/L and chloride exceeding 70 mmol/L) (Pagana & Pagana, 1999). The pancreatic insufficiency results in pancreatic juice that lacks trypsin, an enzyme that must be exogenously replaced throughout life. Chronic lung disease is secondary to recurrent infections resulting from the inability of the ciliated epithelium to secrete excessive mucus. Pulmonary function progressively deteriorates and a large number of affected children die before age 10. Presently, over 50% of children with cystic fibrosis live beyond age 20, and survival depends on the extent of the disease and on additional involvement of body systems (Ferri, 1999). Other symptoms include rectal prolapse, neonatal meconium ileus, cirrhosis of the liver, gallstones, and salivary gland obstruction. Pregnancy for women with cystic fibrosis obviously presents serious risks of increased morbidity and mortality. A classic national survey of cystic fibrosis reported the outcome of 97 pregnancies in women with cystic fibrosis (Cystic Fibrosis "GAP" Conference Report, 1975). According to this survey, the most damaging factor to the success of a pregnancy was a decreasing vital lung capacity secondary to pulmonary disease. Prenatal diagnosis is available.

Mucopolysaccharidoses

This diverse group of mucopolysaccharide accumulation disorders (MPS) encompasses six different syndromes, whose primary types are: Hurler syndrome (type I), Hunter syndrome (type II), Sanfilippo's syndrome (type III), and Morquio syndrome (type IV). All but type II are inherited as autosomal recessive traits. Hunter syndrome is an X-linked recessive disorder.

Individuals with type I disease exhibit coarse facies in infancy, short stature, skeletal and joint deformities, deafness, corneal clouding, umbilical hernia, progressive mental retardation, and death in the second decade of life. Type II (X-linked) is similar to type I, except for later onset, clear corneas, and death in the third decade. Type III is the most common type, with normal facies, stature, and corneas, progressive mental retardation in early childhood, and death in the second decade. Type IV results in normal intelligence, facies, and corneas; short stature with scoliosis; and death in the third decade. Some types of mucopolysaccharidosis can be detected prenatally, since their defective enzymes (listed here in parentheses) have been identified: Hurler syndrome (α-L-iduronidase); Hunter syndrome (α-L-iduronic acid-2-sulfatase); Sanfilippo syndrome (type A: heparin sulfatase; type B: N-acetyl-α-D-glucosaminidase); Morquio's syndrome (chondroitin sulfate-N-acetylhexosamine sulfate sulfatase).

Phenylketonuria

One of the most fascinating genetic diseases, phenylketonuria (PKU) represents a success story in the management of a genetic disorder. PKU results from an enzyme (phenylalanine hydroxylase) deficiency, and the consequent accumulation of the amino acid phenylalanine and its by-products cause mental retardation and other manifestations. Management for PKU consists of removing phenylalanine from the newborn's diet and maintaining a low dietary phenylalanine intake throughout life. If initiated within the first days of life, a low-phenylalanine diet ensures a normal development and life span. However, the offspring of "rescued" (treated) women with PKU are at risk for mental retardation, microcephaly, congenital heart disease, and intrauterine growth retardation. This is not a result of their genetic makeup, since children of homozygous mothers (−/−), except in the rare case of the father being a heterozygous carrier (+/−) for PKU, are unlikely to be homozygous for the mutant allele. Fetal damage is the result of intrauterine exposure to high levels of maternal phenylalanine and its metabolites, and the degree of damage is proportional to the maternal phenylalanine blood level. Placing a rescued woman with PKU on a low-phenylalanine diet before a pregnancy to maintain her blood levels at 120 to 480 µmol/L produces good outcome. Unfortunately, the treatment is often initiated after conception, at times too late to prevent microcephaly and cardiac damage to the fetus. The possibility of preventing malformations and mental retardation among the offspring of rescued mothers with PKU is a strong argument in favor of early identification or disclosure of those women at risk and pre-conceptual counseling. Initiated in the 1960s and now a legal requirement in all states, screening for PKU in newborns has made early initiation of treatment and the prevention of mental retardation possible in most cases. Prenatal diagnosis by means of measuring fetal phenylalanine hydroxylase has been accomplished.

Reflections from a Nurse

J.X. and S.T., a married couple, had just delivered their first child, after an uncomplicated pregnancy. The newborn girl weighed 3500 g at birth and began feeding well. However, 10 days after the delivery, results of biochemical tests indicated that the child had phenylketonuria (PKU). The baby's serum phenylalanine level was 30 mg/dL, the normal level is less than 2 mg/dL. On a subsequent office visit, I informed the parents that PKU is an inborn error of metabolism that prevents the use of an amino acid, phenylalanine, found in most foods. The disorder is inherited as an autosomal recessive trait, which indicates that both parents are heterozygous carriers for the PKU gene. I recommended that the baby be placed on a low-phenylalanine diet to prevent mental retardation and ensure a healthy life. I also told the parents that a low-phenylalanine diet must be observed throughout the child's life span, because an increase in dietary phenylalanine during childhood or adolescence may result in loss of cognitive function and in emotional disorders. While acknowledging the difficulty of maintaining a child on such a strict diet, I also stressed the need for adherence and suggested referrals to counseling and support group activities. In addition, I told the parents that, on reaching child-bearing age, their 'PKU-rescued' daughter would need to be aware that increases in dietary phenylalanine may increase her chances of producing children with mental retardation.

As a nurse working with this family, I found that my ability to provide nursing care was greatly enhanced by a strong procedural knowledge and understanding of the condition and its implications. This prepared me to answer the parents' questions regarding:

- Their risks for transmitting this condition to future offspring
- The consequences of this condition for normal life activities of this child
- The chances of this child passing on the condition to her offspring.

Sickle Cell Disease

Sickle cell disease (SCD) is a serious, chronic hemolytic anemia that results from homozygosity for the mutant allele (−/−) of the *HbS* gene. As a consequence of this genetic imbalance, hemoglobin S (HbS), an abnormal hemoglobin, replaces the normal adult hemoglobin A. HbS has reduced oxygen-carrying capacity and red blood cells have a decreased life span. The affected red blood cells acquire a sickle-shaped appearance, a morphologic change that greatly contributes to obstruction of small vessels and further ischemia. Infarctions of the lungs, kidneys, spleen, and bones are common. The result is a lifelong series of sickle cell crises, with recurrent pneumoccocal infections and salmonellal osteomyelitis, painful leg ulcers, dactylitis, priapism, and other symptoms. Renal failure is a common serious complication. The life span is significantly shortened, even with aggressive management.

The gynecologic and obstetric management of the woman with SCD requires special attention. Complications during pregnancy include aggravation of sickle cell crises and infections, development of other anemias, and toxemia. The prevalence of SCD is extremely high among Blacks and significant among people of Mediterranean origin. The prevalence of homozygotes (−/−) among Blacks is approximately 1 in 400, with a heterozygote carrier frequency of 1 in 10.

Tay-Sachs Disease

Tay-Sachs disease (TSD) is a lipid storage disorder, with accumulation of GM_2 ganglioside in cells of the nervous system, resulting in a progressive neurologic disorder. The genetic defect results in decreased production of the enzyme β-hexosaminidase A (HexA), from a significant reduction in the heterozygote carrier (+/−) to total absence in the homozygote (−/−). During their short life, children with TSD experience a progressive and steady neurologic deterioration in a series of mental and motor deficits, which begin at approximately 6 months of age. Symptoms at various ages include loss of the developmental milestones acquired before the onset of the disease, along with deafness, blindness, seizure activity, and death by age 3 to 5. TSD is highly prevalent among the Ashkenazi Jews (Jews of Central and Eastern European origin), with a frequency of approximately 1:3,600 for homozygotes (−/−), 1:25 to 30 for heterozygote carriers (Jorde, Carey, Bamshad, & White, 1998). By comparison, among Sephardic Jews (Jews of Southern European, North African, and Middle-Eastern origin) and gentiles, the gene is 100 times rarer (1:360,000). Prenatal diagnosis by determination of fetal HexA levels is commonly performed.

X-Linked Disorders

Genetic disorders whose causative gene is located on the X chromosome include Duchenne muscular dystrophy glucose 6-phosphate dehydrogenase deficiency, the hemophilias, and Lesch-Nyhan syndrome.

Duchenne's Muscular Dystrophy

One of two types of X-linked recessive muscular dystrophies (the other being Becker's muscular dystrophy), Duchenne muscular dystrophy (DMD) results in progressive muscle weakening, atrophy, and contractures, beginning in early childhood. In the majority of cases, the age of onset is less than 5 years and the disease is characterized by delayed walking. A pseudo-hypertrophy of the calf (in which muscle is replaced by adipose tissue) may mask the disease to the inexperienced clinician. Affected children are usually unable to run, and 95% of affected children are using a wheelchair by age 12 (Korf, 1996). Mild mental retardation occurs in about 1 of 4 cases. Death, often from respiratory insufficiency, usually occurs in the second decade. Prenatal diagnosis is done by assessing for various mutations that lead to the deficiency of dystrophin, the deficient protein in various muscular dystrophies.

Glucose-6-Phosphate Dehydrogenase Deficiency

This common, self-limiting hemolytic anemia is often used as a prototype for genetic environmental interaction. Glucose-6-phosphate dehydrogenase (G6PD) deficiency is usually asymptomatic until the affected male is exposed to one of many environmental triggers, such as certain drugs (antimalarial agents, aspirin, sulfonamides) or certain foods (especially fava beans, from which the popular name "favism" originates). The hemolytic episode may also be precipitated by infections. In one disease subtype (B variant), affected males suffer from a chronic hemolytic anemia in the absence of environmental triggers. Carrier females (+/−) remain asymptomatic even when exposed to a trigger agent. Homozygote females (−/−) do

exist, as progeny of a carrier female (+/−) and an affected hemizygous (−/−) male. Pregnancy in women with G6PD deficiency (homozygotes) presents several complications. Hemolytic episodes are more frequent; urinary infections, common in pregnancy, cannot be treated with sulpha-based drugs; and exposure of a fetus with G6PD deficiency to maternally ingested trigger substances may result in fetal hemolysis, hydrops fetalis, and death. The incidence of anemia, hyperbilirubinemia, and kernicterus is also increased among newborns with G6PD deficiency.

Hemophilia A

Classic, or type A, hemophilia is a fairly common X-linked recessive disorder of coagulation, resulting from deficiency or defect in clotting factor VIIIc. In 10% of clients, the factor VIIIc level is normal, but its activity is reduced (Jorde et al., 1998). Variable degrees of deficiencies are probably caused by genetic heterogeneity (different mutations). In the presence of severe factor VIIIc deficiency, massive hemorrhages after trauma and surgical procedures (including dental procedures) can occur. "Spontaneous" bleeding frequently occurs in areas subject to trauma (e.g., joints, resulting in hemarthroses). Petechiae and ecchymoses are usually absent. Prenatal diagnosis by measurement of factor VIII is possible.

Lesch-Nyhan Syndrome

Also known as HGPRT deficiency, Lesch-Nyhan syndrome is a rare X-linked recessive disease characterized by a tendency toward self-mutilation, mental retardation, choreoathetosis, spasticity, and hyperuricemia. Prenatal diagnosis is made by determination of fetal levels of HGPRT.

CHROMOSOME ABNORMALITIES

Both the autosomes and the sex chromosomes can experience numerical and structural chromosomal abnormalities that have clinical consequences. Table 8-2 shows the prevalence of chromosomal abnormalities in newborns. Structural chromosomal abnormalities do not alter the total chromosome number, but in some cases, they can cause clinical consequences as devastating as those resulting from numerical changes. As previously mentioned, numerical alterations resulting in hyperploidy (3n, 4n, and so on) produce a wide spectrum of malformations that render them incompatible with life. However, small variations around the normal diploid number (46), such as occurs in trisomies (total chromosome number 47), are often found in clinical practice. The only monosomy compatible with life is a missing X chromosome in persons with Turner's syndrome.

Table 8-2   Incidence of Selected Chromosomal Abnormalities in Newborns

CHROMOSOME ABNORMALITY	INCIDENCE
Numerical, Autosomes	
Trisomy 21 (Down syndrome)	1:650 to 700 live births
Trisomy 16–18 (Edward syndrome)	1:8,000 live births
Trisomy 13–15 (Patau syndrome)	1:20,000 live births
Other autosomal anomalies	1:50,000 live births
Numerical, Sex Chromosomes	
47, XXY (Klinefelter syndrome)	1:1,000 male births
47, XYY (Jacobs syndrome)	1:1,000 male births
Other male anomalies	1:1,350 male births
45, X0 (Turner syndrome)	1:10,000 female births
47, XXX (triple-X female)	1:1,000 female births
Other female anomalies	1:2,700 female births
Structural, Autosomes	
Balanced robertsonian, t(Dq/Dq)	1:1,500 live births
Balanced robertsonian, t(Dq/Gq)	1:5,000 live births
Reciprocal translocations	1:7,000 live births
46, XX or XY, B(5)p cri du chat syndrome	1:20,000 live births
Total Chromosome Abnormalities	**1:160 live births**

Note. Data adapted from *Genetic's in Obstetrics and Gynecology* (2nd ed.), by J. L. Simpson and M. S. Golbus, 1992, Philadelphia: W.B. Saunders.

Numerical Abnormalities of the Autosomes

Numerical alterations of the autosomes include some of the most common trisomies found in humans: trisomy 21 (Down syndrome), trisomy 18 (Edwards' syndrome), and trisomy 13 (Patau syndrome).

Trisomy 21

Down syndrome is the most common aneuploidy compatible with development to full term with a reasonable quality of postnatal life. Physical and mental abnormalities vary enormously in spectrum (Jorde et al., 1998). Mean IQ is 50, with a range of 25 to 70. Multiple physical anomalies include craniofacial abnormalities (brachycephaly, flat occiput, low-set ears, oblique palpebral fissures, epicanthal folds, Brushfield spots on the iris, broad nasal bones and flattened profile, and open mouth with protruding tongue); skeletal abnormalities (broad, short fingers, clinodactyly of fifth finger); cardiac malformations (ventricular and atrial septal defects, patent ductus arteriosus); and various other abnormalities (hypotonia; increased susceptibility to respiratory infections and to acute leukemia; palmar simian crease; and abnormal dermatoglyphics, or fingerprint pattern). In spite of modern medical developments, life expectancy is still shortened, with 22% dying in the first decade and 50% by age 60, mostly from hematologic malignances and cardiac defects. Males with Down syndrome are usually sterile, but a few females have reproduced. About one third of their offspring are also trisomic for chromosome 21.

The chromosomal constitution of Down syndrome is variable, with three possible configurations:

1. Free trisomy, 47, XX or XY, G(21)[+], is the pattern in 95% of all cases of Down syndrome; the extra chromosome 21 is unattached and segregates freely during meiosis. This type of Down syndrome increases linearly in frequency with increasing maternal age (from 1:1,500 live births for mothers age 20, to 1:30 live births by age 45) (Korf, 1996).

2. Translocation Down syndrome, 46, XX or XY, t(Gq/Dq)[+] or t(Gq/Gq)[+], accounts for approximately 4% of all Down syndrome cases. The majority of cases are sporadic (without family history), but about 40% have one balanced-translocation carrier parent. When one such carrier and a normal partner reproduce, their chances of producing a child with Down syndrome range from 33% (for carriers of t(Gq/Dq) and t(21q/22q)) to 100% (for carriers of t(21q/21q)). This latter situation is one of the rare examples in genetics in which an abnormality is passed on to *all* living descendants. The incidence of translocation Down syndrome is slightly elevated (9%) among mothers who are older than age 30 at conception (compare with 2% for mothers younger than age 30) (Gelehrter, Collins, & Ginsburg, 1998).

3. Mosaic Down syndrome, 46, XX or XY/47, XX or XY, G(21)[+]. This rarer type of Down syndrome (about 1% of all cases) results from mitotic nondisjunction that occurs during early embryonic development of a normal zygote. Persons with this type have mixed cell populations, some with the normal karyotype, others with the extra chromosome. Contrary to what might be expected, children with Down syndrome mosaicism do not necessarily have a better developmental outcome than those with the free trisomy syndrome.

Trisomy 18

Edwards' syndrome is a fairly common trisomy affecting mostly chromosome 18. In addition to severe mental retardation, children with this defect present with severe craniofacial abnormalities (dolichocephaly with a prominent occiput, low-set and malformed ears, and micrognathia), skeletal abnormalities (clenched fist with overlapping fingers, flexion deformities, adducted hips, "rocker-bottom" feet), cardiac anomalies (ventricular and atrial septal defects, patent ductus arteriosus), and urogenital malformations ("horse-shoe" kidneys, hydronephrosis, cryptorchidism, prominent genitals). Hypotonia is also common. Although the life span is longer for females (10 months, average), females are more often affected. Mean survival for males is about 3 months. Overall, 30% of these children die in the first month, 50% die in the second month, and few survive 1 year (Simpson & Golbus, 1992).

Trisomy 13

Patau syndrome causes more severe malformations than the previous two trisomies discussed, which is consistent with the increased size of the extra chromosome and a greater gene imbalance. Craniofacial anomalies are much more pronounced: microcephaly, low-set and malformed ears, microphthalmia or anophthalmia, coloboma of the iris, and cleft lip and palate. Skeletal abnormalities include polydactyly and syndactyly; overlapping, flexed fingers; and hypoplasia of the pelvis. Systemic anomalies include cardiac defects (ventricular and atrial septal defects, patent ductus arteriosus) and urogenital malformations (malformed kidneys, hydronephros, polycystic kidneys, cryptorchidism, bicornuate uterus). Mean life expectancy is 4 months, with 45% dying in the first month and fewer than 5% surviving 3 years (Simpson & Golbus, 1992).

Numerical Abnormalities of the Sex Chromosomes

Alterations in number may also involve the sex chromosomes. Some of the most common genetic disorders caused by sex chromosome aneuploidies are Klinefelter, Jacobs, Turner, and the triple-X female syndromes.

47, XXY

Klinefelter syndrome is characterized by multiple X chromosomes and one Y chromosome. The greater the total chromosome number, the more severe the anomalies that result from increased gene imbalance. Physical abnormalities include elements of decreased masculinization, such as gynecomastia; hypogonadism (with sterility caused by degeneration of seminiferous tubules); and increased pubis-to-sole length, reflecting elongated lower limbs. Mental development is normal in most cases; mental retardation, if it occurs, is in the IQ range of 50 to 85. Delayed language skills, however, are common. Chromo-

some mosaicism (46, XY/47, XXY) rarely occurs; when it does, it results in individuals with milder manifestations than their trisomic counterparts.

47, XYY

Jacobs syndrome was reported in the early 1960s by Patricia Jacobs, a Scottish cytogeneticist who detected a higher-than-expected frequency of double-Y males among inmates of penal institutions in Britain. In early reports, an extra Y chromosome was seen as responsible for an individual's increased tendency toward aggression against property (as opposed to aggression against humans). A detailed statistical analysis by Borgaonkar and Shah (1974) of more than 200 cases later revealed that the only correlates with an extra Y chromosome were tall stature (more than 6 feet) and skin disorders, such as persistent adult acne. Mental retardation and aggressive tendency correlations with XYY were not found to be significant in that large study, and the syndrome remains a scientific curiosity. A majority of children produced by XYY fathers have normal chromosomal constitution, probably reflecting a selective advantage of normal haploid gametes over aneuploid ones.

45, XO

Turner syndrome, originally described clinically as ovarian dysgenesis (with gonads consisting of streaks of connective tissue and devoid of germ cells), is an example of a monosomy that is compatible with quasi-normal life. Clinical manifestations include low birth weight and short adult stature (4′6″ to 4′8″); low posterior hairline and webbing of the neck; shield-shaped chest with divergent nipples; short fourth metacarpals; cubitus valgus; coarctation of the aorta; urinary tract abnormalities; lymphedema of hands and feet in the newborn; and fetal cystic hygroma and hydrops. Intellectual development is normal, with verbal IQ exceeding performance IQ. Due to decreased secondary sexual characteristics, administration of female hormones at puberty is a common practice. However, it tends to further stunt growth and must be wisely considered. Treatment for the reduced growth with growth hormone and anabolic steroids is also in practice. Mosaicism also occurs in Turner syndrome (46, XX/45, X0), resulting in milder expression of the phenotype.

47, XXX

Occasionally, triple-X females have been reported in textbooks under the unfortunate term "super females." Whereas this term is valid in fruit flies, where the extra X chromosome intensifies female characteristics, it is totally unjustified in humans. A relatively common condition (1:1,000 live female births), triple-X females display a normal phenotype, with perhaps a slight decrease in mental capacity, when compared to their euploid sisters.

Gynecologic complications include a delayed menarche and a premature menopause. As with XXY males, the offspring of XXX females are largely normal, indicative of a selective advantage of euploid gametes.

Structural Chromosomal Abnormalities

Structural abnormalities include a variety of chromosome defects (e.g., deletions, translocations) that do not alter the total chromosome number. They include the cri du chat (cat's cry) syndrome, fragile X syndrome, and several chromosome instability syndromes, in which the hallmark is chromosome breakage or rearrangement.

46, XX or XY, B(5)p

Cri du chat, or cat's cry, syndrome is a rare (1 in 50,000 live births) (Jorde et al., 1998) chromosome deletion syndrome resulting from loss of the small arm of chromosome B(5). In early infancy, this syndrome presents with a typical but nondistinctive facial appearance, often a "moon-shaped" face, with wide-spaced eyes (hypertelorism). As the child grows, this feature progressively diminishes and by age 2, the child is undistinguishable from age-matched controls. Profound mental retardation persists throughout a short life; most affected children die in infancy from multiple genetic imbalances. Typical of this disease is a crying pattern that is abnormal and cat-like. At times, it sounds like an angry cat; at others, like a soft mewling sound. This is a result of laryngeal atrophy, which improves with age. By age 3, the crying pattern is still abnormal, but it acquires a normal pitch and loses its cat-like quality.

Fragile X Syndrome

Although listed here as a structural abnormality, fragile X syndrome acquired its name from the fact that in in vitro conditions, the X chromosome frequently displays breaks and gaps in its terminal portions. However, this is an X-linked dominant condition with increased prevalence among males (approximately 1 in 1,250 males and 1 in 2,500 females are affected). Clinical features include mental retardation and a typical facial appearance, including an elongated face and long, elf-like ears (Jorde et al., 1998).

Chromosome Instability Syndromes

This is a heterogeneous group of genetic disorders characterized by a high frequency of chromosome breakage that is observed in vitro. They include ataxia-telangiectasia (or Louis-Bar's syndrome), Fanconi anemia, and xeroderma pigmentosum. These syndromes are associated with decreased immune function and an increased incidence of cancer, mostly lymphomas and leukemias.

GENETIC SCREENING

Because of the complexity and magnitude of genetic damage, treatment for genetic disorders is rarely successful. The primary weapon against increases in the prevalence of genetic disease is an aggressive program of genetic screening and counseling. The first corollaries of any such intervention must be *voluntary participation*, *equal access to all*, and *confidentiality* (both in conducting the tests and in handling records and results). In addition, education and counseling about tests and procedures must be an integral part of any screening program. Attention must be paid to ensure quality control of all aspects of testing and laboratory procedures.

Purposes for genetic screening are threefold:

1. To provide early recognition of a disease for which effective intervention and therapy exist, before symptoms occur. Example: PKU.
2. To provide identification of carriers of a genetic disease for the purpose of maximizing parenthood planning options. Example: Tay-Sachs disease.
3. To obtain population data on frequency, spectrum, and natural history of a genetic disease. Examples: chromosomal abnormalities in newborns.

Screening for genetic disorders can occur during various times in a person's life:

- Screening of selected populations for heterozygous carriers (e.g., mass screening of Blacks for sickle cell disease, as it occurred in the 1970s in clinics sponsored by the Black Panther Party)
- Screening of relatives of a known carrier or affected individuals within a family, for the purpose of reproductive decision making
- Preconception screening for carriers (e.g., screening for Tay-Sachs disease among couples contemplating parenthood, as it occurred in synagogues in the United States after development of testing methods)
- Postconception (prenatal) testing (e.g., screening for Tay-Sachs disease in the product of a pregnancy by two heterozygous carriers)
- Newborn testing (e.g., testing for PKU in all newborns, as mandated by law in all U.S. states). The benefits of early detection of PKU and treatment initiation warrant mandatory testing.

An ideal genetic screening test must have high sensitivity (ability to detect true-positive results) and specificity (limited false-negative results); it must yield rapid results and be safe and cost-effective; and it should cause minimum physical and emotional discomfort to all involved. Geneticists and other members of the genetics team must be prepared to weigh favorable and unfavorable consequences of genetic screening before implementing a program or conducting a screening activity.

Among the potential benefits of screening for carriers is the removal of a stigma and restoration of self-esteem when the results do not reveal a carrier status. It also facilitates genetic counseling and reproductive planning and provides useful information to other potentially affected family members. Testing newborns for genetic defects provides for early detection and treatment initiation, maximizing quality of life.

Risks incurred in genetic screening include the potential for stigmatization of those identified as carriers or affected individuals and for the development of feelings of inadequacy and guilt often seen in conjunction with genetic disease. Many are concerned about their ability to obtain health insurance or about their employers knowing about their risks. A positive test result for one family member may result in the disclosure of genetic risks to other family members who did not seek or want to know the outcome of the tests.

GENETIC COUNSELING

In its narrower sense, genetic counseling consists of one or more encounters with the probands and their families with the objective of providing information about their genetic disease. A **proband** is a clinically identified person who displays the characteristics or features of the disease in question. This information includes risk figures, options, and provides a framework for a course of action to be taken by the individual or family. It should also include an assessment of psychosocial family dynamics, which are an integral part of a genetic disease, and an exploration of feelings and perceptions often elicited by the newly obtained knowledge. **Genetic counseling**, in its broader definition, refers to a series of procedures that include processing the initial referral, assessing the needs, deciding on the appropriate tests, interpreting the results, and, finally, communicating these findings to the proband and family.

In the majority of families requesting genetic counseling, the precipitating event is the birth of an affected child. In the case of dominant diseases, usually one of the parents is affected, and there is some degree of preparation for the possibility of an affected child. In recessive disorders, however, the parents are usually clinically normal, which prevents any warning of a potentially negative outcome. Maternal age is another reason clients may request genetic testing.

The counseling process has been referred to as a specialized form of family counseling. However, two factors make genetic counseling a unique process. First, counselors must work with grief and anticipatory grief issues. Even with the knowledge of a potentially negative outcome, a certain amount of hope and denial usually prevails until the birth of the affected child brings the family back to reality. Second, the parents' knowledge that they are biologically responsible for their child's condition is a burden often too heavy to carry without emotional

Critical Thinking

So You Want to Be Part of a Genetic Team?

Until the mid-70s, the field of medical genetics was exclusively in the hands of physicians who did not have a formal education in genetics. Most medical geneticists of the time were self-taught and came from a medical specialty: most were pediatricians (who saw several cases of the same genetic disorder and became interested experts), obstetricians (after observing a recurrent birth defect or fetal loss), endocrinologists (who may have been repeatedly consulted for delayed puberty), and family physicians. Medical genetics was taught in the medical curricula not in comprehensive courses, but as part of specific body systems.

In 1981, the American Society of Human Genetics instituted a Medical Genetics Board with certification in several specialties: M.D. clinical geneticist, Ph.D. medical geneticist, clinical cytogeneticist, or biochemical geneticist, all required clinical or research doctorates. Genetic counselor was the only entry point for a master's degree–prepared genetic counselor. Nurses, at first hesitant in undertaking an activity for which they were not originally trained, soon became invaluable members of medical genetics teams. Several programs in genetic counseling soon followed the pioneer efforts at Sarah Lawrence University.

If you want to know more about applying nursing skills and technology to medical genetics and genetic counseling, visit the Genetics Society of America/American Association for Human Genetics Web site or the University of Kansas Medical Center Web site. Another excellent resource is the International Society of Nurses in Genetics Web site, which contains useful genetics-related hyperlinks (see Resources).

damage. The physical contact with that person, sometimes for a lifetime, is a constant reminder of what may be perceived as "reproductive failure" and "bad seed."

For these reasons, a strong medical-psychological-spiritual support system is essential. These forms of support are usually available to the client through diverse sources. Medical and client care issues are covered by the health care professionals, such as nurses and physicians. The nurse is often in a position to offer initial and ongoing support. Emotional support is provided by family members, counselors, social workers, or even through question-and-answer columns in daily newspapers and on the Internet. Spiritual, religious, and ethical support may be received from a hospital chaplain or family clergy. Unfortunately, in many instances, the helping efforts of these three areas function independently from one another and in an uncoordinated manner. Efforts should be made to ensure effective communication among the services provided by professionals in these three areas. Since no health care provider alone can provide all needed services, the best approach to genetic counseling is a team approach. Members of the team should include a generalist physician, geneticist, medical specialist, nurse, psychologist (psychiatrist, clinical social worker, or therapist), and clergy.

Typically, the genetic counseling process begins when a clinician refers a family in which a genetic disease has been identified. It is important at this point to have a conclusive diagnosis of the condition, as many errors in genetics counseling are a result of mistaken or incomplete diagnoses. Provided with this information, a member of the genetic counseling team (GCT) contacts the family and describes the process that is about to begin. The parents should be informed that they need to collect data about their family, such as previous disease cases, causes of death, degree of closeness of relationships (e.g., consanguinity), and how to secure medical records. In small communities, especially in traditional rural cultures, a family Bible is often a good source of information.

In the first personal interview, the GCT gathers pertinent information from family members. Once a detailed **pedigree (genogram)** chart is generated, the GCT identifies the mode of inheritance and confirms the initial diagnosis. Testing of other family members, if recommended, is initiated at this time, and a second appointment is made. It is important in the first contact that the family members be made to feel at ease, and that ample time be allotted for answering all questions. In the second interview, with all the previous information processed, the GCT discusses with the family all the implications of the findings, presents options, and clarifies possible outcomes. Team mem-

bers should be prepared to handle ethical and religious issues that often surface, such as the possibility of therapeutic abortion or sterilization, in a sensitive and caring manner. It is of topmost importance that genetic counseling remain a nondirective process, with the GCT members refraining from pressuring family members in any possible direction and remaining supportive but neutral about decisions that must be made. At times, this may present a challenge to a health care provider who feels

Critical Thinking

Genetic Counseling Situation

Mrs. B. presents to the emergency service with a broken tibia, the result of a fall. While taking a medical history, the nurse discovers that Mrs. B. is 12 weeks into her fifth pregnancy. The nurse finds out further that, of the previous children, three have osteogenesis imperfecta (OI), as has Mr. B. The nurse calls for an obstetric consult and places the hospital chaplain on alert. The obstetric resident discovers that Mrs. B. is well-informed about OI, its mode of inheritance, and the risk for this pregnancy. Apparently, all of the children are in good shape, as is Mr. B., and the disease seems to present no major concerns to them. However, the resident feels that it is his duty to offer to Mrs. B. a therapeutic abortion and tubal ligation. Mrs. B. refuses both suggestions on the basis of her religious beliefs. The resident is convinced that Mrs. B. is making the wrong decision and presents forceful arguments, accompanied by color photographs of people with severe OI. Mrs. B. is unmoved. The hospital chaplain is called into consultation and, after a long interview, concurs that Mrs. B. is making a well-informed decision that is based on her strong religious convictions. Mrs. B. returns to her small rural community. The obstetrics department is later informed in a follow-up letter from the local physician that Mrs. B. has delivered her fifth child, the fourth to be born with OI.

Do you think that the obstetric resident should have been more forceful and tried to convince Mrs. B. to have an abortion and a tubal ligation? Would you be able to accept Mrs. B.'s decision, given the severity of this disease?

that he or she has the correct answers and that the family is mistaken about the decision they have made. It must be remembered that the family members are the ones who will have to live with their decision, and therefore their decision, once made, must be respected and supported by all health care team members.

Prenatal Diagnosis

One of the commonly used tools in genetic counseling is prenatal diagnosis of genetic disorders. Several approaches for prenatal diagnosis have been developed: screening procedures include a trisomy profile test and an ultrasound-assisted nuchal translucence test. The two main diagnostic procedures are midtrimester amniocentesis and chorionic villi sampling (CVS). In addition, routine ultrasonography provides invaluable information in a noninvasive manner.

Trisomy Profile Test

It has been known since 1984 that maternal serum **alpha-fetoprotein** (MSAFP) levels are, on the average, lower in pregnancies affected by Down syndrome compared with levels in a normal pregnancy. The accuracy of the test was later increased by taking into consideration maternal age. In 1987, it was discovered that maternal serum levels of human chorionic gonadotropin (hCG) were twice as high in Down syndrome pregnancies during the second trimester. In addition, unconjugated estrogen (uE_3) levels in maternal serum were found to be 25% lower in the presence of a Down syndrome pregnancy. The trisomy profile maternal serum test presently includes maternal age, MSAFP, hCG, and uE_3 and has a high rate of identification of common chromosome disorders.

Nuchal Translucency on Intravaginal Ultrasonography

This high-resolution ultrasonography is being used more and more often to detect increased nuchal translucency, as an indicator of Down syndrome. An increased nuchal translucency or the presence of cystic hygromas (septated, fluid-filled sacs in the nuchal region) are common features of several fetal aneuploidy conditions, including the common trisomies 13, 18, and 21. The sensitivity of this test for these trisomies combined is approximately 62%, and for trisomy 21 alone, 54% (Taipale, Hiilesmaa, Salonen, & Ylostalo, 1997). The procedure can be performed earlier in the pregnancy than serum screening, and it may decrease the need for future CVS or amniocentesis.

Midtrimester Amniocentesis

This method was applied for the first time for diagnosis of genetic disorders in the early 1960s and has been widely used since then. The procedure is commonly performed between the 14th and 16th weeks of gestation, under ultrasound guidance, and consists of transabdominally withdrawing approximately 20 mL of amniotic fluid for analysis of cells sloughed off by the developing embryo. The material obtained is then cultured to obtain a large number of cells. Two basic sets of tests are performed: chromosome analysis and biochemical analysis of the fluid (e.g., alpha-fetoprotein measurements for the assessment of neural tube defects) or cell products (e.g., hexosaminidase A determinations for the diagnosis of Tay-Sachs disease). The high accuracy of amniocentesis in detecting chromosomal and biochemical defects has been well established. However, one serious concern still remains: since the test is run as late as the 16th (and sometimes the 17th) week of pregnancy, the results are often returned at a quite advanced phase of pregnancy, making the possibility of a late therapeutic abortion an issue of ethical and medical concern. Potential sources of error include the mistaken analysis of maternal cells (but only if the embryo is female) or when mosaicism masks the presence of aneuploid cells. However, if a sufficient number of cells is studied, the abnormal cells eventually are detected. The risks involved in this procedure are small but measurable, at approximately 0.5%, and include risks for the developing embryo (needle perforations and scratches), for the continuation of the pregnancy ("spontaneous" abortions), and for the mother (immunologic cross-reactions) (Jorde et al., 1998). However small the risk, this is an invasive procedure that should be used only after careful consideration. Indications for amniocentesis include maternal age above 35, previous history of chromosomal abnormalities, family history of genetic disorders that can be diagnosed by amniocentesis, and an increased risk of neural tube defect.

Chorionic Villi Sampling (CVS)

This recently developed prenatal diagnosis technique is rapidly replacing the traditional midtrimester amniocentesis, mostly because it can be performed at an earlier time (usually 9th to 12th week), yields results sooner, and its safety approaches that of the midtrimester test. The test is accurate in 99% of the cases, provided true chorionic villi material is obtained. One major disadvantage of CVS is that alpha-fetoprotein determination for detection of neural tube defects cannot be obtained and must be attempted at a later date, when the concentration of this substance increases.

NURSING IMPLICATIONS

One of the most important advances in biomedical science is the mapping of the human genome. This project has the potential to make dramatic changes in all health care and certainly will affect the care of women and infants. Apart from a few genetic disorders that have a direct expression in disease, the majority of genetic information is more complex and, in many cases, a genetic predisposition to a disease interacts with environmental conditions for expression. The latter has the most implications for nurses because of the need to teach environmental modification through lifestyle modification, risk avoidance, and health management.

The nurse is likely to interact with the client and family in a number of ways related to genetics. The involvement can vary depending on setting and level of education.

The staff nurse should have a general knowledge of genetics and genetic terminology to answer client questions and direct them to resources. There are major implications in supporting couples in reproductive decision making and in coping with potential genetic risks. Additionally, nurses may be in the position to provide education and support for risk management for clients who have their own genetic risk factors, such as breast cancer.

Nurses in advanced practice may function as genetic counselors, provided they have appropriate education in genetics and counseling. They may also work in birth-defect clinics and provide risk screening for normal prenatal or high-risk populations. Advanced practice nurses also are in a position to screen their clients for genetic conditions, even if the appropriate management would include referral to another member of the health care team.

All nurses need to have read and learned from current literature related to genetic information and to be able to provide information to clients about rapidly changing information and technology related to this field. Nurses in any area of practice are likely to be faced with ethical issues regarding the advancing knowledge of genetics. Each new discovery in genetics raises questions about who should have genetic information about individuals and families. Who should be treated for genetic conditions? When should treatment be given and what should be treated? What treatment is appropriate? These questions must be answered. As new treatments evolve, the cost concerns regarding distribution of scarce resources becomes an issue that must be addressed.

WEB ACTIVITIES

••• Visit the National Coalition for Health Professional Education in Genetics at http://www.nchpeg.org. It has care competencies for all health care providers as well as links to other resources.

••• Visit the March of Dimes Web site at http://modimes.org and explore the various resources available to families and health care professionals about birth defects.

••• Visit the Cytogenetics Gallery at the University of Washington (Seattle) Web site at http://www.pathology.washington.edu and explore different karyotypes and their association with diseases processes and clinical manifestations.

••• Visit the Genetic Alliance Web site at http://www.geneticalliance.org and use this resource to guide a family with a genetic disorder.

••• Visit the Human Genome Project Information Web site at http://www.ornl.gov/Tech Resources/Human_Genome and participate in ethical, legal, and social debates on applications of the Human Genome Project. Communicate with experts and peers in a chat room.

••• Visit the Med Help International Web site at http://medhelp.org to retrieve a list of support organizations to assist families with genetic disorders.

••• Visit the Center for Bioethics, University of Pennsylvania Web site at http://www.med.upenn.edu to review articles on discrimination, privacy, and other ethical issues in genetic screening.

Key Concepts

■ An alteration in a single gene may cause multiple physical and mental derangements without changing the gross structure of a chromosome, or altering the total chromosome number of an individual. Therefore, genetic disorders may be classified under gene disorders and chromosome abnormalities.

■ Structural genes encode genetic information for the synthesis of enzymes. A mutation in one gene may result in the synthesis of an abnormal enzyme, thus interrupting a metabolic pathway and causing a genetic syndrome. Many genetic syndromes are single-gene (Mendelian) disorders.

■ Many genes often cooperate to create or modify a given phenotype. Many human characteristics follow this polygenic inheritance pattern.

■ Chromosomal abnormalities may result from alterations in individual chromosomes (structural abnormalities) or from alterations in the total number of chromosomes (numerical abnormalities). Either situation may cause significant phenotypic alterations and pathologic conditions.

■ Genetic screening is the process by which individuals or populations can be assessed for various genetic disorders to detect the presence of a gene before it expresses as a genetic disease or to identify the carrier of a recessive trait.

■ Many genetic disorders are not treatable with conventional techniques. In many instances, the prevention of a genetic disease is only possible through genetic counseling of persons at risk.

Review Questions and Activities

1. The parents of a newborn with Down syndrome (DS) inquire about what could have caused this abnormality. One of the following responses is *not* appropriate:
   a. DS was caused by an accidental chromosomal nondisjunction.
   b. DS is an inborn error of metabolism.
   c. DS is a rare event for the age group of these parents.
   d. DS in this child could have been identified by prenatal chromosome analysis.

   The correct answer is b.

2. The same parents are concerned about the possibility of having other children with DS. What correct information can be conveyed to them?
   a. Free trisomy 21 is not inheritable and therefore is unlikely to recur.
   b. Future pregnancies may be tested prenatally.
   c. Free trisomy is hereditary, and the recurrence risk for future pregnancies is high.
   d. Both *a* and *b* are correct.
   e. Both *b* and *c* are correct.

   The correct answer is d.

3. The parents of a newborn with phenylketonuria (PKU) ask what PKU means. One of the following is *not* a correct response to their question:
   a. PKU is an enzyme deficiency resulting in the inability to metabolize phenylalanine.
   b. PKU is an inborn error of metabolism.
   c. PKU results from a chromosomal abnormality called nondisjunction.
   d. PKU is transmitted as an autosomal recessive disorder.

   The correct answer is c.

4. What information should the same parents be given about the consequences of PKU?
   a. High dietary levels of phenylalanine may help induce enzyme production.
   b. PKU is commonly associated with other congenital anomalies.
   c. Failure to avoid dietary phenylalanine results in progressive mental retardation.
   d. Mental retardation is inevitable.

   The correct answer is c.

5. A woman is heterozygous for an *autosomal dominant* disease. If she mates with a normal man, what are the chances of the coupling producing an affected child in any pregnancy?
   a. 1:4
   b. 1:2
   c. 1:400 ($1/10 \times 1/10 \times 1/4 = 1/400$)
   d. No risk, since she is a carrier and he is not.

   The correct answer is b.

6. Three siblings have a *rare autosomal recessive* disease. Both parents are clinically normal. Which of the following statements apply?

a. Both parents are homozygous for the normal allele.

b. Both parents are homozygous for the defective allele.

c. All three children are homozygous for the defective allele.

d. All three children are heterozygous.

The correct answer is c.

7. The term *autosomal recessive* refers to the mode of inheritance of a disorder:

a. That is always expressed in heterozygotes

b. Whose causative gene is located on an autosome

c. That is always present at birth

d. That cannot be transmitted from mother to son

The correct answer is b.

8. Choose the correct statement about the carrier state

a. The son of a mother with hemophilia has a 50% chance of being a carrier.

b. The son of a woman with achondroplasia has a 50% chance of being a carrier.

c. The son of a man with achondroplasia has a 50% chance of being a carrier.

d. None of the above statements is correct.

The correct answer is d.

9. The son of a man with Y-linked hairy ears marries the daughter of a man with the same condition.

a. All their children will have hairy ears.

b. All their boys will have hairy ears.

c. None of their children will have hairy ears.

d. Half of their boys will have hairy ears.

The correct answer is b.

10. If a man who is affected with an X-linked recessive disorder marries a woman who is phenotypically and genotypically normal:

a. All his sons will be carriers

b. All his daughters will be carriers

c. Half his sons will be carriers

d. Half his daughters will be carriers

The correct answer is b.

References

Borgaonkar, D. S., & Shah, S. A. (1974). The XYY chromosome male or syndrome? In A. G. Steinberg and A. G. Bearn (Eds), *Progress in medical genetics* (Vol. 10, pp. 135–222). New York: Grune & Stratton.

Cox, T. M., & Sinclair, J. (Eds.). (1997). *Molecular biology in medicine.* Boston: Blackwell Scientific.

Cystic Fibrosis "GAP" Conference Report. (1975). *Problems in reproductive physiology and anatomy in young adults with cystic fibrosis.* Atlanta, GA: Cystic Fibrosis Foundation.

Ferri, F. F. (1999). *Ferri's clinical advisor: Instant diagnosis and treatment.* St. Louis, MO: Mosby.

Gabow, P. (1993). Medical progress: Autosomal dominant polycystic kidney disease. *New England Journal of Medicine, 329,* 332–342.

Gelehrter, T. D., Collins, F. S., & Ginsburg, D. (1998). *Principles of medical genetics* (2nd ed.). Philadelphia: Lippincott, Williams & Wilkins.

Godfrey, M. (1993). The Marfan syndrome. In P. Beighton (Ed.), *McKusick's heritable disorders of connective tissue* (5th ed., pp. 51–123). St. Louis, MO: Mosby-Year Book.

Ingram, V. M. (1956). A specific chemical difference between the globins of normal and sickle-cell anemia hemoglobins. *Nature, 178,* 792–794.

Jorde, L. B., Carey, J. C., Bamshad, M. J., & White, R. L. (1998). *Medical genetics* (2nd ed.). St. Louis, MO: Mosby.

Korf, B. R. (1996). *Human genetics: A problem-based approach.* Cambridge MA: Blackwell Science.

McKusick, V. A. (2000). *Online Mendelian inheritance in man (OMIM).* Retrieved November 25, 2003, from http://www.ncbi.nlm.nih.gov/omim.

Pagana, K. D., & Pagana, T. J. (1999). *Diagnostic testing and nursing implications: A case study approach.* St. Louis, MO: Mosby-Year Book.

Seashore, M. R., & Wappner, R. S. (1996). *Genetics in primary care and clinical medicine.* Stamford, CT: Appleton & Lange.

Simpson, J. L., & Golbus, M. S. (1992). *Genetics in obstetrics and gynecology* (2nd ed.). Philadelphia: W. B. Saunders.

Taipale, P., Hiilesmaa, V., Salonen, R., & Ylostalo, P. (1997). Increased nuchal translucency as a marker for fetal chromosomal defects. *New England Journal of Medicine, 337,* 1654–1658.

Suggested Readings

Clarke, A. (Ed.). (1994). *Genetic counselling practice and principles.* New York: Routledge.

Clarke, J. T. R. (1996). *A clinical guide to inherited metabolic diseases.* New York: Cambridge University Press.

Jones, K. L. (1997). *Smith's recognizable patterns of human malformation* (5th ed.). Philadelphia: Saunders.

King, R. C., & Stansfield, W. D. (2002). *A dictionary of genetics* (6th ed.). New York: Oxford University Press.

Kingston, H. (2002). *ABCs of clinical genetics* (3rd ed.). London: British Medical Journal.

Lea, D. H., Jenkins, J. F., & Francomario, C. A. (1998). *Genetics in clinical practice: New directions for nursing and health care.* Boston: Jones and Bartlett.

McKusick, V. A. (2000). *Mendelian inheritance in man. Catalogs of human genes and genetic disorders* (12th ed.). Baltimore: Johns Hopkins University Press.

Pauling, I., Itano, H., Singer, S. J., & Wells, I. C. (1949). Sickle cell anemia, a molecular disease. *Science, 110,* 543–548.

Robertson, J. A. (1994). *Children of choice: Freedom and the new reproductive technologies.* Princeton, NJ. Princeton University Press.

Schardein, J. L. (2000). *Chemically induced birth defects* (3rd ed.). New York: Marcel Dekker.

Simpson, J. L. & Elias, S. (2003). Genetics. In *Obstetrics and gynecology* (3rd ed.). Philadelphia: W.B. Saunders.

Resources

American Society of Human Genetics: http://www.ashg.org

Genetics Society of America/American Association for Human Genetics, http://www.genetics-gsa.org

Human Genome Project Information, http://www.ornl.gov/sci/techresources/Human_Genome/home.shtml

International Society of Nursing in Genetics, http://www.isong.org

Mendelian (after Gregor Mendel) inheritance rules and facts, http://www.mendelweb.org

National Coalition for Health Professional Education in Genetics: Core Competencies in Genetics (2003): http://www.nchpeg.org

National Institutes of Health gene sequencing databases, http://www.ncbi.nlm.nih.gov/blast

Online Mendelian Inheritance in Man (OMIM), http://www.ncbi.nlm.nih.gov/omim

The University of Kansas Medical Center, Genetics Education Center, http://www.kumc.edu/GEC

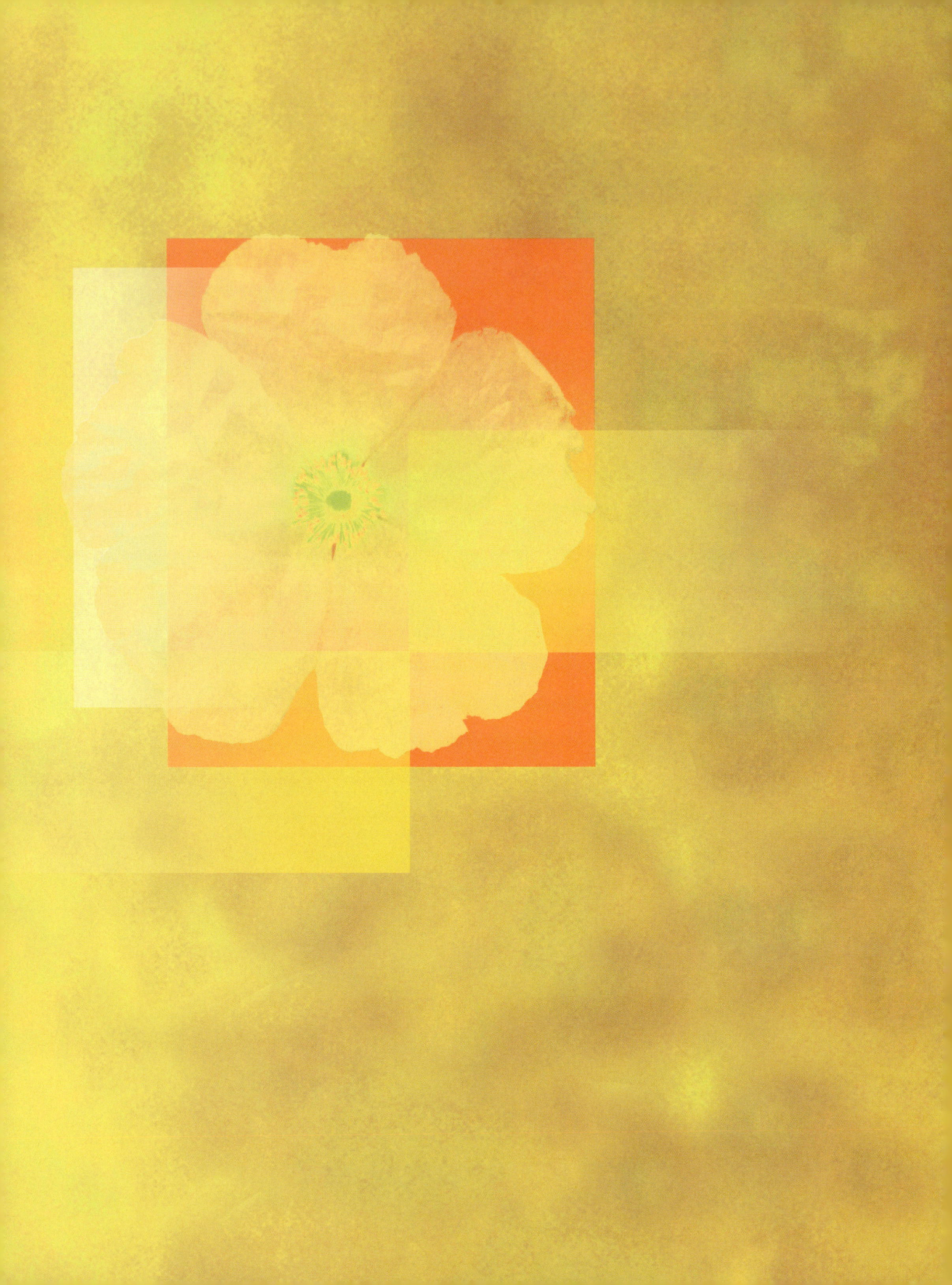

UNIT 4

Pregnancy

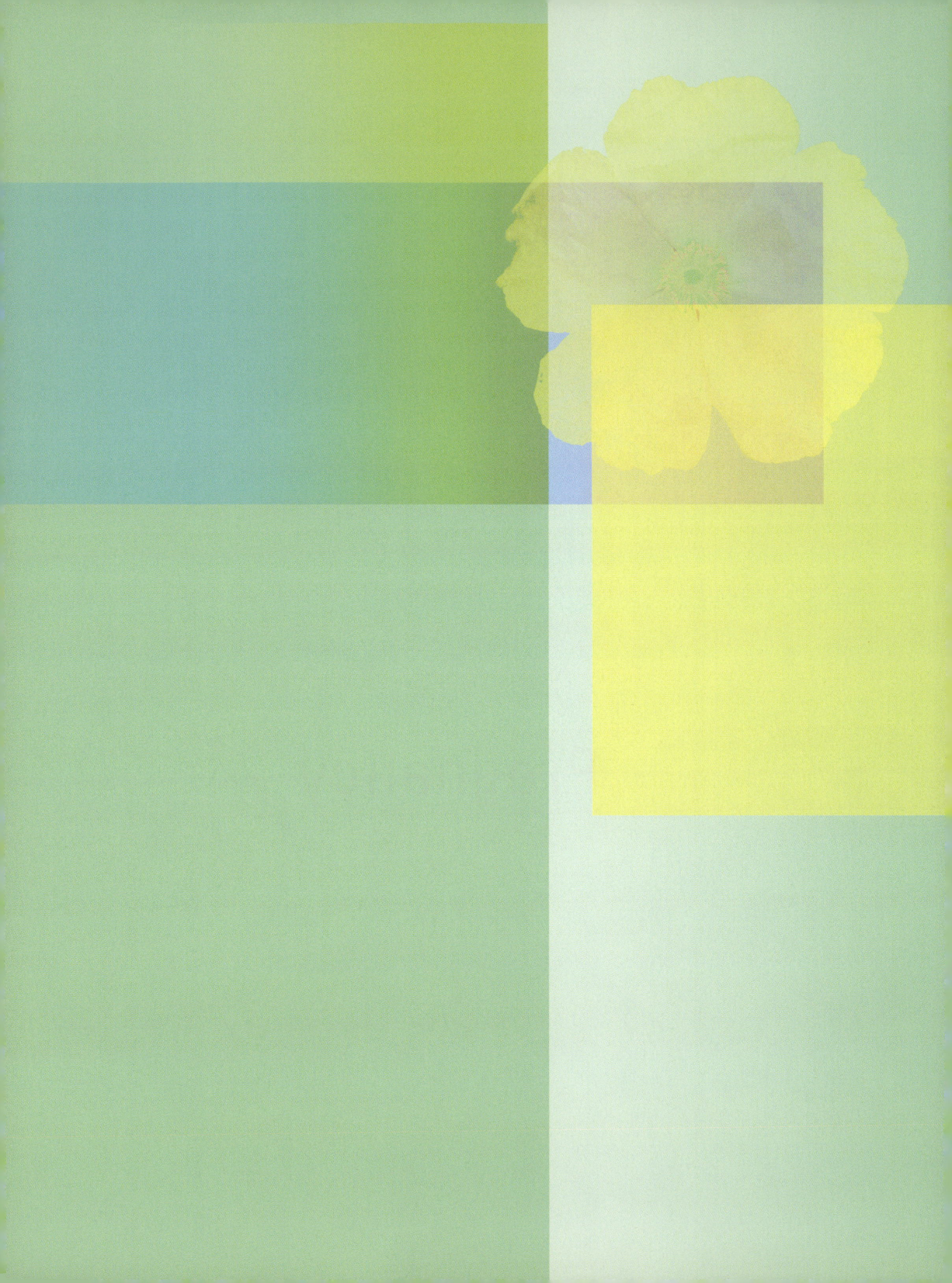

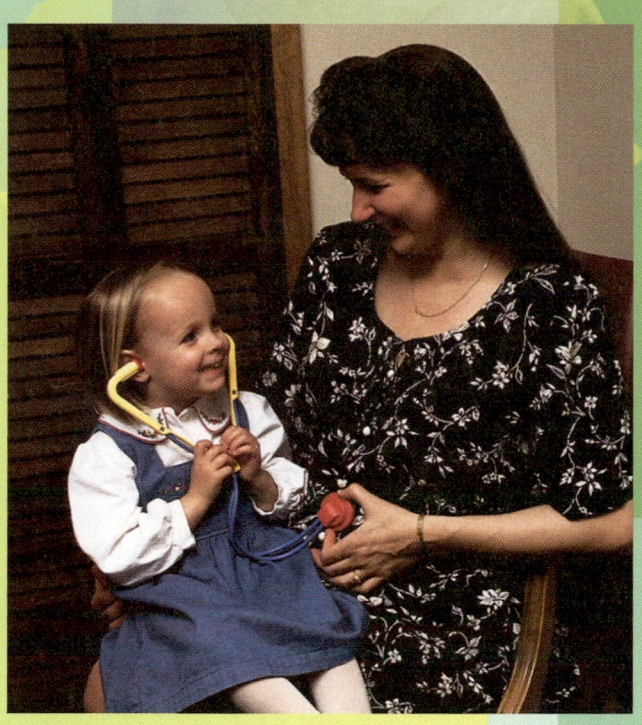

CHAPTER 9

NORMAL PREGNANCY

For a woman, pregnancy is a time of great change and adaptation. Many times, women proceed through the process unaware of the total picture. Nurses can play a vital role in helping a woman achieve a healthy, successful pregnancy by supporting, nurturing, educating, and caring for the pregnant woman and her family. Small gestures, such as always remembering her name, inquiring about family happenings, and being supportive and nonjudgmental, aid the nurse in rendering accurate, effective, and sensitive care. To be a nurse and provide care to a woman during this special life transition and to provide that care with compassion and respect is a great privilege.

Key Terms

Amenorrhea
Ballottement
Braxton Hicks
 contractions
Chadwick's sign
Chloasma
Couvade
Goodell's sign

Hegar's sign
Hyperemesis gravidarum
Linea nigra
Physiologic anemia of
 pregnancy
Quickening
Striae gravidarum
Supine hypotension

Competencies

Upon completion of this chapter, the reader should be able to:

1. List the presumptive, probable, and positive signs of pregnancy.
2. Describe the anatomic and physiologic adaptations to pregnancy.
3. Explain how the anatomic and physiologic adaptations to pregnancy relate to the common discomforts of pregnancy.
4. Outline self-help tips to assist the client in relieving the discomforts of pregnancy.
5. Describe methods of teaching health topics to the pregnant woman.
6. List the developmental tasks that successfully integrate the motherhood role into the woman's personality.
7. Explain how understanding a client's culture can affect her plan of care.

P regnancy is a time of enormous change in a woman's body and mind. These changes affect her physical well-being, self-esteem, interactions with others, daily activities, and future plans. She looks for answers to questions that arise during her pregnancy from many different sources. The nurse's role is uniquely suited to forming a professional bond with the pregnant client and to offering impartial and accurate information that will guide her 9-month journey.

The nurse-client relationship can serve as a "safe haven" for the pregnant woman to ask questions and discuss concerns. Initially, the questions are related to how the pregnancy and birth of the newborn will affect her activities of daily living, her relationship with others, and her interaction with her health care providers. The information may not always be sought by direct questions; therefore, the nurse must be skilled in interviewing and physical assessment techniques with which to meet the woman's needs.

A woman's body changes dramatically to maintain a viable pregnancy. The knowledge and understanding of how these changes occur gives the nurse the ability to assess, make diagnoses, plan, intervene, and evaluate to ensure that the expected outcomes are achieved.

SIGNS OF PREGNANCY

There are many signs of pregnancy. Some signs are suggestive of pregnancy and are referred to as *presumptive* (subjective) signs; these signs could be caused by other conditions, so they do not establish a diagnosis of pregnancy. *Probable* (objective) signs of pregnancy can be documented by physical examination and are signs that are most often characteristic only of pregnancy; these findings could also be caused by other conditions, however, and therefore do not establish a diagnosis of pregnancy. Only three physical findings can establish a diagnosis of pregnancy; these are referred to as *positive* signs. In today's fast-paced world, women are more likely to use an over-the-counter home pregnancy test at the first hint of pregnancy and later seek final confirmation from their health care provider.

Presumptive Signs

Amenorrhea, absence of menses for 3 or more months, is usually the first sign to alert a woman to a possible pregnancy. Other factors, such as excessive exercise, emotional stress, chronic disease states, the onset of menopause, and the use of oral contraceptives, can stop regular periods. The cause of amenorrhea should be assessed and validated.

Nausea and vomiting is another subjective sign that can appear after the first missed period and continue into the fourth month of pregnancy. Women most often report feeling sick in the morning, hence the phrase "morning sickness," but nausea and vomiting may occur at any time of the day. The cause is not clear; it may be the increased levels of hormones. Many women report that emotional factors, noxious smells, irregular eating schedules, and fatigue contribute to the feeling of nausea. Nausea may result from conditions other than pregnancy.

The fatigue of pregnancy can be overwhelming and distressing. The client may voice concerns that she is more tired or drowsy after a normal day during pregnancy than she was after a normal day before she became pregnant; fatigue, however, does not confirm pregnancy.

In the first few weeks of pregnancy, the pressure exerted on the bladder by the enlarging uterus causes urinary frequency. In the second trimester, the uterus grows into the abdomen, somewhat relieving the pressure. Late in pregnancy, as the fetus grows and descends into the pelvis, urinary frequency returns. Do not assume urinary frequency is caused by the changes of pregnancy; assess for signs of infection.

Changes in the breasts are another presumptive sign of pregnancy. Increased amounts of estrogen and progesterone cause the breasts to swell and become tender. The initial changes in the breasts are similar to the changes that occur in the menstrual cycle. As the pregnancy progresses, the tenderness subsides, but growth of breast tissue continues.

A woman's first awareness of fetal movement is called **quickening**. The movement is usually described as a fluttery feeling, similar to being excited and having "butterflies." Quickening is initially felt between 18 and 20 weeks of gestation, but may be felt by the multigravida (woman who is pregnant for at least the second time) as early as 16 weeks. The documented date of the first fetal movement can be used in conjunction with other data in determining the expected date of delivery. Other conditions may mimic quickening; these must be ruled out before a diagnosis of pregnancy may be made.

Probable Signs

At 8 to 10 weeks' gestation the bimanual pelvic examination will document an enlarged and softened uterine body. Uterine enlargement is more definitive if the growth is progressive and predictable. The fundus should be just above the symphysis pubis at 10 to 12 weeks and at the umbilicus at 20 weeks. Abdominal enlargement mirrors the uterine growth and is especially evident earlier in the pregnancy of the multigravida. Other causes for uterine enlargement, such as fibroids or tumors, must be ruled out before pregnancy can be confirmed.

There are other changes that may be noted on physical examination. Softening of the cervix is called **Goodell's sign**; normally the cervix is firm. The color change from pink to bluish-purplish in the mucous membranes of the cervix, vagina, and vulva is identified as **Chadwick's sign**. The increased vascularization in this area causes the color change and is attributed to the increase in the estrogen hormone. **Hegar's sign**, usually evident at 6 to 8 weeks' gestation, is the softening of the isthmus of the uterus, often referred to as the lower uterine segment.

During the fourth or fifth month, if the fetus is pushed upward through the vagina or abdomen, the floating fetus rebounds against the examiner's fingers; this is known as **ballottement** (Figure 9-1). This occurs only while the fetus is small in comparison to the amount of amniotic fluid.

Today, pregnancy tests are available in inexpensive commercial kits that can be done quickly. Tests that are performed by trained personnel are highly accurate and, with correct technique, precise. Most pregnancy tests work on the same premise: they identify human chorionic gonadotropin (hCG) hormone, or a subunit, by detecting an antibody to the hCG molecule in urine or serum. Commercial laboratory tests that measure hCG in the urine are accurate close to 100% of the time and can detect a pregnancy as early as 10 days after conception. The hormone hCG can be detected in maternal blood at 7 days after conception with sensitive assays; the exact level of hCG can

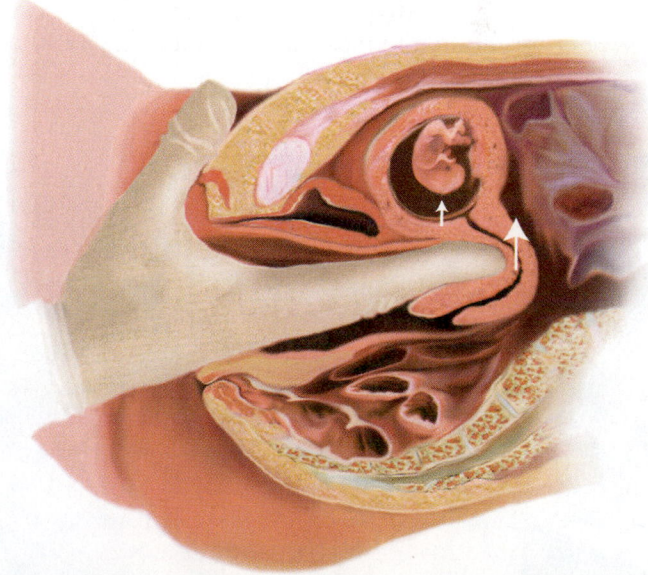

Figure 9-1   Ballottement.

assist in dating the pregnancy. Most sensitive commercial test kits can detect a pregnancy with precision after the first missed period.

For most home pregnancy test kits the number-one concern is operator error. A false-negative result can mislead the woman, who may ignore the presumptive signs of pregnancy and therefore delay seeking prenatal care. A positive test result may cause a delay in seeking follow-up care, because many women feel the first visit to a practitioner is only for diagnosis of pregnancy. Preconception counseling is crucial for educating women on caring for their body before pregnancy. At that time, it is beneficial to share information on the appropriate management of pregnancy, diagnosis and the initiation of prenatal care.

Positive Signs

Positive signs (noted by the examiner) that confirm the pregnancy are fetal heart sounds and fetal movement and visualization of the fetus during ultrasound.

The fetal heartbeat can be auscultated with a fetoscope at 18–20 weeks. The heartbeat can be detected at 10–12 weeks with an electronic Doppler. Normal fetal heart rate is 120 to 160 bpm.

The earlier the fetal heartbeat is detected, the more likely it may be confused with other sounds that can be detected in pregnancy. The uterine souffle is the sound made by the increased amount of blood perfusing the uterus and mimics the maternal pulse, which is a slower rate than the fetal heartbeat. The sound heard as the blood flows through the umbilical cord is called the funic souffle.

Fetal movement detected by a qualified examiner is another sign that is diagnostic of pregnancy. At 18 to 20 weeks' gestation, the movement is felt as a faint flut-

Nursing Tip *Accurate Detection of the Fetal Heart Rate*

To ensure an accurate diagnosis of the fetal heart beat, it must be distinguished from the maternal pulse. To do this, the fetal heartbeat should be auscultated, while simultaneously assessing the maternal radial pulse.

tering and progresses to rolling and kicking in the late second and third trimester. The movement in later gestation can often be seen on visual inspection of the abdomen.

The use of ultrasound is very common in today's obstetric practice. The ultrasound examination is accomplished by placing a transducer on the abdomen above the symphysis pubis (Figure 9-2). A normal pregnancy can be detected at as early as 4 weeks' gestation, using the last menstrual period for dating. The fetal brain and heartbeat can be visualized by 8 weeks' gestation.

The use of a transvaginal transducer placed into the vagina is helpful when using ultrasound to confirm a pregnancy or seek pathology in the obese woman or to detect a pregnancy in a complicated case. The fetal heart rate can be detected via transvaginal ultrasound as early as 4 weeks after conception. A transvaginal ultrasound examination produces better visualization than abdominal ultrasound, and can detect not only an early pregnancy but also extrauterine structures, such as an ectopic pregnancy or ovarian mass (Gabbe, Niebyl, & Simpson, 1996).

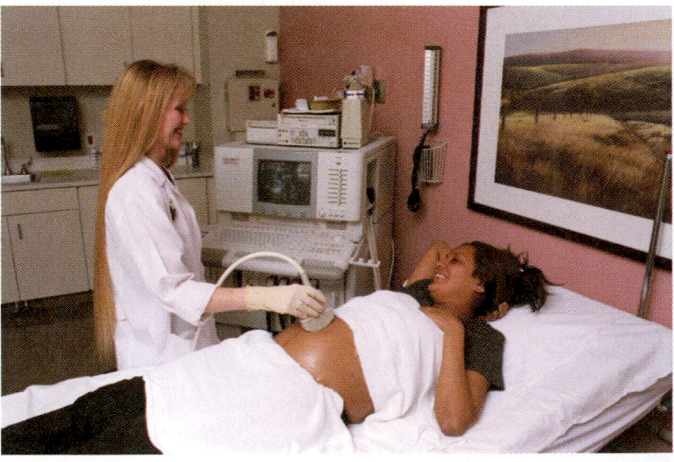

A.

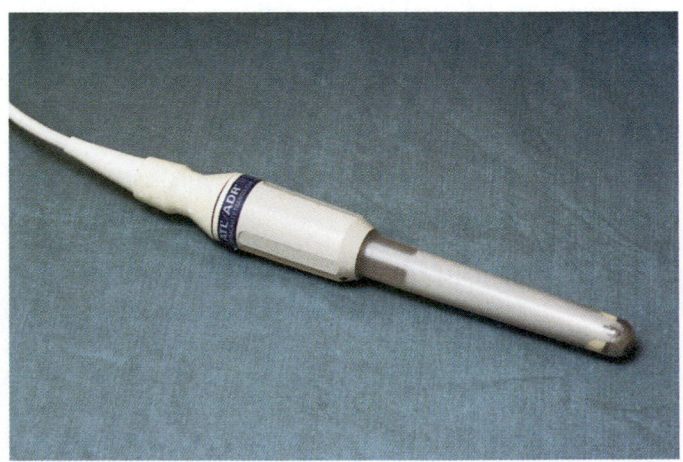

B.

Figure 9-2   A. Abdominal ultrasound. B. Transducer for transvaginal ultrasound.

EXPECTED DATE OF DELIVERY

The mean duration of pregnancy can differ between groups of women by ethnicity, geographical location, or age, but the most common period used as the mean is 280 days, or 40 weeks from the first day of the last period. Naegele's rule is the most commonly used calculation for date of expected delivery. To calculate the gestational or menstrual age, add 7 days to the date of the first day of the last normal menstrual period and count back 3 months.

This date is an estimated date of delivery and it can be inaccurate by 2 weeks. Because gestation, measured in weeks, is so important for the management of the pregnancy, other clinical indicators should be monitored. During the first physical examination, the size of the uterus can be determined; the fetal heart rate can be heard at 10 to 12 weeks by electronic Doppler ultrasound; the first fetal movement can be felt at about 18 weeks; and the measurement of fundal (top of the uterus) height with each prenatal visit can track gestational age (Figure 9-3). If the results of the physical examination do not correspond with the estimated weeks of pregnancy, as determined by calculating the delivery date, an ultrasound examination may be performed between 12 and 18 weeks to obtain fetal measurements that result in a more accurate delivery date.

PHYSIOLOGIC ADAPTATION TO PREGNANCY

Many physiologic changes take place in a woman's body when she is pregnant. The nurse and client must be able to distinguish between those changes that are normal adaptations and responses to the pregnant state and those changes that are outside the realm of normal and require intervention.

Reproductive System

Each organ of the reproductive system undergoes dramatic changes during pregnancy.

Uterus

Although every system in a woman's body changes to adapt to the growing fetus, the uterus undergoes the most dramatic transformation (Figure 9-4). Beginning as an almost solid organ the size of a human fist, the uterus enlarges to a thin-walled, hollow organ that can hold a volume of 15 to 20 liters. The increased production of estrogen and progesterone is thought to initiate the process of uterine growth, but the exact trigger mechanism is unclear.

> **Nursing Tip** *Example of Naegele's Rule*
>
> First day of last period was January 12, 2004.
>
> Calculate: 1/12/2004 + 7 days = 1/19/2004.
>
> Count back 3 months to October. The expected delivery date is 10/19/2005.

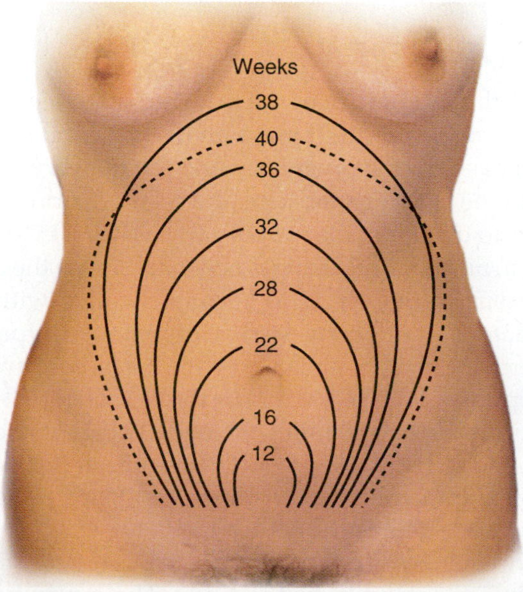

Figure 9-3 Approximate height of the fundus as the uterus enlarges.

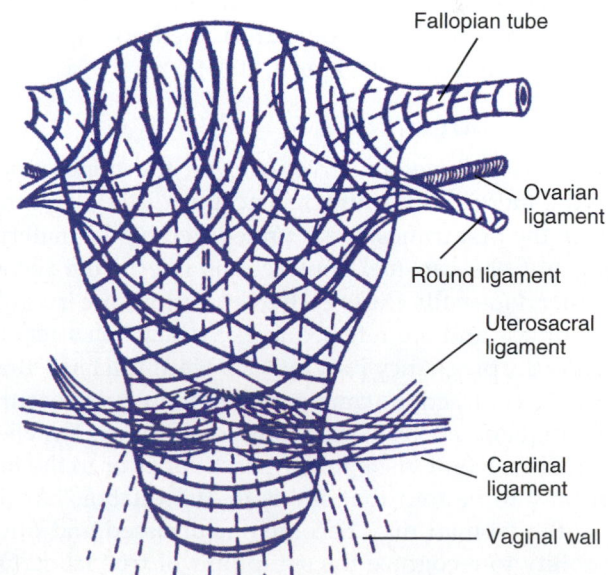

Figure 9-4 The configuration of muscle layers allows the uterus to expand evenly in all directions during pregnancy.

It is not until the 12th week of gestation, when the fetus reaches a crown-to-rump length of 8 to 9 centimeters, that the growth of the uterus can be attributed to mechanical distention. The increase in intrauterine pressure results from the growing fetus, placenta, and increase in volume of amniotic fluid. Growth of the uterus is not symmetrical and occurs predominantly in the fundus. The walls of the uterus become thin but are strengthened by the accumulation of fibrous tissue in the muscle layers and an increase in elastic tissue. At 12 weeks, the fundus rises above the symphysis and begins to displace the intestines. It will continue to grow upward and slightly rotate to the right. When the pregnant woman is upright, the broad and round ligaments anchor the gravid uterus and the anterior abdominal wall provides support. The weight of the uterus may produce tension on these ligaments that causes inflammation and discomfort. In the supine position, the uterus of the pregnant woman falls backward and puts pressure on the vertebral column and the great blood vessels. Uterine growth is predictable, any significant deviation should be investigated.

Uteroplacental Blood Flow

Although not visibly evident to the pregnant woman, the changes that begin at conception progress rapidly. The placenta is mature at 8 to 10 weeks and remains larger than the fetus until 15 to 16 weeks. To achieve adequate exchange of nutrients and waste, there is an increase in the supply of blood to the uteroplacental unit. The body is able to accommodate the necessary volume by increasing the number and diameter of the vessels feeding the uterus. The proportion of the blood volume needed to perfuse the uterus and intervillous space increases over the weeks of gestation. By term, a total of 20% to 25% of the maternal cardiac output is used to supply the uterus and placenta (Blackburn, 2003).

Uterine Contractility

The uterus is never inactive; even in the nonpregnant state the uterus will contract (Blackburn, 2003). Contractions in the first trimester are undetected by the maternal client, but she can feel contractions late in the second trimester. Normally these early contractions are irregular and painless and are referred to as **Braxton Hicks contractions**. As the pregnancy progresses toward full term, Braxton Hicks contractions can become more regular, occur at more frequent intervals, and cause discomfort. The client may make several visits to her practitioner or to the hospital only to be told that she is in "false labor." At this point, the woman may become embarrassed and doubt her ability to recognize the symptoms of true labor. One component of prenatal education is to communicate to the client the symptoms of preterm and term labor and the importance of notifying her health practitioner if she has any questions.

Client Education

True versus False Labor

The following are symptoms of true labor which help to differentiate from symptoms of false labor:

- **Pain begins in the lower back and moves forward across the lower abdomen.**

- **Contractions intensify and do not ease, despite the level of the client's activity.**

- **Contractions most often become progressively more frequent, regular, and painful.**

- **To check for contractions, place your hand on the fundus or top of the uterus; during the peak of the contraction the degree of firmness should be similar to the firmness felt when touching your forehead.**

- **Bloody show from the vagina is present and is pinkish or blood-streaked.**

- **If the membranes rupture, the fluid may either leak or gush from the vagina (about 15% of time the membranes rupture before labor begins).**

Contractions occur throughout the pregnancy and help stimulate blood flow and maintain the muscle tone of the uterus.

Cervix

Although the cervix does not undergo the same dramatic changes as the uterus, it plays an instrumental role in the maintenance of the pregnancy and the delivery of the infant. In the prepregnant state, the cervix is firm and feels similar to the top of the ear. As early as 4 weeks after conception, biochemical changes occur and cause the connective tissue of the cervix to become swollen with water (edematous) and congested with blood (hyperemic). These changes, in conjunction with the hypertrophy and hyperplasia of the cervical glands, demonstrate the characteristic cervical softening of Goodell's sign and cervical cyanosis of Chadwick's sign. At this time, a digital examination of the cervix demonstrates a softened consistency, similar to the feel of the ear lobe.

The changes that occur in the cervix demonstrate the amazing adaptability of the body. The cervix provides support to maintain an intact pregnancy and, as delivery approaches, it softens and opens to allow delivery of the infant.

A mucus plug forms within the cervix and serves to protect the fetus and the membranes from bacteria that may ascend through the vagina during pregnancy. As labor becomes imminent, the mucus plug is expelled (sometimes over a period of time) as the cervix begins to dilate. As the cervix dilates, small arteries may burst and the blood mixes with the normal mucus, producing what is known as bloody show.

Vagina, Perineum, and Vulva

In preparation for the delivery of the neonate, there is increased vascularization, softening of the connective tissue, and hypertrophy of the smooth muscle in the vagina, perineum, and vulva. The vagina turns the characteristic purplish color of Chadwick's sign and vaginal secretions increase as a result of increased vascular engorgement. The walls of the vagina must expand without trauma during the delivery; therefore, the mucosa thicken and the rugae (vaginal folds) become pronounced. Upon vaginal examination, the caregiver may note that the rugae that line the lower portion of the anterior wall of the vagina are so enlarged that they protrude through the vulva.

As the physiologic changes progress, the cells of the vagina contain increasing amounts of glycogen. The cells slough off the walls of the vagina and contribute to the increase in discharge. The *Lactobacillus acidophilus* found in normal vaginal secretions breaks down the glycogen into lactic acid (Cunningham et al., 2001). The environment of the vagina is acidic and prevents the growth of many bacterial infections. If the client complains of increased vaginal discharge, the amount, color, consistency, and odor of discharge must be assessed so that an appropriate diagnosis can be made. One of the most frequent infections in pregnancy is a vaginal yeast infection (candidiasis), which grows readily in the normal acidic discharge.

Ovaries

Once conception has occurred, the production and release of follicles from the ovaries ceases. The corpus luteum is formed within the ovary and secretes progesterone, with production peaking at 8 days. Progesterone is necessary for the maintenance of the pregnancy, so that if implantation occurs, the trophoblast secretes hCG to stimulate the corpus luteum to continue with the production of progesterone (Blackburn, 2003). The placenta begins manufacturing progesterone at 6–7 weeks' gestation. At this time the placenta assumes this function and the involution of the corpus luteum begins.

Breasts

The changes in the physical characteristics of the breasts are caused by the increased production of estrogen and progesterone. Early in pregnancy, the breasts become full and tender. In preparation for feeding the infant, the number of mammary alveoli increase and the breasts become physically larger. As the breasts enlarge, a web of veins may become visible under the skin. The pregnant woman may question the slightly reddened or darkened, depressed streaks that appear on the skin of the breasts. These striations (stretch marks) occur most often on breasts that enlarge significantly. The striae eventually fade to a soft silver color, but do not disappear completely. The areolae broaden and become darker in color as a result of increased pigmentation. The tubercles of Montgomery are sebaceous glands located on the areolae that become more visible through hypertrophic changes. In preparation for lactation, the glands secrete a substance that helps maintain the suppleness of the areolae. Increased sensitivity of the now larger and more erect nipple contributes to the later establishment of lactation. The pregnant woman may notice leaking of colostrum, a protein-rich yellowish fluid, from her breasts after the first few months of pregnancy.

Women with small breasts may welcome the increase in size, but women with large breasts may find it difficult to tolerate. Wearing a properly fitted bra that supports the breasts should be emphasized in early prenatal visits.

Hematologic System

The changes in the hematologic system occur to maintain homeostasis during the pregnancy and the postpartum period. Blood volume increases to nourish the fetus and to protect the mother from excessive blood loss during and after delivery and placental separation. Being aware of these changes and how they affect normal hematologic values helps the nurse in identifying the difference in expected adaptations and pathologic alterations (Table 9-1).

Blood Volume

The blood volume of the pregnant woman is 40% to 50% more than the prepregnant state. Obese women and women who have multiple fetuses or a fetus that is large for gestation age may attain a blood volume that is double their usual blood volume. Progesterone causes the tone of the vasculature to relax and enables the body to accommodate the massive increase in blood volume that is necessary to meet the increased needs of the pregnancy. Hypervolemia of pregnancy is an expected and necessary change and affects the plan of client care.

Plasma volume begins to increase at 6 to 8 weeks' gestation, increases rapidly until about 32 to 34 weeks, and then reaches a plateau until term. The increase in the plasma volume is 40% to 45% and measures 1,200 to 1,600 mL above prepregnant volume. As in most changes that occur during pregnancy, the exact mechanism that triggers this change is not well understood. One influencing factor may be increased hormone production. Another

Table 9-1	Normal Changes in Maternal Laboratory Values	
TEST	**NORMAL VALUE**	**CHANGE DURING PREGNANCY**
Hematocrit	37%–47%	Decreased
Hemoglobin level	12–16 g/dL	Decreased
Platelet count	150,000–350,000/mm³	Increased after delivery
Partial thromboplastin time (PTT)	12–14 sec	Slightly decreased
Leukocyte	6.0 (4.5–11) × 10/mm³	9.2 (6–16) × 10/mm³
Fibrinogen level	250 mg/dL	Increased

Note. From *Medical Complications during Pregnancy* (5th ed.), by G. N. Burrow and T. F. Duffy, 1999, Philadelphia: W. B. Saunders.

Critical Thinking

Physiologic Anemia of Pregnancy

Joan is a 16-year-old woman with a pregnancy at 28 weeks' gestation. She is attending high school and plans on living at home when the baby comes. She is feeling more tired than usual. Laboratory samples are drawn and analyzed; her hemoglobin level is 8.5 mg/dL and hematocrit is 30%. This is lower than the physiologic anemia of pregnancy.

Is this within the range of physiologic anemia of pregnancy or is this iron deficiency anemia? The nurse might want to get the following information:

What are the mainstays of Joan's diet? Has iron supplementation been prescribed? Is she taking the supplement? Is Joan well hydrated? What fluids is she drinking? What other labs would be helpful in determining the cause of Joan's anemia?

close link may be the changes that take place in the fluid balance in the renal and cardiovascular systems.

Blackburn (2003) noted that placental mass and birth weight are positively correlated with plasma volume, demonstrating the close relationship of fetal weight to plasma volume. In pathologic states, such as pregnancy-induced hypertension, there is a decrease in plasma volume related to the changes that occur in the vasculature.

Red Blood Cells

An increase in the number of red blood cells is another significant adaptation to pregnancy. The red blood cell mass increases up to 33% (450 mL) with iron supplementation and increases up to 18% (200 mL) without supplementation (Blackburn, 2003). The volume increase is progressive without the plateau at term that is observed in the plasma volume.

During the pregnancy, the plasma begins to expand earlier and to a volume three times greater than the red blood cell mass. The disproportion of these volumes causes a dilution of the red blood cell mass, thus lowering the hemoglobin of the pregnant woman and resulting in a phenomenon called **physiologic anemia of pregnancy**. Because this anemia is caused by normal physiologic changes in blood volume during pregnancy, it is not considered a true anemia. The average hemoglobin level of the pregnant woman at term is 12 mg/dL, with a mean hematocrit of 33.8%. Although the normal hemoglobin level can drop up to 2 mg/dL with the normal dilution of the red blood cell mass, Blackburn (2003) states that true iron deficiency anemia should always be considered, especially when the hemoglobin level drops to 10.5 mg/dL or less.

Blood Coagulation

Neither bleeding time or clotting time change in the normal pregnant woman. Gabbe et al. (1996) noted that although there are increases in some of the clotting factors, especially fibrinogen, the hypercoagulability of pregnancy is more likely attributable to the higher incidence of thrombus formation and coagulopathies during pregnancy. When evaluating the pregnant woman, remember that the highest incidence of thromboembolism is in the postpartum period.

Cardiovascular System

To maintain a viable pregnancy, the cardiovascular system undergoes major but reversible changes in cardiac function and hemodynamics. These changes are triggered by the increase in circulating hormones: estrogen, progesterone, and prostaglandin.

Heart

The position of the heart is changed by the inability of the diaphragm to fully expand, increasing intra-abdominal pressure. The heart is pushed upward and to the left and rotated slightly, as shown in Figure 9-5. On radiographic film, the heart may appear enlarged. The position is influenced by other anatomic changes, and the varying degrees of these changes in individual pregnancies make it difficult to diagnose cardiomegaly by X-ray studies alone.

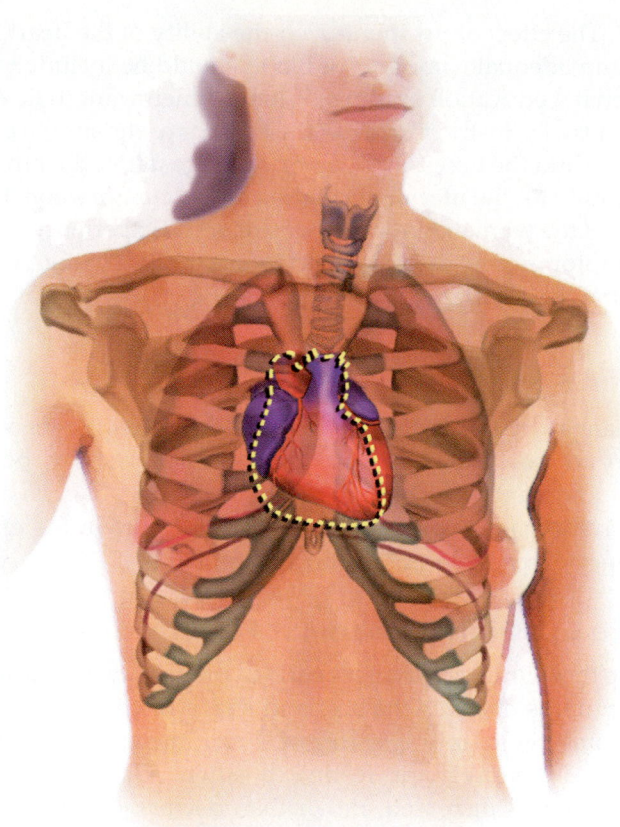

Figure 9-5   The position of the heart is changed during pregnancy. The dotted lines represent the nonpregnant position of the heart. The PMI (point of maximal impulse) is altered and heart sounds may be louder.

There are no significant changes in the electrocardio-gram (ECG) of the pregnant woman. In 90% of pregnant women, a systolic heart murmur can be heard at 20 weeks' gestation and disappears shortly after delivery. Also, in the majority of pregnant women, a third heart sound, or gallop, can be easily detected. Diastolic mur-murs are rare in normal pregnant women and the cause of these sounds should be investigated. A murmur known as the "mammary souffle" can be heard in the left and right side between the first, second, and third intercostal spaces. The increased blood flow to the breasts is believed to be the cause of this continuous murmur.

Cardiac Output

During pregnancy, there is an increase in cardiac output beginning as early as 10 weeks and peaking at 20 at 24 weeks. Cardiac output is calculated by the heart rate times the *stroke volume*, the amount of blood leaving the heart. Early in pregnancy the increase in cardiac output is caused by an increase in the stroke volume, and the heart rate remains at the prepregnant rate. As the pregnancy progresses, the heart rate increases by up to 20 bpm and the stroke volume declines to prepregnant rates. By means

of the increase in the heart rate, the blood volume needed to adequately provide blood flow to the fetus and the ma-ternal vital organs can be maintained. In the nonpregnant woman, average cardiac output is 4.5 L/min with the uterus receiving 2%; at term in the pregnant woman, car-diac output is about 6 L/min with about 20% going to the uterus. The percentage of the cardiac output that is mapped to the other organs remains relatively the same in the nonpregnant and pregnant woman. Because of the overall increase in blood volume, the amount of blood available to most vital organs increases.

Blood Pressure

It would seem logical to assume that the increases in the blood volume and cardiac output of the pregnant woman would lead to elevated blood pressure, but other adapta-tions take place to prevent this from occurring. Both sys-tolic and diastolic blood pressure actually decrease in the first trimester by 5 to 10 mmHg and 10 to 15 mmHg, re-spectively, and begin to rise at 22 to 24 weeks, returning to normal prepregnant readings at term. The decrease in the blood pressure is probably a result of the effect of in-creased circulating hormones, which, in turn, decrease the peripheral vascular resistance. This adaptation must be understood when assessing the blood pressure late in the second and into the third trimester.

The ability of the pregnant body to compensate for the increased blood volume results from the increased ca-pacity and compliance of the vascular system. Venous pressure in the upper extremities is unchanged. In the lower extremities, the pressure may gradually increase as the uterus enlarges and begins to exert pressure on the in-ferior vena cava and pelvic veins. The increase in pressure below the level of the uterus can result in the develop-ment of varicose veins in the legs and perineum. When the pregnant woman is in the upright position, the uterus can interfere with the blood return to the heart. Blood pools in the lower extremities and may contribute to the dependent edema that may occur in the last half of the pregnancy. The lower extremity blood congestion seen in pregnancy can be alleviated by lying in a lateral re-cumbent position (Figure 9-6). Prenatal education should include teaching pregnant women to avoid prolonged standing, use support hose, and take frequent rest breaks.

Nursing Tip   *Assessing Blood Pressure*

Prepregnant blood pressure measurements, instead of first trimester readings, should be used as the baseline when ruling out pregnancy-induced hypertension.

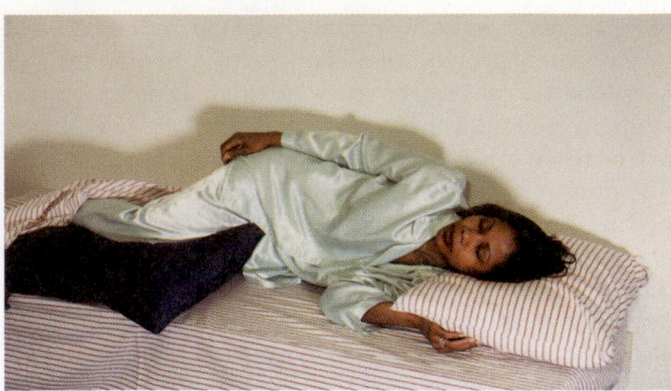

Figure 9-6   Resting in the lateral position helps to alleviate pooling of blood in the lower extremities and reduce vena caval compression by the gravid uterus.

Systemic Vascular Resistance

In pregnancy the increase in cardiac output and the slight decrease in mean arterial pressure results in a decrease in the *systemic vascular resistance*, or total circulatory resistance. Increased hormonal activity relaxes smooth muscle, causing vessels to dilate and thus allowing the body to accommodate the increased blood volume without pressure changes. The uteroplacental circulation provides a new and large capacity organ that diverts a portion of the increased cardiac output. Finally, increased circulating levels of prostaglandin during pregnancy serve to buffer the effects of certain vasoconstrictors. These adaptations allow the pregnant woman to accommodate the larger volume of cardiac output without the injurious side effects expected in a nonpregnant woman.

The Effect of Positioning during Pregnancy

As the pregnant woman approaches term, she may report that lying on her back (supine) causes her to feel lightheaded, dizzy, or faint. The symptoms are a result of the hypotension that occurs when the weight of the gravid uterus partially occludes the vena cava and descending aorta. The occlusion of these vessels may cause a decrease in the blood return from the lower extremities to the heart, therefore causing a decrease in cardiac output and a decrease in blood pressure. If the decrease in cardiac output is prolonged, blood flow to the placenta can be affected and fetal hypoxia may occur.

Supine hypotension, also known as vena cava syndrome, occurs when the pregnant woman is supine. The enlarged, heavy uterus presses on the inferior vena cava causing a reduced blood flow back to the right atrium (Figure 9-7). The pregnant woman experiences dizziness; clammy, pale skin; and lowered blood pressure. The situation is relieved when the pregnant woman lies on her side.

The effect of positioning on the ability of the heart to pump adequate amounts of blood should be included in prenatal education sessions. When women want to lie on their backs, instruct them on the hazards of the supine position and the necessity of using a wedge under the hip to laterally tilt the uterus, alleviating vessel compression. Instruct the woman to turn to her side if she experiences the symptoms of hypotension and to use the side-lying position when resting.

Respiratory System

Changes that occur in the respiratory system are necessary to meet the increased demand for oxygen by both the pregnant woman and her fetus. These changes are both mechanical and biochemical and improve the efficiency of the maternal respiratory function.

Changes in Mechanical Function

The thoracic cavity changes early in pregnancy. The growing uterus changes the size and shape of the abdomen, causing the diaphragm to rise 4 centimeters above the normal nonpregnant resting position. Diaphragmatic excursion is increased, rather than decreased. The chest circumference increases 5 to 7 centimeters, and the transverse diameter increases approximately 2 centimeters (Gabbe et al., 1996). Changes in the structure of the respiratory organs takes place to prepare the body for the enlarging uterus and increased lung volume.

Effects of Progesterone

The level of circulating progesterone increases as the pregnancy progresses. Progesterone works by direct stimulation of the central respiratory system to increase tidal volume and decrease blood P_{CO_2}. The increased awareness of breathing or dyspnea experienced in pregnancy may be related to this change. Progesterone also plays a role in decreasing airway resistance by relaxation of smooth muscle, thus improving the efficiency of breathing.

Lung Volumes and Gas Exchange

Respiratory rate does not change significantly, so lung volume changes are based on mechanical and hormonal or biochemical influences. The greatest change is the 30% to 40% increase in tidal volume, which is the amount of air inspired and expired with each breath. The functional residual capacity, the volume of gas that remains in the lungs at the end of a normal expiration, is decreased by 20% because of the elevated position of the diaphragm. The volume changes help maintain a better mix of air and a more efficient method of gas exchange.

Lung volume changes and the effect of progesterone cause a state of compensated respiratory alkalosis. The

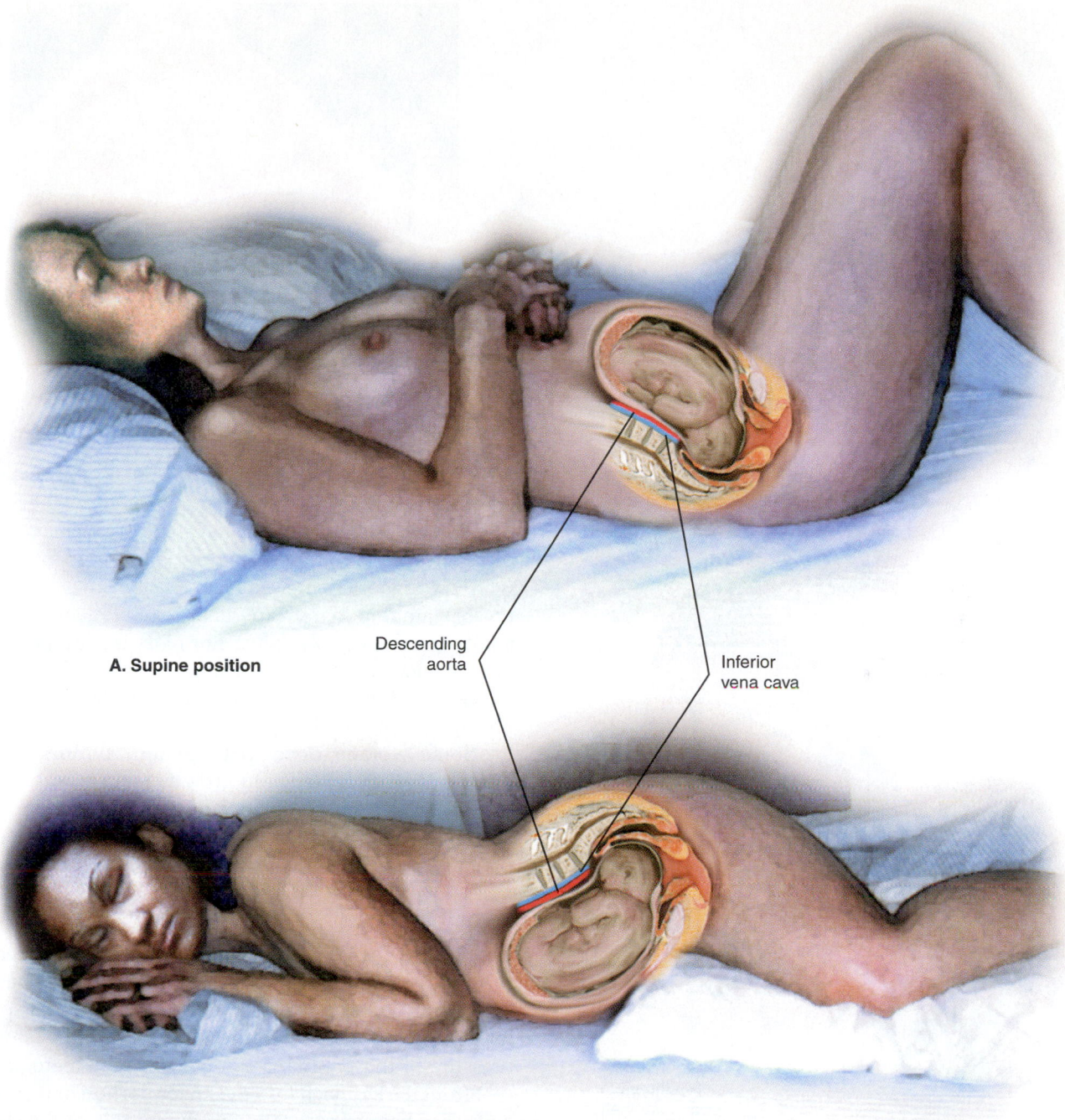

A. Supine position

Descending
aorta

Inferior
vena cava

B. Right lateral position

Figure 9-7   A. Supine hypotension can occur when the woman is in the supine position. The weight of the gravid uterus may partially occlude the descending aorta and vena cava. B. Maintaining a lateral position alleviates the compression.

purpose of the increased Pao_2 and the decreased Pco_2 of maternal circulation is to facilitate the removal of carbon dioxide from the fetus. The decreased maternal Pco_2 level is compensated by increased renal secretion of bicarbonate, allowing the maternal arterial pH to remain within normal limits. Many women also experience increased nasal congestion.

Gastrointestinal System

There are anatomic and physiologic changes that occur in the gastrointestinal and hepatic system. These changes are necessary to support maternal and fetal nutrition but are also the changes most often associated with the common discomforts of pregnancy. As shown in Figure 9-8, many organs of the gastrointestinal system are displaced or compressed by the gravid uterus.

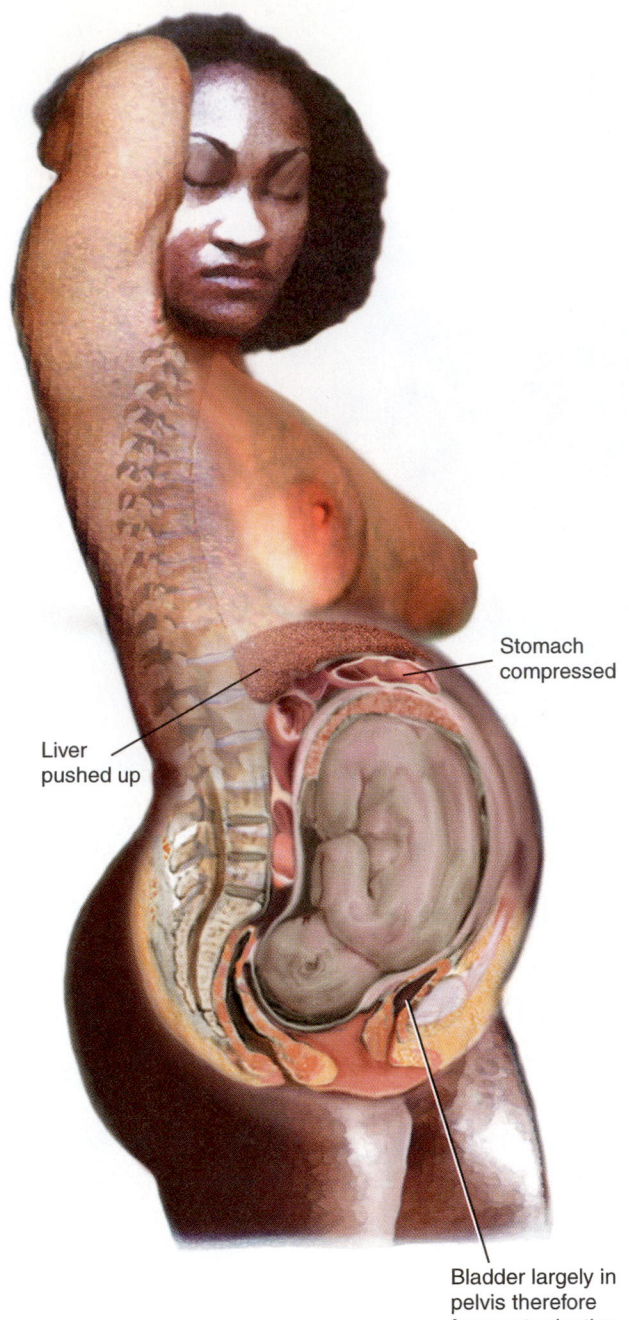

Figure 9-8   Crowding of abdominal contents by gravid uterus.

Liver pushed up

Stomach compressed

Bladder largely in pelvis therefore frequent urination

Mouth

Estrogen causes increased proliferation of blood vessels and connective tissue in the gums, causing them to become soft and edematous. The tissue is friable and may bleed easily. Chewing can cause discomfort and make meeting nutritional demands more difficult. Poor oral hygiene, periodontal disease, and increased maternal age may increase the incidence of gingivitis. Contrary to folk beliefs, there is no evidence that pregnancy increases the incidence of dental caries or tooth loss. However, some

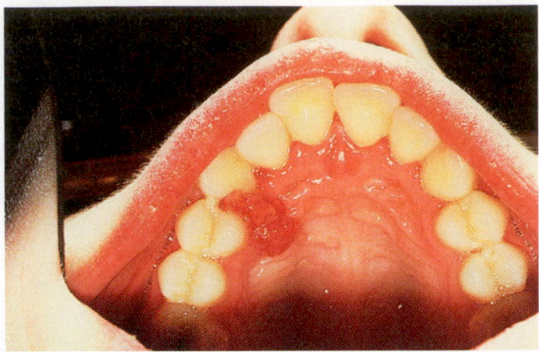

Figure 9-9   Pregnancy tumor. (Courtesy of Dr. Joseph L. Konzelman, School of Dentistry, Medical College of Georgia)

women may be more prone to gingivitis. Good dental hygiene is important to prevent this.

The saliva becomes more acidic, but an increase in the amount of saliva is not a normal change in pregnancy. There is an unusual condition called ptyalism, or an increase in saliva, that usually occurs in pregnant women who are experiencing nausea. Gabbe and colleagues (1996) state that many experts believe ptyalism is the inability to swallow the saliva normally during periods of nausea and vomiting. Pytalism can begin as early as 2 to 3 weeks and occurs most frequently in the daytime and disappears after delivery.

Some women develop pregnancy tumors in their mouths (Figure 9-9). These growths are usually benign. The vascular proliferation occurs secondary to hormonal changes. These changes may not resolve at the end of pregnancy.

Esophagus

Changes in the esophagus are caused by the effects of progesterone on smooth muscle. Peristalsis of the esophagus decreases and relaxes the lower esophageal sphincter. These changes and the increase in the stomach pressure of the pregnant woman can potentiate acid reflux from the stomach into the lower portion of the esophagus. The burning sensation in the middle of the chest is called pyrosis, or heartburn.

Stomach and Intestines

When assessing the stomach and intestines, some physical findings may be changed because of the displacement of these organs by the enlarging uterus. Bowel sounds may not be evident in the four normal quadrants of the abdomen, and the appendix may be found as high as the right flank. Changes in the tone of the stomach and delayed stomach emptying may contribute to the early nausea and vomiting that sometimes accompany pregnancy.

Acid production in the stomach is decreased in the first and second trimester, gradually returning to normal prepregnant levels at term. Because normal acid production returns at term and stomach emptying is slowed during labor, the oral intake of the pregnant woman must be assessed for 6 to 8 hours before labor, because vomiting and aspiration are major risks during the administration of general anesthesia, should that be necessary.

The progressive slowing of intestinal motility correlates with the increase in the production of progesterone as pregnancy moves to term. The slowing progression of the intestinal contents allows more efficient absorption of nutrients and fluids but also contributes to constipation. Another annoying problem, flatulence, results from the slowing of contents through the intestinal tract and the bowel compressed by the gravid uterus.

Gallbladder

The effect of progesterone on smooth muscle also decreases the tone and motility of the gallbladder. The cholesterol in the bile of the pregnant woman is more likely to crystallize, resulting in gallstones being more frequently retained.

Liver

The liver is physically displaced by the enlarging uterus, which can make the diagnosis of hepatomegaly difficult. Blood flow to the liver is not markedly changed, although the proportion of the cardiac output sent to the liver is decreased.

The most remarkable changes are in the laboratory and clinical signs that stem from the changes in the liver of the pregnant woman. These findings are commonly seen in clients who have liver disease, but in pregnancy these changes are normal. Findings include spider angiomata and palmar erythema, found in 70% to 90% of normal pregnant women. These physical findings disappear after delivery. Although liver function remains unchanged, the normal changes seen in laboratory findings of the pregnant woman are also seen in clients with liver disease. These changes include a serum albumin concentration that is decreased by 30% at term; a serum alkaline phosphatase level that is increased to two to three times normal levels; and a serum cholesterol level that is twice the level of the nonpregnant woman (Gabbe et al., 1996).

Endocrine System

Changes in the endocrine system are manifested in many ways.

Thyroid

The thyroid gland enlarges slightly from increased vascularity and hyperplasia of the tissue. The gland does not enlarge to the extent that was once thought, and, there-

fore, any extraordinary growth should be assessed. The normal relationship of the hypothalamus, pituitary, and thyroid glands is believed to remain intact and the pregnant woman remains with normal thyroid function. Cunningham and colleagues (2001) state that the changes that occur in the regulation of thyroid hormone production are related to high estrogen levels, effects of the placenta on function, and decreased availability of iodide resulting from increased renal clearance. These complex alterations in thyroid regulation do not dramatically change laboratory analysis but do cause a progressive increase in the *basal metabolic rate* (BMR). There is a 25% increase in the BMR, which is defined as the amount of oxygen consumed by the body over a unit of time (mL/min). The increase may be characterized by an increased pulse rate, heat intolerance, and elevated level of cardiac output.

Parathyroid

The parathyroid glands secrete parathyroid hormone, which is responsible for calcium and phosphorus metabolism. In pregnancy, the secretion of parathyroid hormone increases to meet the demands of the growing fetus for calcium. Total circulating calcium levels are decreased in pregnancy, probably resulting from fetal demands, the increase in glomerular filtration rate (GFR), and increased plasma volume.

Pituitary

The pituitary gland enlarges, with the most significant growth in the anterior pituitary. During pregnancy, the production of hormones responsible for ovulation is suppressed in the anterior pituitary; the production of prolactin is increased. Prolactin works in conjunction with other hormones for breast development in preparation for lactation. Oxytocin is produced in the hypothalamus, and the posterior pituitary stores and secretes the hormone. Oxytocin produces the uterine contractions during labor and is necessary for the ejection of breast milk. There is increased sensitivity by the myometrium (muscle layer of the uterus) to the effects of oxytocin as the pregnancy advances, probably a result of the increasing levels of estrogen.

Adrenal Glands

The adrenal glands do not change appreciably in size during pregnancy. Cortisol and aldosterone are two hormones secreted from the adrenal cortex that are important in pregnancy.

Cortisol

Cortisol works at multiple sites in the body to promote the metabolism of carbohydrate, protein, and fat. When the body needs more energy, cortisol activates gluconeogenesis to increase blood levels of glucose. Although the secretion of cortisol is decreased in pregnancy, it is hypothesized that the metabolic clearance of the hormone is slowed, thus maintaining higher than normal levels of circulating cortisol.

Aldosterone

During pregnancy the secretion of aldosterone increases, as does that of renin and angiotensin II. Renin is released from the kidneys in response to decreased perfusion pressure in the kidney. At this time, angiotensin II levels rise and act upon the maternal adrenal glands to secrete higher levels of aldosterone. It has been hypothesized that the increased circulating levels of aldosterone may protect the pregnant woman from the excessive sodium loss that is attributed to elevated progesterone levels during pregnancy.

Pancreas

The pancreas, an endocrine gland, secretes insulin from the beta cells of the islets of Langerhans. During pregnancy these beta cells increase in number and enlarge in size and cause the changes that occur in carbohydrate metabolism during pregnancy.

Placenta

Endocrine activities of the placenta are important to preserving a viable pregnancy and to the metabolic adaptations that must take place for the fetus to develop.

Human Chorionic Gonadotropin

Human chorionic gonadotropin (hCG) is secreted by a mass of trophoblastic tissue surrounding the embryo. The detection of hCG is used to confirm pregnancy. In early pregnancy, the corpus luteum increases progesterone and estrogen levels that are necessary to maintain the pregnancy. The function of hCG is to maintain the corpus luteum until the placenta is sufficiently developed to produce the needed hormones. As the pregnancy advances, hCG is involved in the suppression of the immunologic response of the maternal body to the fetus.

Human Placental Lactogen

Production of human placental lactogen (hPL) begins soon after implantation; levels gradually rise and peak at about 36 weeks. This hormone is involved in the process of making adequate glucose available for fetal growth, through the alteration of the maternal carbohydrate, fat, and protein metabolism. The hPL lowers the sensitivity of maternal cells to the action of insulin and then improves the ability of the body to metabolize and use fatty acids for energy. Therefore, as glucose levels decrease, the levels of hPL increase to allow the available glucose to be used for fetal development and growth.

Estrogen

Estrogen levels increase rapidly early in pregnancy, slow between 24 and 32 weeks' gestation, and increase again toward term. The production of estrogen is dependent on the interaction between the maternal and fetal components of the placenta. Estrogen plays an integral role in:

- Increasing blood flow to the uterus by promoting vasodilation
- Changing the sensitivity of the respiratory system to carbon dioxide
- Softening of the cervix, initiating uterine activity, and maintaining labor
- Developing the breasts in preparation for lactation and secretion of prolactin by the pituitary gland

Progesterone

Progesterone is produced by the corpus luteum in the first 5 weeks of pregnancy and then by the placenta until term. Elevated levels of progesterone ready the uterus for implantation, relax the smooth muscle of the uterus to prevent spontaneous abortion, and work to prevent a maternal immunologic response to the fetus. Progesterone, along with relaxation, play key roles in preterm labor. This hormone also relaxes smooth muscle of the gastrointestinal tract to decrease motility and improve absorption of nutrients. Relaxation of the smooth muscle of the urinary tract enlarges the ureters and bladder to increase capacity. Progesterone also plays a role in development of the alveoli and ductal system to prepare the breasts for lactation.

Changes in Metabolism

The metabolic changes that occur in pregnancy are all directed at providing the needs of the developing fetus, meeting the increased physiologic demands of the pregnancy, and providing energy for the woman throughout her pregnancy, labor, and delivery.

The metabolism of carbohydrates in the pregnant woman adapts to provide a constant source of glucose for the growing and developing fetus. In a fasting state, the pregnant woman experiences hypoglycemia, and a state of ketosis develops more quickly than in the nonpregnant woman. The speed at which this maternal response occurs is probably a result of the constant need of the fetus for glucose and the ability of the pregnant woman to more quickly utilize fat for energy. In contrast, a pregnant woman who eats a normal meal produces more glucose, insulin, and triglycerides than a nonpregnant woman does. The increased amounts of glucose and the decreased sensitivity to insulin by the cells therefore produces high amounts of circulating available glucose for the fetus. This

Nursing Alert

Signs of Diabetic Ketoacidosis

- Elevated blood glucose level >200
- Polydipsia and polyuria
- Nausea and vomiting
- Headache and malaise

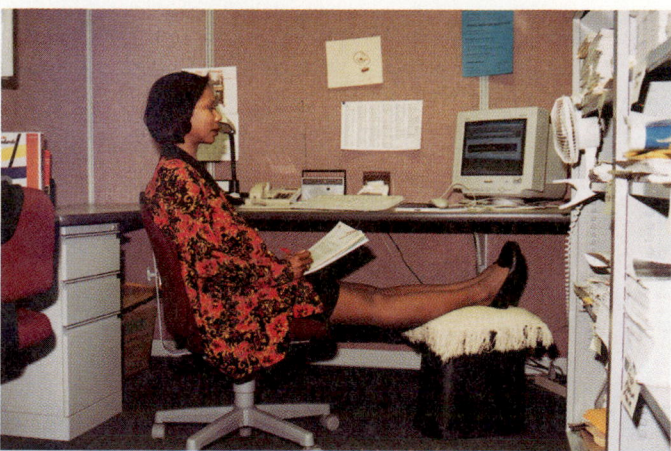

Figure 9-10 *Elevating the feet while seated can help relieve edema of the ankles and feet.*

adaptation is sometimes called the diabetogenic effect of pregnancy.

Gestational diabetes results from the inability of the pancreas of the pregnant woman to produce enough insulin to move the necessary glucose into the cells for energy production. When this happens, hyperglycemia may need to be regulated by changes in diet. Ketoacidosis may occur in a pregnant woman in whom diabetes has just been detected. Gabbe and colleagues (1996) state that because the pregnant woman is naturally in a state of insulin resistance with lipolysis and ketogenesis, ketoacidosis can occur in pregnant women with a blood glucose level as low as 200 mg/dL. To treat this disorder, the quick return of metabolic and fluid levels to normal values is necessary.

In the first two trimesters, there is an increase in triglyceride synthesis and the storage of fat at central sites. Later in the third trimester, there are more nutritional demands, both for glucose and fatty acids, by the fetus, and fat stores begin to decrease. The ability to more readily use fat as an energy source is a way to conserve glucose for the fetus and high-priority maternal needs.

Iron is necessary for the formation of hemoglobin, the oxygen-carrying component of the red blood cell. With red blood cell volume increasing by 30%, there is an increased need for iron. The intestinal tract increases its ability to absorb iron, but dietary intake and maternal stores are usually not adequate to meet all of the needs. The transport of iron across the placenta to the fetus, especially in the third trimester, takes place at the expense of maternal iron stores. Iron supplements are usually prescribed to maintain the maternal iron stores and decrease the chance of iron deficiency anemia.

Retention of water is a natural and expected part of pregnancy, resulting from changes in water metabolism. According to Cunningham and colleagues (2001), it occurs mainly because of several factors:

1. The plasma osmolality is lowered in pregnancy, mainly because of the reduced serum levels of sodium and protein.
2. The intravascular pressure and permeability increase.
3. The fetus, placenta, and amniotic fluid increase the demand for fluid.

The total average volume retained can be as much as 6.5 liters. Normal water retention causes the dependent edema seen in the lower legs and ankles, most often at the end of the day. Edema that is not relieved by the elevation of the legs or excessive edema in the face, hands, or sacral area deserves further assessment (Figure 9-10).

Weight Gain

Weight gain in pregnancy is variable and recommendations should be individualized. The prepregnant weight and the pattern of weight gain that occurs over time are important factors. Tulman, Moren, and Fawcett (1998) note women with extreme prepregnancy body weights, either low or high, plus pregnancy weight gain have an increased risk for maternal and neonatal complications.

Nursing Tip **Grading Dependent Edema**

The severity of edema is documented by grading and noticing trends in the changes.

1+ Slight pitting

2+ A somewhat deeper pit than in 1+

3+ The pit is noticeably deep; the dependent extremity is swollen and full

4+ The pit is deeper yet and lasts when the finger is removed; the dependent extremity is shiny, with extremely taut skin

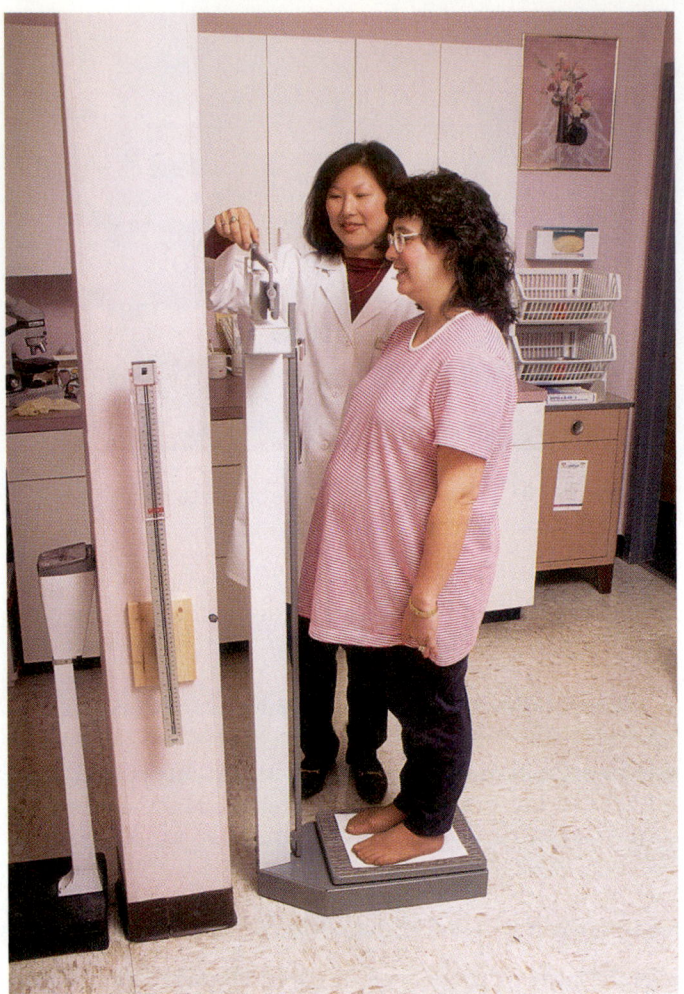

Figure 9-11 Monitoring weight gain at each prenatal visit helps the client to maintain a healthy pregnancy.

Except at the extreme ends of the scale, a good clinical outcome is possible within a wide range weight gain. The average weight gain for healthy primigravidae is 12.5 kg (27.5 lb). Of this, the fetus, placenta, amniotic fluid, uterus, increase in maternal blood volume, breasts and the retention of water account for 9 kg (Figure 9-11). The National Academy of Science (1990) recommends the following weight gain: 12.5 to 18.0 kg (27.5 to 39.6 lb) for underweight women, 11.5 to 16.0 kg (25.3 to 35.2 lb) for normal-weight women, and 7.0 to 11.4 kg (15.4 to 25 lb) for overweight women.

Urinary System

Changes in the urinary system, both anatomic and physiologic, are necessary for the adaptations that occur in other body systems. The key to assessing the renal system is remembering that the parameters of normal renal function are changed and that an awareness of these changes is necessary to make appropriate clinical judgments.

Anatomic Changes

As early as 16 weeks, the kidneys change in size and shape, resulting from the dilation of the renal ureters and pelvices. The right kidney and ureter are larger than the left, probably because of the structural changes in other organs. Early in pregnancy, the enlargement may be caused by the effect of hormones that cause increased tone and decreased motility of the smooth muscle. After 20 weeks gestation, the ureters are compressed at the pelvic brim by the growing uterus. Above the pelvic brim, the ureters are elongated and twisted, with a capacity to increase urine volume as much as 25-fold. Pooling of the increased volume of urine can lead to: (1) an increased incidence of pyelonephritis, (2) difficulty in the interpretation of radiographic studies of the renal system, and (3) interference with the accuracy of diagnostic studies, such as a 24-hour urine sample analysis.

By the end of the second trimester, the bladder is displaced upward and forward by the gravid uterus. The structural changes that occur with this displacement can lead to urinary frequency and incontinence. In most women, this is the first experience with incontinence, or involuntary loss of urine, and many will mistake it for the rupture of placental membranes late in pregnancy. The tone of the bladder is relaxed and capacity and the pressure within the bladder increases. These changes, along with the edema of the bladder mucosa, make this area susceptible to infection and trauma.

Physiologic Changes

Blood flow to the kidneys increases by 35% to 60%, as a result of the increase in cardiac output. In turn, this leads to an increase in the glomerular filtration rate (GFR), or the rate that water and solutes filter through the glomeruli, as much as 50% by 12 weeks' gestation. The increase in the GFR leads to the following changes:

1. Increased urine flow and volume
2. Decreased serum blood urea nitrogen (BUN), creatinine, and uric acid levels
3. Increased nutrients delivered to the kidneys
4. Increased filtration and excretion of water and solutes
5. Altered renal excretion of drugs, resulting, at times, in subtherapeutic blood levels

Urinalysis

The alterations that occur in tubular function increase the reabsorption of sodium, chloride, glucose, potassium, and water to prevent the depletion of these solutes. Because of the increased perfusion rate, at times reabsorption is not complete and there is a loss of glucose in the urine. Levels

Nursing Alert

Urinary Tract Infection

The changes that occur in the urinary tract make the pregnant woman more susceptible to infection. Symptoms include urinary frequency, urgency, dysuria (painful or difficult urination), and pyuria (pus in the urine). If untreated, the infection can ascend and pyelonephritis, a serious medical complication of pregnancy may develop. Urinary tract infections can also lead to premature labor, if left untreated.

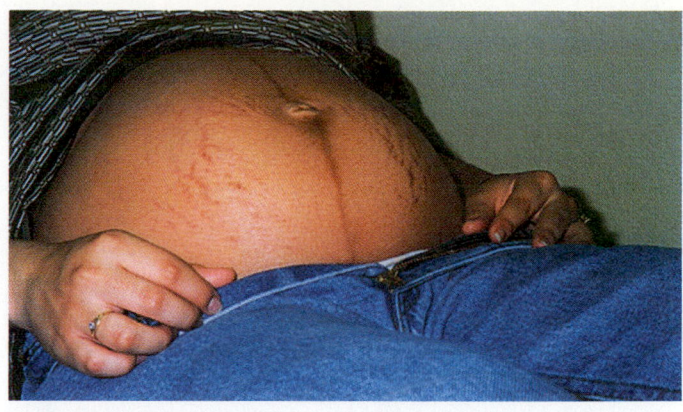

Figure 9-12   Dark line of pigmentation, called linea nigra, may appear in midline of abdomen, from symphysis pubis to umbilicus.

of glucose in the urine vary day to day and slightly elevated levels are not uncommon, but an assessment for gestational diabetes should be considered if glycosuria is recurrent. In normal pregnancy, small amounts of protein may occasionally spill into the urine. Proteinuria levels above 300 mg in 24 hours warrant further investigation, especially when accompanied by hypertension.

Glucose and protein in the urine lead to a higher susceptibility to urinary tract infections.

Integumentary System

The skin undergoes many changes that rarely cause significant physiologic problems. It is the emotional distress caused by the cosmetic alterations (that may persist until after delivery) that are problematic. Most of these skin changes disappear or lessen after the delivery of the newborn.

The vascular changes include spider angiomas and palmar erythema, which usually occur together. Spider angiomas or nevi usually appear between 8 and 20 weeks' gestation in about 75% of pregnant women. The nevi are central dilated arterioles that are visible or raised, with radiating branches. Appearing most often on the face, neck, throat, and arms, they may be distressing to the pregnant woman. Most often the nevi fade or disappear after delivery. There is a familial tendency for palmar erythema, which appears during the first half of the pregnancy. This skin change causes a mottling of the fleshy portion of the palm and redness of the fingers.

Hyperpigmentation, caused by elevated hormones, is usually visible primarily on the nipples, areolae, umbilicus, perineum, and axillae. The dark line in the midline of the abdomen is called **linea nigra** (Figure 9-12). Women may also experience dark blotching on the face (Figure 9-13), similar to that seen in women who take birth control pills. This condition, **chloasma**, is commonly called the

Client Education

Preventing and Coping with Chloasma: "Pregnancy Mask"

1. **Wear sunscreen in the daytime and protect yourself from direct sunlight.**

2. **If skin is very dark, seek the advice of a professional dermatologist.**

3. **Use a cover stick to neutralize the dark skin before applying makeup.**

4. **Darkened pigment usually fades once delivery occurs.**

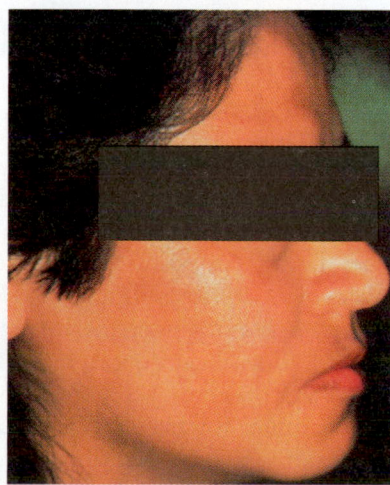

Figure 9-13   Blotches on face during pregnancy are known as chloasma. (Courtesy of Timothy Berger, MD, Chief, Department of Dermatology at San Francisco General Hospital)

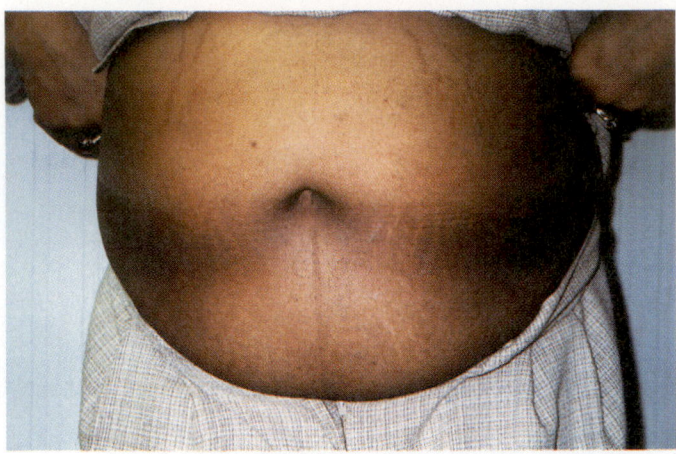

Figure 9-14   Striae gravidarum (stretch marks) are pink to purple streaks on skin. Marks are a result of linear tears in connective tissue of skin as body enlarges.

Eyes

Changes that occur in the eye normally do not affect vision, other than the transient loss of accommodation (the power of the eye to alter the convexity of the lens according to the nearness or distance of an object) that has been reported (Blackburn, 2003). The cornea becomes thicker, probably caused by edema. If the woman wears contact lenses, she may notice that her normally comfortable lenses are now bothersome.

DISCOMFORTS OF PREGNANCY

An important nursing responsibility during the prenatal period is educating the client regarding the discomforts that occur during pregnancy and how to remedy these, or feel better. Information on why the woman feels the way she does and self-help remedies usually assist in

"mask of pregnancy." The condition may be a concern to the pregnant woman because of the cosmetic effect. Chloasma may disappear after pregnancy but often only fades. Preexisting nevi may also be affected and become darker during pregnancy. The management of these nevi should include close observation and the removal of nevi that change rapidly.

Changes that occur in the connective tissue during pregnancy can lead to the formation of **striae gravidarum**, which occurs in approximately 50% of all pregnant women. Women who have a genetic disposition may develop pink-to-purple lines on the skin from the stretching that occurs during growth of the fetus. These lines, as seen in Figure 9-14, usually appear on the breasts, lower abdomen, and upper thighs and fade to a silver color with time. "Stretch marks" do not ever completely disappear, and there is no prophylactic skin treatment to prevent them.

Musculoskeletal System

To maintain balance with the shift in weight from the growing uterus, the lumbar spine forms an exaggerated forward, convex curve (lordosis) (Figure 9-15). The body adjusts the center of gravity over the lower extremities and, unfortunately, this adjustment is often the cause of low back pain in later pregnancy. Ligaments in the pubic symphysis and sacroiliac joints soften from the effects of the hormone relaxin. This adaptation is necessary to ready the body for vaginal delivery but can also cause pelvic discomfort and an unsteady gait as the pregnancy nears term. Falls are a common occurrence; women should be instructed to wear flat, well-fitting shoes.

Nursing Alert

Signs of Potential Problems in Pregnancy

Immediate assessment and referral to a health care provider is required for:

Problem	Possible Cause
Persistent vomiting	Hyperemesis gravidarum
Bright red vaginal bleeding	Abruptio placentae, placenta previa
Edema of the hands and face	Pre-eclampsia, hypertension
Body temperature above 101°F (38.3°C)	Infection
Persistent abdominal pain, with or without a rigidity	Abruptio placentae
Epigastric pain, unrelieved by comfort measures	Pre-eclampsia
Dysuria	Urinary tract infection
Intermittent back pain, pelvic pressure, or abdominal pain or pressure	Preterm labor
Visual disturbances	Pre-eclampsia, hypertension
Changes in fetal movement	Potential fetal stress

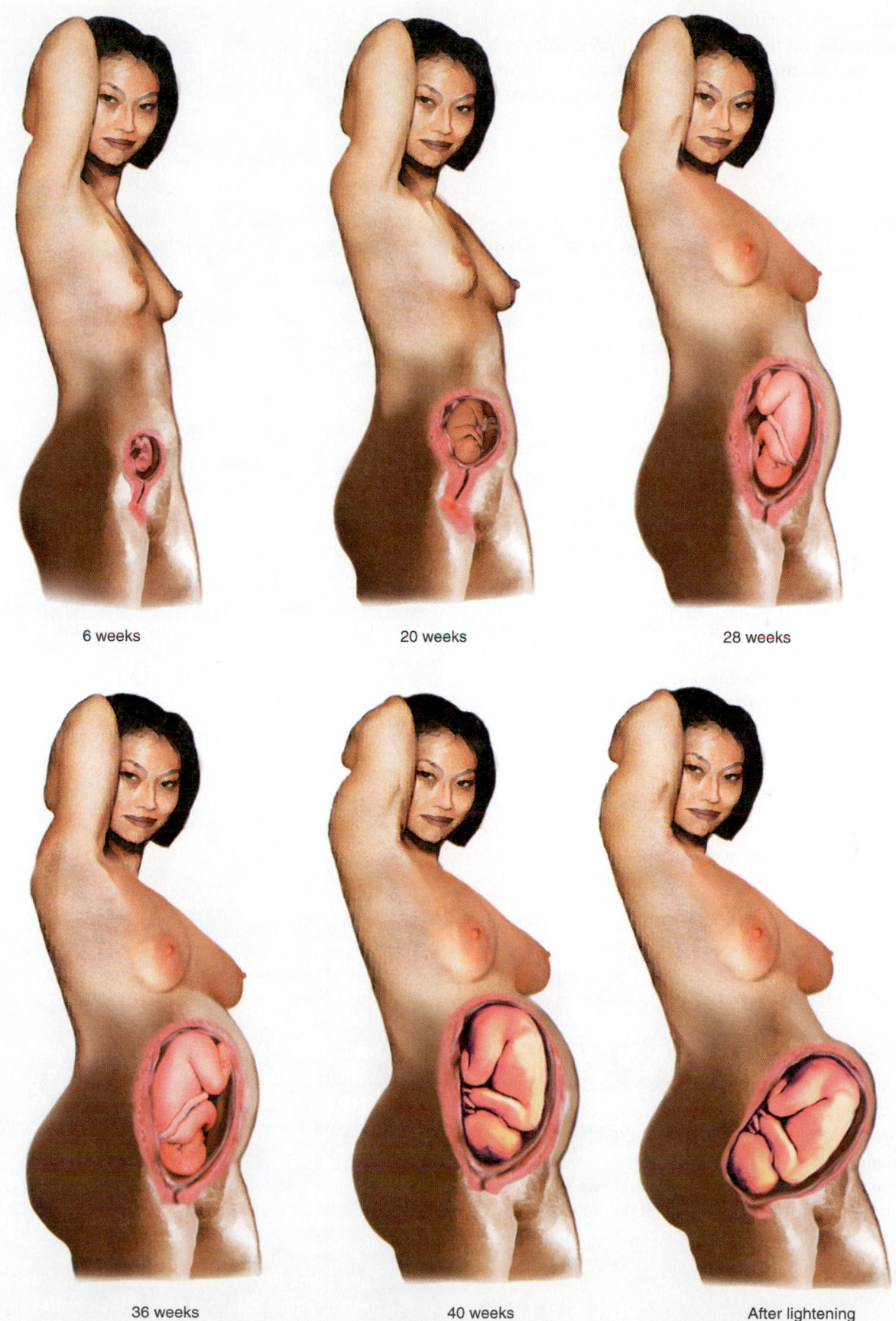

6 weeks   20 weeks   28 weeks

36 weeks   40 weeks   After lightening

Figure 9-15   As pregnancy advances, changes in posture are obvious. Exaggerated curve in the back is called lordosis.

making this time more comfortable. Another important aspect of counseling on the discomforts of pregnancy is to help the pregnant woman distinguish between a normal discomfort and a sign that may signal a real problem in the pregnancy.

Nausea and Vomiting of Pregnancy

The discomfort of nausea and vomiting of pregnancy (NVP) can range from mild nausea (with or without vomiting) to severe vomiting (hyperemesis gravidarum) that occurs throughout the day. Although NVP is referred to as morning sickness, episodes can occur throughout the day. The cause of NVP is not known, but it is speculated to be related to increased levels of hCG and estrogen. Emotional factors and irregular eating habits have also been cited as possible contributors to this discomfort. The discomfort of NVP cannot be completely eliminated, but can be minimized by self-help measures. Recent research suggests that there may be a protective benefit of NVP in that it shields the fetus from potentially harmful pathogens, such as those found in undercooked meat.

Hyperemesis gravidarum is a serious complication of pregnancy and must be managed under the close observation of a health care provider. Dangerous sequelae of hyperememsis gravidarum can include weight loss, dehydration, electrolyte imbalance, and starvation.

Heartburn

Heartburn is a frequent complaint throughout pregnancy and results from the reflux of gastric acid contents into the esophagus and sometimes into the mouth. The changes

Client Education

Nausea and Vomiting in Pregnancy

- Drink plenty of fluids, 6 to 8 glasses of water daily, to maintain hydration.
- Avoid fluids that contain caffeine or carbonation.
- Eat a diet that is high in protein and carbohydrates, in 5 to 6 small meals daily.
- Eat crackers throughout the day to avoid an empty stomach.
- Pay attention to your senses; avoid noxious odors, such as tobacco smoke, and tastes that may nauseate you.
- Limit stressful events and get plenty of rest; avoid being in a hurry, especially in the morning.
- Consider acupuncture or acupressure to assist in relieving nausea.
- Do not take any medication for this or any other condition without consulting your health care provider.

Client Education

Heartburn in Pregnancy

- Monitor your diet for foods that cause upset. Keep a list.
- Avoid drinking large amounts of liquid with meals; instead, spread fluid intake throughout the day.
- Remain sitting upright for at least 30 minutes after a meal and sleep with an extra pillow at night to keep the head elevated.
- Don't bend at the waist, always bend at the knees, maintaining a more upright abdominal posture.
- Try lying on your right side and using relaxation techniques to calm your stomach and promote digestion.
- Take commercial calcium-containing low-sodium antacids just before meals; check with your practitioner for brand preferences.

Critical Thinking

Nausea and Vomiting of Pregnancy

Two weeks ago Mehalia purchased a home pregnancy test, which gave positive results after she missed one of her regular periods. She has called the clinic and is experiencing nausea and vomiting.

Formulate questions for Mehalia that will help you determine the severity of her NVP and the potential for hyperemesis gravidarum, centering on:

- Frequency of vomiting
- Pain or fever
- Tolerance for food and fluids

that occur in the gastrointestinal system, such as decreased stomach and intestinal motility, softening of the cardiac sphincter and esophagus, and displacement of the stomach by the uterus, seem to contribute to the burning sensation that is felt behind the sternum and in the epigastric area. Instruct the client to call her health care provider if self-help measures or antacids do not relieve persistent heartburn. Epigastric pain or right upper quadrant pain, especially when associated with edema of the hands and face, proteinuria, and elevated blood pressure, could indicate a problem in the liver, and the client should be referred to her health care provider.

Constipation

Constipation is another discomfort related to the changes that occur in the gastrointestinal tract. Increased levels of progesterone cause the relaxation of intestinal smooth muscle, which leads to decreased motility and increased capacity, allowing more time for the absorption of nutrients. Although this process benefits the nutrition of the mother and fetus, it can cause bloating, increased flatulence, and hard stools that aggravate hemorrhoids. Assess the frequency of bowel movements in women taking iron supplements, because iron supplements may cause constipation.

Fatigue

The fatigue that pregnant woman feel in the first trimester is real and sometimes distressing for the "superwoman" of today. The tiredness is legitimate and may seem overwhelming but is of no special medical significance. The best advice for the busy pregnant woman is to give in and rest when she feels the need. She may need to take shortcuts in her daily life, and she should know that the fatigue usually disappears by the fourth month. Alleviating stress through meditation or relaxed breathing may assist in coping with the feeling of being tired.

Frequent Urination

Urinary frequency ranks at the top of the list of the most common complaints of pregnancy. In the first trimester, before the uterus ascends above the symphysis, the weight of the enlarging uterus irritates and puts pressure on the bladder. Frequent urination diminishes slightly in the second trimester, returning near term. When talking with clients, differentiate between urinary frequency and the symptoms of a urinary tract infection. If the woman has symptoms such as pain, burning, or urgency when urinating, a health care provider should be notified. Kegel exercises (contracting the muscles of the pelvic floor) help to prevent urinary stress incontinence.

Client Education

Constipation in Pregnancy

If you are constipated and taking iron, do not stop taking your supplement. Try these self-help tips first:

- Increase the fiber in your diet by eating fruits and vegetables raw (or vegetables slightly steamed). Whole grains are also a good source of fiber.

- Drink plenty of fluids, avoiding caffeine; keep in mind that increasing your fiber without increasing your fluid can worsen constipation.

- Exercise to stay regular; walking, swimming, or cycling 3 to 4 times per week for 20 to 30 minutes is recommended.

- Try to establish a regular time for your bowel movement and never ignore your body's signals.

Client Education

Fatigue in Pregnancy

Find a comfortable and reasonably quiet place and try meditation. Close your mind to external sensation and outside stimulation. Pick one of the following five methods to achieve a single focus:

1. **Meditative repetition:** repeat a rhythmic chant, most commonly called a mantra, that is chanted over and over.

2. **Visual concentration:** stare at an image, such as a candle, flower, or fruit.

3. **Repetitive sounds:** listen to a sound, such as a drum, chimes, or waterfall.

4. **Physical repetitive motion:** perform motions such as rhythmic breathing or a rhythmic aerobic exercise.

5. **Repeated tactile motion:** hold or manipulate a small object, such as a rosary or tumble stone.

Client Education

How to Perform Kegel Exercises

1. In the first 3 months of pregnancy, lie on your back with both knees bent to perform this exercise; after the third month, sitting or standing is a better position.

2. Contract the muscles that surround the vagina and anus and hold for 5 seconds, then slowly release. These are the same muscles you would use to stop urination. Isolating these muscles requires practice.

3. Do at least 25 to 50 repetitions. You may want to space them out during the day.

Client Education

Varicose Veins in Pregnancy

- Maintain good circulation in your legs; avoid sitting, standing, or crossing your legs for long periods, and wear maternity support hose during the day.

- Elevate your legs as often as you are able or flex your feet several times every few minutes while sitting.

- Take breaks and short frequent walks when performing intense, stationary work.

- Wear clothes that fit loosely and avoid wearing knee-high hose that may constrict the blood vessels in the legs.

Epistaxis and Nasal Congestion

The capillaries inside the nose become engorged with blood during pregnancy, leading to edema and hyperemia of the nasal passages. These changes can lead to *epistaxis*, or nosebleed, and nasal congestion, which can worsen in the winter months when conditions are dry and the use of home heaters is prevalent. The congestion and dryness of the nose may lead to more frequent blowing of the nose. With mucous membranes engorged with blood, blowing the nose gently may prevent epistaxis. The nurse can recommend that the client sleep with a cool mist humidifier and use commercially prepared saline spray. If the congestion becomes severe enough to interfere with activities of daily living, the client should consult her practitioner.

Varicosities

Varicosities are dilated veins that occur most often in women who have a genetic predisposition for them. The valves in the veins can become incompetent, allowing a reverse of blood flow. In pregnancy, these veins may be more pronounced because of the increased blood volume, the changes in venous pressure that occur because of the enlarged uterus, and increased time in the standing position. On assessment, changes may be noted that range from mild discomfort after long periods of standing to severe tortuous and bulging blue veins that require long periods of rest with the legs elevated. Occurring most often in veins of the lower extremities, varicosities may also be present in the veins of the vulva and rectum (hemorrhoids).

Hemorrhoids

Hemorrhoids are varicosities of the rectum, which may occur outside the anal sphincter or inside the anal sphincter. Typically, hemorrhoids that are already present are exacerbated by the changes that occur in the body during pregnancy. Other factors that may exacerbate hemorrhoids are prolonged sitting or standing, straining at stool, and

Client Education

Hemorrhoids in Pregnancy

- Maintain healthy and regular bowel habits.

- Try a sitz bath: sit for about 20 minutes in a tub filled with warm water to which you have added a half-cup of baking soda.

- Apply cool compresses or cotton balls soaked with witch hazel to the swollen hemorrhoids. Commercial preparations that contain witch hazel or anesthetic compounds are also available.

- If hemorrhoids are protruding from the anus, gently push them back into the rectum. Using a glove and lubricant, gently press the hemorrhoid back through the anus and hold for a few seconds. This may be most comfortably achieved after a sitz bath.

Client Education

Back Pain in Pregnancy

- Be aware of your posture; be sure your neck, shoulders, and back are straight and your pelvis is tilted slightly forward.

- Bend at the knees, never at the waist.

- Wear comfortable, low-heeled shoes.

- Elevate one foot when standing for extended periods of time (Figure 9-16).

- Practice deep breathing and relaxation exercises that focus on the upper body.

- Get a massage to relax tired muscles.

pushing in the second stage of labor. Hemorrhoids may continue to be problematic into the postpartum period.

Back Pain

The back pain of pregnancy usually occurs in the lumbar region and becomes more problematic as the uterus enlarges. Low back pain is a common complaint in pregnancy and results from the changes in posture as the uterus grows. Obesity and previous problems with back pain are also risk factors. The degree of pain is closely linked to the strain of bending, lifting, and walking. The use of good body mechanics when performing these activities limits the potential for severe injury.

Leg Cramps

Leg cramps are thought to be the result of an imbalance between the electrolytes calcium and phosphorus. During pregnancy, the ratio of calcium to phosphorus is difficult to maintain because of changes in renal absorption and diet. The decreased circulation to the lower extremities produced by the pressure of the uterus may also contribute to painful cramps. The woman may awaken at night with painful knots in the calf muscles. When the cramp occurs, getting out of bed and walking usually relieves the pain. If the pain is too severe to walk, the woman should be instructed to sit with her legs and knees straight, grab her toes, and flex her foot. A partner can also assist in relieving leg cramps by flexing the foot forward (Figure 9-17). Instruct the client to do flexibility or stretching exercises before going to bed.

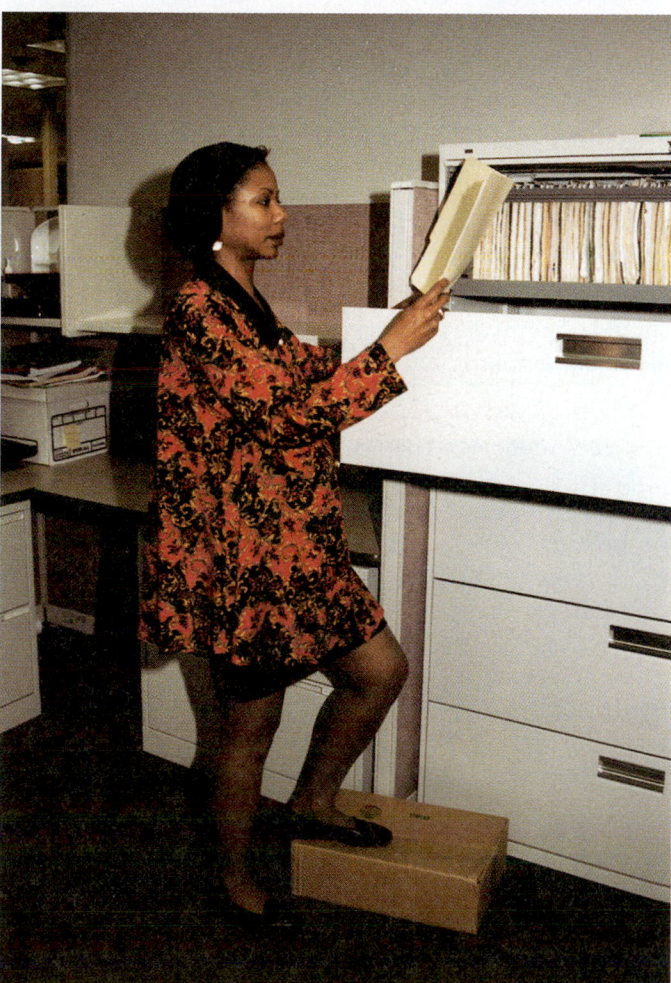

Figure 9-16   Keeping one foot elevated during prolonged periods of standing can help relieve back pain.

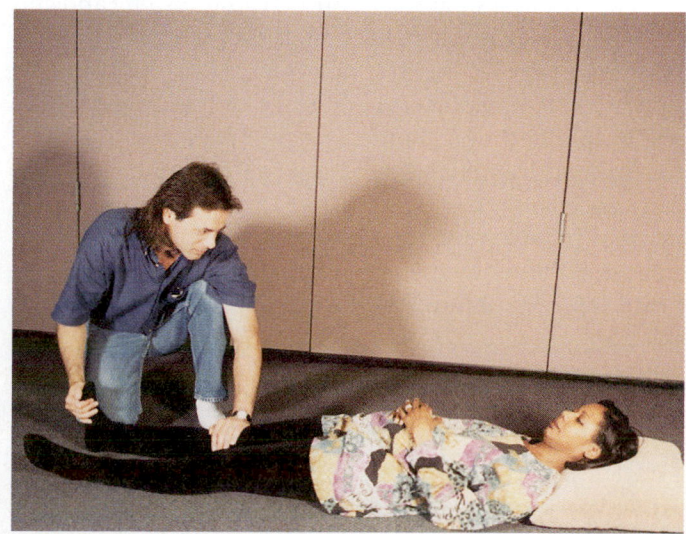

Figure 9-17   Leg cramps can be relieved by flexing the foot toward the knee.

Critical Thinking

Health Promotion

Formulate responses to these comments made by nurses that help nurses understand the importance of avoiding making assumptions about clients when instructing them on changing health behavior.

1. "The health change is obviously the right thing to do and everyone is motivated to change if good health is the outcome."

2. "I understand the problems concerning not changing, but why does the client not understand?"

3. "The time for change is now and if the client is not ready, then this session is over. I can only give her the advice, she has to decide to change."

Health Promotion

When considering health behavior changes, remember what it is like to be the individual attempting to change what may be long-standing habits. The nurse, as the health care provider, understands the need to change certain behaviors to achieve and maintain wellness, but the client is the person who must be ready to change.

Many women must make changes in their daily lives to achieve and maintain a healthy pregnancy. When planning education for women concerning the lifestyle changes that may need to be made, make sure she has had a complete physical examination, but also understand the woman's educational background, value system, and cultural beliefs. To implement change, there must be a readiness to change. If this is a new idea to the woman, she may need to complete several stages of readiness before she is able to think about changing a behavior. Relaying the importance of the change and convincing her that she can successfully make the change are also necessary. The manner in which the information is presented can either motivate the woman to change or build a wall of resistance. As a health care provider, the nurse must be sensitive to the fact that communication techniques can either make the process more difficult or can assist in the adjustments that need to be made.

Employment

At least one-half of the women of childbearing age in the United States are in the workforce. Cunningham and associates (2001) noted that women now have the legal right to work during pregnancy, and employers cannot deny any job to a woman because she is pregnant. If a job requires excessive standing (more than 8 hours), frequent rest periods or intermittent walking should be included in the work day. Women should be instructed to avoid any work or play that may cause severe physical strain or fatigue. Women should also avoid environmental toxins.

Travel

Travel during pregnancy has not been shown to be harmful to the pregnant woman or her fetus. Most airlines have requirements for the woman who is traveling close to her expected date of delivery. Instruct the woman to discuss travel plans with her health care provider.

When traveling in a car, it is appropriate to use a properly positioned three-point safety restraint. The woman should be instructed to adjust the lap belt so that it is positioned under her abdomen and low across her hips and the shoulder harness so that it is snug between her breasts (Figure 9-18). With any mode of travel, frequent rest periods are advantageous. Pregnant women should not sit for extended periods as they are at risk for deep venous thrombosis (DVT), especially later in pregnancy.

Smoking

The effect of smoking on the fetus is well-documented. Newborns born to mothers who smoke have lower birth weights, a higher incidence of sudden infant death syndrome (SIDS), a higher incidence of premature birth, and are more likely to have episodes of apnea (Cunningham et al., 2001). The discussion concerning smoking cessation should occur in the preconception period. The nurse should assess for smoking in every client of childbearing age, re-

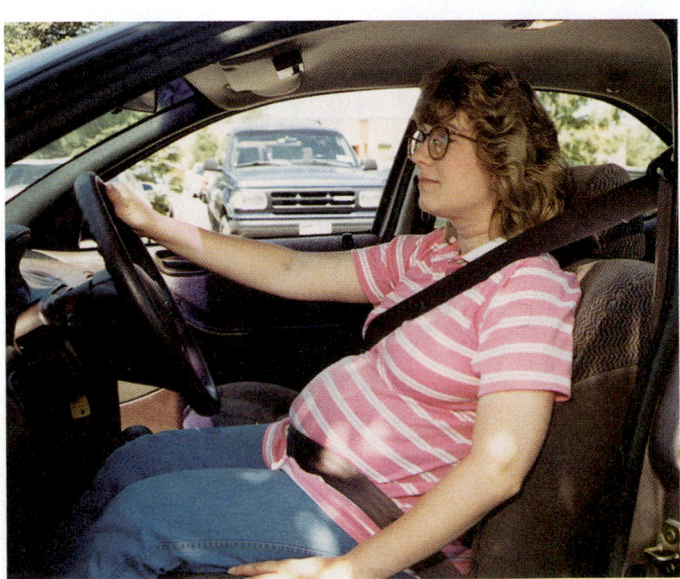

Figure 9-18   Car seatbelts should be secured low and snug under abdomen and across hips.

Reflections from a Nurse

I cannot understand. I had just explained how detrimental smoking was to her baby, and in the her next breath, she wanted to go smoke a cigarette. What should my response as a concerned health care provider be?

view the negative effects of smoking on the fetus, and suggest ways to assist the client in quitting the smoking habit. The nurse should first understand the long-term addiction of cigarette smoking and then work with the woman to assist in identifying her motivation to smoke. From this assessment, a plan of care can be outlined to begin the process of changing health behavior.

Alcohol Use

Women who are pregnant or are considering becoming pregnant should abstain from consuming alcohol. Experts have been unable to identify exactly how much alcohol is too much, but alcohol may have a teratogenic effect on the fetus. Again, the time to identify an alcohol problem is before the woman becomes pregnant. Explaining the deleterious effects of alcohol on the developing fetus may be enough motivation for the social drinker to stop, but women who are addicted to alcohol need professional assistance and may benefit from a referral to a treatment program.

Illicit Drug Use

Large doses of illicit drugs or street drugs, such as opium derivatives, amphetamines, or barbiturates, can cause low birth weight and fetal distress (Cunningham et al., 2001). A health care provider team that has an established program should manage the pregnant woman with a drug addiction. The newborn needs special care if the mother has remained on drugs throughout her pregnancy. If the nurse identifies a woman who has a drug addiction, quick referrals are the best avenue to obtaining a reasonably positive outcome.

Medication Use

During preconception counseling the health care provider should assess the medications that the woman may routinely consume. Almost all drugs that affect the mother systemically cross the placenta and affect the fetus. Therefore, the best advice to the pregnant woman is to avoid taking any medications or herbal preparations without consulting her provider. If a drug is prescribed during pregnancy, the risk-benefit ratio should be weighed and discussed with the woman.

PSYCHOSOCIAL ADAPTATIONS TO PREGNANCY

There are developmental challenges that must be met to move to the next stage of life. Pregnancy is a maturational crisis that causes a developmental shift for the woman and her family members. To successfully move into the new role of parenting, both the woman and her partner must complete certain tasks. The movement through this journey is affected by many variables, both internal and external. In the role of the nurse, understanding the psychological adaptations that are necessary in moving into the parenting role helps with supporting and caring for the family unit.

Psychological Responses to Pregnancy

Because pregnancy is an event that happens over time, the woman's responses are episodic in nature. Her response to certain changes may be somewhat exaggerated, while other changes are accepted with little concern. Being able to provide unbiased counsel to these women and their families is important and assists in the smooth transition from a childless couple to a family.

Acceptance of the Pregnancy

The nurse should not automatically assume that every woman has planned her pregnancy. Approximately 31% of births in the 5 years preceding 1995 were reported as unintended (Henshaw, 1998), with unintended pregnancy defined as one in which the woman did not want to have the infant or had decided not to have more children. The definition does not suggest that she will be unsuccessful in her progress through the adaptation and acceptance of her pregnancy. In fact, ambivalence to the pregnancy is a very normal initial response, and discussion concerning this topic is a productive intervention. Many women express concern over the timing of the pregnancy, wishing that planned goals or criteria had been met before becoming pregnant. Other women worry about how an infant will affect their career or their relationships with family and friends. These feelings can be confusing for the woman who feels conflict instead of elation. Even when the pregnancy was planned, and the woman is eagerly looking forward to motherhood, acceptance of the pregnancy is an important psychological aspect of the pregnancy. As her pregnancy progresses, the physical changes of an enlarging abdomen and fetal movement bring reality to her situation. As she accepts this reality, she becomes tolerant of

Reflections from a Mother

In my second year of graduate school, while working part-time, I was shocked and disappointed to learn that I was pregnant. My initial reaction was, "Oh no, not now!" I was so ashamed by the way I was feeling toward being pregnant. We had always planned to have a baby, but there were so many things we still wanted to accomplish before starting a family.

the discomforts she may be experiencing. At this time, reassurance that what she is feeling is normal and that her conflicting feelings about the pregnancy will resolve are appropriate.

Time for Reflection

During the first trimester the woman often turns inward and reflects on what "being pregnant" means. There are few physical signs of an impending newborn, so the unstable moods that sometimes accompany early pregnancy may be unnerving to the woman and her partner. As the pregnancy advances, the focus becomes the growing fetus. Many women disengage from familiar outside activities and focus on issues that result in a safe and healthy pregnancy. At times, the plans for the newborn may completely monopolize her attention, and her partner may feel neglected or left out of the planning. The introversion that occurs is a normal psychological adaptation to the journey to motherhood. The nurse can discuss these issues with the couple and assist in providing suggestions to maintain the focus on the family.

Body Image Changes

The initial changes that occur in the woman's body validate her pregnancy, and she may demonstrate pride in her changing body. As the pregnancy progresses, her increasing size, waddling gait, and posture changes may become distressing. The discomforts of pregnancy that accompany the physical changes may add more distress to an already stressful time. Women who are experiencing difficulty adapting to the pregnancy because of real or imagined issues, such as single parenthood, marital problems, financial issues, dread of the future, or an uninterested or absent partner, typically have a more difficult time accepting the physical changes of pregnancy. The nurse and client can discuss the issues and look for solutions. It may be helpful to focus the client on the idea of pregnancy as a time-limited event.

Becoming a Mother

As the woman moves toward the maternal role, she has hopefully accomplished previous life transitions, has adequate role models, has an interpersonal support system, and the acceptance of others. During the transition, the woman is in a state of internal disequilibrium and may demonstrate disorganized behavior. The behavior may result in mood swings and changes in normal roles and relationships. Pregnancy and role changes are a developmental crisis. During a crisis, the woman and her family may be more open to the health care provider's expert advice and guidance. It is an important time because the change that occurs in the newly pregnant woman is integrated into her personality as her maternal identity. The incorporation of the maternal identity into the woman's life is a process that leads to the acceptance of the new infant as her child.

Development of the Maternal Role

Rubin (1984) describes the steps that must be accomplished to successfully move into the maternal role and the tools the new mother uses to accomplish this transition.

Mimicry

The pregnant woman uses mimicry in role transition when she seeks out other women who are pregnant or have been pregnant and asks to share their stories and customs. She solicits the different opinions of these experts and tries to obtain consensus before deciding which aspects of motherhood she will incorporate into her new role. Wearing maternity clothes before they are necessary, or imitating the waddling gate of other pregnant women demonstrates a trying on of the role. The role models also serve to plot a course for the expected sequence of events or changes during pregnancy. The woman finds comfort in knowing what to expect, although information that does not seem pertinent to her stage of pregnancy may be temporarily disregarded. An example of premature information would be showing a woman in her first trimester how to bathe or feed the baby. The information is stored in her memory and will be reviewed when it is more pertinent to her stage of pregnancy.

The woman's mother is the model most closely mimicked. She has an expectation that she will experience the same prenatal course and delivery as her mother experienced. When this sequence of events does not progress as anticipated, the woman may become distressed and worried. At this point, it is important to discuss with the client the differences that occur in every woman's pregnancy.

Role Play

Role play happens intermittently and is the woman's opportunity to try on the mother role. When the opportunity arises, she may offer to hold, feed, or play with a child in front of an observer. If she receives a positive response from both the infant and the observer, this encounter bolsters her confidence in successfully becoming a mother. If the infant or the observer rejects the woman, she will feel as if she has failed and will expect rejection with the next encounter. Helping the woman understand that acquiring the skills necessary for motherhood is a process that continues throughout life is a sound approach.

Fantasy

Fantasizing is common in the pregnant woman and involves imagining the infant and how she will fare as a mother. Dreams may initially focus on what the infant will look like or how the infant will look dressed in baby clothes. To test her ability to solve similar issues for her child, the mother may relive, through her dreams, childhood conflicts that may have been left unresolved. As the woman moves closer to delivery, she may have dreams that question her maternal skills or her ability to cope with motherhood and a career. Fantasies are the woman's way of working through conflicts and readying herself for the motherhood role. Offering a listening ear and reassurance that dreams and fantasies are a normal adaptation to her changing role is a positive intervention.

Role Fit

After the woman has acquired a set of maternal role expectations, she matches her expectation to the actions of other mothers. As she "tries on" the different behaviors, she will either accept or reject them as agreeable to her view of the motherhood role. The investigation into the appropriate skills necessary for motherhood suggests that throughout her pregnancy the woman has successfully taken the necessary steps toward the maternal role. In sessions with new mothers, discussing ideas of motherhood and offering informational sources reinforces positive perceptions of the new role.

Maternal Tasks

In the work of Rubin (1984) a list of maternal tasks are discussed. These tasks are identified as developmental milestones that the woman must accomplish to successfully incorporate the maternal identity into her personality.

Safe Passage

The goal of safe passage is to achieve a healthy pregnancy and an intact newborn with no detrimental effects to the mother. In the first trimester, the woman will focus on herself and her pregnancy. Later in the second trimester, she becomes very aware of her responsibility to protect the fetus and does this by adhering to different aspects of her prenatal care. As she moves closer to delivery, her thoughts shift to mother and baby as a couple: what happens to one will happen to the other. The pregnant woman will seek out role models and expert advice on the best way to proceed through the pregnancy and delivery and on to parenting. Expectant women are often very receptive to health education.

Acceptance by Others

The woman's world before pregnancy is dependent on the social interactions of the family and secondary groups, such as community activities, school, or work. Initially, the secondary groups are significant to who the woman is and how she defines her life's meaning. Throughout the pregnancy her family and especially her partner become the motivational force behind her desire to be successful as a mother. To succeed, the mother becomes aware of sacrifices that will need to be made. If she has other children, she will have to assist them in adapting to the growing family.

During this time, the most important role for the nurse is to listen to the woman's concerns and offer assistance, when applicable, in a nonjudgmental manner.

Binding in to the Child

In the first trimester, the woman focuses on herself and maintaining the pregnancy. Once fetal movement is felt, in the second trimester, the fetus becomes real and she begins to feel there is significance in working to meet the challenges of becoming a mother. At this time, the fetus becomes an independent person and all of the mother's being is directed toward the newborn's safe arrival.

Critical Thinking

Successful Role Adaptation

Rosie is a teen who is pregnant with her first baby, and she is approaching her eighth month. She is in the office for her prenatal visit and has brought her girlfriend; they are going to a party at a friend's house later that night.

1. How can you determine if Rosie has accepted her pregnancy?

2. What behaviors would you expect Rosie to report to indicate that she is successfully adapting to her impending role as mother?

3. What questions will you ask to determine if Rosie understands the changes that she will have to make in her lifestyle to care for her infant?

Giving of Oneself

The experience of pregnancy and childbirth would be very difficult to endure without the prospect of a healthy newborn as the outcome. Pregnancy is a time of giving gifts between couples, family, and friends. The grandmother may give the baby a family heirloom and a friend may give a baby book. The partner gives the woman a child and the woman gives the fetus a healthy diet and often eliminates unhealthy habits. The act of giving a gift is not the primary focus for the woman, but the communication of appreciative approval helps the woman to endure the changes and discomforts of the pregnant body. Health care providers who give generously of their time to answer questions and provide guidance reinforce the importance of the sacrifices that must be made to achieve a successful pregnancy and healthy family.

Conflicting Developmental Tasks

Because pregnancy is not always a planned or intended developmental stage of the woman's or her family's life, there may be other developmental tasks that are in the process of being accomplished. These tasks may conflict with or make the accomplishment of the role transition more difficult.

An example would be the teen mother who is working on the developmental aspects of adolescence while attempting the transition to the motherhood role (Table 9-2). Many times, the tasks overlap or conflict. When this hap-

pens, the role of the nurse is to assist in isolating the issues and to assist the teen in working through each one. The nurse may want to enlist the assistance of professionals that specialize in the care of teens or assist the teen in finding a support group for pregnant teens.

Becoming a Father

Traditionally, an assumption was made that the father of the infant was also the husband of the mother. Today, more babies are being born to single mothers, and the situation of caring for a woman without a husband is common.

The transition to fatherhood is made easier when there is a bond or relationship between the man and the woman. It is important to successful fetal attachment for both the mother and the father that the parents are united and their feelings are mutual. Wilson et al. (2000) described mutuality as a close and emotional relationship in which each participant is secure in their own identity. In relationships that foster clear communication and the recognition that different roles are necessary to foster a healthy family, a new being can readily be accepted as a member. In families without a husband-father, the nurse can investigate how other family members may fit into the structure. A female partner, grandfather, or close friend may be the father figure in a particular family. Assisting the woman in identifying her emotional needs as she moves into the motherhood role helps her to adjust to any deficits that may be noted.

Table 9-2 Conflicting Development Tasks		
DEVELOPMENTAL TASKS OF ADOLESCENCE	**DEVELOPMENTAL TASKS OF PREGNANCY**	**CONFLICTS**
Personal value system	Seeking safe passage	• Wants the approval of others, especially peers • May conform to prenatal care only to avoid negative reaction from authority figures • May not readily express concerns about prenatal care
Vocation or career	Acceptance of the reality of the unborn child	• Not future-oriented • Limited means of support • Developing feminine self may assist in focusing on fetus, but role confusion may occur
Body image and sexuality	Acceptance of the pregnancy by self and others	• May be awkward about looking different; still struggling with own identity • Relationship with father of infant may not be as strong as she had hoped • Family may react negatively to her pregnancy
Achievement of a stable identity	Acceptance of the reality of parenthood	• Is attempting to develop the feminine identity; feels pregnancy may assist in her validation as a woman; may feel the conflict
Independence from parents	Giving of oneself	• Teen's parents may replace her as the parent figure, limiting her involvement with the newborn

Transition to Fatherhood

Men have their own unique transition that must take place to incorporate the identity of father into their personality. In accepting the pregnancy, the man needs to perceive that certain goals have been accomplished before the birth of the newborn. Has he thought about becoming a father at some point in his future and has he accepted the end to his childless period? Men are concerned about the financial and emotional stability of the couple and how they will fare with this new individual entering their lives. If these questions are not positively answered, there may be some ambivalence to the pregnancy on the part of the man. The nurse's knowledge of social and community resources is helpful in assisting the couple with role adjustment.

The Stress of the Paternal Role

The adaptation of the male to the fatherhood role is a life crisis, just as it is for the woman accepting the maternal role. The woman needs her partner to be empathic, trustworthy, reliable, and available to assist in the successful completion of pregnancy and childbirth. These responsibilities, plus the change that will occur in the lifestyle of the couple, cause stress in the structure of the family. Often men note that potential financial issues, learning new routines, work conflicts, fewer hours of sleep, and caring for the infant are issues that may block the evolution of the fatherhood role. In a relationship, the woman is usually the man's emotional counselor, and in the parent role, the woman is most often focused on the needs of the newborn and not available to help the man through his challenges. The successful role adaptation of the man to fatherhood is typically closely related to the emotional health of the couple's relationship.

The custom of taking on symptoms of pregnancy and childbirth by the man is called **couvade**. There are many different theories that identify possible reasons for this condition; these include sympathy and identification with the pregnant woman, being left out, feeling guilty about putting the woman in this condition, or the stress of living in such a unpredictable situation. The symptoms may appear around the third month or at delivery and may include nausea and vomiting, abdominal pain, weight gain, food cravings, fatigue, and mood swings. Of course, these symptoms could signal illness, so a full assessment is necessary. Becoming more involved in the pregnancy, or seeking out knowledge concerning areas that the father feels insecure about, may alleviate the symptoms of couvade.

Bonding between the Father and Infant

Fathers bond in much the same way as mothers do. Looking at and touching their infants, perceiving the infant's characteristics as unique and perfect, being attracted to the infant, and feeling happy are strong indicators of successful attachment. Early physical contact and involvement in the newborn's care are important for future positive father-child adjustment.

The Family

The family is a dynamic and complex unit that adapts to each individual's role changes and crisis resolution. The success of the family depends on the ability to continue to move forward on the developmental course while each individual moves through their own maturational and situational crises. The process of family life now takes on a different look from the families of the early to middle 20th century. Parents may be unmarried, not living together, of the same sex, older, adoptive, or grandparents who are raising the infant.

The participation of caregivers outside the family, that is, day care providers, is a challenge for families. The close extended family that was traditionally relied on for support and help with child care is often not geographically or financially able to assist. Nurses are finding that knowledge of community resources is necessary in assisting many of these families with the challenges of day to day living.

Duvall (1985) has described developmental tasks that are necessary in the successful transition to the family role. They include adapting relationships to the realities of pregnancy; planning for the pregnancy, childbirth, and parenting; and reevaluating financial responsibilities for the impending family. The couple needs to orient themselves to their new roles and have insight into how their relationships with other family members will change. Sexual relations during pregnancy and after childbirth are different from the experience of the past. Dividing the new responsibilities that come with this change in family life, such as who takes the infant for newborn checkups or wakes up in the night for feedings, is a necessary task. Depending on the working status of the couple, making decisions on the physical care of the newborn will rank high on the list of tasks. In general, maintaining the morale of the family and adapting to the rapidly changing environment is most important.

> ## Nursing Tip   *Family Variety*
>
> In providing care to families, remember that the content of the family is the key to assisting members through a crisis and not the form that the family takes.

Siblings

When children are already present in the family, the parents may have questions on how to handle the announcement of the expected newborn. The age of the child may dictate the timing of the announcement. If the sibling is under age 2, it may be best to wait until the fifth or sixth month to explain about a new brother or sister. A 9-month pregnancy progresses slowly for a child this age. If the mother is obviously not feeling well from the discomforts of pregnancy, it may be advantageous to tell the young child about the pregnancy. The young child may be afraid that mother is sick and that something bad will happen to her.

All children should be acquainted with the baby before it is born (Figure 9-19). There will be many questions, and these should be answered in a straightforward age-appropriate manner using the correct terminology. The nurse and the couple can discuss available age-specific books that can be used to explain the growth of the fetus as the pregnancy progresses. Children between the ages of 3 and 12 may want to track the growth of the fetus as the months progress. The older child can accompany the mother on her prenatal visits and listen for the baby's heartbeat. Also, involving siblings in preparing the home for the new baby can help them to feel that this is their baby too. Especially for the younger siblings, advance notice of the hospital stay and helping them to understand that they will be taken care of while the mother is away is extremely important. Including the child in the care of mother and baby can help with the transition once the infant is born. The nurse can assist the family in understanding that the sibling may not be immediately elated to have to share the parent's attention with this little stranger. The parents need to provide a smooth transition by keeping the sibling informed of coming events. The nurse can advise the family to monitor the attention that is showered on the new arrival and to provide a similar level of celebration for the brother or sister.

Grandparents

The grandparents' level of involvement in the pregnancy and birth of their grandchild is dependent on many variables. Today, geographic distance to the new family may not allow the level of involvement that was experienced by their grandparents. Grandparents today are typically expected to be available for the young family if an emergency arises. The new parents may call and ask advice or seek counsel from the experienced older parents. The financial situation, health, mental capacity, and working status influence the grandparents' ability to assist the new parents.

In today's family, both grandparents may be involved in careers and be focused on a retirement goal. The younger grandparent may have difficulty adjusting to the connotation of aging when they are called grandmother or grandfather. Grandparents with an active business and social life may resist being involved at the level others feel is appropriate. The conflict between reality and expectations can cause discord between family members. Nurses can discuss these issues during prenatal visits to assist the new parents in planning the involvement of the grandparents in ways that fit into everyone's lifestyle.

A growing phenomenon in the United States is the increasing number of grandparents who are raising their grandchildren. In 1997, Thomson, Minkler, and Driver (2000) reported that 3.7 million grandparents had taken their grandchildren into their homes to raise; of these, 2.3 million were single grandmothers. Many times, the parents are not living in the home with the family, which places great stress on the unprepared guardians. Grandparents are attempting to accomplish their own developmental tasks and the new role of late parenting may cause confusion and social and financial concerns.

CULTURAL CARING

What is a culture? The word is used to describe the intellectual, social, and artistic styles of a group of people, but for this discussion, we are referring to the customs, beliefs, and behaviors that have been learned through association with a particular group of people (Galanti, 1997).

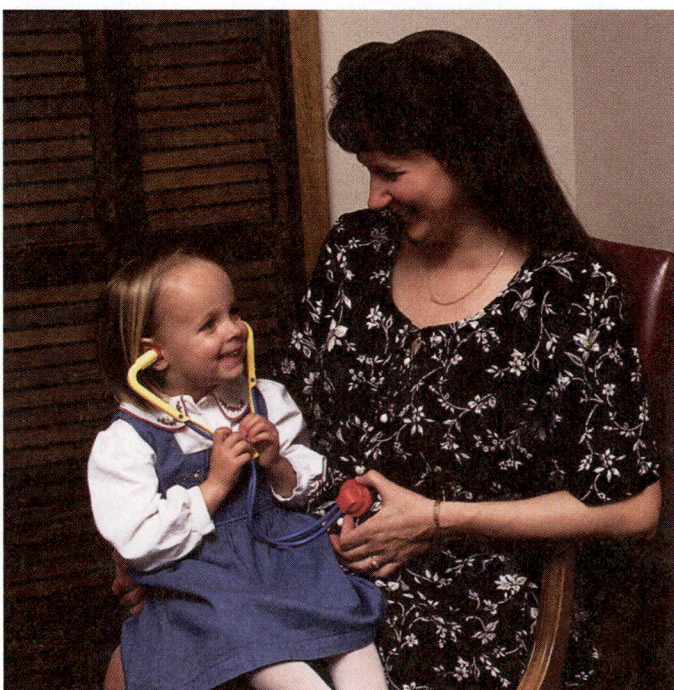

Figure 9-19 Young children can be encouraged to be involved in the pregnancy to develop a connection with the baby before birth.

The learned behaviors of individual cultures are shared within the group and passed down to future generations. But there are factors that can dilute the culture and cause members to stray from their specific culture. When an individual has lived among people of another culture, especially since childhood, or has achieved a different social or economic class, their behaviors may deviate from their cultural heritage. The dilution or absence of the original culture is the reason why individuals should not be stereotyped. For example, the nurse assumes that because a woman appears to be from Mexico that she has or wants a large family. If the woman was born and raised in the United States in a predominantly Caucasian environment, a large family may not be a priority. It is acceptable to generalize concerning cultural behaviors, if this is used only as the beginning of an assessment to ascertain the true feelings of the individual client.

Because each person has values that are important to them, there are values that different cultures view as important. In the United States, freedom, independence, and autonomy are values that many people feel are important. In many cultures, remaining in the family home where members can assist each other with day-to-day activities is far more acceptable than obtaining independence from the family. The view of family involvement sometimes causes conflict with the American health care system's values of efficiency and self-control. Some cultures want the involvement of their family members in decision making and care and as intermediaries. Nurses must avoid ethnocentrism, that is, the view that a certain culture's way of doing things is the only appropriate way, and attempt to be open-minded concerning the individual's values, beliefs, and behaviors, the view that is called cultural relativism (Galanti, 1997).

A person may see illness differently from the dominant health care community norms. Most medical models in the United States rely on the belief that germs, viruses, and environmental toxins cause disease and that health can be maintained through diet and exercise. Galanti (1997) states that, in some cultures, the worldview is focused on the belief that these aspects of life are out of human control and in the hands of a greater being. Some cultures also relate to the natural aspect of all things and strive to obtain harmony with the earth. These individuals may prefer to treat ailments with herbal medicine or through prayer, touch, or meditation. There are cultures that do not view pregnancy as a medical condition, so the pregnant woman may not see the necessity of prenatal care. In these situations, it is necessary to explain the importance of health teaching and maintenance and not assume that everyone views healthy behaviors in the same way.

Another aspect of cultural differences that often becomes evident in pregnancy is the relationship of the father and mother. Most Americans believe that the man or partner should be involved in every aspect of the pregnancy and delivery. In some Middle Eastern families the man is present during the pregnancy and delivery to protect the woman's virtue, not to assist the woman with the birth. The woman of Mexican heritage may prefer her mother to attend her delivery, and the man may feel that his presence is inappropriate.

Nurses have an opportunity to act as advocates to the women of different cultures that make up the American population. Nurses can design and implement programs that integrate the customs and values of the culture into the care of pregnant women. Mayberry, Affonson, Shibuya, and Clemmens (1999) described a health care program, *"Malama Na Wahine,"* or Caring for Pregnant Women for the native Hawaiian, Filipino, and Japanese women living in Hawaii. Mayberry and associates designed the program to acknowledge the value and self-esteem of the women they served by incorporating their customs and beliefs into every aspect of their care. Examples of cultural interventions that were used in the program included:

1. Enlisting the assistance of local cultural healers to participate in the program as recruiters and caregivers

2. Using "talk story," a form of communication that is used by the women in this culture to deliver knowledge

3. Helping women choose a name for their newborn that honors their culture

4. Providing *lomilomi* massage, which demonstrates health promotion, as part of the care of the woman and newborn

---

Nursing Tip   *Preparation for the Infant*

A lack of preparation for the birth of the baby may indicate a problem in meeting the task of role transition. However, some cultures or families do not actually purchase any items for the baby until after birth, because purchasing gifts for the baby before birth is believed to bring bad luck. Nurses must be sensitive to cultural practices different from his or her own and not assume that the couple who has not established a nursery before the birth is not eagerly awaiting the new baby's arrival.

The nurse's role in caring for clients of different cultures is to develop an individualized plan of care for each woman that supports her beliefs and customs and, at the same time, provides healthy and safe interventions for a positive outcome.

COMPLEMENTARY THERAPIES

Consumers of health care are turning to complementary therapies in large numbers. The odds that a pregnant client is practicing some type of complementary therapy are high. Strasen (1999) defines "complementary medicine" as any practitioner or practice that is not in the realm of traditional-Western or academic medicine. This definition opens up a wide range of healing methods to consumers as a complement to what may be viewed as usual health practices. Assisting clients to feel good on emotional, spiritual, and physical levels is a common goal of complementary therapists. Frequently, complementary practitioners may view their role much the same as the holistic role of the nurse, that is, to assist the client in bringing optimal health to the body, mind, and spirit.

In pregnancy, most of the complementary therapies practiced today can be beneficial in assisting the woman with easing the discomforts of pregnancy and providing mental calm in the midst of a fast-paced world. The area in which caution may be necessary is that of herbal medicine. Research into the effects of these supplements on pregnancy is just beginning. Women who request information on the use of herbs during pregnancy should be advised to avoid using them in any form during the first trimester and to seek the advice of their health care practitioner concerning the use of herbs in later pregnancy. Ginger tea for nausea is the exception.

Because a large number of women are using complementary therapies, the nursing assessment should include questions concerning these practices. The information enables the nurse to advise the woman on the continuation of these therapies or to seek further consultation concerning the safety of the practice during pregnancy.

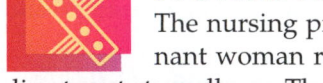

NURSING PROCESS

The nursing process in the care of the pregnant woman represents a map for the most direct route to wellness. The steps included in the nursing process operate in a continuum to provide a framework for individualizing the client's care.

Assessment

In performing the client assessment, there are many tools available to the nurse. Prerequisites for a thorough assessment include being nonjudgmental, open-minded, empathic, and a skilled interviewer; having a knowledge of physical assessment skills and parameters; and exhibiting the ability to communicate therapeutically and to collaborate. As the assessment is continuous, every time the nurse has contact with the client, her family, her friends, or other health care professionals, a synthesizing process should take place.

Interviewing is a skill that is essential to the nurse's data collection. The data that are collected should come directly from clients and their families. An important aspect of interviewing is to listen in an unbiased manner, understanding that the client and her family are the experts in this portion of the data collection. The questions should explore biophysical, psychosocial, cultural, and spiritual aspects of the client's well-being. The interview is an opportunity to begin to develop a relationship with the client and accumulate a primary list of needs.

The nurse caring for the pregnant woman must remember that there are two clients, the woman and her fetus; each requires an assessment that entails specific parameters. During the prenatal course, the nurse plans and organizes the care process over a period of time, documenting the outcomes clearly. The assessment data that are contained in the prenatal record provide a basis for the prenatal needs assessment for the family and also for the intrapartum and postpartum needs assessment.

Data obtained from diagnostic studies are included in building the database. Studies that are completed in the prenatal period are used to identify client care needs throughout pregnancy, labor, and delivery. Computerized documentation that can be shared between the prenatal provider's office and hospital or birthing center is invaluable because of easy access at all hours of the day or night.

Nursing Diagnoses

Nursing diagnoses provide a uniform method of communicating the pregnant client's concerns and needs. The nursing diagnoses reflect the nurse's clinical judgment concerning actual or potential problems for the client, the family, or the community. When prioritizing needs of the pregnant woman, the nurse should involve the client, family, and other disciplines to be sure the plan is correctly focused and realistic.

Critical Thinking

Additional Nursing Diagnoses

Refer to the case study of 16-year-old Rhonda. Develop a care plan that includes these additional nursing diagnoses:

- Compromised family coping
- Risk for impaired parenting
- Deficient knowledge (infant care)
- Home maintenance management, risk for impaired

Nursing Tip *Successful Planning*

Because the plan of care is a communication tool to organize and prioritize the client's care, all entries should be timed, dated, and initialed.

client, and the role of the nurse may be coordination or delegation. It remains the nurse's responsibility to ensure that the plan of care is updated as the interventions are completed; this is accomplished through complete documentation at each prenatal visit.

Outcome Identification

For the pregnant woman, outcomes are typically centered on nursing diagnoses relating to a healthy pregnancy, successful adaptation to new family roles, and preparation for motherhood. In identifying desired outcomes, the nurse should make every effort to involve the pregnant client's partner or family, according to client wishes, and to incorporate the client's personal goals for her pregnancy.

Planning

Once the nursing diagnoses and outcome statements have been developed, the nurse and client should plan care that will result in an achievable and desired response of the client and family, to the nursing interventions. Planning should take into account such factors as quality of life, acuity of medical condition, resources, time, finances, and situation. Working with the client to establish an individualized plan of care is important, because both the client and the nurse are accountable for accomplishing the planned outcomes.

Nursing Intervention

Interventions are derived from the nurses' knowledge base and through consultation with other disciplines. The interventions should be based on scientific principles and implemented with an understanding of where the pregnant client is on the continuum of wellness. Other health care providers may complete some of the interventions that are included in the plan of care for the pregnant

Evaluation

The nurse must assess the pregnant client's response to the interventions, and then make adjustments to the plan of care. By interviewing the client at each prenatal visit, the nurse can ascertain the client's comfort level with the plan of care and make adjustments as new diagnoses present or other factors change.

Nursing Tip *Successful Evaluation*

Questions that the process of evaluation will answer are:

1. Were the diagnoses correct?
2. Have the outcomes been met?
3. Should the interventions be changed?
4. Have new problems occurred?
5. Should new health care providers be involved?
6. What interventions were most effective and should other interventions be included?
7. Are new outcome criteria required?

The evaluation process should be thought of as a flowchart of the client's care with ongoing assessment of the client's needs.

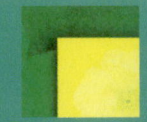

CASE STUDY/CARE PLAN
ADOLESCENT PREGNANCY

Rhonda is a 16-year-old female at 26 weeks' gestation. Her vital signs are within normal limits and her weight gain is at 17 pounds. She states she is still smoking because she is concerned about gaining too much weight. She presents to the clinic for only the second time, complaining of difficulty having a bowel movement. Rhonda has stopped taking her prenatal vitamins because one of her friends told her they could make her constipated. She is living with the father of her baby. She continues to wear the clothes she wore before she was pregnant, although they appear tight and uncomfortable.

Assessment

- Age 16 at 26 weeks' gestation
- Vital signs normal
- Risk for fetal injury results from maternal smoking and lack of prenatal care
- Constipation
- Body image disturbance

Nursing Diagnosis

Risk for fetal injury related to cigarette smoking and limited prenatal care

Expected Outcomes	The client will:
	Verbalize understanding of the risk to the fetus from cigarette smoking
	Verbalize importance of prenatal visits to maintain a healthy pregnancy
	Demonstrate lifestyle changes that reduce the risk to the fetus
Planning	Collaborating with client, determine desired means of delivering necessary information, based on client's learning style and preferences.
NOC	Knowledge: Child and personal care
NIC	Health education

Nursing Interventions	**Rationales**
1. Stress the importance of ongoing prenatal care to monitor the growth of the fetus and to prevent maternal complications.	1. Many teens feel well and do not understand the necessity of prenatal visits.
2. Explain the hazards to the fetus from maternal cigarette smoking.	2. Smoking can cause growth retardation and an increased incidence of SIDS.
3. Help client to identify her motivation to smoke and her motivation to stop smoking.	3. Teen mothers are more receptive to changing health habits if the reasons are outlined in a nonjudgmental manner. Offering the option of cutting down and then quitting may soften the request.
4. Refer her to a support group or find another teen who has successfully stopped smoking to discuss options with her.	4. Engaging Rhonda in group or peer support sessions may help her to feel less socially isolated.

Evaluation	At Rhonda's next visit, she was able to verbalize the necessity to stop or at least curtail her smoking. She had cut her smoking down to three cigarettes a day and was working to completely stop smoking. She still appeared doubtful that the prenatal visits were necessary. Refer Rhonda to the clinic's teen childbirth classes.

(continues)

Nursing Diagnosis

Constipation related to smooth muscle relaxation, slowed intestinal motility, ingestion of iron supplements, and diet.

Expected Outcome	Rhonda will maintain her normal pattern of bowel function.
Planning	Determine with client her usual bowel patterns and what routine would make her comfortable.
NOC	Bowel elimination
NIC	Bowel management

Nursing Interventions	**Rationales**
1. Assess for prepregnant elimination patterns.	1. With appropriate diet, usual elimination patterns should be maintained.
2. Assess for dietary history and make recommendations based on nutritional needs.	2. A dietary history tells the practitioner what modifications need to be made.
3. Instruct on the benefits of increasing fiber intake. Consult the dietitian to identify high-fiber foods that are acceptable to a teen (fruit and salads may be the most acceptable).	3. Adequate bulk and fiber assists in regulating bowel movements; a teenager's eating habits are influenced by peer pressure.
4. Advise client to increase fluid intake, avoiding drinks with caffeine. Encourage water, flavored water, fruit juices, or sports drinks.	4. An increase in fiber without an increase in fluids may compound the elimination problem.
5. Encourage mild exercise, such as brisk walking or riding a bicycle.	5. Exercise promotes peristalsis and may help to prevent constipation.
6. Encourage client to continue taking prenatal vitamins and, if constipation remains a problem after dietary adjustments, contact the health care provider.	6. Remind the client that prenatal vitamins are important to a healthy pregnancy and to the proper development of the baby.
7. Caution against the use of stool softeners or laxatives.	7. Never take medications that have not been approved by a health care provider.

Evaluation	The nurse called Rhonda at home 5 days after her visit. She had increased her fluid intake to 6 to 8 glasses per day of water or a sports drink. She was eating fresh and dried fruit and salads. She continued to take her prenatal vitamins and her bowel movements had returned to her normal pattern.

Nursing Diagnosis

Disturbed body image related to pregnancy, as evidenced by wearing of prepregnancy clothing.

Expected Outcome	Client will: verbalize understanding and acceptance of body image changes that are occurring Demonstrate a positive self-image by maintaining an appropriate appearance
Planning	Collaborate with client to understand her self-image and what she is or is not willing to change.
NOC	Body image
NIC	Body image enhancement

(continues)

Nursing Interventions	Rationales
1. Determine Rhonda's attitude toward her pregnancy, changing body image, and her peers' and significant other's reactions. Suggest that her significant other accompany her to her next prenatal visit.	1. Her views on her pregnancy affect how she feels about her body and about becoming a mother. The father of the baby is a strong influence on health behaviors.
2. Identify Rhonda's sense of self-esteem in relationship to her pregnancy and her new role. Assess her relationship with her mother and the availability of other female role models.	2. Honest, nonjudgmental, respectful treatment facilitates interactions with the client. Female role models are helpful in the transition to the motherhood role.
3. Review the physiologic changes of pregnancy and why these changes are necessary for the development of her fetus; assure her that mixed feelings are normal.	3. Show her that the changes in her body are normal and beneficial to the growth of the fetus. Talking through her feelings helps to decrease the stress she may be feeling.
4. Assess her ability to purchase or borrow comfortable maternity clothes. Make a referral to social services or targeted case management for assistance.	4. Embarrassment concerning financial issues may prevent her from purchasing or borrowing appropriate clothing.

Evaluation

The case manager made a visit to Rhonda's home with several maternity outfits that were appropriate for a teenager. She discussed the role of parenthood with both Rhonda and her significant other. While in the home, she assessed the couple's plans for caring for the infant and adapting to the changes they need to make in their lifestyle. Rhonda had new questions about the changes occurring in her body and felt comfortable discussing these with the case manager.

WEB ACTIVITIES

••• What resources can you locate that give mothers self-help tips on alleviating the discomforts of pregnancy? Do they offer resources to download?

••• What types of organizations offer this information?

••• Would you encourage your clients to use the Web? If so, what type of advice would you give concerning the use of Web resources?

Key Concepts

- The presumptive signs of pregnancy are the subjective signs noted by the woman and include amenorrhea, nausea and vomiting, urinary frequency, changes in the breast, and quickening. Probable signs of pregnancy are the objective signs noted by the examiner, such as uterine enlargement, Goodell's sign, Chadwick's sign, Hegar's sign, and positive results on pregnancy tests. Detecting the fetal heart rate and fetal movement and visualization of the fetus by ultrasound are the positive signs of pregnancy.

- There are anatomic and physiologic changes that occur in virtually every body system of the pregnant woman. These changes are necessary to accommodate the growing fetus.

- Plasma volume increases by 50%; red blood cell volume increases by 18% to 30%. The disproportionate increases in volume cause a dilution of the red blood cell volume that results in the physiologic anemia of pregnancy.

- Maternal cardiac output increases from 4.5 L/min to 6.0 L/min. The uteroplacental unit requires approximately 17% of this volume to achieve adequate perfusion.

- In preparation for lactation, the number of mammary alveoli increase, the breasts become physically larger, areolae broaden, nipples become firmer and more erect, and the tubercles of Montgomery, sebaceous glands, begin to secrete a substance that keeps the areolae supple.

- The position of the heart is changed; it is pushed upward to the left and rotated. These changes mimic cardiomegaly on normal radiographic films. In 90% of pregnant woman, a systolic heart murmur can be heard at 20 weeks' gestation.

■ When the woman lies in the supine position, the gravid uterus may compress the vena cava and descending aorta. The compression can cause maternal hypotension and decrease the blood return to the heart.

■ Many of the discomforts of pregnancy can be linked to changes that occur in the body systems to accommodate a pregnancy.

■ Blood flow to the kidneys is increased, which in turn increases the glomerular filtration rate. Because of this increase, absorption is not always complete and glucose periodically spills into the urine. Protein may also be detected in the urine, but proteinuria of more than 300 mg in 24 hours warrants further investigation, especially when accompanied by hypertension and edema.

■ Individuals, as well as families, are challenged to successfully accomplish developmental tasks that move them toward role adaptation.

■ Siblings need assistance in dealing with the changes that occur when a new individual is brought into the family.

■ An assessment to identify cultural values, customs, and beliefs should be completed for every client. The information gathered should be incorporated into the client's plan of care.

■ The involvement of the client and her family is the key to planning a realistic and achievable plan of care.

Review Questions and Activities

1. All of the following are considered presumptive (subjective) signs of pregnancy except:
   a. Nausea and vomiting
   b. Urinary frequency
   c. Fetal heart beat
   d. Fatigue

   The correct answer is c.

2. During pregnancy, the plasma volume increases by 50% and the red blood cell volume increases by 18% to 30%; the disproportionate increases results in the following:
   a. Iron deficiency anemia
   b. Sickle cell anemia
   c. Thalassemia
   d. Physiologic anemia of pregnancy

   The correct answer is d.

3. An assessment to determine what aspects of the client's culture may affect her plan of care should include:

   a. Traditional customs and behaviors related to preparation for birth
   b. Beliefs related to who should be present at the birth
   c. Values related to congenital defects
   d. All of the above

   The correct answer is d.

4. A new baby affects the family unit, especially the newborn's siblings. What measures should be avoided in helping siblings adjust to the transition?
   a. Involve the sibling in planning the nursery.
   b. Answer questions in a honest and straightforward manner.
   c. Use age-specific books to inform the sibling of the fetus' growth.
   d. Avoid telling the sibling when it is time to go to the hospital for delivery.

   The correct answer is d.

5. Maternal cigarette smoking can be hazardous to the growing fetus. Which of the following is not a common risk of maternal cigarette smoking?
   a. Heart defects
   b. Increased incidence of SIDS
   c. Low birth weight
   d. Increased incidence of apnea

   The correct answer is a.

6. When a pregnant woman lies in the supine position, what potentially harmful physiologic processes occur?
   a. Increased edema in the hands and face
   b. Maternal hypotension
   c. Decreased blood return to heart
   d. After a prolonged period, decreased oxygen to the fetus

   The correct answer is d.

7. During adaptation to the role of motherhood, the woman must accomplish all but which of the following developmental tasks?
   a. Giving of oneself
   b. Binding in to the child
   c. Fantasizing or dreaming
   d. Shift her affections and alliance from her partner to the developing infant.

   The correct answer is d.

8. Complementary therapy is becoming more accepted in the United States. Which of the following therapies would you as the nurse be cautious about suggesting to the pregnant woman?
   a. Reflexology
   b. Meditation
   c. Herbal therapy
   d. Imagery

   The correct answer is c.

References

Blackburn, S. T. (2003). *Maternal, fetal and neonatal physiology: A clinical perspective* (2nd ed.). Philadelphia: W. B. Saunders.

Burrow, G. N., & Duffy, T. F. (1999). *Medical complications during pregnancy* (5th ed.). Philadelphia: W. B. Saunders.

Cunningham, F. G., MacDonald, P. C., Gant, N. F., Leveno, K. J., Gilstrap, L. C., Hankins, G. D. V., et al. (1997). *Williams obstetrics* (20th ed.). Stamford, CT: Appleton & Lange.

Duvall, E. M. (1985). *Marriage and family development* (6th ed.). New York: Harper & Row.

Gabbe, S. G., Niebyl, J. R., & Simpson, J. L. (1996). *Obstetrics: Normal & problem pregnancies* (3rd ed.). New York: Churchill Livingstone.

Galanti, G. A. (1997). *Caring for patients from different cultures* (2nd ed.). Philadelphia: University of Pennsylvania Press.

Henshaw, S. K. (1998). Unintended pregnancy in the United States. *Family Planning Perspectives, 30*(1), 24–29, 46.

National Academy of Science, Institute of Medicine. (1990). *Nutrition during pregnancy: Weight gain and nutrients.* Washington, DC: National Academy Press.

Mayberry, L. J., Affonson, D. D., Shibuya, J. & Clemmens, D. (1999). Integrating cultural values, beliefs, and customs into pregnancy and postpartum care: Lessons learned from a Hawaiian public health nursing project. *The Journal of Perinatal and Neonatal Nursing, 13*(1), 15–26.

Rubin, R. (1984). *Maternal identity and maternal experience.* New York: Springer.

Strasen, L. (1999). The silent health care revolution: The rising demand for complementary medicine. *Nursing Economics, 17*(5), 246–251.

Thomson, E. F., Minkler, M., & Driver, D. (2000). A profile of grandparents raising grandchildren in the United States. In C. B. Cox (Ed.), *To grandmother's house we go and stay* (pp. 20–31). New York: Springer.

Tulman, L., Mortin, K. H., & Fawcett, J. (1998). Prepregnant weight and weight gain during pregnancy. Relationship to functional status, symptoms, and energy. *Journal of Obstetric, Gynecologic & Neonatal Nursing, 27*(6), 629–631.

Wilson, M. E., White, M. A., Cobb, B., Curry, R., Greene, D., Popovich, D. (2000). Family dynamics, parental-fetal attachment and infant temperment. *Journal of Advanced Nursing 31*(1), 204–210.

Suggested Readings

Acevedo, M. C. (2000). The role of acculturation in explaining ethnic differences in the prenatal health-risk behaviors, mental health, and parenting beliefs of Mexican American and European American at-risk women. *Child Abuse & Neglect, 24*(1), 111–127.

Allaire, A. D., Moos, M. K., & Wells, S. (2000). Complementary and alternative medicine in pregnancy: A survey of North Carolina certified nurse-midwives. *Obstetrics & Gynecology, 95*(1), 19–23.

Belew, C. (1999). Herbs and the childbearing woman: Guidelines for midwives. *Journal of Nurse-Midwifery, 44*(3), 231–252.

Charlish, A. (1996). *Your natural pregnancy: A guide to complementary therapies.* Berkeley, CA: Ulysses Press.

Doenges, M. E., & Moorhouse, M. F. (1999). *Maternal/newborn plans of care* (3rd ed.). Philadelphia: F. A. Davis.

Doswell, W. M., & Erlen, J. A. (1998). Multicultural issues and ethical concerns in the delivery of nursing care interventions. *Nursing Clinics of North America, 33*(2), 353–361.

Drake, P. (1996). Addressing developmental needs of pregnant adolescents. *Journal of Obstetric, Gynecologic, & Neonatal Nursing, 25*(6), 518–524.

Eisenberg, A., Murkoff, H. E., & Hathaway, S. E. (1996). *What to expect when you're expecting* (2nd ed.). New York: Workman.

Gorrie, T. M., McKinney, E. S., & Murray, S. S. (1998). *Foundations of maternal-newborn nursing* (2nd ed.). Philadelphia: W. B. Saunders.

Lederman, R. P. (1996). *Psychosocial adaptation to pregnancy.* New York: Springer.

Malnory, M. E. (1996). Developmental care of the pregnant couple. *Journal of Obstetric, Gynecologic, & Neonatal Nursing, 25*(6), 525–532.

National Safety Council. (1995). Stress management. Boston: Jones & Barlett.

Sawyer, L. M. (1999). Engaged mothering: The transition to motherhood for a group of African American women. *Journal of Transcultural Nursing, 10*(1), 14–21.

Sears, W., Sears, M., & Hole, L. H. (1997). *The pregnancy book.* Boston: Little, Brown.

Tiller, C. M. (1995). Father's parenting attitudes during a child's first year. *Journal of Obstetric, Gynecologic, & Neonatal Nursing, 24*(6), 508–514.

Resources

American Botanical Council, 6200 Manor Rd., Austin, TX 78723 512-926-4900, http://www.herbalgram.org

American College of Nurse-Midwives, 8403 Colesville Rd., Suite 1550, Silver Spring, MD 20910, 240-485-1800, http://www.acnm.org; http://www.midwife.org

American College of Obstetrics and Gynecology (ACOG), 409 12th St. SW, P.O. Box 96920, Washington, DC 20024-2188, http://www.acog.org

Association of Women's Health, Obstetric and Neonatal Nurses, 2000 L Street, NW, Suite 740, Washington, DC 20036, 800-673-8499 (USA), 800-245-0231 (Canada), http://www.awhonn.org

March of Dimes, 1275 Mamaroneck Avenue, White Plains, NY 10605, 888-MODIMES (663-4637), http://www.modimes.org

CHAPTER 10

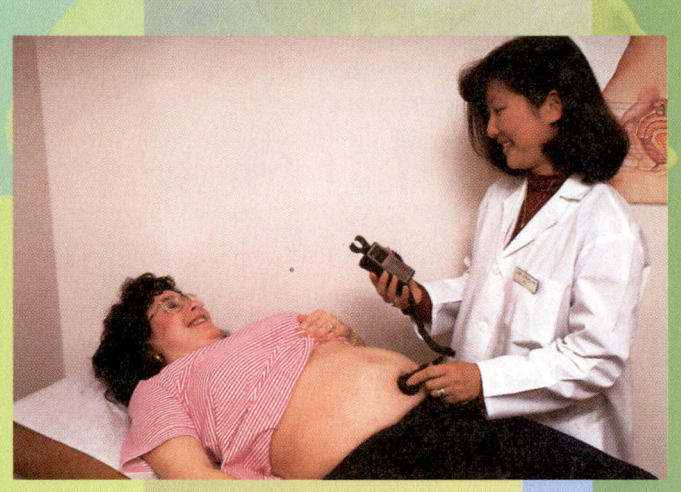

NURSING CARE OF THE PREGNANT WOMAN

Nursing care centered around health promotion and health maintenance during pregnancy presents an excellent opportunity for nurses to teach expectant mothers about normal changes expected and alert them to a variety of risk factors. You may be in contact with clients who have thoughts, values, feelings, and circumstances that are different from your own. Examine your feelings and values elicited by the following questions:

- How do I feel about my own past or potential future experiences with pregnancy? Would my feelings be different about a planned compared with an unintentional pregnancy?
- How would I feel about the changes of pregnancy happening to my body?
- Do I value prenatal care? How do I feel toward people who do not value prenatal care?
- How do I feel about families having several babies while they are receiving public assistance or welfare? What are my feelings as I see them for prenatal care?
- What would I need to do to prepare for motherhood?
- How would my eating patterns support a healthy pregnancy?
- How do I think a pregnancy would change the relationship between the pregnant woman and her partner and family?

Key Terms

Biischial diameter
Childbirth education
Cleansing breath
EDB
EDC
EDD
Gravida
GTPAL
Health maintenance
Health promotion
Interspinous diameter
LMP
Midpelvis
Modified-paced
   breathing

Multipara
Naegele's rule
Obstetrical conjugate
Paced breathing
Para
Patterned-paced
   breathing
Pelvic inlet
Pelvic outlet
Perinatal education
Pica
Preconception care
Pregnancy-induced
   hypertension (PIH)
Primipara

Competencies

Upon completion of this chapter, the reader should be able to:

1. Discuss the advantages of preconception care and counseling for a woman and her partner who are planning a pregnancy.
2. Discuss factors related to access to prenatal care.
3. Discuss nutritional consideration for the pregnant woman.
4. Describe areas of physical and psychosocial assessment that are covered in an initial prenatal visit and in subsequent visits.
5. Describe risk-assessment measures recommended for routine prenatal visits in uncomplicated pregnancies.
6. Discuss the educational principles of adult learning and the group process as they relate to perinatal education.
7. Describe the major approaches to childbirth education.
8. Discuss different strategies to enhance relaxation, such as biofeedback, imagery, touch, meditation, and music.
9. Explain nursing interventions and teaching points used to assist clients in dealing with the commonly occurring discomforts of pregnancy.
10. List eight danger signs for which clients should be taught to seek immediate medical attention.

The goal of prenatal care is the delivery of a healthy infant by a healthy mother at the end of a healthy pregnancy. *Healthy People 2010* has goals for increasing prenatal care and reducing maternal-infant-mortality.

Pregnancy and childbirth are normal physiologic processes that change from conception to delivery. The nurse has a unique opportunity to reinforce the normalcy of these processes and at the same time, assess clients for possible problems that require intervention. Additionally, the nurse can teach clients about the changes that are taking place and provide valuable guidance for clients and their families about when to seek guidance from health care providers.

Early contact between the health care team and the pregnant client provides the opportunity to address the concepts of health promotion and health maintenance. **Health promotion** consists of education and counseling activities that help enhance and maintain health and healthy behaviors. **Health maintenance** is the concept of prevention or early detection of particular health deviations through routine periodic examinations and screenings. Part of this process is the identification of risk factors.

BENEFITS OF EARLY CARE

The healthier the client before pregnancy and the better her nutritional state, the better the pregnancy outcomes, especially in terms of the baby's health. Although this may be accepted as an accurate statement, the nurse must not overlook the elements involved here. It is unlikely that a state of good health "just happened" for those particular women. Closer examination usually reveals that a conscientious self-help effort took place to produce this healthy state. Good nutritional patterns, regular exercise, avoidance of known deterrents to good health, and seeking routine periodic health examinations all contribute to a healthy pregnancy.

PRECONCEPTION CARE

Preconception care, or consultation with health care professionals before pregnancy, facilitates optimal pregnancy outcomes (Figure 10-1). The most critical and vulnerable time for a developing fetus is the interval of days 17 to 56 after fertilization. Hazards encountered during this time frequently translate into high infant morbidity or mortality. Many women seek prenatal care after that time is past, especially if the pregnancy was unplanned. Preconception care involves a team approach including a physician, nurse practitioner, Certified Nurse Midwife, or other health care professionals. Early counseling may indicate the need for referral to other specialized providers. For example, an endocrinologist can provide valuable input for a client who has diabetes, or a geneticist may clarify risk factors for a client with a family history of genetically transmitted disorders.

In the absence of an available specialized team, nurses in primary care settings (particularly in the community) can initiate preconception care and distribute literature during routine health screenings or during group classes for health promotion (Perry, 1996).

The components of preconception care include systematic identification of pregnancy risks, individualized educational materials, and referral to complementary and supplementary services such as special nutritional counseling or smoking cessation programs. Nutritional counseling and avoidance of exposure to teratogenic substances are included. Additional medications may need to be adjusted for a safe pregnancy.

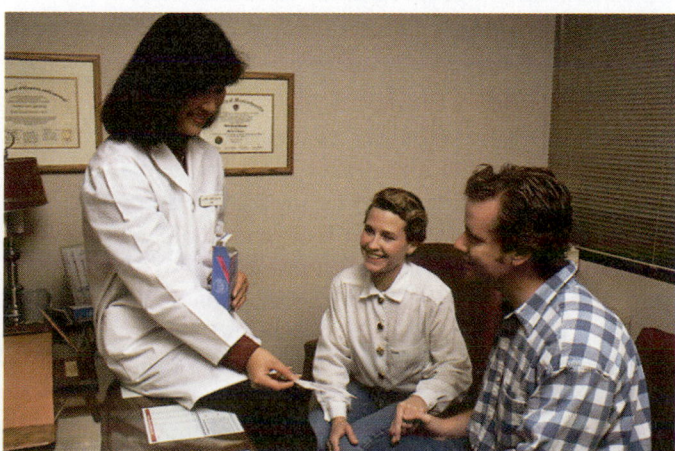

Figure 10-1   Many couples visit their health care provider for preconception counseling.

Critical Thinking

Congenital Anomalies as a Major Cause of Infant Deaths in the United States

You may work with clients who give birth to infants who have congenital anomalies with known causes. Examine your feelings about the client's responsibilities for a birth anomaly.

- Did they knowingly risk exposure to any teratogens?
- Were they innocent victims of exposure?
- Are your feelings toward these clients different from those towards couples with a normal pregnancy?
- Is the quality of your care influenced when you feel a client has been careless in taking care of herself and her developing fetus?

PRENATAL CARE

Early prenatal care provides benefits to the client, her partner, her family, and the health care team assuming responsibility for her care. Numerous teaching opportunities arise, especially regarding interpretation of normal physiologic and psychological changes. Psychological concerns can be addressed early to avoid stress and undue concern. In summary, early prenatal care allows psychological, physiologic, cultural, and social concerns to be addressed while maternal and fetal well-being and the overall pregnancy status are monitored simultaneously.

 ### COLLABORATIVE CARE

The Prenatal Health Care Team

The nurse is a valuable member of the health care team. In prenatal care the nurse is likely to be working with physicians, Certified Nurse Midwives, nurse practitioners, nutritionists, social workers, childbirth educators, and radiology and ultrasound technicians to meet the health care needs of the pregnant family. In some settings, the team may include community health workers, geneticists, psychologists, and others. With multiple providers, good verbal and written communication is essential.

Facilitation of Client Access to Care

Approaching the health care system can provoke fear in many clients, especially those with language or cultural differences. Additionally, concerns about costs and lack of knowledge regarding affordable resources can be deterrents for clients needing prenatal care. Good access to health care is a goal of *Healthy People 2010*.

Public education programs can be very effective in facilitating early and consistent use of prenatal care. The nurse can make a valuable contribution to these programs by participating in public service announcements or becoming active in organizations, such as the March of Dimes, whose efforts are directed toward formal educational programs and development of professional and lay literature.

As poor pregnancy outcomes have become associated with late or limited prenatal care, more research has emerged related to the reasons for limited care. Numerous studies report typical, predictable barriers: finances; transportation; disparities of language; clinic hours and location; and work schedule problems. More recently, clients have reported concerns about the possibility of being asked to have an abortion, having their baby taken away, or facing deportation because of their lack of citizenship.

Some clients may attach little value to prenatal care, yet value the health of their children. The value of prenatal care can then be presented in terms of a healthy start for their baby at birth.

Components of Prenatal Care

Prenatal care is designed to promote the health and well-being of mother and fetus and to prepare the family for birth and care of the infant. Education of the childbearing family is one of the most important aspects of prenatal care. Prenatal education incorporates anticipatory guidance related to pregnancy, childbirth, and care of the newborn, as well as modifying risk factors. An important aspect of prenatal health is the nutrition of the childbearing woman. Prenatal visits are established and scheduled to monitor the progress of pregnancy, assess risk factors, and provide interventions when necessary.

Prenatal care requires assessment of maternal and fetal well-being from all aspects: physiologic, psychologic, economic, and sociocultural. Depending on the findings for each individual case, the monitoring may vary slightly at each prenatal visit. For example, a client with prepregnancy diabetes may receive more frequent or closer monitoring for complications associated with diabetes. Other clients would receive routine screening for glucose in the urine.

Nutrition in Pregnancy and Lactation

The nutritional status of women entering the reproductive phase of life plays a direct role in the development of the fetus as well as the health of the woman. All women in their teens and throughout their 40s should be cognizant of their potential to conceive and, therefore, optimize their nutritional status prior to conception. Health professionals in any setting should try to help women in all age groups form sound, lifetime nutritional practices.

The first 6 weeks after conception are extremely important for optimum fetal development. Therefore, the woman must be aware of and avoid nutritional risk factors and ingestion of teratogenic substances. These include consumption of alcohol, tobacco, and prescription, over-the-counter, and illegal drugs. Currently, the recommendation is for supplementation of folic acid, 4 mg daily prior to conception to lower the risk of neural tube defects (Cuskelly, McNulty, & Scott, 1999). A well-planned pregnancy should ideally include an initial health examination 8 to 12 weeks before conception. This period is critical for establishing a prepregnancy baseline weight.

Weight Gain in Pregnancy

At the first prenatal visit, the health professional should measure height and weight, determine the prepregnancy BMI and compare with current BMI, and explain the importance of adequate weight gain during pregnancy. The weight gain of the pregnant woman should be recorded, plotted, and monitored at each prenatal visit. Weight gain during the first half of the pregnancy is reflective of increasing maternal stores. In the second half of gestation, the weight gain is primarily attributable to fetal growth (Box 10-1).

Under no circumstances should a woman lose weight during her pregnancy. If this happens, or if an excess rate of weight gain occurs, the cause should be assessed and referral made to a registered dietitian. During the second

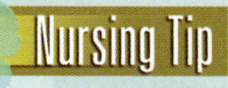

Nursing Tip

Encourage the Client to Keep All Appointments for Prenatal Care

- Provide the client with a schedule of frequency of visits by trimester.
- Emphasize the timing of various screening and monitoring activities at each visit. Explain why the time of the monitoring is so important.
- Point out the importance of all screening and monitoring activities scheduled. Indicate which tests are for the mother's benefit and which are for the baby's benefit.

Table 10-1   Recommended Total Weight Gain Ranges for Pregnant Women in Second and Third Trimesters According to Prepregnancy BMI

PREPREGNANT BMI	TOTAL WEIGHT GAIN (KG)	GAIN IN 4 WEEKS (KG)	TOTAL WEIGHT GAIN (LB)	GAIN IN 4 WEEKS (LB)
Underweight (BMI < 19.8)	12.7–18.2	2.3	28–40	5.0
Normal (BMI = 19.8–26.0)	11.4–15.9	1.8	25–35	4.0
Overweight (BMI = 26.1–29.0)	6.8–11.4	1.2	15–25	2.6
Obese (BMI > 29.0)	6.8	0.9	<15	2.0
Twin gestation	15.9–20.4	2.7	35–45	6.0

BMI, body mass = weight (kg)/height (m^2)

Note. From *Nutrition during Pregnancy* by the Institute of Medicine, 1990, Washington, DC: National Academy Press.

and third trimesters of pregnancy, underweight women (prepregnancy BMI of less than 19.8) should gain slightly more than 1 pound per week. Women with normal or moderate prepregnancy BMI of 19.8 to 26.0 should gain about 1 lb/wk. Women with a high prepregnancy BMI of 26.1 to 29.0 are encouraged to gain two-thirds of a pound per week. Very obese women (prepregnancy BMI of more than 29.0) should have their total weight gain determined on an individual basis (Table 10-1). The date of the office visit, the weeks of gestation, the mother's weight, and any significant findings should be recorded at each visit. Weight should be plotted at each visit to ensure no weight loss is occurring and, if it does, an explanation for the loss can be found. A copy of this information should also be given to the mother, if she also wants to keep track of this.

Box 10-1

Weight Gain Distribution During Pregnancy

5.0 kg (11 lb)	Fetus, placenta, and amniotic fluid
0.9 kg (2 lb)	Uterus
1.8 kg (4 lb)	Increase in blood volume
1.4 kg (3 lb)	Breast tissue
2.3 to 4.5 kg (5 to 10 lb)	Maternal stores

Total = 11 to 13 kg (25 to 30 lb) gained

For women at their ideal BMI at conception

Note. Adapted from *Williams Obstetrics* (21st ed.), by F. G. Cunningham, N. E. Gant, K. J. Leveno, L. C. Gilstrap III, J. Hauth, & K. Wenstrom, 2001, Stamford, CT: Appleton-Lange.

In 1992 the Committee on Nutritional Status during Pregnancy and Lactation proposed eight recommendations in its book, *Nutrition Services in Perinatal Care*, 2nd edition (Institute of Medicine, 1992). These key recommendations are relevant today and are listed below.

1. Basic, client-centered, individualized nutritional care should be integrated into the primary care of every woman and infant—beginning prior to conception and extending throughout the period of breastfeeding.
2. All primary care providers should have the knowledge and skills necessary to screen for nutritional problems, assess nutritional status, provide basic nutritional guidance, and implement basic nutritional care.
3. Nutritional care should be documented in the permanent medical record.
4. When health problems that benefit from special nutritional care are identified, there should be consultation with and often referral to an experienced registered dietitian or other appropriate specialists.
5. Attention should be directed toward aspects of nutritional care that have been seriously neglected in the past: providing care prior to conception and in support of breastfeeding and ensuring the continuity of nutritional care despite changes in providers.
6. Action should be taken to make appropriate policy and structural changes for the promotion and support of breastfeeding.
7. Where not already in place, mechanisms should be established to pay for basic and special nutrition services in both the public and the private sectors.
8. Cost-effective strategies for implementing the nutritional care recommended in the report should be developed and tested.

Table 10-2 Recommended Daily Prenatal Multivitamin and Mineral Supplement for Pregnant Women at Increased Nutrient Risk

Iron	30–60 mg	Vitamin B$_{12}$	2 µg
Zinc	15 mg	Folate	400 µg
Copper	2 mg	Vitamin C	50 mg
Calcium	250 mg	Vitamin D	10 µg (400 IU)
Vitamin B$_6$	2 mg		

Note. From *Fundamentals of Clinical Nutrition* (2nd ed.), by S. L. Morgan and R. L. Weinster, 1998, St. Louis, MO: Mosby.

Dietary Supplements in Pregnancy

For pregnant women a daily multivitamin and mineral preparation containing the nutrients listed in Table 10-2, is recommended. Pregnant women who are considered to be at high risk for vitamin and mineral deficiency would include the following: those who smoke or are alcohol or drug abusers; those who have frequent, closely spaced, or multiparous births; those who are carrying more than one fetus; those who experience hyperemesis gravidarum; those who have an eating disorder or are obese or underweight; and those who are adolescents or strict vegetarians.

Over-the-counter prenatal vitamin and mineral supplements are readily available. Generic brands should be compared with name brands for price and nutrients.

Ingestion of Harmful Substances

Many ingested substances pose a risk to the mother or fetus during pregnancy and should therefore be avoided.

Mercury. If mercury contamination is suspected, the pregnant woman should wash all vegetables and fruits (if the skin is eaten) with a weak soap solution and scrub the skin with a brush and rinse well. Otherwise, the skin should be peeled and disposed of before consumption. Likewise, raw fish (e.g., sushi) or fish caught in contaminated waters should be avoided during pregnancy.

Toxic Doses of Vitamin A. Excessive intake (over 10,000 IU per day of vitamin A) from food and supplements as well as medications should be avoided.

Alcohol. Women should avoid alcohol consumption during pregnancy. All alcoholic beverages display the Surgeon General's warning regarding the possible ill effects on the fetus. An absolutely safe minimum limit has not been established. Alcohol increases the urinary excretion of zinc.

Caffeine. There is no specific medical recommendation about caffeine consumption levels for pregnant women. However, The FDA recommends that pregnant women reduce their caffeine intake from coffee, tea, colas, and cocoa to not more that two to three servings per day, for a total of 300 mg of caffeine per day. More than 1,000 over-the-counter drugs have caffeine as an ingredient, in addition to prescription drugs that contain caffeine.

Artificial Sweeteners. Moderation in the consumption of artificial sweeteners is recommended for pregnant and lactating women. Use of saccharin is not recommended because studies have been inconclusive about its safety.

Herbal Supplements. The key concern with herbal medicine is the lack of consistent potency in the active material in any given batch of product. The reputable manufacturers try to ensure quality, purity, safety, and reliability. "Natural" does not always mean "safe."

Nursing Tip · Herbal Medicines

The German Federal Health Agency established scientific commissions to review various categories of drugs in 1974. Commission E was charged with reviewing herbal medicines to determine the safety and effectiveness of each (Blumenthal et al., 1998). Their monographs have recently been translated into English. These can serve as a useful tool for the health care professional to use in evaluating herbal supplements taken by clients. Because some herbal products may be harmful during pregnancy, or may interact with medication, it is very important for health providers to always ask what herbal products the client is taking.

Nursing Tip · Morning Sickness

For treatment of motion sickness or morning sickness, if there is no history of miscarriage, the following may be tried, with the approval of the obstetrician:

A 12-ounce glass of ginger ale, provided it contains ginger and not artificial flavor, or a prescribed preparation of 500 to 2,000 mg ginger, taken 30 minutes before travel. Ginger may be used in the form of capsules, ginger tea infusions, or ginger ale. For ginger tea, add 2 teaspoons of powdered or grated ginger root to 1 cup of boiling water. Steep 10 minutes.

Ginger has been shown to be safe in the treatment of morning sickness, at a dose of less than 1 g, but causes uterine contractions and triggers menstruation when given at a dose that is 20 times the stomach-settling dose. Women who are attempting to conceive and pregnant women may use culinary amounts of digestion-enhancing herbs but must have the approval and supervision of their obstetrician or health care provider for any herb used medicinally.

Over-the-Counter Drugs. Drugs taken during pregnancy can cause serious congenital malformations. Potentially more than 500,000 over-the-counter drugs are on the market. Health care providers should be made aware of all such drugs taken intermittently or on a regular basis by women desiring to conceive and after conception.

The effects of these substances on the fetus include low birth weight, CNS disturbances, pulmonary hypertension, neonatal bleeding, renal failure, growth and mental retardation, inhibition of bone growth, discoloration of teeth, drug addiction fetal alcohol syndrome (FAS), congenital malformations, spontaneous abortions, and fetal death.

Pica. Pica, a psychobehavioral disorder, is the persistent ingestion of substances having little or no nutritional value or the craving for nonfood articles as food (Rainville, 1998). Pica may indicate anemia, for which the client should be evaluated if the behavior is known to the practitioner, but it is more likely to be a consequence of family traditions.

Commonly ingested nonfood substances include dirt or clay; laundry starch or cornstarch; lead paint flakes; ice or ice frost; and chalk, mothballs, baking soda, coffee grounds, or cigarette ashes. Some of these items contain toxic compounds or untolerated substances. Eating these items usually displaces the intake of nutritious foods or interferes with nutrient absorption.

When evaluating a pregnant client's dietary intake, inquiring about pica behavior is essential. The health care practitioner should always inquire about unusual nonfood cravings, even if there is no suspicion of pica. Being culturally sensitive and nonjudgmental when discussing this topic is key to obtaining information about the practices of clients. It is important to know if a woman is consuming these substances to enhance safety for herself and her unborn child.

Nursing Alert

Medication and Pregnancy

Pregnant women must use extreme caution in taking or using any herb, over-the-counter or prescription drug; illicit drug; excessive amounts of caffeine; or alcohol or nicotine immediately before conception and throughout the pregnancy. Use of any of the above should be discussed with the health care provider.

Client Education

Relieving Nausea and Vomiting

Women experiencing nausea and vomiting in early pregnancy could try a few of the following ideas:

- Eat small, low-fat meals and snacks, every 2 to 3 hours.
- Eat slowly.
- Drink soups and liquids between meals, rather than with meals, to avoid dehydration.
- Slowly sip a carbonated beverage when nauseated.
- Avoid citrus and tomato products, spearmint, peppermint, and caffeine. For some, peppermint is not nauseating and helps to alleviate nausea.
- Avoid or limit intake of spicy and high-fat foods; avoid greasy or fried foods.
- Avoid eating or drinking for 1 to 2 hours before lying down.
- Avoid aromatic foods and cooking odors that may trigger nausea.
- Avoid drinking coffee or tea.
- Inhale the scent of fresh-cut lemon to refresh the senses.
- Get plenty of fresh air and rest.
- When rising from the bed or couch, get up slowly.
- Eat more pasta, bread, and potatoes.
- Eat a few bites of a soda cracker before getting out of bed in the morning.
- Take a walk after meals to help with digestion of food.
- Wear loose-fitting clothing.
- Sleep or rest with the head elevated.
- Never take medicines for nausea without first consulting with a health care professional.
- Ginger capsules or herbal tea infusions help some clients with nausea. Consult a health care professional on type, quantity, and safety. Do not exceed 1 g/day.

Constipation and Hemorrhoids. Constipation has been associated with the smooth-muscle relaxation of the gastrointestinal tract, increased progesterone levels, and pressure of the fetus on the intestines. Other causes may include inadequate fluid and fiber intake or a decrease in physical activity. Iron supplements may also contribute to constipation. Constipation often causes gastrointestinal discomfort, a bloated feeling, exacerbated hemorrhoids, and, sometimes, decreased appetite. Strategies to combat constipation and hemorrhoids include increasing fluid intake to 2 to 3 quarts per day; eating high-fiber cereals, whole grains, legumes, fruits, and vegetables daily; and engaging in physical activity. Laxatives and herbal products with laxative effects should be used only with a physician's approval.

The Initial Prenatal Visit

The initial prenatal visit, especially in the absence of preconception care and counseling, can be rather lengthy. At this time a detailed medical history and physical examination are completed. Accuracy of these baseline data is particularly important because health care providers will be referring back to them throughout the pregnancy. Nurses can assist clients through this time-consuming process by pointing out the importance of each step and by emphasizing that subsequent visits should be briefer. Nurses should congratulate clients for seeking early prenatal care and encourage early prenatal care for subsequent pregnancies.

Pregnancy Confirmation

Many times clients and partners appear at a prenatal clinic for one distinctive purpose: to find out for sure if they are pregnant or not. Some clients may have already conducted an at-home pregnancy test and are seeking validation of the results. The availability and affordability of over-the-counter test kits have made them increasingly popular. However, the accuracy of the results is highly dependent on proper use of the kits, a point emphasized in the manufacturers' instruction sheets. Home pregnancy tests can be valid 10–14 days post conception. Confirmation of pregnancy in the office or clinic setting usually is by means of a urine test for the presence of human chorionic gonadotropin (hCG). If necessary, a blood test for the hCG placental hormone can be performed (Cunningham et al., 2001).

Estimation of Due Date

After confirmation of a pregnancy, the next logical query from prospective parents is to estimate the date the baby is due to be born. This is commonly and historically referred to as the **EDC**, or expected date of confinement. Other terms in common use are **EDD** for expected date of delivery, or **EDB** for expected date of birth. Clients usually refer to the EDB as their due date.

The EDC usually is calculated from the menstrual history, using a method called **Naegele's rule**. The calculation begins with the *first* day of the last normal menstrual period (or **LMP**); from this date, 3 months are subtracted and then 7 days are added. For example, if the first day of the LMP was September 15: LMP – 3 months + 7 days = EDC 9/15 (– 3 months) = 6/15 (+7 days) = 6/22.

The resulting calculated EDC is based on the presumption of ovulation occurring 14 days *before* the next anticipated period rather than 14 days *after* the last period began. This calculation usually is confirmed by a second method, measurement of uterine size, particularly as the pregnancy progresses. Neither method alone is deemed to be exact; however, the correlation of the findings of the two methods is fairly reliable. In clients with irregular menses, uterine size can be helpful in either confirming or redating the duration of the pregnancy and may be confirmed by ultrasound.

Pregnancy wheels (Figure 10-2) are used to determine the EDC by aligning the arrow of the first day of the LMP and then reading off the date that corresponds with the 40-week mark. Aside from the dates, pregnancy wheels usually contain other information, such as corresponding weight and length of the fetus and height of the fundus at various weeks' gestation.

Determination of Gravidity and Parity

Gravidity and parity are used much like a shorthand way of recording pregnancy history. **Gravida** is the number of pregnancies, regardless of duration or outcomes. A client who is pregnant for the first time thus is a gravida 1, a client experiencing her second pregnancy is a gravida 2, and so on. Sometimes the gravida 1 client is referred to as a *primigravida*, meaning this is her first pregnancy. **Para** is

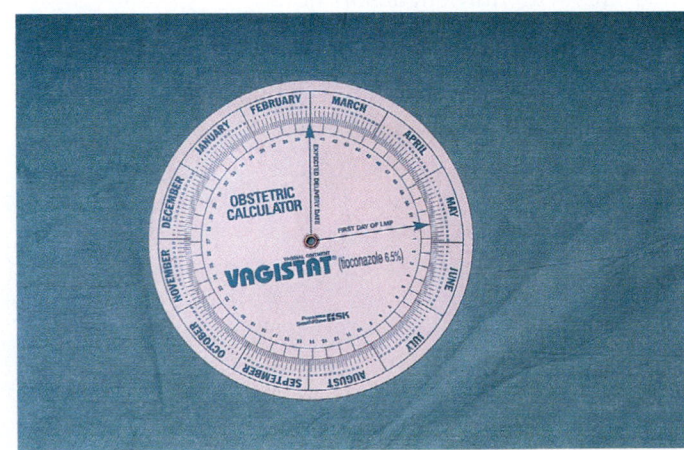

Figure 10-2   Gestation wheel. Place arrow labeled *first day of LMP* on date of LMP. Read data at arrow labeled *expected delivery date.*

the number of births after 20 weeks' gestation, whether live births or stillbirths.

A five-digit system is commonly used to give more detailed information about past deliveries. This system refers only to past pregnancies and their outcomes; it does not reflect the current pregnancy. The five digits **GTPAL** indicate the following in this order: the number of conceptions, the number of full-term deliveries (usually considered to be 37 to 40 weeks' gestation), the number of premature or preterm deliveries (between 20 and 36 weeks' gestation), the number of abortions (induced or spontaneous terminations of pregnancy before 20 weeks' gestation), and the number of children born to the client who are alive at the time of data collection. As an example, a woman who has had three term pregnancies, delivered three live infants, but suffered the loss of her 6-year-old son in an accident would be considered a 3-3-0-0-2. It is helpful to remember that the first three digits are in order of time in utero, from longest to shortest.

Other commonly used terms to describe the parity status of clients are **primipara**, a woman who has experienced only one birth after 20 weeks' gestation, and **multipara**, a woman who has had two or more births after 20 weeks' gestation.

Medical History and Family Medical History

Comprehensive medical histories for the client and her partner should be obtained. Age, race, ethnic background, and even address may not be viewed as crucial information, yet each can provide the health care professional with important information. Age, such as teens and women of advanced age, are associated with pregnancy risks. Certain genetic conditions, such as the sickle cell trait, anemia, or Tay Sachs disease, are associated with specific racial groups. The client's or partner's work and residence addresses may be related to known contaminants or pollution associated with disease and birth defects.

All entries in a client's records are purposeful and should be explored accordingly with the client and her partner. The medical history provides an excellent starting point for the nursing process, particularly the sharing of expert knowledge and analysis and interpretation of information. The mutuality of data exploration cannot be overemphasized. Clients and their partners often have information readily available but are unaware of its significance to their health status without interpretation by health care professionals.

The medical history provides an excellent database to identify risk factors to be monitored as the pregnancy progresses. A psychosocial history can be helpful in making an assessment of readiness for parenting. Other areas to be assessed from this history are whether the pregnancy was planned, and the client's expectations about the pregnancy and the social history of the client and her partner regarding use of alcohol, tobacco, or drugs.

The Physical Examination

The initial prenatal visit includes a physical examination that, with some exceptions, follows the systematic approach seen in routine physical assessments. A complete physical examination usually is performed only at the time of the first visit. Thereafter, the elements of the repeat visits are very much abbreviated, yet specific to the progress of the pregnancy and the well-being of the mother and fetus.

Nursing Alert

Immunizations Contraindicated in Pregnancy

- Immunizations with live (attenuated) viruses should not be given during pregnancy because of potential damage to the fetus.
- Preconception care encompasses assessment of immunization status with the opportunity to update immunizations, assuming avoidance of pregnancy in the near future.

Immunizations may be given in the postpartum period with emphasis on the use of contraception (for at least 3 months) to avoid an immediate pregnancy with possible fetal harm.

Client Education

Prenatal Visits

For a client to understand her time commitment and plan ahead for prenatal visits, she should know how often her return visits typically will be scheduled:

- Up to 28 weeks' gestation (covers first and second trimesters), every 4 weeks
- 29 to 36 weeks' gestation, every 2 weeks
- 37 to 40 weeks' gestation, every week

Clinical Pathway for Prenatal Care

	Initial Visit	Subsequent Visits
Assessment/Monitoring		
Physical Examination	Complete Examination	Monitoring Examination
Lab Work and Testing	CBC, UA, serology, blood typing and RH, rubella titer, HepB screen, HIV, Chlamydia and GC; 1-hour glucose (if appropriate)	Triple screen @ 14–22 weeks; 1-hour glucose @ 24–28 weeks; group B strep screen @ 35–37 weeks; monitor CBC for hgb, HCT, and platelets; ultrasound @ ~18–20 weeks
Functional Assessment		
Nutritional	Height; weight; exercise 24-hour recall; and caloric, iron, folate, and protein intake	Continue to monitor diet in relation to weight gain and adequate intake
Elimination	Assess bowel and bladder function	Continue to monitor and counsel pregnancy-related changes
Rest/Activity	Assess sleep, rest, and exercise status	Continue to monitor and counsel regarding pregnancy-related changes
Comfort	Discern normal discomforts of pregnancy from other discomforts	Continue to monitor and counsel regarding pregnancy-related changes
Psychosocial/Family	Assess family structure and dynamics, reaction to pregnancy, and economic and social impact of pregnancy	Continue to monitor family dynamics and adaptation to the pregnancy, preparation for birth of the infant, and parenting
Developmental/Pregnancy Progress	Determine EDC	Monitor progress of the pregnancy
Spiritual	Assess spiritual implications of pregnancy	Monitor for any emergent spiritual needs
Risk Assessment	Assess for actual and potential risk factors for the health of the mother and the pregnancy	Management of existing risk factors and monitor for emergent risk factors
Interventions		
Medications	Assess for Rx medications, OTC medications, and other herbal, alternative/complementary, or dietary supplements	Treatments for conditions based on laboratory findings; note all Rx and nonRx medications
Treatments	Treat existing conditions, if necessary	Treat existing conditions
Anticipatory Guidance/ Teaching and Support	See Box 10-2	See Box 10-2
Referral	Nutritionist; WIC; social worker, if needed; other referrals as indicated	Childbirth education, educator, or CB/parenting classes; other referrals as indicated

Note. Refer to appendix for abbreviations and their definitions.

Changes occur from trimester to trimester that vary from the baseline but still are normal anticipated findings. An example of the latter are the hemoglobin and hematocrit values. Assuming a normal baseline of 12 to 15 g/dL and 35% to 45%, respectively, the nurse would not be alarmed to see these values (especially hemoglobin) decrease slightly in the third trimester. As the circulating blood and fluid volume increases with the progression of the pregnancy, the number of erythrocytes is essentially the same; however, the erythrocytes are suspended in a larger amount of fluid, thereby yielding a smaller percentage value. This effect is sometimes referred to as physiologic anemia of pregnancy.

Laboratory Tests. Comprehensive prenatal care indicates specific laboratory tests that need to be performed at the initial visit and periodically throughout the pregnancy. The timing of some laboratory testing is crucial for an accurate assessment. If blood is collected too early or too late in the pregnancy, the values will not be very reliable. For example, initial hemoglobin and hematocrit testing at 30 weeks' gestation certainly provides information to the nurse; however, without an early baseline for comparison, assessment of normal compared with abnormal changes is difficult. In addition, some laboratory testing is time-sensitive within a tighter time frame. An example is the glucose testing in which the glucose level is mea-

Nursing Tip *Laboratory Tests at the Initial Visit*

1. Blood work: complete blood count, hemoglobin, hematocrit, Rh status, and blood type. Screening for sickle cell trait, as indicated. Serology for syphilis, rubella titer, human immunodeficiency virus (HIV), and hepatitis screening, as indicated or as per department policy or client request. Glucose screening if the first visit is at 24 to 28 weeks' gestation. Alpha-fetoprotein screening if the first visit is at 16 to 18 weeks' gestation.

2. Urinalysis (with culture, if indicated): examine for glucose, protein, erythrocytes, leukocytes, and bacteria.

3. Pelvic laboratory tests: Pap smear, cultures for gonorrhea and chlamydia. Presence of group B *Streptococcus* is often tested if the first visit is after 24 weeks' gestation.

sured from a blood sample drawn 1 hour after the client drinks a glucola preparation.

Ultrasonography. In addition to a urine or blood test for pregnancy confirmation, ultrasonography is often used, depending on the length of gestation. This technology has been refined throughout the years to a very high level of sophistication. It can be used to identify a yolk sac, a fetal heart before it is audible with Doppler ultrasonography, the sex of the fetus, and internal structures of the developing fetus. Routine use usually is limited to pregnancy confirmation; assessment of fetal development for determining gestational age and well-being, as indicated; sex determination, if indicated or desired; and overall fetal size as term approaches.

Further use of ultrasonography is indicated in cases of unusual findings that suggest deviations from a normal prenatal course. Examples of these situations include a fundal height inconsistent with calculated dates of pregnancy (larger, often with multiple gestation or some known fetal anomalies, or smaller, which may indicate poor fetal growth), or inability to find the fetal heartbeat using routine methods.

Pelvic Examination. The pelvic examination, including collection of pelvic cultures and smears and the performance of the bimanual examination, usually is the last part of the initial physical examination. The pelvic laboratory specimens are collected first. Some of these (e.g., for chlamydia and gonorrhea) may be by DNA probe or culture. The bimanual examination is done to determine the uterine size and to assess for deviations in expected shape or size. Normal cervical and uterine changes expected in pregnancy (see Chapter 9) also are noted.

Assessment of the Bony Pelvis. Assessment of the bony pelvis is necessary to determine the probability of a fetus of normal size being delivered vaginally. A client who has already delivered an infant of 7 pounds or larger is said to have a "tried" pelvis, one with large enough measurements for delivery of another infant of normal size. True measurement of the pelvic structure usually is done using X-ray films; however, a reliable indirect measurement is possible with a pelvic examination by a skilled nurse or physician. Borderline or questionable measurements are cause for either further evaluation or careful monitoring for labor progression.

The pelvis consists of four bones: two os innominate (or os cocci), the sacrum, and the coccyx. The ischium, ilium, and symphysis pubis are anatomic regions of the bones and should not be confused with actual bones. The joints formed by the four bones are the symphysis pubis, two sacroiliac joints (junction of the sacrum and each os innominate), and the sacrococcygeal joint (connection of the sacrum and coccyx). The status of these joints takes on greater significance as the pregnancy progresses and these joints "soften."

The pelvis is visually divided into three planes. The first plane is the **pelvic inlet**, with the transverse segment being corresponding points on the brim of the true pelvis and the anterior-posterior points being the back side of the symphysis pubis and the sacral promontory. This anterior-posterior diameter of the pelvic inlet is the smallest diameter. This is called the **obstetrical conjugate**; it is measured indirectly by the diagonal conjugate (Figure 10-3). The

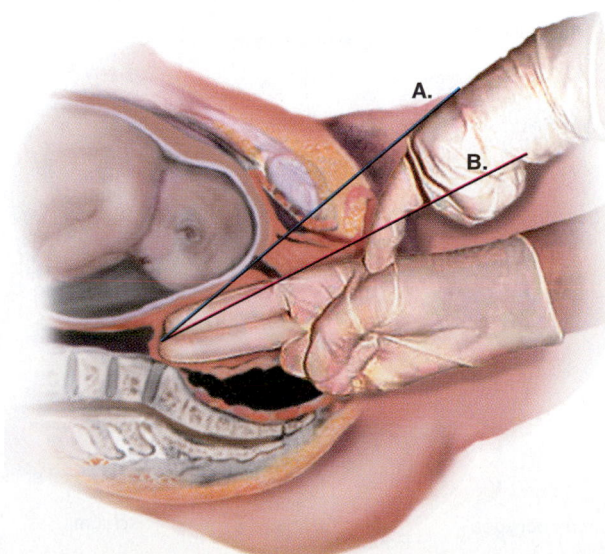

Figure 10-3 Diameters of the (A) pelvic inlet and (B) pelvic outlet.

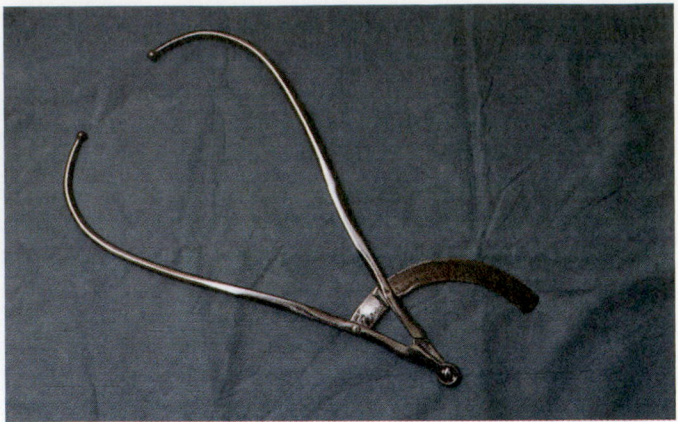

Figure 10-4 Obstetrical caliper.

Nursing Tip

Teaching Partners How to Help Prevent Client Accidents and Falls

The client's partner can assist in avoiding falls or near-falls by stooping and lifting for her, assisting her over irregular surfaces, helping her in and out of the car, and assisting her with stair steps. Partner attention is more likely with understanding of the physiologic changes that produce the risks.

examiner inserts the middle and index fingers of the examining hand and touches the tip of the middle finger to the sacral promontory. At this point, notation is made of where the examining hand touches the symphysis pubis. The measurement of this distance on the examiner's hand can be done with an obstetrical caliper (Figure 10-4).

From this diagonal conjugate, the obstetrical conjugate (smallest diameter) can be estimated fairly accurately by subtracting 1.5 or 2 cm. The resulting measure should be at least 10.5 cm, assuming normal thickness and tilt of the symphysis pubis. A smaller measurement requires further evaluation.

The second pelvic plane is known as the **midpelvis**. The smallest diameter of the midpelvis or midplane is the transverse or **interspinous diameter** (between the two ischial spines). The ischial spines are evaluated by palpation for their prominence or flatness (Figure 10-5). Prominent converging spines can compromise this diameter or, in the least, cause a "tight fit" for the fetal head, with possible tis-

sue damage to the mother during delivery. The sacral curvature (or flatness) is evaluated. A curved sacrum allows more room in the midpelvis than does a flat sacrum, thus becoming somewhat of a compensatory mechanism for a marginal interspinous measurement.

The third plane, the **pelvic outlet**, is the plane of greatest compensation. The smallest measurement is the distance between the two ischial tuberosities; this measurement usually is called the intertuberous or **biischial diameter**. The size is estimated by the knuckles of the examiner's fist being placed across the perineum at the level of the tuberosities (Figure 10-6). Assuming a fist size of at least 8 cm, the knuckles usually do not touch both tuberosities simultaneously, indicating a diameter of 8 cm or greater. The anterior-posterior measurement is from the bottom of the symphysis pubis to the tip of the sacrum, at the sacrococcygeal joint, which usually is about 10 to 11.5 cm. The coccyx is evaluated for mobility by examination through finger touch. A mobile nonprominent coccyx allows for some flexibility in the pelvic outlet plane. The angle of the subpubic arch is evaluated as part of the pelvic outlet. In the normal female pelvis, this angle is about 90 degrees and allows room for the upward extension of the fetal head at delivery (see Chapter 13).

Subsequent Visits

A schedule of future visits is given to each client. This time is an excellent opportunity to explain what is done at each visit, to give printed instructions and educational materials, and to anticipate client concerns. The client should be given thorough instructions regarding nutrition and fluid intake (at least eight glasses of water a day plus other fluids), the normal changes of pregnancy, recommendations regarding exercise and general hygiene, and recommended treatment of various discomforts she may encounter as the pregnancy progresses. This is also an appropriate time to give the client printed materials about designated danger signs for which she should seek immediate assistance (Figure 10-7). Although these signs usually are not seen until the last trimester, it is still not too early to give clients these materials.

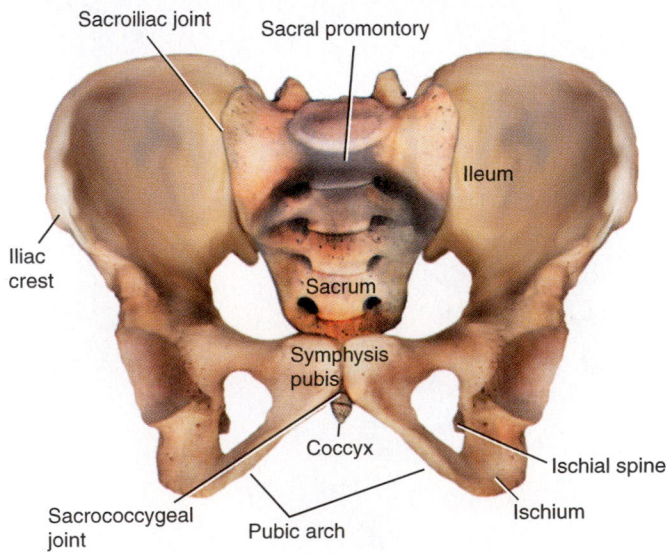

Figure 10-5 Anterior view of the female pelvis.

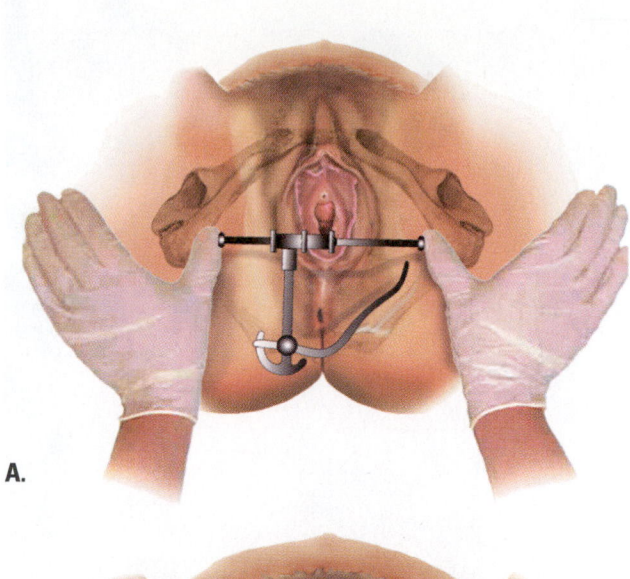

A.

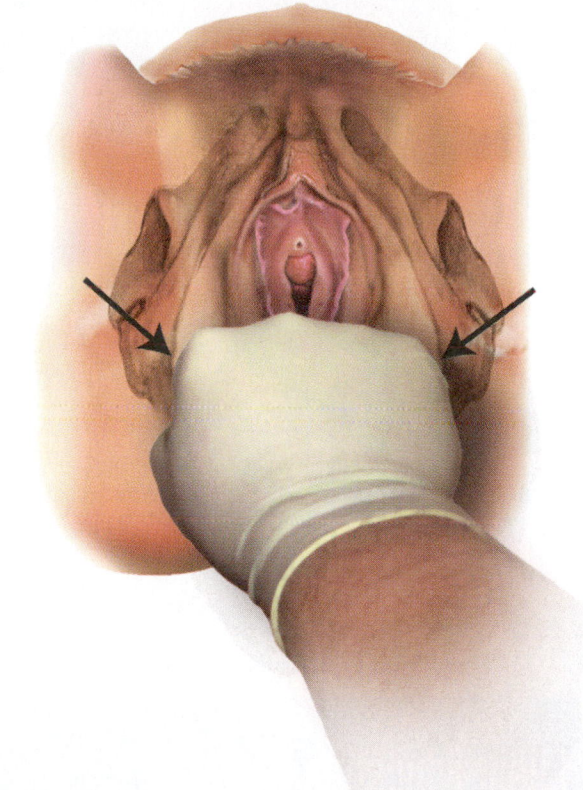

B.

Figure 10-6   Measurement of the biischial diameter with (A) caliper or (B) clenched fist.

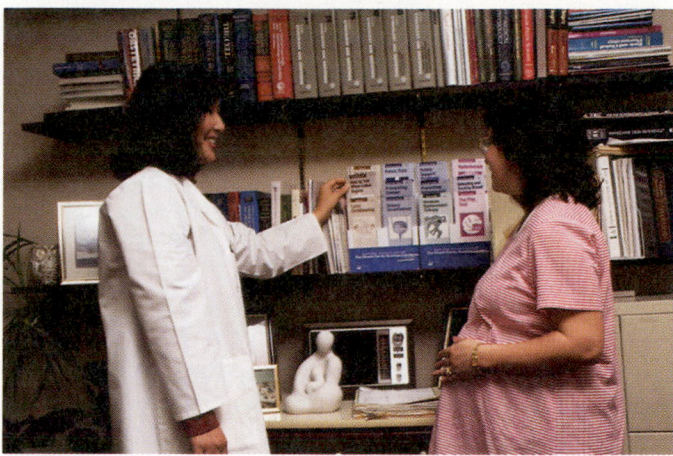

Figure 10-7   Supplying clients with information on a healthy pregnancy and potential risks and danger signs is an important nursing responsibility.

Each Subsequent Visit

To assist in proper monitoring of the pregnancy, the following are evaluated in each visit.

■ Blood pressure. Blood pressure is evaluated for any increase from baseline (Figure 10-8). An increase may be an alert to the onset of **pregnancy-induced hypertension (PIH)**, also referred to as pre-eclampsia or

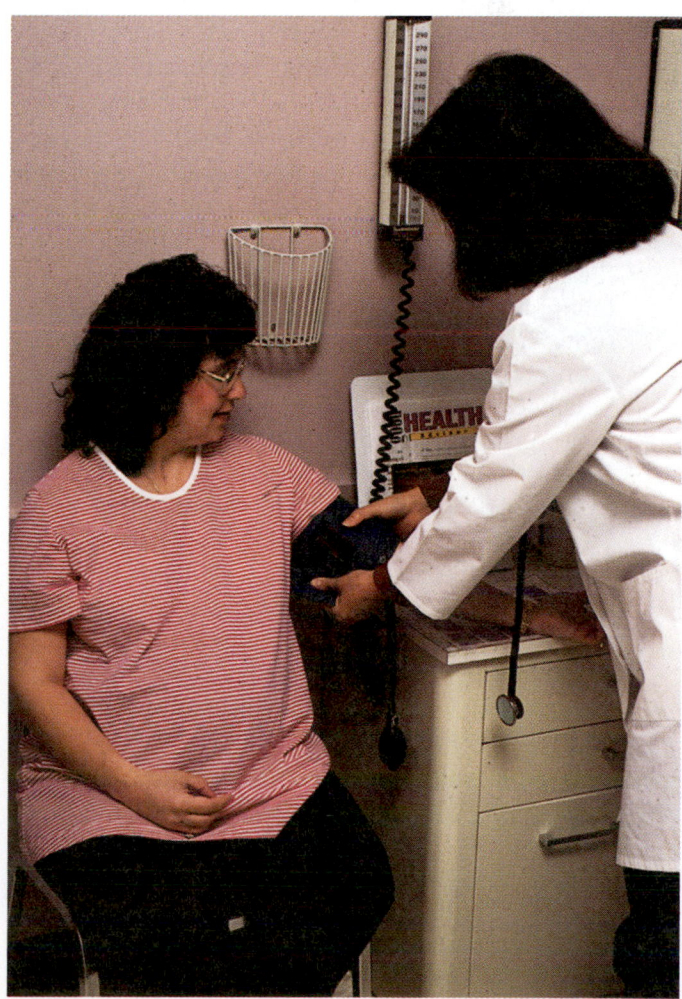

Figure 10-8   Blood pressure is measured at each prenatal visit.

Nursing Alert

Attention to Baseline Blood Pressure

At each prenatal visit the blood pressure finding should be compared with the baseline value. A client may have a blood pressure reading that seems to be within normal limits but is actually a significant increase for her. This is especially true for very young clients whose normal blood pressure values are around 90–92/58–60 mmHg. In these cases, a seemingly normal blood pressure value of 120/82 mmHg may be a caution flag for the need to monitor for further signs of PIH.

toxemia of pregnancy. Typically, PIH is characterized by elevated blood pressure, persistent edema, and proteinuria. Guidelines for signs and symptoms that should be reported to the nurse or physician are included in the danger signs listed below.

- Weight. Weight is assessed for appropriate weight gain (Figure 10-9). Too little or too much gain requires further assessment and counseling. Either may be indicative of a high-risk pregnancy.

- Fundal height. Fundal height should be consistent with dates. The uterus is palpable above the symphysis at about 12 weeks' gestation; is midway between the symphysis pubis and umbilicus at 16 weeks' gestation; and at the umbilicus at 20 weeks' gestation (now measuring 20 cm). Overall fundal height changes generally are reflective of fetal growth. Small uterine size for dates may indicate a fetus that is not growing appropriately; large uterine size for dates may be associated with a multiple pregnancy (more than one fetus), congenital anomaly, or another complication to be assessed. Measurement is by flexible tape measure (McDonald's method; Figure 10-10A,B) held by the examiner at either a curved pattern from the symphysis pubis to the fundus (top of the uterus), or a straight pattern from the symphysis pubis to the point where the examiner's hand is directly above the fundus at a 90-degree angle. Either method is acceptable but should not be interchanged because slightly different readings are obtained. Fundal height in centimeters correlates very closely with the number of weeks of pregnancy after 18 weeks' gestation to 36 weeks. Discrepancies call for further evaluation.

- Fetal heart tones. Fetal heart tones are assessed for rate and rhythm (Figure 10-11). Normal rate is 120 to 160 bpm.

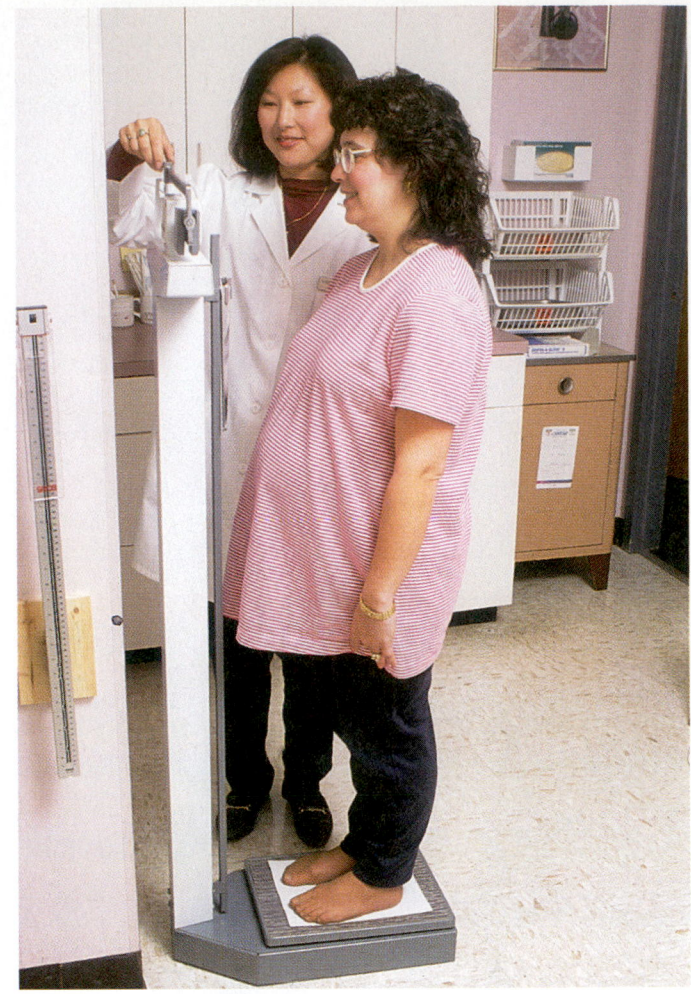

Figure 10-9   Weight gain is tracked throughout the pregnancy.

Client Education

Weight Gain

Clients should be instructed in the importance of and necessity for a recommended weight gain of about 25 to 35 lb in a pattern similar to the following:

- First trimester: approximately 3 to 5 lb
- Second trimester: approximately 12 to 15 lb
- Third trimester: approximately 12 to 15 lb

Remind clients that pregnancy is not a time for weight loss.

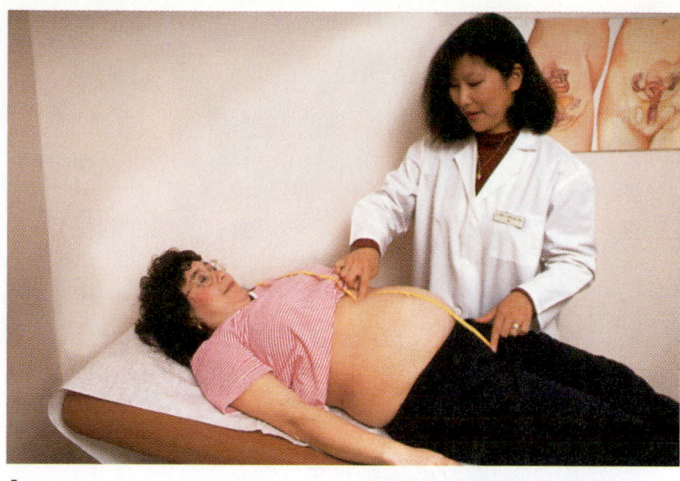

A.

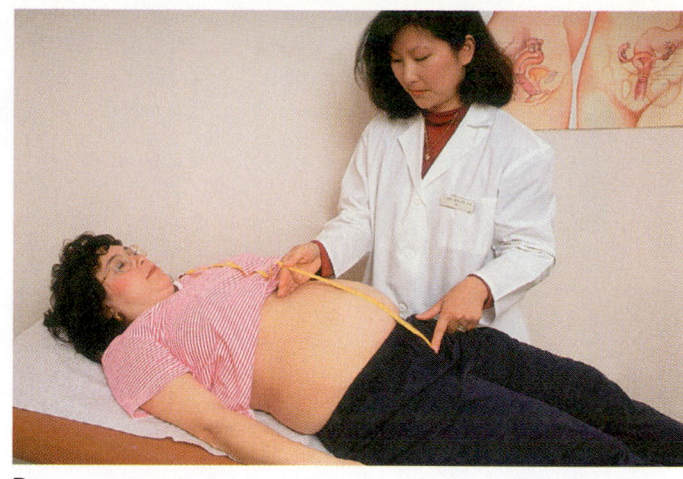

B.

Figure 10-10   Fundal height is measured by placing the end of the tape measure at the symphysis pubis and extending it in either a curved (A) or straight (B) pattern to the fundus.

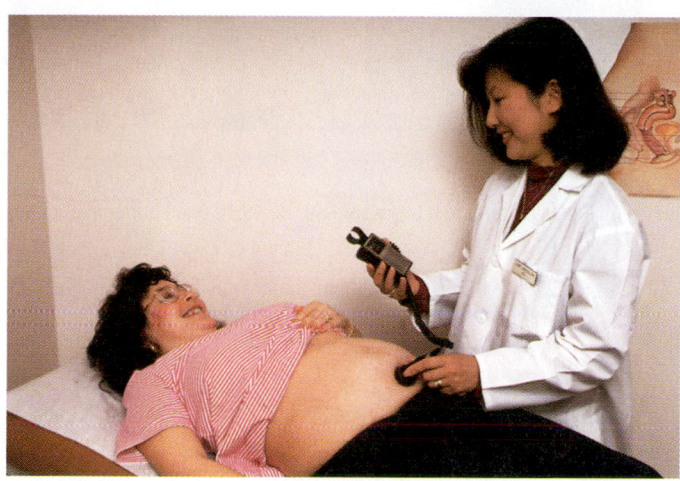

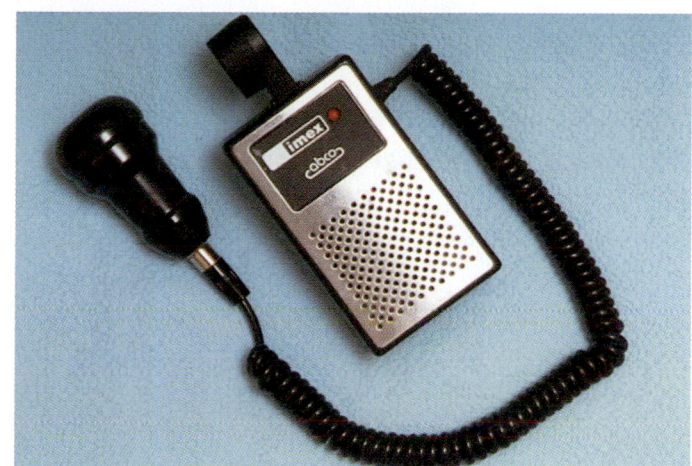

Figure 10-11   Fetal heart tones are measured with a handheld Doppler.

■ Urine. Urine is tested for the presence of glucose or protein (albumin) (Figure 10-12). Clients should be instructed in obtaining a clean-catch urine specimen to avoid a positive protein caused by mucoid vaginal secretions in the specimen. Proteinuria may be indicative of PIH, especially if seen in the presence of elevated blood pressure and edema. Glucose in the urine may reflect the relatively normal change in glomerular filtration that allows the larger glucose molecule to be excreted. Further evaluation is still needed. Serum glucose screening usually is done between 24 and 28 weeks' gestation. If blood glucose is elevated, a glucose tolerance test usually is scheduled.

■ Edema. Edema is evaluated at each visit. Dependent edema of the feet and legs is not unusual toward the

end of pregnancy. A ring sizer can be used to screen for edema in the fingers. Edema of the face is more ominous; when this is noted, the client should be evaluated for other signs and symptoms of PIH. All edema should be assessed for pitting.

■ Other. Each visit should include an opportunity for the client to ask questions and share concerns. Time should be allotted to explore her adaptation to the pregnancy as well as that of her partner. It should not be assumed that the client who has a history of alcohol, tobacco, or other drug use before pregnancy is not using that drug during pregnancy. Screening for abuse should be done during pregnancy because initial abuse may appear during pregnancy. Assessment and referral should be provided as indicated.

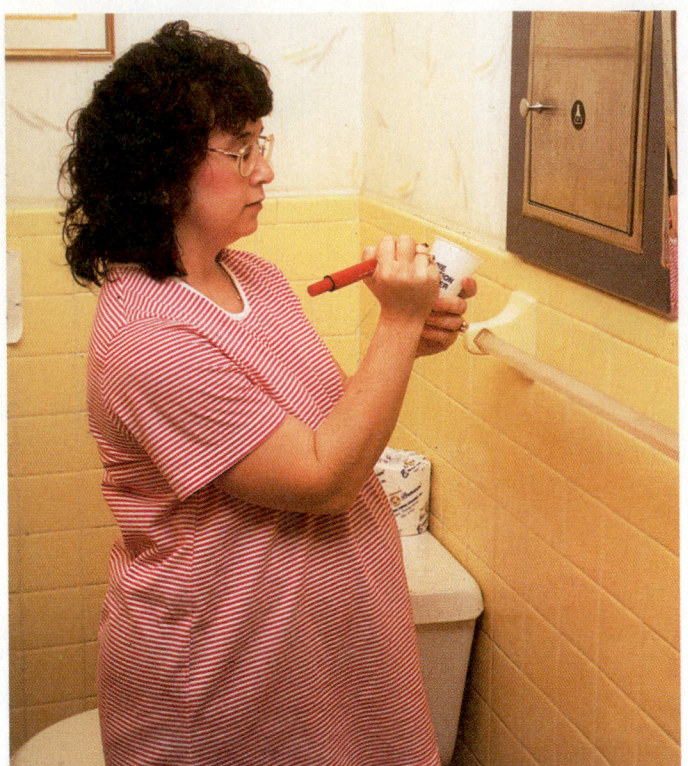
A.

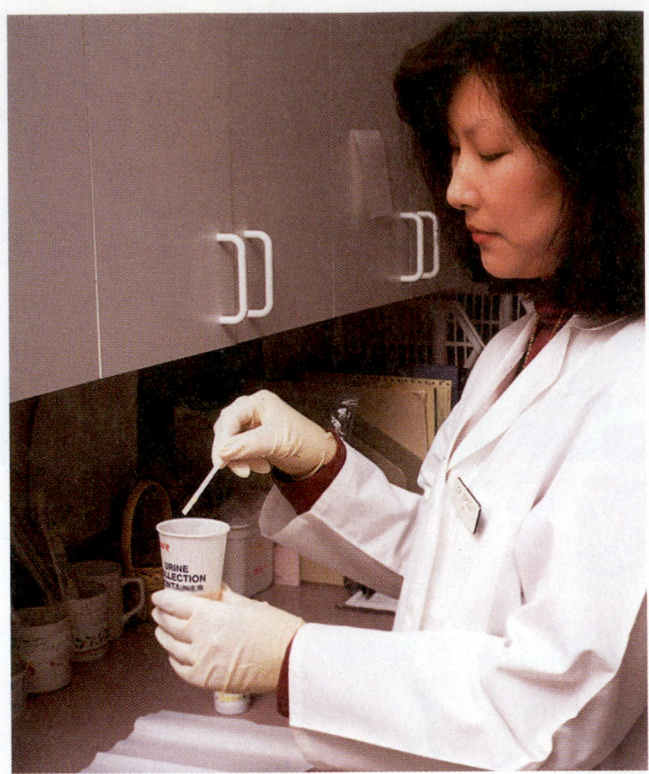
B.

Figure 10-12   Urine is tested at each visit for glucose and protein. A. Client provides a clean-catch urine sample. B. Nurse uses urine dipstick to measure glucose and protein.

PROCEDURE 10-1

Assessing Fetal Heart Tones with a Doppler Device

PURPOSE

To evaluate fetal well-being through auscultation of the fetal heart rate to determine rate and rhythm.

Equipment

Fetoscope or mini-dop
Lubricant.

Actions and Rationales

1. Determine the fetal lie, position, and presentation using Leopold's maneuvers to locate the back of the fetus (see Figure 10-13). *This is the ideal position to best hear the fetal heart rate.*

2. Place the lubricated mini-dop transducer over the area previously identified as the fetus's back. *The lubricant provides a seamless medium through which the sound can travel.*

3. Determine the number of heartbeats per minute. *The fetal heart rate is an important indicator of fetal well-being.*

(continues)

PROCEDURE 10-1 *(continued)*

4. Clean the transducer and the mother's abdomen with clean tissue. *Ensures comfort for the client. Always clean equipment between clients.*

5. Document the heart rate in an appropriate place in the client's record. *All nursing activities should be accurately documented in the client's record.*

Follow-up

Fetal heart tones should be auscultated on each prenatal visit. Any questionable fetal heart reading should be verbally reported to the physician, Certified Nurse Midwife, or nurse practitioner immediately.

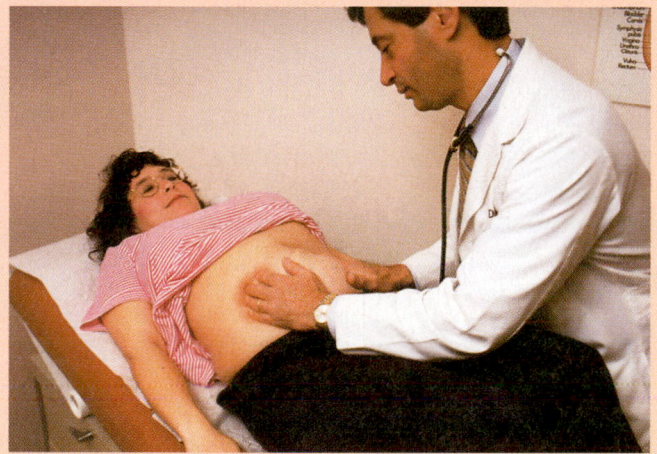

A.

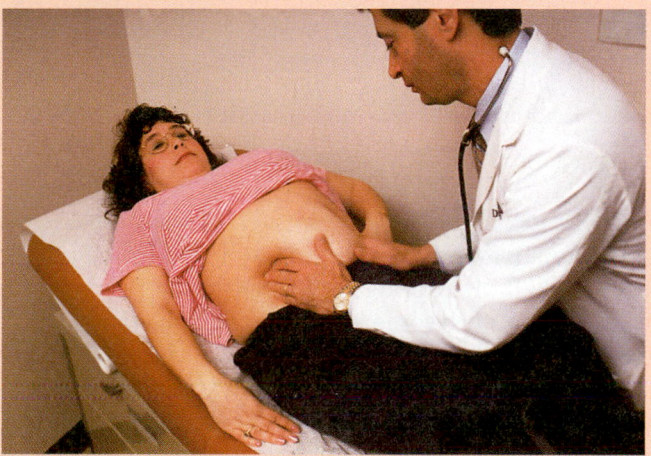

B.

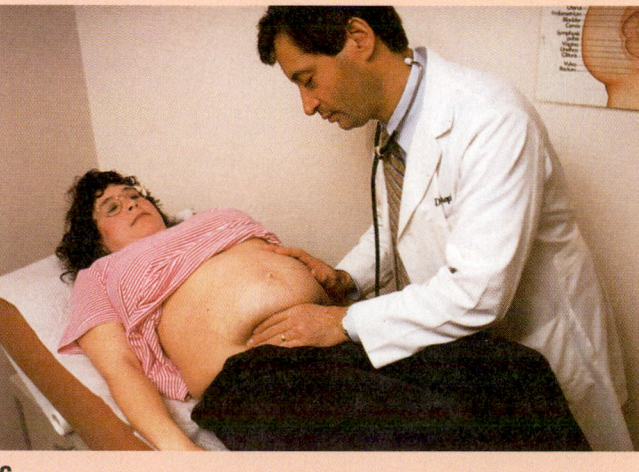

C.

D.

Figure 10-13   Leopold's maneuvers. A. First, the examiner palpates to determine which fetal part is in the fundus. Generally, it is the buttocks. B. Second, the examiner moves hands to the sides of the uterus and determines on which side of the mother the fetal back is located. C. Third, the examiner's hand is placed above the symphysis pubis to note whether the head or breech is near the pubic symphysis (this should correlate with the first maneuver). D. Fourth, the examiner changes position to face the client's feet, and palpates the sides of the abdomen to determine on which side the cephalic prominence presents.

Client Education

Teaching Materials

A large variety of educational materials is available from a number of sources: books, pamphlets, brochures, videos, calendars with pregnancy tips and advice, and Internet sites increasing in number daily. Before recommending any particular materials or sources, be sure you have checked out the accuracy and thoroughness of the contents. Be familiar with the contents of all educational materials available from your work setting. Surf the Internet periodically to become familiar with available sites and their suitability for clients. Aside from recommending and interpreting educational materials, your professional responsibilities also include tactfully pointing out inaccuracies or inadvisable elements of such materials.

Selected Subsequent Visits

As previously noted, the first prenatal visit usually is the most detailed. Monitoring activities continue throughout the pregnancy, with some less frequent than others. In the absence of abnormal findings or the identification of risk factors that necessitate closer scrutiny, other evaluations are done only at selected visits or at particular times during the pregnancy. Some examples of periodic evaluations are as follows:

- Additional pelvic examinations usually are not necessary until the time of weekly visits, which usually occurs in the last 3 to 4 weeks of an uncomplicated pregnancy. The cervix can be evaluated for softening, thinning, and dilation. An assessment can be made of the fetal presenting part and status of descent after lightening (see Chapter 9) Prior to this time, Leopold's maneuvers can be used to evaluate the size and position of the fetus (Figure 10-13).

- Laboratory tests. In the absence of anemia at the initial screening or development of signs and symptoms subsequently, hemoglobin and hematocrit screenings usually are not repeated until 28 to 34 weeks' gestation (third trimester) and again immediately before delivery. Alpha-fetoprotein screening is done at 16 to 18 weeks' gestation, glucose screening for gestational diabetes at 24 to 28 weeks' gestation, and vaginal culture for group B *Streptococcus* (GBS) at 35 to 37 weeks' gestation. Antibody titer for clients who are Rh negative is done at 22 weeks' gestation and as indicated. Triple screening (maternal serum alpha-fetoprotein, hCG, and estriol) sometimes is

done at 16 to 18 weeks' gestation or 16 to 20 weeks' gestation as a combined evaluation of fetal well-being and for predictors of genetic or congenital anomalies. In some areas of the United States, triple screenings are used routinely; in other areas, they are used more on an as indicated basis (Table 10-3).

Table 10-3	Screening Tests in Pregnancy
TEST	**RESULTS**
Complete Blood Count	
RBC	3.75 million/mm^3 due to hemodilution.
WBC	Rises to 18,000/mm^3 by late pregnancy. Mostly an increase in neutrophils.
Hemoglobin (Hgb)	May decrease to 11.5g/dL later in pregnancy due to hemodilution. Repeat at 28 and 36 weeks.
Hematocrit (Hct)	33% lowest acceptable, due to hemodilution.
Blood Type	A, B, AB, or O
Rh factor	Positive or negative. If negative, do indirect Coomb's test. Check father's Rh.
Coomb's Test	Should remain negative. Retest Rh negative woman at 28 weeks.
Rubella Titer (HAI)	> 1:10 indicates immunity, < 1:10, immunize after birth of infant.
Blood Glucose	Should be 60–110 mg/dL. Retest at 24 and 32 weeks.
VDRL or RPR (Syphilis)	Should be negative.

Cervical/Vaginal Culture
  Gonorrhea
  Chlamydia
  Group B *Streptococcus*
	Should be negative.

Hepatitis B Surface Antigen (HB$_s$Ag)	Positive indicates either active hepatitis or carrier state.
Antibody Titer HB$_s$Ag	Positive indicates immunity to hepatitis.
HIV (many states mandate that it be offered)	Should be negative.
Tuberculosis skin tests: Mantoux or Tine	Should be negative. If positive, do chest X-ray.
Urinalysis Color, specific gravity, pH, ketones, albumin, glucose	Same as nonpregnant. Repeat at 28 weeks. Trace of glycosuria may occur in pregnancy.
Alpha-fetoprotein (AFP)	Check with laboratory for normal range for each week of gestation. If elevated, may have neural tube defects. If decreased, may have Down syndrome.

EDUCATION OF THE CHILDBEARING FAMILY

Nurses are in an excellent position to influence pregnancy outcomes and family adaptation through interaction with clients. Women and their families are particularly interested in promoting health when anticipating childbearing. Often the nurse is the primary person the client will contact both at clinic visits and telephone calls. The nurse should take every opportunity to look for teachable moments. Many nurses have outlined specific topics to cover individually with clients throughout the pregnancy. Nurses generally teach prenatal classes and many other health-related topics.

Cultural Considerations in Childbirth Preparation

Childbirth is enmeshed in cultural beliefs and values. These beliefs direct behaviors from conception through childrearing. Cultural beliefs and traditions also dictate a great deal of maternal behavior during pregnancy, especially about activities that might have a negative effect on the baby. Cultural practices also determine the place or setting for birth; who should be present at the birth; and in many cases, much of the process of birth and ceremonies surrounding the birth.

Many traditions also exist related to particular foods that should or should not be eaten during pregnancy or when approaching labor. One example of a culturally adaptive way of delivering health care occurred in Chiapas, Mexico. When the Indian women in the town would not give birth in the newly built hospital, a local medicine woman was hired to set up an altar in a birthing room and deliver babies in the hospital (Shilling, 2000).

Expression of pain during labor reflects culturally appropriate ways of managing pain and the meaning of

Client Education

Health Care Providers

A number of health care providers are available to clients who are pregnant. Nurses may be asked to provide information about the credentials of various providers.

- **Obstetricians:** Licensed medical doctors who have specialty preparation in obstetrics.
- **Family practice physicians:** Medical doctors who are generalists and provide prenatal care and delivery services for uncomplicated pregnancies and referrals to specialists for high-risk pregnancies.
- **Nurse practitioners:** Nurses who specialize in women's health and provide prenatal and postpartal care. They generally work in collaboration with obstetricians who supervise the delivery.
- **Certified Nurse Midwives:** Licensed nurses certified to provide prenatal and postpartal care and perform uncomplicated deliveries. They also generally collaborate with physicians for high-risk care.
- **Lay midwives:** Unlicensed women who see clients and deliver infants in the home or community setting. In some states they are required to register with the health department.

pain related to childbirth. Culture affects women's behavior during the postpartum period, for instance, the amount of activity she should engage in, her personal hygiene, and her relationship to other family members. Some families may not want the mother or infant to wear white because it is the color of mourning. In some cultures, a woman who does not appear to pay much attention to her infant is protecting it from bad luck; whereas in others, it may be important for the mother to take the infant to bed with her (Shilling, 2000).

Nurses should continually develop their cultural awareness and understand that much variation exists within cultural groups and between ethnic groups. Open-minded approaches to diverse ways of thinking and acting to accommodate their clients are the first steps in developing cultural competence. Astute nurses will incorporate cultural awareness into their assessments of individual families and endeavor to adapt their nursing care according to the family's cultural beliefs and practices.

Critical Thinking

Considerations in Childbirth

Examine your own cultural beliefs about birth. Imagine that you or your partner are pregnant and in an unfamiliar culture.

- Which things would you feel are necessary for a safe pregnancy?
- Who would you want to be present at the birth?
- Where and with whom would you want to give birth?

Perinatal Education and Preparation for Childbirth

Childbirth education, more recently referred to as perinatal education, began as a consumer movement to humanize the birth experience and promote an active role by women in the birth process. The increasing involvement of the expectant woman's partner has changed the hospital environment and now is an integral part of health care for childbearing women.

The Association of Women's Health, Obstetrics, and Neonatal Nurses (AWHONN), developed guidelines for childbirth education (AWHONN, 1993). These guidelines provide recommendations for improving the quality of perinatal education to promote healthy birth outcomes and emotionally satisfying birth experiences (AWHONN, 1993).

Many couples are motivated to learn and attend classes because they want strategies to cope with impending labor and ensure a healthy baby. Expectant parents often have a heightened interest in health-promoting behaviors during pregnancy. Application of the nursing process assists the nurse to identify and meet the needs of expectant families. Evaluation of family outcomes leads to continued improvement in the approaches nurses use to prepare families for childbirth.

Childbirth Preparation

Early childbirth education classes were focused entirely on developing and practicing techniques for use in managing pain and facilitating the progress of labor. More recent developments in perinatal education have broadened the focus to incorporate family adaptation to the pregnancy and parental roles for the newborn. Family adaptation also includes the adaptation of siblings and the entire family unit. Additional content has been added to childbirth education curricula that includes breastfeeding, infant care, transition to parenthood, relationship skills, family health promotion, marital intimacy, and sexuality; some curricula have added the role of perinatal bereavement counselor (Humenick, 1999; 2000).

Across cultures, women have been assisting other women in preparing for childbirth and the maternal role and have been informally handing down these traditions. By the mid-1900s, most births occurred in hospitals, and midwives were used only in remote areas. In the 1960s the prepared childbirth movement began. The emphasis on preparation and a more natural approach to birth has decreased many of the risks from unnecessary medical interventions and allowed a birth experience that better addresses the psychological, cultural, social, and spiritual aspects of the experience.

Methods of Childbirth Preparation

Early childbirth classes were held by the Red Cross and the Maternity Center Association in the early 1900s to teach women about birth and infant care. The notion that pain could be controlled by psychological preparation became the foundation for childbirth education and preparation. The most common contemporary methods are Lamaze and Dick-Read.

Lamaze Method of Psychoprophylaxis.
Fernand Lamaze, a French physician, developed a version of psychoprophylaxis, using body conditioning exercises, education, and relaxation techniques (Lamaze, 1972). This method became very popular throughout Western Europe. Through training and repetition the client learns to respond to pain with breathing and relaxation. The Lamaze approach to childbirth is taught through Lamaze International, Inc. This organization has certified programs and childbirth educators in the Lamaze method since 1965.

Most childbirth preparation classes offered in North America today provide content and instruction based on the Lamaze method. The fundamental techniques for instruction are conditioning, discipline, and concentration (Figure 10-14). Conditioning teaches the mother to adapt her responses to the physical and emotional demands of labor by becoming skillful in tuning into her body. Discipline enables the person to stick to the program or regimen. Concentration breaks the flight or fight response by substituting muscle release and deep oxygenation for tension and breath holding.

Practice during pregnancy allows the woman to build up a discipline of concentration. The couple practices using verbal and other cues to recondition the tension response to pain. For example, the partner might touch her

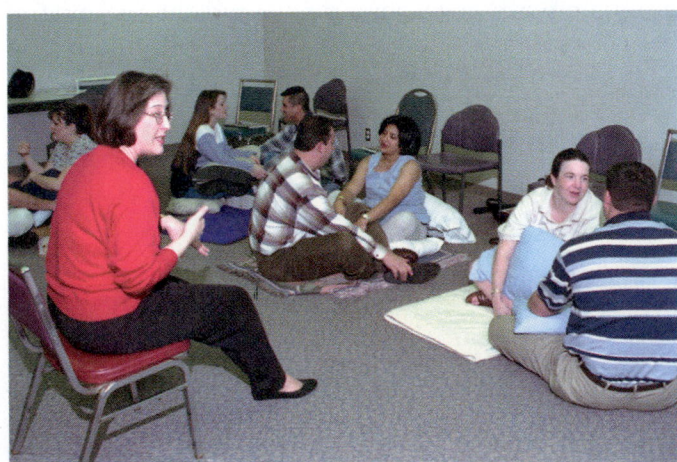

Figure 10-14 Couples practice conditioning and concentration techniques during childbirth preparation classes.

on her neck and, through practice, she would develop a conditioned response of relaxation to that stimulus. Thereby the usual response to pain, which is tension, would be replaced by relaxation. Basic breathing patterns were taught to class attendees and practiced frequently in preparation for labor. The more time devoted to practice of the patterns, the more automatic they will become and the more likely they will be used during childbirth. As research advanced regarding the physiology of breathing and the understanding of relaxation during labor, paced breathing became more individualized and the centrality of relaxation became more important than were the specific breathing techniques.

Dick-Read Method.
British obstetrician Dr. Grantly Dick-Read (1979) promoted the belief that the degree of fear could be diminished with increased understanding of the normal physiologic response to labor. Select physical conditioning exercises were included in the program to strengthen the muscles. Relaxation techniques were taught that interrupt the circular pattern of fear, tension, and pain (Figure 10-15). Breathing and relaxation techniques during labor are the key features of the Dick-Read approach to childbirth.

Strategies for Labor Management

Prenatal or childbirth education may be with individuals, families, or groups. Nurses can design educational content using trimesters as guidelines, allowing for standardized content. Many agencies have designed specific classes for various topics and stages of pregnancy. Adaptations always must be made to accommodate individual family needs.

Relaxation Techniques.
Relaxation is central to many of the techniques for coping with labor. Relaxation is a systemic response that reduces fear and tension during labor. Reduction in fear and tension facilitates the body's efficient use of energy for labor, thereby reducing fatigue and thus making labor more effective. Tense abdominal muscles form resistance to uterine contractions and use oxygen, resulting in less oxygen available to the fetus. Tension increases lactic acid buildup, which increases pain. Relaxation during pregnancy results in increased oxygen to tissues and organs and fewer stress hormones reaching the fetus (Figure 10-16). Relaxation skills also are helpful after delivery in coping with the demands of a new baby and in helping establish breastfeeding. Developing relaxation skills promotes the health of the entire family (Humenick, Shrock, & Libresco, 2000).

Melzak and Wall (1965) proposed the gate-control theory of pain in 1965. This theory states that pain stimuli can be modified as they travel on small-diameter nerve fibers along the ascending pathway through the spinal

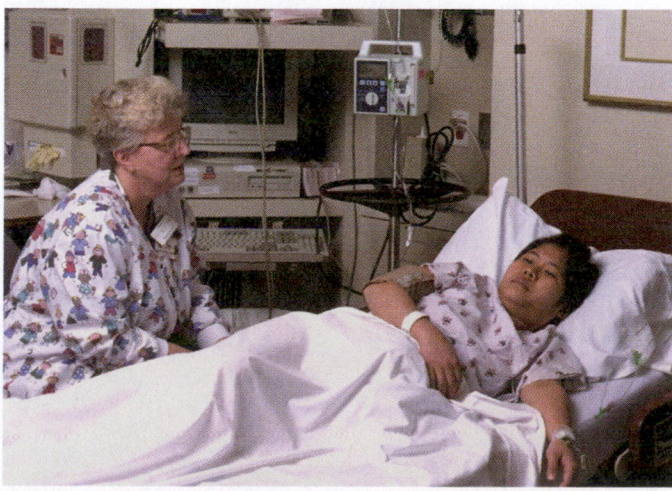

Figure 10-15   The nurse knows that her encouraging words and soothing voice will help this first-time mother to relax as her labor progresses.

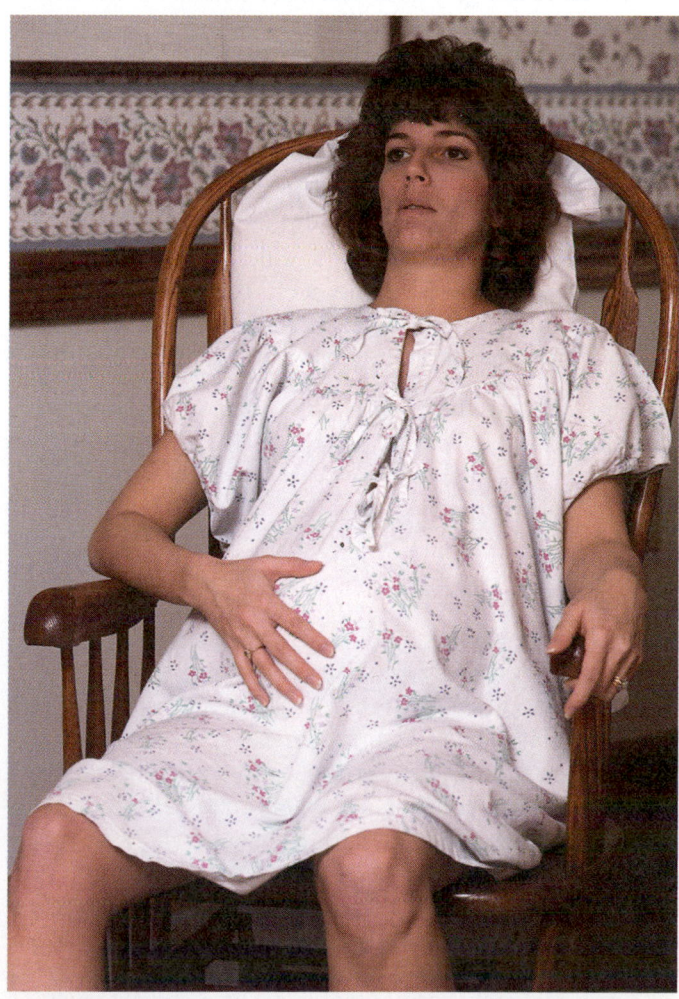

Figure 10-16   Using paced breathing, the laboring woman controls and regulates her breathing patterns.

Nursing Tip *Relaxation*

"Relaxation is the foundation of all childbirth preparation techniques" (Nichols, 2000).

Nursing Alert

Slow-Paced Breathing

The rate of slow-paced breathing should be no less than half of the woman's normal respiratory rate. Less than this rate may not provide adequate ventilation.

cord. A gating mechanism can be activated by sensations traveling through large-diameter fibers, which transmit messages more quickly than do the small-diameter fibers. This gating mechanism is activated by massage and by heat and cold. Habituation may occur in 15 to 20 minutes and may be mistaken for an increase in actual pain rather than in perception. Changing the site or type of stimulus can reactivate the "gate" (Jimenez, 2000).

Several techniques are employed to promote relaxation; these are discussed below.

Paced Breathing. **Paced breathing** decreases stress and pain and increases relaxation. The term *paced breathing* now is used to describe the research-based breathing techniques used to decrease stress responses and thus decrease pain. This type of breathing also implies self-regulation. In 1983, Lamaze International adopted the standards for prepared childbirth. Paced breathing techniques use a slow rate and individualized and flexible approaches to promote relaxation of the laboring woman.

A **cleansing breath** is a deep relaxed breath, such as a sigh, designed to signal relaxation and provide deep ventilation. This breath often is used to signal the beginning

of a contraction and separates the stimulus of the contraction that usually has a response of alarm and tension. Cleansing breaths often have been used along with a focal point to help the woman in labor concentrate and focus on relaxation.

Slow-Paced Breathing. Slow deep breathing is associated with relaxation. Research has shown that slow-paced breathing is associated with increased relaxation and decreased anxiety, pain, psychological response to threats, and stress (Nichols, 2000). The rate of breathing should be comfortable for the woman and provide adequate ventilation for the mother, fetus, and work of labor. A rate of half the woman's normal rate is appropriate during the early part of labor. Often, couples will learn the woman's normal rate and practice slowing breathing in preparation for labor (Figure 10-17). Abdominal or chest breath-

Nursing Alert

Effleurage

Light touch, such as effleurage, travels along the same small-fiber pathways as do pain stimuli and, therefore, can increase pain perception. Many women prefer a harder massage as labor progresses.

Relaxation and stress reduction are beneficial for many physical conditions and pain control. Positive effects also may be related to the special attention and support the laboring woman receives from the nurse, her labor partner, or a doula. This positive effect can reduce fear and pain. Other mechanisms may be related to the benefits of spiritual connection with the supportive presence of others who have intent to help.

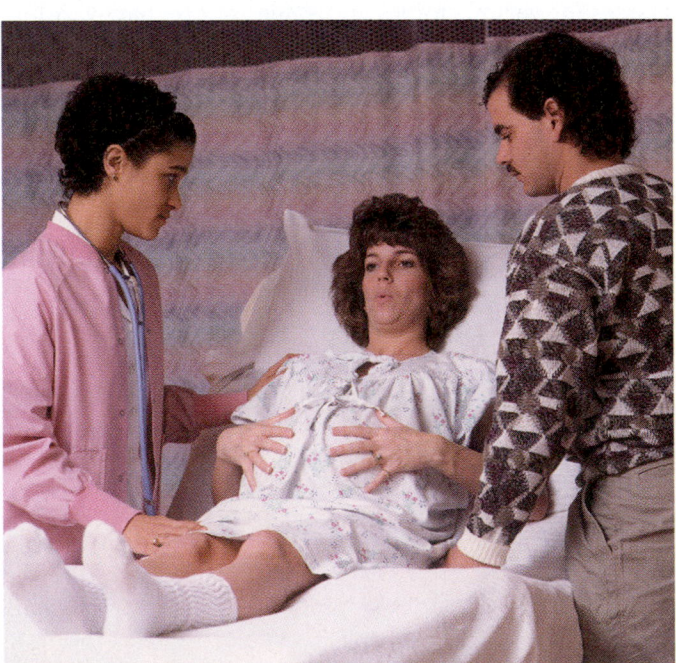

Figure 10-17 Slow-paced breathing provides comfort to the mother and adequate ventilation to both mother and fetus during labor.

Nursing Tip   *Effective Breathing*

Always work with the woman to help her breathe at her comfort level. Avoid complicated breathing techniques that interfere with relaxation. Remember that relaxation is the key.

ing may be used. If mouth breathing is used, moisture in the woman's mucous membranes will need to be replenished during labor. The woman should be encouraged to use the slow-paced breathing pattern for as long as possible.

Modified-Paced Breathing.   During increased work or stress, the respiratory rate increases. **Modified-paced breathing** paces this increase at a controlled rate. These techniques are learned and are best practiced during pregnancy for optimal use during labor.

Patterned-Paced Breathing.   **Patterned-paced breathing** is similar to modified-paced breathing but with the addition of a rhythmic pattern. One of the rhythms that frequently is taught in childbirth classes is 4—1, which means four light breaths plus one similar inspiration followed by an exhalation, such as that used when blowing out a candle. Different patterns may be used, such as 4—1, 6—1, 4—1. Many couples use pyramids or other patterns. The patterns sometimes help the woman to focus. Any pattern is encouraged as long as the basic principles of rate and relaxation are met.

Progressive Muscle Relaxation or Neuromuscular Relaxation.   The technique of progressive muscle relaxation or neuromuscular relaxation uses the client's ability to recognize muscle tension and relaxation in her own body. The client thus learns to release muscle tension and relax through systematic contraction and relaxation of specific muscle groups. This technique generally is done with a partner who observes the tension in the

Nursing Tip   *Maintaining Mouth Moisture*

Offer a laboring woman sips of water, clear liquids, or crushed ice to help keep her mouth moist, per physician or institution policy.

muscle groups and cues the woman into achieving overall relaxation.

Neuromuscular Dissociation.   Neuromuscular dissociation focuses on differentiating tension from relaxation. The woman practices by tensing some muscles while simultaneously relaxing other muscle groups. Eventually, couples may practice substituting a relaxation response rather than tension to painful stimuli.

Touch.   Various techniques of touch are used with women in labor that range from gentle comforting touch to massage and acupressure (Figure 10-18).

Imagery.   Imagery has been used in childbirth, starting with the focal point for concentration and using pleasant images for relaxation training. Use of these images transforms pain into a less stressful sensation. Imagery in childbirth is used alone or in combination with other relaxation techniques. For example, Lamaze (1972) suggested that the laboring woman visualize contractions like waves in the rising tide and waning of contractions as the ebbing tide. Some childbirth educators encourage women to visualize their cervix dilating during labor. Most people self-select and use the type of relaxation technique most comfortable for them.

Support during Labor

Around the world, women support other women in childbirth. Since the 1970s in the United States, husbands or partners have moved into this role as a result of the childbirth movement. Currently, fathers are encouraged to accompany their partners through labor if the couple wishes.

In addition to midwives and nurse midwives, a new group of health providers has emerge as labor companions. They have many names. Some are called birth assistants or labor assistants, who often are laypersons with some midwifery skills. Doulas are labor companions trained and experienced in childbirth. They provide continuous emotional support, physical comfort, and informational support. A montrice is a nurse who can provide nursing care and assessment in addition to labor support.

The support person works with the laboring woman to make sure she understands the physical changes of labor, encourages distracting activities and relaxation activities, and assists in finding comfortable positions throughout labor. (Some of these positions are illustrated in Figure 10-19.) Often, the nurse, nurse midwife, doula, or montrice works with the family before delivery and thus applies the types of relaxation techniques the couple has been practicing.

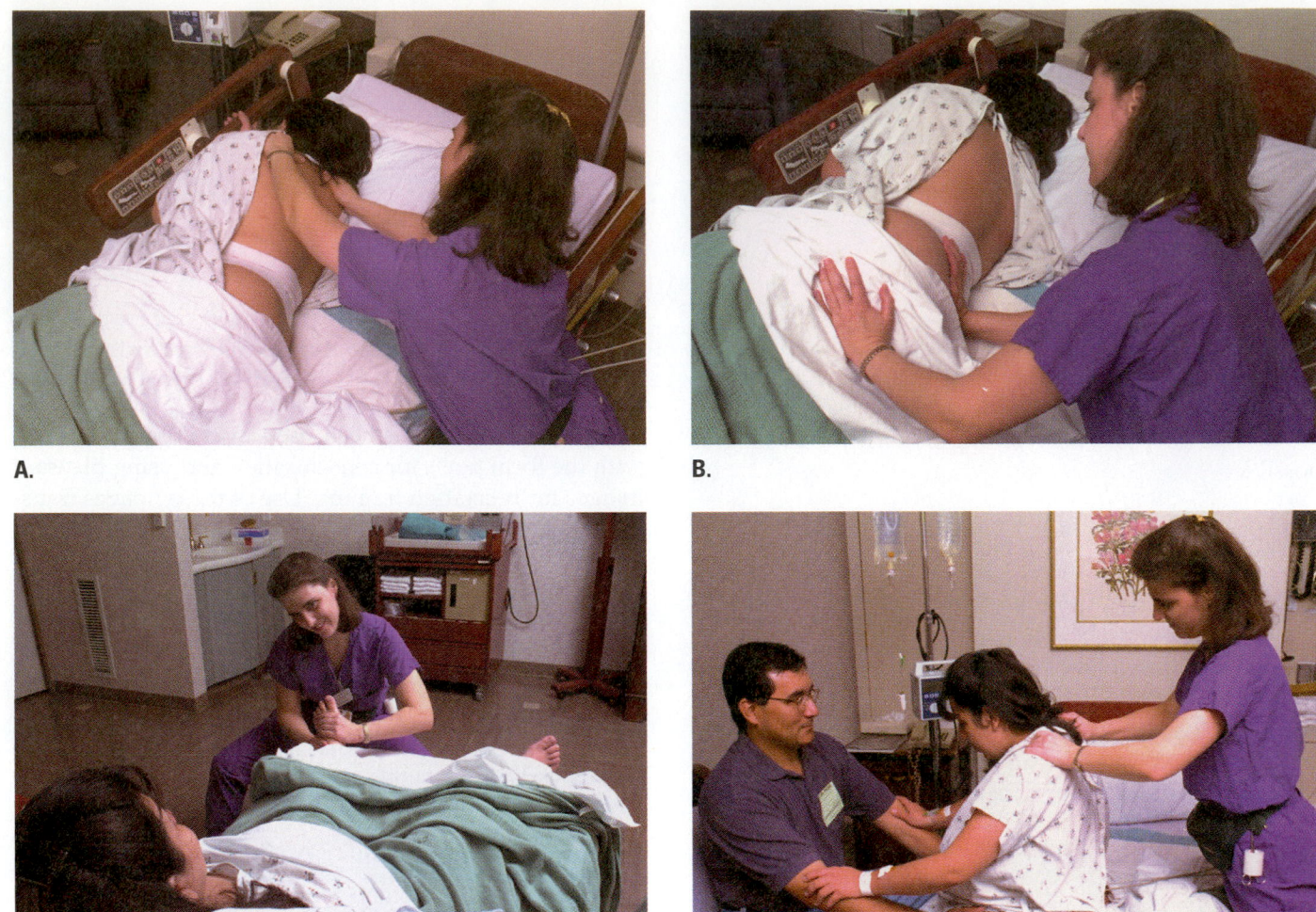

Figure 10-18 Touch therapy for the woman in labor may include the following. A Shoulder massage. B. Low back pressure to relieve the pain of back labor. C. Foot massage. D. Partner-supported touch.

Parenting, Role Transition, and Family Adaptation

The perinatal educator approaches childbearing in a broader sense than the focus on the birth, incorporating education about family adjustment to the pregnancy and the new infant. Infant feeding and infant care are major components of client education.

Additional Classes Offered to Childbearing Families

Special classes may need to be adapted for families. The following may need to be taken into consideration: cesarean birth, vaginal birth, vaginal birth after cesarean section, parents, grandparents, siblings, single parents, specific cultural groups, high-risk pregnancies, pregnant adolescents, parents with handicaps, parents with med-

ical problems, communication barriers, and preconceptual classes (AWHONN, 1993). Specific content for prenatal education is outlined in, Box 10-2.

Preparation for the Perinatal Educator Role

Nurses and laypersons may be certified as perinatal educators. The position statement of the International Childbirth Education Association (ICEA) states that no single training or academic background is necessary to become a child-birth educator (ICEA, 1999). AWHONN (1993) guidelines for nurses specify that perinatal educators are expected to have completed appropriate previous education and training and have experience in both general nursing practice and teaching techniques. For nurses, some experience working in obstetrics or women's health

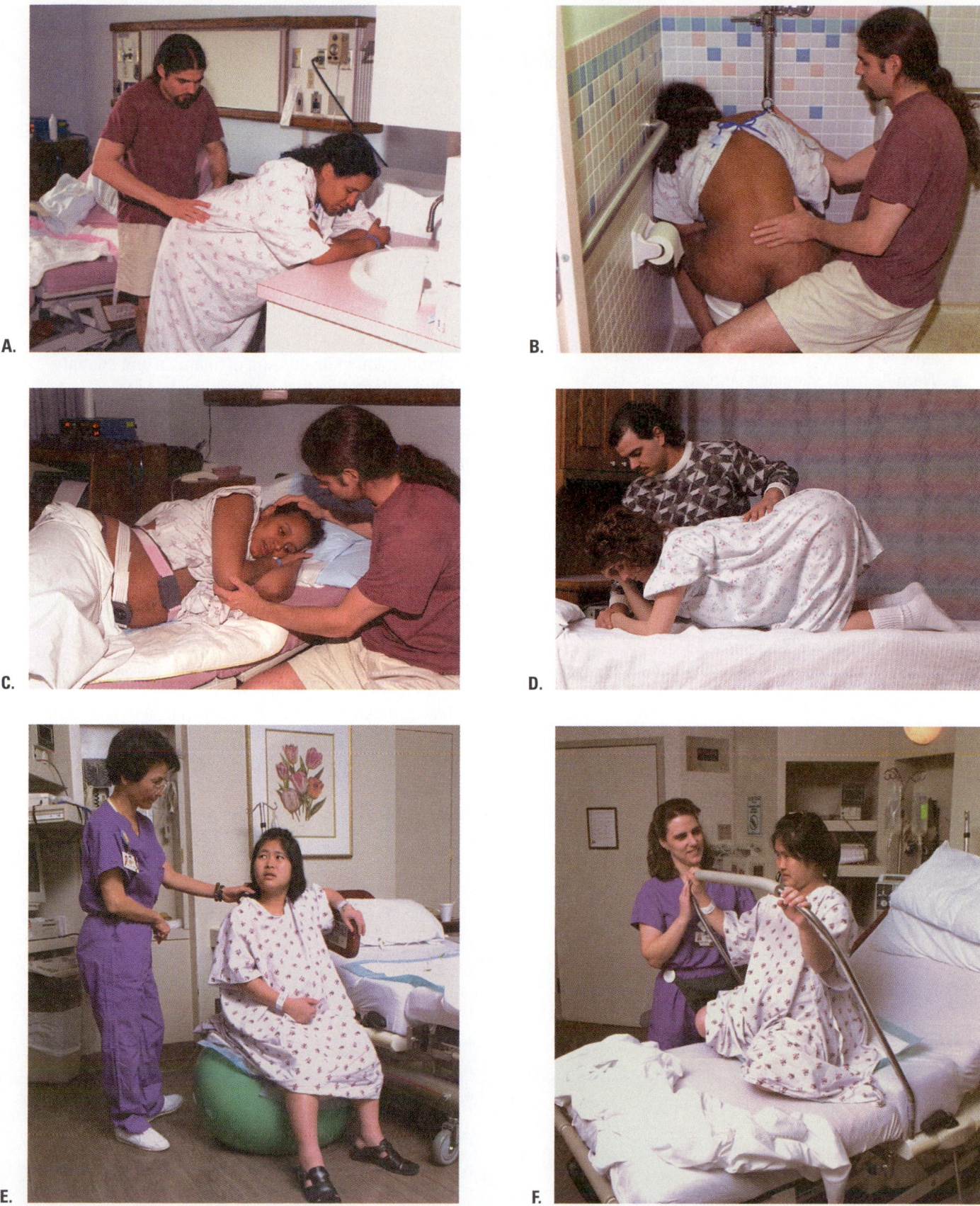

Figure 10-19   Various positions can ease the discomforts of and assist in the progress of labor. A. Standing. B. Sitting on toilet. C. Side-lying position. D. Hands and knees position. E. Sitting on birthing ball. F. Squatting with birthing bar.

Box 10-2

Specific Educational Content for Each Trimester

First Trimester

Knowledge of the Pregnancy

- Anatomy and physiology of pregnancy
- Physical and emotional changes related to pregnancy
- Fetal development
- Importance of prenatal care
- Diagnostic tests, such as chorionic villus sampling, amniocentesis, and ultrasonography
- Warning signs of complications
- Dangers of substance abuse and exposure to toxins and teratogenic hazards

Management of Pregnancy

- Morning sickness
- Sleep disturbances
- Libido changes
- Urinary frequency
- Fatigue
- Emotional lability

Relaxation Techniques

- Awareness of the stress response: breathing patterns, muscle tension, and other physical symptoms of stress in contrast with relaxation
- Awareness of stimuli for tension and relaxation
- Introduction to relaxation techniques
- Slow-paced breathing
- Body awareness

Exercise and Nutrition

- Nutritional needs
- Vitamin supplements
- Exercise
- Body mechanics
- Stretching
- Kegel exercises
- Pelvic tilt exercises
- Toning and aerobic exercises

Family Adaptation

- Choices of provider and birth setting
- Response to emotional and physical changes of pregnancy
- Sexuality
- Infant feeding method
- Exploring maternal and paternal roles
- Communication skills to discuss adaptive changes in the family
- Introduction of discussion of financial and spatial family adaptation to the expanding family

Second Trimester

Builds on previous teaching or incorporates previous trimester teaching if necessary

Knowledge of Pregnancy

- Physiologic changes of pregnancy
- Fetal development and characteristics
- Fetal movement
- Review of warning signs and complications

Management of Pregnancy

- Management of heartburn, back pain, and discomforts
- Changes in body and body image
- Comfort and hygiene measures

Relaxation Techniques

- Explore and identify techniques, such as imagery, massage, music, touch, visualization, and so on
- Work together as a couple (client and support person) to elicit relaxation to stimuli
- Practice slow-paced breathing, modified-paced breathing, and patterned-paced breathing

Exercise and Nutrition

- Continue good nutrition and monitor weight gain
- Increase repetitions of exercise
- Modify activity related to physical changes

Family Adaptation

- Identity of the fetus as a separate individual and building maternal-fetal attachment

(continues)

Box 10-2

Specific Educational Content for Each Trimester *(continued)*

Family Adaptation (cont.)

- Financial considerations; may include a discussion of working or career in relation to the pregnancy
- Paternal concerns: role in labor, role as father, financial concerns, and provision of safety for the mother and fetus
- Sibling preparation
- Preparation of the home for the infant
- Discussion of feeding choices for the infant
- Selection of a pediatric provider

Third Trimester

Often the time for formal classes and need to include all of the above if not already covered

Knowledge of Pregnancy

- Anatomy and physiology of late pregnancy
- Mechanisms and signs of labor
- Additional testing or medical information related to specific conditions
- Medications and anesthesia
- Policies and practices of the facility chosen for delivery
- Postdelivery physical and emotional changes
- Signs and symptoms of labor
- Warning signs of complications
- Progress of labor

Management of Pregnancy

- Preparation for labor
- Comfort measures
- Sleep patterns

Relaxation Techniques

- Practice relaxation techniques
- Practice all methods of breathing for labor
- Practice additional relaxation techniques

Exercise and Nutrition

- Continue good eating patterns
- Monitor appropriate weight gain
- Watch body mechanics, safety, and comfort
- Prepare for delivery: tailor sitting, pelvic tilt, and Kegel exercises
- Perform walking and other conditioning exercises
- Introduce postpartum exercise

Family Adaptation

- Rehearse preparation for delivery and role of support person
- Evaluate family and extended family's preparation for birth
- Discuss normal appearance, care, and feeding of the infant
- Discuss breast-feeding techniques and preparation
- Discuss parental roles
- Discuss sexual adjustment

---

serves as a good background for the educator role. The guidelines describe teaching and content competencies.

Formal preparation for the perinatal educator role is available from several professional organizations, including the International Childbirth Education Association (ICEA), the Bradley method, ASPO/Lamaze, Prepared Childbirth Educators, Inc., and other organizations. Perinatal educators must be able to clearly communicate the following: scientific bases of pregnancy and the birth process, psychosocial and cultural aspects of childbearing, and the most current information for promoting health throughout the pregnancy and preparation for birth. According to AWHONN (1993) guidelines, the educator should work as a team member and demonstrate a philosophy of perinatal education that honors pregnancy as a state of wellness and respects the beliefs and attitudes of families. Specific content includes health education regarding pregnancy and childbirth, specific coping and relaxation strategies for childbirth, preparation of support persons, and provision of anticipatory guidance for the family in the postpartum period.

The AWHONN provides guidelines for nurses engaged in perinatal education. This organization also provides guidelines and information across the spectrum of perinatal nursing. *The Journal of Obstetric, Gynecologic, and Neonatal Nursing* (JOGNN) is the official journal of AWHONN. The AWHONN Web site also contains many publications related to guidelines for nurses in perinatal education.

Client Education

Good Posture during Pregnancy

- Standing: head should be held erect with chin tucked, shoulders relaxed, and knees slightly bent (Figure 10-20A).

- Sitting: knees should be level with or higher than hips; a pillow may be placed behind the lower back for comfort (Figure 10-20B).

- Lying on your side: a pillow should be placed under the upper leg, keeping the leg slightly flexed. A pillow also may be placed under the abdomen for support (Figure 10-20C).

- Lying on your back: A pillow should be placed under the knees to elevate the legs (Figure 10-20D); a pillow under the right hip displaces the uterus and prevents vena cava syndrome. This position should not be used after the fourth month of pregnancy.

Exercises for Pregnancy

Specific exercises can be taught to clients to help strengthen muscle tone in preparation for birth.

- The pelvic tilt reduces back strain and strengthens the abdominal muscles. Figure 10-20E illustrates how to perform the pelvic tilt in both a standing and kneeling position. Exhale, roll the hips and buttocks forward, hold for a count of five, then inhale and relax.

- Abdominal muscle tightening with every breath increases abdominal muscle tone. This exercise can be done anywhere in any position. While slowly taking in a deep breath, expand the abdomen. Then exhale slowly while pulling the abdomen in until the muscles are completely contracted. Relax a few seconds and repeat the exercise.

- Kegel exercises strengthen and tighten the perineal muscles. Tighten these muscles and pull them up toward the vagina as if trying to stop urination midstream. This exercise also can be done anytime, anyplace (see Chapter 9).

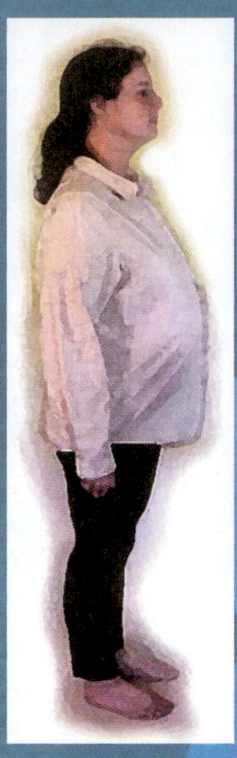
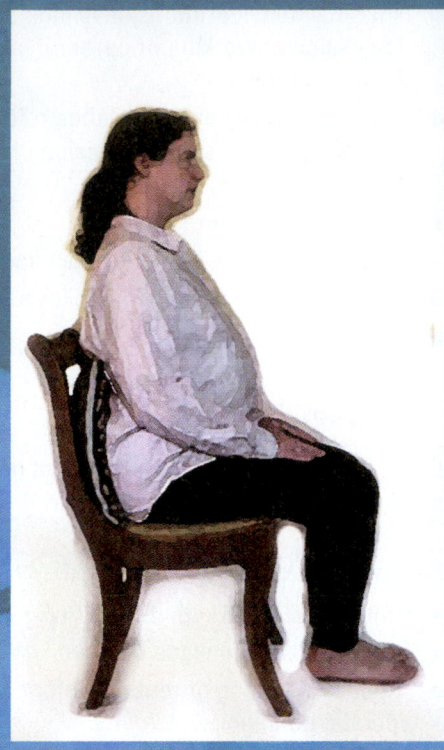

Figure 10-20A   **Figure 10-20B**

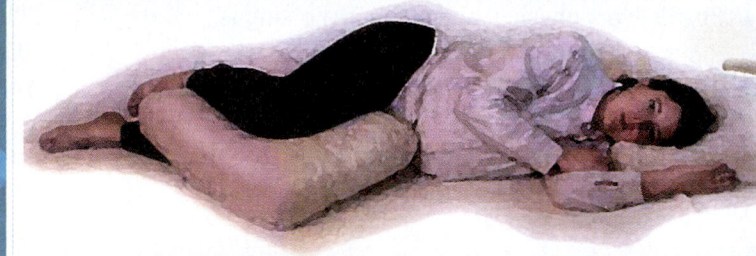

Figure 10-20C

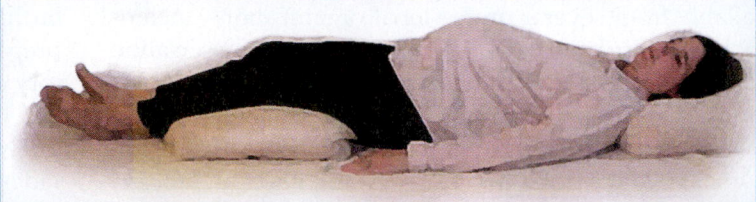

Figure 10-20D

(continues)

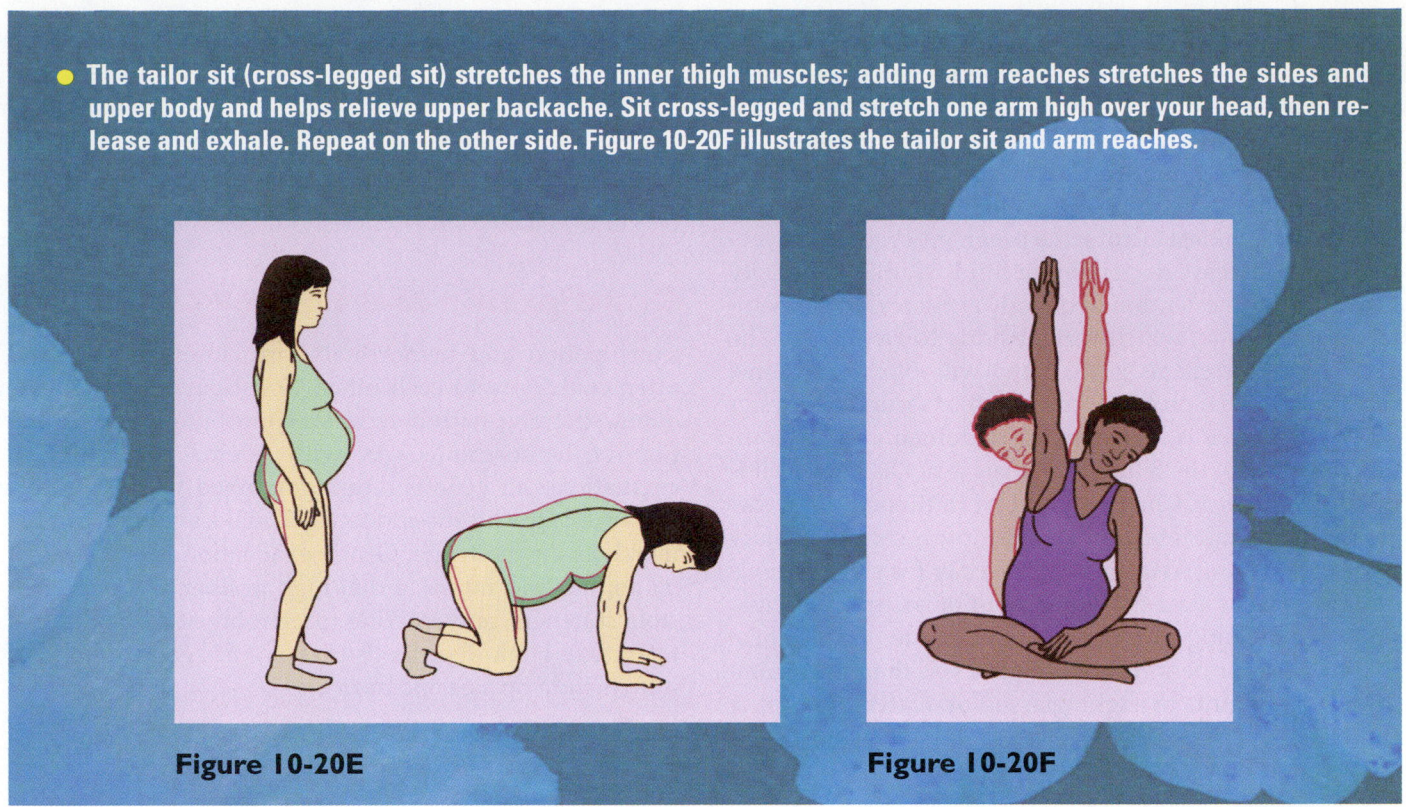

● The tailor sit (cross-legged sit) stretches the inner thigh muscles; adding arm reaches stretches the sides and upper body and helps relieve upper backache. Sit cross-legged and stretch one arm high over your head, then release and exhale. Repeat on the other side. Figure 10-20F illustrates the tailor sit and arm reaches.

Figure 10-20E   Figure 10-20F

MANAGING THE DISCOMFORTS OF PREGNANCY

The normal progression of a pregnancy to produce a healthy infant requires, by necessity, a variety of physiologic changes within the mother. Several of these changes have a cascading effect and subsequently produce conditions of discomfort. Whereas some clients view these as annoyances to be dealt with, others perceive them to be interferences that are sometimes intolerable. In most cases, a detailed explanation of what is happening and suggestions for alleviation are sufficient, especially when clients have a social support system in place. For the other category of clients, further exploration of their feeling about and attitude toward the pregnancy is warranted.

Recommendations to clients should be made with sensitivity to the client's cultural background. The nurse should listen when clients want to discuss home remedies or alternative interventions for various problems. A sensible approach calls for ruling out known harmful practices (with careful explanations) and exploring all options that are within the realm of the client's social, cultural, or spiritual preferences and background. When clients are taught to blend cultural mores and self-care practices with specific basics of routine prenatal considerations (e.g., avoidance of alcohol, caffeine, and certain medications), they will be empowered to make wise choices for themselves and the unborn infant. Furthermore, clients can share their new knowledge with others in their community. In doing so they foster the idea that clients can be proactive in their care, using health care professionals for joint decision-making and establishing mutual goals.

Some women have round ligament discomfort during pregnancy. Typically, they describe a sharp pain below the umbilicus on one or both sides of the uterus. This discomfort, along with leg cramps, may be relieved by calcium supplementation. Good body mechanics also may help in relief of other musculoskeletal discomforts.

The following are some commonly encountered discomforts, their causes, and some recommended interventions. Nurses are encouraged to review resources (such as the Internet) that are available and to assess information for accuracy and advisability, especially before referring clients to a particular website. All information should be consistent with normal, routine, and mainstream prenatal care protocols.

Urinary Frequency

The physical sensation of needing to void frequently, sometimes accompanied by a feeling of urgency, is encountered primarily in the first and last trimester. The gravid, growing uterus presses on the bladder, and the fetus puts direct pressure on the bladder. In addition to these mechanical factors, the pregnant client also experiences an increase in circulating fluid volume, especially in the third trimester, and frequently an increased glomerular filtration rate, which further adds to frequency. The good news for clients is that they will experience some relief from this problem during the second trimester when the uterus is higher in the abdomen and the combined weight of the fetus and uterus is not as great as it is in late pregnancy. Clients should be cautioned not to decrease their fluid intake in an attempt to control urinary frequency. Doing so is appropriate only for short periods of time, such as a car trip for an hour or so, or in anticipation of a meeting of a similar time frame. Fluid intake for any 24-hour period should not be less than the recommended amount, or eight glasses of water plus other fluids.

Nausea and Vomiting

Nausea and vomiting are problems usually associated with the first trimester. Although sometimes referred to as morning sickness, the nausea and vomiting may occur at any time of the day. A variety of stimuli, such as certain smells and, the sight of some foods, can produce the sensations. Nausea seems to be more of a problem than does vomiting. Many clients experience nausea, with minimal vomiting. The hormones of pregnancy are the generally acknowledged basis for morning sickness. General guidelines for prevention call for eating dry toast or crackers without liquids before getting out of bed. Avoidance of known offenders, such as spicy foods and acidic citrus fruit on an empty stomach, is recommended. Other measures may include favorite decaffeinated teas. Peppermint tea is preferred by many clients because it tends to calm a queasy stomach. Ginger tea may also help with controlling nausea.

Indigestion

Indigestion is a common annoyance that shares some common causes with nausea. Also, the hormones progesterone and relaxin are implicated because they relax the cardiac sphincter and allow reflux to occur. Many clients have identified specific offending foods and beverages that caused them problems, even before pregnancy. Obviously, these foods should be avoided as much as possible. If reflux is a problem at bedtime, the use of an extra pillow may be helpful in overcoming the gravity factor that can enhance reflux. Caution clients about the use of antacids, especially those with a high sodium content. Mild herbal teas of the client's preference should be encouraged.

Constipation and Hemorrhoids

Constipation and hemorrhoids are closely related and often contribute to each other. Constipation and subsequent straining with defecation contribute to the formation of hemorrhoids. As with edema, the sluggish circulation and venous return combined with the direct pressure of the uterus and fetus all make avoidance of hemorrhoids a challenge. Gentle evacuation is encouraged by ample fluid intake, a diet high in fiber, use of certain stool softeners, and walking (preferably at a brisk rate, if tolerated). High-fiber foods that also are good sources of iron include prunes and apricots.

Edema of Lower Extremities

Swelling of the feet and lower legs is most commonly seen later in pregnancy, with several factors coming together to cause it. The increased circulating fluid volume, relaxed blood vessels, sluggish venous return, and mechanical obstructive nature of the heavy uterus and fetus on vessels of the lower extremities all contribute to the problem. Avoidance of long periods of standing without walking around helps to prevent edema. Clients should be advised to have their feet and legs elevated as much as possible while sitting. Clients also should be cautioned to avoid sitting with the hips at a sharp angle when the feet are elevated because doing so will further impede venous return and aggravate the original problem. Moderate walking is of great help in controlling edema (contracting muscles facilitate venous return) and preventing constipation (walking increases peristalsis). Walking is also an excellent exercise for pregnant women, especially when done at a sensible pace, avoiding fatigue and extreme weather conditions. For clients fortunate enough to live near a seashore, wading in the surf is very therapeutic. Not only does this improve venous return from lower extremities but it does so at pressures that are ideal; that is, the pressure of the water is greatest at the bottom (feet) and decreases toward the surface (farther up the legs). Also, the psychological benefits of reflective thinking and clearing the mind while wading in the water contribute to the client's overall well-being.

Danger Signs to Be Reported

With the availability of so much educational materials from a variety of sources, many clients are very knowledgeable about pregnancy and the various changes that occur. Even though information sources caution clients about the need for medical care and supervision, it remains the responsibility of the nurse to provide certain information without the assumption that clients have access to it elsewhere.

There are a number of possible events in pregnancy that reflect one or more complications; at best, these require assessment to rule out a problem. Whereas it may sound overreactive to refer to these as danger signs, and the policy of a clinic or facility may be to avoid use of the term danger for fear of alarming clients, it is imperative that clients be made aware of events that require immediate reporting to their health care provider. The nurse must reinforce the importance of reporting any of these things immediately, rather than making a note to report them at the next scheduled visit. A detailed explanation of the physiology and implications is not necessary for the client unless she requests it; however, she should know that immediate assessment is for the good of her health and her baby's health. Signs and symptoms that require immediate attention are the following:

- Any vaginal bleeding. The only exception to this is if a vaginal examination has been done within the past 24 hours and the examiner has told the client to expect some slight spotting of old blood. This phrase should be carefully explained, complete with a pencil drawing of how much spotting is acceptable. Some practitioners and physicians do not even mention the exception; they want to be notified of any spotting so they can assess it at that time.

- Swelling of the face and fingers. As a general rule, the higher the edema above the feet and ankles, especially in the face, coupled with suddenness of onset, the more ominous. This finding is usually associated with PIH.

- Severe headache that is continuous. Headache may be caused by a dangerously elevated blood pressure and associated with the onset of PIH. Other causes are possible.

- Vision changes, such as blurring or dimming of vision, or spots or flashes of light before the eyes. These changes also may be associated with PIH.

- Abdominal pain. There is no need to differentiate the epigastric pain of PIH from the onset of labor for the client; both require evaluation.

Reflections from Families

During my last pregnancy the nurse gave me a list of things called "Topics to Report Right Away." One of the things listed was "Rupture of membranes or escape of fluid from the vagina." My neighbor, Rhonda, and I were out shopping. I was in my last month, with delivery about 3 weeks away. Just as we went back to the car and I reached to open the door, it happened. Fluid ran down my leg to about my knees. It wasn't a lot, but it was there. I just wanted to go home and clean myself up. Rhonda asked me if this wasn't one of the things I was supposed to report right away to my doctor. I called the office from her car phone. The nurse told me to come straight to the doctor's office, which was about 2 miles from the mall. So we went. They checked me out right away and tested the fluid. It turned out to be urine! Can you imagine? I was so embarrassed. I told the nurse I'd never be back for that again. She told me that this happens a lot, and that I shouldn't be embarrassed. She said I did the right thing. I felt better. And Rhonda didn't laugh at me. Thank goodness she didn't call my husband to meet us at the hospital!

- Chills and fever. Instruct the client to report these and not to wait for other "flu" symptoms to appear.

- Persistent vomiting. Even though client may have read "somewhere" that nausea and vomiting are common in pregnancy, she should not dismiss persistent vomiting as normal.

- Sudden gush of fluid from the vagina. This usually signals spontaneous rupture of membranes and requires assessment for possible cord prolapse, prevention of infection, and evaluation for the onset of labor.

In instances in which the client, after receiving these instructions, reports events or symptoms that are subsequently evaluated as nonemergencies or not indicative of a complication, the nurse must be very tactful with and sensitive to the client. The nurse must not allow the client, or the client's family, to feel as though she has acted inappropriately. She should not be intimidated by thoughts of future false alarms.

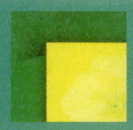

CASE STUDY/CARE PLAN
CLIENT WITH A NORMAL PREGNANCY

Susan M. is a 30-year-old gravida 3, para 1, who is 20 weeks pregnant. She has a 5-year-old daughter at home. She experienced an early spontaneous abortion before her daughter was born. She works full-time in a large downtown investment firm.

Susan and her husband bought a house in an adjacent rural area. They discussed the length of the daily commute for each of them but decided it was worth it to live in their dream house.

This pregnancy was planned and has thus far progressed uneventfully. During her last prenatal visit she expressed a strong desire to avoid constipation with this pregnancy and to prevent hemorrhoids. She has been told by some coworkers that the more constipation she had, the more certain she was to develop hemorrhoids. Constipation had been a problem for her with the last pregnancy. Her nutritional status is good. She is taking a daily prenatal vitamin with iron primarily because of her irregular eating habits at lunch. Weight is normal for height. Weight gain has been minimal. Immunizations are complete and current. She has no difficulty getting time off from work for prenatal appointments.

Assessment

Healthy 30-year-old with a 20-week intrauterine pregnancy. She has had no difficulties with this pregnancy. She is concerned about the health of herself and her family. She has strong family support from her husband and extended family. She works at a desk job 40 hours a week.

Nursing Diagnosis

Health-seeking behaviors: self-care of pregnancy related to the desire to prevent constipation and development of hemorrhoids, as evidenced by her expressed wish to avoid a previous experience with constipation.

Expected Outcomes	After nursing interventions, Susan will:
	■ Recall examples of foods and fluids recommended for their properties of constipation prevention.
	■ Report a pattern of regular bowel movements that do not require straining.
	■ Remain free of the signs and symptoms of hemorrhoids for the remainder of the pregnancy.
Planning	Because Susan has had a previous experience with constipation in pregnancy, it is important to explore with her those approaches that worked in resolving the problem. These approaches should be incorporated with any new recommendations. With her previous pregnancy, Susan did not understand the role of walking in preventing constipation; this intervention should be explored with this pregnancy.
NOC	Knowledge: health promotion
NIC	Health education

Nursing Interventions	Rationales
1. Review with Susan the major areas involved in prevention and resolution of constipation: diet, exercise, and fluid consumption.	1. An accurate knowledge base is essential for clients to make informed decisions in caring for themselves.
2. Discuss things Susan did to alleviate constipation with her last pregnancy.	2. Healthy self-care practices should be encouraged; others should be modified as indicated. Clients can be empowered in self-care with sensitive guidance and instructions.
3. Encourage fluid intake of eight glasses of water daily, above other fluid intake.	3. Water is essential to prevent dry, hard stools. Fluids containing sugars and caffeine usually are excreted by the kidney without contributing to fluid content of the lower intestine.

(continues)

Nursing Interventions	Rationales
4. Review and encourage intake of high-fiber foods. Focus on Susan's favorite foods as well as those she found helpful in her last pregnancy.	4. High-fiber foods, when combined with adequate fluid intake, form sufficient bulk in the stool to stimulate peristalsis. High-fiber dry foods, such as cereals, in the absence of adequate fluid intake can cause or contribute to constipation.
5. Encourage walking as a daily exercise.	5. Walking helps to stimulate peristalsis and to stimulate the general circulation. Hemorrhoids are prevented by avoidance of constipation and prevention of sluggish pelvic circulation.
6. Explore Susan's perception of iron supplement relative to constipation in the past pregnancy.	6. Whereas iron tends to contribute to constipation in some clients, it may be responsible for loose stools or diarrhea in others.
7. Review the list of stool softeners recommended for use as needed by Susan's physician and nurse practitioner.	7. Some laxatives and oil-based stimulants can interfere with nutrient absorption and may cause harsh evacuations. The potential for dependence also exists.

Evaluation

Susan was able to verbalize the role of fluids, diet, and exercise in preventing constipation and hemorrhoids. She had tried the recommended dried prunes with her last pregnancy but found that they worked better for her if she cooked them instead. Walking, particularly during her lunch hour, was convenient. She and her friend opted for daily walks around the perimeter of an enclosed ice skating rink located in a building adjacent to her office; this is a safe area where they can walk during any weather conditions. Susan reports having regular soft bowel movements with no straining. No signs of hemorrhoids are noted.

NURSING PROCESS

Care of the pregnant woman is unique in that nursing care must be planned for two individuals, the mother and the fetus, with consideration for the family. The dynamic relationship between the mother and fetus must be the basis for all planning and interventions.

Assessment

Assessment is designed for early detection to facilitate prevention of complications. Assessment is done on the initial visit and includes a thorough maternal history and physical examination. This examination incorporates an assessment of the condition of the fetus and the maternal progress of the pregnancy. During this assessment, the nurse should pay attention to the family's preparation for pregnancy, labor, and parenting. Actual and potential risk factors are identified. The objective of planning nursing care for the maternal-infant dyad is to minimize morbidity and facilitate the most positive birth experience for the mother and family.

Nursing Diagnoses

Nursing diagnoses common to women receiving prenatal care are likely to include the following:

- Deficient knowledge related to inexperience with the physiologic changes of pregnancy
- Pain related to the physiologic changes in pregnancy
- Imbalanced nutrition: more than body requirements, related to excessive caloric intake
- Deficient knowledge related to the importance of prenatal care

Outcome Identification

Outcomes planned for women experiencing an uncomplicated pregnancy may include the following:

- The client is able to remain free from the common discomforts of pregnancy.
- The client incorporates strategies to increase her comfort as the pregnancy progresses.
- Weight gain does not exceed 1 lb/wk in the first 36 weeks of pregnancy and 0.5 lb/wk the last month.
- The client comes to her regular prenatal visits.

Planning

Planning should focus on the physical and emotional needs of the woman in relation to the changes she will

Critical Thinking

Refer to the Case Study

Assessment: Do you think that her job (sitting at a desk, with very little walking) may contribute to Susan's possibly experiencing constipation?

Nursing Diagnosis: What are some other possible nursing diagnoses pertaining to health-seeking behaviors in women who are eager to be in control of their care?

Expected Outcomes: Is there a single outcome listed that is more important than the others? Or, are they all equally important in meeting the goal?

Planning: Which approaches might you take to be sure the planning phase is actually joint decision-making?

Interventions and Rationales: Examine these to see if you can identify any that may be unacceptable to a client who wants to be in control of her self-care activities.

Evaluation: If Susan developed constipation at a later point in her pregnancy, how would you revise the planning? What information would you need or which questions would you ask to say that a revised plan was necessary?

---

experience in each trimester. The client's partner, family, or support system should be included in the planning, as desired by the client.

Nursing Intervention

The client should be taught strategies to deal with the common discomforts of pregnancy, because many of these can be prevented or minimized by lifestyle modifications. Many times it is difficult for a client to discriminate between a benign cause of discomfort and a serious complication; if discomfort does occur, the client should not hesitate to call the health care provider.

The client should also be taught expected weight gain parameters and common dietary pitfalls. The more weight a woman gains above 35 to 40 lb, the greater the risk of maternal-fetal morbidity, as well as health risks related to obesity for the mother after delivery.

The nurse should also be sure to teach the client the importance of early detection and treatment of abnormalities as well as the health-promoting benefits to herself and her baby. During the course of prenatal care, the mother will obtain information about lifestyle choices that ensure better health for her and her infant. Regular prenatal care allows for early detection and intervention for many pregnancy complications.

Evaluation

Each expected outcome must be evaluated with each client-nurse interaction to determine if the current goals have been accomplished or need to be modified.

WEB ACTIVITIES

• • • Visit the Web sites of some nursing organizations, such as the Association of Women's Health Obstetric and Neonatal Nurses (AWHONN) and the American Nurses Association (ANA). What information do they offer regarding nursing care of the women during an uncomplicated pregnancy? Do they also include any information targeted for the client?

• • • Find the sites listed in the Resources for this chapter. Read the information that will be most useful to you as you begin working with pregnant clients and their families.

Key Concepts

- Preconception care is the ideal approach to childbearing. Many risk factors can be identified and dealt with before pregnancy begins.

- Health care communities must develop plans for availability and accessibility of prenatal care for their citizens. Barriers should be minimized.

- Early and consistent prenatal care is essential for proper monitoring of any pregnancy. Prevention of potential complications is possible with monitoring.

- Balancing intake of necessary nutrients and vitamin supplements is important in maintaining a healthy pregnancy.

- The pregnancy experience can be enhanced when clients are aware of changes taking place in their bodies.

- Clients can be empowered with involvement in decision-making about their care.

- Nurses play a key role in the education of the child bearing family to promote healthy pregnancy and prepare for childbirth and family adaptation.

- Relaxation is a key strategy in preparing for childbirth.

- Nurses have a responsibility to review all materials recommended for client information.

- Danger signs in pregnancy may affect the health of the mother, baby, or both. Special attention is needed.

Review Questions and Activities

1. Low birth weight and congenital anomalies remain two problems on which prenatal care has had litle impact in the past 40 years. Explain how preconception care can decrease the incidences of these problems.

2. Design a healthy diet for a pregnant woman.

3. Becky S. is seeing the nurse midwife with her fifth pregnancy. Her first two babies were born prematurely but are healthy youngsters now. Her third pregnancy resulted in a miscarriage at 18 weeks' gestation, and her fourth went to term with delivery of an 8 lb, 6 oz boy. How is her GTPAL status correctly noted?

4. Diane's last normal menstrual period began on May 10th, and her pregnancy test (7 weeks later) was positive. Calculate her EDC. Give the month, date, and year.

5. Explain the physiologic anemia usually seen in pregnancy.

6. List one commonly encountered discomfort of pregnancy for each of the three trimesters. Explain why each is likely to occur in that particular trimester.

7. Discuss comfort measures for each of these three identified common discomforts.

8. What are some examples of pregnancy risk factors that can be identified from a client's psychosocial history? From her partner's medical history?

9. Your neighbor thinks she is pregnant and has made an appointment with her family doctor. How would you respond to her inquiry about what to expect during the visit?

10. Describe three educational topics you would teach to a pregnant woman.

References

Association of Women's Health, Obstetric, and Neonatal Nurses (AWHONN). (1993). *Competencies and program guidelines for nurse providers of perinatal education*. Washington, DC: Author.

Blumenthal, M., Busse, W. R. Goldberg, A., Gruenwald, J., Hall, T., Riggins, C. W., et al. (1998). *The complete commission E monographs: Therapeutic guide to herbal medicines* (S. Klein & R. S. Rister, Trans.). Austin, TX: American Botanical Council; Boston: Integrative Medicine Communications.

Cunningham, F. G., Gant, N. E., Leveno, K. J., Gilstrap, L. C. III, Hauth, J., & Wenstrom, K. (2001). *Williams obstetrics* (21st ed.). Stamford, CT: Appleton-Lange.

Cuskelly, G. J., McNulty, H., & Scott J. M. (1999). Fortification with low amounts of folic acid makes a significant difference in folate status in young women: Implications for the prevention of neural tube defects. *American Journal of Clinical Nutrition, 70*, 234–239.

Dick-Read, G. (1979). *Childbirth without fear*. New York: Harper & Row.

Humenick, S. S. (1999). The versatility of the perinatal educator. *Journal of Perinatal Education, 8*(2), vi–vii.

Humenick, S. S. (2000). The evolution of childbirth educator to perinatal educator. *Journal of Perinatal Education, 9*(1), vi–vii.

Humenick, S. S., Shrock P., & Libresco, M. M. (2000). Relaxation. In F. H. Nichols & S. S. Humenick (Eds.), *Childbirth education: Practice, theory and research* (2nd ed.). Philadelphia: W. B. Saunders.

Institute of Medicine. (1992). *Nutrition during pregnancy and lactation: An implementation guide*. Washington, DC: National Academy Press.

Institute of Medicine. (1990). *Nutrition during pregnancy: Part I—Weight gain; Part I—Nutritional supplements*. Washington, DC: National Academy Press.

Institute of Medicine. (1992). *Nutrition services in prenatal care* (2nd ed.). Washington, DC: National Academy Press.

International Childbirth Education Association (ICEA). (1999). ICEA position paper: The role of the childbirth educator and the scope of childbirth education. *International Journal of Childbirth Education, 14*(4), 33–41.

Jimenez, S. L. M. (2000). Comfort and pain management. In F. H. Nichols & S. S. Humenick (Eds.), *Childbirth education: Practice, theory and research* (2nd ed.). Philadelphia: W. B. Saunders.

Lamaze, F. (1972). *Painless childbirth: The Lamaze method*. New York: Pocketbooks.

Melzak, R., & Wall, P. (1965). *Pain mechanisms: A new theory. Science, 150*, 971–979.

Morgan, S. L., & Weinsier, R. L. (1998). *Fundamentals of clinical nutrition* (2nd ed.). St. Louis, MO: Mosby.

Nichols, F. (2000). Paced breathing techniques. In F. H. Nichols & S. S. Humenick (Eds.), *Childbirth education: Practice, theory and research* (2nd ed.). Philadelphia: W. B. Saunders.

Perry, L. E. (1996). Preconception care: A health promotion opportunity. *Nurse Practitioner, 2*(11), 24–26.

Rainville, A. J. (1998). Pica practices of pregnant women are associated with lower maternal hemoglobin level at delivery. *Journal of the American Dietary Association, 98*, 293–296.

Shilling. T. (2000). Cultural perspectives on child-bearing. In F. H. Nichols and S. S. Humenick (Eds.), *Childbirth education: Practice, theory and Research* (2nd ed.). Philadelphia: W. B. Saunders.

U.S. Department of Health and Human Services. (2000). *Healthy people 2010* (Conference edition, in two volumes). Washington, DC: author. Also available online: http://www.health .gov/healthypeople or call 1-800-367-4725.

Suggested Readings

American Academy of Pediatrics and The American College of Obstetricians and Gynecologists. (1997). *Guidelines for perinatal care* (4th ed.). Washington, DC: Authors.

Association of Women's Health, Obstetrical and Neonatal Nurses (AWHONN). (1999). *Clinical competencies and education guidelines: Limited ultrasound examinations in obstetrics and gynecology/infertility settings.* Chicago: Author.

Brown, S. (Ed.). (1988). *Prenatal care: Researching mothers, reaching infants.* Washington, DC: National Academy Press.

Expert Panel on the Content of Prenatal Care. (1989). *Caring for our future: The content of prenatal care.* Washington, DC: U.S. Department of Health and Human Services.

Jakobi, P., Goldstick, O., Sajov, P., & Itskovitz-Eldor, J. (1996). New CDC guidelines for prevention of perinatal group B streptococcal disease. *Lancet, 348*(9032), 969.

Knuppel, R. A., & Drukker, J. E. (1993) *High risk pregnancy: A team approach.* Philadelphia W. B. Saunders.

Kogan, M. D., Martin, J. A., Alexander, G. R., Kotelchuck, M., & Frigolette, F. (1998). The changing pattern of prenatal care utilization in the United States, 1981–1995, using different prenatal care indices. *Journal of the American Medical Association, 279,* 1623–1628.

LaVeist, T. A., Keith, V. M., & Gutierrez, M. L. (1995). African American/Caucasian differences in prenatal care utilization: An assessment of predisposing and enabling factors. *Health Services Research, 30*(1), 43–58.

Lin, G. G. (1998). Birth outcomes and the effectiveness of prenatal care. *Health Services Research, 32*(6), 805–807.

Murray, M. (1997). *Antepartal and intrapartal fetal monitoring.* Albuquerque, NM: Learning Resources International.

Rosenstein, N. E., & Schuchat, A. E. The Neonatal Group B Streptococcal Disease Study Group. (1997). Opportunities for prevention of perinatal group B *Streptococcal* disease: A multistate surveillance analysis. *Obstetrics & Gynecology, 90*(6), 901–906.

Simpson, K. R., & Creehan, P. A. (1996). *Perinatal nursing.* Philadelphia: Lippincott-Raven.

Taylor, M. C., Mercer, B. M., Engelhardt, K. F., & Fricke, J. L. (1997). Patient preference for self-collected cultures for group B. *Streptococcus* in pregnancy. *Journal of Nurse Midwifery, 42*(5), 410–413.

U.S. Department of Health and Human Services. (1989). *Caring for our future: The content of prenatal care.* Washington, DC: National Institutes of Health.

Youngkin, E. Q., & Davis, M. S. (1994). *Women's health: A primary care clinical guide.* Norwalk, CT: Appleton & Lange.

Resources

Childbirth: http://www.childbirth.org

Fetal Development and Prenatal Diagnosis (Dr. Jason Birnholz): http://www.amnionet.com

Fetal Ultrasound (Greggory R. DeVore, MD): http://www.fetal .com

International Childbirth Education Association: http://www.icea .org

Perinatal Education Associates: http://www.birthsource.com

University of Pennsylvania School of Medicine: http://www.med .upenn.edu

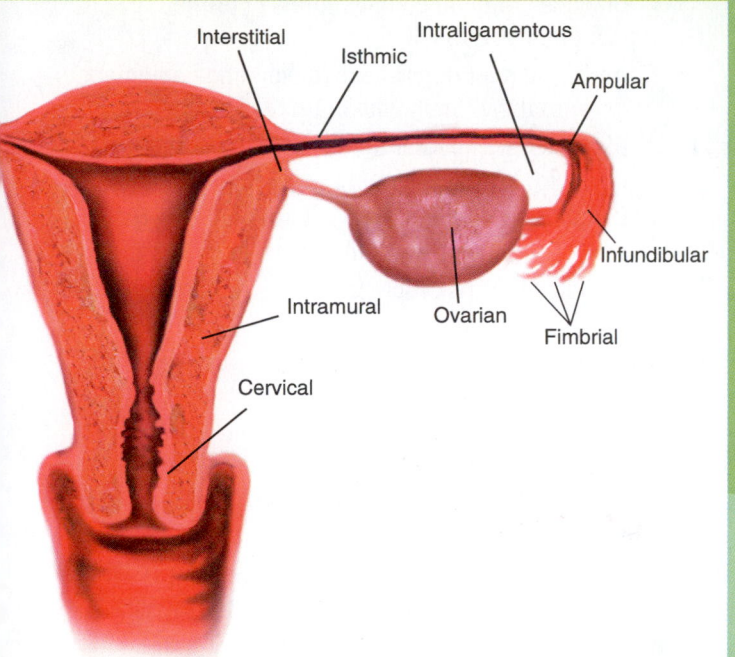

CHAPTER 11

MANAGEMENT AND NURSING CARE OF HIGH-RISK CLIENTS

The birth of a child generally is thought of as a joyous occasion for families. Whereas many women experience an uncomplicated pregnancy and childbirth, complications can develop at any point in the pregnancy, labor and delivery, or postpartum period. These complications can lead to serious illness, injury, and even death for the pregnant woman and her baby and place tremendous stress on the family.

Key Terms

ABO incompatibility
Abortion
Abruptio placentae
Acquired immunodeficiency syndrome (AIDS)
Adolescence
Adolescent pregnancy
Amniocentesis
Amnioinfusion
Antiretroviral therapy
Cerclage
Chronic hypertension
Cognitive development
Developmental tasks
Disseminated intravascular coagulation (DIC)
Dizygotic
Eclampsia
Ectopic pregnancy
Elective abortion
Gestational diabetes
Human immunodeficiency virus (HIV)
Hydramnios
Hydrops fetalis
Incompetent cervix

Induced abortion
Ketoacidosis
Macrosomia
Marginal placenta previa
Monozygotic
Oligohydramnios
Partial previa
Percutaneous umbilical blood sampling (PUBS)
Placenta previa
Polyhydramnios
Postterm pregnancy
Pre-eclampsia
Premature rupture of membranes (PROM)
Preterm labor
Preterm premature rupture of membranes (PPROM)
Seroconversion
Sexual maturation
Spontaneous abortion
Therapeutic abortion
Thrombocytopenia
Thyrotoxicosis
Type I diabetes mellitus
Type II diabetes mellitus
Vertical transmission

Competencies

Upon completion of this chapter, the reader should be able to:

1. Discuss potential complications of pregnancy-induced hypertension.
2. Apply the nursing process to plan and implement care for the woman with diabetes in pregnancy.
3. Discuss nursing interventions for the pregnant client who is experiencing vaginal bleeding.
4. Discuss the psychosocial impact of a high-risk pregnancy on the woman and her family.
5. Identify labor risk factors for the woman with cardiac disease.
6. List the components of client education related to preterm labor.
7. Describe the scope and significance of adolescent pregnancy.
8. Describe the psychosocial and physical risks for pregnant adolescents and their children.
9. Discuss adolescent sexuality and appropriate contraceptive methods.
10. Formulate a nursing care plan for pregnant adolescents.
11. Describe the significance of HIV infection in pregnant women.
12. Discuss the importance of prevention of vertical and perinatal transmission of HIV infection.
13. Discuss the clinical manifestations and medical management of HIV-infected pregnant women and neonates.

The maternal mortality rate in the United States was reported to be 7.5 deaths per 100,000 live births from 1982 to 1996 (Centers for Disease Control and Prevention, 1998a). Identification of common medical and obstetric conditions that place the client and fetus at increased risk for morbidity and mortality is essential in developing a nursing plan of care and achieving optimal outcomes for both. Assessment of family values, available resources, and learning needs also is a critical part of nursing care for these families who are at risk for serious health problems or even loss of a family member.

This chapter provides a broad overview of some common conditions that place mother and fetus at risk and provides guidelines for nursing assessments and interventions.

HEMORRHAGIC DISORDERS

Obstetric hemorrhage is a common cause of maternal mortality occurring in 1.4 per 100,000 live births (Chichakli et al., 1999). In this section some common causes of obstetric hemorrhage are discussed. The most common obstetric hemorrhagic event, postpartum hemorrhage, is discussed in detail in Chapter 17.

Abortion

Abortion is termination of pregnancy before fetal viability. This term usually is applied to pregnancy termination before 20 weeks' gestation. Spontaneous abortion refers to pregnancy termination that occurs naturally and commonly is referred to as miscarriage. Box 11-1 lists categories of spontaneous abortion.

Induced abortion is termination of pregnancy before fetal viability by medical or surgical intervention. Induced abortions may be **therapeutic**, in which case the pregnancy is terminated because of health risks to the mother in continuation of the pregnancy or for fetal disease. The terms **elective abortion** and voluntary abortion are used to describe termination of pregnancy before fetal viability at the request of the client.

Incidence

Most spontaneous abortions occur in the first trimester of pregnancy, possibly before the woman realizes she is pregnant. The exact cause of spontaneous abortion is not always identified. Approximately half of these losses are attributed to chromosomal abnormalities (Cunningham et al., 2001).

Clinical Presentation

Vaginal bleeding or bloody discharge in the first trimester of pregnancy with or without cramping is a sign of threatened abortion, although other causes of vaginal bleeding are possible. The amount of vaginal bleeding may be minimal but may persist for days or weeks. The presence of pain along with vaginal bleeding usually is a poor prognostic indicator for continuation of the pregnancy (Cunningham et al., 2001).

Management

Clients presenting with vaginal bleeding are examined to determine if cervical dilation has occurred, making abortion inevitable. Other potential causes of vaginal bleeding to be considered are cervical lesions and physiologic bleeding at the time normal menses would occur.

The woman with a threatened abortion may be managed expectantly, which may include bed rest and serial laboratory tests to assess for decreasing hemoglobin and hematocrit levels and the presence of infection. Pain medication may be necessary in some cases.

The client who experiences a spontaneous abortion is observed closely for hemorrhage. The health care provider will assess the client, fetus, and placenta to determine if all products of conception have been expelled. In the event of retained tissue or postpartum hemorrhage, curettage (scraping of the endometrial lining) may be performed.

Nursing Care

Nursing care of the client experiencing an abortion or threatened abortion includes assessing for amount (pad count and weight) and character of blood loss, assessing for signs and symptoms of shock or infection, and responding promptly to complications. Immediate measures may be necessary, such as volume and blood replacement, oxygen therapy, and medical and surgical interventions. All procedures and the plan of care should be communicated clearly to the client. The nurse should provide emotional support to the client and family during this difficult experience. Spiritual support, client literature for education, and information about support groups where available may be offered.

Box 11-1

Categories of Abortion

Complete

All products of conception are expelled, and uterine bleeding and cramping cease.

Incomplete

A portion of the products of conception is expelled, and a portion is retained. Bleeding and cramping continue until the uterus is evacuated.

Threatened

Uterine bleeding and cramping occur; however, the products of conception have not been expelled.

Missed

A pregnancy becomes nonviable; no uterine bleeding, cramping, or passage of tissue has occurred.

Recurrent Spontaneous

Situation wherein a woman has three or more successive spontaneous abortions.

Inevitable

Abortion cannot be stopped when membranes rupture and cervix dilates.

Client Education

Clients as Resources

Pregnant women are a very valuable resource in assisting with prenatal care. They are able to help only if they know what to expect. For example, some women can have spotting early in a pregnancy, and it is not serious. In other cases, spotting may suggest a missed abortion or ectopic pregnancy. You should teach clients that even if they think their spotting is not serious, they should notify their health care provider immediately so that the cause can be identified.

Ectopic Pregnancy

Ectopic pregnancy is the implantation of the fertilized ovum in a location other than the endometrial lining (Figure 11-1). The most common implantation site is the fallopian tube, usually in the distal end; however, implantation may occur in numerous locations, including the ovaries, cervix, and abdomen (Hankins, Clark, Cunningham, & Gilstrap , 1995).

Incidence

In the United States, the rate of ectopic pregnancy in women 15 to 45 years of age is about 19.7 per 1,000 pregnancies (Tenore, 2000). Many factors contribute to ectopic pregnancy. Damage to the fallopian tubes from pelvic inflammatory disease (PID) is cited as the most common cause of ectopic pregnancy. *Neisseria gonorrhoeae* and chlamydia are common causative organisms implicated in the development of PID (Kamwendo, Forslin, Bodin, & Danielsson, 2000). A previous surgery, chromosomal abnormalities of the embryo, the use of intrauterine contraceptive devices (IUDs), ovarian hyperstimulation as the result of assisted reproductive technology, delayed or premature ovulation, multiple induced abortions, and peritoneal dialysis also have been implicated as causes of ectopic pregnancy (Hankins et al., 1995; Creasy, Resnick, & Iams, 2004). Maternal age greater than 35 years is another risk factor. Ectopic pregnancy can be a life-threatening event because hemorrhage may occur with rupture if this complication is not diagnosed and treated promptly. Ectopic pregnancy is the leading cause of pregnancy-related deaths during the first trimester in the United States (American College of Obstetricians and Gynecologists [ACOG], 1998a).

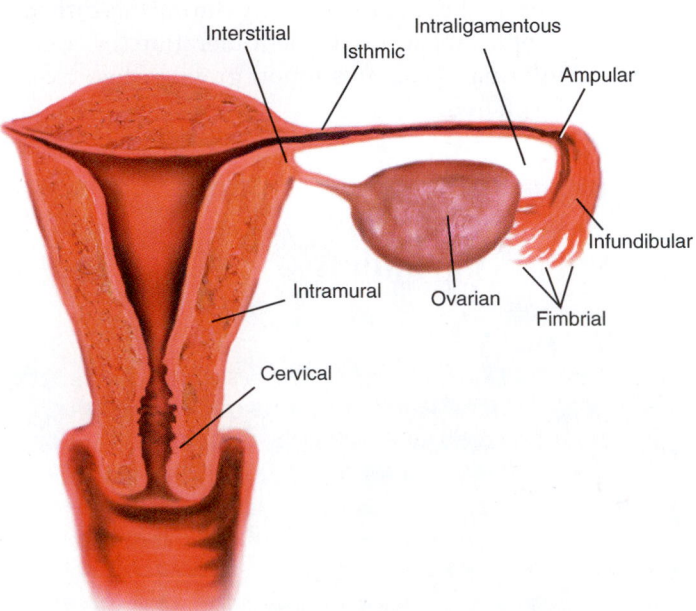

Figure 11-1 Sites of implantation in ectopic pregnancy.

Clinical Presentation

The client with an ectopic pregnancy often presents with vaginal bleeding or spotting, a missed period, severe lower quadrant abdominal and pelvic pain when the fallopian tube bursts, tenderness of the abdomen on palpation, and severe pain on movement of the cervix on pelvic examination. When the tube bursts, there is bleeding into the abdominal cavity. Abdominal bleeding irritates the phrenic nerve, causing radiating pain to the shoulder.

Management

Once an ectopic pregnancy is confirmed, medical management of the client may include surgery or administration of methotrexate, a drug used to resolve the pregnancy. Laboratory assessments include a complete blood count (CBC) to evaluate for blood loss and infection, and a serum pregnancy test. The client also may undergo vaginal or abdominal ultrasonography to determine the location of the pregnancy. The site of implantation helps determine the medical management. A culdocentesis, which involves insertion of a needle into the culdosac to aspirate the contents from the pelvic peritoneum, also may be performed to assess for the presence of nonclotting blood in the peritoneum (Hankins et al., 1995).

Nursing Care

Nursing care for the client experiencing an ectopic pregnancy includes assessment for the amount and character of vaginal bleeding and for signs and symptoms of shock.

Nursing Alert

Signs and Symptoms of Hypovolemic Shock

Early signs and symptoms:

- Tachycardia
- Weak peripheral pulses
- Tachypnea
- Skin cool to touch
- Pale skin and mucous membranes

Late signs and symptoms:

- Hypotension
- Weak, thready pulses (rapid)
- Cyanosis with cold, clammy skin
- Urinary output less than 30 mL/hr
- Mental status change (anxiety, restlessness, irritability, confusion, difficulty following directions)

The nurse obtains laboratory tests and procedures, such as ultrasonography, and reports the findings to the physician promptly. The woman with an ectopic pregnancy often will experience a great deal of pain, and pain medication should be administered as ordered. The nurse prepares the client for the surgical procedure, explaining what the client can expect before and after the procedure. The woman who has an ectopic pregnancy may experience grief as a result of pregnancy loss. The nurse should offer emotional support, spiritual care, client literature for education, and information about support groups when appropriate. If the woman is Rh negative, she will also need to receive RhoGAM (Rh$_o$(D) immune globulin).

PLACENTAL ABNORMALITIES

Abnormalities in placental form and function include placenta previa and abruptio placentae.

Placenta Previa

In placenta previa the placenta lies over or near the cervical os (Figure 11-2). There are three classes of placenta previa (Clark, 1999):

1. **Marginal placenta previa** (also called low-lying placenta previa) in which the placenta lies more than 3 cm from the cervical os.
2. **Partial previa** in which the placenta is within 3 cm of the cervical os but does not completely cover it.
3. **Placenta previa** (also called total placenta previa) in which the cervical os is covered by the placenta in the third trimester of pregnancy.

Incidence

Placenta previa is a fairly uncommon complication of pregnancy; however, the consequences can be very serious for the mother and fetus. The incidence of placenta previa is reported to be from 0.3% to 2.0%, or 1 in 200 deliveries (Hendricks, Chow, Bhagavath, & Singh, 1999).

Previous cesarean section and induced abortion increase the risk for occurrence of placenta previa. The risk increases as the number of previous cesarean sections increases (Castles, Adams, Melvin, Kelsch, & Boulton, 1999; Ananth, Smulian, & Vintzieleos, 1997). Multiparity and advancing age of the woman also are associated with placenta previa, as is maternal smoking (Cunningham et al., 2001; Castles et al., 1999; Ananth, Smulian, & Vintzieleos, 1999). Cocaine use by the mother is an independent risk factor for the development of placenta previa (Macones, Sehdev, Parry, Morgan, & Berlin, 1997).

Clinical Presentation

The diagnosis of placenta previa frequently is made after onset of sudden, painless vaginal bleeding in the second or third trimester of pregnancy. The amount of bleeding varies and may stop spontaneously; however, in some cases, bleeding can be so perfuse as to be life-threatening. The diagnosis of placenta previa is made after ultrasonographic examination.

Management

Management of the woman with placenta previa is determined by the degree of placenta previa present, gestational age of the fetus, and presence and amount of vaginal bleeding.

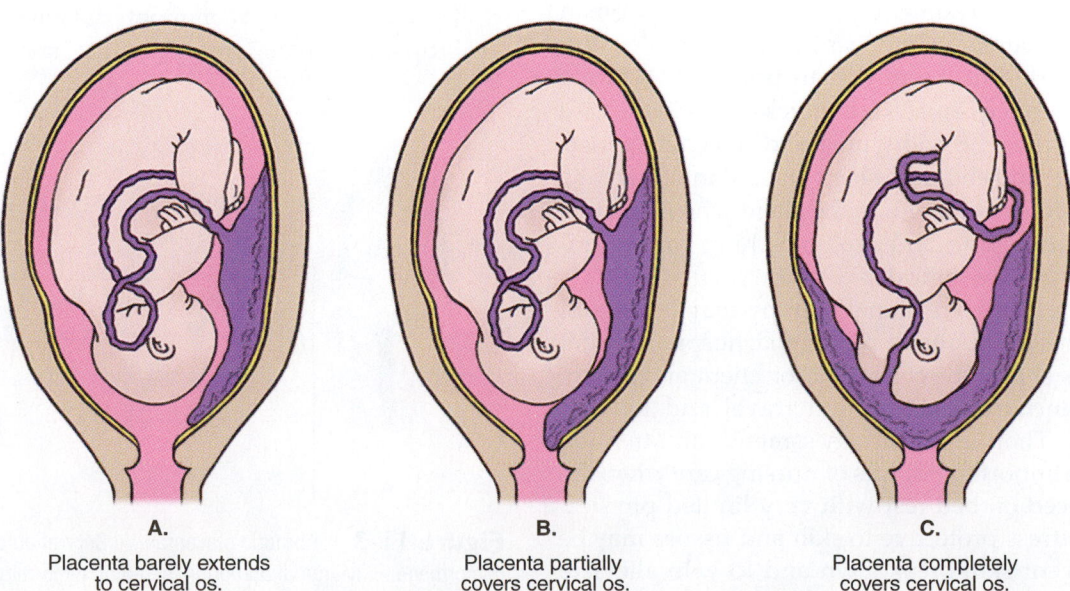

A.
Placenta barely extends to cervical os.

B.
Placenta partially covers cervical os.

C.
Placenta completely covers cervical os.

Figure 11-2   Placenta previa. A. Low implantation (marginal). B. Partial placenta previa. C. Total placenta previa.

In cases of severe hemorrhage, delivery is induced despite the gestational age of the fetus. Volume resuscitation and transfusion of blood products frequently are required. An emergency cesarean section delivery is performed to prevent further blood loss that could occur with disruption of the placenta during vaginal delivery.

Laboring women who present with a diagnosis of placenta previa generally are delivered by cesarean section even in the absence of active bleeding. This decision is determined by the degree of placenta previa present. In the case of a marginal placenta previa, some clients are allowed to labor as long as facilities for an emergency are immediately available (Clark, 1999).

In the woman who is preterm and nonlaboring, delivery may be delayed if the bleeding has stopped or is minimal and the mother and fetus are in stable condition. The physician may order hospitalization until the time of delivery or may allow select clients to remain at home. The decision is individualized according to placental location, physician preference, and the condition of the mother and fetus (Maloni, Cohen, & Kane, 1998).

If placenta previa is suspected, the nurse should not perform a vaginal examination or do anything to stimulate uterine contractions until a health care provider assesses the woman.

Nursing Care

Nursing care specific to the client diagnosed with placenta previa includes assessment for signs and symptoms of vaginal bleeding, performance of laboratory tests as ordered, supportive care, and client education. A peripad count is kept and recorded for clients who have active vaginal bleeding, and the perineum is checked frequently for the presence of bleeding, especially after the woman defecates or urinates. A significant increase in bleeding should be reported to the physician promptly. A large-bore IV catheter often is placed for quick access in the case of acute hemorrhage. Blood typing and screening generally are ordered and should be kept current in the event a blood transfusion is required. In the client who has active bleeding, blood typing and crossmatching for several units of blood may be indicated.

Occupational or recreational therapy may be helpful to the woman who requires prolonged hospitalization. Social services should be consulted for client and family concerns, financial assistance, and travel and lodging arrangements. Thorough skin assessment and attention to hygiene are important aspects of nursing care when the woman is placed on bed rest with very limited physical activity. A mattress protective to skin and tissues may be useful to prevent skin breakdown and to help alleviate client discomfort.

Information should be given to the client and family regarding the proposed plan of care and the potential complications that may arise from this condition. On occasion, vaginal bleeding may begin with no warning and may be hemorrhagic in nature. This emergency situation is very alarming to the woman and family members. The nurse should make an effort to prepare them for this possibility, explain the series of events that would follow in preparation for an emergency cesarean section, and provide reassurance if this should occur. Women who are discharged with placenta previa should receive instructions to return immediately in the event of uterine contractions, vaginal bleeding, or a decline in fetal movement.

Abruptio Placentae

Abruptio placentae (abruption) is separation of the placenta from its implantation site before delivery of the fetus (Figure 11-3). Bleeding associated with a placental abruption may be concealed in a space between the now detached placenta and uterus. More often, external vaginal bleeding is present. Placental abruptions can be total, with ensuing fetal death likely, or partial, in which case a portion of the placenta remains intact and perfusion to the fetus is possible (Cunningham et al., 2001).

Incidence

Abruption occurs in about 1 in 150 deliveries (Cunningham et al., 2001). According to Chichakli, Atrash, Mackay, Musani, and Berg (1999), abruptio placentae was the leading cause of pregnancy-related deaths in the United States from 1979 to 1992. Black women in this study had a threefold increased risk for death compared with Caucasian women.

The condition most commonly associated with placental abruption is hypertension in pregnancy (Hauth et al.,

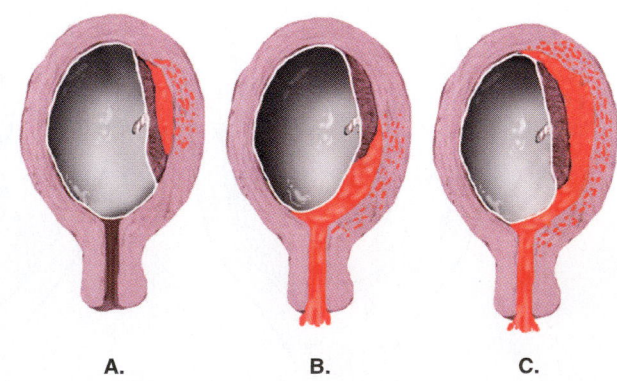

A.   B.   C.

Figure 11-3 Abruptio placentae. A. Central abruption, concealed hemorrhage. B. Marginal abruption, external hemorrhage. C. Complete abruption, external hemorrhage (could also be concealed).

2000). Preterm premature rupture of membranes and maternal trauma, especially associated with high-speed automobile accidents, also have been associated with abruption (Reis, Sander, & Pearlman, 2000). Cocaine use during pregnancy and cigarette smoking also have been associated with a large number of placental abruptions (Cunningham, et al., 2001; Castles et al., 1999; Ananth et al., 1999).

Clinical Presentation

The diagnosis of abruptio placentae may be difficult to make and often is made only after excluding other potential causes of the presenting symptoms, the hallmark of which is pain. Common presenting symptoms are abdominal pain and vaginal bleeding, tenderness, or rigidity. On admission assessment, fetal heart sounds may be absent or there may be a nonreassuring fetal heart pattern and high-frequency uterine contractions on electronic fetal monitoring.

The amount of vaginal bleeding present does not necessarily reflect the extent of abruption. Up to 10% of women who have an abruption present with concealed bleeding. Ultrasonographic examination to assess the presence of an abruption often is not helpful in establishing this diagnosis (Cunningham et al., 2001; Clark, 1999).

Maternal morbidity in abruption is common and can be serious. In a review of pregnancy-related mortality in the United States, placental abruption was the leading overall cause of death as a result of hemorrhage (Chichakli et al., 1999). Acute blood loss from both placenta previa and abruptio placentae can lead to shock in the mother. Decreased perfusion to the kidneys during massive blood loss may cause oliguria, which usually responds to volume resuscitation with intravenous (IV) fluids and blood. Acute tubular necrosis and renal failure are serious complications that can occur when there is a delay in or inadequate treatment for blood loss and hypovolemic shock (Clark et al., 1997; Cunningham et al., 2001).

Abruption is the most common obstetric cause of **disseminated intravascular coagulation (DIC)**. This process occurs as a result of excess consumption of some components of coagulation. With the massive consumption of circulating clotting factors and activation of the fibrinolytic system the client experiences hemorrhage, end-organ ischemia, vascular permeability, and hypotension (Sisson & Ruth, 1999; Clark et al., 1997; Cunningham et al., 2001).

Neonatal complications of placenta abruptio include preterm birth, anemia, and respiratory distress syndrome (RDS) (Crane, van den Hof, Dodds, Armson, & Liston, 1999). The perinatal mortality rate for abruptio placentae is reported to be from 20% to 35%, accounting for a large percentage of third-trimester fetal deaths. Even when infants survive, they may be seriously affected by the decreased perfusion to the placenta and may develop neurologic sequelae (Cunningham et al., 2001).

Management

The treatment for abruptio placentae depends on the condition of the mother and fetus. When bleeding is not severe and the mother is stable, fetal status and gestational age often determine the plan of care. The physician may choose to manage the woman who is stable with a preterm fetus expectantly under close observation and may employ the use of tocolytic agents to stop uterine contractions (Clark, 1999). The viable fetus that is near full term often is electively delivered to avoid a larger abruption that could seriously compromise the fetus or result in fetal death.

In the case of acute hemorrhage, resuscitation with blood transfusion and IV fluids and immediate delivery are indicated. This life-threatening complication usually requires aggressive volume resuscitation with IV fluids, blood pressure support, oxygen therapy, and evacuation of the uterus (Clark et al., 1997).

In the event of an abruption in which there is an intrauterine fetal death, delivery will be induced once maternal stability is achieved, and the woman will be closely observed for complications.

Nursing Care

Nursing care of the client with an abruption includes an assessment of the amount and nature of vaginal bleeding. A peripad count may be indicated in the presence of ongoing bleeding. The nurse should palpate the uterus to assess for tenderness and rigidity, the height of the fundus, and the location and nature of pain. It is sometimes difficult for the client to describe the pain associated with an abruption when she also is experiencing painful uterine contractions. However, pain associated with uterine contractions subsides during the relaxation phase, whereas the pain associated with an abruption is constant.

In an acute bleeding episode, vital signs are monitored closely for signs of hypovolemic shock. The fetus may be compromised as a result of uteroplacental insufficiency, and, therefore, continuous electronic fetal monitoring usually is employed for assessment of the viable fetus. In the event of hemodynamic changes in the client or a nonreassuring fetal heart rate, resuscitative measures should be initiated by the nurse and the physician should be notified immediately.

In the case of acute blood loss, a large-bore IV catheter is indicated for fluid and possibly blood replacement. The nurse obtains ordered laboratory tests that usually include blood typing and screening or blood typing and cross-matching, a CBC, and clotting studies. A Foley catheter is indicated, with hourly intake and output measured and recorded. The nurse may prepare the client for an emergency cesarean section, as indicated.

When induction of labor is ordered as a result of intrauterine fetal loss, the nurse should ensure adequate pain relief according to the client's wishes. The nurse should be familiar with the medications used to induce labor and their potential side effects.

Once stabilized, the client should receive a thorough explanation of her condition and that of the fetus. The potential complications and proposed plan of care should be discussed with the client and family. Grief support and spiritual care should be offered to the woman and family in the event of fetal or neonatal death.

LABOR DISORDERS

Disorders that fall into this category include incompetent cervix, preterm labor, and postterm pregnancy.

Incompetent Cervix

Incompetent cervix describes the often painless dilation of the cervix in which the pregnancy is lost. This condition may result from a congenital cause such as diethylstilbestrol (DES) exposure, or an acquired cause, such as trauma to the cervix from previous gynecologic or obstetric procedures (Creasy et al., 2004).

Incidence

The reported incidence of cervical incompetence varies greatly but may account for 8% to 15% of spontaneous pregnancy losses (Hankins et al., 1995).

Clinical Presentation

The diagnosis of an incompetent cervix may be made after repetitive spontaneous second-trimester pregnancy losses, incidentally on an ultrasonographic examination, or acutely with the advanced cervical dilation and effacement (Creasy et al., 2004). The client may present with complaints such as lower abdominal pressure, bloody show, or urinary frequency. As the bag of water protrudes through the cervix, small frequent contractions may occur.

Management

Management of cervical incompetence is achieved primarily through a surgical procedure, a cerclage, to suture the cervix. The suture is usually removed in the late third trimester of pregnancy. Contraindications to this procedure include active vaginal bleeding, rupture of membranes, active labor, chorioamnionitis, and major congenital abnormalities of the fetus (Creasy et al., 2004). Complications such as rupture of the membranes and ensuing intrauterine

infection and preterm labor may occur with surgical intervention (Hankins et al., 1995).

Nursing Care

Nursing care for the client with an incompetent cervix includes obtaining a complete history of the events of current and past pregnancies. The client should be observed for signs of impending delivery, such as rupture of membranes, active bleeding, and regular painful uterine contractions. Emotional support is a key element of nursing care because these clients and families often are very anxious about the well-being of the fetus. The nurse should explain the plan of care and all procedures to the client and family.

Preterm Labor and Premature Rupture of Membranes

Preterm labor is defined as labor that occurs after 20 weeks and before 37 completed weeks' gestation. Premature rupture of membranes (PROM) is defined as spontaneous rupture of membranes before the onset of labor. Preterm premature rupture of membranes (PPROM) is PROM before 37 weeks' gestation.

Incidence

Preterm births account for approximately 8% to 15% of births in the United States; worldwide, 13 million premature infants are born, accounting for the overwhelming majority of perinatal morbidity and mortality (Althabe, Carroli, Leder, Belizan, & Althabe, 1999).

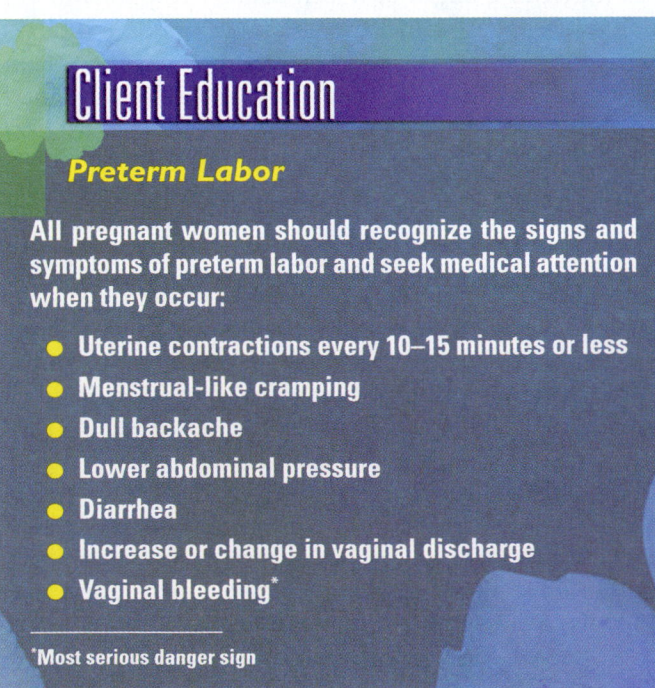

Client Education

Preterm Labor

All pregnant women should recognize the signs and symptoms of preterm labor and seek medical attention when they occur:

- Uterine contractions every 10–15 minutes or less
- Menstrual-like cramping
- Dull backache
- Lower abdominal pressure
- Diarrhea
- Increase or change in vaginal discharge
- Vaginal bleeding*

*Most serious danger sign

Clinical Presentation

Despite vast improvements in obstetric care, the ability to predict which clients will develop preterm labor, and therefore to have an impact on its prevention, has been unsuccessful (Althabe et al., 1999). Numerous risk factors for preterm labor have been cited, including the following: multiple gestation; previous preterm labor; exposure to DES; more than one second-trimester abortion; infectious causes, such as bacterial vaginosis; pyelonephritis; cigarette smoking; poor maternal weight gain; history of cervical conization; maternal age; and maternal parity (Schieve et al., 2000; McGregor & French, 2000; Kyrklund-Blomberg & Cnattingius, 1998). The most frequently cited risk factor is a history of a previous spontaneous preterm delivery. These clients have an increased risk for preterm delivery in their current pregnancy of about 2.5 times that of a normal pregnancy. A previous preterm delivery caused by PPROM and preterm labor are significantly associated with a similar event in the current pregnancy (Mercer et al., 1999).

The client who has preterm labor may present with a variety of complaints. Common sign and symptoms of preterm labor include uterine contractions (felt or unfelt), menstrual-like cramps, continuous dull backache, pressure sensation in the pelvic area or thighs, diarrhea or intestinal cramps, increased vaginal discharge, and vaginal bleeding.

Complications of preterm labor to the mother are related largely to the tocolytic agents used in treatment. See the Nursing Alert for common medications, side effects, and complications.

Infants with birth weights of less than 1,500 g or gestational age under 34 weeks have greatly increased risks for RDS, intraventricular hemorrhage, and necrotizing enterocolitis (NEC). Long-term complications of preterm birth include bronchopulmonary dysplasia, cerebral palsy, developmental delays, blindness, and deafness (Cunningham et al., 2001). Whereas the incidence of these major complications decreases in babies born after 32 weeks' gestation, other complications, such as feeding difficulties and hypothermia, occur frequently until 35 weeks' gestation and can prolong hospitalization (Seubert, Stetzer, Wolfe, & Treadwell, 1999). The preterm low-birth-weight infant generally is not discharged from the hospital until 35 to 37 postconceptional weeks, or approximately the time of the infant's original due date (Rawlings & Scott, 1996).

Nursing Alert

Common Tocolytic Medications and Potential Complications

Magnesium sulfate:
- Respiratory depression or arrest
- Pulmonary edema
- Hypotension
- Cardiac arrest
- Profound hypotension

Beta-adrenergics (ritodrine (Yutopar), terbutaline (Brethine)):
- Hyperglycemia
- Hypokalemia
- Hypotension
- Arrhythmias
- Pulmonary edema/congestive heart failure—this is the most serious side effect
- Myocardial ischemia with chest pain
- Tachycardia (maternal and fetal)—this is a frequent side effect
- Tremors and restlessness

Indomethacin (Indocin):
- Gastrointestinal symptoms
- Renal failure
- Hepatitis
- Premature closure of the ductus arteriosus, necrotizing enterocolitis, and intracranial hemorrhage in the fetus or neonate
- Bleeding (bruises, GI tract, gums, etc.)

Nifedipine (Procardia):
- Profound hypotension
- Possible decrease in uteroplacental perfusion
- Flushing
- Headache

Nursing Alert

Magnesium Sulfate Therapy

Magnesium sulfate is used as a tocolytic for management of preterm labor. It acts as a smooth muscle relaxant by substituting magnesium for calcium at the cellular level.

Management

The treatment for preterm labor is intended to improve outcomes for neonates by prolonging the pregnancy or by affecting their adaptation to the extrauterine environment. Treatment options are highly individualized and depend on physician and client preference, gestational age of the fetus, and additional medical or obstetric complications.

The medical therapies for preterm labor range from nonintervention to the use of tocolytic agents to stop preterm contractions. IV hydration and sedation may be ordered when the client initially presents with signs and symptoms of preterm labor. When labor does not progress the client may be admitted to the hospital for a period of observation. Once discharged, she most likely will be placed on bed rest or asked to modify physical activities. The physician may order antibiotics to treat presumed or confirmed infections that can be causative factors in preterm labor. Corticosteroids may be given to the client to enhance fetal lung maturity after 24 weeks' and before 34 weeks' gestation. The corticosteroid is given weekly until 34 weeks. Betamethasone (Celestone) and dexamethasone (Decadron) worsen diabetes and hypertension and increase the risk of UTIs. In the case of ongoing preterm labor, the client may receive tocolytic medication given in an attempt to stop uterine contractions.

Nursing Care

Nursing care for the woman experiencing preterm labor includes prompt and thorough assessment of the client on presentation to the hospital, obtaining or assisting in collection of laboratory specimens, administration of prescribed medications and therapies, and client education. Nursing assessment should include taking vital signs, including temperature; assessing the fetal heart rate; evaluating uterine activity; and obtaining a history of the pregnancy and events associated with the onset of the current symptoms. The client should be asked about the presence of vaginal bleeding and rupture of membranes. Common laboratory tests specific for assessment of the client who has preterm labor include urinalysis, urine culture and sensitivity, cervical cultures, and CBC. The nurse must be familiar with the actions, contraindications, and potential side effects of common medications administered in the treatment of preterm labor. The tocolytic agents frequently ordered may have serious side effects (Table 11-1).

The client who is at risk for delivering a preterm infant often is very anxious about the risks to the infant and herself and about the medical therapies ordered. Coincidental concerns often exist about separation from family and loss of income during prolonged hospitalization.

Occupational or recreational therapy often is helpful in providing diversional activities during prolonged hospitalization. Social services can be of assistance in financial, housing, and transportation concerns for the client and family.

The nurse should provide information for the client regarding the plan of care for both mother and infant to enable decision making and reduce anxiety. It may be helpful for the client and family to speak to a health care provider from the nursery about the care planned for the neonate in the event of delivery.

Postterm Pregnancy

Postterm pregnancy is defined as a pregnancy that is greater than 42 postmenstrual weeks' gestation (Creasy et al., 2004).

Incidence

Approximately 4% to 14% of pregnancies are postterm and are associated with increased fetal morbidity and

Table 11-1 Side Effects and Complications of Tocolytic Medications		
MEDICATION	**SIDE EFFECT**	**COMPLICATIONS**
Beta-adrenergics (ritodrine, terbutaline)	Tachycardia, shortness of breath, chest pain, nausea and vomiting, diarrhea, anxiety	Pulmonary edema, arrhythmias, hyperglycemia, hypokalemia, hypotension, myocardial ischemia
Calcium channel blockers	Flushing, tachycardia	Profound hypotension, possible decrease in uteroplacental perfusion
Magnesium sulfate	Flushing, drowsiness, muscle weakness, blurred vision, nausea and vomiting	Pulmonary edema, respiratory depression or arrest, cardiac arrest, profound hypotension **Neonate:** hypermagnesemia
Prostaglandin inhibitors	Epigastric pain, nausea and vomiting	Gastrointestinal bleeding, renal failure **Fetus or neonate:** premature closure of the ductus arteriosus, necrotizing enterocolitis, intracranial hemorrhage

mortality (Creasy et al., 2004). Some risks to the fetus include umbilical cord compression because of decreased amniotic fluid (oligohydramnios), meconium aspiration, large for gestational age fetus (macrosomia), and shoulder dystocia. The frequency of labor induction and cesarean section delivery is increased in this group of postterm clients (Cunningham et al., 2001).

Management

The postterm pregnancy may be managed initially with antepartum fetal testing beginning at 41 to 42 weeks' gestation (Creasy et al., 2004). Antepartum fetal surveillance tests include a nonstress test, an oxytocin challenge test, and a biophysical profile and may be scheduled weekly or twice weekly. Clients also are asked to monitor fetal movement and to notify the health care provider if they note a significant decrease in fetal activity. Induction of labor often is ordered when antepartum testing is not reassuring or the pregnancy exceeds 42 weeks' gestation.

Nursing Care

Nursing care specific to the postterm pregnant client usually includes assessing fetal well-being by performance of fetal surveillance testing, and performing induction of labor as ordered by the provider.

Antepartum surveillance tests should be carried out according to unit protocol or physician's order and the results should be reported to the physician.

Induction of labor should be performed according to unit protocol or physician's order. As with administration of any medication, the nurse must be knowledgeable about the actions, contraindications, and potential side effects of the medications that are ordered. Labor can be induced by various medications, hydrophilic agents, or stripping membranes. Medications such as prostaglandins cause cervical ripening and uterine contractions. These agents should be used cautiously with lung, eye, liver, and kidney disorders. Hydrophilic or moisture-attracting absorbent products (such as Laminaria) produce dilation by absorbing moisture from the cervix. Oxytocin (Pitocin), another medication, stimulates uterine contractions and is used for induction and augmentation purposes.

The postterm client and family often are anxious. Client education is a key aspect of nursing care and can provide some reassurance. The plan of care, including tests, procedures, and ordered medications, should be thoroughly explained to the client and family.

DISORDERS OF AMNIOTIC FLUID VOLUME

Disorders of amniotic fluid volume include polyhydramnios and oligohydramnios. Each condition can be a sign of negative fetal outcomes.

Polyhydramnios

The average amount of amniotic fluid at term is approximately 800 mL. **Polyhydramnios**, also referred to as **hydramnios**, is diagnosed when more than 1,500 to 2,000 mL of amniotic fluid has accumulated (Creasy et al., 2004).

Clinical Presentation

Amniotic fluid volume may be affected by a number of factors. During the second trimester of pregnancy the fetus swallows and urinates amniotic fluid. In most cases of severe polyhydramnios a fetal anomaly is present. These anomalies are generally those of the gastrointestinal (GI) system, inhibiting the ability of the fetus to swallow fluid, or the central nervous system (CNS), wherein increased volumes of amniotic fluid can be transferred from the spinal defect into the amniotic cavity (Cunningham et al., 2001).

The largely overdistended uterus may put pressure on the surrounding organs. In cases of excessive polyhydramnios the pregnant woman may experience dyspnea secondary to pressure on the lungs and edema of the lower extremities and vulva because of decreased venous return. The client with polyhydramnios is at increased risk for preterm delivery secondary to contractions occurring with uterine distension.

Management

The client who has mild to moderate polyhydramnios usually does not require treatment. In severe cases of polyhydramnios that cause dyspnea or pain the client may be hospitalized. In these cases an amniocentesis may be performed to relieve these symptoms. In this procedure a catheter is placed through the maternal abdomen into the amniotic cavity and is attached to a IV tubing set, which drains amniotic fluid into a container placed at floor level. The rate of fluid drainage is controlled to avoid rapid decompression (Cunningham et al., 2001). This procedure can provide immediate symptomatic relief for the client.

Nursing Care

Nursing care for the client with polyhydramnios includes monitoring the client for symptoms of dyspnea, abdominal pain, uterine contractions, and severe edema of the lower extremities and vulva. When a therapeutic amniocentesis is performed, the nurse assists the physician in the procedure by positioning the client and helping with the mechanism of the drainage apparatus. The nurse monitors the rate of fluid drainage, amount and characteristics of the fluid, and response of mother and fetus. The nurse ensures that the client has an opportunity to ask questions and understands the procedure. FHR is measured before, during, and after the procedure.

Oligohydramnios

Oligohydramnios can occur as a result of premature rupture of membranes or may not have a clear cause. Regardless of the cause, the condition may require a decision regarding whether the fetus should remain in utero.

Clinical Presentation

When the amniotic fluid volume decreases to as little as 500 mL, the condition is termed **oligohydramnios** (Creasy et al., 2004). Any condition that prevents the fetus from making urine or that blocks the entry of urine into the amniotic sac can cause oligohydramnios. Leaking of the bag of water or frank rupture of membranes also may cause oligohydramnios. Hypertension in pregnancy, uteroplacental insufficiency, and diabetes also are factors associated with oligohydramnios in late pregnancy (Cunningham et al., 2001). The diagnosis of oligohydramnios is made by ultrasonographic examination because the client will have no presenting symptoms.

Oligohydramnios more frequently develops late in pregnancy. The volume of fluid normally is diminished after 35 weeks' gestation. The development of oligohydramnios in early pregnancy may be an ominous sign (Cunningham et al., 2001; Creasy et al., 2004).

The risks of oligohydramnios to the fetus can be quite serious. Umbilical cord compression may occur, diminishing perfusion to the fetus. Adhesions can develop between the fetus and the amnion, which can cause serious fetal deformities and possibly amputation of fetal parts. The fetus also may suffer from musculoskeletal deformities as it is compressed in utero (Cunningham et al., 2001). Pulmonary hypoplasia possibly related to mechanical restriction of the fetal chest can occur in the presence of very low amniotic fluid levels (Creasy et al., 2004).

Management

The client who has oligohydramnios may be managed outside the hospital setting with serial ultrasonographic evaluations and fetal surveillance testing. Once delivery is inevitable and the membranes have ruptured, an **amnioinfusion** may be performed to replace fluid in the amniotic cavity (Creasy et al., 2004). In this procedure crystalloid fluid is infused through an intrauterine catheter placed through the cervix into the uterine cavity. The infusion is administered in a controlled manner to prevent overdistension of the uterus.

Nursing Care

The client who has oligohydramnios and a viable fetus and is not hospitalized will require periodic evaluation of fetal well-being. Nursing care may include fetal surveillance testing, such as a nonstress test or contraction stress test. In the intrapartum period the nurse observes for fetal intolerance of labor and may assist in the performance of amnioinfusion. When amnioinfusion is ordered the nurse infuses fluid into the client's uterus by way of an intrauterine catheter at a prescribed rate. The return of amniotic fluid onto the bed linen and maternal and fetal tolerance of the procedure should be observed and documented. The FHR is measured before, during, and after the procedure. The nurse should provide an explanation of the plan of care to the client and family.

HIGH-RISK FETAL CONDITIONS

Fetal conditions that increase the risk for negative fetal outcomes include multiple gestation, Rh isoimmunization and ABO incompatibility, and nonimmune hydrops fetalis, severe edema of the fetus that is not the result of isoimmunization.

Multiple Gestation

Multiple gestation increases pregnancy risks because of the high risks for preterm labor and delivery and conditions related to prematurity.

Incidence

The incidence of multiple births in the United States is relatively infrequent yet represents a large proportion of poor pregnancy outcomes. Multiple gestation pregnancies are at increased risk for preterm delivery and intrauterine fetal demise. Maternal morbidity is significantly increased in these pregnancies (Creasy et al., 2004).

The incidence of twins, triplets, and higher-order multiples has dramatically increased because of the widespread use of fertility drugs and advanced reproductive techniques (ACOG, 1998). Twins frequently are the result of two separate ova, called **dizygotic** or "fraternal" twins. The incidence of this type of twinning is highly variable according to maternal age, race, parity, and heredity. Twins resulting from a single fertilized ovum that then divides are called **monozygotic** or "identical" twins; the incidence of identical twins is about 1 in 250 births (Cunningham et al., 2001). The process is the same in higher-order multiples, with quadruplets being the result of either one or four fertilized ova.

Clinical Presentation

In the second trimester a discrepancy between the measured fundal height and gestational age of the fetus often is the first clue that there may be a multifetal pregnancy. The diagnosis of a multiple gestation pregnancy generally is made or confirmed by ultrasonographic examination.

Multiple gestation pregnancies are at increased risk for many complications. Early pregnancy loss is more common in a multifetal pregnancy. Multiple gestations also have a greater incidence of low birth weight secondary to intrauterine growth restriction or preterm delivery (ACOG, 1998b).

Maternal complications in a multiple gestation pregnancy can be significant. The incidence of pregnancy-induced hypertension (PIH), gestational diabetes, postpartum hemorrhage, anemia, urinary tract infections (UTIs), endometritis, and need for cesarean delivery are increased in multifetal pregnancies. Among parous women, multiple gestation is associated with a twofold increase in risk of death compared with a singleton pregnancy (Conde-Agudelo, Belizan, & Lindmark, 2000; Myatt & Miodovnik, 1999).

Significant weight differences can develop in twins in the second or third trimester of pregnancy, with one twin being growth restricted. The incidence of fetal death in these discordant twin pregnancies is greatly increased (Cunningham et al., 2001).

Management

The client with a multifetal pregnancy likely will be followed throughout her pregnancy with serial ultrasonographic examinations to assess for fetal growth and development. Fetal surveillance testing often is initiated late in the second trimester. The client who develops signs and symptoms of preterm labor and whose fetus develops complications often will be managed in the hospital setting, which allows for closer and more frequent observation.

The intrapartum period can be a particularly risk-filled time in the multifetal pregnancy. These pregnancies are at increased risk for complications, such as fetal malpresentation, dysfunctional labor, PIH, abruptio placentae, umbilical cord prolapse, cesarean delivery, and endometritis (Conde-Agudelo et al., 2000; Myatt & Miodovnik, 1999). In the intrapartum period, electronic fetal monitoring is employed to evaluate for fetal tolerance to labor or evidence of cord prolapse. After vaginal delivery of the first twin the client is reassessed to determine if vaginal delivery of the second twin is possible and imminent. Vaginal delivery of the second twin may be minutes to hours after the first delivery. The client may require cesarean section for the second twin if it is in a nonvertex position (Creasy et al., 2004).

Nursing Care

Outpatient nursing care for the client with multifetal pregnancy focuses on assessment of the client at each visit for signs and symptoms of possible complications, such as threatened abortion, PIH, and preterm labor. Once the decision is made to initiate fetal surveillance testing, the nurse performs nonstress tests or contraction stress tests.

Clients who are admitted to the hospital for complications such as PIH or preterm labor receive care as discussed in the applicable sections of this chapter. The client admitted for labor and planned vaginal delivery usually receives continuous electronic fetal monitoring to provide assessment data for both uterine activity and fetal tolerance to labor. Adequate personnel to attend to the mother and to each neonate should be available at the time of delivery. The client and family should be informed of the potential for cesarean delivery and all questions should be answered.

Rh Isoimmunization and ABO Incompatibility

Immunization, or sensitization, occurs when fetal blood enters the maternal circulation, causing antibodies to be formed in the maternal blood. Once formed, these antibodies are able to cross the placenta into the fetal circulation and attack fetal erythrocytes, with resulting hemolysis. Rh sensitization is the most common and most significant cause of maternal immunization and hemolysis in the fetus or newborn (Bowman, 1999). In this process an Rh-negative mother, or a mother with absent $Rh_o(D)$ antigen, who is carrying an Rh-positive fetus forms anti-D antibodies whenever fetal erythrocytes enter the maternal bloodstream. A very small amount of Rh-positive fetal blood in the maternal bloodstream can result in the formation of antibodies (Duffy, 1999). The amount of hemolysis that results varies, with severe hemolysis causing fetal anemia. The severely affected fetus develops **hydrops fetalis** in which the fetus and placenta have severe edema; the fetus also may develop pleural and cardiac effusions, cardiac enlargement, hepatomegaly, and splenomegaly (Cunningham et al., 2001).

Clinical Presentation

The injection of fetal blood into the maternal circulation occurs most commonly at the time of delivery but may occur during the course of the pregnancy. A significant number of women who become Rh immunized do so at about 28 weeks' gestation or within 3 days after delivery. Approximately 75% of women have some evidence of a transplacental hemorrhage during the pregnancy or in the immediate postpartum period (Bowman, 1999). Sensitization may occur in the antepartum period after abortion; after an invasive procedure, such as amniocentesis; or in the disruption of the placenta with abruption or placenta previa (Cunningham et al., 2001). Once antibodies are formed, subsequent pregnancies are at risk for hemolytic disease of the fetus and newborn.

ABO incompatibility is a less serious form of isoimmunization that may occur when a mother who has type O blood is pregnant with a fetus who has type A or B blood. The mother may form antibodies that can lead to hemolysis in the fetus and neonate. These infants may develop hyperbilirubinemia, requiring phototherapy (Bowman, 1999).

Management

Pregnant women undergo routine screening for sensitization at the first prenatal visit when blood is drawn for blood typing, determination of Rh factor, an antibody titer test, or indirect Coombs test (ACOG, 1996b). The presence of anti-Rh_o(D) antibodies on the laboratory test results indicates sensitization has occurred and alerts the clinician to the possibility of an affected fetus. The fetus is monitored throughout the pregnancy, and the mother has repeated titer tests. A titer of 1:8 or higher usually indicates the need for further testing and evaluation (Cunningham et al., 2001).

The client who has titer values that are increasing will undergo repeated ultrasonography to evaluate fetal growth, amniocentesis, or percutaneous blood sampling to evaluate fetal condition. In an **amniocentesis** fluid is withdrawn from the uterus with a needle to evaluate for the presence and amount of bilirubin, which is evidence of hemolysis. Amniotic fluid with high levels of bilirubin may indicate a fetus who needs immediate treatment to survive.

Percutaneous umbilical blood sampling (PUBS) is a direct sampling of fetal blood from the umbilical cord guided by ultrasonography. PUBS is typically performed only in a regional perinatal center with a level 3 nursery. The severely affected fetus may undergo intrauterine fetal transfusion. This is accomplished by transfusion of blood into the fetal peritoneal cavity or directly into the umbilical vein (ACOG, 1996b). Intravascular transfusion into the umbilical vessels is associated with good long-term outcomes (Grab, Paulus, Bommer, Buck, & Terinde, 1999).

Preterm delivery may be necessary for the severely affected fetus. The neonate is evaluated at birth for severity of hemolytic disease of the newborn and may require treatment ranging from phototherapy to exchange transfusion.

The client with negative indirect antibody test results on entry into prenatal care usually is retested at 28 weeks' gestation. If the test results remain negative, at that time the mother is given a prophylactic dose of Rh_o(D) immune globulin (RhoGAM) (ACOG, 1999a). Administration of this Rh antibody can prevent an active antibody response by providing passive immunity to the mother (Bowman, 1999).

In the postpartum period, clients who are Rh-negative are considered for postpartum administration of RhoGAM. Mothers of infants who are Rh-positive will receive RhoGAM as prophylaxis within 72 hours after delivery. Women experiencing a first-trimester pregnancy loss or those undergoing invasive procedures, such as amniocentesis or fetal blood sampling, also should receive RhoGAM (ACOG, 1999a).

Nursing Care

In the antepartum period the nurse should evaluate routine maternal laboratory tests and alert the primary care provider of the maternal blood type in the Rho(D)-negative client. It is very important that RhoGAM be administered as ordered at approximately 28 weeks' gestation. The administration of RhoGAM should be documented in the client's medical records.

Clients who are determined to be sensitized will need thorough explanation of the implications of Rh isoimmunization and the plan of care for the pregnancy. The invasive procedures described previously that may be performed in the severely affected fetus are very anxiety-provoking for most clients. The nurse should provide support to the mother and family as the mother undergoes these procedures.

In the postpartum period the nurse obtains maternal and neonatal laboratory values, assesses the need for RhoGAM, and administers the prophylactic dose as ordered by the primary care provider.

HYPERTENSION

Terminology used in describing hypertension in pregnancy has changed over many years of studying this disease process. Hypertension as defined by the National High Blood Pressure Education Program Working Group on High Blood Pressure in Pregnancy (2000) is a blood pressure 140 mmHg systolic or higher or 90 mmHg diastolic or higher. The classifications of hypertension are as follows:

- **Chronic hypertension** is defined as hypertension that occurs before pregnancy or is diagnosed before 20 weeks' gestation. Hypertension diagnosed for the first time during pregnancy that persists beyond the postpartum period also is classified as chronic hypertension.

- **Pre-eclampsia**-eclampsia is a pregnancy-specific syndrome usually occurring after 20 weeks' gestation. The diagnosis is determined by (1) increased blood pressure, over 140 mmHg systolic or over 90 mmHg diastolic in a woman who has had normal blood pressure before 20 weeks' gestation; and (2) proteinuria, which is defined as more than 0.3 g of protein in a 24-hour urine collection. **Eclampsia** is the occurrence of seizures in a pregnant woman who has pre-eclampsia that cannot be attributed to another cause.

Reflections from a Family

I was really excited to find out I was pregnant. My husband and I had planned a family for a long time. Then my wonderful pregnancy turned into a horror show when I developed pre-eclampsia. The doctor was not able to control my condition at home. I was admitted to the hospital at 32 weeks' gestation and was told I would need to stay in the hospital on bed rest until my due date. I cannot explain how that changed my life. I went from being happy and excited to being full of dread and fear. Luckily, the nurses on the unit where I was hospitalized were able to teach me what to expect. It reduced my fear tremendously.

Table 11-2   Potential Complications of Pregnancy-Induced Hypertension

ORGAN OR SYSTEM	POTENTIAL COMPLICATIONS
Maternal	
Cardiopulmonary	Pulmonary edema, hypertensive crisis, stroke
Hematologic	Thrombocytopenia, hemorrhage, disseminated intravascular coagulation
Hepatic	Hematoma, rupture
Neurologic	Retinal detachment (rarely), cerebral edema, seizures, cerebral hemorrhage, coma
Renal	Decreased glomerular filtration, increased plasma uric acid and creatinine, necrosis (rarely)
Fetal	Intrauterine growth restriction, hypoxia, intrauterine death, prematurity

■ Pre-eclampsia superimposed on chronic hypertension is "highly likely" with the findings of (1) women with hypertension and no proteinuria before 20 weeks' gestation that have new onset of proteinuria; and (2) women who have hypertension and proteinuria before 20 weeks' gestation who develop any of the following: (a) sudden increase in proteinuria, (b) sudden increase in blood pressure, (c) thrombocytopenia, (d) increase in alanine aminotransferase or aspartate aminotransferase.

■ Gestational hypertension is used to describe blood pressure elevation occurring for the first time after midpregnancy and without proteinuria. This diagnosis may change to that of pre-eclampsia if other symptoms develop. The definitive diagnosis of gestational hypertension can only be made if the hypertension has resolved after 12 weeks postpartum.

Incidence

Hypertension occurs in 6% to 8% of pregnancies and is the second leading cause of maternal mortality in the United States, accounting for 15% to 18% of deaths (ACOG, 1996a; Berg, Atrash, Koonin, & Tucker, 1996). Complications of PIH are outlined in Table 11-2.

Clinical Presentation

Many theories regarding the cause of PIH have been proposed but none proven. PIH has been shown to occur more commonly in the primipara, in women with pregestational diabetes mellitus, in multiple gestation pregnancies, and in older women who have an increased incidence of chronic hypertension (Abu-Heija, Jallad, & Abukteish, 2000). The only known "cure" for PIH is delivery of both fetus and placenta.

Pre-eclampsia is a disease characterized by generalized vasospasm, a significant decrease in circulating blood volume, and an activation of the coagulation system. The end result of these changes is hypertension, decreased perfusion, and resultant ischemia particularly to the placenta, kidneys, liver, and brain (National High Blood Pressure Education Program Working Group, 2000).

The fetus may be significantly impacted by decreased uteroplacental perfusion. In cases of long-standing hypertension the fetus is at increased risk for mortality and morbidity, such as intrauterine growth restriction. The additional complication of superimposed pre-eclampsia significantly increases the risk to the fetus (National High Blood Pressure Education Program Working Group, 2000). Delivery of the fetus may be indicated by worsening maternal or fetal condition, placing the fetus of the client who has pre-eclampsia at increased risk for low birth weight and prematurity.

Renal blood flow and the glomerular filtration rate are decreased in pre-eclampsia. Proteinuria is a common finding in pre-eclampsia but is highly variable from hour to hour and, thus, is not a sensitive marker for severity of the disease process. Oliguria may occur in severe disease. Renal insufficiency is rarely severe enough to cause permanent damage, and the client usually will have complete recovery of renal function after delivery (Creasy et al., 2004).

The coagulation effects of pre-eclampsia may include thrombocytopenia, a decrease in platelets to less than 100,000, placing the client at increased risk for hemorrhage. This coagulation problem may occur at any time during pregnancy. Symptoms may antecede blood pressure elevation.

HELLP syndrome is a complication of pre-eclampsia/eclampsia. In 1982, Weinstein first described 29 cases of severe pre-eclampsia/eclampsia complicated by hemolytic anemia, elevated liver enzymes, and low platelet counts. This syndrome was given the acronym HELLP to describe its clinical presentation of Hemolysis of red blood cells, Elevated Liver enzymes, and Low Platelet count. Since 1982, numerous cases of this syndrome have been reported.

Barton and Sibai (2001) discuss a classification system for HELLP syndrome. Class 1 is the most severe and occurs when the platelet count reaches a low of <50,000 per mm³. Class 2 occurs when the platelet count reaches a low between 51,000 and 100,000 per mm³. Class 3 occurs when the platelet count reaches a low of 101,000 to 150,000 per mm³. These classes are used to predict postpartum disease recovery, risk of recurrence of HELLP syndrome, perinatal outcome, and the need for plasmaphoresis.

At the University of Tennessee in Memphis, where much research has been done related to PIH and its complications, they have developed the following criteria for the diagnosis of HELLP syndrome. The criteria for hemolysis are abnormal peripheral blood smear; a total bilirubin of 1.2 mgd/L or greater; and lactic dehydrogenase (LDH) of 600 U/L. To meet the criteria for elevated liver enzymes requires serum aspartate aminotransferase of ≥ 70 U/L; and an LDH of >600 U/L (Barton & Sibai, 2001).

The incidence of HELLP syndrome is significantly higher in the Caucasian population and multiparous women as well as among pre-eclamptics who are being managed conservatively (Barton & Sibai, 2001).

Clinical manifestations of HELLP syndrome include remoteness from term with right upper quadrant pain, nausea and vomiting, and nonspecific flu-like symptoms. Clients with HELLP syndrome usually exhibit significant weight gain and generalized edema. They usually have severe hypertension.

Pathophysiology of HELLP syndrome involves hemolytic anemia; this type of anemia can occur in other conditions besides HELLP syndrome and may confuse the diagnosis. The elevated liver enzymes are a result of

Magnesium Sulfate (MgSO₄)

Pharmacologic Class	Pregnancy category A
Therapeutic Class	Anticonvulsant
How Supplied	50% (4 mEq/mL)
Indications for Use	Prevents or controls seizures in pre-eclamsia/eclampsia (primary action); smooth muscle relaxant for preterm labor (secondary action)
Chemical Effect	Blocks release of acetylcholine at the myoneural junction
Therapeutic Effect	CNS depressant
Dosage	Loading dose of 4–6 g IV, followed by a maintenance infusion of 2–4 g/h
Side Effects and Adverse Reactions	Flushing, sweating, nausea, vomiting, hypotension, muscle weakness, CNS depression
Contraindications	Heart block or myocardial damage
Nursing Considerations	Position client in left lateral position and maintain electronic fetal monitoring to assess fetal status. Monitor blood pressure, respiratory rate, and deep tendon reflexes. Observe closely for signs of magnesium toxicity as evidenced by absent deep tendon reflexes and/or respiratory rate less than 12 breaths/minute. Monitor intake and output, especially in clients with decreased renal function. 10% calcium gluconate should be readily available for emergency use.
Client Teaching	Teach about side effects and importance of bed rest.
Laboratory Finding	Monitor magnesium levels (therapeutic range is 4–6 mEq/L). Therapeutic serum levels are 4–6 mEq/L.

liver involvement. The most common liver lesion is liver necrosis. Periportal hemorrhage is associated with fibrin deposition. Steatosis or fat degradations is associated significantly with abnormalities in platelet count (Barton & Sibai, 2001).

Management of HELLP syndrome involves stabilization of the maternal condition, evaluation of fetal well-being, and estimation of fetal lung maturity. Management may be aggressive or conservative. Aggressive management includes delivery of the infant by cesarean section as quickly as the maternal condition is stabilized.

Conservative management includes use of antihypertensives and MgSO$_4$. The predominant reason for terminating the pregnancy is fetal distress or fetal demise. Usually the pregnancy is not terminated due to maternal conditions. Potential risks associated with conservative management are abruption of the placenta, pulmonary edema, acute renal failure, eclampsia, perinatal death, and maternal death (Barton & Sibai, 2001).

Complications of HELLP syndrome may include delayed wound closure, eclampsia, and hematoma or infarction of the liver. If a hepatic hematoma occurs, there is potential for liver rupture. Other severe complications include DIC, acute renal failure, severe ascites, pulmonary edema, pulmonary effusions, cerebral edema, retinal detachment, and laryngeal edema (Barton & Sibai, 2001).

HELLP syndrome can occur in the antepartum or postpartum period. If the woman survives this complicated pregnancy, there is a 19–27% risk of developing recurrent HELLP syndrome in future pregnancies (Barton & Sibai, 2001).

Management

Clients who develop mild elevation of blood pressure in pregnancy may be managed conservatively by the physician and placed on bed rest at home, with increased frequency of office visits and laboratory evaluations (National Heart, Lung and Blood Institute, 2000). Once the client is admitted to the hospital for evaluation and management of pre-eclampsia, the course of treatment is highly individualized and based on disease severity. A client with mild pre-eclampsia may be managed on an antepartum unit, with evaluation for signs and symptoms of worsening disease, fetal evaluation, and laboratory testing. In the case of worsening or severe pre-eclampsia the client often is managed with administration of magnesium sulfate (see drug box), frequent targeted assessments, laboratory tests, electronic fetal monitoring if indicated by the gestational age, and possibly the induction of labor. Those clients who are more severely affected are likely to be found on the labor and delivery unit where they can receive more intensive nursing care.

Hydralazine (Apresoline)

Pharmacologic Class	Pregnancy category A
Therapeutic Class	Vasodilator
How Supplied	10, 25, 50, 100 mg tablets and IV use
Indications for Use	Controls high blood pressure
Chemical Effect	Directly dilates arterioles
Therapeutic Effect	Decreases arteriolar spasms to produce vasodilation and a decrease in blood pressure.
Dosage	5–10 mg by IV push over 10 minues. Repeat doses may be ordered according to levels of blood pressure decrease.
Side Effects and Adverse Reactions	Tachycardia, hypotension, dizziness, headache, tingling of the extremities, and disorientation
Contraindications	Pheochromocytoma or aortic aneurysm
Nursing Considerations	Position client in left lateral position and maintain electronic fetal monitoring to assess fetal status. Check maternal blood pressure every minute for the first 5 minutes following administration and then every 5 minutes for 30 minutes.
Client Teaching	Explain the need for monitoring heart rate and blood pressure and maintaining a low-stimulus environment.
Laboratory Finding	None

Nursing Tip — Targeted Assessments in Clients with Pre-eclampsia

- Blood pressure measurement
- Intake and output measurements
- Physical assessments for:

    Presence and location of edema

    Deep tendon reflexes

    Presence of headache and visual changes

    Presence of nausea, vomiting, and epigastric or right upper quadrant pain

- Fetal evaluation appropriate for gestational age and fetal well-being
- Proteinuria is most accurately monitored with 24-hour urine collections. Urine dipsticks are unreliable for evaluating proteinuria related to pre-eclampsia.

Nursing Care

Skilled nursing assessments are necessary for the pregnant woman with pre-eclampsia. A thorough physical assessment should be performed at the start of each shift, followed by frequent targeted assessments. See Procedure 11-1 for assessment of deep tendon reflexes. Magnesium sulfate, antihypertensive agents such as hydralazine (Apresoline) (see Drug box), and medications for cervical ripening and induction of labor are administered as ordered. The nurse must be familiar with the actions of, side effects of, and complications that may arise from the use of these medications. Laboratory tests should be obtained as ordered, and abnormal results should be reported to the physician promptly. Significant findings from nursing assessments also should be reported promptly (see the Nursing Tip on targeted assessments).

Client and family education should begin as soon as the diagnosis is made. Education should include an explanation of the disease process; signs and symptoms of worsening disease; proposed course of treatment, including physical and laboratory assessments; medications; potential complications for the client and fetus; and the plan for delivery, as indicated. If the infant is to be delivered

PROCEDURE 11-1

Assessing Deep Tendon Reflexes (DTRs) during Magnesium Sulfate Therapy

Purpose

To assess the level of CNS depression associated with magnesium sulfate therapy.

Equipment

Reflex hammer

Action and Rationale

Hold the knee in a slightly flexed and very relaxed position. Briskly tap the patellar tendon with a reflex hammer just below the kneecap. Grade the response as 0 (no response), 1+ (sluggish), 2+ (normal), 3+ (brisk), or 4+ (hyperreflexic). *A decrease in response or absence of DTRs could indicate magnesium toxicity.*

Follow-up

Along with assessment of DTRs the nurse should assess blood pressure, pulse, respirations, and serum magnesium levels as ordered.

preterm, it is very important for the client and family to be made aware of the proposed plan of care for the baby.

ENDOCRINE DISORDERS

Endocrine disorders may predate pregnancy or be precipitated by pregnancy. Either way, these disorders can have profound effects on the pregnant woman and her fetus.

Diabetes

Diabetes has serious implications for the mother and fetus even though survival rates for both have improved dramatically over the past few decades.

Incidence

Diabetes results in complications in 2% to 3% of all pregnancies in the United States and is the most common medical complication in pregnancy (ACOG, 1994). Pregnancy outcomes for women with diabetes have improved dramatically since the beginning of the 20th century. Prediction of pregnancy outcome and timing of the delivery on an individual basis improved perinatal survival rates to about 85% by the late 1950s (Cunningham et al., 2001). The improvement in survival rates has now reached mortality rates similar to those in normal pregnancy after accounting for fetal malformations, which occur approximately four times more often in women with pregestational diabetes (ACOG, 1994). A decrease in the occurrence of perinatal demise is related to the ability to manage glucose levels within normal limits. Although death in the pregnant woman with diabetes is rare, the mortality rate is greatly increased compared with that of the general population. Death often is the result of diabetic ketoacidosis, concomitant hypertension or PIH, and complications associated with pyelonephritis (Cunningham et al., 2001).

Clinical Presentation

Diabetes is classified into three categories: **Type I diabetes mellitus**, or insulin-dependent diabetes; **Type II diabetes mellitus**, or non–insulin-dependent diabetes; and **gestational diabetes**, or diabetes diagnosed during pregnancy. Type I diabetes is an immune disorder in which the beta cells of the pancreas are destroyed, resulting in a lack of insulin secretion. This type of diabetes is most often diagnosed before the age of 30 years and requires lifelong insulin therapy and dietary management. Type II diabetes is characterized by abnormal insulin secretion and insulin resistance and most often is found in persons over the age of 40 years and in overweight individuals. This type of diabetes may be managed by diet alone or with oral hypoglycemic agents, although oral hypoglycemic agents are contraindicated during pregnancy. Gestational diabetes is the onset of abnormal carbohydrate metabolism diagnosed during pregnancy.

In general, pregnant women with any form of diabetes are at increased risk for additional maternal, fetal, and neonatal complications. Women with pregestational Type I diabetes are at increased risk for the development of pre-eclampsia and adverse neonatal outcomes, and the rates of these complications increase with disease severity. Hypoglycemia generally occurs with greater frequency and severity in early pregnancy (Inzucchi, 1999). This increase in hypoglycemia may be related to the strict glycemic control attempted in this population but also may be induced by nausea and vomiting associated with pregnancy and an increased sensitivity to insulin in the first trimester (Kendrick, 1999).

The pregnant woman who has diabetes has an increased incidence of UTIs. Screening for asymptomatic bacteriuria may reduce the impact of this complication. The incidence of hydramnios also is more common in women who have diabetes (Creasy et al., 2004).

Approximately 1% of diabetic pregnancies are affected by ketoacidosis. This complication is more common in the pregnant woman who has diabetes (Inzucchi, 1999). **Ketoacidosis** is diagnosed when glucose levels are greater than 300 mg/100 mL, positive serum ketones are at a level of 1:4, and metabolic acidosis is present (Creasy et al., 2004). This life-threatening condition may result from poor compliance, hyperemesis gravidarum, infection, or use of beta-sympathomimetic drugs or corticosteroids (Creasy et al., 2004). Diabetic ketoacidosis carries a perinatal mortality rate of approximately 20%, making prompt recognition and treatment critical (Cunningham et al., 2001).

The major causes of fetal death are congenital malformations, RDS, extreme prematurity, and unexplained stillbirth during the antepartum period (Creasy et al., 2004). Perinatal mortality, especially late fetal death, is significantly increased for the fetus of the woman with Type II diabetes.

From 15% to 45% of infants of mothers who have diabetes may be at increased risk for **macrosomia,** defined as a fetal weight of 4,000 g or higher and, therefore, may be at increased risk of a difficult delivery (Creasy et al., 2004).

Hypoglycemia occurs in approximately 30% to 50% of neonates and may be manifested immediately after delivery and for the next 24 hours of life. The incidence of hypoglycemia is increased significantly in infants of mothers with poor glucose control in the antepartum period and elevated glucose levels during labor (Inzucchi, 1999). Infants of mothers who have diabetes also may develop significant hypocalcemia in the first few days of life, the cause of which has not yet been clearly determined (Creasy et al., 2004). Hyperbilirubinemia is common, occurring in 20% to 25% of infants born to mothers who have diabetes.

Management

Screening for gestational diabetes is a routine test in pregnancy that usually is performed at 26 to 28 weeks' gestation. A serum glucose level of 140 mg/dL is considered abnormal and is followed up with a 3-hour glucose tolerance test.

Management of the pregnant woman who has diabetes is focused on tight glycemic control and evaluation of fetal well-being throughout the pregnancy. Prenatal visits are scheduled with greater frequency than in a normal pregnancy. Control of diet is an essential aspect of client management, and nutritional counseling regarding a diabetic diet is critical in this effort. The goals for glycemic control include fasting blood glucose levels consistently less than 105 mg/dL and 2-hour postprandial levels of less than 120 mg/dL (ACOG, 1994). The woman is asked to monitor her blood glucose levels several times daily and to record her dietary intake. Insulin therapy usually is begun when the prescribed diabetic diet does not result in a consistent fasting glucose level of less than 105 mg/dL or a 2-hour postprandial glucose of less than 120 mg/dL (ACOG, 1994). Women with poorly controlled diabetes or concomitant hypertension usually are hospitalized.

In the antepartum period the pregnant woman who has diabetes typically receives serial ultrasonographic evaluations of fetal growth and additional fetal surveillance testing, beginning at about 28 to 34 weeks' gestation (Creasy et al., 2004). Fetal surveillance may be ordered earlier than 26 weeks' gestation for clients with uncontrolled diabetes or those with additional complications (ACOG, 1994).

Delivery timing is individualized and ideally occurs around term. Maintaining maternal glucose levels within the normal range during the intrapartum period is important to avoid stimulation of the fetal pancreas with resulting fetal or neonatal hypoglycemia. In the client who has Type I diabetes, long-acting insulin is avoided during labor and an infusion of regular insulin along with an IV glucose infusion may be ordered to be administered by way of infusion pump (Creasy et al., 2004). Blood glucose is checked frequently during this period, and adjustments are made to the infusion. Additional boluses of insulin may be ordered as needed.

The increased insulin resistance occurring in the pregnant woman who has diabetes often resolves in a matter of a few hours after delivery. The insulin infusion generally is discontinued at the time of delivery, and many women will not require insulin during the first 24 hours. Because clients with Type I diabetes can have sharp decreases in insulin requirements during the first 24 hours after delivery, the insulin dose is titrated to measured blood glucose levels in the immediate postpartum period (Inzucchi, 1999).

Pregnant women who develop gestational diabetes may be counseled about the strong possibility of developing overt diabetes in the next 20 years (Buchanan & Kjos, 1999). It is important that a 1-hour glucose tolerance test be performed 6 to 8 weeks postpartally to ensure return to normoglycemia.

Nursing Care

Antepartum nursing care of the pregnant woman who has diabetes may include reviewing blood glucose values obtained between prenatal visits and obtaining blood glucose values at the time of the visit. All pregnant women should have routine screening of blood glucose levels. Nursing care also often will include performance of fetal surveillance testing, such as a nonstress test or an oxytocin challenge test, as ordered. Nonreassuring test results should be reported to the physician promptly.

In the intrapartum period the frequency of vital sign and fetal assessments is individualized based on the client's condition and the stage of labor. The nurse should be alert for signs of fetal intolerance to labor and report these to the physician promptly. A continuous insulin infusion may be ordered and serum or capillary blood glucose levels monitored as ordered by the physician during labor. The nurse should assess the client frequently for signs and symptoms of hypoglycemia and institute prompt administration of glucose according to unit protocol or physician's order. Hourly intake and output monitoring usually is initiated during the intrapartum period.

Education of the diabetic gravida and her family members is critical for the successful management of diabetes. The diagnosis of diabetes can be very frightening, and the volume of information needed to be imparted to the woman and family can be overwhelming. The plan of care for antepartum management should be reviewed carefully. Teaching regarding a culturally appropriate diabetic diet is very important and may need to be reinforced periodically. The dietician is a valuable member of the health care team and can assist in tailoring the diet for the client's preferences. Clients and family members also will need thorough instruction on blood glucose test-

Critical Thinking

Labor Assessment Skills

A woman with uncontrolled gestational diabetes is in labor at 39 weeks' gestation. The labor nurse should be alert for which maternal and newborn complications? Develop a plan of care for these scenarios.

ing, goals for blood glucose values, insulin administration, and common signs and symptoms of hypoglycemia and hyperglycemia. In addition to these self-management principles the potential maternal, fetal, and neonatal complications should be addressed.

Hypothyroidism

Hypothyroidism is a condition frequently encountered in women of childbearing age. This condition has been associated with difficulty in conception and other negative outcomes.

Incidence

Thyroid disease occurs more commonly in women than in men (Burrow, 1999). Hypothyroidism occurs in about 1 of every 1,600 to 2,000 pregnancies (Montoro, 1997). Clients with severe hypothyroidism often have difficulty conceiving, and women with hypothyroidism are at increased risk for pregnancy loss (Burrow, 1999).

Clinical Presentation

Hormonal and metabolic changes that occur in pregnancy may stress thyroid function. Clients who have mild or moderate hypothyroidism generally are able to achieve pregnancy, and the disease does not significantly impact the pregnancy in most cases (Glinoer, 1999).

In general, the client who has hypothyroidism may present with complaints of cold intolerance, coarse hair, and dry skin. Hypothyroidism rarely is first diagnosed during pregnancy. Women who are pregnant and have hypothyroidism may complain of increased fatigue in addition to the above-mentioned complaints. Laboratory assessments may reveal an elevated level of serum thyroid-stimulating hormone (TSH) and a low serum level of free thyroxine, or T_4 (Creasy et al., 2004).

Congenital hypothyroidism is difficult to diagnose clinically and is found in about 1 in 4,000 to 7,000 infants (Cunningham et al., 2001). Because of the risk of severe neurologic deficits as a result of a deficiency of thyroid hormone, screening of neonates is strongly recommended (Creasy et al., 2004).

In regions where there is dietary deficiency of iodine, fetal brain damage may result. The severe manifestation of this damage is referred to as cretinism, which is characterized by marked developmental retardation, deaf mutism, spasticity, strabismus, and abnormal sexual development (Creasy et al., 2004).

Management

Replacement thyroxine is given to the pregnant woman, with dosages titrated until thyroid function tests are within the normal range. The dosage usually is increased approx-

imately every 4 weeks until TSH levels are within the normal range (Creasy et al., 2004). Clients who have received thyroxine replacement therapy before pregnancy often require higher dosages during pregnancy (Brent, 1999).

Nursing Care

Antepartum nursing care for the client with hypothyroidism includes monitoring for signs and symptoms of worsening disease, such as increased fatigue, dry skin, and coarse hair. The nurse should provide education to the client regarding the disease process and the medical management plan. There are no specific nursing care issues in the intrapartum period. In the postpartum period, clients may not have thyroid hormone replacement therapy until thyroid function studies can be evaluated several weeks after delivery.

Hyperthyroidism

Hyperthyroidism can cause menstrual irregularities but usually does not affect fertility, and pregnancy does not alter the disease (Major & Nageotte, 1999). The primary maternal concern is uncontrolled disease called thyroid storm, which is a medical emergency. Heart failure also is of concern. Hyperthyroidism has been associated with adverse fetal outcomes.

Incidence

Hyperthyroidism, or **thyrotoxicosis**, is common in the general population, affecting approximately 2% of women and 0.02% of men (Gittoes & Franklyn, 1998). Similar to hypothyroidism the diagnosis of hyperthyroidism rarely is made during pregnancy, and the disease causes complications in about 0.2% of pregnancies.

Clinical Presentation

The classic signs of hyperthyroidism include heat intolerance, diaphoresis, warm skin, fatigue, anxiety, emotional lability, tachycardia, and vomiting, which also are found frequently in a normal pregnancy. A lack of weight gain, unanticipated weight loss, and increased heart rate above the norm for pregnancy may be signs that would help differentiate hyperthyroidism from the symptoms of a normal pregnancy. Laboratory values in the diagnosis of hyperthyroidism indicate an elevated serum level of free thyroxine and a low TSH level (Creasy et al., 2004).

Approximately 95% of cases of hyperthyroidism are caused by Graves' disease, which is an autoimmune process (Creasy et al., 2004). Perinatal outcomes in hyperthyroidism are largely dependent on control of the disease state in pregnancy. Adverse outcomes associated with hyperthyroidism include an increased risk for PIH, preterm labor, congestive heart failure, and intrauterine fetal demise

(Burrow, 1999). Rarely, clients will undergo thyroid storm, which is a potentially life-threatening complication resulting in cardiac failure (Cunningham et al., 2001).

Rarely, fetal and neonatal hyperthyroidism may result from transplacental passage of thyroid-stimulating immunoglobulins. Fetal hyperthyroidism may increase the risk for intrauterine growth retardation, nonimmune hydrops, and intrauterine fetal death (Zimmerman, 1999). The neonate born to a client who has hyperthyroidism also may have hyperthyroidism that may require medical treatment. These infants may demonstrate hyperkinesis, irritability, poor feeding, vomiting, diarrhea, poor weight gain, jaundice, ophthalmopathy, cardiac failure, hypertension, and thrombocytopenia up to 5 to 10 days after delivery (Zimmerman, 1999; Creasy et al., 2004). A neonate who has been exposed to antithyroid medication in utero also may develop hypothyroidism with development of a goiter and exophthalmos.

Management

Hyperthyroidism usually is managed with thionamide drugs, such as propylthiouracil (PTU) (Propacil). The dosage of this medication is titrated until the free thyroxine levels are within the normal range for pregnancy and the clinical symptoms appear to be improved. The drug is administered at the lowest possible dosage to maintain normal serum levels. In many cases, PTU can be discontinued at about 32 to 36 weeks' gestation (Creasy et al., 2004). In rare cases during pregnancy, a thyroidectomy may be performed when medical management fails (Cunningham et al., 2001).

Nursing Care

The nursing care of the client with hyperthyroidism includes monitoring for signs and symptoms of worsening disease and client education regarding the disease process and medical plan of management. The nurse also may perform fetal surveillance testing as ordered. The client with thyroid storm or cardiac failure will need intensive nursing care, the discussion of which is beyond the scope of this chapter.

CARDIOVASCULAR DISORDERS

Cardiovascular disease in pregnant women is either congenital or acquired. The consequences of heart diseases for the mother and fetus depend on disease type and severity.

Clinical Presentation

In the recent past, many women with congenital or acquired heart disease were counseled to avoid pregnancy and in some cases did not survive to childbearing age themselves. Advances in health care have allowed for surgical repair of structural defects and have vastly improved outcomes for this group of women. Women with existing heart disease can present a challenge to the health care team because many significant cardiovascular changes occur during pregnancy.

Most pregnant women with significant cardiovascular disease are diagnosed before pregnancy. Some cases of heart disease are first detected during pregnancy when the hemodynamic changes of pregnancy begin to place stress on the heart. Normal symptoms found in pregnancy, such as palpitations, tachypnea, fatigue, edema, and syncope, are similar to symptoms of cardiovascular disease. A careful evaluation of existing symptoms is needed for the pregnant woman and any new or additional symptoms, or an increase in symptoms with exertion, should be cause for further evaluation. Symptoms that should prompt further evaluation include severe dyspnea, syncope with exertion, hemoptysis, paroxysmal nocturnal tachycardia, and chest pain on exertion (Creasy et al., 2004).

Many specific cardiovascular structural defects may be affected by pregnancy. The discussion of these defects is beyond the scope of this chapter because each one would require a discussion of the specific defect and a detailed discussion of the medical management. Cardiovascular conditions that are specific to or common in pregnancy or that need special consideration include peripartum cardiomyopathy, cardiac arrhythmias, and myocardial infarction (MI).

Pregnancy generally is contraindicated in clients who have experienced an MI before becoming pregnant and who have severe left ventricular damage and heart failure (Creasy et al., 2004). When pregnancy occurs accidentally, the woman may be asked to consider terminating the pregnancy if her condition is severe.

Management

Each client with cardiovascular complications should have an individualized plan of care determined by a multidisciplinary team and based on her underlying disease process or structural defect. Certain principles in the management of the pregnant woman with cardiovascular disease can be applied to most all types of disease. These clients generally should have frequent prenatal visits and consultation with a specialist. They also may need to be placed on bed rest at any point in the pregnancy as they become symptomatic or as cardiac function is impaired (Creasy et al., 2004). The physician may choose conservative management of clients who are stable and not hemodynamically compromised, including observation and bed rest.

The woman who has experienced an MI previously is counseled to wait 1 year before becoming pregnant

(Creasy et al., 2004). Once pregnant, women often will be placed on bed rest during pregnancy. The client whose delivery occurs within 2 weeks of the MI has an increased risk for death, and, therefore, adequate rest during this time is very important (Clark et al., 1997; Creasy et al., 2004). In the intrapartum period, efforts are made to minimize hemodynamic changes and optimize perfusion. The client is labored in a lateral position, provided with adequate pain relief, and given oxygen (Clark et al., 1997). Invasive hemodynamic monitoring may be necessary (Clark et al., 1997; Creasy et al., 2004).

The specific cardiovascular complications and the condition of the client will help determine the method of delivery. In general, the mode of delivery usually is decided based on obstetric indications. The second stage of labor may be shortened by the use of forceps or vacuum extraction to avoid the prolonged Valsalva maneuver in pushing (Cunningham et al., 2001). In some specific cardiac complications, to avoid the strain of labor an elective cesarean section may be performed. The stress of major surgery, the potential for infection, and increased blood loss as compared with vaginal delivery is taken into consideration in planning the method of delivery (Clark et al., 1997).

Clients with cardiovascular complications who will undergo labor and anticipated vaginal delivery often need special considerations. During the intrapartum period attempts are made to minimize changes in blood pressure and pulse, including placing the client in a lateral position, adequate pain management, and the avoidance of hemorrhage. The avoidance of infection is an important consideration because an infection can have a detrimental effect on the client's overall condition. Supplemental oxygen and antibiotics frequently are prescribed (Clark et al., 1997).

Nursing Care

Nursing care of clients who have cardiovascular disease can be very challenging. In some cases, nurses from the obstetric, cardiovascular, or critical care service may need to collaborate in the care. Thorough physical assessments should be performed, and any change in cardiopulmonary status should be reported to the physician promptly. Meticulous care should be given to aseptic technique to avoid an infection because infection could have a serious impact on the client's overall condition. Intake and output should be monitored closely in most clients with cardiovascular disease to avoid volume overload. The nurse should have a thorough understanding of the pathophysiology of the specific cardiovascular disease and be familiar with any vasoactive drugs that may be used.

Clients and families are often very anxious and need thorough explanations regarding the plan of care. Emotional support is an essential piece in the care of these clients, and spiritual needs should be considered.

PULMONARY DISORDERS

Pulmonary disorders that can complicate pregnancy include asthma and tuberculosis (TB). The impact these diseases have on the mother and fetus is related to the severity of the disease process.

Asthma

Asthma is considered to be an obstructive pulmonary disease.

Incidence

Asthma affects about 1% to 4% of pregnancies, which is a lower incidence than in the general population in which the reported incidence is 3% to 5% (Kurinczuk, Parsons, Dawes, & Burton, 1999; Weinberger & Weiss, 1999).

Clinical Presentation

Bronchospasm and increased mucus production cause airflow to be limited, especially during expiration. Exacerbation of asthma may be related to specific events or "triggers," such as dust, animal dander, exercise, and respiratory infection; in contrast, there may be no obvious precipitating event. Symptoms of exacerbation of asthma, or an "attack," include coughing, wheezing, and dyspnea. Maternal and perinatal outcomes in clients with asthma depend on disease severity and treatment adequacy throughout pregnancy (Weinberger & Weiss, 1999).

Asthma usually begins in childhood but can occur at any age. The course of asthma in pregnancy is unpredictable; some clients experience worsening of the disease, some improve, and an equal number remain unchanged (Weinberger & Weiss, 1999). Pregnant clients rarely will experience an asthma attack during pregnancy, although the reason for this is not clear (Creasy et al., 2004).

Management

Treatment for pregnant asthmatics is aimed at preventing and relieving bronchospasm. Undertreatment of pregnant women with asthma is common and based on fears about the effects medications used to treat asthma may have on the fetus. Most medications used for treatment of asthma in the general population are safe for use in pregnancy (Creasy et al., 2004). The risks to the client of leaving severe asthma untreated are greater than are the risks of using medication to control asthma during pregnancy (Schatz, 1999).

Clients with mild or occasional asthma attacks are generally managed outside the hospital setting with inhaled beta-agonist agents, such as albuterol (Proventil, Ventolin). Clients experiencing several attacks a week may be placed on scheduled doses of inhaled anti-inflammatory medications as a preventive measure. Inhaled corticosteroids also are used to prevent airway inflammation in clients who have moderate or severe asthma (Creasy et al., 2004; Cunningham et al., 2001). In very severe cases of asthma, parenteral or oral steroids may become necessary. The treatment is usually converted to inhaled steroids over time (Cunningham et al., 2001).

In a severe asthma attack the goals are to correct maternal hypoxia, relieve bronchospasm, ensure adequate ventilation, and support uteroplacental perfusion. Intubation and mechanical ventilation may be necessary for clients who are unresponsive to medical therapy (Clark et al., 1997).

Nursing Care

Client education is a key part of nursing care for the pregnant woman who has asthma. The client should be counseled that her asthma might possibly improve, worsen, or remain unchanged during pregnancy. The importance of using inhalers and other prescribed medications as ordered by the primary care provider should be stressed. Many pregnant women are fearful of taking any type of drug during pregnancy and should be reassured about the safety of these medications.

The technique of inhaler use should be evaluated because proper dosing depends on adequate use of the device. Clients who have difficulty with traditional inhalers can be offered the use of a spacer, an additional device that helps deliver accurate doses.

A severe asthma attack is a medical emergency. A pregnant woman who is experiencing a severe asthma attack should be observed closely and receive a thorough physical assessment. The client should be placed in a lateral recumbent position to optimize ventilation and uteroplacental circulation. The client's response or lack of response to medications should be noted and reported to the physician. The client experiencing an asthma attack will exhibit anxiety and often will be anxious about the fetal condition and her own. Reassurance should be offered to the client and family as should thorough explanations about procedures, medications, and the medical plan of management.

Tuberculosis

Tuberculosis is a worldwide health concern and a major cause of illness and death. The prevalence of TB is increasing worldwide. Many causes have been implicated in the resurgence of TB in recent years in the United States: presence of the human immunodeficiency virus (HIV), development of drug-resistant strains of TB, an increase in the number of immigrants, difficulty accessing medical care in the population with TB, and lack of adequate resources to handle the increasing number of cases (Saade, 1997; Hageman, 1997; Anderson, 1997).

Clinical Presentation

The lung is the major site of involvement. Some clients, however, will have extrapulmonary disease, including endometrial, lymphatic, intestinal, skeletal, renal, meningeal, and genital TB (Jana, Vasishta, Saha, & Ghosh, 1999; Soussis, Trew, Matalliotakis, Margara, & Winston, 1998). The diagnosis of TB generally is made by isolation of the organism *Mycobacterium tuberculosis* from involved sites. The organism is cultured from a sputum specimen in the case of pulmonary TB. Infection is caused by inhalation of the *M. tuberculosis* organism. Clients can be asymptomatic at the time of primary infection. TB may lie dormant for long periods of time before reactivating. Clinical manifestations include symptoms of pneumonia, such as fever and a cough that may be nonproductive, pleuritic chest pain, hemoptysis, and weight loss. Outcomes for clients who have TB during pregnancy are related to disease severity and treatment adequacy.

Management

The tuberculin skin test is a routine but important screening test for TB that may be performed in high-risk women during pregnancy (Nolan, Espinosa, & Pastorek, 1997; Riley, 1997). Clients at high risk include those who have HIV, those with close contact with persons known to have TB, persons who recently have immigrated to the United States, and clients who are incarcerated or in long-term care facilities (Cunningham et al., 2001). A chest radiograph may be performed in the client who has a positive result on a skin test and who previously has had a negative test result, or in the client whose medical history or physical examination is suggestive of TB. When a chest radiograph is indicated, it should be delayed until after the first trimester if possible to avoid exposing the rapidly developing fetus to radiation. Shielding also can be used to reduce fetal exposure.

Pregnant women who test positive for TB but do not have clinical evidence of active disease may delay treatment until after delivery (Cunningham et al., 2001). Treatment of pulmonary TB in pregnant women is similar to that in women who are not pregnant (Saade, 1997). Treatment consists of daily doses of Isoniazid (isonicotinic acid hydrazide [INH]), rifampin (Rifamate), pyrazinamide, and ethambutol (Myambutol) over a 6-month period. These first-line agents appear to have minimal risks for the development of congenital anomalies and may be started as soon as the diagnosis of TB is made (Brost &

Newman, 1997). Clients who have HIV and TB are placed on extended regimens. Hepatitis is a major side effect of INH; therefore, clients may require serial liver enzyme testing (Cunningham et al., 2001).

Neonatal infection is uncommon if the mother has received adequate treatment for at least 2 weeks before delivery. The neonate is at greatest risk for the development of TB shortly after birth because the newborn is susceptible to TB infection (Starke, 1997). The newborn is isolated from the mother for up to 2 weeks if she has active disease (Creasy et al., 2004).

Nursing Care

Clients who are in high-risk groups should be screened for TB in pregnancy. A thorough medical history will include information on potential exposure to TB and any signs and symptoms of the disease. The client will often need education about the disease process, potential complications, and management plan. Compliance to the medication regimen, if prescribed, is key to optimal outcome in the mother and fetus and should be stressed.

The pregnant client who has TB will need emotional support in dealing with the implications of the disease. The client who must be isolated from her newborn may be very distraught. She should be made aware of the rationale for isolation and offered the opportunity to verbalize her concern and grief.

HEMATOLOGIC DISORDERS

Hematologic disorders in pregnancy range from idiopathic thrombocytopenic purpura to sickle cell disease.

Immunologic Idiopathic Thrombocytopenic Purpura

Immunologic thrombocytopenic purpura (ITP), also referred to as idiopathic thrombocytopenic purpura, is a process in which antibodies are directed against platelets and usually is an immune response to drugs or viral infections (Duffy, 1999).

Clinical Presentation

Acute cases of thrombocytopenia often follow a viral infection and usually resolve spontaneously (Cunningham et al., 2001). Chronic cases of ITP are most common in young women and occur in about 7% to 8% of pregnancies. The initial diagnosis of ITP sometimes is made during pregnancy when a routine CBC reveals a decreased platelet count (ACOG, 1999b). It is unclear what impact pregnancy could have on chronic ITP.

Antibodies are able to cross the placenta and cause thrombocytopenia in the fetus and neonate. Concern exists that the fetus with thrombocytopenia is at risk for intracranial hemorrhage during labor and delivery, prompting direct measurement of fetal platelet count by PUBS or fetal scalp sampling (Cunningham et al., 2001). The actual incidence of moderate to severe neonatal thrombocytopenia and intracranial hemorrhage is low (Song, Lee, Kim, & Choi, 1999). It is estimated that significant neonatal thrombocytopenia occurs in 10% of babies born to clients with ITP (Bussel, 1997).

Management

Once thrombocytopenia is diagnosed, secondary causative factors are investigated, such as lupus, leukemia, and lymphoma. Clients whose very low platelet counts persist (less than 50,000) are usually treated with steroids. The goal of therapy is to decrease the incidence of hemorrhage. Improvement usually occurs within 2 to 3 weeks. More than 70% of clients will have an increase in platelet count, and the steroid dose is tapered as the platelet count is normalized (Creasy et al., 2004). Clients who continue to have persistent severe thrombocytopenia and who are bleeding despite steroid therapy may require a splenectomy; however, this is rarely required in pregnancy (Duffy, 1999). Women who are asymptomatic and have ITP and a platelet count greater than 50,000 usually do not require treatment.

Clinicians have attempted to predict fetal and neonatal thrombocytopenia based on maternal characteristics without much success. Some clinicians will opt to deliver the baby by cesarean section if the fetus has thrombocytopenia (Duffy, 1999). Laboratory tests used to determine fetal platelet count are expensive, and there is a significant risk to the fetus from the procedures (Song et al., 1999). Studies have been performed that have found that neither the determination of fetal platelet count nor performance of a cesarean section significantly impact neonatal outcomes. Although this remains a controversial issue, many clinicians determine the route of delivery based strictly on obstetric indications.

Nursing Care

Clients diagnosed with ITP will need thorough explanations of the disease process and of possible maternal and fetal implications. The medical plan of management, including considerations for the route of delivery, should be discussed with the client and family.

Sickle Cell Disease

Sickle cell disease encompasses several inherited disorders of hemoglobin synthesis, with sickle cell anemia (SS disease), sickle cell–hemoglobin C disease (SC disease), and sickle cell–β-thalassemia (S-β-thalassemia) being the most common forms.

Clinical Presentation

Sickle cell anemia (SS disease) occurs when the gene for S hemoglobin is inherited from both parents. Sickle cell trait, which is the inheritance of one gene for the production of S hemoglobin and one for normal hemoglobin, occurs in 1 of 12 Blacks. SC disease, in which there is a gene for the production of hemoglobin C, occurs in approximately 1 in 2,000 Black women (Cunningham et al., 2001). S-β-thalassemia occurs with the inheritance of an S gene and a β-thalassemia gene. S-β-thalassemia occurs in approximately 1 of every 2,000 women (Cunningham et al., 2001). Pregnancy places a strain on women with sickle hemoglobinopathies, and, accordingly, they have significant maternal and perinatal morbidity and mortality.

The diagnosis of hemoglobinopathies is made by hemoglobin electrophoresis, which identifies the type and percentage of abnormal hemoglobin.

Most of the signs and symptoms of SS disease are a result of hemolysis, vaso-occlusive disease, or increased susceptibility to infection (Creasy et al., 2004). Clients with SS disease experience sickling of erythrocytes and resulting occlusion of the microvasculature precipitated by hypoxemia. Chronic anemia and episodes of "crises" in which there is vaso-occlusion causing ischemia, acute pain, and possible organ failure are characteristic of the disease. These painful episodes of sickle cell crisis may occur in the long bones, abdomen, chest, or back; these episodes are potentially life-threatening and often increase in frequency during pregnancy (Clark et al., 1997; Creasy et al., 2004).

In general, clients who have SS disease are more susceptible to infection. Infections and pulmonary complications are major causes of morbidity and mortality in women who have SS disease and are more common in pregnancy (Cunningham et al., 2001).

During pregnancy women who have SC disease may have an increased incidence of severe bone pain and additional serious complications, even though they often are asymptomatic before pregnancy. Maternal and perinatal mortality rates are higher than in the general population but much lower than in SS disease (Duffy, 1999).

Pregnancy outcomes for clients who have β-thalassemia usually are good. These women may experience mild to moderate anemia during pregnancy (Duffy, 1999).

Management

Hemoglobin electrophoresis may be ordered prenatally as a screening test for Black women. The pregnant woman with a sickle hemoglobinopathy generally will have chronic hemolytic anemia and requires increased folic acid supplementation throughout pregnancy. Disease treatment mainly consists of relieving symptoms, with the objective being to end painful crisis and fight infection (Creasy et al., 2004).

Transfusions of erythrocytes are used in cases of chronic anemia to prevent acute or chronic complications based on the client's symptoms (Simon et al., 1998).

Clients are monitored throughout pregnancy for asymptomatic bacteriuria because women with sickle cell hemoglobin have a greatly increased risk for bacteriuria (Pastore, Savitz, & Thorp, 1999). Infections are poorly tolerated and are managed aggressively to avoid precipitation of a crisis.

The management of sickle cell crisis usually involves hospitalization, evaluation for sources of potential infection, rest, hydration, oxygen therapy, and pain management. IV therapy to correct dehydration is a key aspect of therapy because it can lower the blood viscosity and may help alleviate vaso-occlusion (Creasy et al., 2004). Oxygen therapy is reserved for clients who are experiencing hypoxia, those with a pulmonary infection, and those in labor (Clark et al., 1997). The pain of sickle cell crisis can last for up to a week and is managed according to severity; some clients require narcotic analgesia.

Nursing Care

Clients who have sickle hemoglobinopathies require education about the impact of pregnancy on their disease. Avoidance of infection is an important consideration and should be stressed. Pregnant women are more susceptible to UTIs than are women in the general population, and clients should be instructed to alert their health care provider as soon as the first symptoms of UTI appear. In fact, routine screening is likely to be included in prenatal care because of asymptomatic bacteriuria.

Clients experiencing crisis will require supportive care: a warm restful environment, adequate pain control, IV hydration, and oxygen therapy as ordered. Intake and output should be recorded; however, catheterization should be avoided because of risk of infection. Crisis is an extremely anxiety-provoking event, with the very real threat of death. Clients require emotional support and reassurance from family and health care providers.

NEUROLOGIC DISORDERS

Neurologic disorders, namely epilepsy, can affect the health of the mother and baby.

Seizure Disorders

Seizure disorders may be acquired as a result of trauma, tumors, or metabolic disorders.

Incidence

Most frequently the seizure activity is idiopathic and is known as epilepsy (ACOG, 1996c). Epilepsy is common in the general population and affects an estimated 1 million women of childbearing age (Chang & McAuely, 1998). Seizure disorders are the most common major neurologic complication seen in pregnancy, affecting approximately 0.5% of all pregnancies (Nulman, Laslo, & Koren, 1999; ACOG, 1996c). This section focuses on epilepsy.

Clinical Presentation

Preconceptual counseling for women of childbearing age who have epilepsy is very important. The outcome of the pregnancy is greatly determined by control of the seizure disorder, achieving therapeutic blood levels of the prescribed anticonvulsant, compliance with the medication regimen, and vitamin supplementation.

During pregnancy psychological, hormonal, and pharmokinetic changes can cause an increase in seizure activity. As many as half of women with epilepsy will experience an increase in seizure activity during pregnancy (Cunningham et al., 2001). Status epilepticus is a rare condition in which recurrent generalized seizures occur. This condition is an emergency because the mother and fetus are at risk for hypoxia. This complication seems to occur more frequently in the third trimester (Licht & Sankar, 1999).

Serum levels of anticonvulsant drugs can change dramatically during pregnancy, usually decreasing as the pregnancy progresses. These changes may be related to nausea and vomiting, delayed gastric emptying, increased plasma volume, and altered protein binding. Serum level fluctuations may cause a nontherapeutic level of the anticonvulsant drug or, in some cases, maternal toxicity (Nulman et al., 1999; ACOG, 1996c). Therefore, close monitoring is required during pregnancy.

Most anticonvulsant drugs interfere with metabolism of the essential vitamins folic acid and vitamin K. Folic acid deficiency is associated with an increased incidence of neural tube defects and other major malformations. Interference with vitamin K metabolism places the neonate at increased risk for bleeding because certain clotting factors are dependent on vitamin K (Chang & McAuely, 1998; ACOG, 1996c).

Children born to women without seizure disorders have a 0.5% to 1% risk of developing epilepsy. Children born to a woman with epilepsy are four times more likely to develop epilepsy (ACOG, 1996c). Children exposed to phenytoin in utero are at risk for cleft lip and fetal hydantoin syndrome.

Management

Women of childbearing age who have epilepsy may be started on folic acid supplementation even before conception. Once pregnant, the woman should receive folic acid supplementation throughout the first trimester (Nulman et al., 1999). Some clinicians prescribe vitamin K supplementation during the last month of pregnancy. The infant also receives a vitamin K injection at birth.

The woman with epilepsy should be counseled regarding possible teratogenic effects of uncontrolled seizures and the increased risk for major congenital malformations associated with the anticonvulsant medications (Samren, van Duijn, Christiaens, Hofman, & Lindhout, 1999). There is about a two to three times increased risk for birth defects in infants with mothers who have epilepsy compared with the general population. Seizure control is preferably achieved at least 6 months before conception.

Medical therapy during pregnancy is ideally accomplished with the lowest possible effective dose of a single antiseizure medication (Chang & McAuely, 1998). Because serum levels of drugs considered therapeutic in clients who are not pregnant are not reliable during pregnancy and because of the fluctuations, drug levels are checked periodically as the pregnancy progresses. Clients should be educated regarding the signs and symptoms of drug toxicity.

Some clients are reluctant to take the prescribed anticonvulsant medications because of fear of fetal effects (ACOG, 1996c). They should be strongly advised to adhere to the medical regimen and report increase in seizure activity. Because lack of sleep and stress may cause an increase in seizure activity, the pregnant client should be encouraged to get adequate rest.

During the early antepartum period clients are offered screening for potential neural tube defects using a maternal serum alpha-fetoprotein determination and ultrasonography. If these tests are inconclusive the woman may be offered an amniocentesis for a definitive diagnosis. Frequently, a comprehensive ultrasonography to assess for congenital malformations is performed at approximately 18 to 22 weeks' gestation. Further antepartum surveillance is not always necessary and is determined based on the individual client's condition.

In the event of status epilepticus the physician may order IV phenytoin (Dilantin), which must be administered slowly to avoid significant cardiac dysrhythmias. Phenobarbital or diazepam (Valium) may be ordered alternatively; however, both these drugs may cause respiratory depression. Emergency supplies for endotracheal intubation, oxygen, and suction equipment should be readily available (ACOG, 1996c).

During labor the client may be unable to take prescribed oral medications. Serum drug levels may be evaluated and the client may receive an anticonvulsant parenterally.

In the postpartum period serum levels of anticonvulsants may increase rapidly. When the drug dosage is increased during pregnancy, it frequently needs to be decreased in the postpartum period (Aminoff, 1999). Serum levels are checked frequently to avoid toxic drug levels. Antiepilectic drugs interact with oral contraceptives, making them less effective. Clients should be counseled on the need for increased dosage or a second method of birth control to avoid an unplanned pregnancy (Chang & McAuely, 1998).

Infants born to mothers with epilepsy who are receiving barbiturates may experience withdrawal symptoms beginning about 1 week after birth and lasting 1 to 2 weeks. A breastfed infant may develop withdrawal with abrupt cessation of breastfeeding and may require low-dose phenobarbital with gradual withdrawal (ACOG, 1996c).

Nursing Care

In the antepartum period most clients will need education regarding the effect their pregnancy might have on their disease, medical therapy prescribed, potential complications for the fetus and neonate, and the medical plan of care. Clients diagnosed with epilepsy and their families may be fearful of the effects their disease can have on their babies and will need accurate information about their disease and emotional support throughout the pregnancy.

NURSING IMPLICATIONS

Few events over the course of a lifetime have such a momentous impact on women and their families as do a pregnancy and the eventual birth of the baby. Pregnancy

COLLABORATIVE CARE

Working with Hospitalized Antepartal Clients

Women who are hospitalized during the antepartum period must deal with a variety of physical, emotional, and psychosocial stresses. Nurses who are caring for these women must recognize the importance of a multidisciplinary care plan. In addition to nursing care, the plan would include collaboration among some or all of the following:

- Health care provider
- Physician/nurse midwife
- Specialist related to the woman's diagnosis
- Social worker
- Dietician
- Physical/occupational therapist
- Lactation consultant
- CCU/MICU/NICU staff member
- Chaplain/spirtual advisor
- Psychiatric consultant

Critical Thinking

Significant Findings from Nursing Assessment

Nurses are in a position to detect early signs of obstetrical risks. What might be the significance of the following findings from a nursing assessment?

- Oliguria of less than 30 mL/h
- Significant change in vital signs
- Diastolic blood pressure of 110 mmHg or higher
- Nonreassuring fetal status
- Seizure activity
- Vaginal bleeding
- Severe epigastric or upper right quadrant pain
- Altered mental status
- Signs and symptoms of pulmonary edema
- Abnormal laboratory results

can be a time of great hope and joy or, when complications arise, a time of great concern and even despair. Major advances in obstetric care have been made in the last half of the 20th century that have allowed women with serious medical and obstetric complications to achieve positive pregnancy outcomes. The availability of adequate prenatal care, early identification of risk factors, and an interdisciplinary approach to the management of the high-risk pregnancy is critical to optimize outcomes for the family.

The role of the nurse in caring for the high-risk obstetric client will vary depending on the condition and setting. For the client being managed in the community, the role may be one of counseling, teaching, and case management. It is very important that the client and family understand the pathophysiology of the condition and which self-help measures can be taken. It also is important to teach danger signs and the procedure that should be followed in the event of a change in the woman's condition. The intervention depends not only on the condition but the severity of the condition, with home care used for milder cases in which client compliance is not likely to be an issue.

In a hospital setting, nursing care of high-risk obstetric clients requires close monitoring of both maternal and fetal status. These clients may be hospitalized for several weeks prior to delivery and require a multidisciplinary care approach. In addition, they require psychosocial support to help alleviate the stress and boredom related to lengthy hospital stay as well as the anxiety associated with a premature delivery.

Nurses working with pregnant women and families must be familiar with common complications that can arise during the course of pregnancy. Nurses should be prepared to function as an integral part of the health care team, performing thorough nursing assessments, administering medications and treatments, and providing clients and families with education and support.

PREGNANCY IN HIV-INFECTED WOMEN

Acquired immunodeficiency syndrome (AIDS) is a debilitating and life-threatening condition caused by HIV, a retrovirus. **Human immunodeficiency virus (HIV)** is transmitted by exposure to an infected person's body secretions, including blood, vaginal fluid, semen, breast milk, and saliva.

Incidence and Significance

Women of reproductive age are increasingly affected by HIV infection; many women become HIV-infected during the adolescent years and manifest the symptoms of AIDS as young adults. One in five of all reported cases of AIDS occurs in persons ages 20 to 29, and adolescent minority females are more proportionately represented than adolescent males (King, 1996). Given that the mean time from viral infection to the development of AIDS is approximately 10 years, many of those in the 20 to 29 age category were infected with HIV as adolescents.

The statistics on women with HIV infection and AIDS are alarming. HIV infection is a major cause of morbidity and mortality among women and children in the United States. Infection by HIV and the subsequent development of AIDS is reported as the third leading cause of death for all women ages 25 to 44 and is the leading cause of death among Black women in this age group (CDC, 1996).

Over 90% of the reported cases of pediatric AIDS in the United States are acquired by transmission from an HIV-infected mother. An estimated 7,000 infants are born annually to HIV-infected women and approximately 15% to 30% of these infants would become HIV-infected if no treatment with **antiretroviral therapy** (medications used to suppress HIV replication and reduce viral load) were instituted (CDC, 1996). Approximately 25% to 50% of children with perinatally acquired HIV infection manifest AIDS in the first year of life, and about 80% have clinical symptoms of the disease within 3 to 5 years (Mauskopf, Paul, Wichman, White, & Tilson, 1996).

The most effective way to reduce vertical and perinatal transmission of HIV infection is through prevention of infection of women during their reproductive years. However, despite adequate screening, detection, and educational efforts, the HIV-infection rate among heterosexual women of reproductive age continues to rise.

The young heterosexual female population accounts for an increase in new HIV **seroconversions** (i.e., conversion of the blood serum from negative to positive for HIV infection), primarily from transmission by HIV-infected intravenous drug users to their heterosexual partners (CDC, 1997a). For many young women, the only identifiable risk factor is their male sexual partner. During the 1980s, the proportion of adolescents who reported being sexually active increased significantly, yet many young women remain naive about their partner's history of sexual activity or of intravenous drug use (IVDU). Because adolescents and young adults have proportionately higher rates of STDs, they are more vulnerable to HIV infection. HIV transmission during sexual contact may be facilitated by STDs that cause open genital lesions, such as herpes, syphilis, and chancroid.

Reflections from a New Mother

"I always wanted to have children," states 22-year-old Janice. "I never dreamed that it would end up being like this. Our baby developed pneumonia in the newborn nursery and didn't respond well to treatment, so they tested him for HIV. We thought this was just routine and we were shocked when he was HIV-positive. How could that be? Where could he get HIV? My doctor looked at me and said, 'He got it from you, and both you and your husband need to be tested as soon as possible.' We were stunned. I had sex with different partners in high school and college and my biggest fear was getting pregnant, not getting HIV. I didn't think that anyone I knew could be HIV-positive. I admit I wasn't always as careful as I should have been. I just didn't think this could happen to me. Now my baby is sick, my husband is in shock, and I am so afraid. What will happen to us?"

Screening, Testing, and Diagnosis

Although the cure for AIDS is yet undetermined, the statistics on longevity among women and their children appear promising if antiretroviral therapy is initiated in a timely manner. Until an effective vaccine is developed, early detection and treatment, behavioral risk reduction, and other preventative strategies targeted toward high-risk populations remain the most effective methods of reducing the spread of HIV to noninfected persons and delaying the onset of full-blown AIDS in those who are infected. However, many HIV-infected women are not tested for the virus until symptoms of AIDS are apparent or they deliver a child who has an AIDS-related condition.

Controversy continues about who should be screened for HIV. Because of the availability and efficacy of early antiretroviral treatment and the problems associated with selecting who should be screened, many authorities advocate voluntary prenatal testing of all pregnant women regardless of their actual or perceived risk of infection. Young women, especially teenagers, often believe AIDS to be a disease that occurs only among homosexual men or IVDUs, and therefore feel invulnerable to the disease. Because many women do not receive any prenatal care or receive prenatal care only in the last trimester of pregnancy, counseling and testing are recommended for all adolescents and young adults who use drugs or engage in unprotected sexual intercourse, especially those with multiple partners and those diagnosed with STDs. Broadening the scope of screening and testing may identify those who are infected with HIV before pregnancy or early in an existing pregnancy (CDC, 1999). Box 11-2 identifies women who are considered to be at risk for HIV infection and for whom screening and testing services should be made available. Mandatory pre- and post-test counseling should always be available in a confidential setting.

HIV infection (seroconversion) is identified by the use of the enzyme-linked immunosorbent assay (ELISA), which detects serum antibodies to HIV and is confirmed by the Western blot test. Results of these diagnostic tests are highly reliable; false-positives and false-negatives rarely occur. Seroconversion among adolescents and adults generally occurs from 6 to 12 weeks after transmission of the virus. The diagnosis of HIV infection in infants born to HIV-positive mothers is confounded by the presence of maternal immunoglobulin G (IgG) antibodies to HIV. Detection of HIV DNA and RNA by polymerase chain reaction (PCR), detection of the serum p24 antigen, and viral cultures for the virus are the tests used to confirm HIV in the neonate (Barrett & Sleasman, 1997). A presumptive diagnosis of HIV infection is confirmed by two positive results on PCR tests or viral cultures. Because some HIV-infected neonates have undetectable virus levels, di-

---

Box 11-2

Behaviors of Women at Risk for HIV Infection

- Current or past history of drug use, especially intravenous drug use
- History of prostitution
- Sexual intercourse with multiple partners
- Sexual intercourse under the influence of drugs
- Sexual intercourse with men who also have sex with men
- Current or past history of sexual intercourse with any persons with any of these characteristics

High Risk Criteria

- Residence in an area of the country or travel abroad to a country with high prevalence of HIV infection, particularly in the northeast and southeast areas of the United States
- Received a blood transfusion or blood products before 1985, when HIV screening became available for blood donors

---

Client Education

Pretest Counseling for HIV Infection

- Explain that testing is confidential.
- Assess the client's understanding of HIV risk.
- Obtain a careful sexual history.
- Explain the modes of HIV transmission.
- Explain the relationship between infection and transmission.
- Discuss the prevention of transmission to others, including methods of safe sex.
- Provide age-appropriate reading materials on HIV transmission, detection, and treatment.
- Describe and explain the serologic tests used to confirm HIV infection.
- Discuss what test results mean, including false-negative and false-positive results.
- Make a plan for the client to receive test results and post-test counseling.

Note. Adapted from *HIV Counseling, Testing, and Referral Standards and Guidelines,* by the Centers for Disease Control and Prevention, 1994, Washington, DC: U.S. Department of Health & Human Services.

agnostic tests should be repeated at 1 and 4 months. The HIV ELISA should be used to test for HIV in these infants from 6 months to 18 months of age. In uninfected neonates, the maternal antibodies disappear by approximately 18 months of age, and the child remains asymptomatic.

After HIV is confirmed by screening tests, the level of immunocompetence is measured by counting the CD4+ T-lymphocyte cells and, in research settings, by measuring plasma RNA levels of HIV. Progressive depletion of CD4+ T-lymphocytes and rising plasma levels of HIV RNA are associated with an increased likelihood of clinical disease and opportunistic infections (CDC, 1997b; Carpenter et al., 1997). The average CD4+ T-lymphocyte cell count in healthy individuals is approximately 1,000 cells/µL. HIV-infected persons lose approximately 200 to 300 CD4+ T-lymphocyte cells per microliter of blood in the first year of infection, followed by a subsequent decline of 50 to 80 CD4+ T-lymphocyte cells per microliter yearly thereafter (Stein, Korvick, & Vermund, 1992). Opportunistic infections and clinical symptoms of AIDS generally occur when the CD4+ T-lymphocyte cell count declines to 200/µL or less. While many factors influence the progression of HIV disease, time remains the most significant prognostic indicator of mortality in clients with HIV infection. In 1993, the CDC expanded the AIDS surveillance case definition to include persons with CD4+ T-lymphocyte cell counts of less than 200 cells/µL along with HIV-related wasting syndrome, HIV-related dementia, disseminated tuberculosis (TB), or one of the following conditions: pulmonary TB, recurrent bacterial pneumonia within 12 months, or invasive cervical carcinoma (CDC, 1993).

Clinical Manifestations of HIV Infection in Pregnant Women

While there is no conclusive data that nongynecologic opportunistic infections of HIV differ in men and women, it has been suggested that women present with higher rates of candidal esophagitis as an AIDS-defining condition (Carpenter et al., 1997). HIV-infected women may initially present with complicated gynecologic conditions rather than the traditional AIDS-defining diagnoses. The most frequent manifestation of HIV infection in females is recurrent vaginal candidiasis in otherwise healthy women. As the number of CD4+ T-lymphocyte cells declines, women exhibit (1) candidal vaginitis, (2) pelvic inflammatory disease (PID), which may lead to abscess formation and resistance to antibiotic therapy, (3) genital herpes infections, which are frequent, persistent, and progress to severe ulcerating disease, (4) human papillomavirus (HPV) infection, with an accelerated progression to cervical neoplasia, (5) rapidly progressing cervical neoplasia, and (6) co-infection with syphilis, which has an aggressive progression to neurosyphilis (Eldred and Chaisson,

Client Education

Post-Test Counseling and Education for HIV Infection

HIV-Negative Results

- Inform client of negative results and the need for future testing related to exposure.
- Review pretesting educational materials, the need to screen partners, and avoidance of other risk behaviors.
- Offer contraception information.
- Offer counseling and education to partners.
- Review safe sex practices.
- Identify community resources for health care and substance abuse if necessary.
- Advise client not to donate blood, plasma, or organs until HIV status is firmly established.

HIV-Positive Results

- Offer immediate psychological support.
- Help the client understand what the test result means.
- Review methods of transmission and assess the client's risk of transmitting HIV to others.
- Explain that treatment is available.
- Identify immediate health care resources.
- Identify immediate psychiatric services, as appropriate.
- Assist the client in developing a plan to notify all sexual partners of exposure.
- Help the client develop a plan to notify all others who may need to know about her HIV status.
- Offer counseling and education to partners.
- Offer contraception information.
- Review safe sex practices and other risk reduction strategies.
- Advise client not to donate blood, plasma, or organs.

Note. Adapted from *HIV Counseling, Testing, and Referral Standards and Guidelines,* by the Centers for Disease Control and Prevention, 1994, Washington, DC: U.S. Department of Health & Human Services.

1996). Women rarely exhibit Kaposi's sarcoma but do present with *Pneumocystis carinii* pneumonia (PCP), wasting syndrome, and HIV-related dementia (McDonnell & Kessenich, 2000).

There is no conclusive evidence that maternal HIV infection has an adverse effect on the fetal outcome in pregnancy. Studies conducted in the United States that have been controlled for substance abuse factors have not shown significant obstetrical or perinatal complications. However, poverty, lack of prenatal care, drug abuse, and HIV infection are often concomitant, and the combination is costly in terms of obstetrical and perinatal complications and adverse neonatal outcomes.

Clinical Manifestations of HIV in Neonates

Although studies are inconclusive, it appears that HIV can be transferred from mother to the baby during pregnancy or birth and while breastfeeding and that most perinatal transmission occurs at the time of labor and delivery (Riley and Green, 1999). Many attempts have been made at identifying predictors of HIV transmission, but the results are inconclusive.

Clinical signs of HIV infection in the neonatal period are difficult to identify. In approximately 20% of vertically infected infants, high levels of plasma viral load in the first year of life appear to predict rapid progression of disease (Barrett and Sleasman, 1997). These infants are likely to manifest signs of opportunistic infections such as PCP, interstitial lymphocytic pneumonia (ILP), candidal diaper rash, thrush, diarrhea, and other recurrent bacterial infections. Growth failure, neurologic problems, and developmental delays are also common.

Nursing Implications

Pregnant women who are HIV-positive or who have clinical AIDS should be identified as soon as possible during pregnancy for early intervention (Figure 11-4). Early identification of either pregnancy or HIV status assumes contact with the health care system. However, poor minority women, who are either IVDUs or have unprotected sex with infected persons, are more vulnerable to HIV infection and are less likely to seek health care early.

In 1994, the AIDS Clinical Trials Group Protocol 076 (ACTG 076) demonstrated that zidovudine (azidothymydine, AZT) given to HIV-infected women during pregnancy and labor and delivery plus 6 weeks of oral AZT therapy for the neonate decreased vertical transmission from 25.5% to 8.3% (Connor, Sperling, & Gelber, 1994). The ACTG 076 protocol showed such promising results that the clinical trials using a placebo group were terminated prematurely once the effectiveness of AZT was demonstrated and all participants were offered the drug.

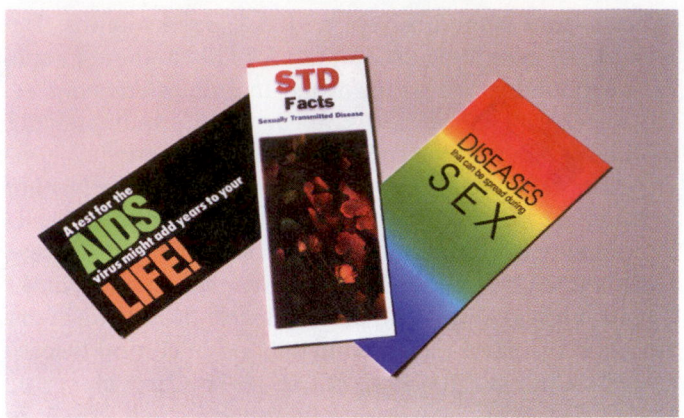

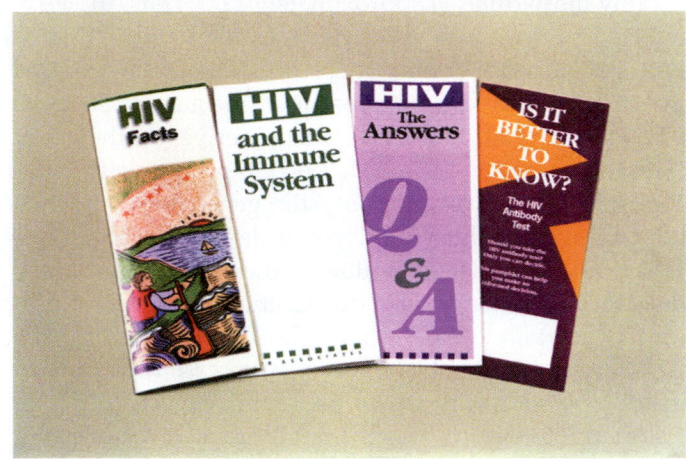

Figure 11-4   Pregnant women at risk for AIDS or other sexually-transmitted diseases should be tested immediately, and information on health promotion and treatment options should be provided.

The efficacy of AZT in decreasing vertical transmission of HIV was a major breakthrough in treatment. Box 11-3 describes the ACTG 076 protocol for administration of AZT in pregnancy. Table 11-3 identifies various clinical situations of women during pregnancy and AZT therapy currently recommended to prevent vertical transmission. In all drug treatment regimens offered to pregnant women with HIV infection, the known and unknown risks and benefits to mother and fetus should be considered and discussed before drug treatment is instituted during pregnancy or at delivery.

In 1996, the final results of the ACTG 076 protocol reported mother-to-baby transmission rates of less than 8% (CDC, 1998b). Research continues on the use of AZT in the treatment of pregnant women, with the emphasis on decreasing the frequency of dosing to increase drug compliance among clients and the use of combination therapy (i.e., AZT and other antiretroviral agents). In 1998, the U.S. Public Health Service Task Force on antiretroviral medications during pregnancy recommended the use of combination therapy for HIV-positive pregnant women. The

Box 11-3

ACTG-076 Protocol for Administration of Zidovudine during Pregnancy

Client Eligibility Criteria

- Confirmed pregnancy of 14–34 weeks' gestation
- No antiretroviral drug treatment during current pregnancy
- No clinical indication for antiretroviral drug therapy during the antenatal period
- CD4+ T-lymphocyte count ≥ 200 μL at initial assessment

Zidovudine Regimen for Mother and Baby

- Zidovudine (ZDV), 100 mg orally, 5 times daily, begun at 14–34 weeks' gestation and continued throughout pregnancy
- During labor, an intravenous loading dose of ZDV of 2 mg/kg over 1 hour, followed by continuous infusion of 1 mg/kg/hr until delivery
- For the neonate, ZDV syrup orally 2 mg/kg, every 6 hours for 6 weeks, beginning 8–12 hours after delivery

Note. Adapted from, "Zidovudine for the Prevention of HIV Transmission from Mother to Infant," by the Centers for Disease Control and Prevention, 1994b. Morbidity and Mortality Weekly Report, 43(16), p. 286.

Table 11-3   Recommended Zidovudine Therapy for Prevention of Vertical HIV Transmission

CLINICAL STATUS	RECOMMENDATIONS
HIV-infected pregnant women, no previous antiretroviral therapy	Clinical, immunologic, viral evaluation. Risk/benefits of therapy discussed. Three-part zidovudine (ZDV) chemoprophylaxis (ACTG Protocol) initiated at 10–12 weeks' gestation.*
HIV-infected pregnant women receiving antiretroviral therapy during pregnancy	Continue antiretroviral therapy if identified after first trimester. If identified during first trimester, risks/benefits of therapy should be discussed and continuation of therapy should be considered. If drug therapy is discontinued during first trimester, drugs should be simultaneously reintroduced to avoid development of drug resistance. If current drug regimen does not contain ZDV, it should be added after 14 weeks' gestation. ZDV is recommended for the pregnant woman during the intrapartum period and for the newborn according to the ACTG Protocol.
HIV-infected pregnant women in labor with no previous antiretroviral therapy	ACTG Protocol 076 for intrapartum and postpartum period along with the 6-week regimen for the newborn. Woman should be evaluated to determine if antiretroviral therapy should be recommended.
Infants born to HIV-infected women who received no antiretroviral therapy during pregnancy or delivery	The ACTG Protocol for neonates should be discussed with the mother and offered for the newborn. ZDV should be initiated as soon as possible after delivery— preferably within 12–24 hours after birth. Woman should be evaluated to determine if antiretroviral therapy should be recommended.

*Dosing of ZDV has changed from the original ACTG Protocol, which recommended 100 mg five times daily to 200 mg three times daily, or 300 mg twice daily.

Note. Adapted from "Public Health Service Task Force Recommendations for the Use of Antiretroviral Drugs in Pregnant Women Infected with HIV-1 for Maternal Health and for Reducing Perinatal HIV-1 Transmission in the United States," by the Centers for Disease Control and Prevention, 1998, *Morbidity and Mortality Weekly Report, 47*(No. RR-2), pp. 1–31.

Nursing Tip

Assessment of the HIV-Positive Client

Client history

- Age
- Parity
- Complete health history
- Risk level for HIV infection
   Drug history (particularly injected-drug use)
   Sexual exposure
   Environmental or occupational exposure
- Subjective symptoms of HIV infection
- Perceptions of HIV status and anxiety level
- Social support system

Physical examination

- Review results of complete physical examination, especially any physical findings related to HIV infection

Diagnostic studies

- Enzyme-linked immunosorbent assay (ELISA) and confirmatory Western blot test
- CD4+ T-lymphocyte cell count, if the client is HIV-positive

long-term effects of the ACTG 076 protocol AZT regimen on women and children is currently unknown, although there appear to be no immediate adverse consequences to the mother or infant or to child development during the first 2 years after therapy (CDC, 1998b).

The most promising strategy for reducing perinatal transmission is the combination of elective cesarean section and AZT therapy. The combined approach reduces the transmission rate to 2% (Read, 1999). However, elective cesarean section is not financially possible for all women, and women undergoing a cesarean section have more complications than those delivering vaginally (Mofenson, 1998).

Pregnant women who are HIV-infected and already on antiretroviral therapy should immediately inform their health care provider of their pregnancy and continue medications as directed. Treatment of HIV-infected pregnant women should be considered in the context of optimal health care for the mother and pregnancy termination may be considered as an option. Because AZT is the only drug that has been shown to significantly reduce vertical HIV transmission, AZT should be included in any regimen of antiretroviral therapy during pregnancy whenever possible. Currently, if pregnant women are taking combinations of antiretroviral drugs that have reduced their plasma levels of HIV to undetectable levels, these women should be encouraged to continue the drug regimen, especially if treatment with AZT alone has failed (Carpenter et al.,

1997). More research is needed on combination antiretroviral therapy in pregnancy before recommendations can be made relative to efficacy (CDC, 1998b).

In addition to antiretroviral therapy, pregnant women with HIV infection may also be taking prescribed drugs for treatment or prophylaxis for opportunistic infections or clinical symptoms of AIDS. The management of pregnancy in HIV-infected women can be complex and referral to special health care providers is usually indicated.

Contraception for HIV-infected pregnant women should always be addressed in the antepartum period. All methods of contraception should be discussed and selection should focus on methods that are highly effective and fit into the client's lifestyle. Effective contraception, including the concepts of potential sterilization and abstinence, is of great importance, because women who are HIV-infected are often at high risk for unplanned pregnancies. In addition to contraception, HIV-infected women should use latex condoms with every episode of sexual intercourse to prevent transmission of the virus to others. Nurses are in an excellent position to counsel women regarding effective contraception and safe sexual practices.

PREGNANCY IN ADOLESCENCE

The period known as **adolescence** spans ages 11 to 19 and is defined as the biologic and psychologic transition from childhood to adulthood. Pregnancy in adolescence is not a new phenomenon but is of increasing concern because childbearing during the teenage years has profound socioeconomic and physical consequences for both the teen mother and her offspring. **Adolescent pregnancy** (the state of pregnancy in young females ages 11 to 19) is a complex, multifaceted problem with no easy or obvious solutions. The burden of an unintended pregnancy is especially heavy for young teens who are still in high school and are trying to juggle their education, their own identity formation, and the physical and emotional changes occurring with pregnancy (Stevens-Simon, 1997).

Incidence and Significance

Approximately 1,000,000 teen pregnancies occur in the United States annually (Alan Guttmacher Institute, 1999). The majority (about 82%) of teen pregnancies are unplanned (Stevens-Simon, 1997) and most teens (about 79%) who had a baby in 1998 were unmarried (National Center for Health Statistics, 1999).

According to the 1999 data from the National Center for Health Statistics (NCHS), the worldwide rate of adolescent pregnancy is declining, although the adolescent pregnancy rate in the United States remains among the highest in the industrialized world. Reasons for the decline in teen pregnancy rates include decreased sexual activity, increased

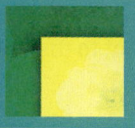

CASE STUDY/CARE PLAN
HIV TESTING AND COUNSELING

Because Janice and her husband have recently learned that their newborn has HIV-related pneumonia, they are referred for testing, for HIV and counseling before and after testing. Refer back to "Reflections from a New Mother."

Assessment

Janice is crying and asking "Does this mean I have HIV?" "And if so what do I do?" "What does it mean if I test positive?" Her husband is visibly agitated and is asking similar questions. "How could the baby get HIV?" "Does this mean we both have HIV?"

Nursing Diagnosis

Anxiety related to unknown HIV status and fear of a positive result.

Expected Outcome	Client will identify support systems and experience a reduction in anxiety.
Planning	With clients, make a list of potential support persons with whom they can share their news.
NOC	Anxiety self-control; coping
NIC	Anxiety reduction

Nursing Interventions	Rationales
1. Assure Janice that test results and any information she shares is confidential.	1. Clients are more likely to share sensitive information if confidentiality is assured.
2. Encourage Janice to vent her feelings related to a possible HIV-positive test result.	2. Allowing Janice to express her fears will assist her in coping with the testing process.
3. Provide Janice with information about the HIV testing process and what the laboratory test results mean.	3. Providing Janice with factual information will allow her to set her expectations relative to the testing procedure and assist her in understanding what a positive result means for herself and her family.
4. Assist the client in appropriate disclosure of HIV status with others who need to know.	4. Disclosing HIV status is a difficult and sensitive matter. Discrimination against HIV-positive individuals does exist. However, disclosure is important in obtaining appropriate medical and psychosocial support.
5. Encourage Janice to identify immediate support systems within her family and community.	5. Social support increases coping and assists the client in initial problem solving.

Evaluation	After discussing her feelings of fear with the nurse, Janice identified her parents, her family physician, and the pastor at her church as a support system for herself and her family. The nurse encouraged Janice to role-play to help decide how and what she would disclose about her HIV status with others, and Janice felt more prepared to share her uncertainty at this difficult time. Factual knowledge of the testing procedure assisted Janice in making an appointment for learning the test results and identifying a support person when obtaining the test results. Although still fearful of a positive result, Janice has identified an initial plan for coping with the test results.

Nursing Diagnosis

Deficient knowledge related to HIV disease process.

Expected Outcome	Client will increase understanding of disease process and treatment.

(continues)

Planning	Gather materials, resources, and referrals to ensure that the couple can react to the news from a base of knowledge.
NOC	Knowledge: Treatment regimen
NIC	Teaching: Disease process

Nursing Interventions	Rationales
1. Assess the client's understanding of HIV risk.	1. Before the nurse can begin client education about HIV, it is important to identify what is known.
2. Provide information on HIV transmission and effective measures to decrease transmission.	2. If the client understands the basis for transmission of HIV, appropriate precautions can be taken to prevent the spread of the disease.
3. Encourage the client to avoid breastfeeding.	3. Current literature suggests that HIV can be transmitted in breast milk. If the infant is HIV-positive, repeated exposure to the virus can increase viral load.
4. Discuss sexual abstinence and the use of latex condoms if the client is sexually active.	4. Female-to-male transmission is less common than male-to-female transmission. Latex condoms help to decrease viral transmission to either HIV-positive or HIV-negative partners. Repeated exposure to the HIV virus can increase viral load.
5. Encourage the client to refrain from the use of drugs and alcohol.	5. Because of a compromised immune system in HIV-positive individuals, drugs and alcohol should be used in limited quantities or not at all.
6. Advise client not to donate blood, plasma, or organs.	6. Blood, blood products, and body organs may contain HIV and thus be transmitted to others.
7. Assure client that if test results are positive, treatment and counseling are available.	7. Although there is currently no cure for HIV infection, effective treatment can decrease viral load to undetectable levels in the blood. If viral load remains low, opportunistic infections are less likely to occur. Because a diagnosis of HIV can be psychologically devastating, counseling should be made available for the family.

Evaluation	Janice has expressed understanding of the disease process and is encouraged that effective treatment is available. She denies other risky behaviors, such as drug and alcohol use and recent exposure to partners other than her husband. If she is HIV-infected, she will seek the nurse's assistance in identifying a plan to notify partners before her marriage. Janice is open to referral to an HIV specialist if her test result is positive.

condom use, and the use of injectable and implantable contraceptives (Ventura, Mosher, Curtain, Abma, & Henshaw, 1999). While these statistics may initially appear encouraging, the facts suggest that teen birth rates have remained relatively stable over the past decade. Reasons for the stability in birth rates are the decrease in spontaneous abortions (miscarriages) and elective abortions among adolescents.

Infant and Child Outcomes

Costs related to adolescent pregnancy are often measured in terms of negative infant and child outcomes (Table 11-4). Infants born to adolescents are often premature (less than 37 weeks' gestation) or low birth weight (less than 2,500 grams), constituting the two most common and serious risks associated with adolescent pregnancy. Infants born to adolescents under the age of 16 are twice as likely to be of low weight at birth, which is largely the result of the adolescent mother's smaller body and the lack of appropriate nutrition and prenatal care during pregnancy (Stevens-Simon & McAnarney, 1992).

In addition, untreated sexually transmitted diseases (STDs), smoking, and substance abuse are factors that contribute to preterm labor, prematurity, intrauterine growth retardation (IUGR), and low-birth-weight infants. Cigarette smoking among pregnant women of all ages has been shown to have a significant relationship to delivery of low-birth-weight infants.

Table 11-4 Negative Infant and Child Outcomes Indirectly Related to Adolescent Pregnancy

INFANT	CHILD
Blindness/deafness	Chronic behavioral problems
Cerebral palsy	Chronic cognitive defects
Infant death	Chronic runaway
Low birth weight	Developmental delays
Mental retardation	Foster/alternative placement
Prematurity	Neglect and abuse
Serious respiratory problems	School failure/withdrawal

Note. Data from *Kids Having Kids: A Robin Hood Foundation Special Report on the Costs of Adolescent Childbearing*, by R. Maynard, 1996, New York: The Robin Hood Foundation; and "Teenage Childbearing," by C. Stevens-Simon and R. Lowry, 1995, *Archives of Pediatric and Adolescent Medicine, 149*, pp. 912–915.

In the postneonatal period, the mortality rate of infants born to adolescent mothers, age 17 and younger, is twice as high as that of infants born to more mature women. The lack of knowledge about child development, appropriate discipline, supervision, level of maturity, and adequate health care are thought to contribute to the increased incidence of illness, injury, and mortality among infants and young children of teenage parents (Stevens-Simon & McAnarney, 1991).

Adolescent Psychosocial Development

The physical and psychosocial consequences for adolescent mothers and their offspring are substantial. To understand the context of adolescent pregnancy, a knowledge of adolescent psychosocial development and acquisition of developmental tasks is necessary. **Developmental tasks** of adolescence include the competencies in psychosexual development related to identity formation, sexual and vocational identity, and independence. In the search for their personal identity, adolescents try on many new roles until they discover a role that fits and an identity is formed. Having completed identity formation, the adolescent is emancipated from the family and becomes independent. The adolescent achieves autonomy by the use of abstract reasoning, which allows analytical thinking, problem solving, and planning for the future. Other developmental tasks include the formation of a sexual and vocational identity (Box 11-4).

There is a wide developmental age span between early and late adolescence (ages 11 to 19). Each age group has unique reactions to the developmental tasks, which

Client Education

Teen Pregnancy and Smoking

You may wish to provide and discuss information with expectant teen mothers on the adverse effects of cigarette smoking during pregnancy, including the following points.

- There is a clear association between maternal smoking and perinatal loss.
- Smokers have three and one-half to four times more risk for small-for-gestational-age babies than nonsmokers.
- The average weight of infants born to smokers is 170 to 200 grams less than infants born to nonsmokers.
- Studies have shown increased premature rupture of membranes in smokers.
- Newborns of smokers are smaller at every gestational age.
- Infants who are born to women who have stopped smoking early in their pregnancy are of normal weight at birth.
- There may be an increase in sudden infant death syndrome (SIDS) among infants born to mothers who smoke.

Note. Data from *Smoking and Women's Health* by American College of Obstetricians and Gynecologists, 1997, *ACOG Educational Bulletin*, No. 240, copyright 1997 by American College of Obstetricians and Gynecologists.

are influenced by the adolescent's cognitive thinking and are tied to the adolescent's sexuality (Table 11-5).

Cognitive development, or the age-related development of intellectual reasoning and perception, influences every aspect of adolescent psychosocial development. According to Piaget (1969), cognition moves from concrete to abstract

Box 11-4

Adolescent Developmental Tasks

- Formation of identity/self-perception
- Acquisition of education/vocation
- Emancipation from family/independence
- Formation of sexual identity
- Development of social network of peers

Table 11-5   Stages of Cognition and Aspects of Adolescent Sexuality and Pregnancy

	EARLY ADOLESCENCE (AGES 11–14) CONCRETE THINKING	MIDDLE ADOLESCENCE (AGES 14–16) EARLY ABSTRACT THOUGHT	LATE ADOLESCENCE (AGES 16–19) ABSTRACT REASONING
Cognitive Thinking	Limited abstract thought Appreciates the here and now Little sense of later consequences	Use of inductive and deductive reasoning Ability to understand later consequences of actions Ability to connect separate events and to project into the future Introspective/narcissistic	Ability to abstract and conceptualize Ability to analyze and plan for the future Consider another's needs above their own Concern for society as a whole
Issues in Sexuality	Changing body image Sexual fantasy Sexual vocabulary Sexual abuse/incest Masturbation Menstruation Nocturnal emissions Limited sexual experimentation Same sex peers	Sexual experimentation Peer pressure for sex activity Self-esteem issues and sexuality Over-the-counter contraception Sexual abuse/incest Homosexuality/safe sex practices Sexually transmitted diseases Responsible decision-making related to sexual issues Adequate/effective contraception Sexual preference may still be in flux Short-term commitments to partners Peer acceptance at peak	Responsible sexual decision making Correct use of contraceptive Sexual preference may be set Greater intimacy/long-term commitments Pregnancy/parenting Some continuation of sexual experimentation More realistic expectation of partner's role Peers of less influence
Issues in Pregnancy	Failure to recognize signs of pregnancy Denial of pregnancy if recognized Fear of telling partner, parents, or other adults about pregnancy Delay in seeking pregnancy diagnosis Delay in seeking prenatal care Disturbed about body changes Family upset about pregnancy Ambivalence about pregnancy Other coexisting risk-taking behaviors (drugs, etc.) Conflict in maternal role Lacks problem-solving abilities re: pregnancy Fears related to labor and delivery Lack of ability to plan for the future Partner often not involved	Same Same Same Seeks pregnancy diagnosis from over-the-counter test kits May seek professional diagnosis of pregnancy Ambivalent about body changes Same Same or desires pregnancy May be the same Same Some problem-solving skills present re: pregnancy Able to learn about labor and delivery but still may fear experience May be able to plan for pregnancy and consider future consequences Partner sometimes involved	Recognizes signs of pregnancy Confirms pregnancy Tells partner and/or parents about pregnancy Seeks professional diagnosis of pregnancy Seeks prenatal care early Accepts body changes Family ambivalent or accepts pregnancy Realistic decisions about pregnancy Less risk-taking evident although risk-taking may still occur Accepts maternal role if pregnancy is desired Able to solve problem re: pregnancy Realistic about labor and delivery Able to plan for future Considers options to pregnancy Partner may be involved, especially for older adolescent/young adult

thinking during the three phases of adolescent development (i.e., early, middle, and late adolescence). Concrete thinking focuses on the present, with little thought to later consequences; abstract thinking in early adolescence encompasses inductive and deductive reasoning and the ability to connect separate events and to understand later consequences; and abstract thinking, in late adolescence, is increasingly logical and complex. Some older adolescents

Critical Thinking

Counseling and Cognition

You need to consider the adolescent's cognitive capacity when doing any counseling or education. Counseling a group of teens about birth control may be ineffective if the consequences of their behavior are tied to the future, when their thinking focuses only on the present. What other aspects of the adolescent's behavior would you need to consider in relation to cognitive capacity?

Nursing Tip *Assessment and Sexual Abuse*

You should always consider aspects of sexual abuse in any health care encounter as young teens begin to reach physical and sexual maturation. Questions relative to the adolescent's sexuality should be included in the health history. For example, you may begin a discussion of the teen's sexuality by stating: "Many young people your age begin to think about sexual behavior, tell me what you think." Consider what your responsibilities are in asking teens about sexually sensitive information.

remain concrete thinkers because of low intellect, lack of education, or chronic substance abuse.

Issues Related to Adolescent Sexuality, Pregnancy, and Parenting

Adolescence is a period of transition: Pregnancy at any stage of adolescent development, but particularly in early and middle adolescence, poses an additional transition that makes identity formation more difficult. Sadler and Catrone (1983) describe adolescent pregnancy as a "dual developmental crisis" and describe major areas of potential conflict (Table 11-6).

The change in body image is particularly distressing to young adolescents who may find labor, delivery, and lactation not only frightening but unpleasant and undesirable. The father-to-be may also find his partner's body changes unattractive, throwing the young expectant

mother into despair over her rapidly changing appearance. Because relationships are relatively short during early and middle adolescence, partners may terminate the relationship before the baby's birth (Figure 11-5). Approximately two-thirds of teen relationships in which pregnancy occurs end before delivery.

Adolescents who give birth may actually have little understanding of their own body functions or their own sexuality. Nurses are in an excellent position, in both the prenatal and postpartum periods, to explore these areas

Nursing Tip *Negotiating with Teens*

Whenever possible, you should negotiate choices with teens and always consider how teens are judged by their peers. Knowledge of specific peer group norms is essential and limits should appear reasonable and acceptable to teens. For example, when educating pregnant teens about the importance of prenatal nutrition, you should be sensitive to food preferences and develop a diet plan that is realistic for teens to follow. Adequate intake of calcium can be obtained by a variety of products, such as yogurt, ice cream, and cheese. Diet planning also should include meals consumed outside the home, such as those at school and teen social events.

Table 11-6 Dual Developmental Tasks of Adolescent Mothers

ADOLESCENCE	VERSUS	PARENTHOOD
Narcissistic and egocentrist/ introspective, self-absorbed; focus on own needs		Empathy with the child; place child's needs before own
Ambivalent attachment to child		Mutuality between mother and child; mother's needs met through parenting
Identity formation through role experimentation; no firm commitment to a specific role		Maternal role identification and definition
Sexual identity formation/ body image development		Body image changes of pregnancy, delivery, and postpartum
Emancipation from family		Family role reassignments: from child to mother
Cognitive development: transition from concrete to abstract thinking		Problem-solving and decision-making skills necessary for raising child

Note. Adapted with permission from "The Adolescent Parent: A Dual Developmental Crisis," by L. Sadler and C. Catrone, 1983, *Journal of Adolescent Health Care, 4,* p. 102.

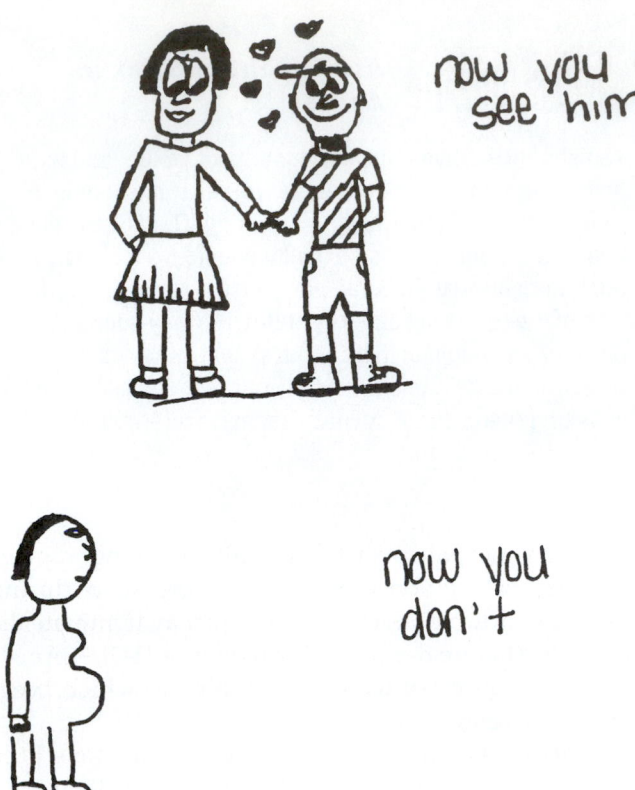

now you
see him

now you
don't

Figure 11-5 Teen pregnancy: now you see him, now you don't.

with teen mothers. Pregnancy and subsequent parenthood limit the teen's time, mobility, and ability to experiment with new roles because the responsibilities of child care must be assumed. Conflicts may arise regarding whose needs are being met as the adolescent mother attempts to differentiate her needs from her infant's needs during the normal adolescent transition period. Emancipation issues may become an area of conflict for the teen mother and her family. Developmentally, the teen mother needs to move away from the family and become autonomous, but realistically, she may be dependent on the family for financial and child care assistance.

Who's in charge and how the infant is raised is a likely area for disagreement. It is not uncommon to see the young adolescent mother step aside as her own mother takes over decisions related to the child's health and welfare. Finally, all aspects of parenting are influenced by the mother's cognitive development. Adolescent parents who lack the cognitive skills to understand their child's behavior and development may have unrealistically high expectations for their infants and young children and may be harsh disciplinarians who use physical punishment frequently. A young mother who does not realize that a toddler has a limited memory may become easily frustrated and angry when the child fails to follow her commands. The mother's ability to understand

the principles of child development and to project and plan for the future has a definitive effect on the child's well-being.

Adolescent Sexual Activity

The scenario in the "Reflections" box is not uncommon among teen mothers, and yet, after over 30 years of effective and available birth control measures, adults often ask, why. The path to teen pregnancy is influenced by many factors. Experimentation with sexual relationships, the need to love and be loved, peer pressure, sexually explicit media, promotion of self-esteem, partner pressure, and the need to feel grown up are reasons cited by teens as motivation for early sexual activity (Moore, 1996). Furthermore, teens state that loneliness, lack of understanding childcare responsibilities, poor self-respect, lack of knowledge about their bodies and birth control, drinking and drug use, and a general dissatisfaction with their lives contribute to an early, unplanned pregnancy (Chassler, 1997).

On a national level, the use of drugs and alcohol among adolescents has risen steadily, the family structure and social mores that discouraged unwed motherhood have diminished, and religious affiliations have declined. Responsible sexual behavior and the consequences of sexual risk-taking are not taught consistently. Some adolescents view having a child as their only real accomplishment, when even a high school diploma doesn't guarantee a job.

The age at which adolescents initiate sexual activity has declined as the age of **sexual maturation** (the establishment of menstruation and ovulation in females and the development of spermatogenesis in males) has declined. Unfortunately, emotional maturity develops later than physical maturity, and many adolescents who engage in

Reflections from a Teen Mother

"I never expected to get pregnant," says 15-year-old Alyce, "It just sort of happened. Now I'm struggling with school, and I have to get up a lot earlier just so I can get the baby ready, take him to daycare, and make it to class. It's getting harder to stay in school as he gets older; he wants my attention all the time. I wish my mother would just take care of him so I could get on with my life."

Nursing Tip *Confidentiality and Referral*

You should know the laws of confidentiality in your state for providing care to adolescents and have resources available for all adolescents, including minors, who are pregnant or are engaging in high-risk sexual behaviors.

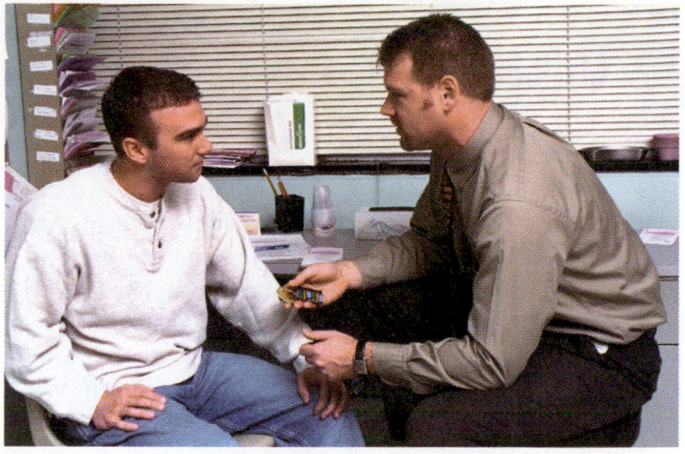

Figure 11-6   A straightforward, friendly approach when taking a health history from a teen facilitates a discussion about sexuality and birth control.

sexual relations to meet their biologic needs do not think of future consequences. Young people are confronted with sexual feelings and opportunities for sexual activity for which they may be cognitively and emotionally unprepared.

Taking an accurate sexual history from adolescents during routine health care visits is an opportunity to discuss the adolescent's sexuality and to assist her or him in selecting a method of contraception or help prepare for the initiation of sexual intercourse (Figure 11-6). Adolescents respond best to direct, open questions that are stated clearly and in terms they understand. It is necessary to be sincere and to demonstrate empathy, support, and understanding when questioning the adolescent about such sensitive issues (Box 11-5). The nurse should be comfortable and knowledgeable with the subject, not appear hesitant, and maintain good eye contact.

Box 11-5

Taking the Adolescent Sexual History

- Many young people your age begin to have sexual thoughts and feeling. Tell me about yours.
- What age did you start menstruation/ejaculation? Tell me how you are feeling about this development.
- You do have a choice about whether or not you want to have sex. Do you feel that you have a choice? Tell me something about what choices you have made.
- Are you having sex now? (*If yes*) With females/males/both? Oral or anal sex? With the same partner or different partners? At what age did you have your first sexual experience? Is having sex pleasurable for you? Tell me about the last time you had sex. Are you or your partner using anything to prevent pregnancy or sexually transmitted diseases (STDs)? What methods do you use?
- Have you ever been pregnant? Tell me about it.
- Have you ever had a sexually transmitted disease? How was this treated? Was your partner(s) treated also? What do you understand about this disease?
- What would you do if you (or your partner) became pregnant?
- Would you like to know about methods to prevent pregnancy?
- Tell me what you know about HIV/AIDS. Do you know what it means to have "safe sex"? Have you ever used (or practiced using) a condom? What would you like to know about condoms?
  (*If no to sex now*) Have you had sex in the past? Tell me how you felt about it.
- Are your friends having sex? Having babies?
- Before having sex, would you talk to your parent(s) about making that decision? Perhaps to a friend or another adult? How do you feel about using condoms? Have you considered what method of birth control you would use? How do you feel about becoming pregnant now?
- Have you ever been sexually assaulted? Sexually abused? Touched in a private way that you did not want? (*If yes*) Tell me about what happened to you. How did you feel about this? Who supported you after this happened? Did you have any counseling? (*If yes*) Describe how you felt about the counseling. (*If no*) Would you consider counseling now?

Critical Thinking

The Nurse and Sexuality

Nurses who are open, honest, and comfortable with their own sexuality are the most likely to gain the adolescent's trust and confidence and to interact with adolescents in a confidential atmosphere. How comfortable are you with your own sexuality and discussing sexual issues with teens? How do you feel about maintaining confidentiality with information that you think an involved parent might want to know?

Nursing Implications

Early diagnosis of an adolescent pregnancy is important for counseling purposes and for early entry into prenatal care. Many adolescents delay diagnosis and have no prenatal care in the first trimester of pregnancy. Early and consistent prenatal care is known to decrease the negative outcomes to the fetus, especially those born to women under the age of 16 (Stevens-Simon & White, 1991). Pregnant adolescents may initially present for confirmation or diagnosis of pregnancy with a variety of complaints. Some present with typical signs and symptoms of pregnancy, others present with vague complaints that may or may not be helpful in establishing a diagnosis of pregnancy. Teens who are in denial may be vague with respect to their last menses and complain of fatigue, headache, or abdominal pain. Because adolescents often do not know when they became pregnant, pelvic ultrasound is helpful in estimating gestational age. Approximately one-third of adolescents have vaginal bleeding during the first trimester and may mistake this for regular menses, denying the possibility of a pregnancy. The adolescent's sense of invulnerability may be in full operation and denial is common. "I thought I was too young to get pregnant" and "I had sex a lot and I didn't get pregnant so I thought I couldn't" are frequent comments when pregnancy is confirmed.

The use of a good sexual history is essential in obtaining information that leads to the confirmation of pregnancy. Once the pregnancy is confirmed, the adolescent should be counseled regarding her options and appropriate referrals should be made. Pregnant adolescents may have difficulty in solving problems and making decisions related to the pregnancy. Because adolescents need a great deal of support they should be strongly encouraged to share their pregnancy with their parents or another adult who can help them solve problems. Young women should also be encouraged to share confirmation of their pregnancy with the father of the baby. Teens who have short-lived relationships are often reluctant to share pregnancy information with the father of their child. Roles for the adolescent father can include taking responsibility for the pregnancy, participating in the decision-making process related to the pregnancy, and offering financial and emotional support if possible (Figure 11-7).

Prenatal Care, Labor and Delivery, and Postpartum Care

If the adolescent decides to continue the pregnancy, she should be referred to a comprehensive adolescent maternity program. Such programs are best at providing age-appropriate care and for offering prenatal education that is developmentally appropriate. Young teens who are concrete thinkers are best taught by simple, graphic instruction and demonstration. Videotapes, role modeling, interacting with other teen mothers, parenting exercises, and a hands-on approach to prenatal care are methods of instruction that are more effective than just providing verbal and written materials to pregnant teens. Being in a similar peer group assists the pregnant adolescent in adjusting to the pregnancy and becoming engaged in the activities necessary for a successful outcome. School-based clinics and programs, such as Communities in Schools (CIS), that provide prenatal education for pregnant couples are effective in preparing young teens for pregnancy, labor, delivery, and parenting. Prenatal education should include anatomy and physiology of the mother's body, the developing fetus, and the physiologic aspects of labor and delivery. Young women are particularly interested in

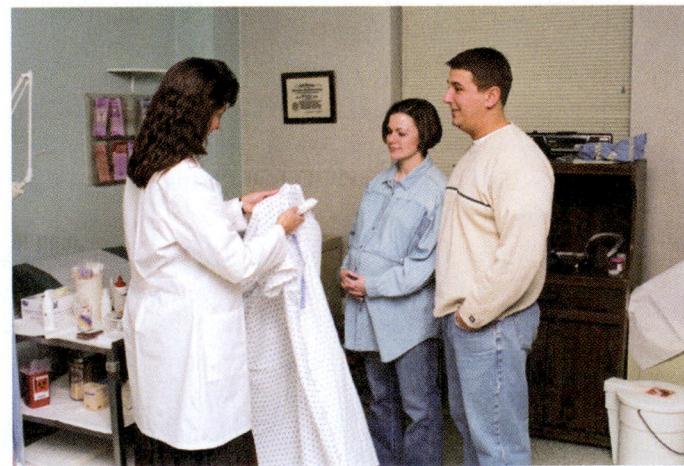

Figure 11-7 Expectant fathers who participate in prenatal visits gain a better understanding of pregnancy and the imminent responsibilities of parenthood.

seeing pictures of the developing fetus and graphic illustration (such as videotapes) of labor and delivery. Graphic illustrations provide the adolescent with a visual experience and help to decrease the misconceptions about body changes and what to expect during labor and delivery.

Other aspects of prenatal care should include the importance and frequency of:

- Prenatal visits
- Prenatal diet and exercises
- Treatment of STDs
- Immunizations
- Use of medications and abstinence from cigarettes, alcohol, and other drugs
- Preparation for labor and delivery
- Recognition of signs of labor, who to call, and where to go
- Discharge planning and postpartum follow-up

Prenatal education involving the infant would include:

- Information on breastfeeding, formulas, and infant nutrition
- Identification and acquisition of the necessary clothing and equipment for the newborn
- The need for and identification of appropriate resources for well childcare
- Basic skills such as bathing, diapering, and feeding newborns
- How to take a temperature
- Recognition of urgent and emergent conditions in newborns
- Identification of emergency resources
- Automobile and child safety
- Infant and child development with particular emphasis on age-appropriate discipline
- Educational goals and resources available

Ideally, comprehensive maternity programs include the baby's father and offer classes with other young expectant couples over a series of weeks or months in preparation for the baby's birth. Adolescents should be strongly encouraged to remain in school during the pregnancy, and school-based maternity programs are particularly supportive to that outcome. Community- or school-based programs designed especially for teens also emphasize issues in the transition to parenting and offer guidance for couples in maintaining relationships and dealing with conflicts related to their change in lifestyle. Negotiating an intimate relationship is often difficult enough for teen couples; the additional stress of finances and child-rearing

can be devastating given the tenuous nature of many adolescent relationships. More children of teen mothers grow up in a single-parent household than any other group in the United States (Maynard, 1996).

Pregnant teens under the age of 16 years are at greatest risk for obstetric complications. These complications are thought to be less causally related to physiologic factors but strongly linked to factors associated with teen pregnancy, such as poverty, poor nutritional habits, and inadequate and late prenatal care. Pregnant teens are at greater risk for iron-deficiency anemia that is secondary to poor nutritional intake. Teens need help in selecting iron-rich foods that are palatable and acceptable; most maternity services refer to a nutritionist to assist teens in developing diet plans that are nutritionally sound but include "fast foods" that are popular with teens. For low-income families with a pregnant adolescent, federal- and community-supported food resources are generally available. Body changes may be disturbing, and pregnant teens may restrict their caloric intake to maintain a prepregnant figure. Information on the increased nutritional needs of the body and the developing fetus is important. Assurances that diet and exercise after birth will return the teen to her prepregnant weight are encouraging.

Pregnancy-induced hypertension appears to be related to parity and weight gain. In multiparous adolescents, blood pressure and weight gain should be monitored frequently after baseline data have been established (Figure 11-8). Cephalopelvic disproportion (CPD) is common only in very young adolescents (ages 11 to 13) who have not

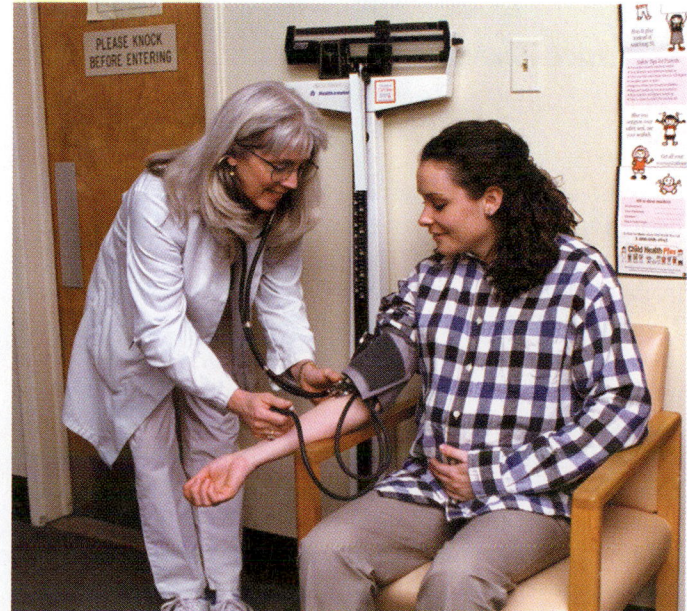

Figure 11-8   The adolescent's blood pressure should be carefully monitored throughout a pregnancy.

themselves and the developing fetus. Teens with a casual drug habit are more inclined to discontinue or decrease drug use during pregnancy. Teens who are addicted are more likely to remain addicted during pregnancy; crack cocaine is frequently the drug of choice. Referral to substance abuse treatment may be a viable option.

Although the postpartum period most often focuses on maternal identity and infant care, ongoing primary care for the mother and the baby should be identified early and become well-established. Adolescent mothers often seek care for their baby but lack care for themselves. Clinics that offer health care for both the mother and child are more successful in delivering services that support child health and consistent contraceptive practices, thus decreasing repeat pregnancy and encouraging education and vocation (Figure 11-9). Young couples with multiple social problems are best referred to comprehensive adolescent parenting classes that are designed to meet their social, psychological, and health care needs. Such programs are generally available through state and federal maternal-child health services at low cost or free to the participants.

Client Education

Home Visit Guidelines for Adolescent Parents

- Assess the social support system (parents, relatives, friends, neighbors, community agencies) for the adolescent parents.

- Encourage ongoing contact with the health care system for parents and infant, including community agencies such as the Visiting Nurse Service (VNS).

- Review the parents' knowledge of child development and expectations for their child.

- Identify school- and community-based services that would encourage continuing education for the parents and enhance infant development.

- Provide support to adolescent couples who may experience stress in the parenting role.

- Include the baby's father in all aspects of infant care, when possible.

- Identify referral sources for social, educational, and vocational needs.

- Provide information on reproductive physiology and family planning.

- Provide support for future plans, if adolescent parents choose to stay together.

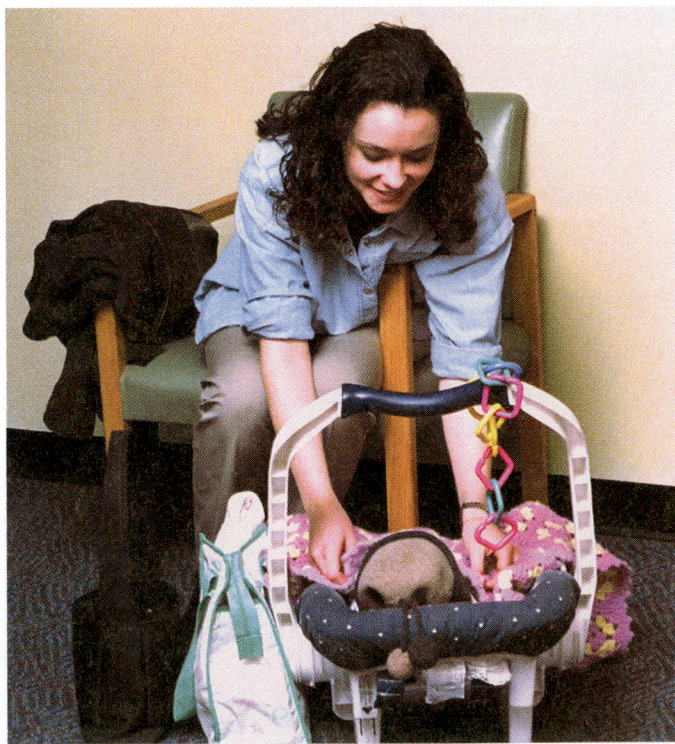

Figure 11-9   Postpartum and newborn health checkups are especially important for new teenage mothers who are learning to care for themselves and their new infants.

---

established complete pelvic growth and is more causally related to body type than to maternal age. STDs and substance abuse are known to be common co-existing factors in adolescents who exhibit other high-risk behaviors. Therefore, STDs and substance abuse must be considered in any adolescent pregnancy. Adolescents with a history of multiple partners and drug abuse should be counseled and tested for HIV infection. Specific and consistent follow-up is extremely important in decreasing the **vertical transmission** of HIV from the mother to the fetus during pregnancy or delivery and to the neonate during breastfeeding. STDs should be treated appropriately for both partners. Pregnant teens should also receive education regarding the effects of smoking, alcohol, and drugs on

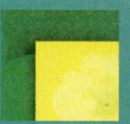

CASE STUDY/CARE PLAN
ADOLESCENT PREGNANCY

Shannon, a 10th grader, is an average student yet outgoing and popular. It seems that she always has a new boyfriend and is hopelessly romantic. She talks on the phone to her friends for hours about boys and dreams that someday she will become an actress. Shannon is 15 years old and presents to the school-based clinic complaining of nausea and a headache. Shannon's symptoms are vague, but she says that she has had nausea and some vomiting in the morning off and on for the past couple of months. After doing a complete health history and a brief physical examination, the nurse asks Shannon if she thinks she might be pregnant. Shannon denies being pregnant and tells the nurse that she can't possibly be pregnant because she broke up with her boyfriend over 6 weeks ago and she is having regular periods. On further questioning, Shannon admits the couple only used condoms "sometimes." She further adds that her periods are a little different, and she hasn't had as much bleeding as she usually does. She's also noticed that her breasts are tender and somewhat enlarged. After a positive result on a urine pregnancy test and a pelvic examination, she is estimated to be approximately 10 to 12 weeks pregnant. Shannon begins to cry and says, "What am I going to do? My parents will kill me! They were so glad when I broke up with my boyfriend and now this! Please, don't tell my mother," she sobs.

Assessment

- Single, pregnant adolescent
- High school student
- Lives with parents
- Unplanned pregnancy
- Unknown date of conception
- Concrete thinker
- Emotionally upset at confirmation of pregnancy
- Inadequate support at present

Nursing Diagnosis

Ineffective individual coping related to confirmation of unplanned pregnancy and parental notification.

Expected Outcome	Shannon will receive support and assistance from the health care staff and her family in problem solving, planning, and decision making regarding the current pregnancy.
Planning	Encourage Shannon and help her to outline the steps she feels are necessary to come to terms with this pregnancy.
NOC	Coping
NIC	Coping enhancement

Nursing Interventions	Rationales
1. Encourage Shannon to verbalize her fears related to the pregnancy and notification of her parents and the baby's father.	1. Decreases anxiety level and encourages beginning to solve problems.
2. Encourage Shannon to tell her parents immediately about the pregnancy and also encourage her to tell the baby's father.	2. Adolescent mothers need family support and also support from the baby's father, if possible. If the baby's father cannot support Shannon, he should be encouraged to assume some responsibilities related to the pregnancy.
3. Offer to assist Shannon in parental notification of the pregnancy but assure her of confidentiality if she refuses.	3. In developing a therapeutic relationship with adolescents, confidentiality is of utmost importance. Some teens welcome assistance in notifying their parents of an unplanned pregnancy and others prefer to tell them on their own. Nurses and other health care staff can assist adolescents with decisions about notification and provide support in this process.
4. Have Shannon identify who will be her immediate support person regarding the pregnancy today.	4. An immediate support person can decrease Shannon's anxiety about the pregnancy confirmation and parent and partner notification and assist her in immediate decision making.

(continues)

Evaluation   Shannon identified her best friend as an immediate support person and, with her assistance, notified her parents of her pregnancy. She chose not to notify the baby's father at this time. Shannon's anxiety decreased and she is considering her options regarding the pregnancy.

Nursing Diagnosis

Deficient knowledge related to lack of experience with the normal signs and symptoms of pregnancy.

Expected Outcome   Shannon will demonstrate a basic understanding of the signs and symptoms of pregnancy.

Planning   Gather materials for Shannon that outline the normal indicators of pregnancy.

NOC   Knowledge: Pregnancy

NIC   Health education

Nursing Interventions	Rationales
1. Discuss the signs and symptoms of pregnancy in the first trimester.	1. Providing information related to the normal physiologic and emotional changes of pregnancy allows Shannon to adjust to the pregnancy and decrease her anxiety about what is normal. Simple graphic instruction, in terms Shannon understands, will not overwhelm her in this time of crisis.
2. Encourage Shannon to ask any questions related to the pregnancy and provide anticipatory guidance. Provide written information for Shannon about the signs and symptoms of pregnancy during the first trimester.	2. Adequate knowledge about the pregnancy will assist Shannon to set immediate expectations and decrease her anxiety about the pregnancy.

Evaluation   After discussion with the nurse, Shannon understood how she got pregnant, approximately when, and why she still had minimal monthly bleeding and other signs of pregnancy.

Nursing Diagnosis

Deficient knowledge regarding decisions about pregnancy alternatives.

Expected Outcome   Shannon will make an informed decision about the alternatives regarding her pregnancy.

Planning   Gather materials and information appropriate to her level of understanding to share with Shannon the different pregnancy options.

NOC   Knowledge: Health resources

NIC   Decision-making support

Nursing Interventions	Rationales
1. Discuss all the possible alternatives relative to the pregnancy: termination, adoption, and keeping the baby.	1. Although many adolescents know of alternatives to pregnancy, they are often unaware of the timing of pregnancy termination, available resources, how to access resources, and costs. Health care providers can assist the adolescent and their support persons through this decision-making process in a nonjudgmental manner.
2. Encourage Shannon to discuss her feelings, values, and needs related to each alternative presented.	2. It is important to allow Shannon to discuss the consequences of all possible outcomes of the pregnancy and to support her in the decision she makes.

(continues)

3. Encourage Shannon to discuss her decision regarding pregnancy alternatives with her parents.

3. Shannon needs support from her parents in whatever decision she makes. Cultural mores and family and religious values often play a part in the decision to terminate or retain a pregnancy.

Evaluation

After an ultrasound examination which established an estimated 10-week pregnancy, Shannon elected to undergo pregnancy termination. Shannon's ex-boyfriend was not consulted about this decision, and Shannon has continued with school. She is currently unattached and is not sexually active, but she says that she will seek a birth control method before becoming sexually active in the future. Shannon's parents have remained supportive and have encouraged Shannon to concentrate on school and set realistic expectations for the future.

WEB ACTIVITIES

- Use a search engine such as PubMed or Ovid to search for a specific condition discussed in this chapter.

- Visit the Web site of the American College of Obstetricians and Gynecologists for clinical guidelines on managing pregnant clients with hypertensive and cardiovascular disorders.

- Visit the Web sites listed above. What types of information do they provide? Is the material targeted to the client or the health care provider?

- What other Internet resources can you find for pregnant teens (i.e., chat rooms, adoption services)?

- Visit nursing and government Web sites to find their guidelines on optimum ages for pregnancy.

- What does the CDC's site say about pregnancy, HIV infection, and AIDS?

Key Concepts

- Pregnancy is considered a normal process with minimal risks. However, the potential exists for development of risks.

- The best practice is to anticipate and attempt to reduce risks or prevent the occurrence of complications.

- A pregnant woman has the potential for changing from being normal to being high risk very quickly.

- Adolescent pregnancy is of increasing concern because childbearing during the teenage years has profound socioeconomic and health consequences for teen mothers and their children. The burden of an unintended pregnancy is especially heavy for young teens who are still in high school and are trying to manage their education, develop their own identity, and adapt to the physical and emotional changes occurring with pregnancy.

- The factors contributing to adolescent pregnancy are multifaceted and complex; they are influenced by the adolescent's cognitive and psychosocial development as well as cultural mores and socioeconomic status.

- The psychosocial and physical risks of pregnancy in adolescence are closely related to the adolescent's health and psychosocial well-being and the achievement of normal adolescent developmental tasks. Age, degree of substance abuse, level of nutrition, use of prenatal care, level of family support, and socioeconomic factors greatly influence maternal and neonatal outcomes.

- HIV infection has a significant physical and emotional impact on pregnant adolescents and young adults. Early detection and treatment of HIV infection is essential. With current antiretroviral therapy, vertical and perinatal transmission of HIV can be dramatically reduced and the outlook for greater longevity for mothers and children is promising.

Review Questions and Activities

1. Why is it important for you to differentiate the following: complete abortion, threatened abortion, and missed abortion?

2. Which signs and symptoms would alert you to a potential ectopic pregnancy?

3. When providing care for a woman who is in the third trimester of pregnancy and bleeding, what should you include in emergency preparations?

4. When magnesium sulfate is given to the pregnant woman, which complications or adverse effects will you need to monitor?

5. Why is it important to identify the blood type and Rh factor of all pregnant women?

6. Why is gestational diabetes a health problem for the pregnant woman? For the neonate?

7. What are the differences between chronic hypertension and pregnancy-induced hypertension?

8. Which of the following socioeconomic factors contributes to the high incidence of adolescent pregnancy in the United States?
   a. The lack of adequate birth control
   b. Poverty
   c. The lack of information on safe sex
   d. The availability of public assistance for unmarried mothers

   The correct answer is b.

9. Which of the developmental tasks listed is most affected by an unplanned pregnancy in early to middle adolescence?
   a. Identity formation
   b. Sexual identity
   c. Vocational identity
   d. Emancipation

   The correct answer is a.

10. When is HIV passed from mother to infant?
    a. Prenatal period
    b. Intrapartum period
    c. Postpartum period via breastfeeding
    d. All of the above

    The correct answer is d.

11. Which of the following groups in the United States is experiencing an increase in the rate of HIV infection?
    a. Homosexual men
    b. Heterosexual men
    c. Intravenous drug users
    d. Heterosexual female adolescents and young adults

    The correct answer is d.

References

Abu-Heija, A., Jallad, M., & Abukteish, F. (2000). Maternal and perinatal outcomes after the age of 45. *Journal of Obstetrics and Gynaecology Research, 26*(1), 27–30.

Alan Guttmacher Institute. (1999). *Special report U.S. Teenage pregnancy statistics with comparative statistics for women 20–24.* New York: Author.

Althabe, F., Carroli, G., Lede, R., Belizan, J., & Althabe, O. (1999). Preterm delivery: Detection of risks and preventative treatment. *Pan American Journal of Public Health, 5*(6), 373–385.

American College of Obstetricians and Gynecologists. (1994). *Diabetes and pregnancy* (ACOG Technical Bulletin No. 200). Washington DC: Author.

American College of Obstetricians and Gynecologists. (1996a). *Hypertension in pregnancy* (Technical Bulletin No. 219). Washington, DC: Author.

American College of Obstetricians and Gynecologists. (1996b). *Management of isoimmunization in pregnancy* (ACOG Educational Bulletin No. 227). Washington, DC: Author.

American College of Obstetricians and Gynecologists. (1996c). *Seizure disorders in pregnancy* (ACOG Technical Bulletin No. 231). Washington, DC: Author.

American College of Obstetricians and Gynecologists. (1997). *Smoking and women's health.* (ACOG Educational Bulletin. No. 240). Washington, DC: Author.

American College of Obstetricians and Gynecologists. (1998a). *Medical management of tubal pregnancy* (ACOG Practice Bulletin No. 3). Washington, DC: Author.

American College of Obstetricians and Gynecologists. (1998). *Special problems of multiple gestation.* (ACOG Educational Bulletin No. 253). Washington, DC: Author.

American College of Obstetricians and Gynecologists. (1999a). *Prevention of Rh D alloimmunization* (ACOG Practice Bulletin No. 4). Washington, DC: Author.

American College of Obstetricians and Gynecologists. (1999b). *Thrombocytopenia in pregnancy* (ACOG Practice Bulletin No. 6). Washington, DC: Author.

Aminoff, M. (1999). Neurologic disorders. In R. Creasy & R. Resnik (Eds.), *Maternal fetal medicine* (pp. 1091–1119). Philadelphia: W. B. Saunders.

Ananth, C., Smulian, J., & Vintzileos, A. (1997). The association of placenta previa with history of cesarean delivery and abortion: A meta-analysis. *American Journal of Obstetrics and Gynecology, 177*(5), 1071–1078.

Ananth, C., Smulian, J., & Vintzileos, A. (1999). Incidence of placental abruption in relation to cigarette smoking and hypertensive disorders during pregnancy: A meta-analysis of observational studies. *Obstetrics and Gynecology, 93*(4), 622–628.

Anderson, G. (1997). Tuberculosis in pregnancy. *Seminars in Perinatology, 21*(4), 328–335.

Barrett, D., & Sleasman, J. (1997). Pediatric AIDS: So now what do we do? *Contemporary Pediatrics, 14*(6), 111–124.

Barton, J. B., & Sibai, B. M. (2001). HELLP syndrome. In B. M. Sibai (Ed.), *Hypertensive disorders in women*, Philadelphia: W. B. Saunders.

Bowman, J. (1999). Hemolytic disease (erythroblastosis fetalis). In R. Creasy & R. Resnik (Eds.), *Maternal fetal medicine* (pp. 736–767). Philadelphia: W. B. Saunders.

Brent, G. (1999). Maternal hypothyroidism: Recognition and management. *Thyroid, 9*(7), 661–665.

Brost, B., & Newman, R. (1997). The maternal and fetal effects of tuberculosis therapy. *Obstetrics and Gynecology Clinics of North America, 24*(3), 659–673.

Buchanan, T., & Kjos, S. (1999). Gestational diabetes: Risk or myth? *Journal of Clinical Endocrinology, 84*(6), 1854–1857.

Burrow, G. (1999). Thyroid diseases. In G. Burrow & T. Duffy (Eds.), *Medical complications during pregnancy* (pp. 135–161). Philadelphia: W. B. Saunders.

Bussel, J. (1997). Immune thrombocytopenia in pregnancy: Autoimmune and alloimmune. *Journal of Reproductive Immunology, 37*(1), 35–61.

Carpenter, C., Fischl, M. A., Hammer, S. M., Hirsch, M. S., Jacobson, D. M., Katzenstein, D, A., et al. (1997). Antiretroviral therapy for HIV infection in 1997. *Journal of the American Medical Association, 277*(24), 1962–1969.

Castles, A., Adams, E., Melvin, C., Kelsch, C., & Boulton, M. (1999). Effects of smoking during pregnancy: Five meta-analyses. *American Journal of Preventative Medicine, 16*(3), 208–215.

Centers for Disease Control and Prevention. (1993). 1993 revised classification system for HIV infection and expanded surveillance case definition for AIDS among adolescents and adults. *Morbidity and Mortality Weekly Report,* 411–19.

Centers for Disease Control and Prevention. (1994a). *HIV counseling, testing, and referral standards and guidelines.* Atlanta, GA: U.S. Department of Health & Human Services.

Centers for Disease Control and Prevention. (1994b). Zidovudine for the prevention of HIV transmission from mother to infant. *Morbidity and Mortality Weekly Report, 43*(16), 286.

Centers for Disease Control and Prevention. (1996). HIV testing among women aged 18–44 years—United States, 1991 and 1993. *Morbidity and Mortality Weekly Report, 45*(34), 733–736.

Centers for Disease Control and Prevention. (1997a). *AIDS cases in male and female adolescents and young adults by heterosexual contact through 1996, United States.* AIDS Surveillance in Adolescents [L265 Slide Series]. Retrieved November 20, 1999, from http://www.cdc.gov/nchstph/hiv__aids/graphics/adolesnt.htm

Centers for Disease Control and Prevention. (1997b). 1997 revised guidelines for performing CD4+ T-cell determinations in persons infected with human immunodeficiency virus (HIV). *Morbidity and Mortality Weekly Report, 46*(RR-2), 1–3.

Centers for Disease Control and Prevention. (1998a). Maternal Mortality, United States, 1982–1996. *Morbidity and Mortality Weekly, 47*(34), 705–707.

Centers for Disease Control and Prevention. (1998b). US Public Health Service Task Force recommendations for the use of antiretroviral drugs in pregnant women infected with HIV-1 for maternal health and for reducing perinatal HIV-1 transmission in the United States. *Morbidity and Mortality Weekly Report, 47*(No. RR-2), 1–31.

Centers for Disease Control and Prevention. (1999). *Status of perinatal HIV prevention: U.S. declines continue.* National Center for HIV, STD, and TB Prevention-Divisions of HIV/AIDS Prevention. Retrieved January 23, 2000, from http://www.cdc.gov/nchstp/hiv__aids/pubs/facts/perinatl.htm

Chang, S., & McAuely, J. (1998). Pharmacotherapeutic issues for women of childbearing age with epilepsy. *Annals of Pharmacotherapy, 32*(7-8), 794–801.

Chassler, S. (1997, February 2). What teenage girls say about pregnancy. *Parade Magazine,* 4–5.

Chichakli, L., Atrash, H., Mackay, A., Musani, A., & Berg, C. (1999). Pregnancy-related mortality in the United States due to hemorrhage: 1979–1992. *Obstetrics and Gynecology, 94*(5, Pt. 1), 721–725.

Clark, S. (1999). Placenta previa and abruptio placentae. In R. Creasy & R. Resnik (Eds.), *Maternal fetal medicine* (pp. 616–631). Philadelphia: W. B. Saunders.

Clark, S., Cotton, D., Hankins, G., & Phelan, J. (Eds.), (1997). *Critical care obstetrics* (3rd ed.). Malden, MA: Blackwell Science.

Conde-Agudelo, A., Belizan, J., & Lindmark, G. (2000). Maternal morbidity and mortality associated with multiple gestation. *Obstetrics and Gynecology, 95*(6, Pt. 1), 899–904.

Connor, E., Sperling, R., & Gelber, R. (1994). Reduction of maternal-infant transmission of human immunodeficiency virus type 1 from mother to infant. *New England Journal of Medicine, 331* 1173.

Crane, J., van den Hof, M., Dodds, L., Armson, B., & Liston, R. (1999). Neonatal outcomes with placenta previa. *Obstetrics and Gynecology, 93*(4), 541–544.

Creasy, R., Resnik, R., & Iams, J. (Eds.). (2004) *Maternal fetal medicine* (5th ed.). Philadelphia: W. B. Saunders.

Cunningham, F., Gant, N., Leveno, K., Gilstrap, L., Hauth, J., & Wenstrom, K. (Eds.). (2001). *Williams obstetrics* (21st ed.). Stamford, CT: Appleton and Lange.

Duffy, T. (1999). Hematologic aspects of pregnancy. In G. Burrow & T. Duffy (Eds.), *Medical complications during pregnancy* (pp. 79–95). Philadelphia: W. B. Saunders.

Eldred, L., & Chaisson, R. (1996). The clinical course of HIV infection in women. In R. Faden & N. Kass (Eds.), *HIV, AIDS, and childbearing* (pp. 15–25). New York: Oxford Press.

Gittoes, N., & Franklyn, J. (1998). Hypothyroidism. Current treatment guidelines. *Drugs, 55*(4), 543–553.

Glinoer, D. (1999). What happens to the normal thyroid during pregnancy? *Thyroid, 9*(7), 631–635.

Grab, D., Paulus, W., Bommer, A., Buck, G., & Terinde, R. (1999). Treatment of fetal erythroblastosis by intravascular transfusion: Outcome at 6 years. *Obstetrics and Gynecology, 93*(2), 165–168.

Hageman, J. (1997). Congenital and perinatal tuberculosis: Discussion of difficult issues in diagnosis and management. *Journal of Perinatology, 18*(5), 389–394.

Hankins, G., Clark, S., Cunningham, G., & Gilstrap, G. (Eds.). (1995). *Operative obstetrics.* Stamford, CT: Appleton Lange.

Hauth, J., Ewell, M., Levine, R., Esterlitz, J., Sibai, B., Curet, L., et al. (2000). Pregnancy outcomes in healthy nulliparas who developed hypertension. Calcium for Preeclampsia Prevention Study Group. *Obstetrics and Gynecology, 95*(1), 24–28.

Hendricks, M., Chow, Y., Bhagavath, B., & Singh, K. (1999). Previous cesarean section and abortion as risk factors for developing placenta previa. *Journal of Obstetrics and Gynaecology Research, 25*(2), 137–142.

Inzucchi, S. (1999). Diabetes in pregnancy. In G. Burrow & T. Duffy (Eds.), *Medical complications during pregnancy* (pp. 25–51). Philadelphia: W. B. Saunders.

Jana, N., Vasishta, K., Saha, S., & Ghosh, K. (1999). Obstetrical outcomes among women with extrapulmonary tuberculosis. *New England Journal of Medicine, 341*(9), 645–649.

Kamwendo, F., Forslin, L., Bodin, L., & Danielsson, D. (2000). Epidemiology of ectopic pregnancy during a 28 year period and the role of pelvic inflammatory disease. *Sexually Transmitted Infections, 76*(1), 28–32.

Kendrick, J. (1999). Diabetes in pregnancy. In L. Mandeville & N. Troiano (Eds.), *High-risk and critical care intrapartum nursing* (pp. 224–255). Philadelphia: J. B. Lippincott.

King, P. (1996). Reproductive choices of adolescent females with HIV/AIDS. In R. Faden & N. Kass (Eds.), *HIV, AIDS, & childbearing* (pp. 345–363). New York: Oxford Press.

Kurinczuk, J., Parsons, D., Dawes, V., & Burton, P. (1999). The relationship between asthma and smoking during pregnancy. *Women & Health, 29*(3), 31–47.

Kyrklund-Blomberg, N., & Cnattingius, S. (1998). Preterm birth and maternal smoking: Risks related to gestational age and onset of delivery. *American Journal of Obstetrics and Gynecology, 179*(4), 1051–1055.

Licht, E., & Sankar, R. (1999). Status epilepticus during pregnancy. A case report. *Journal of Reproductive Medicine, 44*(4), 370–372.

Macones, G., Sehdev, H., Parry, S., Morgan, M., & Berlin, J. (1997). The association between maternal cocaine use and placenta previa. *American Journal of Obstetrics and Gynecology, 177*(5), 1097–1100.

Major, C. A., & Nageotte, M. P. (1999). Thyroid disease. In D. K. James, P. J. Steer, C. P. Weiner, & B. Gonik (Eds.), *High-risk pregnancy: Management options.* Philadelphia: W. B. Saunders.

Maloni, J., Cohen, A., & Kane, J. (1998). Prescription of activity restriction to treat high-risk pregnancies. *Journal of Women's Health, 7*(3), 351–358.

Mauskopf, J., Paul, J., Wichman, D., White, A., & Tilson, H. (1996). Economic impact of treatment of HIV-positive pregnant women and their newborns with zidovudine. *Journal of the American Medical Association, 276*(2), 132–138.

Maynard, R. (1996). *Kids having kids: A Robin Hood foundation special report on the costs of adolescent childbearing.* New York: The Robin Hood Foundation.

McDonnell, M., & Kessenich, C. (2000). HIV/AIDS and women. *Primary Care Practice: HIV-Related Illness, 4*(1), 66–73.

McGregor, J., & French, J. (2000). Bacterial vaginosis in pregnancy. *Obstetrical and Gynecological Survey, 55*(Suppl. 1), s1–s19.

Mercer, B., Goldenberg, R., Moawad, A., Meis, P., Iams, J., Das, A., et al. (1999). The preterm prediction study: Effect of gestational age and cause of preterm birth on subsequent obstetric outcome. *American Journal of Obstetrics and Gynecology, 181*(5, Pt. 1), 1216–1221.

Mofenson, L. (1998). *Simplified ZDV prophylaxis against mother-to-child transmission.* Medscape Conference News Online. Retrieved November 1999 from http://www.medscape.com/Medscape/CNO/1998/AIDS/06.29/p11/aids.p11.html

Montoro, M. (1997). Management of hypothyroidism during pregnancy. *Clinical Obstetrics and Gynecology, 40*(1), 65–80.

Moore, R. (1996). Overview of developmental physical milestones and psychosocial issues. *Current Practice Issues in Adolescent Gynecology,* 4–7.

Myatt, L., & Miodovnik, M. (1999). Prediction of preeclampsia. *Seminars in Perinatology, 23*(1), 45–57.

National Center for Health Statistics. (1999). Declines in teenage birth rates, 1991–98: Update of national and state trends. *Monthly Vital Statistics Report, 47*(26), 1–12.

National Heart, Lung, and Blood Institute. (2000). *Working group report on high blood pressure in pregnancy.* Washington, D.C.: National Institutes of Health.

National High Blood Pressure Education Program Working Group on High Blood Pressure in Pregnancy Report. (2000). *American Journal of Obstetrics and Gynecology, 183*(1), S1–S22.

Nolan, T., Espinosa, T., & Pastorek, J. (1997). Tuberculosis skin testing in pregnancy: Trends in a population. *Journal of Perinatology, 17*(3), 199–201.

Nulman, I., Laslo, D., & Koren, G. (1999). Treatment of epilepsy in pregnancy. *Drugs, 57*(4), 535–544.

Pastore, L., Savitz, D., & Thorp, J. (1999). Predictors of urinary tract infections at the first prenatal visit. *Epidemiology, 10*(3), 282–287.

Piaget, J. (1969). *The theory of stages in cognitive development.* New York: McGraw-Hill.

Rawlings, J., & Scott, J. (1996). Postconceptual age of surviving preterm low-birth-weight infants at hospital discharge. *Archives of Pediatrics and Adolescent Medicine, 150*(3), 260–262.

Read, J. (1999). The mode of delivery and the risk of vertical transmission of human immunodeficiency virus, type 1. *New England Journal of Medicine, 340*(13), 977–987.

Reis, P., Sander, C., & Pearlman, M. (2000). Abruptio placentae after auto accidents. A case control study. *Journal of Reproductive Medicine, 45*(1), 6–10.

Riley, L. (1997). Pneumonia and tuberculosis in pregnancy. *Infectious Disease Clinics of North America, 11*(1), 119–133.

Riley, L. E., & Greene, M. F. (1999). Elective cesarean delivery to reduce transmission of HIV [Editorial]. *The New England Journal of Medicine, 13* 1032–1033.

Saade, G. (1997). Human immunodeficiency virus (HIV)-related pulmonary complications in pregnancy. *Seminars in Perinatology, 21*(4), 336–350.

Sadler, L., & Catrone, C. (1983). The adolescent parent: A dual developmental crisis. *Journal of Adolescent Health Care, 4*(2), 100–105.

Samren, E., van Duijn, C., Christiaens, G., Hofman, A., & Lindhout, D. (1999). Antiepileptic drug regimens and major congenital abnormalities in the offspring. *Annals of Neurology, 46*(5), 739–746.

Schatz, M. (1999). Interrelationships between asthma and pregnancy: A literature review. *Journal of Allergy and Clinical Immunology, 103*(2, Pt. 2) s330–s336.

Schieve, L., Cogswell, M., Scanlon, K., Perry, G., Ferre, C., Blackmore-Prince, C., et al. (2000). Prepregnancy body mass index and pregnancy weight gain: Associations with preterm delivery. *Obstetrics and Gynecology, 96*(2), 94–200.

Seubert, D., Stetzer, B., Wolfe, H., & Treadwell, M. (1999). Delivery of the marginally preterm infant: What are the minor morbidities? *American Journal of Obstetrics and Gynecology, 181*(5, Pt. 1), 1087–1091.

Sisson, M., & Ruth, D. (1999). Disseminated intravascular coagulation. In L. Mandeville & N. Troiano (Eds.), *High-risk and critical care intrapartum nursing* (pp. 214–223). Philadelphia: J. B. Lippincott.

Song, T., Lee, J., Kim, Y., & Choi, Y. (1999). Low neonatal risk of thrombocytopenia in pregnancy associated with immune thrombocytopenic purpura. *Fetal Diagnosis and Therapy, 14*(4), 216–219.

Soussis, I., Trew, G., Matalliotakis, I., Margara, R., & Winston, R. (1998). In vitro fertilization treatment in genital tuberculosis. *Journal of Assisted Reproduction and Genetics, 15*(6), 378–380.

Starke, J. (1997). Tuberculosis: An old disease but a new threat to the mother, fetus, and neonate. *Clinics in Perinatology, 24*(1), 107–127.

Stein, D., Korvick, J., & Vermund, S. (1992). CD4+ lymphocyte cell enumeration for prediction of clinical course of human immunodeficiency virus disease: A review. *Journal of Infectious Diseases, 165,* 352–363.

Stevens-Simon, C. (1997). Reproductive health care for your adolescent female patients. *Contemporary Pediatrics, 14*(2), 35–69.

Stevens-Simon, C., & Lowy, R. (1995). Teenage childbearing. *Archives of Pediatric and Adolescent Medicine, 149,* 912–915.

Stevens-Simon, C., & McAnarney, E. (1991). Adolescent pregnancy: Continuing challenges. In D. Greydanus & M. Wolraich (Eds.), *Behavioral Pediatrics.* New York: Springer-Verlag.

Stevens-Simon, C., & McAnarney, E. (1992). Adolescent pregnancy. In W. McAnarney, R. Kreipe, D. Orr & G. Comerci (Eds.), *Textbook of adolescent medicine* (pp. 689–695). Philadelphia: W. B. Saunders.

Stevens-Simon, C., & White, M. (1991). Adolescent pregnancy. *Pediatric Annals, 20*(6), 322–331.

Tenore, J. (2000). Ectopic pregnancy. *American Family Physician, 61*(4), 1080–1088.

Ventura, S., Mosher, W., Curtain, S., Abma, J., & Henshaw, S. (1999). Highlights of trends in pregnancies and pregnancy rates by outcome: Estimates of the United States, 1976–96. *Monthly Vital Statistics Report, 47*(29), 1–10.

Weinberger, S., & Weiss, S. (1999). Pulmonary diseases. In G. Burrow & T. Duffy (Eds.), *Medical complications during pregnancy* (pp. 363–400). Philadelphia: W. B. Saunders.

Weinstein, L. (1982). Syndrome of hemolysis, elevated liver enzymes, and low platelet count: A severe consequence of hypertension in pregnancy. *American Journal of Obstetrics and Gynecology, 142*(2), 159–167.

Zimmerman, D. (1999). Fetal and neonatal hyperthyroidism. *Thyroid, 9*(7), 727–733.

Suggested Readings

Aziz, T., Burgess, M., Acladious, N., Campbell, C., Rahman, A., Yonon, N., el al. (1999). Heart transplantation for peripartum cardiomyopathy: A report of 3 cases and a literature review. *Cardiovascular Surgery, 7*(5), 565–567.

Becker, K., & Walton-Moss, B. (2000). Young women with recurrent yeast infections. *Primary Care Practice, 4*(1), 125–131.

Berg, C., Atrash, H., Koonin, L., & Tucker, M. (1996). Pregnancy-related mortality in the United States, 1987–1990. *Obstetrics and Gynecology, 88*, 161.

Bode, J. (1999). *Kids still having kids: Talking about teen pregnancy.* Boston: Horn Book.

Bowman, J. (1997). The management of hemolytic disease of the fetus and newborn. *Seminars in Perinatology, 21*(1) 39–44.

Bragg, E. J. (1997). Pregnant adolescents with addictions. *Journal of Obstetrical and Neonatal Nursing, 26*(5), 577–584.

Brauch, D. W., & Porter, T. F. (1999). Autoimmune disease. In D. K. James, P. J. Steer, C. P. Weiner & B. Gonik (Eds.), *High risk pregnancy: Management options*. Philadelphia: W. B. Saunders.

Brown, C., & Bertolet, B. (1998). Peripartum cardiomyopathy: A comprehensive review. *American Journal of Obstetrics and Gynecology, 178*(2), 409–414.

Busen, N. (1997). The adolescent. In J. Ashwill & S. Droske (Eds.), *Nursing care of children: Principles and practice* (p. 168). Philadelphia: W.B. Saunders.

Castro, W., Mayden, B., & Annitto, M. (1999). *First talk: A teen pregnancy prevention dialogue among Latinos*. Washington, DC: Child Welfare League of America.

Contraception and adolescents. (1995, July). *The Contraception Report,* 5–12.

Cox, J., & Bithoney, W. (1995). Fathers of children born to adolescent mothers. *Archives of Pediatric and Adolescent Medicine, 149* 962–966.

Cundy, T., Gamble, G., Townend, K., Henley, P., MacPherson, P., & Roberts, A. (2000). *Diabetic Medicine, 17*(1), 33–39.

Cunningham, F. G., & Leveno, K. (1995). Childbearing among older women: The message is cautiously optimistic. *New England Journal of Medicine, 333*(15), 1002–1003.

Cydulka, R., Emerman, C., Schreiber, D., Molander, K., Woodruff, P., & Camargo, C. (1999). Acute asthma among pregnant women presenting to the emergency department. *American Journal of Respiratory and Critical Care Medicine, 160*(3), 887–892.

Ellers, D., Patterson, C., & Webb, G. (1997). Maternal and fetal implications of anticonvulsant therapy during pregnancy. *Obstetrics and Gynecology Clinics of North America, 24*(3), 523–524.

Endersbe, J. (2000). *Teen fathers: Getting involved*. Mankato, MN: Capstone Press.

Erikson, E. (1968). *Identity: Youth and crisis*. New York: W. W. Norton.

Friedman, S. A., Lubarsky, S. L., & Lim, K. H. (2001). Mild gestational hypertension and pre-eclampsia. In B. M. Sibai (Ed.), *Hypertensive disorders in women*. Philadelphia: W. B. Saunders.

Gilbert, E. S., & Harmon, J. S. (1998). *Manual of high risk pregnancy and delivery*. St. Louis, MO: Mosby.

Gilchrist, L., Hussey, J., Gillmore, M., Lohr, M., & Morrison, D. (1996). Drug use among adolescent mothers: Prepregnancy to 18 months postpartum. *Journal of Adolescent Health, 19* 337–344.

Gladman, D., & Urowitz, M. (1999). Rheumatic disease in pregnancy. In G. Burrow & T. Duffy (Eds.), *Medical complications during pregnancy* (pp. 415–438). Philadelphia: W. B. Saunders.

Gordon, C. (1998). Use of intravenous immunoglobulin therapy in pregnancy in systemic lupus erythematosus and antiphospholipid antibody syndrome. *Lupus, 7*(7), 429–433.

Haddow, J., Palomaki, G., Allen, W., Williams, J., Knight, G., Gagnon, J., et al. (1999). Maternal thyroid deficiency during pregnancy and subsequent neuropsychological development of the child. *New England Journal of Medicine, 341*(8), 549–555.

Haddow, J., Palomaki, G., Knight, G., Cunningham, G., Lustig, L., & Boyd, P. (1994). Reducing the need for amniocentesis in women 35 years or older with serum markers for screening. *New England Journal of Medicine, 330*(16), 1114–1118.

Haffner, D. W. (1995). *Facing facts: Sexual health for America's adolescents: The report of the national commission on adolescent sexual health*. New York: SIECUS.

Hatcher, R., Stewart, F, Trussell, J., Kowal, D., Guest, F., Stewart, G., et al. (1998). *Contraceptive technology* (17th ed.). New York: Irvington.

Heider, A., Kuller, J., Strauss, R., & Wells, S. (1999). Peripartum cardiomyopathy: A review of the literature. *Obstetrical and Gynecological Survey, 54*(8), 526–531.

Hershberger, P. (1998). Smoking and pregnant teens. *Association of Women's Health, Obstetric, and Neonatal Nurses Lifelines, 2*(4), 27–31.

Hibbard, J., Lindheimer, M., & Lang, R. (1999). A modified definition for peripartum cardiomyopathy and prognosis based on echocardiography. *Obstetrics and Gynecology, 94*(2), 311–316.

Holmes, L., Rosenberger, P., Harvey, E., Khoshbin, S., & Ryan, L. (2000). Intelligence and physical features of children of women with epilepsy. *Teratology, 61*(3), 196–202.

Hutti, M. H., dePacheco, M., & Smith, M. (1998). A study of miscarriage: Development and validation of the perinatal grief intensity scale. *Journal of Obstetric, Gynecologic, and Neonatal Nursing, 27*(5), 547–555.

Jamiolkowski, R. (1997). *A baby doesn't make the man: Alternative sources of power and manhood for young men*. New York: Rosen.

Joffe, G., Esterlitz, J., Levine, R., Clemens, J., Ewell, M., Sibai, S., et al. (1998). The relationship between abnormal glucose tolerance and hypertensive disorders of pregnancy in healthy nulliparous women. *American Journal of Obstetrics and Gynecology, 179*(4), 1032–1037.

Joglar, J., & Page, R. (1999). Treatment of cardiac arrhythmias during pregnancy: Safety considerations. *Drug Safety, 20*(1), 85–94.

Katz, V., Farmer, R., & Kuller, J. (2000). Preeclampsia into eclampsia: Towards a new paradigm. *American Journal of Obstetrics and Gynecology, 182*(6), 1389–1396.

Koonin, L., Ellerbrook, T. V., Atrash, A. K., Rogers, M. F., Smith, J. C., Hogue, C. J., et al. (1989). Pregnancy-associated deaths due to AIDS in the United States. *Journal of the American Medical Association, 261*, 1306–1309.

Lewis, D., Van Dyke, D., Stumbo, P., & Berg, M. (1998). Drug and environmental factors associated with adverse pregnancy outcomes. Part I: Antiepileptic drugs, contraceptives, smoking, and folate. *Annals of Pharmacotherapy, 32*(7-8), 802–817.

Lindsay, J., Schilling, M., & Enright, S. (1997). *Books, babies and school-aged parents: How to teach pregnant and parenting teens to succeed.* Buena Park, CA: Morning Glory Press.

Lindsay, J. W. (1997). *Pregnant? Adoption an option.* Buena Park, CA: Morning Glory Press.

Lu, J., & Nightengale, C. (2000). Magnesium sulfate in eclampsia and preeclampsia: Pharmokinetic principles. *Clinical Pharmokinetics, 38*(4), 305–314.

Luke, B., Bigger, H., Leurgans, S., & Sietsema, D. (1996). The cost of prematurity: A case-control study of twins vs singletons. *American Journal of Public Health, 86*(6), 809–814.

Luker, K. (1996). *Dubious conceptions: The politics of teenage pregnancy.* Cambridge, MA: Harvard University Press.

Luskin, A. (1999). An overview of the recommendations of the Working Group on Asthma and Pregnancy. *Journal of Allergy and Clinical Immunology, 103*(2, Pt. 2), s350–s353.

Lynch, M., & Pugh, K. (2000, January). Uneven ground: HIV in women of color. *Advance for Nurse Practitioners,* 45–48.

Malone, F., & D'Alton, M. (1997). Drugs in pregnancy: Anticonvulsants. *Seminars in Perinatology, 21*(2), 114–123.

Mashburn, M. (1994). Levonorgestrel implant use among adolescents. *Journal of Pediatric Health Care, 8*(6), 255–260.

Meng, C., & Lockshin, M. (1999). Pregnancy in lupus. *Current Opinion in Rheumatology, 11*(5), 348–351.

Mestouan, J. H. (1997) Perinatal thyroid dysfunction: Prenatal diagnosis and treatment. *Medscape Womens Health 2*(7), 2.

Morrell, M. (1998). Guidelines for the care of women with epilepsy. *Neurology, 51*(5, Suppl. 4), S21–S27.

Mucrow, C. D., Chiquette, E., Ferree, R. C., Sibai, B. M., Stevens, K. R., Harris, M., et al. (2000). *Management of chronic hypertension during pregnancy.* Bethesda, MD: Agency for Healthcare Research and Policy.

Panting-Kemp, A., Nguyen, T., Chang, E., Quillen, E., & Castro, L. (1999). Idiopathic polyhydramnios and perinatal outcome. *American Journal of Obstetrics and Gynecology, 181*(5, Pt. 1), 1079–1082.

Pauker, S., & Pauker, S. (1994). Prenatal diagnosis—why is 35 a magic number? *New England Journal of Medicine, 330*(16), 1151–1152.

Payne, S., Resnik, R., Moore, T., Hedriana, H., & Kelly, T. (1997). Maternal characteristics and risk of severe neonatal thrombocytopenia and intracranial hemorrhage in pregnancies complicated by autoimmune thrombocytopenia. *American Journal of Obstetrics and Gynecology, 177*(1), 149–155.

Putnik, J. (1996, August 19). Welfare bill: Legislating morality? *New York Times,* B1.

Rabinerson, D., Gruber, A., Kaplan, B., Lurie, S., Peled, Y., & Neri, A. (1997). Isolated persistent fetal bradycardia in complete A-V block: A conservative approach is appropriate. A case report and review of the literature. *American Journal of Perinatology, 14*(6), 317–320.

Rahman, P., Gladman, D., & Urowitz, M. (1998). Clinical predictors of fetal outcome in systemic lupus erythematosus. *Journal of Rheumatology, 25*(8), 1526–1530.

Raines, C. (2000). Antiretroviral treatment in HIV infection. *Primary Care Practice, 4*(1), 83–100.

Reichlin, M. (1998). Systemic lupus erythematosus and pregnancy. *Journal of Reproductive Medicine, 43*(4), 355–360.

Reuters News Service. (1997, October, 28). Teen pleads not guilty in prom baby case. *The Houston Chronicle,* 7A.

Roach, V., Hin, L., Tam, W., Ng, K., & Rogers, M. (2000). The incidence of pregnancy-induced hypertension among patients with carbohydrate intolerance. *Hypertension in Pregnancy, 19*(2), 183–189.

Rodis, J., Borgida, A., Wilson, M., Egan, J., Leo, M., Odibo, A., et al. (1998). Management of parvovirus infection in pregnancy and outcomes of hydrops: A survey of members of the Society of Perinatal Obstetricians. *American Journal of Obstetrics and Gynecology, 179*(4), 985–958.

Rogowski, J. (1998). Cost-effectiveness of care for very low birth weight infants. *Pediatrics, 102*(1), 35–43.

Samuels, L., Kaufman, M., Morris, R., & Brockman, S. (1998). Postpartum coronary artery dissection: Emergency coronary bypass with ventricular assist device support. *Coronary Artery Disease, 9*(7), 457–460.

Sauer, M., Paulson, R., & Lobo, R. (1995). Pregnancy in women 50 or more years of age: Outcomes of 22 consecutively established pregnancies from oocyte donation. *Fertility and Sterility, 64*(1), 111–115.

Shellhaas, C., & Iams, J. (1998). Ambulatory management of preterm labor. *Clinical Obstetrics and Gynecology. Ambulatory Obstetric Management, 41*(3), 491–502.

Sibai, B. (2000). Risk factors, pregnancy complications, and prevention of hypertensive disorders in women with pregravid diabetes mellitus. *Journal of Maternal-Fetal Medicine, 9*(1), 62–65.

Sibai, B., Caritis, S., Hauth, J., Lindheimer, M., VanDorsten, J., MacPherson, C., et al. (2000a). Risks of pre-eclampsia and adverse neonatal outcomes among women with pregestational diabetes mellitus. *American Journal of Obstetrics and Gynecology, 182*(2), 364–369.

Sibai, B., Hauth, J., Caritis, S., Lindheimer, M., MacPherson, C., Klebanoff, M., et al. (2000b). Hypertensive disorders in twins versus singleton gestation. National Institute of Child Health and Human Development Network of Maternal-Fetal Medicine Units. *American Journal of Obstetrics and Gynecology, 182*(4), 938–942.

Silver, R., & Branch, D. (1997). Autoimmune disease in pregnancy. Systemic lupus erythematosus and antiphospholipid syndrome. *Clinics in Perinatology, 24*(2), 291–320.

Silver, R., Branch, D., & Scott, J. (1995). Maternal thrombocytopenia in pregnancy: Time for a reassessment. *American Journal of Obstetrics and Gynecology, 173*(2), 479–482.

Silverman, N., Rohner, D., & Turner, B. (1997). Attitudes toward health-care, HIV infection, and perinatal transmission interventions in a cohort of inner-city, pregnant women. *American Journal of Perinatology, 14*(6), 341–346.

Simon, T., Alverson, D., AuBuchon, J., Cooper, E., DeChristopher, P., Glenn, G., et al. (1998). Practice paramenters for the use of red blood cell transfusions: Developed by the Red Blood Cell Administration Practice Guideline Development Task Force of the College of American Pathologists. *Archives of Pathology and Laboratory Medicine, 122*(2), 130–138.

Spratto, G. R., & Woods, A. L. (2004). *PDR nurse's drug handbook.* Clifton Park, NY: Delmar Learning.

Stevens-Simon, C. (1998). Providing reproductive health care and prescribing contraceptives for adolescents. *Pediatrics in Review, 19*(12), 409–417.

Stevens-Simon, C., Kelly, L., Singer, D., & Cox, A. (1996). Why pregnant adolescents say they did not use contraceptive prior to conception. *Journal of Adolescent Health, 19*, 48–53.

Szal, S., Croughan-Minihane, M., & Kilpatrick, S. (1999). Effect of magnesium prophylaxis and preeclampsia on the duration of labor. *American Journal of Obstetrics and Gynecology, 180*(6, Pt. 1), 1475–1479.

Temmerman, M., Chamba, E. N., Ndinya-Achola, J., Plumer, F. A., Coppens, M., & Piot, P. (1994). Maternal human immunodeficiency virus-1 infection and pregnancy outcome. *Obstetrics and Gynecology, 83*(4), 495.

Trapani, M. (1997). *Listen up!: Teenage mothers speak out.* New York: Rosen.

Ventura, S., Martin, J., Taftel, S., Mathews, T., & Clarke, S. (1995). Advance report of final natality statistics, 1993. *Monthly Vital Statistics Report, 44*(Suppl.), 1–88.

Webber, M., Halligan, R., & Schumacher, J. (1997). Acute infarction, intracoronary thrombosis, and primary PTCA in pregnancy. *Catheterization and Cardiovascular Disease, 42*(1), 38–43.

Wolbrette, D., & Patel, H. (1999). Arrhythmias and women. *Current Opinion in Cardiology, 14*(1), 36–43.

Yancy, M., & Richards, D. (1994). Effect of altitude on the amniotic fluid index. *Journal of Reproductive Medicine, 39*(2), 101–104.

Resources

American Academy of Pediatrics, http://www.aap.org

Interactive teen Web site, http://www.cyberisle.org

International Childbirth Education Association, http://www.icea.org

Sidelines National Support Network for pregnant women on bed rest, http://www.sidelines.org

Society for Adolescent Medicine, http://www.adolescenthealth.org

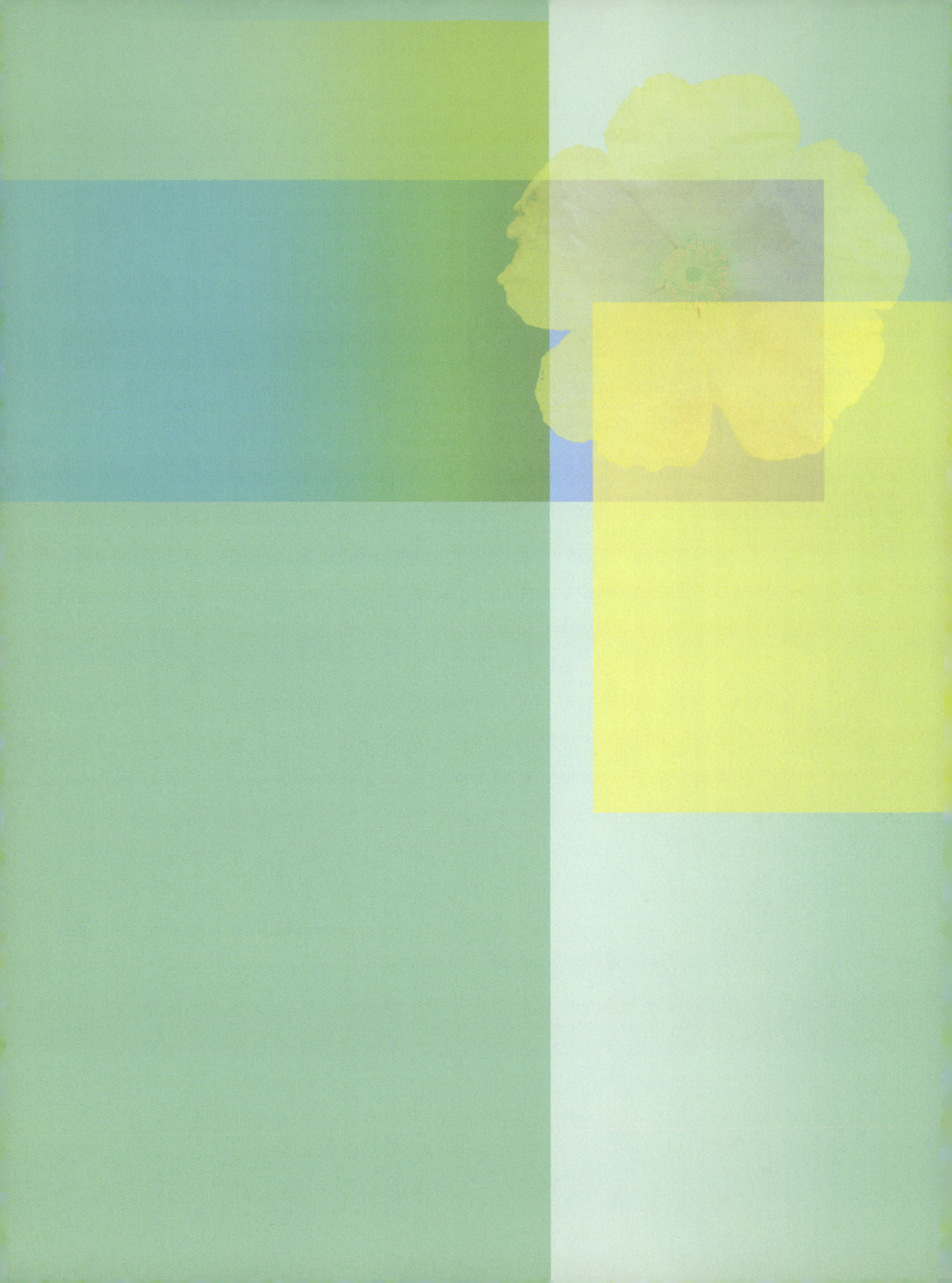

CHAPTER 12

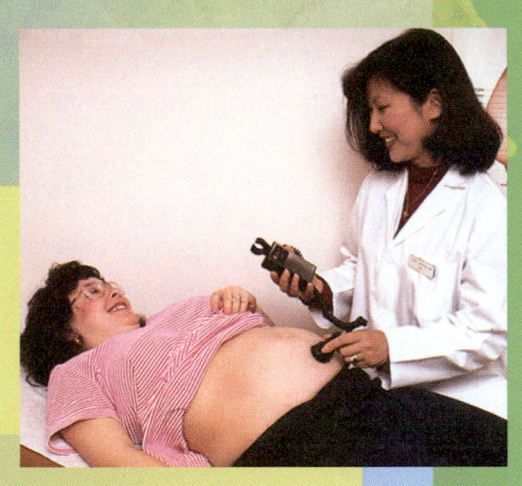

FETAL DEVELOPMENT AND WELL-BEING

Have you ever considered what a baby looks like at various stages of fetal development? Some organs and systems are almost totally completely developed at the end of the first trimester of pregnancy. Other systems, such as the nervous system, are not fully developed.

- What implications does fetal development have for your nursing practice?
- If I were pregnant and my job increased my risk of miscarriage, would I stop working even if I were the only wage earner in my family?
- What is the difference between screening and diagnostic tests for fetal well-being?
- What would I want to know about the well-being of my fetus if I were pregnant?

Key Terms

Amniocentesis
Amnion
Amniotic fluid
Biophysical profile (BPP)
Blastocyst
Chorion
Chorionic villi
Chorionic villus sampling (CVS)
Contraction stress test (CST)
Decidua
Decidua basalis
Decidua capsularis
Decidua parietalis
Doppler blood studies
Embryo
Fertilization
Fetal alcohol syndrome
Fetal fibronectin (fFN) testing
Fetal movement counting (FMC)
Fetal tissue sampling
Heavy metal
Herbicide
Human chorionic gonadotropin (hCG)

Human placental lactogen (hPL)
Hyperthermia
Implantation
Lanugo
Magnetic resonance imaging (MRI)
Maternal serum—α-fetoprotein (MS-AFP)
Meiosis
Mitosis
Morula
Neonatal abstinence syndrome
Nonstress test (NST)
Percutaneous umbilical blood sampling (PUBS)
Pesticide
Spermatozoa
Teratogen
TORCH
Trophoblast cells
Ultrasonography
Wharton's jelly
Zygote

Competencies

Upon completion of this chapter, the reader should be able to:

1. Describe the process of fertilization, implantation, and cell differentiation.
2. Delineate the structure and function of the placenta, amniotic fluid, and umbilical cord.
3. Identify the major stages of fetal development.
4. Discuss threats to fetal well-being found in the home and some workplaces.
5. Discuss how chemical dependency can pose a threat to fetal well-being.
6. Describe infections that can pose threats to fetal well-being.
7. Discuss the clinical applications of ultrasonography.
8. Identify the criteria for interpreting a nonstress test.
9. Differentiate between screening and diagnostic procedures.
10. Teach the client how to perform fetal movement counts.
11. Describe a method to evaluate fetal maturity.

There is no process as amazing as the development of a human being from two single cells. In about 40 weeks, a fertilized egg grows from a single cell to a fully developed fetus able to survive the birthing process. This chapter gives an overview of the developmental process of risk to and assessment of fetal well-being

CELL DIVISION

This section presents an overview of fertilization through embryonic and fetal development. A new life starts from small cells. A fertilized egg grows from a single cell carrying all the required genetic material. Human development occurs through two cell division processes: mitosis and meiosis. During **mitosis** the body cells duplicate into two separate daughter cells. This is how the human body grows and increases in size. Mitosis is a continuous process whereby the cell material duplicates and divides and enables the growth of the fetus. The distinct stages of mitosis are illustrated in Figure 12-1. **Meiosis** is the process by which the ovum and sperm divide and mature. In contrast to mitosis, meiosis results in a reduction in the number of human chromosomes. All human cells normally have 46 chromosomes, except the sex cells (ovum and sperm). These chromosomes are paired, thus, each cell contains 22 pairs of autosomes and one pair of sex chromosomes. The ovum and sperm undergo the process of meiosis (reduction in total number of chromosomes). In the meiotic process (see Figure 12-1) each gamete receives

Cell Division

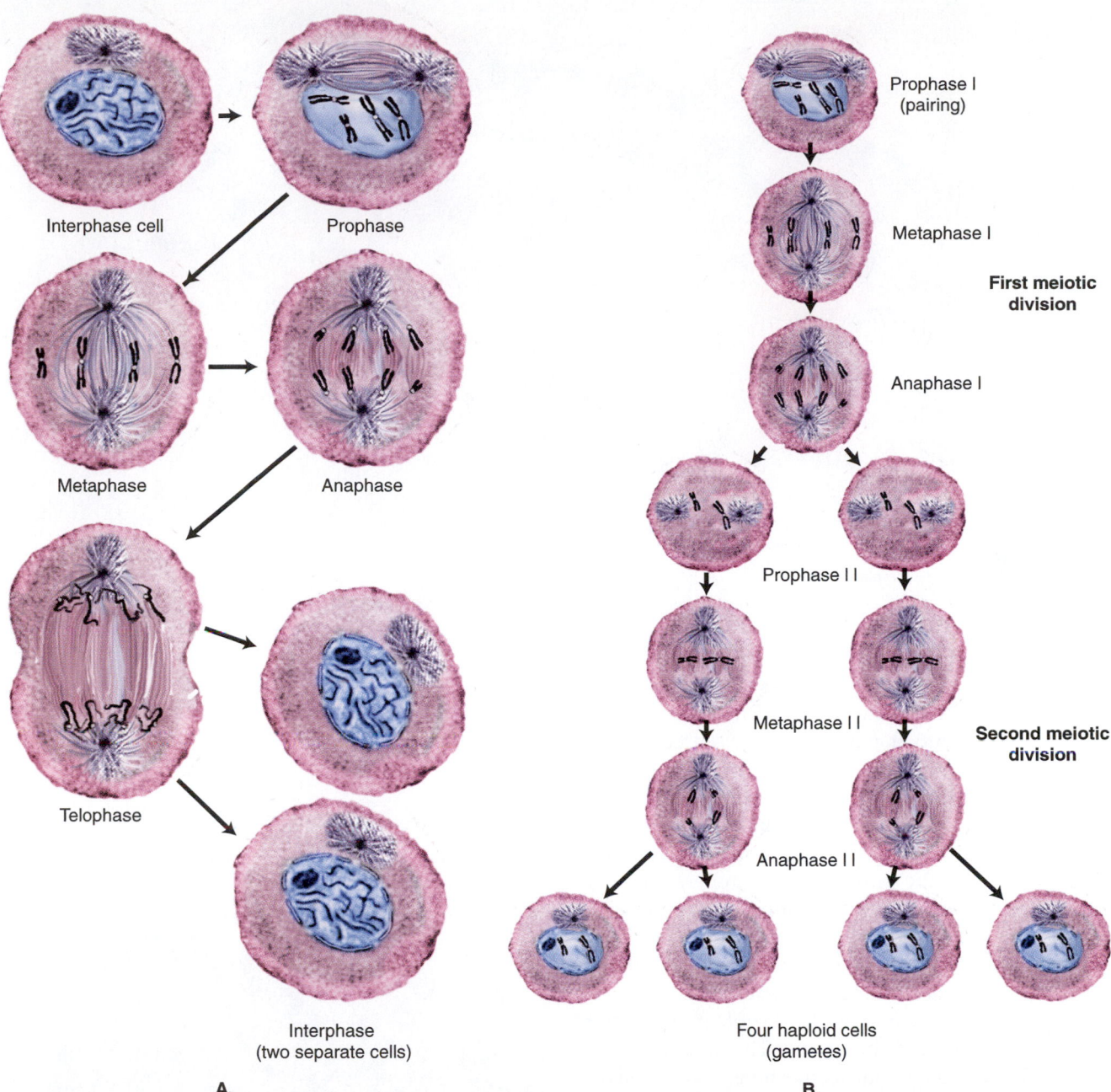

A.
    B.

Figure 12-1 Cell division. A. Mitosis; B. Meiosis.

only one chromosome from each pair. Thus, each mature ovum and spermatozoon has 23 chromosomes.

IMPLANTATION AND FERTILIZATION

Human development begins before **implantation**, which is the embedding of the fertilized ovum into the endometrium. During ovulation in the female, the mature ovum emerges from the ovary and is swept up into the fallopian tube (Figure 12-2). The ovum is propelled through the fallopian tube. **Fertilization** (Figure 12-3) of the ovum (uniting with the sperm) occurs within the first 24 to 48 hours after the release of the ovum into the fallopian tube. If the ovum is not fertilized within this time, the ovum wastes away and becomes nonfunctional. Since the life of **spermatozoa** is approximately 48 to 72 hours, the total time span during which fertilization may occur depends on ovulation occurring during the life of the deposited sperm.

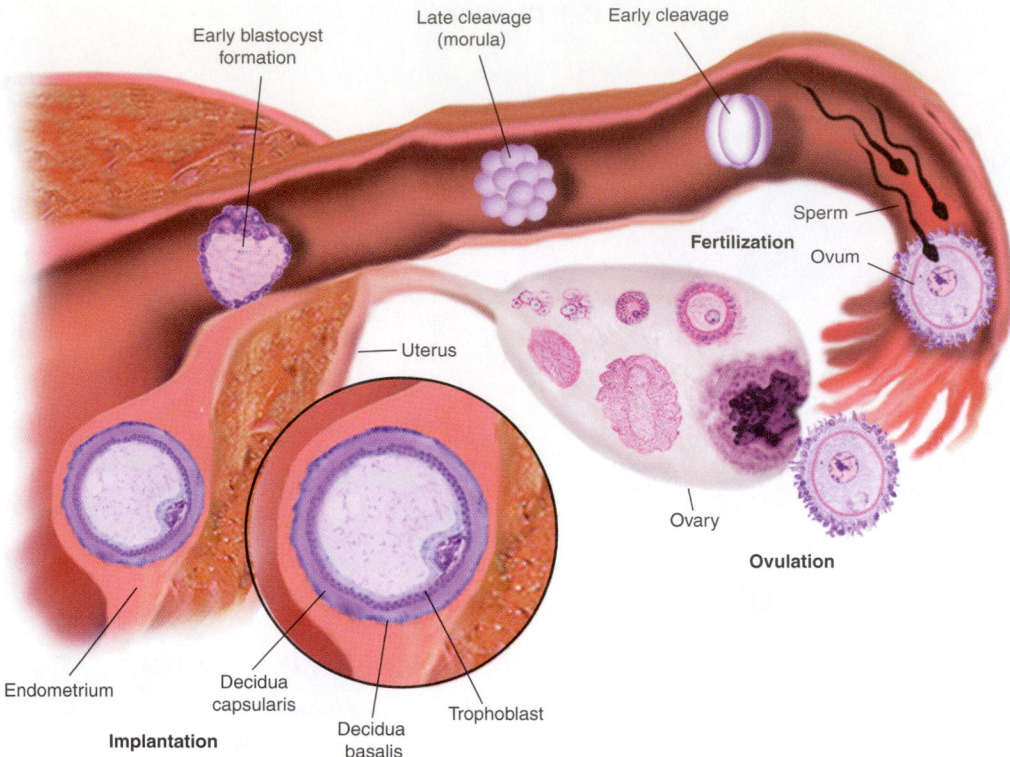

Early blastocyst formation

Late cleavage (morula)

Early cleavage

Fertilization

Sperm

Ovum

Uterus

Ovary

Ovulation

Endometrium

Decidua capsularis

Decidua basalis

Trophoblast

Implantation

Figure 12-2   Ovulation, fertilization, and implantation.

At ejaculation during coitus, 200 to 600 million spermatozoa are deposited in the vagina. The spermatozoa propel themselves into the uterus and eventually into the fallopian tube. Only a few sperm survive to reach the ovum. To penetrate the ovum, the sperm must undergo a process of changes in the plasma membrane of the sperm head in order to penetrate the ovum. Immediately upon entering the ovum, the chromosomal material of the ovum and spermatozoon fuse, resulting in a **zygote**. The fertilized ovum not only forms the fetus but also the accessory structures (placenta and yolk sac) that the fetus will need to support itself during intrauterine life.

Once fertilization is complete, the zygote travels along the fallopian tube toward the uterus. This journey takes approximately 3 to 4 days. During this time, mitotic cell division, or cleavage, occurs. By the time the zygote reaches the uterus, it should consist of 16 to 64 cells. This mass of cells is referred to as a **morula** because of its resemblance to a mulberry. The morula continues to multiply for about 4 more days. During this time, large cells (**trophoblast cells**) cluster on the perimeter of the morula, resulting in a fluid-filled space surrounding the inner cluster of cells, called a **blastocyst**. The outer layer of cells (trophoblast) is part of the structure that forms the placenta, while the inner cluster of cells (blastocyst) develops into the embryo.

On the seventh day after fertilization, the trophoblast becomes embedded into the endometrium of the uterine wall.

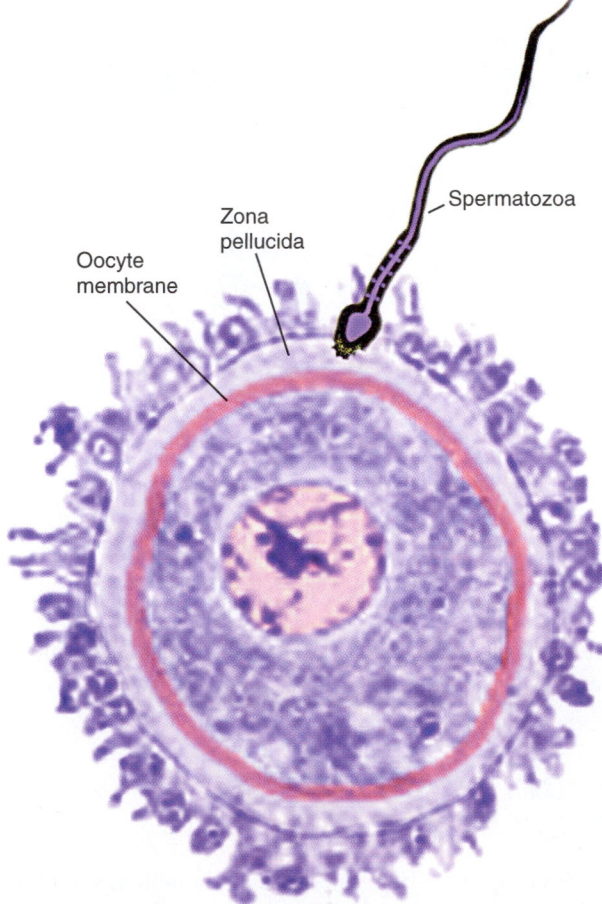

Oocyte membrane

Zona pellucida

Spermatozoa

Figure 12-3   Fertilization.

Implantation generally occurs high in the uterus. If the implantation occurs lower in the uterus, the growing placenta may obstruct the cervix (a situation referred to as placenta previa). Probably one-third of fertilized eggs never implant because there is a major defect in the zygote or the endometrium is not receptive to the invading blastocyst. Of those zygotes that do implant, fewer than one-third progress to establish a productive pregnancy (Moore & Persaud, 2003).

The corpus luteum in the ovary continues to function producing estrogen and progestin, because of the influence of **human chorionic gonadotropin (hCG)**, produced by the trophoblast cells. This allows the endometrium to continue to grow and sustain the pregnancy. At this stage, the endometrium is called the **decidua**. The decidua has three regions: (1) the part resting directly between the embryo and the uterine wall under the **embryo** (**decidua basalis**), (2) the portion of the endometrium that surrounds the surface of the trophoblast (**decidua capsularis**), and (3) the remaining portion of the uterine lining (**decidua parietalis**) (Figure 12-4) (Larsen, 1997).

Once implantation occurs, the trophoblastic layer of cells begins to mature. By the 12th day, **chorionic villi** form and begin to expand into the uterine endometrium.

PLACENTA

After implantation, the placenta begins to develop. The placenta develops from the trophoblast cells at the site where the developing embryo attaches to the uterine wall. The placenta eventually serves as the lungs, kidneys, endocrine system, and gastrointestinal tract for the fetus. Placental development and circulation begins around the third week of embryonic development. The placenta continues to grow in size until the 20th week of gestation, at which time it covers nearly one-half of the uterine wall. After the 20th week, the placenta becomes thicker but not larger in diameter. At term, the placenta is about 6 to 8 inches (15 to 20 cm) in diameter, with walls 1 to 1.5 inches (2.5 to 3.0 cm) in thickness, and weighs approximately 14 to 21 ounces (400 to 600 g).

The placenta has two parts: the maternal portion and the fetal portion. The maternal portion consists of the decidua basalis and its circulation. The fetal portion consists of the chorionic villi and the surface is covered by the amnion, which gives it a shiny, gray appearance.

Functions of the Placenta

The placenta begins to function shortly after implantation and is involved in the metabolic, transport, and endocrine activities necessary for fetal development (Carlson, 1999).

Metabolic

The placenta produces glycogen, cholesterol, and fatty acids for fetal use and hormone production and numerous enzymes required for fetoplacental transfer. It also stores glycogen and iron.

Transport

The placenta controls the exchange of several substances by five mechanisms: simple diffusion, facilitated transport, active transport, pinocytosis, and hydrostatic and osmotic pressure.

Other mechanisms of transfer also exist; for example, fetal red blood cells may pass into the maternal circulation through breaks in the placental membrane. Due to the possibility of tears in the semipermeable membrane, there may be some mixing of fetal and maternal blood. As the maternal blood picks up waste products and carbon dioxide from the fetus, it drains back into the maternal circulation. The transfer of substances, the ratio of blood on either side of the placenta, and the binding abilities of certain molecules in the blood affect changes in blood flow between the fetus and the maternal intervillous spaces.

Endocrine

The placenta produces hormones that are vital to the survival of the fetus. These include hCG, human placental lactogen (hPL), and estrogen and progesterone.

The hormone hCG prevents the normal involution of the corpus luteum at the end of the menstrual cycle. If the

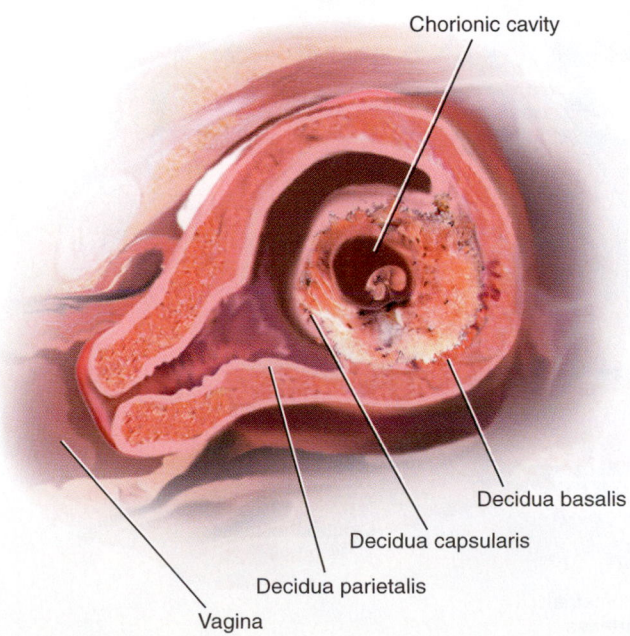

Chorionic cavity

Decidua basalis

Decidua capsularis

Decidua parietalis

Vagina

Figure 12-4 Decidua.

corpus luteum stops functioning before the 11th week of pregnancy, spontaneous abortion occurs. The hCG stimulates the corpus luteum to secrete increased amounts of estrogen and progesterone. hCG and hPL also play a role in preventing the rejection of the placenta and embryo by the mother's body.

After the 11th week, the placenta produces enough progesterone and estrogen to maintain pregnancy. Progesterone is essential for the maintenance of the pregnancy because it provides appropriate nutritive elements for the developing morula and blastocyst. Progesterone also decreases the contractility of the uterus, thus preventing uterine contractions, which could result in spontaneous abortion. After the 10th week, the placenta takes over the production of progesterone and estrogen, which has a generating function on the uterus, the breasts, and the breast glandular tissue.

Placental Circulation

After the blastocyst implants, the cells differentiate into fetal cells and trophoblastic cells. The trophoblast invades the decidua basalis of the endometrium (Figure 12-5). At the same time, the chorionic villi continue to grow and eventually form the fetal vessels. On about the 12th day, maternal blood pools in the intervillous spaces surrounding the chorionic villi. By the end of the 21st day, oxygen, glucose, and other nutrients diffuse from the maternal blood to the chorionic villi and are transported to the developing embryo.

In the fully developed umbilical cord, fetal blood flows through two umbilical arteries to the capillaries of the villi and oxygen-enriched blood flows back through the umbilical vein to the fetus.

Maternal blood, rich in oxygen and nutrients, spurts from the uterine arteries into the intervillous spaces.

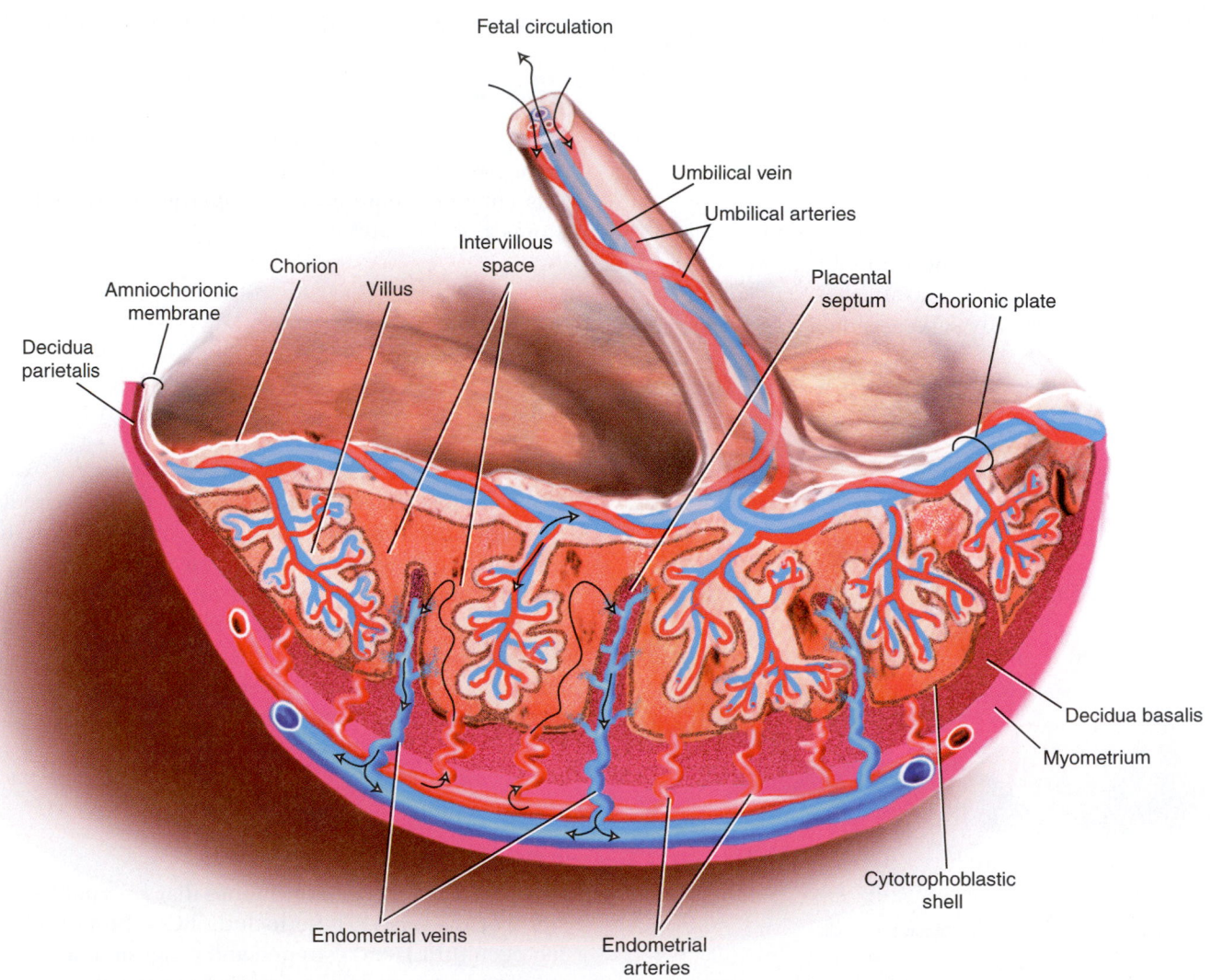

Figure 12-5   Placental circulation.

Fetal Circulation

The blood circulation after birth is much different from that of the fetus. During fetal development, the lungs are collapsed and do not function. The placenta performs the role of supplying oxygen to the blood and removing carbon dioxide. This requires that there be unique structures (i.e., foramen ovale, ductus venosus, and ductus arteriosus) that play major roles in fetal circulation and disappear after birth.

The blood from the placenta flows through the umbilical vein, which penetrates the abdominal wall of the fetus at the site of the umbilicus (Figure 12-6A). It divides into two branches, one of which circulates a small amount of blood through the fetal liver and empties into the inferior vena cava through the hepatic vein. The second and larger branch, called the ductus venosus, empties directly into the fetal vena cava. This blood then enters the right atrium, passes through the foramen ovale into the left atrium, and pours into the left ventricle, which pumps it into the aorta. Some blood returning from the head and upper extremities by way of the superior vena cava is emptied into the right atrium and passes through the tricuspid

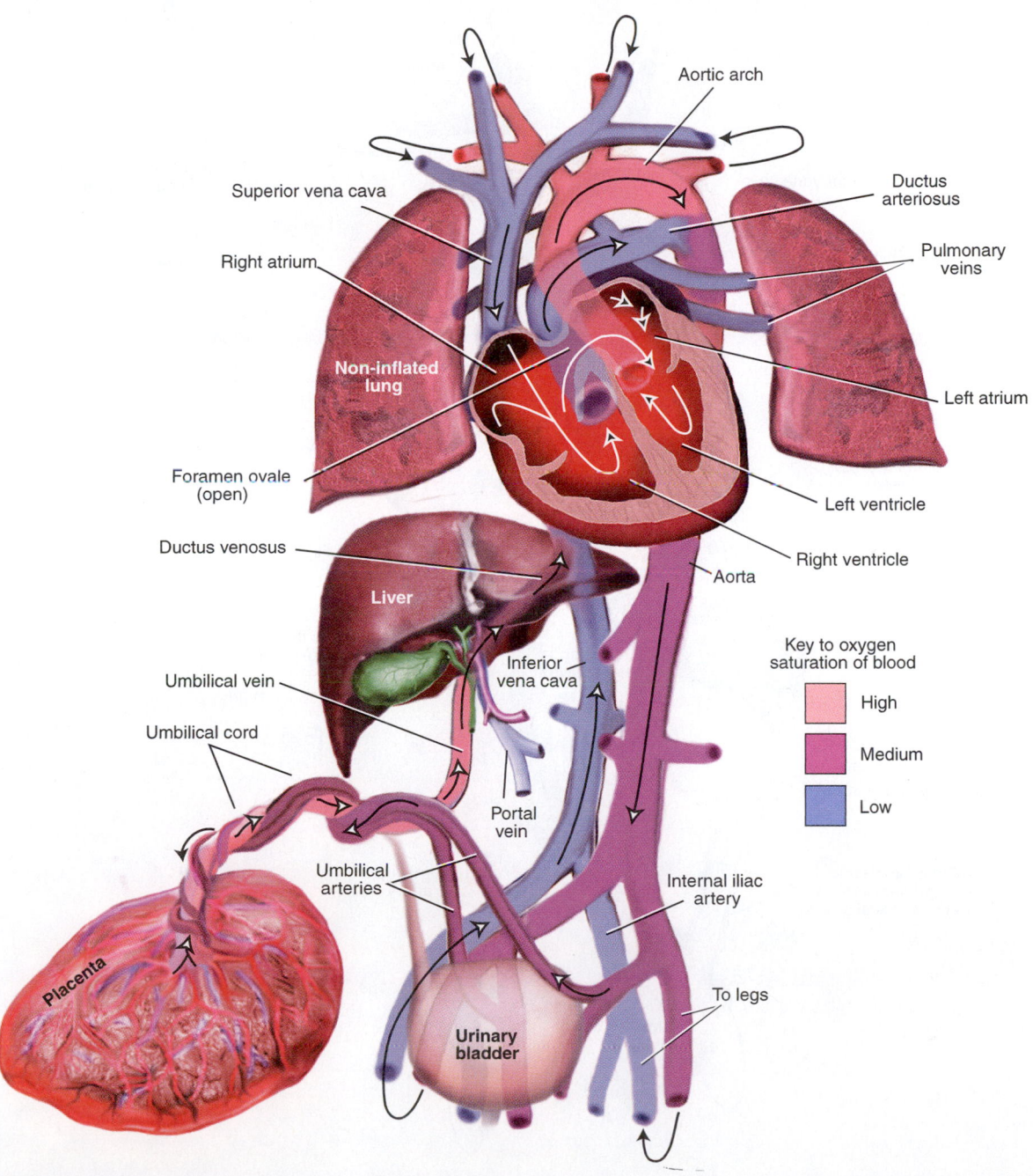

Figure 12-6   A. Fetal circulation.

valve into the right ventricle. This blood is pumped into the pulmonary artery, and a small amount passes to the lungs and provides nourishment only. The larger portion of blood passes from the pulmonary artery through the ductus arteriosus and into the descending aorta, bypassing the lungs. Finally, blood returns to the placenta through the two umbilical arteries, and the process is repeated.

The fetus receives oxygen via diffusion from the maternal circulation. Fetal hemoglobin facilitates obtaining oxygen, since it carries as much as 20% to 30% more oxygen than adult hemoglobin. Fetal circulation delivers the highest available oxygen concentrations to the head, neck, brain, and heart and a lesser amount of oxygenated blood to the abdominal organs and the lower body. This circulatory pattern leads to cephalocaudal (head-to-tail) development of the fetus.

Newborn Circulation

Fetal circulatory shunts are not necessary after birth because the baby is able to oxygenate the blood through the lungs rather than the placenta (Figure 12-6B). As the new-

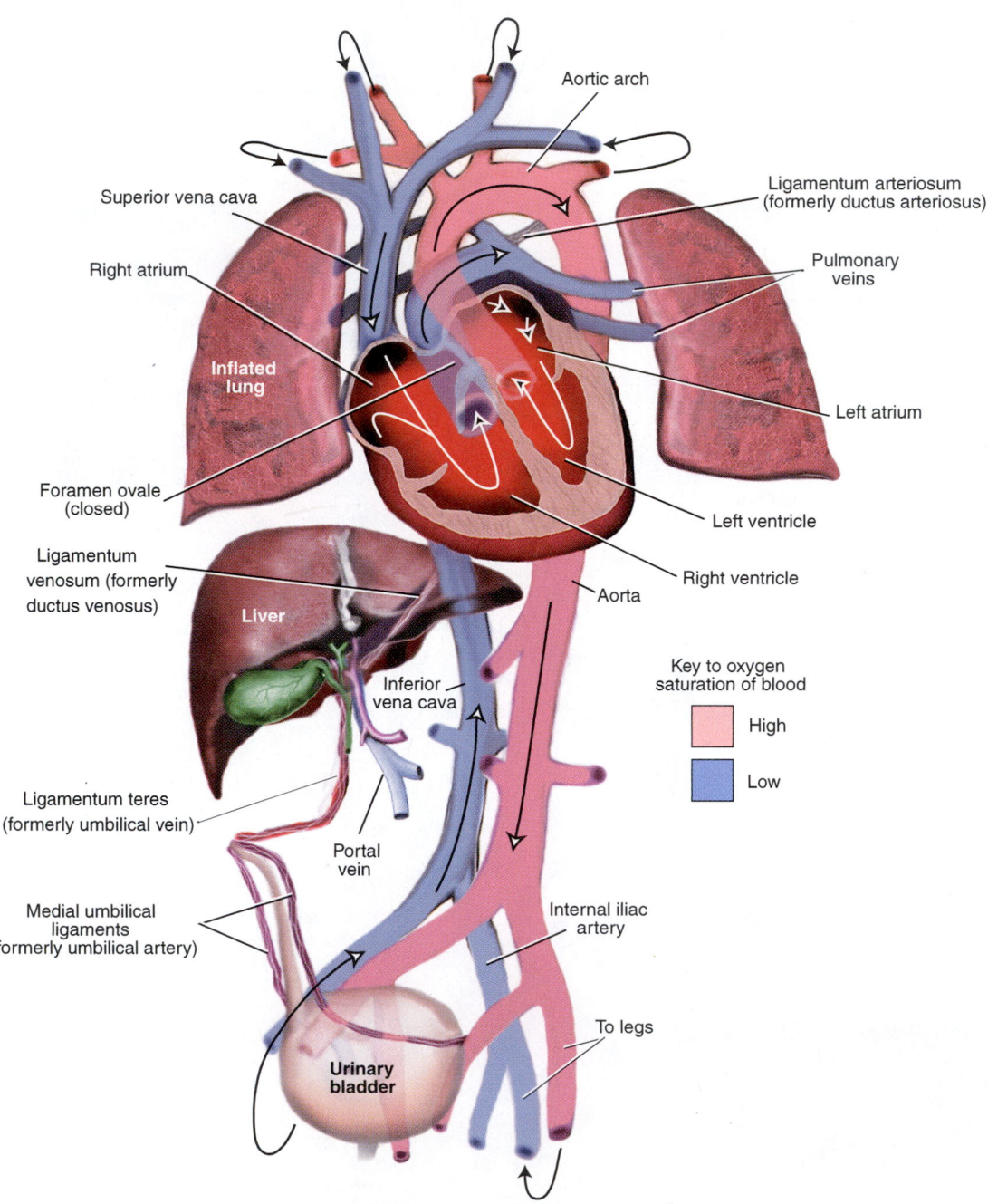

Figure 12-6   (continued) B. Newborn circulation.

born breathes, the foramen ovale closes as a result of the increased blood flow to the lungs and the decreased pressure in the right side of the heart. The ductus venosus closes when the blood from the umbilical cord stops. The ductus venosus and the foramen ovale are permanently closed as tissue develops in these structures. The ductus areteriosus, a fetal shunt that connects the pulmonary artery to the descending aorta, closes after birth.

UMBILICAL CORD

While the placenta is developing, the umbilical cord is also being formed. The body stalk, which attaches the embryo to the yolk sac, contains blood vessels that extend into the chorionic villi. As the body stalk elongates, the vessels in the cord contract into one large vein and two smaller arteries. The larger vein brings the oxygenated blood from the placenta to the fetal circulatory system. The two small arteries carry deoxygenated blood and waste products back to the placenta. A specialized connective tissue (**Wharton's jelly**), which is an extension of the amnion, surrounds the blood vessels in the umbilical cord. This tissue, plus the high volume of blood in the vessels, prevents compression of the umbilical cord. The major function of the cord is to transport oxygen and nutrients to the fetus and to return waste products from the fetus to the placenta. At term, the cord is almost 1 inch (2 cm) across and about 22 inches (55 cm) long. Deviation from this may suggest a fetal anomaly. The cord can attach itself to the placenta at various sites. Central insertion into the placenta is considered the norm. Umbilical cords can look twisted or spiraled; this is most likely caused by fetal movement. A true knot in the umbilical cord is rare, because of the high pressure and rapid blood flow in the cord.

MEMBRANES AND AMNIOTIC FLUID

The fetal membranes include the **amnion** and the chorion; both surround the fetus. The amnion is the inner of the two fetal membranes (the outer is the **chorion**). The amnion begins to appear in the second week of gestation. The sac formed by the amnion and chorion contains an opaque fluid (**amniotic fluid**). The fluid surrounds the embryo and, as the pregnancy progresses, the amount of fluid increases. The composition of the fluid changes as pregnancy advances. The volume of amniotic fluid increases as the pregnancy progresses. Amniotic fluid volume reaches a peak of approximately 1 L at 38 weeks and then stabilizes or decreases slightly until delivery.

Amniotic fluid's main function is to provide an optimal environment for the fetus. The fetus begins to swallow the fluid in the fourth month, and, thus, it may be important to fetal metabolism. Amniotic fluid helps to dispose of secretions from the kidneys and the respiratory tract, allows the fetus to move with ease in the uterus, equalizes the pressure from sudden external forces, and keeps the fetus at a uniform temperature.

EMBRYONIC STAGE

The stage of the embryo begins about the 14th day and continues until approximately the eighth week of development. The embryonic stage is a period of tissue differentiation, forming of essential organs, and development of external features (Table 12-1). During this period, the embryo is vulnerable to **teratogens**. Teratogens are environmental substances that may cause adverse effects on the developing fetus. A teratogen has the greatest effect on an organ during that organ's period of differentiation and development. Brain development occurs throughout the pregnancy, and teratogens can affect mental development throughout gestation.

Client Education

Healthy Pregnancy

Help your clients achieve a healthy pregnancy.

- Educate parents on critical stages of embryonic development; this helps the client understand the importance of maintaining a healthy lifestyle to ensure optimal fetal growth and development and the importance of early prenatal care to ensure adequate nutrition for both mother and fetus.

- Ascertain the client's knowledge level of dietary needs; fetal and maternal well-being depend on maternal nutrition during pregnancy and, in certain conditions, for approximately 2 years before the pregnancy (folic acid). Also ascertain iron intake; increased levels of iron are necessary during pregnancy for developing maternal and fetal tissue and fetal iron stores.

- Provide general information about antepartum testing that may be ordered and the specific times during pregnancy when these tests are most accurate. Many clients want to know how safe the tests are and how much discomfort they may cause. Review the procedures and explain why some tests may need to be repeated. Provide simple and clear explanations of what the tests measure.

Table 12-1 Stages of Fetal Development

	STAGE	FETAL DEVELOPMENT
	Embryonic or Germinal Stage Weeks 1 and 2	Rapid cell division and differentiation. Germinal layers form.
	Embryonic Stage Week 3*	Primitive nervous system, eyes, ears, and RBCs present. Heart begins to beat on day 21.
 4 weeks	Week 4* Wt 0.4 g L 4–6 mm (crown–rump, C–R)	Half the size of a pea. Brain differentiates. GI tract begins to form. Limb buds appear.
	Week 5* L 6–8 mm (C–R)	Cranial nerves present. Muscles innervated.
	Week 6* L 10–14 mm (C–R)	Fetal circulation established. Liver produces RBCs. Central autonomic nervous system forms. Primitive kidneys form. Lung buds present. Cartilage forms. Primitive skeleton forms. Muscles differentiate.
	Week 7* L 22–28 mm (C–R)	Eyelids form. Palate and tongue form. Stomach formed. Diaphragm formed. Arms and legs move.
 8 weeks	Week 8* Wt 2 g L 3 cm (1.2 in) (C–R)	Resembles human being. Eyes moved to face front. Heart development complete. Hands and feet well formed. Bone cells begin replacing cartilage. All body organs have begun forming.
	Fetal Stage Week 9	Finger and toenails form. Eyelids fuse shut.
	Week 10 Wt 14 g ($\frac{1}{2}$ oz) L 5–6 cm (2 in) crown–heel (C–H)	Head growth slows. Islets of Langerhans differentiated. Bone marrow forms, RBCs produced. Bladder sac forms. Kidneys make urine.
	Week 11	Tooth buds appear. Liver secretes bile. Urinary system functions. Insulin forms in pancreas.

*Vulnerable to teratogenic effects.

(continues)

Table 12-1   Stages of Fetal Development *(continued)*

	STAGE	FETAL DEVELOPMENT
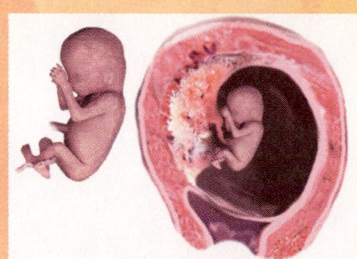 12 weeks	**Week 12** Wt 45 g (1.5 oz) L 9 cm (3.5 in) (C–R) 11.5 cm (4.5 in) (C–H)	Lungs take shape. Palate fuses. Heart beat heard with Doppler ultrasound. Ossification established. Swallowing reflex present. External genitalia. Male or female distinguished.
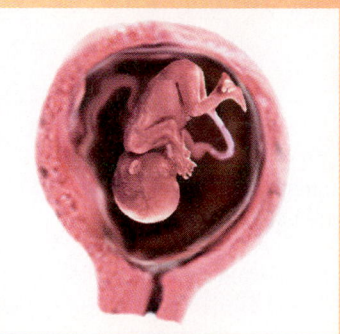 16 weeks	**Second Trimester** **Week 16** Wt 200 g (7 oz) L 13.5 cm (5.5 in) (C–R) 15 cm (6 in) (C–H)	Meconium forms in bowels. Scalp hair appears. Frequent fetal movement. Skin thin. Sensitive to light. 200 mL amniotic fluid. (Amniocentesis possible.)
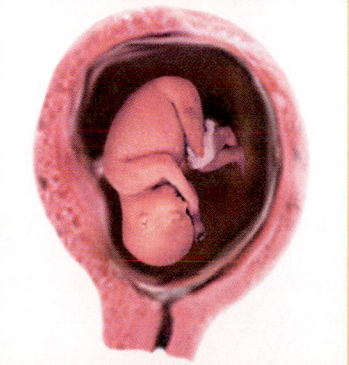 20 weeks	**Week 20** Wt 435 g (15 oz) L 19 cm (7.5 in) (C–R) 25 cm (10 in) (C–H)	Myelination of spinal cord begins. Peristalsis begins. Lanugo covers body. Vernix caseosa covers body. Brown fat deposits begun. Sucks and swallows amniotic fluid. Heartbeat heard with fetoscope. Hands can grasp. Regular schedule of sucking, kicking, and sleeping.
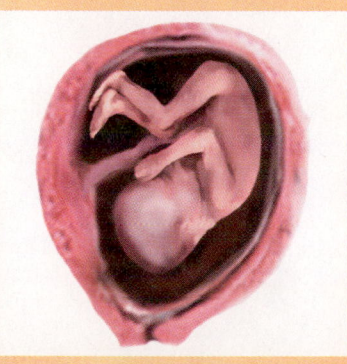 24 weeks	**Week 24** Wt 780 g (1 lb, 12 oz) L 23 cm (9 in) (C–R) 28 cm (11 in) (C–H)	Alveoli present in lungs, begin producing surfactant. Eyes completely formed. Eyelashes and eyebrows appear. Many reflexes appear. Chance of survival if born now.

(continues)

Table 12-1   Stages of Fetal Development *(continued)*

	STAGE	FETAL DEVELOPMENT
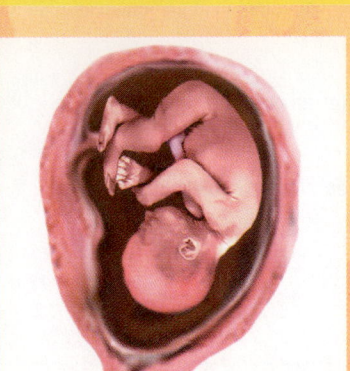 28 weeks	**Third Trimester** Week 28 Wt 1200 g (2 lb, 10 oz) L 28 cm (11 in) (C–R) 35 cm (14 in) (C–H)	Subcutaneous fat deposits begun. Lanugo begins to disappear. Nails appear. Eyelids open and close. Testes begin to descend.
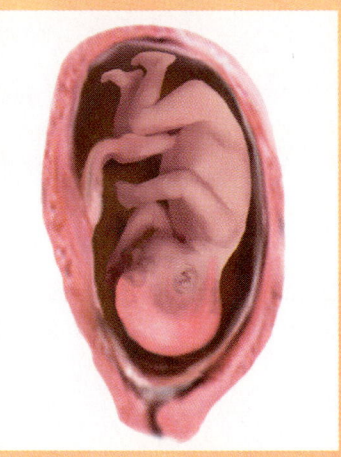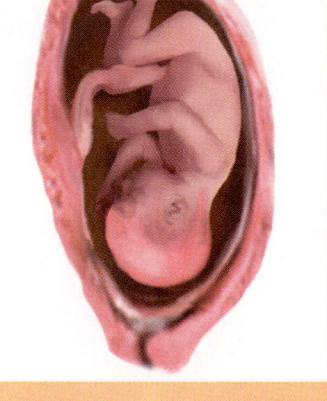 32 weeks	Week 32 Wt 2,000 g (4 lb, 6.5 oz) L 31 cm (12 in) (C–R) 41 cm (16 in) (C–H)	More reflexes present. CNS directs rhythmic breathing movements. CNS partially controls body temperature. Begins storing iron, calcium, phosphorus. Ratio of the lung surfactants lecithin and sphingomyelin (L/S) is 1.2:2.
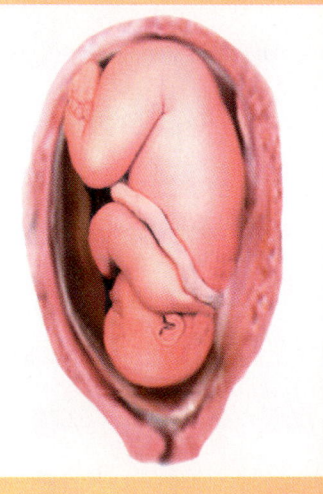 36 weeks	Week 36 Wt 2,500–2.750 g (5 lb, 8 oz) L 35 cm (14 in) (C–R) 48 cm (19 in) (C–H)	A few creases on soles of feet. Skin less wrinkled. Fingernails reach fingertips. Sleep-wake cycle fairly definite. Transfer of maternal antibodies.

(continues)

Table 12-1   Stages of Fetal Development *(continued)*

	STAGE	FETAL DEVELOPMENT
	Week 38	L/S ratio 2:1
	Week 40 Wt 3,000–3,600 g (6 lb, 10 oz–7 lb, 15 oz) L 50 cm (20 in) (C–H)	Lanugo only on shoulders and upper back. Creases cover soles. Vernix mainly in folds of skin. Ear cartilage firm. Less active, limited space. Ready to be born.

40 weeks

3 Weeks

In the third week, the embryonic disk becomes elongated and pear-shaped, with a broad cephalic end and a narrow caudal end. The ectoderm forms a long cylindrical tube called the notochord, from which brain and spinal cord develop. The most advanced organ is the heart, which appears as a single tube outside the embryo's body cavity. The heart muscle is able to contract, and peristaltic waves pass along the heart tube. The cardiovascular system begins to form and blood begins circulating in the primitive heart. The gastrointestinal tract, created from the endoderm, appears as a tube-like structure that communicates with the yolk sac.

4 Weeks

By the end of 28 days, the tubular heart is beating at a regular rhythm, and the contractions are efficient enough to produce circulation through the main fetal blood vessels.

5 Weeks

The embryo has a marked C-shaped body, accentuated by the rudimentary tail and the large head that is folded over a protuberant trunk. By day 35, the arm and leg buds are well developed, with paddle-shaped hand and foot plates.

Critical Thinking

Medical History

Review obstetric and medical history for risk factors (detrimental lifestyle, abusive relationship, inappropriate use of medications, and potential teratogens, such as alcohol or nicotine). Which of these factors is most likely to produce birth defects, and why?

Client Education

Drug Use

Assess fetal gestational age and counsel clients regarding drug use to prevent teratogenic problems in the developing embryo and fetus.

6 Weeks

At six weeks, the head structures are more developed, and the trunk is straighter than in earlier stages. The heart now has most of its definitive characteristics, and fetal circulation begins. The liver starts to produce blood cells. The arms have begun to extend ventrally across the chest, and both arms and legs have digits, although they may be webbed. There is a slight bend in the arms, which are more advanced in development than the legs.

7 Weeks

During the seventh week, the head of the embryo is rounded and nearly erect. At this point the beginnings of all essential external and internal structures are present.

8 Weeks

At eight weeks, the embryo is approximately 1.2 inches (3 cm) long and resembles a human being. External genitals appear, but the embryo's sex cannot be determined visually.

FETAL STAGE

By the end of the eighth week, the embryo is sufficiently developed to be called a fetus. Every organ system and external structure that is found in the full-term newborn is present (England, 1996). The remainder of gestation is devoted to refining structures and perfecting function.

9 to 12 Weeks

By 12 weeks, the fetus reaches 3.2 inches (8 cm) in length and weighs about 1.6 ounces (45 g) (Figure 12-7). Ossification centers begin to form in the bones. The legs are still shorter and less developed than the arms. Ultrasonographic devices can easily ascertain spontaneous movements between 6 and 12 weeks.

13 to 16 Weeks

At 13 weeks, the fetus weighs 2 to 2½ ounces (55 to 60 g) and is about 3.6 inches (9 cm) in length. Fine hair (**lanugo**) begins to appear, especially on the head. The skin is transparent and the blood vessels are clearly visible. Active movements are present; the fetus stretches and exercises its arms and legs.

17 to 19 Weeks

This is a period of somewhat slower growth, but the fetus becomes more active. The mother may feel fetal movements. Rapid brain growth occurs during this time. The fetal heart tones may be heard through a stethoscope.

20 to 23 Weeks

The fetus now measures about 8 inches (19 cm). Fetal weight is between 15.2 to 16.3 ounces (435 and 465 g). Fetal movement is now strong enough to be felt by the mother.

Nursing Tip *Fetal Tests*

Be aware of available fetal tests and support the family in preparing for the tests (ultrasound, amniocentesis, triple-marker screening [analysis of maternal serum for abnormal levels of alpha-fetoprotein, hCG, and estriols]) that may predict chromosomal and neural tube defects.

Nursing Tip *Community Resources*

Inform the clients of the resources in the community that assist clients who need further support and information regarding problems identified through antepartal testing.

Nursing Tip *Fetal Development*

To provide clients with education and support, you must know and understand the stages of embryonic and fetal development, such as when fetal heart tones (FHTs) can first be heard. FHTs confirm the presence of a fetus and rule out gestational trophoblastic disease (hydatidiform mole).

Reflections from a Client

I really didn't even realize I was pregnant until I heard my baby's heartbeat. Then I saw her heart beating on ultrasound and found out it was a girl. I'm amazed to think my baby has all her systems developed and functioning so early.

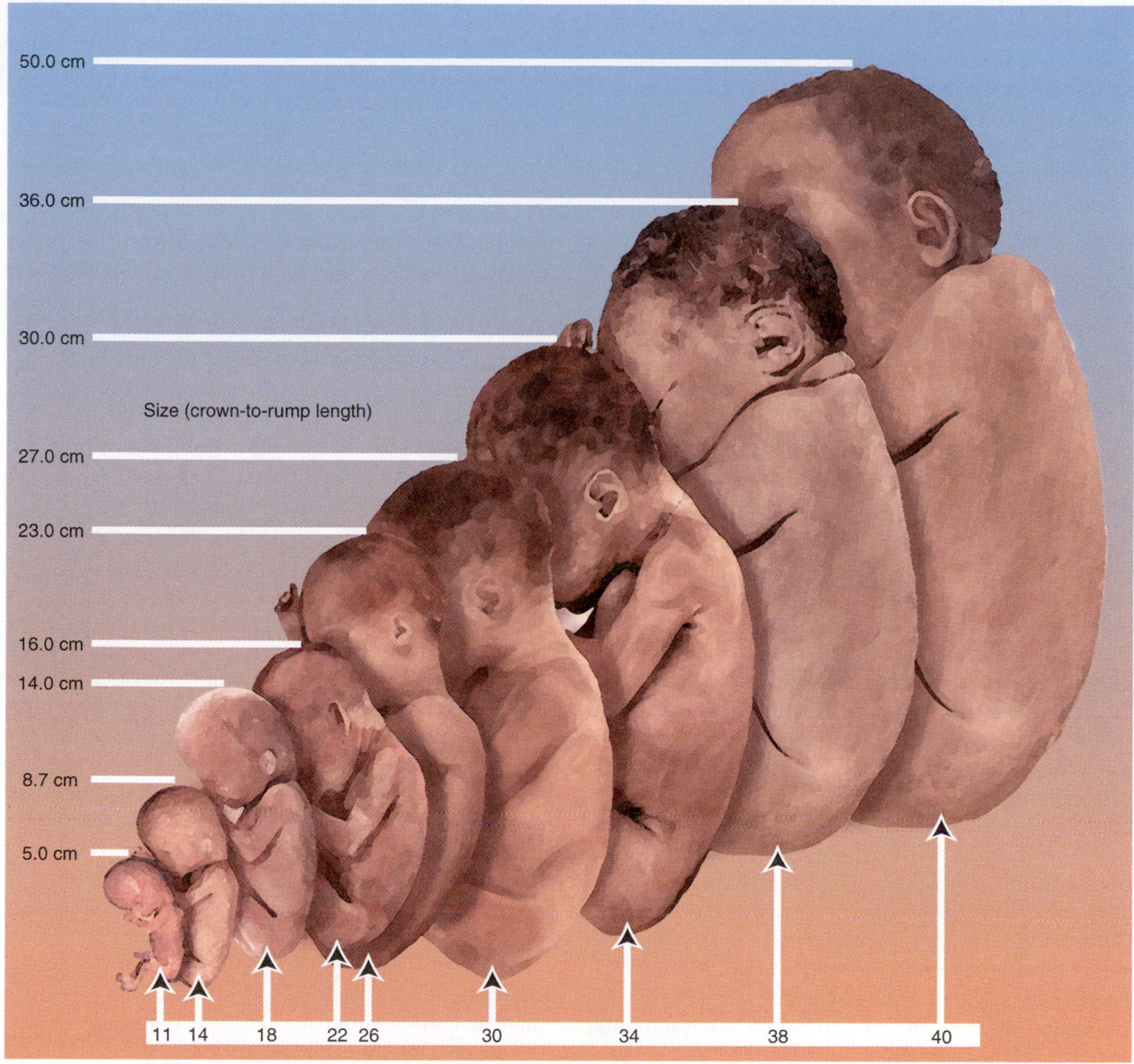

Figure 12-7   Fetal size by gestational age.

24 Weeks

The fetus is considered viable at 24 weeks, though infants born at this age often experience high mortality and morbidity. The fetus at 24 weeks reaches a length of 11 inches (28 cm) and weighs about 1 lb, 10 oz (780 g). The skin over the entire body is covered with a protective cheese-like, fatty substance secreted by the sebaceous glands, called vernix caseosa. Meconium is present in the rectum. If the fetus is a male, the testes begin to descend into the scrotal sac. A fetus born at this time requires immediate and prolonged intensive care to survive.

25 to 28 Weeks

The fetus at 28 weeks is about 14 to 15 inches long (35 to 38 cm) and weighs 2 lb, 10 oz to 2 lb, 12 oz (1200 to 1250 g).

29 to 32 Weeks

The fetus is gaining weight from an increase in body muscle and fat and weighs about 4 lb, 6 oz (2000 g) with a length of about 15 to 17 inches (38 to 43 cm).

33 to 36 Weeks

The fetus is less wrinkled because of increasing deposits of subcutaneous fat. At 36 weeks, the fetal weight is usually 5 lb, 12 oz to 6 lb, 11.5 oz (2500 to 2750 g), and the crown-heel length of the fetus is about 16 to 19 inches (42 to 48 cm). Lanugo is beginning to disappear, and the nails reach the edge of the fingertips. An infant born at this time has a good chance of surviving but may require some special care.

38 to 40 Weeks

The fetus is considered full term at 38 weeks after conception. The length can vary from 19 to 21 inches (48 to 52 cm). The weight at term is approximately 6 lb, 10 oz to 7 lb, 15 oz (3000 to 3600 g) (see Figure 12-7).

RISKS AFFECTING FETAL WELL-BEING

Although most pregnancies proceed normally and result in healthy newborns, some substances and events in the environment can increase the risk of death or injury to the developing fetus. Many chemicals diffuse readily from the maternal bloodstream into that of the fetus. Radiation and heat reach fetal tissue and can affect fetal development. Violent injury to a mother also may injure her fetus. Fetal growth and development are intimately affected by the mother's geographic location; chemical exposures; stresses at work and at home; use of medications and other substances, some of which are illegal; and infections, some of which may have been acquired by risky behavior.

Approximately 3% to 5% of newborns have some form of congenital anomaly. More than half of congenital malformations have an unknown cause. Genetic defects and inherited tendencies brought on by environmental risks taken together explain about a third of all defects.

Environmental Risks

Pesticides are chemicals designed to kill insects or rodents. **Herbicides** are chemicals designed to kill unwanted plant life. Humans are exposed to these chemicals through contact with contaminated air, soil, and water, and through consumption of foods treated during planting and cultivation. Humans also may eat fish or livestock that have ingested the chemicals from contaminated environments. Pesticides and herbicides are widely used not only in the agricultural industry but in homes, lawns, and gardens to destroy insects and weeds. Environmental pesticides are associated with anencephaly.

Teratogens are substances that have been found to interfere with the formation or normal development of the human fetus.

Heavy metals, chemical substances such as lead or mercury, are by-products of industry that may be found in the environment. Methylmercury, when released accidentally, can be present in low levels in lakes. These low levels of mercury in lake water can accumulate in the tissues of fish. Swordfish, shark, and tuna steaks can contain high levels of mercury.

Lead has been known to cause reproductive problems since the early 20th century. Lead exposure can occur as a result of water or air pollution; from exhausts of cars using leaded gasoline; and in workplace exposure in industries such as smelting, battery and paint manufacturing, and typesetting. Exposures to high levels of lead during pregnancy can cause miscarriage, fetal demise, and prematurity and can lead to later developmental and growth delays in children (Needleman & Bellinger, 1994). Women whose male partners are exposed to lead also face increased risks of fetal malformations (Sever, 1994).

Risks Related to Employment

Most pregnant women are employed outside the home. Work itself does not appear to increase pregnancy risks; in fact, in one California county, employed Black women at all income levels were less likely than were unemployed Black women to deliver low-birth-weight infants (Poerksen & Petitti, 1991). Work may increase women's access to health care, sense of well-being, physical fitness, and financial autonomy and may have other healthy effects. However, work also may bring women into contact with harmful substances and physical dangers.

Many jobs require women to stand for long periods, lift heavy objects, climb stairs, bend over for long periods (as in picking vegetables), and perform other physical exertion. Simply standing or sitting for an 8-hour workday can cause significant fatigue. Strenuous activity also results in increased body temperature and thus creates concerns about **hyperthermia**, which is a dangerous elevation in body temperature resulting from fever or external heat sources.

The activities most likely to cause preterm birth and low birth weight are prolonged standing, long working hours, and lifting heavy objects (Simpson, 1993).

In response to studies such as these, the American Medical Association has published guidelines for work limitations during pregnancy (AMA Council on Scientific Affairs, 1984) that suggest prolonged standing (for more than 4 hours), repeated stooping and bending (more than twice an hour), climbing ladders, climbing stairs more than 4 times per shift, and repeated lifting of over 25 pounds should be restricted after 20 to 28 weeks' gestation. Nurses should make an individualized assessment of each pregnant woman's work-related risks as well as the personal beneficial factors related to work.

Client Education

Reducing the Risks of Work in Pregnancy

Women who are employed outside the home during pregnancy or who have strenuous responsibilities within the home or family farm can reduce the risks of having infants with birth defects, preterm infants, or low-birth-weight infants by:

- Becoming aware of hazardous chemicals in the workplace and obtaining protective clothing or a work reassignment if exposure is unavoidable. At most companies, the Human Resources Department keeps a listing of and information about hazardous substances.

- Limiting heavy lifting and carrying at work and home after 20 weeks' gestation, including avoiding carrying children and heavy grocery bags up several flights of stairs. Request work reassignment and use family or home health aid assistance in the home.

- Reducing prolonged standing or sitting. A pregnant woman should take breaks in which she can change position, get up, and walk around if her job involves sitting, or rest with her feet up if her job involves standing. Women who stand at factory assembly lines or cash registers can request a high stool to sit on and a low stool to rest one foot on while standing. If this is not possible, work reassignment should be requested.

- Maintaining adequate food and fluid intake. Pregnant women should have access to drinking water in the workplace and should have at least one meal break and two snack breaks during an 8-hour shift.

Risks Related to Home Environment and Lifestyle

Although industrial workplaces probably have the most intense concentrations of hazardous substances, the products produced in industry may also be used in the home. Foods are another source of harmful exposures. Medications and illicit drugs used in the home also can place the fetus at risk. Nurses can reduce some of the pregnancy risks related to home and lifestyle through teaching and ongoing support.

Medications

Medications are one of the many possible forms in which pregnant women may be exposed to teratogens. It was once thought that the placenta served as a barrier between the fetus and harmful substances in the mother's system. Now it is known that most medications pass to the fetus to some degree (Figure 12-8). Of the many thousands of medications available today, only a few drugs or certain drug classes have been proven to be teratogens: aminopterin; androgens (Megace); angiotensin-converting enzyme (ACE) inhibitors; busulfan (Myleran); cocaine, when abused; coumarin derivatives (Coumadin); cyclophosphamide (Seromycin); diethylstilbestrol (DES); etretinate; isotretinoin (Accutane); lithium (Lithane); methotrexate (MTX); tetracycline (Tetracyn); thalidomide (Thalomid); the antiseizure medications carbamazepine (Tegetrol), paramethadione, trimethadione, phenytoin (Dilantin), and valproic acid (Depakene); and dosages of vitamin A over 18,000 IU/day (Briggs, 1995). Other drugs and drug classes have been

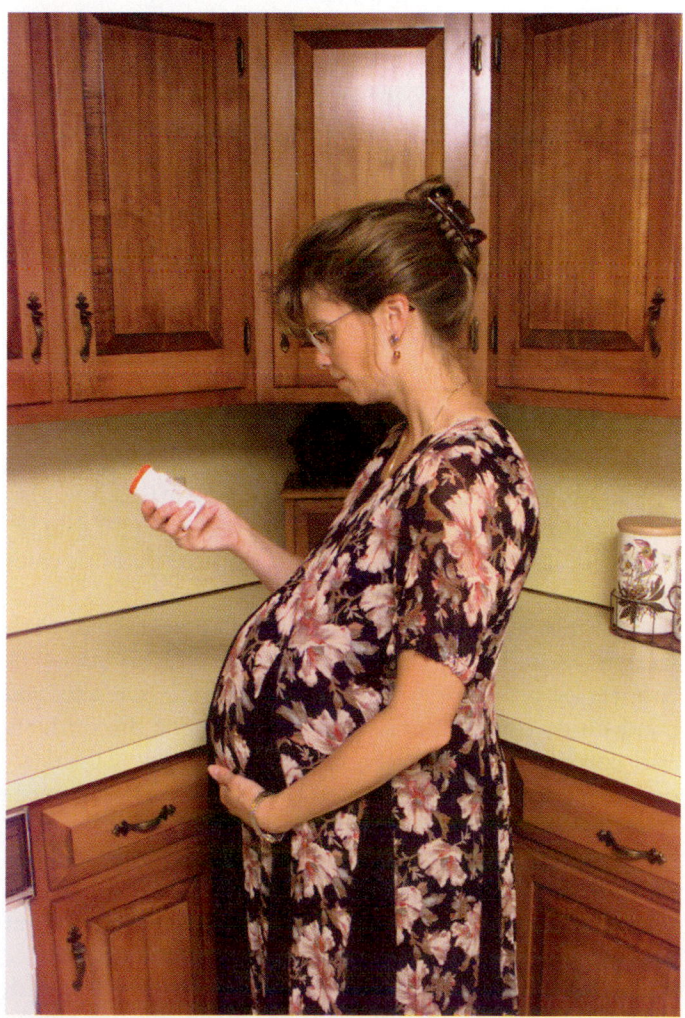

Figure 12-8 Nurses can help pregnant women recognize which over-the-counter medications are safe for use in pregnancy.

Table 12-2 Teratogenic Risks of Drugs: FDA Categories

CATEGORY	RISK
A	Controlled studies in women fail to demonstrate a risk to the fetus in the first trimester or later trimesters. Possibility of fetal harm appears remote.
B	Animal reproduction studies have not demonstrated a fetal risk, but there are no controlled studies in pregnant women. *Or* Animal studies have shown an adverse effect but the risk is not confirmed in human studies in the first trimester (and there is no evidence of risk in later trimesters).
C	Studies in animals have revealed adverse effects on the fetus, and there are no controlled studies in pregnant women. *Or* Studies in women and animals are not available. Drugs should be given only if the potential benefit justifies the potential risk to the fetus.
D	There is positive evidence of human fetal risk, but the benefits from use may be acceptable despite the risk.
X	Studies in animals or humans have demonstrated fetal abnormalities. *And/or* There is evidence of fetal risk based on human experience. The risk of use in pregnant women clearly outweighs any possible benefit. The drug is contraindicated in women who are or may become pregnant.

Note. Adapted from *PDR Nurses' Handbook,* by G. Spratto and A. Woods, 2004, Clifton Park, NY: Delmar Learning.

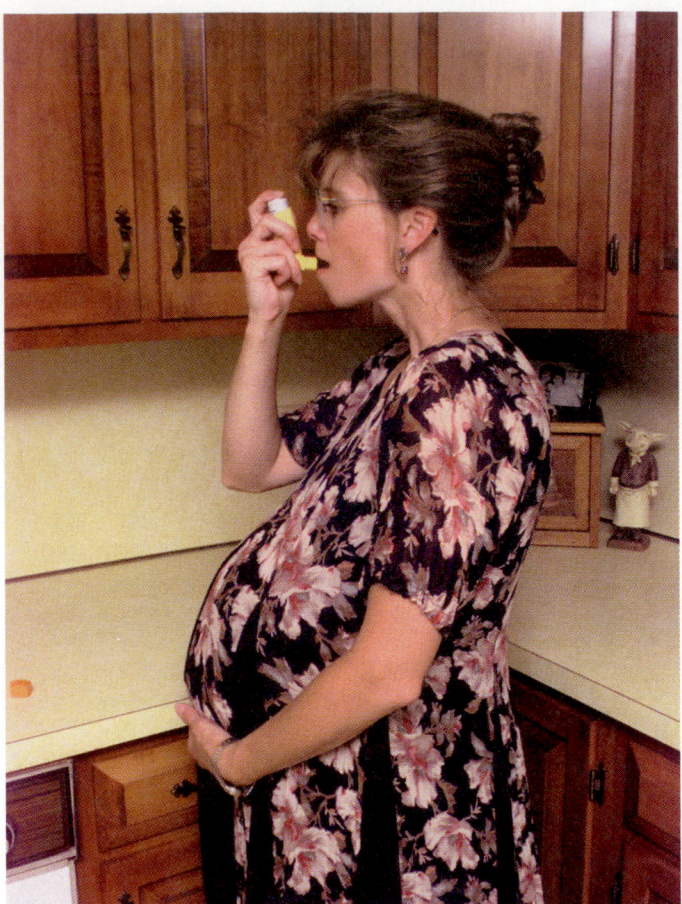

Figure 12-9   Pregnant women with asthma should continue to take their medications to prevent respiratory distress, which may also reduce oxygen to the fetus. Most asthma medications are safe in pregnancy.

linked only anecdotally to fetal problems. (Ethanol, also called grain or ethyl alcohol, also is a teratogen.) Table 12-2 lists teratogenic risks of drugs according to FDA categories.

Although it is wise to be cautious about taking medications, some pregnant women may require over-the-counter or prescription medications for chronic medical conditions, complications of pregnancy, or discomforts and common illnesses (Figure 12-9). Nurses should always caution pregnant women to check with their physicians before taking any medication.

Immunizations

Pregnant women may need immunizations to protect against viral infections that threaten health during pregnancy. The oral polio vaccine, now most commonly used, has no known harmful effects to the fetus.

Because rubella is a live vaccine, its use is avoided in pregnancy, and it is given in the postpartum period

Client Education

Medications for the Common Cold

Time, fluids, humidification of indoor air, rest, and good nutrition are perhaps the best medicines for a common cold. If these measures do not bring relief, you can suggest the following medications:

- For fever, body aches, and headache: acetaminophen (Tylenol)

- For cough: syrup or lozenges containing dextromethorphan and guaifenesin (Robitussin DM). Lozenges are preferred because they do not contain alcohol.

- For nasal and sinus congestion: pseudoephedrine (Sudafed), an over the counter (OTC) decongestant. Do not exceed labelled use.

instead. Influenza vaccines from live viruses should be avoided; however, newer inactivated virus forms may be safe and should be offered to pregnant women who are immunocompromised and others who may receive important benefits (Briggs, 1995). Likewise, the hepatitis vaccine may be given during pregnancy when a mother is at high risk of exposure to the disease, although immunization during the first trimester should be avoided whenever possible. Vaccines given for travel to tropical countries may be risky during pregnancy; the pregnant woman should consult a specialist in tropical medicine.

In general, few problems are reported with immunizations. However, they should be administered during pregnancy only when the benefits outweigh the risks. "Risk to a developing fetus from vaccination of the mother during pregnancy is primarily theoretical. No evidence exists of risk from vaccinating pregnant women with inactivated virus or bacterial vaccines or toxoids. Benefits of vaccinating pregnant women usually outweigh potential risks when the likelihood of disease exposure is high, when infection would pose a risk to the mother or fetus, and when the vaccine is unlikely to cause harm" (ACIP, 1994).

Alcohol Use

Although public concern tends to focus on illegal drug use during pregnancy, alcohol and tobacco use are much more common and are more common causes of harm to the fetus. Many women who use illicit drugs also use alcohol and tobacco, making it difficult to separate the effects caused by illegal drugs from those caused by the more commonly ingested legal substances. In the 1980s and 1990s, nurses and other health care professionals began to take seriously the risks of alcohol and tobacco use in pregnancy and to become involved in helping their clients to stop using these substances.

Prenatal alcohol use is the leading cause of childhood mental retardation, surpassing Down syndrome (Streissguth, Barr, Sampson, & Bookstein, 1997). Yet prenatal care providers probably spend more time counseling and testing women for fetal abnormalities such as Down syndrome than they do in assessing for and intervening in alcohol use. The National Institute for Drug Abuse has estimated that 18% of newborns are exposed to some alcohol during gestation (Young, 1997).

Heavy alcohol use throughout pregnancy (two or more drinks per day) has a 10% risk of producing **fetal alcohol syndrome** (FAS), which is a collection of physical and behavioral problems seen in children of women who drink heavily during pregnancy. Alcohol-related birth defects may include physical defects such as growth retardation; microcephaly; facial malformations, such as a flat midface, thin upper lip, and low or wide nasal bridge; malformations of joints and organs, such as the heart and kidney; and eye anomalies. FAS may also cause mental retardation, which is associated with microcephaly, and seizure disorders. Behavioral problems such as learning and attention difficulties and hyperactivity also have been associated with FAS. Fetal alcohol effect is a less severe form of alcohol-related problems.

A newborn exposed to alcohol during gestation with normal appearance and weight at birth still may have suffered brain damage. Newborns with low birth weight from maternal alcohol intake usually reach normal size by 8 months of age; however, CNS damage does not improve over time. Large amounts of alcohol cause physical malformations. Even small amounts consumed during pregnancy—so-called social drinking—can cause problems that persist into the teenage years and beyond: CNS damage; subtle cognitive delays; and motor, attention, and learning deficits (Streissguth et al., 1997). Thus, pregnant women and those planning pregnancy should be strongly advised to abstain from all alcohol use, because there is no known safe amount of alcohol consumption during pregnancy.

Tobacco Smoking and Passive Smoke

Approximately 20% to 30% of pregnant women report they smoke cigarettes with an average intake of about 14 cigarettes per day (Lawrance & Gruchow, 1996) (Figure 12-10). Tobacco use of over five cigarettes per day in pregnancy doubles a woman's risk of delivering a low-birth-weight infant (Lieberman, Gremy, Lang, & Cohen, 1994)

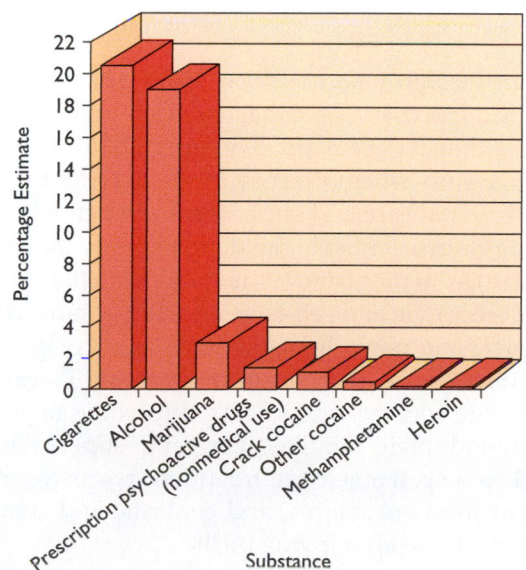

Figure 12-10 Estimated percentage of women who used selected substances in pregnancy, 1992. (Data from National Institute on Drug Abuse, 1996. *National Pregnancy and Health Survey: Drug use among women delivering live births: 1992.* Rockville, MD: Author. NIH Pub. No. 96-381 9, p. 36.)

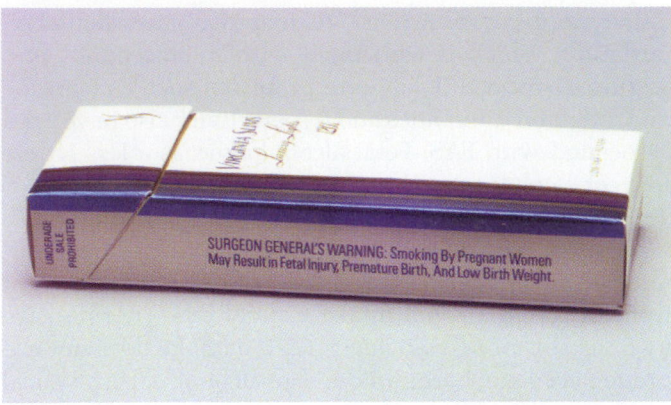

Figure 12-11   Warnings of risk to pregnant women on packages of cigarettes and alcoholic beverages must be supplemented by nursing advice and support.

(Figure 12-11). From 21% to 39% of low birth weights in infants are believed to be related to maternal smoking, and the effect on birth weight is proportional to the amount of tobacco used. The greatest effect is an increased risk of newborns who are small for gestational age; however, prematurity, infant mortality, and other pregnancy complications (such as spontaneous abortion, placenta previa, placental abruption, and premature rupture of fetal membranes) also are increased (Lieberman et al., 1994). There is some evidence that prenatal tobacco exposure causes learning and attention problems in children but less consistently than does alcohol exposure (Streissguth et al., 1997).

Illicit Drug Use

Pregnant women who use illicit drugs often feel unwelcome in nursing care settings such as prenatal clinics. They fear they will be shamed or reported to legal or child protective authorities (Kearney, 1995). In order to provide nonjudgmental care and support for women who use illicit drugs, nurses must understand not only the effects of illicit drugs in pregnancy but how addiction affects a woman's lifestyle and self-concept. Nurses must conduct a complete and nonjudgmental assessment of each pregnant woman's use of all forms of legal and illegal drugs and provide accurate and unbiased teaching to pregnant women and their families. Ongoing support will be needed to help women use treatment resources, remain abstinent from substances, and continue and commit to avoiding relapse after giving birth.

Marijuana

Marijuana, also known as cannabis, is the illegal drug most commonly used in pregnancy. Marijuana is not believed to be physically addictive or to cause withdrawal symptoms during periods of abstinence. Psychological

dependence is possible, however. The effects of marijuana smoking on pregnancy are not yet fully understood.

Cocaine and Other Stimulants

Cocaine causes excitement, euphoria, and anorexia. Amphetamines, also known as "speed," "crack," or "ice," are other stimulants that can be injected, smoked, or taken orally. Their effects are believed to be similar to those of cocaine.

Cocaine is not physically addictive, meaning that use can be stopped without the risks of seizures or other life-threatening physical problems associated with withdrawal. Cocaine causes vasoconstriction, increased blood pressure, and tachycardia. Cocaine reduces placental blood flow. Chronic use in the second and third trimesters can lead to low birth weight, the most common effect of cocaine use in pregnancy (Bateman, Ng, Hansen, & Heagarty, 1993). Sudden decreases in placental blood flow may result in placental abruption. Scattered, rare reports link cocaine to congenital anomalies. Some infants exposed to cocaine in

Critical Thinking

Caring for Pregnant Women Who Abuse Substances

When caring for clients who abuse substances in prenatal or perinatal care, you may be faced with conflicting emotions. As a nurse, you spend your career working for healthy mothers and babies. When a mother places a child at risk, you may feel anger, dislike, or impatience. You may even wish the court system would place the mother under surveillance to prevent substance use. This is not currently legal in any state in the United States because a fetus does not have full legal status as a person with rights of its own.

You are facing a conflict among three ethical principles important in providing health care: *beneficence*, doing good; *paternalism*, taking care of those who are unable to use good judgment for themselves; and *autonomy* (self-determination), the right of an adult to make personal decisions about her own behavior even when it places a fetus at risk. Forcibly controlling a woman's behavior may further diminish her ability to make good decisions on her own.

To promote the health of the fetus while building the mother's confidence and self-esteem, think about how you could form a respectful and interested professional relationship with her. This will help her feel worthwhile and competent, and she may be more likely to continue in prenatal care and seek alternatives to substance abuse.

Nursing Tip · *Asking Clients about Substance Use in Pregnancy*

The most important point to remember is to ask *all* pregnant women about substance use. Do not make assumptions about which women are likely to be smokers or to use illicit drugs. Practice asking these kinds of questions and use them in assessment of all pregnant clients.

Keep these ideas in mind as you assess substance use:

1. Create a private setting to do a social assessment. The presence of other clients or family members may restrict the woman's willingness to discuss stigmatizing conditions such as substance use or domestic violence.

2. Ask about substance use in the part of the assessment that covers family, home life, and social environment. Linking these behaviors to the environment reduces the implication that they are personal failings of the woman. Ideally, ask them after you have established rapport with the client.

3. Consider asking, "Are you exposed to cigarette smoke in your home?" Then ask, "Who are the smokers in your home? Are you a smoker?" Inquire how many cigarettes the woman and her family members smoke each day and whether they have made any changes since the pregnancy began.

4. Use the same calm, warm tone of voice to inquire about alcohol use and then other drug use. Do not simply ask, "Do you use any other drugs?" Be specific: name illicit drugs, including heroin, cocaine, and marijuana.

5. Watch your body language. If you hurry through the questions, shake your head "No," or look away when asking these questions, the woman may assume you do not want to hear the answer.

6. If the woman admits substance use during pregnancy, do not give in to the urge to immediately explain all the risks of these substances and advise her to quit, which may alienate her. Unless she indicates a desire to continue to discuss it, simply say, "Thank you for sharing this, it is important to the health of you and your baby. We'll talk about this more later."

7. Complete the assessment, and then inquire, "You mentioned (substance use) earlier. I would like to review some of the effects of (this substance) during pregnancy and perhaps make some suggestions. Are you interested in discussing this?" If she declines, reply, "I will be happy to go over this information at any time." Offer printed literature on the topic.

8. Continue to treat her warmly and offer support and encouragement so that she develops trust in you. Over time, your positive relationship may enable you to revisit the topic. Your goal is to build her confidence and self-esteem, which will aid in her willingness to try to change her behavior.

9. Remember that she may be focusing on other personal priorities that seem much more urgent to her, such as surviving a violent relationship or keeping a job that her family depends on. She may value the stress reduction and sense of autonomy she gets from smoking more than protecting her fetus from a risk that seems small. Nurses are most effective when they work within the client's personal goals, helping clients see how improving health behaviors will help them meet their other goals as well.

---

utero show increased irritability, difficulty in soothing, and changes in orientation and motor processes.

Heroin

Heroin is a highly addictive narcotic related to morphine that causes sedation, relaxation, and euphoria. When pregnant women who are addicted to heroin withdraw use suddenly or sharply reduce their use, intrauterine fetal demise can occur.

The most common harmful effect of heroin on newborns is withdrawal, or **neonatal abstinence syndrome**. This collection of symptoms may include sneezing, vomiting, diarrhea, irritability, and seizures and is seen in newborns

withdrawing from prenatal exposure to narcotics. In a few studies, heroin has been linked to anomalies and low birth weight. In some cases, children who are exposed to heroin or methadone in utero have shown deficits in developmental and cognitive testing; however, poor maternal-child interaction and other factors of the home environment probably contributed to this effect (Richardson, Conroy, & Day, 1996).

Injection drug use—whether of cocaine, heroin, amphetamines, or other drugs—increases a woman's risk of exposure to the human immunodeficiency virus (HIV) through contaminated needles. Illegal drug use also carries the risk of acquiring a sexually transmitted disease (STD) because women may trade sex for drugs, provide sexual favors to earn money for drugs, or maintain relationships with drug users (Henderson, Boyd, & Mieczkowski, 1994).

Infections

Infections during pregnancy can be acquired from humans, animals, or the natural environment. They fall into two broad categories: STDs, acquired through intimate sexual contact; and other infections, including rubella, *E. coli*, and hepatitis, that may be acquired through casual exposure to infected persons or animals or through food or water. Maternal infections, mainly rubella, toxoplasmosis, and cytomegalovirus, account for approximately 2% of major congenital malformations occurring during pregnancy (Briggs, 1995).

Sexually Transmitted Diseases

One potent route of infection during pregnancy is sexual exposure, which introduces harmful organisms into the maternal system by way of the genital tract (Figure 12-12).

Syphilis

Syphilis infection, caused by the spirochete *Treponema pallidum*, increases the risks of spontaneous abortion, stillbirth, and live birth with congenital syphilis. Congenital syphilis affects about 250 infants annually in the United

States (Sweet & Gibbs, 1995). The longer the mother has been infected, the greater the risk to the fetus.

All pregnant women should receive a blood serology test for syphilis as early as possible in pregnancy. Syphilis can be effectively treated during pregnancy using penicillin.

Gonorrhea and Chlamydia

Gonorrhea, caused by *Neisseria gonorrhoeae*, and chlamydia, caused by *Chlamydia trachomatis*, are transmitted sexually and cause no symptoms in 85% of infected women. Adolescent women and women of color are disproportionately affected by these infections (CDC, 1996).

Gonorrhea and chlamydia infections can cause neonatal conjunctivitis and blindness, and chlamydia infection can cause neonatal pneumonia. Blindness can be prevented by prophylactic treatment of the newborn with ointment applied to the eyes at birth; however, prevention of pneumonia requires that chlamydia infection be treated during pregnancy (CDC, 1996).

Herpes Simplex Virus

The herpes simplex virus (HSV) is a common one that causes painful, pruritic blisterlike lesions and is carried by 0.1% to 4% of pregnant women. Herpes is a chronic recurrent infection. The virus is shed heavily during the primary infection as well as during recurrences (Sweet & Gibbs, 1995). Fetal and neonatal risks from HSV occur mainly when a primary infection occurs in pregnancy.

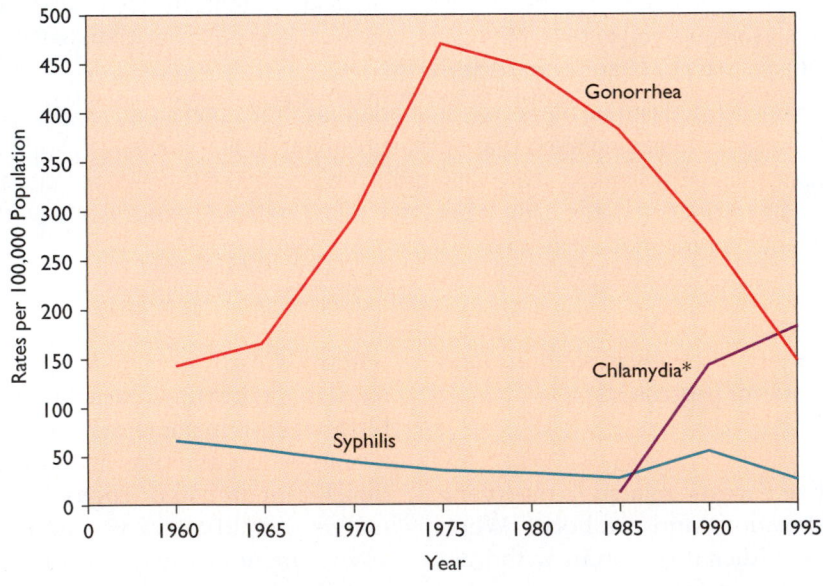

*statistics on chlamydia were not collected until 1984

Figure 12-12   Estimated rates of sexually transmitted diseases per hundred thousand population, 1960–1995. (Data from Centers for Disease Control and Prevention. 1996. *Sexually transmitted disease surveillance, 1995*. Atlanta, GA: CDC, U.S. Department of Health and Human Services, Public Health Service.)

Nursing Tip — Reducing Risks Related to the Herpes Simplex Virus

Isolation in a private room is no longer considered necessary for mothers and full-term newborns when the mother has HSV. Practicing and teaching good handwashing technique are very important. The mother, all family members, and all visitors should wash their hands thoroughly before handling the newborn. The infant should be protected from exposure to herpes lesions. This includes advising the family not to kiss the infant if they have orofacial HSV lesions. Face masks may be worn by persons with orofacial herpes lesions to reduce the risk of spreading the virus in droplet form.

Protecting the newborn and other clients is important, as is treating the family with respect and understanding. The family will feel stigmatized if nurses avoid them or demonstrate a lack of enthusiasm in caring for them.

When the nurse has an orofacial herpes lesion, scrupulous handwashing and coverage of the lesion with a dressing is essential. Lesions are less contagious when crusted over, about 5 to 7 days after onset. Some institutions temporarily reassign nurses with herpes lesions to an area of the unit away from newborns.

The most common route of transmission to the fetus is genital contact during vaginal delivery when the mother has a primary genital HSV infection. In this situation, neonatal HSV infection may occur in 25% to 50% of newborns; 40% to 60% of these newborns are at risk for death, and the remainder are likely to suffer CNS damage.

During a primary infection when the membranes are intact or have been ruptured for less than 4 hours, cesarean delivery may be recommended to reduce the exposure of the neonate to the virus. During a recurrent infection, the risk of transmission to the neonate is estimated at 0% to 4%; however, cesarean delivery may be performed as a precaution. Neonates also can be infected by hospital personnel or visitors with HSV lesions, and, occasionally, a newborn will develop an infection when the mother has no history of lesions but has a positive result on culture for HSV (Sweet & Gibbs, 1995).

Human Immunodeficiency Virus
For childbearing women, a major concern is transmission of HIV to the fetus. Without antiviral therapy, approximately 25% of newborns of women infected with HIV will become infected with HIV (CDC Fact Sheet, 1996).

Nursing Tip — HIV Testing in Pregnancy

Although some practitioners believe that all pregnant women should be tested for HIV, regardless of consent, this practice would be contrary to the ethical principle of autonomy for health care clients. Voluntary counseling and testing has resulted in increased use of zidovudine therapy during pregnancy and reduced transmission of HIV to newborns (CDC Fact Sheet, 1996).

You must provide information and counseling on voluntary testing for HIV to all pregnant women. Explain that this testing will enable the detection of infection early enough to provide zidovudine (AZT) and other important treatments. Advise women diagnosed with other STDs that they may also have been exposed to HIV. Repeated testing over 6 to 12 months is necessary to detect recent infection.

Nursing Alert — Preventing the Spread of HIV and Other Infections

You must maintain standard infection control precautions during prenatal and perinatal procedures to minimize the risk of contamination of the environment with blood or body fluids containing the HIV virus and other pathogens. These precautions apply to all pregnant and postpartum women, not only those known to be infected with HIV.

You must remember that HIV and other infections may be present in any woman, including those whose HIV status was negative at the last test. If the infection is recent, antibodies may not have yet developed that can be detected with testing. Some women may have refused testing because of fear of stigma or loss of employment or insurance coverage if they are found to be HIV-positive. Others may never have been offered the HIV test. You should refrain from making judgments about which women are likely to be infected with HIV and use standard precautions for all clients.

Other Infections

Pregnant women may acquire infections from contaminated food, water, or nonsexual contact with infected persons. Although many kinds of infections may be contracted from these sources, some are known to have harmful effects on the fetus and newborn.

Hepatitis B

This viral infection is transmitted through blood and body fluids and predominantly affects the liver. The acute infection can be fatal or cause permanent liver damage or carcinoma. Infection in pregnancy may cause spontaneous abortion and has been linked to preterm labor. Maternal-infant transmission can occur transplacentally, through intrapartum or postpartum contact with contaminated surfaces, or through breast milk or colostrum.

The neonate of a mother with hepatitis B should receive hepatitis B immune globulin and the first of three injections of hepatitis B vaccine before being discharged from the hospital. Most states require that all parents be offered the opportunity to have their newborns receive the first hepatitis B immunization injection during the nursery stay (Sweet & Gibbs, 1995).

Varicella Zoster

The varicella virus causes the chickenpox infection. Chickenpox is a common childhood disease causing fever, malaise, and pruritic pustules.

In pregnancy, however, varicella can be extremely harmful. Varicella infection in the first trimester of pregnancy has approximately a 10% risk of causing congenital varicella syndrome, which includes limb and digit hypoplasia, eye anomalies, mental retardation, and growth retardation. Infection of the mother late in pregnancy can cause preterm labor and stillbirth and places the newborn at risk for life-threatening neonatal varicella infection. The risk of death can be averted by giving exposed newborns varicella-zoster immune globulin (VZIG), although some may still show signs of infection (Sweet & Gibbs, 1995).

Cytomegalovirus

Cytomegalovirus (CMV) has been linked to serious neonatal infection and malformations. CMV causes mild flulike symptoms in the healthy adult or no symptoms at all, and as many as 75% of adult women have antibodies to CMV (Sweet & Gibbs, 1995). CMV can be transmitted to the fetus transplacentally and at the time of birth.

Newborns infected with CMV have a 10% risk of symptomatic disease at birth. The infection can cause hepatosplenomegaly, jaundice, deafness, and eye problems. Mental retardation, chorioretinitis, cerebral calcifications, and microcephaly or hydrocephaly are long-term effects. Unfortunately, although antiviral treatments are used to limit the extent of disease, no fully effective treatments are available.

Pregnant women can be tested for immunity or current infection using the **TORCH** serum screening panel (see Nursing Tip). For an asymptomatic disease such as CMV, expensive serial titer testing would be needed to detect the presence of primary infection; however, no effective treatments are known for women diagnosed with primary CMV. Nurses should be prepared to counsel pregnant women about this difficult situation and provide

---

Nursing Tip — Standard Precautions

When following Standard Precautions, you must:

1. Wear gloves to prevent transmission of bloodborne infections, such as HBV and HIV, when you are at risk of coming into contact with any bodily fluids that contain blood or amniotic fluid from the client, bedding, or instruments. You must also change gloves between clients. Do not reuse gloves.

2. Wear a mask, eye protection, a face shield, and a fluid-resistant gown in all situations in which bodily fluids are likely to be splashed or propelled onto you.

3. Wear a gown and gloves when handling newborns until all blood and amniotic fluid have been removed by bathing.

4. Do not recap, bend, or break needles. Do not remove needles from syringes. Store all sharps safely for disposal.

5. Perform resuscitation and suctioning using protective equipment rather than by mouth-to-mouth contact or use of a DeLee catheter.

Nursing Tip — TORCH Screening

To collect data prenatally or in the postpartum period when viral infection is suspected you can use the TORCH screening panel, which tests for antibodies to certain infections that have been linked to fetal or neonatal harm. This includes testing for:

1. **T**oxoplasmosis
2. **O**ther infections, including hepatitis
3. **R**ubella
4. **C**ytomegalovirus
5. **H**erpes

support. Some women who have CMV infection may choose to terminate the pregnancy even though the likelihood of a healthy outcome is 90% (Sweet & Gibbs, 1995).

Toxoplasmosis

Toxoplasma is an intracellular parasite that is found in animals, including sheep and mice. It is transmitted in the feces of cats who have consumed infected mice and in meat from infected animals. The disease in humans may have no symptoms or may cause lymphadenopathy, fever, fatigue, sore throat, eye pain, and rash. It may be mistaken for influenza or mononucleosis.

When infection occurs, spontaneous abortion, preterm delivery, and intrauterine growth retardation may result. Toxoplasmosis can be treated with antibiotics if infection is diagnosed early; however, some neonatal disease may still occur. Nurses play an important role in home assessment and prenatal teaching to prevent this infection.

This preventive advice has significantly reduced the incidence of toxoplasmosis in areas where it has been used systematically (Sweet & Gibbs, 1995).

Other Parasitic Diseases

Nurses should counsel pregnant women who travel to tropical and undeveloped areas to avoid exposure to insects, bodies of water, water that has not been treated for drinking, and meat that is not fully cooked. Women who come to prenatal care from these areas should be assessed for signs of parasitic disease and treatment provided when appropriate. Blood and stool cultures can be used to detect many parasites. It is important for the nurse to teach women about the low risk to the fetus of many parasitic conditions and to provide emotional support and instructions on hygiene if treatment must be delayed until after childbirth.

Client Education

Preventing Toxoplasmosis Infection

You should advise clients who are pregnant and those planning pregnancy to:

- Avoid undercooked meat.
- Wash hands after handling cats.
- Have someone else change the cat's litterbox daily.
- Prevent cats from eating wild animals or raw meat.
- Avoid contact with stray animals.

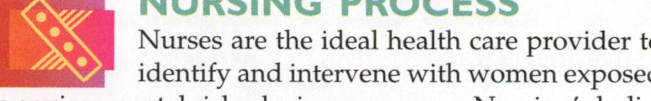

NURSING PROCESS

Nurses are the ideal health care provider to identify and intervene with women exposed to environmental risks during pregnancy. Nursing's holistic focus on clients within the context of their families and environments promotes sensitivity to factors in addition to medical and obstetrical risks that may threaten the well-being of pregnant women and their fetuses.

Assessment

When providing care for pregnant women in acute, ambulatory, or home care settings, the nurse must be aware of and assess for environmental and lifestyle risks that may endanger the mother and fetus.

Nursing Diagnoses and Outcome Identification

Nursing diagnoses, along with expected outcomes, are listed in Table 12-3.

Planning

For each nursing and medical diagnosis that applies to a pregnant woman and her family, you should work with the client to develop a plan of care that addresses health needs within the goals, capabilities, and context of the family. In planning to address each health issue, you should:

1. Consider the values behind the health goal, and clarify that the values are compatible with the client's choices. For example, a pregnant woman who smokes a pack of cigarettes per day may not value prevention of low birth weight as much as she values the autonomy and stress reduction of smoking.

2. Provide the education needed to convey the benefits of behavior or lifestyle changes. For example, if a pregnant woman works in an agricultural environment, explain the relative risks of harm from pesticide exposure and heavy lifting, and the reduction in risk that would be achieved if she were able to eliminate these exposures and activities.

3. Select interventions to reduce risks that are feasible within the client's unique situation and context. These may be client-initiated or nurse-initiated, or initiated by referral to another helping professional. For example, referral-initiated interventions could include providing information about Alcoholics Anonymous (AA) meetings.

Table 12-3   Common Nursing Diagnoses, Causes, and Outcomes

NURSING DIAGNOSIS	CAUSE	EXPECTED OUTCOMES
Risk for (or present) infection	Unsafe sexual practices, preexisting sexually transmitted disease, lack of immunity to childhood diseases that place the fetus at risk, environmental hazards such as parasites	Fetus is protected from infection by immunization, maternal antibiotic treatment, maternal safer sex practices and lifestyle precautions, and safe food handling and preparation.
Risk for injury (fetal)	Industrial waste, employment conditions that expose pregnant woman to dangerous chemicals or activities	Fetus is protected from injury by removing hazards from environment, protecting pregnant woman from exposure, and modifying of employment or household conditions.
Ineffective tissue perfusion (placental)	Cigarette smoking, cocaine use, stress	Placental perfusion is adequate, as demonstrated by appropriate fetal growth and reassuring fetal assessments.
Impaired gas exchange (placental-fetal)	Cigarette smoking, carbon monoxide exposure, maternal anoxia from seizures	Fetus demonstrates adequate oxygenation by reactive nonstress tests and other assessments. Risk is reduced by reduction in maternal cigarette smoking and maintenance of therapeutic level of anticonvulsants.
Delayed growth and development (fetal)	Inadequate nutrition or malformations from chemical or drug exposure	Alterations are diagnosed promptly. Chemical exposures are minimized or eliminated. Pregnant woman and family are informed of risks and supported in decision-making. Pregnant woman and family have adequate support and preparation for birth of an infant with possible altered development.
Imbalanced nutrition, less than body requirements	Substance abuse and consequent anorexia, cognitive alterations, lifestyle disruption	Pregnant woman who abuses substances demonstrates adequate weight gain and fetal growth. Adequate support and teaching are provided to reduce substance abuse and promote healthful lifestyle.
Fatigue	Strenuous employment demands	Pregnant woman demonstrates moderation in physical activity and adequate rest periods.
Ineffective role performance	Role burdens (work and home), changing roles	Employment conditions and role expectations are modified to promote prenatal health.
Fear	Possible birth of damaged infant from exposure to a hazardous substance or infection	Pregnant woman and family report reduction in fear, and demonstrate knowledge of likelihood of fetal harm and measures to minimize fetal damage.
Deficient knowledge	Lack of information about pregnancy, hazards, risk reduction strategies	Pregnant woman and family can state potential risks of their environmental conditions for fetal health, and describe and demonstrate risk reduction strategies.
Ineffective individual and family coping	Substance abuse	Pregnant woman and family demonstrate improved safety in behavior and home management and increased motivation toward healthful behaviors.

Nursing Intervention

Nurses should focus on the whole pregnancy, and follow-up is extremely important. Behavioral changes such as stopping smoking are extremely difficult to sustain; therefore, it is important to let the pregnant woman know that support is always available. Family and community resources can be incorporated in discharge planning.

Evaluation

Interim evaluations should be made of client knowledge, behavior, environmental conditions, and maternal and fetal physical and psychosocial well-being. The ultimate outcome of nursing care to reduce risks during pregnancy is the birth of a healthy infant.

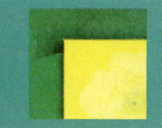

CASE STUDY/CARE PLAN
SUBSTANCE USE IN PREGNANCY

Janice Lord is a 31-year-old (gravida 3, para 1) single Caucasian woman who arrives for her first prenatal visit. She is 16 weeks pregnant. Her first pregnancy ended with delivery of a healthy full-term male infant who is now 3 years old. Her second pregnancy ended in a spontaneous abortion at 18 weeks owing to placental abruption. She has no chronic diseases or known exposures to industrial chemicals or radiation. She lives with her son in a public housing project where gang fighting and public intoxication is common. She is employed full-time as a house cleaner.

Janice smokes 20 cigarettes per day, drinks two or three 12-ounce beers each night to relax after work, and smokes crack cocaine on weekends with her boyfriend. Her mother, also a cigarette smoker, watches Janice's son during the day. Her boyfriend does not live with her but spends most of each weekend in her apartment.

Janice was originally ambivalent about continuing the present pregnancy and also was delayed in seeking prenatal care because she did not have health insurance. She tells you that she believes the previous pregnancy loss was due to a cocaine binge, and she wants to do her best to protect the present fetus from harm. She hopes to move out of public housing sometime soon and relocate to a suburban area with less street violence.

Janice's initial physical examination is within normal limits, with the exception of a foul-smelling vaginal discharge and mild hypertension (140/90 mmHg). Wet prep slide of discharge reveals Trichomonas infection; other culture results are negative. Fetal heart tones are normal, and fetal activity is palpated.

Assessment

Based on nursing knowledge of obstetrical, public health, and psychosocial risks, the nurse determined that the following assessments indicated need for nursing intervention:

- History of late spontaneous abortion, violent home area, smoking by both Janice and her mother, cocaine use, and hypertension, all of which may increase the risk of vasoconstriction and inadequate blood supply to the placenta and fetus
- Reported alcohol and cocaine use in early pregnancy, suggesting an increased risk of fetal injury from these substances
- Trichomonas infection, suggesting unsafe sex practices and risks of other STDs and HIV
- Self-reported substance use, indicating ineffective coping strategies

Nursing Diagnosis

Ineffective tissue perfusion (placenta) related to vasoconstriction from cigarette smoking, cocaine use, hypertension, and chronic stress.

Expected Outcomes	Maintain adequate fetal-placental perfusion, as demonstrated by appropriate fetal activity and growth; absence of drugs in maternal urine; and self-reported reduction in cigarette smoking.
Planning	Adequate perfusion demonstrated by stable activity counts and reactive nonstress tests.
	Normal fetal growth demonstrated by fundal height and ultrasonography.
	Reduced risk, as measured by absence of substance in urine screening sample and self-reported reduction in substance use.
	Pregnancy continues to term without evidence of preterm labor or placental abruption.
NOC	Tissue perfusion: Placenta
NIC	Circulatory care: Placental insufficiency

(continues)

Nursing Interventions	Rationales
1. Educate about effects of cigarettes, neurologic and vaso-constrictive effects of cocaine in pregnancy, and effects of passive smoking on her and her son's health. Offer referrals to stop-smoking and substance abuse treatment programs. Provide ongoing emotional support to maintain behavior change. Engage mother and boyfriend in educational and stop-smoking programs.	1. Information about health risks along with a referral to resources are important to begin change.
2. Monitor placental function with activity counts and nonstress tests. Monitor blood pressure.	2. Monitoring the pregnancy is part of prenatal care.
3. Provide letter to employer requesting activity limitations as recommended by the American Medical Association, and follow-up with phone call, if needed.	3. Interventions may need to be taken at the workplace to facilitate a healthy environment.

Evaluation   Janice describes reduction in smoking to 5 cigarettes per day and abstinence from alcohol and cocaine. Her partner and mother attend stop-smoking classes sporadically. Janice expresses appreciation for support from the nurse as she continues to work on making changes at home and work. Activity counts and nonstress tests are within normal limits. Blood pressure decreases to normal levels as smoking decreases. Janice denies preterm contractions, uterine pain, and vaginal bleeding.

Nursing Diagnosis

Risk for fetal injury; risk factors include prenatal alcohol and cocaine exposure.

Expected Outcomes   Minimize risk to fetus of further substance exposure, as demonstrated by Janice's understanding of the risks of drugs and alcohol use in pregnancy, her reports of abstinence from alcohol and drugs, and negative urine screening.

Planning   Client will be able to state risks to fetus of alcohol and cocaine use in pregnancy.

Alcohol and cocaine intake will stop for remainder of pregnancy, as demonstrated by negative urine screening results and client self-reporting.

NOC   Risk control

NIC   High-risk pregnancy care

Nursing Interventions	Rationales
1. Educate client and family about effects of cocaine and alcohol, as well as impairment of parenting interactions when intoxicated.	1. Knowledge of effects of substance abuse on family and parenting abilities may motivate client to modify behaviors.
2. Refer to AA or Narcotics Anonymous for peer support; refer to formal drug and alcohol treatment, if desired.	2. Education and referral provide the client the tools to make lifestyle changes.
3. Provide ongoing support and encouragement.	3. Client may be more inclined to adopt healthy behaviors if nurse is a strong supporter and change agent.
4. Discuss advantages of regular screening for substances.	4. Knowledge of the benefits of regular screening may encourage client to have frequent contact with a health care provider, resulting in better and more consistent prenatal care.
5. Provide assessment and intervention for newborn alcohol and cocaine effects, if present.	5. Continued assessment and monitoring of newborn risks allows for early intervention and treatment.

Evaluation   Janice reports abstinence from alcohol and cocaine since the time of committing to continue the pregnancy. She attends AA meetings weekly where she has met another pregnant woman who has become a friend. Janice's boyfriend continues to drink and use drugs but not in her apartment. Ultrasonography shows no apparent anomalies.

(continues)

Nursing Diagnosis

Risk for fetal and maternal infection; risk factors include maternal exposure to STDs.

Expected Outcomes	Complete treatment for current infection, consider HIV testing for self and partner, and use safer sex to prevent future infection.
Planning	Client will complete treatment for documented infection. Client will report safer sex practices to prevent future infection. Client will report her decision regarding HIV testing in pregnancy.
NOC	Risk control: Sexually transmitted diseases
NIC	Infection protection

Nursing Interventions	**Rationales**
1. Educate client about implications of Trichomonas infection—not harmful in itself but a sign of other possible STD exposure. 2. Provide treatment with metronidazole (Flagyl) (safe after first trimester), and recheck for cure after completion of treatment. 3. Discuss with client and partner importance of safer sex practices and merits of testing for HIV and other STDs. Advise partner to be treated.	1. Client needs to understand the risks and implications of STDs on her health and that of her developing fetus. 2. Complete course of medication is effective in fighting the infections. 3. Treatments will be most effective if involved partner also undergoes treatment and therapy.

Evaluation	Janice reports she took all medication. Repeat testing is negative for Trichomonas infection. Boyfriend obtained medication, but Janice is unsure about his completion of therapy. Janice reports she has insisted on condom use since learning of risks of STDs in pregnancy. Other STD tests and HIV test are negative. Boyfriend has not yet agreed to HIV testing.

Nursing Diagnosis

Ineffective coping related to lack of alternatives to harmful substances, environmental prevalence of substance use, fatigue, and lack of social support.

Expected Outcomes	Replace ineffective coping strategies (substance use) with alternative activities.
Planning	Client will demonstrate abstinence from substance use or progress toward abstinence and can describe alternative methods of coping with fatigue and stress.
NOC	Risk control: Substance use
NIC	Environmental management

Nursing Interventions	**Rationales**
1. Provide reading materials and refer for counseling to uncover alternative means of recreation and relaxation such as walking, movies, games, playing with her son, and naps in late afternoon while grandmother watches her son. 2. Discuss new sources of social support such as women's groups, religious groups, family, or clubs.	1. Client may need help in identifying alternatives to substance use as a means of recreation; activities that involve her son and family may help strengthen family bonds. 2. Offering client an array of choices will allow her to choose those options most appealing to her, thereby increasing the likelihood of compliance.

Evaluation	Janice remains abstinent from all substances except cigarettes. She has found a friend at a local AA meeting held in a church. She and her son have discovered friends at a playground of a local public library and have begun to go there in the evenings. She describes some distance between herself and her boyfriend but hopes that he will see the benefit of this healthier lifestyle.

EVALUATION OF FETAL WELL-BEING

Technology and science have become prominent components of obstetrical care. Technology can provide useful information about the status of the pregnancy and condition of the fetus; however, it is imperative to balance technologic capabilities with responsiveness to the human needs of the woman and her family. Many of the fetal evaluation techniques described in this chapter are performed in outpatient settings. In addition, many of these procedures, especially those performed during the first half of pregnancy, are technically oriented and have minimal direct care responsibilities for the nurse during the procedure itself. However, the nurse does have a major role in identifying, preparing, counseling, supporting, and educating clients regarding the implementation and understanding of fetal evaluation throughout the period of gestation. Fetal evaluation is an interdisciplinary endeavor involving physicians, sonographers, laboratory technicians, and nurses. However, the nurse often is the only care provider who can establish a therapeutic and holistic relationship with the client and who has the opportunity to interact with the client before, during, and after the procedure. Consequently, nurses need to have a good knowledge base of fetal diagnostic and screening technologies; the disease processes that warrant fetal evaluation; and the meaning of the findings of these procedures to the woman, the pregnancy, and the family. The counseling, support, and education provided by the nurse are vital interventions to assist the woman during the experience of fetal evaluation.

Screening and Diagnostic Tests

A variety of diagnostic techniques and monitoring parameters is used to evaluate *fetal well-being*, that is, the growth and health of the developing fetus as well as its ability to tolerate the physiologic stresses of pregnancy, labor, and birth.

The average duration of human pregnancy is 40 weeks, or 280 days after the first day of the last menstrual period. The gestational period is divided into the period of the embryo (the first 8 weeks) and the period of the fetus (9 weeks to birth). The embryonic period is a time of growth, differentiation, and organization of the cellular components of the developing being. During the embryonic period, evaluation is done primarily to assess for normal implantation, viability, and abnormalities with a genetic base. By the end of the eighth week of gestation, all body systems are present in at least a rudimentary form. During the remainder of the gestational period, the fetal period, the body systems grow, change, and evolve into specialized tissues and organs. During this period of

Nursing Tip

Prenatal Screening

When considering whether prenatal screening should be done, ask the following questions:

1. Is the screening procedure justified in this population?
2. What is the risk to the pregnancy?
3. What is the risk to the woman?
4. What will the results reveal about the status of the pregnancy?
5. Which options are available to the woman and her family if the results indicate increased risk?
6. Which resources are available to support the woman and her family?

pregnancy fetal well-being can be assessed and monitored using a number of biochemical, physical, and physiologic surveillance techniques.

Routine assessment of fetal well-being has included auscultation of fetal heart rate, measurement of fundal height, and maternal perception of fetal movement. These parameters provide indirect measures of fetal condition (Figure 12-13). Three areas of particular concern to nurses regarding fetal surveillance techniques have emerged: purpose, process, and consequences.

Purpose

The purposes of the fetal evaluation technologies are for diagnostic testing, screening procedures, and reassurance procedures. Some of the testing modalities described in this chapter are diagnostic, for example, amniocentesis and chorionic villus sampling to determine the presence or absence of specific genetic conditions. Screening procedures identify a fetus as being at greater risk than other fetuses but do not confirm or rule out the condition in either group. Examples of screening procedures used during the prenatal period are MS-AFP and fetal fibronectin measurements. A third group of evaluation technologies is reassurance procedures. These procedures include the nonstress test. This test provides data predictive of fetal health and well-being; however, when the results are abnormal, no concrete evidence of danger to the fetus is provided. The client must understand the purpose or goal of a particular fetal evaluation technology in order to provide consent to undergo the procedure.

Table 12-4 outlines certain risk factors and the related recommended assessment techniques. Prenatal determination of fetal gender is a valid indication for prenatal

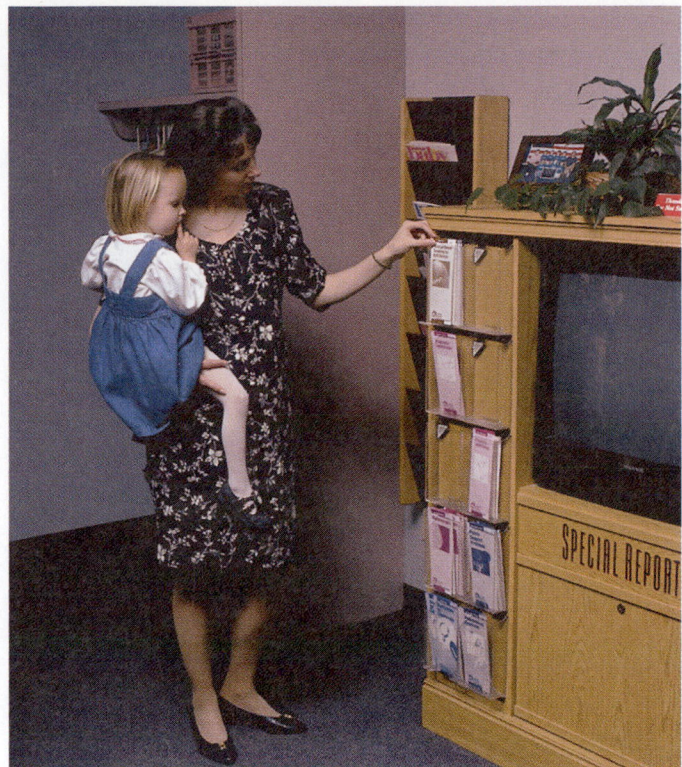

Figure 12-13 Literature should be made available to the expectant parents who will be undergoing fetal evaluation testing. The nurse should also help the client understand and interpret information and be ready to answer questions.

Critical Thinking

Gender Selection

How do you respond to a 36-year-old client (gravida 6, para 5) (all boys) who tells you she wants genetic testing done because if this baby is not a girl, she wants to terminate the pregnancy?

surveillance only when the possibility exists of the presence of an X-linked disorder.

Process

The overriding goal of fetal evaluation is to obtain information about the growth, development, and well-being of the fetus; however, it is impossible to do so without invading the woman's bodily integrity. Table 12-5 provides an overview of the types of fetal surveillance procedures available.

The woman and her family need a clear and thorough explanation of all the problems and potential outcomes of the current pregnancy. They then need to examine the information in view of their personal, social, religious, cultural, and familial beliefs and values. The client needs

Table 12-4 Assessment for Increased Risk of a Genetic Disorder		
RISK FACTORS	**RELATED RISKS**	**ASSESSMENT TECHNIQUES**
Maternal age	At the age of 35, the risk of fetal loss from invasive prenatal testing equals the risk of having a child with a chromosomal anomaly.	Collection of demographic data Interview and general survey
Ethnic background	Certain genetic diseases are found in populations with a specific ethnic background, e.g., • Tay-Sachs disease: Eastern European Jews • Thalassemia: Mediterranean descent • Sickle cell trait: Blacks	Interview Pedigree or genogram to analyze patterns
Family history	The presence of certain diseases (hemophilia, Huntington's chorea, and cystic fibrosis), birth defects (neural tube defects and abdominal wall defects), or mental retardation in the family history increases the risk for future offspring.	Careful family history Pedigree or genogram to analyze patterns
Reproductive history	Previous poor perinatal outcomes, e.g., • Stillbirths • Repeated spontaneous abortions • Children with birth defects or disorders	Careful family history Medical record review
Maternal disease	Some diseases have the increased risk of transmission from mother to fetus.	Careful review of past medical history, current health status, and medication ingestion
Environmental hazards	Exposure to chemicals, radiation, hot tubs, nutrition, or other potential teratogens	Behavior evaluation Preconception education about hazard exposure

Table 12-5	Types of Fetal Surveillance Procedures	
SCREENING	**DIAGNOSTIC**	**REASSURANCE**
Estriol	Amniocentesis	Biophysical profile
Fetal fibronectin screening	Chorionic villus sampling	Contraction stress test
Human chorionic gonadatropin	Fetal cell isolation	Fetal movement counting
Human placental lactogen	Fetal tissue sampling	Nonstress test
Maternal serum–alpha-fetoprotein	Percutaneous umbilical blood sampling	

time to think carefully about the potentially serious implications of pregnancy screening and fetal testing, without feeling pressured to make a decision.

The nurse often is in the position of being the client's advocate and is a key person in assisting the client in accessing and synthesizing the information necessary to make decisions. Also, as with any technical procedure, it is incumbent on the nurse to ensure that the appropriate equipment and resources are available in the event a complication necessitating emergency intervention arises.

Consequences

As with any procedure that generates information, one must think about how that information will be used. Considering the consequences of fetal evaluation when a

Critical Thinking

Client Preparation for Fetal Evaluation

When preparing a client for fetal evaluation procedures, be sure you are prepared to respond to all of the following questions:

- Why is the procedure being done?
- Is the procedure safe?
- How accurate is the test?
- What information will the test provide?
- Who will perform the procedure?
- Is any physical preparation necessary?
- What does the procedure involve?
- How much time will the test take?
- What will I feel?
- What is the recovery time after the procedure?
- Who will interpret the results?
- When will I be informed of the results?
- Who will talk with me about the results?
- Who will answer my questions and address my concerns about the test and the results?
- What other options are available?

problem is detected is as important as considering the impact of fetal evaluation when the postulate condition is not confirmed. A "good" result from fetal evaluation technologies can result in a false sense of security. Fetal evaluation technologies do provide data about a wide variety of fetal conditions; however, many other conditions and factors exist that can impact pregnancy outcome. Fetal evaluation does not guarantee a perfect baby; it only provides data that confirm the presence or absence of a specific condition for which the testing modality was searching (Raines, 1996).

Reflections from a Nurse

My client, Svetlana, received early and consistent prenatal care. She had no complications during her pregnancy. She had a CVS and two ultrasound examinations, and she performed daily fetal movement counts from 28 weeks on. All test results were within normal parameters. When her infant was born, however, he had a rare congenital anomaly. Svetlana and her family were devastated, and as her primary nurse, I was surprised and saddened. She and her family asked again and again, "How can this happen?"

Critical Thinking

Difficult Choices

What are the psychosocial implications of choosing to have prenatal diagnosis and the implied consideration of pregnancy termination on the development of family bonds and trusting relationships?

GENETIC AND BIOCHEMICAL EVALUATION

Genetic and biochemical testing is a means of detecting potentially harmful alterations in chromosomal number, change in molecular structure, metabolic deviation, and hematologic variation (Table 12-6). Biochemical analysis also can provide information related to fetal maturity and placental function that, in turn, can provide the critical data needed to develop a therapeutic treatment plan for managing a high-risk pregnancy. Genetic and biochemical evaluation of pregnancy status can be grouped into either invasive fetal diagnostic studies or maternal serum studies.

Invasive Fetal Diagnostic Studies

Invasive fetal procedures involve violating the integrity of the fetal-placental-uterine environment and include amniocentesis, chorionic villus sampling, percutaneous umbilical blood sampling, and other tests.

Specific concerns, both maternal and fetal, related to the possible risks and complications are discussed for each testing modality. However, a general concern relevant to all invasive fetal procedures is the risk of maternal-fetal hemorrhage. Therefore, blood type should be obtained for all pregnant women undergoing invasive fetal testing procedures. Women who are Rh-negative are candidates for $Rh_o(D)$ immune globulin (RhoGAM). Prophylactic RhoGAM minimizes the potential for maternal sensitization and prevents antibody formation in the event of minor maternal-fetal bleeding.

Nursing Alert

Preventing Antibody Formation

Women who are Rh-negative undergoing invasive fetal evaluation techniques such as CVS, amniocentesis, or PUBS should receive RhoGAM after the procedure to prevent antibody formation in the event of maternal-fetal bleeding.

Amniocentesis

Amniocentesis is one of the oldest invasive methods of fetal evaluation. Amniocentesis is used to obtain amniotic fluid for the diagnosis of a variety of disorders through enzymatic analysis and DNA testing (Reece, 1997).

Amniocentesis is the removal, collection, and analysis of a sample of amniotic fluid from the amniotic sac. Amniotic fluid is fetal in origin. It contains a variety of chemical substances and electrolytes. Amniotic fluid also contains a mixture of cells shed by the fetus. The cellular and biochemical components of amniotic fluid change with gestational age and fetal maturation. Consequently, amniotic fluid analysis is useful to determine chromosomal disorders early in pregnancy and to evaluate fetal health and maturity later in pregnancy.

Table 12-6 Areas of Genetic and Biochemical Evaluation

TYPE OF CONDITION	EXAMPLE
Alteration in chromosomal number	Trisomy 21 (Down syndrome) Trisomy 18 (Edward's syndrome) Trisomy 3, Petau syndrome Klinefelter's syndrome Monosomy: Turner's or Noonan's syndrome
Hematologic	Sickle cell disease β-Thalassemia
Metabolic	Tay-Sachs disease Gaucher's disease
Molecular structure	Cystic fibrosis Hemophilia Duchenne's muscular dystrophy

Nursing Tip

Indications for Amniocentesis in the First Half of Pregnancy

1. Maternal age over 35 years
2. Previous offspring with abnormal chromosomal pattern
3. Altered chromosomal pattern, including a balanced translocation, aneuploidy, or mosaicism in either parent
4. Trisomy 21 (Down syndrome) or other chromosomal abnormality in close family members
5. Pregnancy after three or more spontaneous abortions
6. Elevated MS-AFP level
7. Personal or family history leading to increased risk for a neural tube defect

Timing and Indications

Amniocentesis can be performed at different times during pregnancy for a variety of indications. Amniocentesis was originally used and continues to be most commonly performed between 15 and 17 weeks' gestation. Amniocentesis performed at this time usually is referred to as a mid-trimester procedure and is relatively safe (Davis 1993). One of the major disadvantages of mid-trimester amniocentesis is the need to wait until 15 weeks' gestational age. Combined with the time necessary to culture and grow cells, test results may not be available until the pregnancy is physically evident to others and the woman has felt fetal movement. Early amniocentesis (< 14 weeks) is technically more difficult because the uterus is still positioned within the pelvis and a smaller volume of amniotic fluid is present.

Before 18 weeks' gestation, analysis of amniotic fluid samples is used to provide information about genetic risks. The list of conditions identifiable through amniotic fluid analysis includes chromosomal disorders, such as translocation, aneuploidy, and trisomy; autosomal recessive disorders; X-linked disorders; metabolic diseases; enzyme defects; hematopoietic diseases; and immunodeficiencies. As the number of genes identified by the Human Genome Project continues to grow, the list of conditions identifiable through amniotic fluid analysis also will continue to grow and may include individual traits and attributes as well as medical conditions or syndromes.

Nursing Alert

Potential Complications of Amniocentesis

- Pain, bruising, infection of the puncture site
- Uterine contractions, usually self-limited but may progress to labor
- Occasional spontaneous abortion
- Premature rupture of membranes
- Placental abruption
- Fetal injury
- Cord or placental blood vessel injury/hemorrhage
- Uterine infection
- Rh isoimmunization
- Fluid lead

Note. From *Pfenninger and Fowler's Procedures for Primary Care* (2nd ed.) by J. L. Pfenninger and Grant C. Fowler (Eds.), 2004, St. Louis, MO: Mosby.

In the second half of pregnancy, amniotic fluid analysis can be used to identify fetal hemolytic disease caused by maternal red blood cell (RBC) antigens, for example, Rh incompatibilities.

Amniotic fluid values also can be used to evaluate fetal well-being through the use of gram-staining techniques to identify infections and measurement of creatinine levels reflective of fetal kidney development and fetal muscle mass.

A common use of amniotic fluid analysis in late pregnancy is to evaluate fetal surfactant production and respiratory system maturity. Evaluation of the lecithin-to-sphingomyelin ratio (L/S ratio) is the most widely used method of fetal lung maturity assessment. Pulmonary maturity is established when the lecithin-to-sphingomyelin ratio is 2:1 or greater. A specific phospholipid, phosphatidylglycerol (PG), found in the amniotic fluid also is an indicator of fetal lung maturity. The presence of PG almost ensures pulmonary maturity. A newer technique for evaluating lung maturity is counts of lamellar bodies. Fetal pulmonary maturity is associated with counts of lamellar bodies of over 30,000 particles/μL (Fakhoury, Daikoku, Benser, & Dubin, 1994).

Client Preparation

Amniocentesis usually is performed as an outpatient procedure. Informed consent procedures include a dialogue outlining the risks, benefits, and limitations of the procedure as needed. When amniocentesis is done in early pregnancy, the bladder may be filled to elevate the uterus and increase visualization of a fluid pocket. In the second half of pregnancy, the bladder is emptied to prevent confusion between it and the uterine sac. Maternal vital signs and fetal heart tones are evaluated before the procedure. During the procedure, the client is placed in a supine position. In late pregnancy, a hip roll may be used to prevent supine hypotensive syndrome. The client needs to know that some women experience a sensation of pressure, cramping, or both during the procedure.

Before and during amniocentesis, the nurse is a support person and client advocate. The need for the procedure and the potential outcome are sources of anxiety and uncertainty for most women. Anticipating the client's anxieties and feelings and responding verbally and nonverbally are critical components of client preparation by the nurse.

Procedure

Amniocentesis is performed after ultrasound examination to identify an adequate pocket of amniotic fluid (Figure 12-14). The maternal abdominal wall is cleansed with an antiseptic solution and prepared and draped as a sterile field. In some situations, a local anesthetic may be used

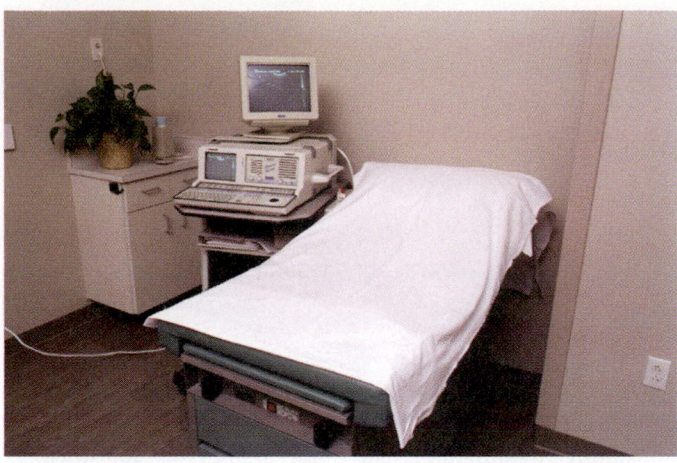

A.

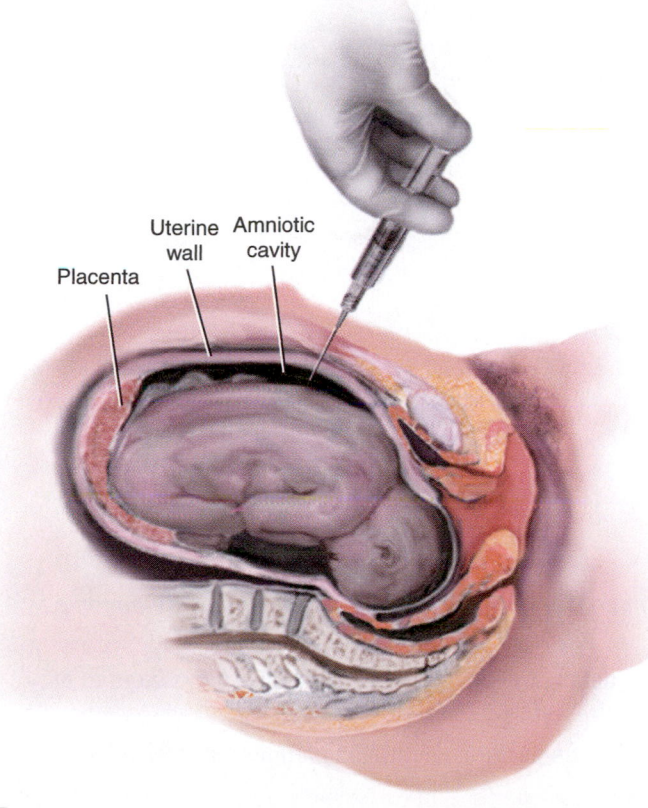

Placenta   Uterine   Amniotic
wall   cavity

B.

Figure 12-14   A. An amniocentesis setup. B. During amniocentesis, a sample of amniotic fluid is aspirated for evaluation.

before amniocentesis is performed. Using an ultrasound probe with a sterile cover, the physician introduces a 20- or 22-gauge spinal needle through the abdominal wall and uterus and into the pocket of amniotic fluid. The amount of fluid withdrawn depends on the stage of gestation and the types of tests to be performed. After with-

drawal the fluid is placed in culture tubes, labeled, and sent to the laboratory for analysis. Culture tubes sometimes require special handling to protect the specimen. For example, specimens for bilirubin analysis must be placed in tubes covered with an opaque material to prevent breakdown of the bilirubin by light rays. After fluid collection the needle is withdrawn, pressure is applied to the site, and the site is dressed.

Follow-up

Maternal vital signs and fetal cardiac activity are documented at the conclusion of the procedure. When amniocentesis is performed before the age of viability, cardiac activity is an indicator of fetal survival. As gestational age of the pregnancy advances, monitoring of fetal tolerance to the procedure is increased and may incorporate other evaluations of fetal well-being, such as a nonstress test.

Many women experience mild cramping for a few hours after the procedure. Women should be instructed to rest until the cramping subsides and then resume normal activity. However, women should refrain from sexual intercourse, heavy lifting, and strenuous physical activity for 24 hours. The abdominal puncture site should be kept clean, and no special skin care is required.

Maternal complications after amniocentesis, including vaginal spotting, fluid leaking, and uterine contractions, are uncommon and usually self-limiting (Tabor et al., 1986; Reece, 1997). Although rare, an amniocentesis can result in excessive bleeding, infection, and fetal loss. Women need to report any vaginal discharge, severe or persistent uterine cramping, and increased temperature to the health care provider.

Women need emotional support and education during the interval between the procedure and availability of the results, especially when the purpose of the testing is for identification of a condition that may threaten the well-being and continuation of the pregnancy. The client needs to be informed of when the results will be available, who will contact her, and how she will learn the outcome. Ongoing support during this period of uncertainty is a critical role for the nurse.

Critical Thinking

"I Feel So Guilty"

How do you respond to a woman who, after having amniocentesis, states, "I feel so guilty. This test makes it seem as if I won't love this baby unless it is perfect"?

PROCEDURE 12-1

Amniocentesis

Removal of amniotic fluid abdominally under local anesthesia with ultrasound visualization to avoid fetal injury.

Purpose

Genetic testing, screening for neural tube defects; testing for fetal hemolytic disease; identification of intra-amniotic infection source; evaluation of fetal kidney development; evaluation of fetal lung maturity.

Equipment

Antiseptic for skin

Local anesthetic (1–2% lidocaine without epinephrine)

Ultrasound with sterile probe

Fetal monitor

Sterile towels for drapes

Sterile gloves

Commercial amniocentesis tray

> 3 plain sterile specimen tubes (10–15 ml)
> 20- or 22-gauge spinal needle
> 22- or 23-gauge x 1.5 needle
> 20 cc syringe
> 5 cc syringe
> Sterile 4 x 4 gauze pads

Actions and Rationales

1. Obtain informed consent. *Signed consent is necessary for legal purposes and should be accompanied by a discussion of risks and benefits.*
2. When the procedure is performed early in pregnancy, the bladder may be filled. *This is done to elevate the uterus out of the pelvis and aid in visualization.*
3. In the second half of pregnancy, the procedure can be performed with the bladder empty. *This is necessary to prevent confusion with the uterine sac.*
4. Maternal vital signs and fetal heart tones are evaluated prior to the procedure. *Monitoring vital signs of fetus and mother ensures attention to adverse effects.*
5. The client is placed in a supine position. A hip roll can be placed under the client's hips in later pregnancy. *This is to prevent positional hypotension.*
6. The nurse is a client advocate during the procedure. *This is done to attend to physical and emotional needs of the client.*

(continues)

PROCEDURE 12-1 *(continued)*

Follow-up

Rest for the remainder of the day.

Avoid heavy lifting, yard work, or gardening for 24 hours.

Abstain from intercourse for 24 hours.

Notify the physician immediately if any of the following occurs:

Abdominal pain or bleeding from the puncture site or vagina
Leaking of fluid from the vagina
Chills or fever
Feelings of weakness or faintness
Lack of fetal movement when stimulated

From Amniocentesis for Antenatal Diagnosis of Genetic Disorders, by M. I. Evans, M. P. Johnson, and A. Drugan, in Current Therapy in Obstetrics and Gynecology *(5th ed., pp. 226–232) by E. J. Quilligan and F. P. Zuspan (Eds.), 2000, Philadelphia: W. B. Saunders.*

Chorionic Villus Sampling

Chorionic villus sampling (CVS) is an alternative to amniocentesis. The primary stimulus for the development of CVS technology was its use in earlier diagnosis, during the first trimester.

Chorionic villus sampling is a prodedure to obtain fetal cells in the first trimester. Chorionic villi cells are living cells fetal in origin, thereby reflecting the genetic content of the fetus. However, unlike amniocentesis, CVS cannot determine the presence of a neural tube defect because the level of α-fetoprotein can only be tested using serum or amniotic fluid.

Timing and Indications

Chorionic villus sampling is usually performed between 10 and 12 weeks' menstrual age of gestation or between 8 and 10 weeks of fetal gestation (American College of Obstetricians and Gynecologists, 1997; Beall, 2000). A small tissue aspiration device is inserted into the developing placenta, allowing the chorion frondosum (which ultimately will form the placenta) to be biopsied.

The greatest benefit of CVS is earlier diagnosis of fetal disorders and a shorter interval between test performance and availability of the results. If the woman chooses to end the pregnancy based on the diagnosis, a first-trimester termination procedure, with a lower risk of complications and lower cost, is an option.

The risks associated with CVS include spontaneous pregnancy loss. While there is possibility of risk, the American College of Obstetricians and Gynecologists (1995) has made the following statement related to the use of CVS in the clinical setting.

Chorionic villus sampling is a relatively safe procedure when performed at 10–12 weeks and is an acceptable alternative to amniocentesis. Chorionic villus sampling is not recommended prior to nine weeks' gestation.

Client Preparation

Chorionic villus sampling usually is performed in an outpatient setting and takes approximately 20 minutes. However, the preparation and recovery time may require approximately 2 hours in the clinical setting. Before the procedure, the client and her family should receive genetic counseling and be informed about its benefits, risks, and limitations. Informed consent must be obtained. The client needs to know what to expect during the procedure. A full bladder is necessary. Some women experience discomfort during the procedure as a result of bladder fullness and pressure from the ultrasound transducer.

Procedure

Two techniques are used for performing CVS: the transcervical catheter aspiration technique and the transabdominal needle aspiration technique (Figure 12-15). The choice of a transvaginal or transabdominal approach usually is based on client preference and provider skill. Both approaches require two practitioners, one performing the sampling and one providing the ultrasound guidance.

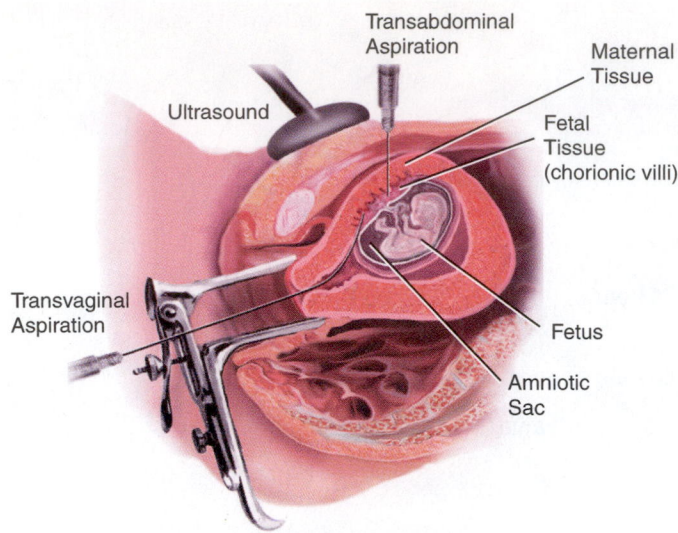

Figure 12-15   During chorionic villus sampling, a small tissue sample is aspirated from the fetal side of the placenta. Needle insertion is made either transabdominally or transvaginally.

If the transcervical technique is selected, the woman is placed in lithotomy position, and a sterile speculum is inserted. Under real-time ultrasound guidance, the physician passes the transcervical catheter through the cervix and into the chorion frondosum and fluid is aspirated. The presence of fetal cardiac activity, appearance of the amniotic sac, and the chorion frondosum are verified.

Ultrasound verification of fetal viability, gestational age, and location of the chorion frondosum is the first step in transabdominal CVS. The maternal abdomen is then draped and prepared with an antiseptic solution similar to the amniocentesis procedure. Under ultrasound guidance, an 18- or 20-gauge needle is inserted through the abdominal and uterine wall and guided into the chorion frondosum and fluid is aspirated. The specimen from either procedure is placed in a sterile medium for transport and cytogenic analysis.

Follow-up

After the procedure the woman's vital signs are evaluated and assessment of uterine status is completed. Uterine cramping should not occur. Vaginal spotting may occur after the transcervical approach, and usually resolves within 3 days. Heavy bleeding or passage of clots, tissue, or amniotic fluid is abnormal and should be reported to the health care provider. After the CVS procedure, the client is advised to avoid sexual activity and strenuous physical activity until all vaginal spotting has resolved. The client also needs to be informed to contact the physician if cramping, vaginal bleeding, or flulike symptoms are experienced within the week. Women usually have follow-up ultrasonography a week after the procedure

and at 16 weeks' gestation to reconfirm integrity of the products of conception.

Percutaneous Umbilical Blood Sampling

Percutaneous umbilical blood sampling (**PUBS**), also known as cordocentesis, is an evaluation technique that provides direct access to the fetal circulation and involves direct aspiration of fetal blood. The most common site for needle placement is the umbilical cord, within 2 cm of the placental insertion site. Alternative sites include the fetal intrahepatic vein and the cardiac ventricle.

Timing and Indications

Percutaneous umbilical blood sampling can be performed any time after 17 weeks' gestation and is useful in diagnosing a variety of conditions, including chromosomal alterations; intrauterine infections; coagulopathy; hemoglobinopathies and RBC disorders; immunodeficiency states; and platelet disorders, including RBC counts for identifying isoimmune disease and fetal thrombocystis levels. In cases of suspected intrauterine growth retardation, PUBS can be used to evaluate fetal hypoxia and determine fetal acid-base status. PUBS also can be used for intrauterine transfusion and fetal drug therapy.

Client Preparation

Percutaneous umbilical blood sampling can be performed in either an outpatient or inpatient setting. The actual sampling procedure takes approximately 10 minutes for specimen collection. Women must give informed consent because of the invasive nature of the procedure. The client needs to understand the reason, risks, benefits, and nature of the follow-up of the PUBS procedure. Depending on uterine size, a full bladder may be necessary. The client can be informed that physical discomfort during the procedure is minimal and similar to the pressure and cramping sensations experienced during other intrauterine procedures such as amniocentesis. Physical care of the woman includes documenting baseline vital signs and fetal cardiac activity. When PUBs is performed after the fetus is viable, preparation for a cesarean birth in the event of fetal distress must be discussed and considered by the client before the procedure is implemented. Preparation also involves ensuring that emergency equipment and personnel are available.

Procedure

Percutaneous umbilical blood sampling is performed under ultrasound guidance to identify the target sampling site. Antiseptic preparation of the maternal abdomen is completed and a local anesthetic may be used. A 20- or 22-gauge spinal needle is inserted through the abdominal and uterine walls and is directed into the umbil-

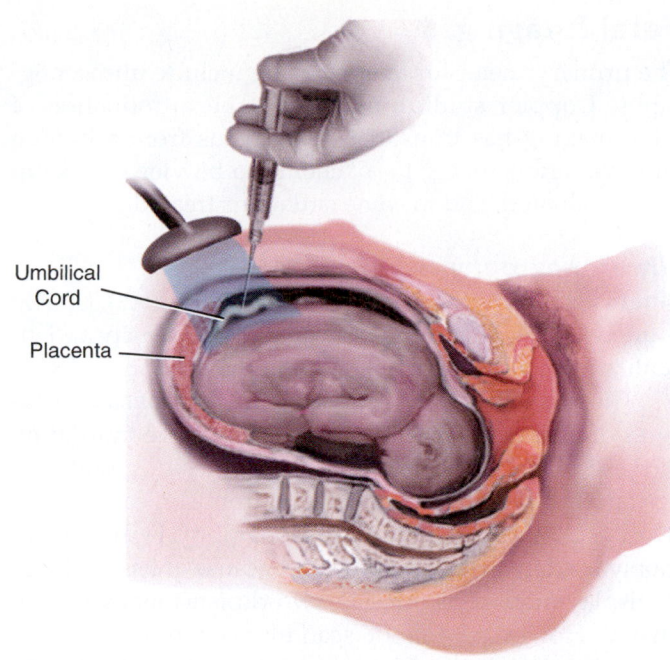

Figure 12-16   The percutaneous umbilical blood sampling technique is performed using ultrasound guidance and transabdominal aspiration of a sample from the fetal umbilical vessel.

Umbilical Cord

Placenta

ical vessel, most commonly the umbilical vein (Figure 12-16). A site approximately 1 to 2 cm from the insertion of the cord into the placenta is desirable. This site minimizes the risk of cord injury and the chance of obtaining maternal blood from the placenta. If fetal movement interferes with the procedure, a sedative can be administered intravenously to the mother, or intravenously or intramuscularly to the fetus.

Percutaneous umbilical blood sampling, or cordocentesis, also provides an access site for administration of medications or blood transfusion to the fetus. After the blood specimen is obtained or the infusion completed, the needle is removed, the site is inspected for bleeding, and fetal cardiac activity is confirmed by ultrasonography.

Follow-up
Postprocedure care includes monitoring maternal vital signs, fetal heart rate, and uterine activity. The fetal heart rate is evaluated for signs of reactivity and the absence of distress. Because of the increased risk of infection, some providers prescribe prophylactic antibiotics. The client also should be instructed to monitor her temperature twice a day to detect temperature elevation.

Other Genetic and Biochemical Evaluations
Fetal tissue sampling and fetal fibronectin are two of the lesser used modalities for evaluation of the status of a pregnancy.

Fetal tissue sampling involves a direct biopsy of fetal tissue using biopsy forceps. Fetal tissue sampling is a highly invasive procedure and is not widely used in the clinical setting.

Fetal fibronectin (fFN) testing is a screening procedure for the prediction of preterm labor. The test for fFN involves obtaining a swab of vaginal and cervical secretions. It is believed that fetal fibronectin leaks into the cervix when the interaction between the fetal membranes and the uterine wall weakens. Consequently, a positive finding may predict the onset of labor. The more useful finding may be a negative result, which is correlated with a low incidence of labor onset in the next 7 to 14 days (Weismiller, 1999).

Maternal Serum Studies
The interaction of the maternal-placental-fetal unit forms the basis for maternal serum studies. Maternal serum testing technologies examine by-products of the gestational state found in the maternal system but do not invade the integrity of the uterine-placental-fetal unit. This method is recognized as a valuable tool in screening women for high-risk pregnancies. Maternal serum studies measure maternal hormone levels, MS-AFP levels, and fetal cell isolation, with MS-AFP measurement being the most widely used prenatal screening modality today. In contrast, many of the invasive fetal studies described previously are diagnostic of specific conditions. Screening procedures simply identify pregnancies at risk for complications or alterations, whereas diagnostic procedures confirm the presence or absence of specific conditions. Therefore, maternal serum screening techniques, if the results are altered, lead to more invasive diagnostic techniques.

Maternal Hormone Levels
Human chorionic gonadotropin, estrogen and estriol, and human placental lactogen are hormones associated with the state of pregnancy. Levels of these hormones can be measured in a sample of maternal venous blood. Maternal serum hormones are used in the diagnosis of pregnancy, differential diagnosis of intrauterine and ectopic pregnancies, and prediction of poor perinatal outcomes.

Human Chorionic Gonadotropin
Human chorionic gonadotropin (hCG) is detectable in maternal serum 8 days after conception. hCG is exclusively produced during pregnancy and, therefore, is the basis for many pregnancy tests. Maternal plasma levels of hCG increase rapidly and then rapidly decline. Values that deviate from the expected pattern suggest an abnormally developing pregnancy.

Estrogen and Estriol

Maternal estrogen levels increase progressively over the course of pregnancy. The increased estrogen level is due primarily to estriol.

Human Placental Lactogen

Human placental lactogen (hPL) levels also increase progressively over the course of pregnancy. The level of hPL peaks at 35 weeks' gestation. hPL promotes fetal and placental growth. The level of hPL in the maternal circulation is directly related to fetal and placental weight. Therefore, alteration in maternal serum levels of hPL may indicate altered placental function, providing a basis for screening for complications.

Maternal Serum–α-Fetoprotein Screening

Maternal serum–α-fetoprotein (MS-AFP) testing is the basis for screening for neural tube defects (elevated levels) and trisomy 21 (decreased levels) during the second trimester of pregnancy. Normal ranges have been identified for each week of pregnancy. The optimal time for testing is 16 to 18 weeks' gestation (Cunningham et al., 2001). The American College of Obstetricians and Gynecologists (1996) recommends that all pregnant women be offered MS-AFP screening. When abnormal levels persist, the client is referred for both ultrasonography to examine for structural anomalies and amniocentesis to further quantify AFP levels and obtain chromosomal analysis.

Several nonpathological variables can affect the level of AFP. Before obtaining a specimen for MS-AFP analysis, informed consent needs to be obtained. Clients need to understand the nature of this procedure (a screening test, not a diagnostic test), the potential outcomes of the test, and the procedures that will be followed if the results are altered. Because of the wide variation of "normal levels" among healthy women, fetuses, and pregnancies, the possibility of a false-positive result should be discussed.

Physical and Psychological Surveillance

Visualization of the physical size, structure, and movement of the fetus is possible with the use of ultrasonography, Doppler flow studies, and magnetic resonance imaging (MRI). Physiologic integrity of the placenta and of fetal compensatory mechanisms can be measured with electronic fetal monitoring and biophysical profile evaluation. Through the use of these technologies, practitioners can gather information about the physical status and structural anatomy and about the physiologic status and functional behavior of the fetus, respectively. Some of these tests are used for reassurance of fetal well-being.

Fetal Imaging

The primary means of fetal imaging include ultrasonography, Doppler studies, and MRI. The introduction of fetal imaging has transformed the fetus from a hidden and mysterious being to a "client" to be viewed, examined, evaluated, and in some situations treated.

Ultrasonography

Ultrasonography is the use of high-frequency (>20,000 Hz) sound waves to detect differences in tissue density and visualize outlines of structures within the body.

Therefore, ultrasonography provides physical measures of tissue density, size, and location. The translation of these physical measures into estimates of gestational age or fetal weight is based on data from clinical research (Docker, 1992). Real-time ultrasonography is most commonly used in obstetrical practice because of its capability to display motion-picture-like two-dimensional sectional images. However, M-mode scan ultrasonography, or static images, is valuable in gaining information about individual structures, such as the dynamic changes occurring in the fetal heart.

Timing and Indications. According to the American College of Obstetricians and Gynecologists (1993) the ultrasound examination may take one of three forms: basic, or level I, examination; comprehensive, or level II, examination; and limited, or targeted, examination.

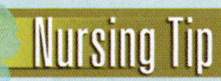

Nursing Tip

Indications for Ultrasound Diagnosis in the Second Trimester

1. Estimation of gestational age for women with uncertain clinical dates
2. Evaluation of fetal growth
3. Estimation of fetal weight
4. Vaginal bleeding of unknown cause
5. Suspected multiple gestation
6. Adjunct to amniocentesis or PUBS
7. Adjunct to cervical cerclage placement
8. Significant uterine size or clinical dates discrepancies
9. Suspected uterine abnormality
10. Suspected alteration in amniotic fluid volume
11. Premature labor
12. Abnormal AFP level
13. Serial evaluation of fetal growth in multiple gestation

Level I, or basic, ultrasonography is used to:

- Detect the gestational sac as early as 5 weeks after the last menstrual period.
- Identify the number of fetuses.
- Document fetal life.
- Detect gross fetal structural anomalies.
- Estimate gestational age.
- Determine fetal position.
- Locate the placenta.
- Estimate amniotic fluid volume.
- Evaluate maternal pelvic masses.

The basic examination takes approximately 20 minutes and is a component of the obstetrical standard of care. The basic examination is the most common use of ultrasonography in obstetrical practice (Tucker, 2004).

A level II, or comprehensive, ultrasound examination is done when the provider suspects a client is carrying an anatomically or physiologically abnormal fetus. Indications for level-II ultrasonography include abnormal findings on clinical examination, history of an abnormal fetus, and validation of information obtained in the level-I examination. The focus of a comprehensive examination is to survey fetal anatomy for specific malformations. A level II, or comprehensive, ultrasound examination is used to:

- Evaluate gestational age.
- Measure fetal growth.
- Perform specific examinations of the brain, heart, kidney, and cord insertion.
- Quantify amniotic fluid volume.
- Determine placental location.

A level II examination usually is performed after 18 weeks' gestation and is done by a perinatologist.

The third type of examination, limited or targeted, is performed when specific information is needed but a complete survey of the fetus and intrauterine environment is not needed. Limited examination usually is performed in conjunction with another procedure or event. Limited ultrasound examinations are performed during amniocentesis, PUBS, or a biophysical profile to confirm fetal cardiac activity as a result of decreased fetal movement, and identify fetal presentation or locate the placenta after the onset of spontaneous bleeding or labor.

Client Preparation. As with any procedure the client needs to be informed about its purpose, content, and limitations. Before transabdominal examination, the client will need to fill her bladder. To establish adequate bladder filling the client should drink 1 to 2 quarts of water 1 hour before the procedure. Maintaining a full bladder can be a source of discomfort for many clients, especially in late pregnancy. When a transvaginal examination is planned, the client will be asked to empty her bladder before the procedure to minimize obscuring the view into the pelvic cavity.

Procedure. Obstetrical ultrasonography can be performed using either a transabdominal or transvaginal scanning approach (Figure 12-17). Transabdominal scanning is the more

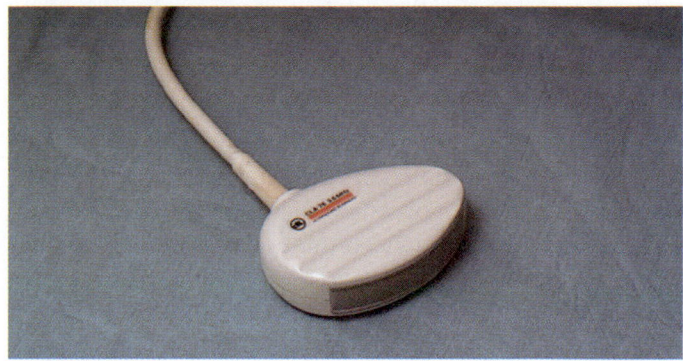

A.

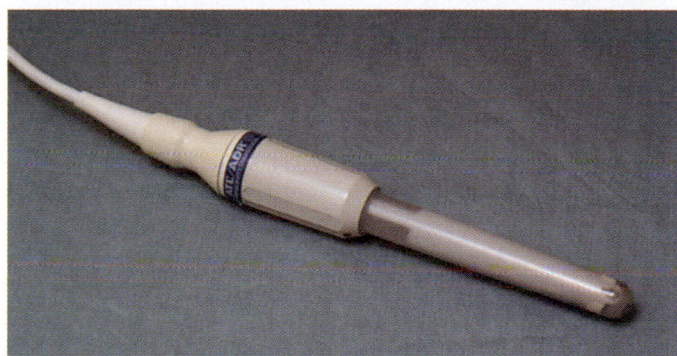

B.

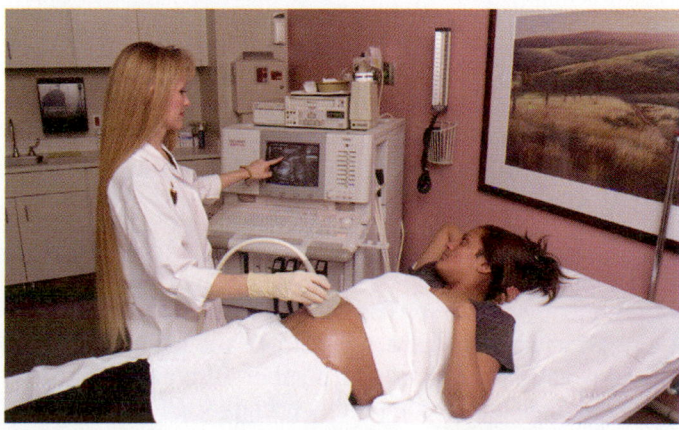

C.

Figure 12-17 A. Transabdominal scanner. B. Transvaginal scanner. C. The nurse and client look at the features of the fetus, as shown on the monitor during transabdominal ultrasonography.

traditional approach and can be used throughout gestation but is most useful in the second and third trimesters. Transabdominal ultrasonography provides a clear view of the fetus and placenta. During transabdominal ultrasonography, a lubricating gel is applied to the abdomen and the probe is moved over the abdominal surface. The lubrication reduces friction and enhances transmission and reception of the sound waves by the probe.

Transvaginal ultrasonography is most useful in the first trimester of pregnancy. During this procedure, a handheld probe is inserted into the vagina, allowing detailed examination of the pelvic anatomy and earlier diagnosis of intrauterine pregnancy (Cunningham et al., 2001).

The findings of an obstetrical ultrasound examination can provide valuable data to influence the management plan during the course of gestation. In addition to data about the physical status of the fetus (e.g., number of fetuses, presentation, and anatomical survey), data obtainable from an ultrasound examination include fetal cardiac activity, gestational dating and fetal growth, placental position and function, and amniotic fluid volume.

Ultrasonography can be used to obtain gestational dating of a pregnancy. During the first 20 weeks' gestation, normal fetuses grow at approximately the same rate.

In the second half of pregnancy, accurate determination of fetal age is enhanced by serial measurements. When three composite measures are obtained at least 2 weeks apart, between 24 and 32 weeks' gestation, a highly accurate estimate of actual age is achievable (Manning, 1999). Determining the exact relationship of the placenta to the internal cervical os is possible after 27 weeks' gestation in the diagnosis of placenta previa.

Placental grading and classification of placental maturity are accomplished by ultrasound scanning. A relationship has been established between placental grade and fetal pulmonary maturity (Manning, 1999).

Critical Thinking

Is Ultrasonography a Routine Procedure?

A study by Berkowitz (1993) concluded that routine ultrasound screening for low-risk women did not improve pregnancy outcome. The author suggested that savings for prenatal care could total about $1 billion if there was a decrease in the number of screening ultrasound examinations in routine pregnancy.

- Do you agree with this position?
- In your opinion, what are the risks of discontinuing routine ultrasounds?

Amniotic fluid volume (AFV) can be objectively quantified using ultrasound technology. Values of 5 to 19 cm are considered normal, whereas values under 5 cm indicate oligohydramnios and over 20 cm indicate hydramnios (Gabbe, Gabbe, & Simpson, 2002).

Follow-up. Ultrasonography is a noninvasive procedure. Follow-up care is primarily education, counseling, and support as referral for additional testing or treatment based on ultrasound findings is implemented.

Doppler Studies

Doppler blood studies is the measurement of blood flow velocity and direction in major fetal and uterine structures. Doppler ultrasonography is used to measure blood flow velocity.

Timing and Indications. Velocity waveforms can be detected as early as 15 weeks' gestation. Decreased umbilical vessel flow is found in fetuses with intrauterine growth retardation (IUGR) and in pregnancies complicated by pregnancy-induced hypertension (PIH) or postdates, when a pregnancy exceeds its EDC, usually 42 weeks. In addition, exposure to nicotine from maternal smoking has been shown to decrease blood flow velocity (Schulman, 1990).

Client Preparation. From the client's perspective, physical preparation is similar to the preparation for imaging ultrasonography. Additional counseling and education are needed specific to the indications.

Procedure. The technique of transabdominal ultrasound is used to obtain blood flow velocity measurements. Color-enhanced flow imaging is an extension of Doppler velocimetry. With color-flow instrumentation, multiple samples of blood flow velocity are obtained.

Follow-up. Follow-up care includes providing information and support to the client and her family, explaining the management plan, and making referrals as needed.

Magnetic Resonance Imaging

Magnetic resonance imaging (MRI) is a noninvasive diagnostic tool that provides high-resolution cross-sectional images of fluid-filled soft tissues. Unlike sonography, there is no interference from skeletal, fatty, or gas-filled structures and a full bladder is not necessary for imaging structures deep in the pelvis.

Timing and Indications. In pregnancy, MRI has been used as early as 10 weeks' gestation to demonstrate placental location and biparietal diameter, and the results are comparable with ultrasound imaging. However, MRI is specifically suited for the detection of soft-tissue abnormalities not easily identifiable on ultrasonography, such as hydatiform mole and fetal anomalies (e.g., cystic hygroma, urethral obstruction, and hydronephrosis) (Fischbach, 2004).

Client Preparation. During the procedure, which can take 20 to 60 minutes, the client must lie completely still.

Procedure. The client is placed in a supine position on a table that is then moved into the bore of the main magnet. Because it takes a significant amount of time to produce magnetic resonance images, the probability of fetal movement during image generation is high. Movement leads to image distortion. MRI is advantageous in situations that are not conducive to ultrasound examination, such as maternal obesity and oligohydramnios. The overall cost and length of time required to complete imaging has reserved the use of MRI in pregnant women to situations in which the results of other imaging modalities are unacceptable.

Fetal Heart Rate Monitoring

Fetal heart rate monitoring is integral to fetal surveillance. Auscultation of the fetal heart rate has been a standard component of each prenatal visit (Figure 12-18). The goal of fetal evaluation with electronic fetal monitoring in late pregnancy is to determine whether the intrauterine environment continues to be supportive of the fetus.

Fetal heart rate variability or rhythmic change in baseline heart rate values is a reassuring indicator of a supportive intrauterine environment. Variability is designated as a nonperiodic fetal heart rate change because it is not related to changes in fetal or uterine activity. Periodic fetal heart rate changes are defined as alterations in the fetal heart rate pattern in response to fetal movement or uterine contraction. The major designations of periodic changes are accelerations and decelerations. An acceleration is a responsive or stimulated increase of fetal heart rate by a minimum of 15 bpm with a duration of at least 15 seconds. A deceleration is a decrease in fetal heart rate in response to fetal or uterine activity. Decelerations in response to uterine contractions are further differentiated by their relationship to the onset, peak, and resolution of the contraction. Analysis and classification of the fetal heart rate pattern are the foundation of antenatal fetal heart monitoring evaluation. The methods of electronic fetal monitoring used for fetal evaluation include nonstress tests with or without the addition of fetal acoustic stimulation (FAS) and contraction stress tests (CST).

Nonstress Test

A **nonstress test (NST)** is the evaluation of fetal heart rate in response to an increase in either spontaneous or stimulated fetal activity. It is a noninvasive method that combines detection of fetal heart rate accelerations and presence of spontaneous or evoked fetal movement. An NST is a relatively inexpensive procedure and has no known contraindications. NSTs are performed by nurses in a variety of settings including outpatient, inpatient, and home environments.

Timing and indications. Nonstress testing can be reliably performed after 28 weeks' gestation. In the healthy fetus with a functional central nervous system (CNS), 90% of fetal body movements are associated with accelerations in fetal heart rate (Tucker, 2004).

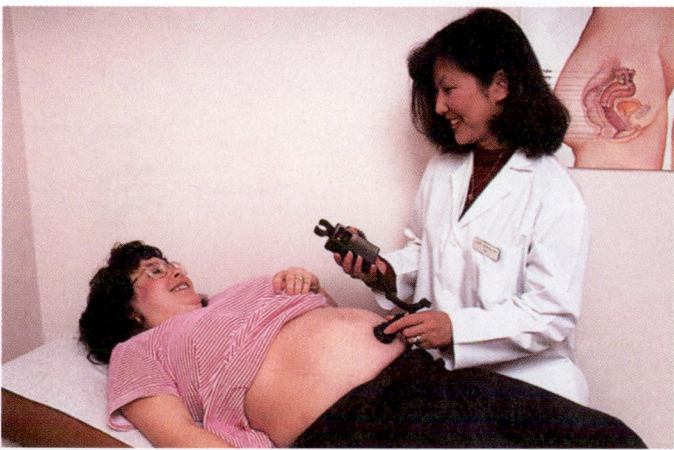

Figure 12-18   Fetal heart rate monitoring is a routine factor in each prenatal visit.

> ## Nursing Tip   *Indications for the NST*
>
> 1. Suspected postmaturity
> 2. Maternal diabetes mellitus
> 3. Maternal hypertension: chronic and pregnancy-related disorders
> 4. Suspected or documented intrauterine growth restriction (IUGR)
> 5. Sickle cell disease
> 6. History of previous stillbirth
> 7. Isoimmunization
> 8. Older gravida
> 9. Chronic renal disease
> 10. Decreasing fetal movement
> 11. Severe maternal anemia
> 12. Multiple gestation
> 13. High-risk antepartal conditions: premature rupture of fetal membranes, preterm labor, bleeding

Client Preparation. The client's blood pressure is taken and documented. The woman is placed in a reclining position or a semi-Fowler position with a lateral tilt to avoid supine hypotension. An external mode of fetal monitoring is placed on the abdomen. The woman may be instructed to depress an event button to mark episodes of fetal movement on the monitoring strip (Figure 12-19).

Procedure. The fetal heart rate is detected and recorded. Fetal movement is documented either by the event button or use of the tocotransducer to document fetal movements as intermittent changes in uterine pressure. The test usually is completed in 20 minutes but may take longer if the fetus is in a sleep state.

The criteria for a reactive NST are two accelerations in a 20-minute test period and a normal baseline fetal heart rate. A nonreactive result is the absence of accelerations during the test period (Figure 12-20). The 40-minute time frame for observation accounts for fetal sleep-wake cycles. A third result is an inconclusive, or equivocal, test result. An inconclusive test result is the finding of less than two accelerations in the 20-minute test window, accelerations that do not meet the criteria of an amplitude increase of 15 bpm for a duration of 15 seconds, or a poor-quality recording that is inadequate for interpretation.

When the NST is reactive, it is highly predictive of fetal health and well-being. However, the use of the NST in identifying the fetus at risk for a poor perinatal outcome is less reliable. NSTs have a significantly high false-positive rate of over 75%; in other words, more than 75% of fetuses with nonreactive NSTs are in fact healthy (Gauthier, 1979; Smith, 1995).

In an attempt to reduce the incidence of false-positive results on NSTs and to differentiate a healthy fetus at rest from one who is sick or asphyxiated, vibroacoustic stimu-

Reflections from a Nurse

I recently worked with a woman who was 33 weeks pregnant and eager to see the end of a rough pregnancy marked by daily nausea, a great deal of back pain, and swollen feet. After a nonreactive NST, the woman emphatically stated, "I want to have a cesarean birth right now, so the nursery can take care of my baby!" Being a mother of three myself, I empathized with her plight, but took it upon myself to gently remind her of the benefits of seeing a pregnancy through to at least 38 weeks. I also made some suggestions for exercise and diet changes, which I thought could help relieve some of her discomforts.

lation has been used. To provoke fetal activity, the stimulation is applied to the maternal abdomen for 1 second. The stimulus startles the fetus, causing a behavioral state change, and generates a state of reactivity. If the fetus does not respond, the stimuli can be repeated twice. After stim-

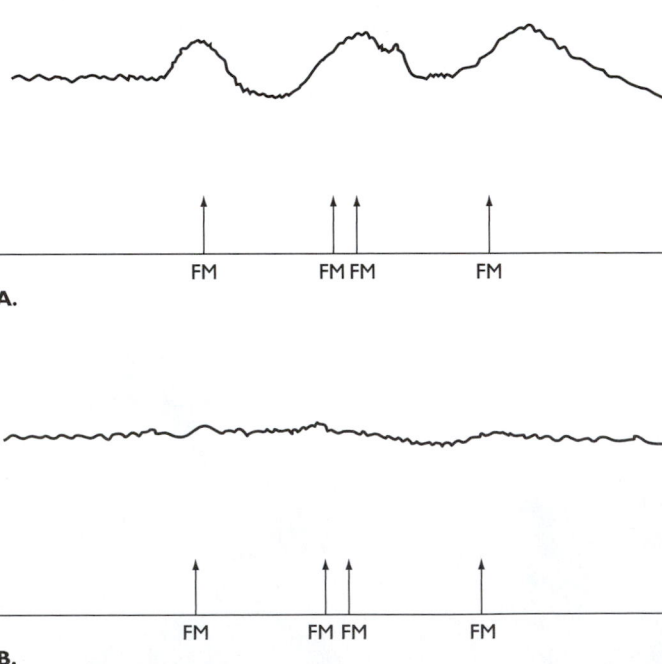

A.

B.

Figure 12-20 A. A reactive nonstress test pattern shows fetal heart acceleration with movement. B. The nonreactive pattern shows absence of accelerations during the test period.

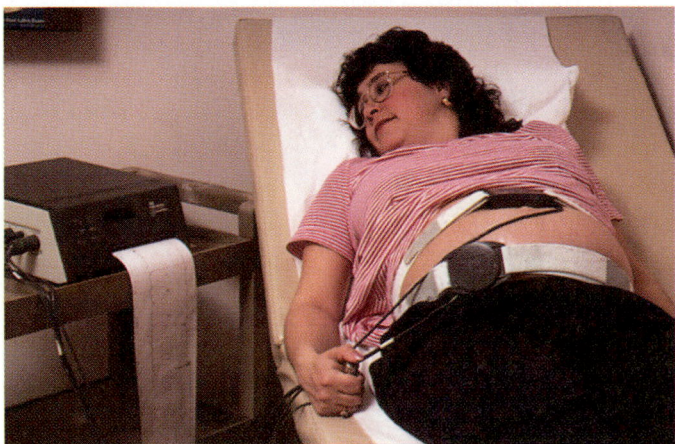

Figure 12-19 A client undergoing a nonstress test is asked to depress a button when fetal movements are felt.

ulation, the fetus is observed until a reactive pattern is attained or until 40 minutes have elapsed. Fetuses exposed to vibroacoustic stimulation exhibit more movements and, therefore, are more likely to have a reactive test pattern (Marden, McDuffie, Allen, & Abitz, 1997).

Follow-up. When the NST is reactive, most practitioners will repeat the examination twice weekly. The pregnancy is continued if the results remain reassuring. When the results are inconclusive or equivocal, either the NST is repeated within 12 to 24 hours or further testing is scheduled, based on the evaluation of the clinical situation. A nonreactive test result is followed by a decision to perform a contraction stress test or a biophysical profile to further evaluate fetal well-being.

Contraction Stress Test

A **contraction stress test (CST)** is performed to evaluate the response of the fetus to the stress of contractions. A CST stimulates uterine contractions for the purpose of assessing fetal response. It evaluates the presence or absence of fetal heart rate decelerations in the presence of uterine contractions (Figure 12-21). The presence of a late deceleration pattern of the fetal heart rate during a uterine contraction is indicative of uteroplacental insufficiency and

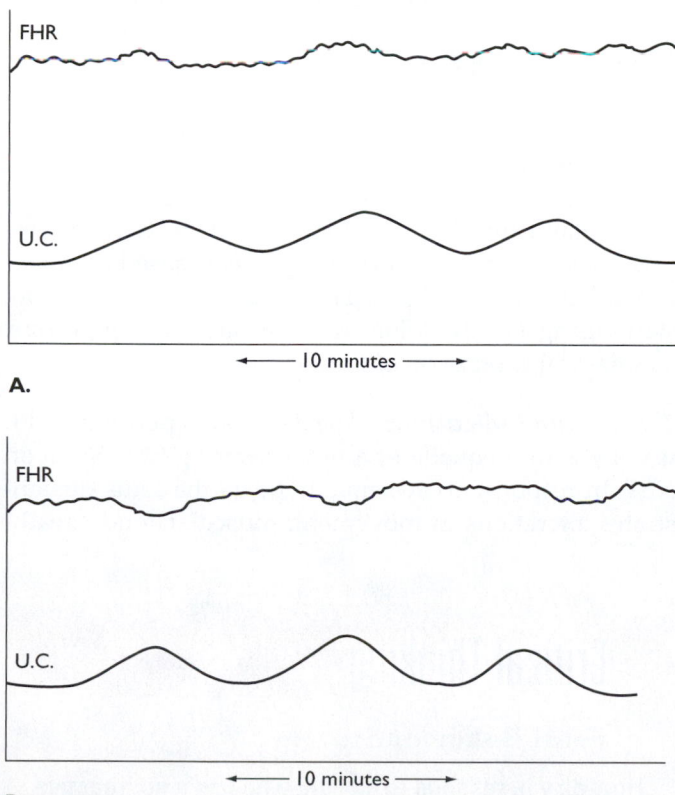

A.

B.

Figure 12-21   A. Negative contraction stress test. B. Positive contraction stress test.

altered fetal cardiorespiratory reserves. In a healthy fetus, cardiorespiratory reserves are adequate to tolerate the decreased or interrupted intravillous blood flow associated with uterine contraction whereas inadequate fetal cardiorespiratory reserves lead to decreased tolerance of altered uteroplacental blood flow that is manifested as late decelerations.

Timing and Indications.   A CST usually is performed after a nonreactive finding on an NST. Although an NST is noninvasive, with no known contraindications, the CST is not. The potential for preterm labor after a CST has led to it being contraindicated in clients with a predisposition to preterm labor or a gestation age at which the risk for preterm birth is greater that is the benefit of the information provided.

Client Preparation.   Because the CST is an invasive procedure, informed consent must be documented. A CST is a potentially dangerous procedure that can stimulate labor or tetanic contractions. It must be performed in a hospital in the event that an emergency C-section becomes necessary.

Procedure.   A CST is an invasive procedure because it stimulates uterine contractions. To perform a CST, the client is placed in a semi-Fowler position and baseline maternal vital signs and fetal heart rate tracings are obtained. Uterine contractions can be induced by either nipple stimulation or administration of exogenous oxytocin. The results of a CST are documented as follows:

- Negative: no late decelerations with three adequate uterine contractions in a 10-minute window, normal baseline fetal heart rate, and accelerations with fetal movement
- Positive: Late decelerations with more than half the uterine contractions
- Suspicious: Late decelerations with fewer than half the uterine contractions
- Unsatisfactory: Inadequate fetal heart rate recording or less than three uterine contractions in 10 minutes

A CST is a lengthy procedure, averaging 90 minutes. It also is an invasive surveillance measure that carries the risks of labor and premature delivery of the pregnancy as a result of stimulation of the uterus. Consequently, these risks must be considered in the decision to undertake a CST. Similar to the NST, the CST also has a high false-positive rate of 50% to 75% (Gauthier, 1979; Paul & Miller, 1995). Therefore, external fetal monitoring as a surveillance technique identifies the healthy well-oxygenated fetus but is of limited use in identifying the at-risk or compromised fetus.

Follow-up. If the CST is negative, the oxytocin source is discontinued. Intravenous fluids are continued until uterine activity has returned to preprocedure status. A negative CST is reassuring that the fetus is likely to survive labor should it occur within 1 week if there are no other changes in either maternal or fetal condition. Immediate retesting is needed if any change in maternal condition occurs. If the CST is positive, continued monitoring and assessment of fetal well-being are needed. A positive result may lead to a decision to end the pregnancy and care for the newborn in the nursery.

Fetal Behavior Studies

Documenting the woman's perception of fetal movement is the traditional method for evaluating fetal behavior. Whereas maternal perception of fetal activity provides valuable data, the addition of ultrasound technology has provided direct measurements of fetal behavior.

Fetal Movement Count

Fetal movement counting (FMC) is the daily maternal assessment of fetal activity by counting the number of movements within a specified time period.

Timing and Indications. The American College of Obstetricians and Gynecologists (ACOG, 1999) recommends daily fetal movement counting beginning at 28 weeks' gestation for pregnant women at increased risk for antepartal fetal death.

Maternal perception of fetal movement usually is related to motion of the trunk or limbs and total body movements, such as flips. During the second half of pregnancy, fetal movement becomes more organized and movements become stronger. The frequency of fetal movement peaks at 32 weeks' gestation and gradually decreases as the pregnancy approaches 40 weeks' gestation (Rayburn, 1995). A number of other factors can influence fetal movement: time of day, glucose loading, and maternal smoking, alcohol, or medication consumption.

Client Preparation. Fetal movement counting after 28 weeks is a no-cost noninvasive method used to heighten the pregnant woman's awareness of fetal activity and behavior.

Procedure. A variety of counting methods exist. Two of the most widely used are the following:

- Record a start time. Place the hands over the abdomen to palpate fetal movement. Count until 10 movements are palpated, and record the time.
- Select a predetermined time interval. Place the hands on the abdomen to palpate fetal activity. Count the number of movements within the selected time period.

To perform fetal movement counts, the woman should be in a relaxing environment and a comfortable position, that is, semi-Fowler, reclining, or side-lying. A side-lying position promotes placental circulation and increases detection of fetal movements. Fetal movement counting should be done at the same time each day, preferably after a meal or when the fetus is most active.

Follow-up. Neither an ideal number of fetal movements nor an ideal interval for fetal movement counting has been established. A trend toward decreasing motion should be reported. In general, a count of less than three fetal movements within 1 hour necessitates further evaluation, usually with an NST or biophysical profile.

Biophysical Profile

The **biophysical profile (BPP)** is a noninvasive dynamic assessment of the fetus and fetal environment. The BPP consists of five parameters: fetal heart rate reactivity, fetal breathing movements, gross body movement, fetal tone, and amniotic fluid volume (Manning, 1995). Each area receives a score of 0 (absent) or 2 (present) based on established criteria (Table 12-7). Therefore, BPP evaluates fetal status using a methodology modeled after the *Apgar score*, a numerical expression of the condition of a newborn.

Timing and Indications. The decision to perform a BPP usually is the sequella of a nonreassuring finding on an NST. In response to systemic hypoxia the fetus demonstrates alterations in movement, muscular tone, breath-

Critical Thinking

Development of Mothering

What is the impact of multiple fetal evaluation procedures on the developmental experience of pregnancy and mothering?

Critical Thinking

Fetal Behavior Studies

How do you respond to a client who has a nonreactive NST and BPP score of 4, but is refusing a cesarean birth because she is afraid of having surgery?

Table 12-7   Biophysical Profile Variables and Scoring Criteria

VARIABLE	NORMAL (SCORE = 2)	ABNORMAL (SCORE = 0)
Fetal breathing movements	One or more episodes of 30 seconds' duration during the 30-minute test period	Absent or breathing movement is <30 seconds' duration
Gross body movement	A minimum of three discrete body or limb movements during the 30-minute test period (active continuous movement is considered one movement)	Less than three fetal movements during the test period
Fetal tone	One or more episodes of active extension with return to flexion of fetal limbs or trunk, or opening and closing of the hand	Slow extension with return to flexion, movement of limb in full extension, or absence of fetal movement
Amniotic fluid volume index	One or more pockets of amniotic fluid measuring ≥1 cm in two perpendicular planes	Pockets of amniotic fluid are <1 cm or absent
Nonstress test	Reactive	Nonreactive

Note. Adapted from "Dynamic Ultrasound-Based Fetal Assessment: The Fetal Biophysical Profile Score," by F. A. Manning, 1995, *Clinical Obstetrics and Gynecology, 38,* pp. 26–44.

ing, and heart rate pattern. Therefore, normal biophysical activities are a proxy measure of a functional CNS (Manning, 1995).

Client Preparation.   The BPP is indicated as a result of a nonreassuring finding from a previous fetal surveillance technique. Therefore, a primary area of client preparation is emotional support, education, and counseling in the face of a potential pregnancy crisis.

Procedure.   Level II, or comprehensive, ultrasonography is used to examine the variables of fetal breathing movements, gross body movements, fetal tone, and amniotic fluid volume. An NST is completed before the ultrasound examination.

A BPP score of 8 to 10 is normal, a score of 6 is equivocal, and a score of 4 or less indicates fetal compromise. The biophysical activities of the fetus provide a reflection of CNS activity because the CNS is among the tissues most sensitive to altered oxygen supply. Based on the gradual hypoxia principle, therefore, progressive fetal hypoxia is manifested as loss of biophysical function. The multiple-variable input of the BPP scoring system improves the specificity and sensitivity of the technique compared with the use of a single surveillance variable. BPP has a low false-negative rate of less than 1 infant per 1,000 (0.726 per 1,000) pregnancies with adequate BPP scores. Therefore, the incidence of fetal compromise is not underestimated with BPP testing. Thus, the BPP is an accurate indicator of impending fetal crisis and should be acted on (Manning, 1995).

Follow-up.   When the BPP score is low, induced labor is considered. When the BPP score is normal, intervention is indicated only for specific obstetrical or maternal factors.

NURSING PROCESS

In the area of fetal evaluation interdisciplinary collaboration and coordination of the client's care is a significant component of nursing care. Some of the fetal evaluation technologies discussed in this chapter are not within the scope of nursing practice; however, the nurse's role in the care of the client surrounding the procedure is essential and needs to be a component of the nursing management plan for the woman's pregnancy.

Assessment

A comprehensive nursing assessment is completed during the initial prenatal contact. The nursing assessment needs to include physical and physiologic factors as well as cultural and emotional ones that influence the woman's need for and perception of fetal evaluation technologies.

Once the need for a fetal evaluation procedure has been identified, the nurse often is the primary liaison between the pregnant client, testing facility, and associated specialist and staff.

A significant component of the nursing assessment is to evaluate the client's psychosocial status to identify the levels of stress and anxiety being experienced. Stress and anxiety also can impact the client's level of understanding and decision making. When faced with the crisis of a

Client Education

Fetal Evaluation

To encourage critical thinking by the client, the nurse may ask the following questions:

- What do you know about the status of your pregnancy and fetus?

- How did you learn this information?

- How do you explain this concern to yourself?

- What do you think will help you to deal with your concern?

- How does this situation affect your daily life?

- If you could have one question answered, what would it be?

- How much control do you think you have over this situation?

problem pregnancy, clients may be unable to absorb information about the procedure, diagnosis, follow-up, and options for alternative modes of evaluation and interventions (Figure 12-22).

The woman's individual belief system also is an integral component of the assessment. Racial, ethnic, and cultural differences are particularly important in assessing clients. It is important to avoid cultural stereotyping, however; that is, the nurse must recognize that not all clients of a specific cultural origin will hold the same values and beliefs. A comprehensive holistic assessment is

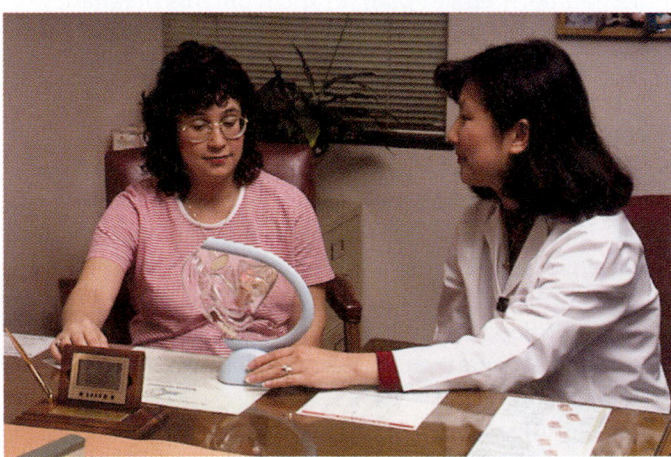

Figure 12-22 Part of the nurse's responsibilities during fetal evaluation procedures is to ensure the client is fully informed and able to participate in the decision-making process.

essential to identifying the client's need for fetal evaluation and to developing an individualized plan of care.

Nursing Diagnoses

A list of nursing diagnoses is provided to give some insight into the types of health care needs typically associated with fetal evaluation testing. The following nursing diagnostic labels can be applied to most of the procedures discussed in this chapter. The cause and supporting data components of the diagnostic statement, however, must be individualized based on the context of the testing situation and client-specific assessment data.

- Risk for injury related to the invasive diagnostic technique

- Powerlessness related to feeling inadequate to properly care for the fetus, inability to control events impacting fetal well-being, and inability to protect the fetus

- Pain related to manipulation during the diagnostic procedure

- Anxiety related to the possibility of an abnormal test result and uncertainty

- Fear related to possible complications of the procedure and possible pregnancy loss

- Ineffective coping related to stress and the inability to control or influence events

- Spiritual distress related to the possibility of a negative outcome of the testing procedure and association of the outcome with pregnancy termination

- Anticipatory grieving related to the loss of a "perfect" pregnancy

Outcome Identification

The outcomes reflect the needs and desired goals for the woman, fetus, and family. Possible outcomes for the client experiencing fetal evaluation include the following:

- The woman and fetus experience no injury or complication from the procedure.
  - The fetal heart rate is audible and within normal parameters based on gestational age.
  - The client has no uterine cramping, or uterine cramping resolves within 24 hours.

- The fetus maintains a state of well-being.
  - Fetal movement level is unchanged.
  - Fetal heart rate is consistent with the norms for gestational age, and accelerations are present.

- The compromised fetus is identified, and timely referral for follow-up is made.

- The woman participates in the decision-making process related to the selection and use of fetal evaluation procedures.
  — She verbalizes the meaning of the fetal evaluation testing results.
  — She states her options based on the testing results.
- The woman and family psychologically adapt to the process and results of fetal evaluation procedures.

Planning

An important component of planning is ensuring that the persons significant to the client are included in the procedure and decision-making process, as desired by the client.

A growing number of nurses are performing ultrasound scans, BPPs, and other fetal evaluation procedures. Only nurses who have training and competence, usually in the form of additional education, can perform these

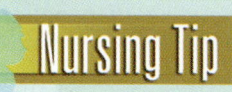

Nursing Tip

Recommendations of the U.S. Preventive Services Task Force: Strategies in Health Education and Counseling

1. Frame the teaching to match the client's perception.
2. Fully inform clients of the purpose and expected effects of the intervention and when to expect these effects.
3. Be specific.
4. Use a combination of strategies.
5. Involve others.
6. Refer.
7. Monitor progress through follow-up contacts.

Ask yourself:

- How do you feel about women who come for prenatal care but refuse to undergo fetal evaluation testing?
- How do your personal values and beliefs about pregnancy, children, and disability influence your interactions with these clients?

Note. From *Guidelines to Clinical Preventive Services* (2nd ed.), by U. S. Preventive Services Task Force, 1996, Philadelphia: Williams & Wilkins.

procedures if it is within the scope of practice as defined in the practice act of their state (Treanor, 1998).

Nursing Intervention

Nursing interventions are concentrated primarily in the area of counseling, support, and education. Before the procedure, nursing interventions encompass explaining the indications, risks, accuracy, technical aspects, rationale, and limitations of the specific evaluation modality. Performance of fetal evaluation procedures such as CVS, amniocentesis, PUBs, and MRI are not within the scope of nursing practice. The nurse is integrally involved in preparing the client, however, and may be present during the procedure. In these situations the nurse plays a vital role in explaining the technical and sensory aspects of the procedure. When the nurse is present during the performance of the procedure, her role is twofold: assisting the physician and supporting the client. During the procedure, the nursing activities may include assisting with skin preparations, positioning the woman, and specimen collection and labeling. The more significant role of the nurse, however, is as client advocate and a source of support. During the procedure, the nurse should be in continuous contact, verbal or nonverbal as appropriate, with the client. The nurse can provide anticipatory guidance about what will happen next, provide comfort measures, use anxiety reduction techniques, and monitor for potential and real problems.

After the procedure, nursing interventions include monitoring the pregnancy for complications that include amniotic fluid leakage; bleeding; uterine irritability; fetal distress, including changes in fetal cardiac activity; and maternal physiologic parameters of distress, such as fever, pain, and changes in baseline vital signs. Facilitating the client's verbalization of her perception of the experience, her concerns, and her coping strategies and support systems while awaiting the results are vital interventions.

Some fetal evaluation procedures, such as fetal movement counts, are completely within the scope of nursing practice. Nurses can initiate the procedure by teaching the client the purpose and process of fetal movement counting. When a decrease in fetal movement is detected, the nurse collaborates with and refers to the physician or certified nurse-midwife for further evaluation and testing.

Evaluation

Depending on the results of the testing procedure, evaluation of nursing interventions and achievement of nursing care goals may lead to formulation of a new nursing care plan focused on promoting a healthy pregnancy or adapting to and coping with an affected fetus, a high-risk pregnancy, or perinatal loss.

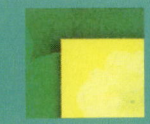

CASE STUDY/CARE PLAN
CLIENT IN A SECOND PREGNANCY

Maria presents for her first prenatal visit. Maria, who is 40 years old, is accompanied by her husband of 14 years, Alex. Maria is a loan officer and Alex is a 43-year-old stockbroker. Both Maria and Alex are very religious. They have not used contraceptive methods during their marriage. They had begun to explore adoption during the past year, with the belief that pregnancy was not in God's plan for their lives.

This is Maria's second pregnancy. Her first pregnancy was at age 16 and produced a 3-pound male infant at 39 weeks' gestation. The infant was placed for adoption, and Maria has had no contact with him.

Assessment

The client reports she has missed two menstrual periods and has had a positive home pregnancy test.

Both Maria and Alex are excited about this pregnancy and the prospect of being parents. They state that they desire this baby and are certain everything will be okay since they have waited so long.

Family history is significant because Maria's older sister gave birth to a stillborn infant with an "open sore on her back" 20 years ago. Alex's family history is without evidence of genetic or birth-related conditions.

Maternal vital signs and prepregnancy weight are within normal limits.

Maria is referred for an amniocentesis for karyotyping and evaluation of AFP level. Maria and Alex tearfully agree to the procedure stating, "We love this baby. There can't be anything wrong. Please tell us everything will be okay."

Nursing Diagnosis

Deficient knowledge related to unfamiliarity with the testing procedures and lack of understanding of genetic predisposition

Expected Outcomes	Client will understand importance of family history related to risk factors. Client will understand general parameters of the procedure. Client will feel empowered during the procedure.
Planning	Referral for comprehensive ultrasonography specifically to examine for neural tube closure, movement of lower extremities, and bladder filling. In later pregnancy, Maria will need to be monitored for IUGR based on a previous history of a low-birth-weight infant and a family history of a stillbirth.
NOC	Knowledge: Disease process
NIC	Teaching: Disease process

Nursing Interventions	Rationales
1. Teach the client about the indications, risks, benefits, and limitations of amniocentesis for fetal karyotype and AFP analysis.	1. Client acceptance of the procedure is based partly on an understanding of how it works and what it does.
2. Provide emotional support during the procedure.	2. The client's fears and feelings of loss of power can be kept in check with thoughtful and sensitive nursing care.
3. Encourage consultation with clergy or presence of religious article, as desired by the client.	3. Show respect for the client's preferences by considering factors that are important to her during the decision-making process.

Evaluation   The client is able to state the purpose, process, and alternatives to the chosen procedure. The client's spiritual needs are met consistent with her beliefs and values.

WEB | ACTIVITIES

• • • These Web sites have information concerning assessment of fetal status:

• • • Visit the March of Dimes Web site to review fetal growth and development.

• • • Fetal Ultrasound: http://www.fetal.com

• • • University College of London, Dept. of Medical Physics and Bioengineering: http://www.medphys.ucl.ac.uk

• • • Amnionet: http://www.amnionet.com

• • • University of Pennsylvania: http://www.med.upenn.edu

• • • Center for Prenatal Diagnosis: http://www.cpdx.com

tant for women who must take medications to control chronic illnesses.

■ Most fetal evaluation procedures have benefits and risks to both mother and fetus. There are limitations to the amount of information provided from these testing modalities.

■ Reactive NST and negative CST are reassuring signs of fetal well-being.

■ A BPP is an evaluation of fetal well-being and condition of the intrauterine environment.

■ Ultrasonography is a commonly used imaging modality during pregnancy with no known side effects.

■ Amniocentesis is performed throughout pregnancy for differing indications: from 15 to 18 weeks' gestation for identification of chromosomal alteration or altered AFP level, in the second trimester for elevated bilirubin levels, and in the third trimester for a lung maturity profile.

■ MS-AFP is a screening test that identifies pregnancies at increased risk for a neural tube defect.

Key Concepts

■ Fertilization occurs in the fallopian tube within 24 hours after ovulation, and implantation occurs approximately 6 days after fertilization.

■ Organ systems and external features develop during the embryonic period (between third and eighth week after fertilization). The embryo is now most vulnerable to teratogenic exposure.

■ Refinement of organ structures and function occurs from 10th week to the time of birth.

■ The placenta carries out two major functions: transport and exchange of products between the fetus and the mother and hormone production.

■ Fetal circulation is supported by the umbilical cord, ductus venosus, placenta, foramen ovale, and ductus arteriosus, and it is dependent on maternal placental circulation.

■ Fetal development proceeds in a pattern of cephalocaudal and proximal to distal.

■ Many substances found in air, soil, food, and water, as well as prescribed and over-the-counter medications, have potential effects on fetal development.

■ Behaviors such as substance abuse may be hazardous to the developing fetus. Alcohol and tobacco use are responsible for widespread fetal risks.

■ Pregnant women must be educated to avoid all medications until advised by a health professional. They also can be reassured that most food additives are not harmful. Preconceptual counseling is impor-

Review Questions and Activities

1. When does implantation occur?

2. When is the embryo susceptible to damage from teratogens?

3. What is the difference between the time of fertilization and implantation? Which time is used in calculating gestational age?

4. How does fetal development progress? Describe the sequence.

5. What is the function of amniotic fluid?

6. View the film *Miracle of Life*, produced by WGBH for "NOVA."

7. Visit an AA meeting. (Some are specified as open, and others may be limited to clients who abuse substances or restricted to specific members.) Note the personal circumstances and family histories of persons who disclose their past experiences. Analyze the difficulties and obstacles to substance abuse recovery. Explore other local resources for pregnant women who want to begin recovery from substance abuse.

8. Research the safety of use during pregnancy of medications commonly prescribed for chronic illnesses such as hypertension, asthma, epilepsy, diabetes, or multiple sclerosis.

9. Identify nonreassuring fetal heart rate patterns using electronic fetal monitoring and discuss the physiology and nursing interventions for each pattern.

10. What are the characteristics of a reassuring fetal heart rate pattern?

11. What is the difference between a screening test and a diagnostic test? Provide examples of each type of test used in the care of the pregnant woman.

12. What are the indications for an NST and how are the results interpreted?

13. What is the purpose of a CST?

References

Advisory Committee on Immunization Practices (ACIP). (1994). *Morbidity and Mortality Weekly Report, 43*(RR-1), 1–38.

AMA Council on Scientific Affairs. (1984). Effects of pregnancy on work performance. *Journal of the American Medical Association, 251,* 1995–1997.

American College of Obstetricians and Gynecologists. (1993). Ultrasound in pregnancy (Tech. Bulletin No. 187). Washington, DC: Author.

American College of Obstetricians and Gynecologists: Committee on Genetics. (1995). Chorionic villus sampling [Committee Opinion No. 169]. Washington, DC: Author.

American College of Obstetricians and Gynecologists: Committee on Educational Bulletins. (1996). Maternal serum screening. *ACOG Educational Bulletin, 28,* 1–9.

American College of Obstetricians and Gynecologists (ACOG). (1997). *Guidelines for perinatal care* (4th ed.). Elk Grove Village, IL: Author.

American College of Obstetricians and Gynecologists (ACOG). (1999). *Antepartum fetal surveillance* (Practice Bulletin No. 9 [replaces Tech. Bulletin No. 188, January 1994]). Clinical Management Guidelines for obstetricians-gynecologists.

Bateman, D., Ng, S., Hansen, C., & Heagarty, M. (1993). The effects of intrauterine cocaine exposure in newborns. *American Journal of Public Health, 83,* 190–193.

Beall, M. H. (2000). Chorionic villi sampling for prenatal diagnosis. In E. J. Quilligan & F. P. Zuspan (Eds.), *Current therapy in obstetrics and gynecology* (5th ed., pp. 736–737). Philadelphia: W. B. Saunders.

Berkowitz, R. L. (1993). Should every pregnant woman undergo ultrasonography? *New England Journal of Medicine, 329,* 874–880.

Briggs, G. (1995). Teratogenicity and drugs in breast milk. In L. Y. Young & M. Koda-Kimble, (Eds.), *Applied therapeutics: The clinical use of drugs* (6th ed., pp. 45/1–45/39). Vancouver, WA: Applied Therapeutics.

Carlson, B. M. (1999). *Human embryology and developmental biology* (2nd ed.). St. Louis, MO: Mosby.

Centers for Disease Control and Prevention (CDC) Fact Sheet. (1996). *Mother-to-child HIV transmission decreases in the US but challenges remain for perinatal prevention.* Retrieved July 1999 from http://www.cdc.gov.

Centers for Disease Control and Prevention (CDC). (1996, September). *Sexually transmitted disease surveillance 1995.* Atlanta, GA: Division of STD Prevention, CDC, U.S. Department of Health and Human Services, Public Health Service. Also available online at http://www.cdc.gov.

Cunningham, F. G., Gant, N. F., Leveno, K. L., Gilstrap, L. C., Hauth, J., & Wenstrom, K. (2001). *Williams obstetrics* (21st ed.). Stamford, CT: Appleton & Lange.

Davis, J. G. (1993). Reproductive technologies for prenatal diagnosis. *Fetal Diagnosis and Therapy, 8*(Suppl. 1), 29–38.

Docker, M. F. (1992). Ultrasound imaging techniques. In D. J. H. Brock, C. H. Rodeck, & M. A. Ferguson-Smith (Eds.), *Prenatal diagnosis and screening* (pp. 69–81). London: Churchill Livingston.

England, M. A. (1996). *Life before birth* (2nd ed.). London: Mosby-Wolfe.

Evans, M. I., Johnson, M. P., & Drugan, A. (2000). Amniocentesis for antenatal diagnosis of genetic disorders. In E. J. Quilligan & F. P. Zuspan (Eds.), *Current therapy in obstetrics and gynecology* (5th ed., pp. 226–232), Philadelphia: W. B. Saunders.

Fakhoury, G., Daikoku, N. H. Benser, J., & Dubin, N. H. (1994). Lamellar body concentrations and the prediction of fetal pulmonary maturity. *American Journal of Obstetrics and Gynecology, 170,* 72–76.

Fischbach, F. (2004). *A manual of laboratory and diagnostic tests* (7th ed.). Philadelphia: Lippincott-Raven.

Gabbe, S., Gabbe, S., & Simpson, J. (Eds.). (2002). *Obstetrics: Normal and problem pregnancies* (4th ed.). New York: Churchill Livingstone.

Gauthier, R. J. (1979). Antepartum fetal heart rate testing II: Intrapartum fetal heart rate observations and newborn outcome following a positive contraction stress test. *American Journal of Obstetrics and Gynecology, 133,* 34–39.

Henderson, D., Boyd, C., & Mieczkowski, T. (1994). Gender, relationships, and crack cocaine: A content analysis. *Research in Nursing & Health, 17,* 265–272.

Kearney, M. (1995). Damned if you do, damned if you don't: Crack cocaine users and prenatal care. *Contemporary Drug Problems, 22,* 639–662.

Lawrance, L., & Gruchow, H. (1996). Adequacy of prenatal care and pregnancy outcomes in cigarette smoking and nonsmoking mothers. *Journal of Women's Health, 5,* 609–614.

Lieberman, E., Gremy, I., Lang, J., & Cohen, A. (1994). Low birthweight at term and the timing of fetal exposure to maternal smoking. *American Journal of Public Health, 84,* 1127–1131.

Manning F. (1999). General principles and application of ultrasound. In R. Creasy & R. Resnik (Eds.), *Maternal-fetal medicine* (4th ed.). Philadelphia: W. B. Saunders.

Manning, F. A. (1995). Dynamic ultrasound-based fetal assessment: The fetal biophysical profile score. *Clinical Obstetrics and Gynecology, 38,* 26–44.

Marden, D., McDuffie, R. S., Jr., Allen, R., & Abitz, D. (1997). A randomized controlled trial of a new fetal acoustic stimulation test for fetal well-being. *American Journal of Obstetrics and Gynecology, 176*(6), 1386–1388.

Moore, K. I., & Persaud, T. V. (2003). *Before we are born: Essentials of embryology and birth defects* (6th ed.). Philadelphia: W. B. Saunders.

National Institute on Drug Abuse. (1996). *National pregnancy and health survey: Drug use among women delivering live births: 1992.* [NIH Pub. No. 96-381, 9, p. 36]. Rockville, MD: Author.

Needleman, H., & Bellinger, D. (Eds.). (1994). *Prenatal exposure to toxicants; Developmental consequences.* Baltimore: Johns Hopkins University Press.

Paul, R. H., & Miller, D. A. (1995). Nonstress test. *Clinical Obstetrics and Gynecology, 38,* 3–10.

Pfenninger, J. L., & Fowler, G. C. (Eds.). (2004) *Pfenninger and Fowler's procedures for primary care* (2nd ed.). St. Louis, MO: Mosby.

Poerksen, A., & Petitti, D. (1991). Employment and low birth weight in African American women. *Social Science & Medicine, 33*, 1281–1286.

Raines, D. A. (1996). Fetal surveillance: Issues and implications. *Journal of Obstetric, Gynecologic, and Neonatal Nursing, 25*, 559–564.

Rayburn, W. (1995). Fetal movement monitoring. *Clinical Obstetrics and Gynecology, 38*, 59–67.

Reece, E. A. (1997). Early and midtremester genetic amniocentesis. *Obstetric and Gynecologic Clinical of North America, 24*, 71–81.

Richardson, G., Conroy, M., & Day, N. (1996). Prenatal cocaine exposure: Effects on the development of school-age children. *Neurotoxicology and Teratology, 18*, 627–634.

Schulman, H. (1990). Doppler ultrasound. In R. Eden & F. Boehm (Eds.), *Assessment and care of the fetus: Physiological, clinical and mediolegal principles*. Norwalk CT: Appleton & Lange.

Sever, L. (1994). Congenital malformations related to occupational reproductive hazards. *Occupational Medicine: State of the Art Reviews, 9*, 471–494.

Simpson, J. (1993). Are physical activity and employment related to preterm birth and low birth weight? *American Journal of Obstetrics and Gynecology, 168*, 1231–1238.

Smith, C. V. (1995). Vibroacoustic stimulation. *Clinical Obstetrics and Gynecology, 38*, 68–77.

Spratto, G., & Woods, A. (2004). *PDR nurses handbook*. Clifton Park, NY: Delmar Learning.

Streissguth, A., Barr, H., Sampson, P., & Bookstein, F. (1997). Prenatal alcohol and offspring development: The first fourteen years. *Drug and Alcohol Dependence, 36*, 89–99.

Sweet, R., & Gibbs, R. (1995). *Infectious diseases of the female genital tract*. Baltimore: Williams & Wilkins.

Tabor, A., Philip, J., Madsen, M., Bang, J., Obel, E. B., Norgaard-Pedersen, B. (1986). Randomised controlled trial of genetic amniocentesis in 4604 low-risk women. *Lancet, 1*(8493), 1287–1293.

Treanor, C. (1998). Exploring nurses' role in limited ultrasound. *Lifelines, 2*, 13–14.

Tucker, S. (2004). *Pocket guide to fetal monitoring and assessment* (5th ed). St. Louis, MO: Mosby.

U. S. Preventive Services Task Force. (1996). *Guidelines to clinical preventive services* (2nd ed.). Philadelphia: William & Wilkins.

Weismiller, D. G. (1999). Preterm labor [Review]. *American Family Physician, 59*(3), 593–602.

Young, N. (1997). Effects of alcohol and other drugs on children. *Journal of Psychoactive Drugs, 29*, 23–42.

Suggested Readings

American Nurses Association. (1996). *Compendium of ANA position statements*. Washington, DC: Author.

Association of Women's Health, Obstetrics, and Neonatal Nursing. (1999). *Clinical competencies and education guide: Limited ultrasound examinations in obstetrics and gynecology/infertility settings*. Chicago: Author.

Briggs, G. (Ed.). (1994). *Drugs in pregnancy and lactation: A reference guide to fetal and neonatal risk* (6th ed.). Baltimore: Williams & Wilkins.

Cook, D., Peacock, J., Feyerabend, C., Carey, I., Jarvis, M., Anderson, H., et al. (1996). Relation of caffeine intake and blood caffeine concentrations during pregnancy to fetal growth: Prospective population-based study. *British Medical Journal, 313*, 1358–1362.

Feinstein, N., Sprague, A., & Trepanier, M. J. (1999). *Fetal auscultation*. Washington, DC: Association of Women's Health Obstetric and Neonatal Nurses.

Feldman, R. G. (1992). *Occupational and environmental neurotoxicity*. Baltimore: Williams & Wilkins.

Gilbert, E. S., & Harmon, J. S. (2002). *Manual of high risk pregnancy and delivery* (3rd ed.). St. Louis, MO: Mosby.

Kellogg, B. (2000). Fetal development. In S. Mattson & J. Smith (Eds.), *Core curriculum for maternal-newborn nursing* (2nd ed.). Philadelphia: Saunders.

Mori, A., Iwabuchi, M., & Makino, T. (2000). Fetal haemodynamic changes in fetuses during fetal development evaluated by arterial pressure pulse and blood flow velocity. *British Journal of Obstetrics and Gynecology, 107*(5), 669–677.

Murray, M. (1997). *Antepartal and intrapartal fetal monitoring*. Albuquerque, NM: Learning Resources International.

Simpson, K. R., & Creehan, P. (1996). *Perinatal nursing*. Washington, DC: Association of Women's Health Obstetric and Neonatal Nurses.

Smith, C. (1994). Amniocentesis. In J. L. Pfenninger & G. C. Fowler (Eds.), *Procedures for primary care physicians*. St. Louis, MO: Mosby.

Resources

Videotape

"A Challenge to Care: Strategies to Help Chemically Dependent Women and their Children." Association for Women's Health, Obstetric, and Neonatal Nursing (AWHONN), 1990.

World Wide Web

American Baby, http://www.americanbaby.com

Association for Women's Health, Obstetric, and Neonatal Nursing (AWHONN), http://www.awhonn.org

Centers for Disease Control and Prevention (CDC), http://www.cdc.gov

Environmental Protection Agency (EPA), http://www.epa.gov

Food and Drug Administration (FDA), http://www.fda.gov

National Human Genome Research Institute, http://www.genome.gov

National Institute for Occupational Safety and Health (NIOSH), http://www.cdc.gov/niosh

OBGYN.net, http://www.obgyn.net

TOXNET: National Library of Medicine database of toxicology research, http://www.nlm.nih.gov

Telephone Resources

Teratology Information Services: Hotlines for clinicians are available in each geographic area.

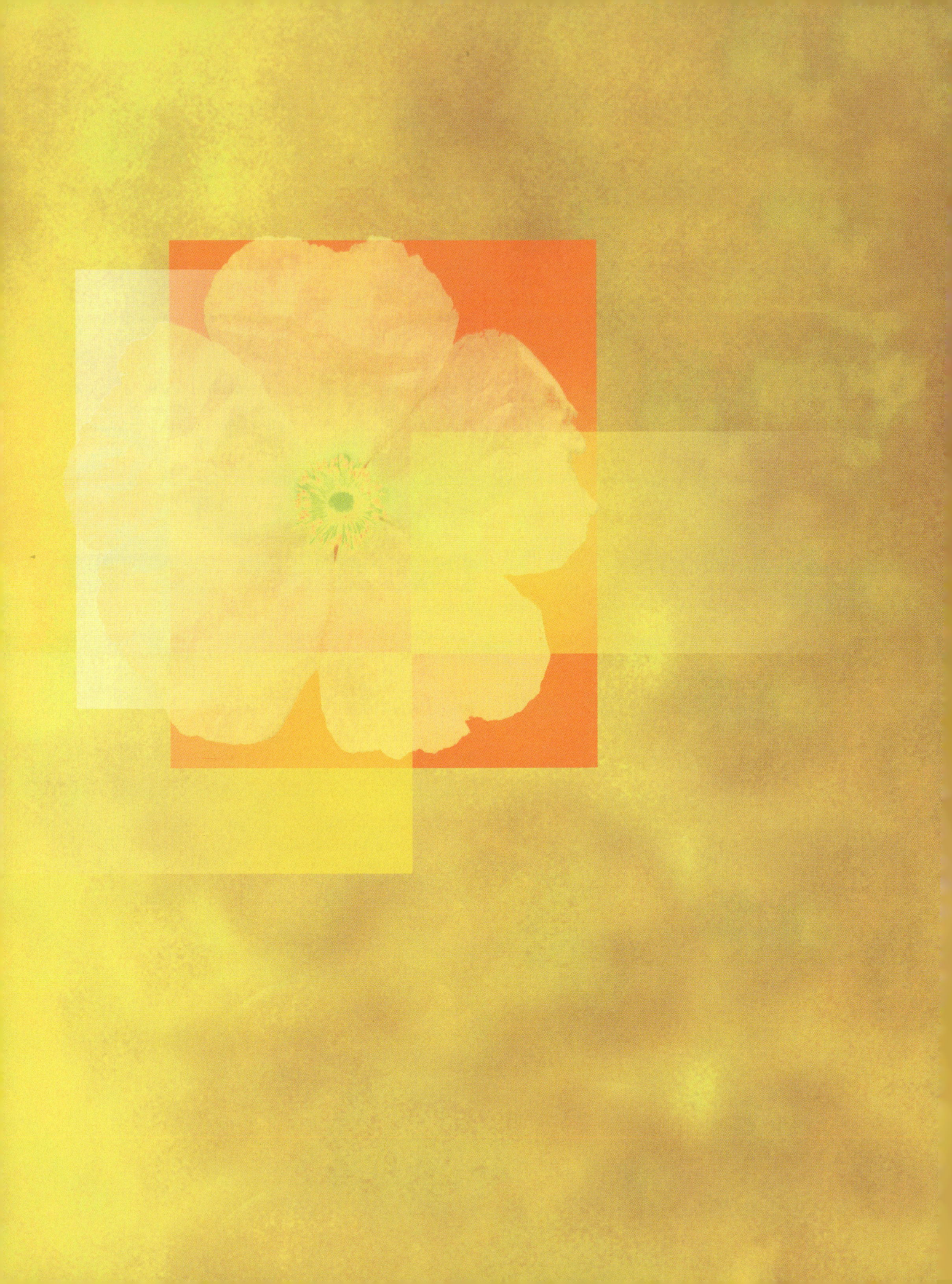

UNIT 5

Childbirth

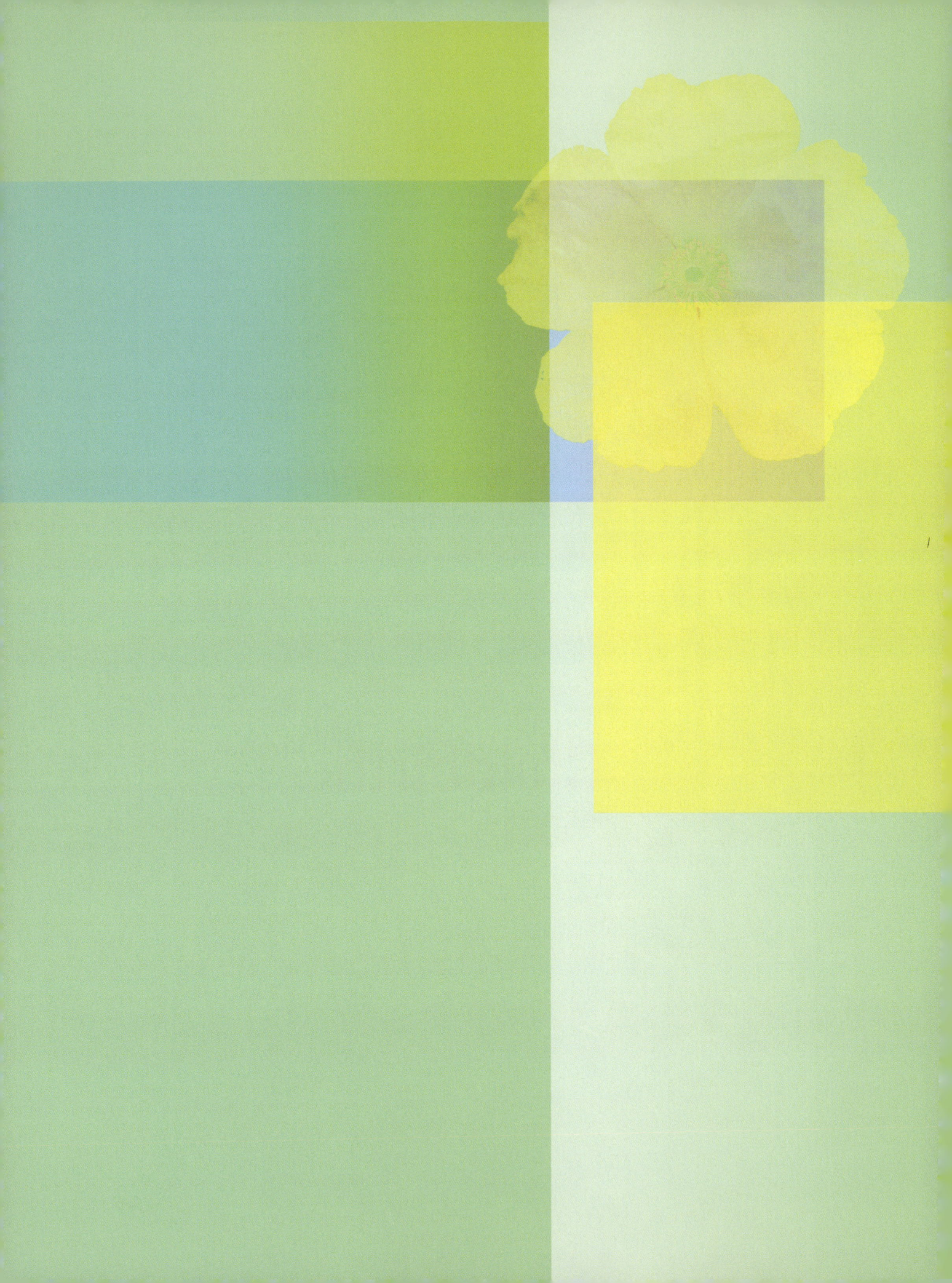

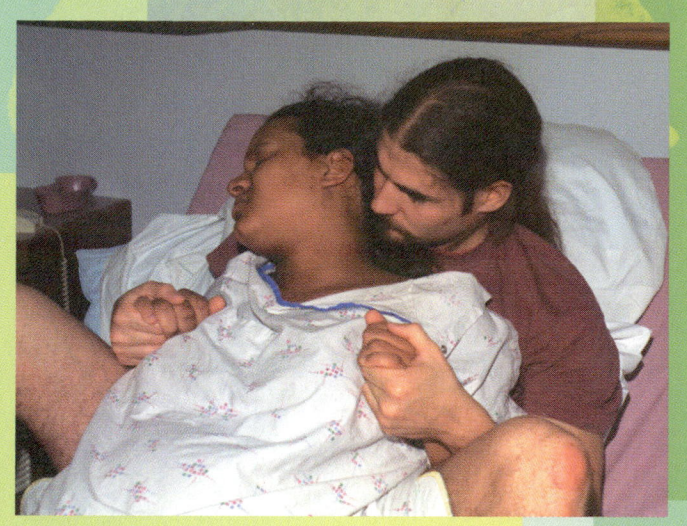

CHAPTER 13

PROCESSES OF LABOR AND DELIVERY: ANALGESIA AND ANESTHESIA

One evening, a group of women began talking about their labor experiences. Each woman could clearly remember the details. It did not matter if it was her first or her fourth child, she could recall many of the details of the labor and delivery, even when the events had occurred decades before. This fact represents how significant the process is and how important it is for the nurse to have a thorough understanding of the physiologic and psychologic changes that occur during labor. Because the labor nurse often is the person who has the most contact with the client during labor, this knowledge can help assist the nurse in making the experience a positive and safe one for both mother and baby. The labor and delivery process is a pivotal point in a woman's life, a time when she is making the transition to her role as mother. A positive experience can have major effects on the key people in the woman's life, such as her spouse or partner, other children, parents, and friends.

Key Terms

Active phase
Amniotomy
Analgesia
Anesthesia
Augmentation of labor
Bloody show
Braxton Hicks
  contraction
Cervical dilation
Cesarean section
Crowning
Dermatome
Descent
Dystocia
Effacement
Fetal attitude
Fetal lie
Fetal position
Fetal presentation
First stage of labor
Flexion
Fontanels
Forceps
Fourth stage of labor
General anesthesia

Labor
Labor induction
Latent phase
Leopold's maneuvers
Lightening
Local anesthetic
Local infiltration
  anesthesia
Maternal role attainment
Molding
Nesting
Oxytocin
Parenteral
Parturition
Placental stage
Primary powers
Pudendal block
Pushing stage
Recovery stage
Regional anesthesia
Second stage of labor
Secondary powers
Station
Third stage of labor
Transition

Competencies

Upon completion of this chapter, the reader should be able to:

1. Define the signs and symptoms of impending labor.
2. Define the five Ps of labor.
3. Describe the psychologic response of the mother during labor.
4. Define the four stages of labor.
5. Explain the maternal adaptations to labor.
6. Define and differentiate analgesia and anesthesia.
7. Describe three main types of anesthesia.
8. Explain the different options of analgesia for labor, and the advantages and disadvantages of each.
9. Describe the nursing actions necessary to prepare a client for placement of an intrathecal narcotic, epidural catheter, or both.
10. Indicate the common side effects of intrathecal and epidural analgesia, and their treatment.

Labor is the bridge between pregnancy and motherhood, and for the laboring woman it often is the most intense experience of the pregnancy. Most nulliparous women can readily visualize themselves as pregnant and their future role as a mother; however, many women cannot or do not visualize what labor is or can be. Labor is both a physical process for the mother and an emotional passage. Family members and friends often are involved in the labor process, introducing additional emotional experiences for all those participating in the labor experience. Finally, the neonate is going through the transition between intrauterine and extrauterine life.

In this chapter we explore the physiologic and psychologic processes of labor, the various stages associated with childbirth, and how labor affects both mother and child. The signs and symptoms of impending labor are examined and the maternal and fetal adaptations reviewed. The medical and surgical interventions and indications for labor induction, augmentation, and cesarean sections are discussed. Analgesia and anesthesia options are also presented.

Because the nurse often is the caregiver who spends the most time with the laboring woman, it is important for the nurse to understand fully the physiologic process of labor and how it affects both the woman and neonate. Knowing the normal process, the nurse can assist the woman and her support group through the experience, ensuring the well-being of all involved.

PHYSIOLOGY OF LABOR

The physiologic process by which the fetus, placenta, and membranes are expelled from the uterus is called **labor** or **parturition**. Labor has four stages. Stage I begins with the onset of labor and continues until full cervical dilation occurs, typically lasting 12 hours for primigravidas (first-

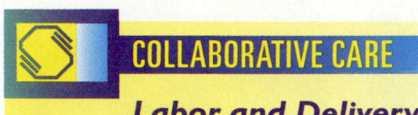

COLLABORATIVE CARE

Labor and Delivery

The nurse in labor and delivery is a very important member of the health care team. Primary care providers are usually not present throughout the labor. Therefore, they depend on the nurse's assessment skills and clinical judgment to make sure they are updated on the client's condition and notified when their presence is needed.

time mothers) and 8 hours for multigravidas. Stage II begins at the point of complete dilation of the cervix and is complete when the fetus is expelled, usually lasting 50 minutes (although it may last up to 2 hours) in primigravidas and 20 minutes in multigravidas. Stage III begins with the delivery of the fetus and ends with delivery of the placenta and membranes, usually within 8 to 10 minutes of delivery of the neonate. Stage IV begins when the placenta and membranes are delivered and is complete 4 hours later.

Theories for the Onset of Labor

Blackburn and Loper (2003) emphasize that the exact cause of the onset of labor still is not completely understood but no doubt involves both maternal and fetal factors. Progesterone withdrawal or binding, increased estrogen levels, prostaglandins, and oxytocin sensitivity are believed to have a part in the onset of labor. Fetal factors such as cortisol levels also are thought to play a role in the onset of labor.

Maternal Factors

Maternal hormone levels are partly responsible for initiation of labor. Estrogen, progesterone, prostaglandins, and oxytocin are the primary hormones involved.

Estrogen and Progesterone

It is believed that progesterone causes relaxation of the myometrium, whereas estrogen stimulates myometrial contraction. Estrogen levels begin to increase at about 34 to 35 weeks' gestation; a decrease in uterine responsiveness to progesterone also occurs, changing the effect of the estrogen-progesterone ratio. The changes in these steroid levels are responsible for the increased number of myometrial gap junctions. *Gap junctions* are proteins that connect cell membranes, facilitating coordinated uterine contractions and myometrial stretching (Ulmsten, 1996). Estrogen also stimulates the production of prostaglandin in the decidua and fetal membranes, which increases stimulation of smooth muscle contraction of the uterus.

Prostaglandins

Increases in prostaglandin production occur late in pregnancy and are thought to play an important role in the onset of labor. The two most important prostaglandins associated with parturition are PGE_2 and $PGF_{2\alpha}$. Prostaglandins are produced in the myometrium, cervix, fetal membranes, and placenta. $PGF_{2\alpha}$ exerts a stimulatory effect on the myometrium, whereas PGE_2 has a stimulatory effect on the cervix. The effect of PGE_2 on the cervix causes remodeling of the connective tissue in the cervix, allowing the cervix to soften, efface, and dilate during labor.

Oxytocin

Produced in the posterior pituitary, **oxytocin** is a hormone that plays a major role in the onset and maintenance of labor. Maternal oxytocin levels increase throughout pregnancy. As a gestation nears term the number of oxytocin receptors in the uterus increases, creating increased sensitivity to oxytocin. Estrogen also increases myometrial sensitivity to oxytocin. In the absence of these end-organ changes, even external administration of oxytocin will not be successful in precipitating labor. Fetal production of oxytocin also occurs, which is thought to stimulate prostaglandin production (Blackburn & Loper, 2003).

Fetal Factors

An increase in fetal adrenocorticotropic hormone levels at term is speculated to have an effect on uterine sensitivity to oxytocin and prostaglandins, thus stimulating the onset of labor (Ulmsten, 1996). Increased cortisol levels also decrease the production of progesterone by the placenta, therefore aiding in the relaxation of the myometrium.

Components of Labor

Five important factors affect the process of labor:

1. Passageway, or the birth canal
2. Passenger, the fetus and placenta
3. Powers, the uterine contractions
4. Position of the mother
5. Psychologic response of the mother (Box 13-1)

Passageway

The bony pelvis is an important structure in the birthing process. It is composed of four bones, two innominate (each consisting of the ilium, ischium, and pubis), the sacrum, and the coccyx. The effects of hormones associated with pregnancy, relaxin and estrogen, are to soften cartilage and increase the strength and elasticity of the pelvic ligaments. These changes cause the pelvic joints to separate slightly, allowing some movement of the pelvic

Box 13-1

The Five Ps of Labor

- **P**assageway
- **P**assenger
- **P**owers
- **P**osition
- **P**sychologic response

joints. As the pregnancy progresses, the symphysis pubis separates slightly, allowing room for the fetal head.

The pelvis is divided into the false pelvis and true pelvis. The *false pelvis* is the shallow upper section of the pelvis. The *true pelvis* is the lower curved bony canal, including the inlet, cavity, and outlet, through which the fetus must pass in the birth process (Seidel, Ball, Dains, & Benedict, 2003).

Station refers to the relationship between the ischial spines in the passage and the presenting part of the fetus (Figure 13-1). The ischial spines are station 0 and in the normal pelvis signify the narrowest diameter the fetus encounters during a vaginal birth. *Engagement* is a term which indicates that the largest diameter of the presenting part has passed through the inlet into the true pelvis. This usually corresponds to station 0.

There are four types of female pelvis: gynecoid, android, anthropoid, and platypelloid. These various pelvis types can play a large role in determining the ease of a vaginal delivery. The most common type of female pelvis is the gynecoid pelvis, found in about half of women. The least common type of female pelvis is the platypelloid pelvis, found in about 3% of women. Figure 13-2 compares

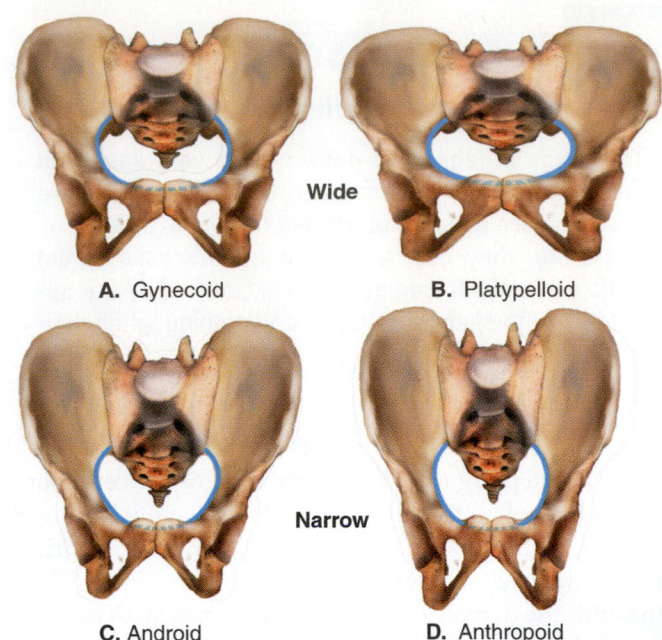

Figure 13-2   Female pelvis types.

A. Gynecoid
B. Platypelloid
Wide
C. Android
D. Anthropoid
Narrow

the four female pelvis types. Wide suprapubic arches (gynecoid and platypelloid) tend to allow normal vaginal delivery, whereas narrow arches (android and anthropoid) increase the likelihood of forceps and cesarean deliveries.

Passenger

The ease with which the passenger goes through the pelvis is determined by many fetal factors: head size, presentation, lie, attitude, and position.

Fetal Head Size

The fetal head is composed of bony parts consisting of a frontal bone, two parietal bones, two temporal bones, and an occipital bone. The skull bones are united by membranous sutures, and the points of intersection of these are called **fontanels**. The two most important fontanels for delivery are the anterior and posterior fontanels (Figure 13-3). The diamond-shaped anterior fontanel is the largest of the two and lies at the juncture of the sagittal, coronal, and frontal sutures. This fontanel generally stays open until about 18 months of age, allowing brain growth. The posterior fontanel is triangular shaped and is formed by the intersection of the sagittal and lambdoid sutures; it closes about 6 to 8 weeks after birth. During a vaginal examination, the fetal presentation can be determined by locating these fontanels.

The fontanels are important during the birth process because they allow molding to occur. **Molding** is the overlapping of the fetal skull that helps the fetal head to adapt

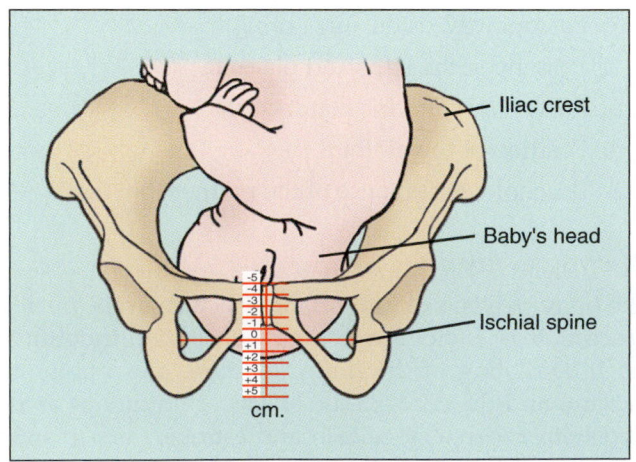

Iliac crest

Baby's head

Ischial spine

cm.

Figure 13-1   Station, or relationship of the fetal presenting part to the ischial spines. The station illustrated is +2.

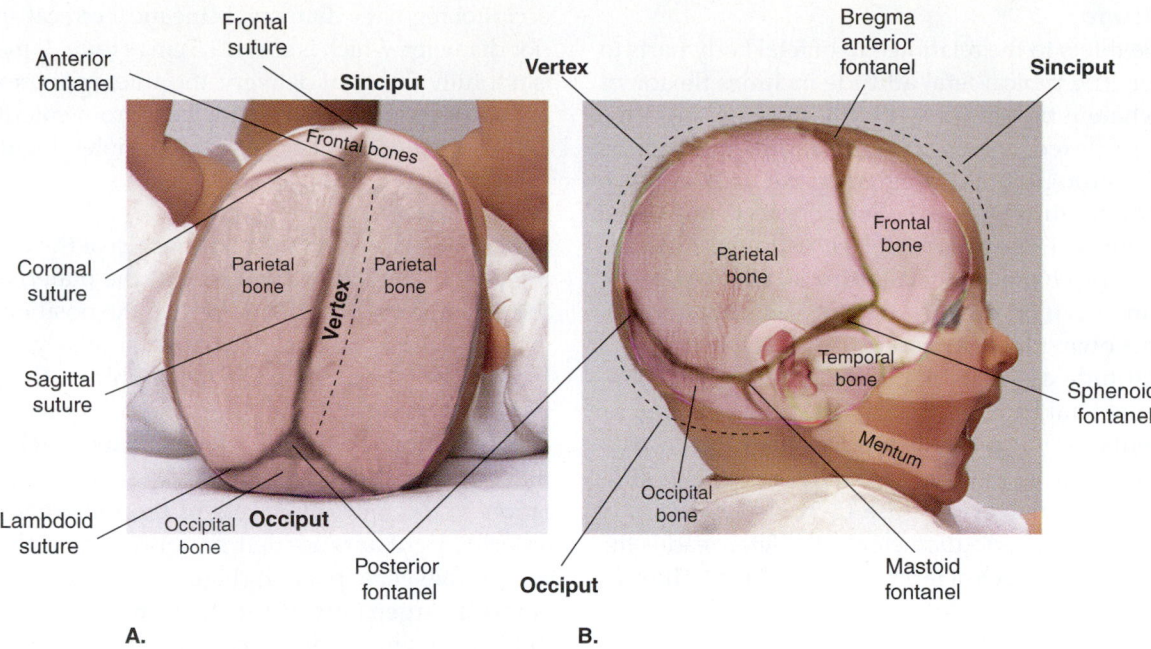

Figure 13-3 Fetal skull—sutures and fontanels. A. Superior view. B. Lateral view.

to the size and shape of the maternal pelvis. Molding can be extensive, causing the fetal head to appear misshapen at birth. The effects of molding on the shape of the head usually resolve completely in 3 days.

Fetal Presentation

Fetal presentation refers to the anatomic part of the fetus that is either in or closest to the birth canal. Presentation is determined by performing a vaginal examination and feeling the part through the cervix. There are three major presentations. Cephalic or fetal head presentation is the most common, occurring in 96% of births, and is most likely to lead to a vaginal birth. Breech or buttock presentation occurs in 3% of births. Shoulder presentation occurs in the remaining 1%. These last two presentations are associated with a complicated birthing process and often require cesarean section.

Fetal Lie

The **fetal lie** describes the relationship of the fetal long (head to foot) axis to that of the maternal long axis or spinal cord (Figure 13-4). In a breech or cephalic presentation, the lie is longitudinal. With a shoulder presentation, the lie is transverse, making vaginal birth unlikely. An oblique lie indicates the fetus is at a 45-degree angle to the maternal long axis and is considered an unstable lie; the oblique lie often converts to longitudinal or transverse lie during labor.

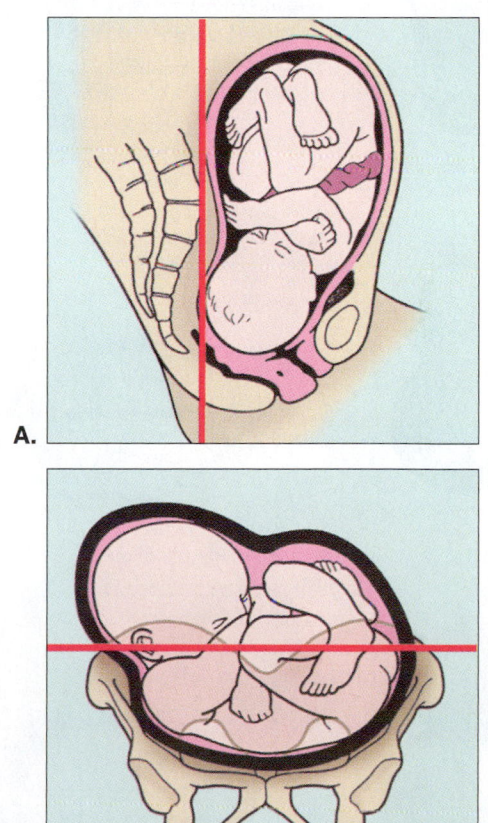

Figure 13-4 Fetal attitude and fetal lie. A. Fetal attitude flexion, fetal lie longitudinal. B. Fetal attitude flexion, fetal lie transverse.

Fetal Attitude

Fetal attitude refers to the relationship of fetal body parts to one another. The typical fetal attitude includes flexion of the head wherein the chin rests on the sternum, the arms and legs are flexed against the chest, and the back is bowed out. Throughout the pregnancy, the fetus assumes various attitudes through movement and stretching of the fetal extremities. The available space within the uterine cavity can cause changes in fetal attitude; large for gestational age infants tend to be flexed more than are normal-sized infants owing to lack of room inside the uterus.

Fetal attitude can affect the birth process. For example, when the fetal head is slightly extended (sinciput or brow presentation), it presents a larger diameter to pass through the maternal pelvis and thus increases the difficulty of labor and delivery (Figure 13-5).

The largest transverse diameter of the fetal head is the biparietal diameter, which at term is about 9.25 cm. The sub-

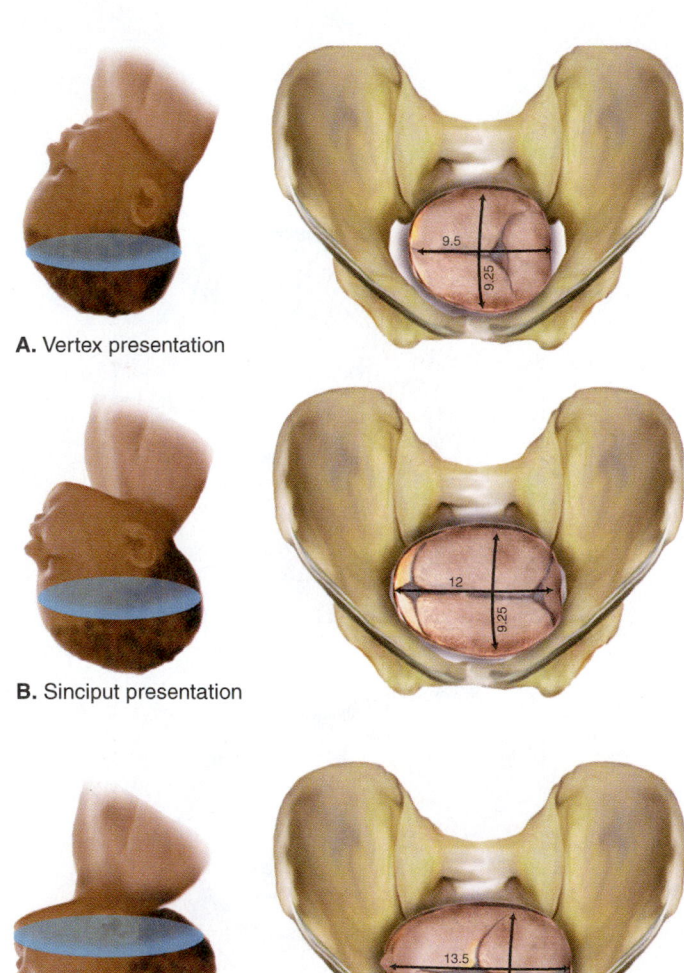

A. Vertex presentation

B. Sinciput presentation

C. Brow presentation

Figure 13-5   Diameter of presenting part in vertex, sinciput, and brow presentations.

occipitobregmatic diameter is the most critical anteroposterior diameter, which is about 9.5 cm at term. If the fetal head is not fully flexed at delivery, the anteroposterior diameter increases and may prevent the head from entering the true pelvis or the deeper cavity below the inlet (Figure 13-6).

Fetal Position

Fetal position refers to the relationship of the fetal presenting part to the left or right side of the maternal pelvis. If the cephalic presentation is vertex, the position landmark is the posterior fontanel or occiput; similarly, in a cephalic face presentation, the mentum or chin is the presenting part. In breech and shoulder presentations, the sacrum and acromion are the landmarks, respectively. The landmark of the presenting part of the fetus is described in relation to the four quadrants of the maternal pelvis (left anterior, right anterior, left posterior, and right posterior) or the transverse portion (Figure 13-7). In a posterior position, a larger part of the head must pass through the pelvis, causing a long labor and often more back pain owing to increased pressure on the sacral nerves.

Assessment of Fetal Presentation and Position

There are two primary means for determining the presentation and position of the fetus. The first and less invasive way is through Leopold's maneuvers; the more invasive way is through a vaginal examination.

Leopold's Maneuvers or Abdominal Palpation. **Leopold's maneuvers** refer to a method of abdominal palpation to determine fetal presentation and position. These maneuvers need to be performed in a consistent and systematic fashion to be as reliable as possible. These maneuvers are a reliable method to determine position and presentation but are very limited in the obese client or the client with an anterior placenta. The examiner should stand at the side of the bed that is most convenient and face the client's head for the first three maneuvers and the client's feet for the last maneuver (Figure 13-8).

First Maneuver

With both hands, the examiner outlines the shape of the uterus, gently palpating the fundus with the fingertips to determine which fetal pole is present in the fundal area. The fetal buttocks give the sensation of a large nodular body, whereas the head is more firm, round, and ballottable.

Second Maneuver

After determining the fetal part in the fundus, the examiner's palms are placed on either side of the client's abdomen, exerting deep but gentle pressure. In a vertex or breech presentation, one side will feel smooth and firm, indicating the back; whereas the other side will have numerous small irregular mobile parts, indicating the fetal

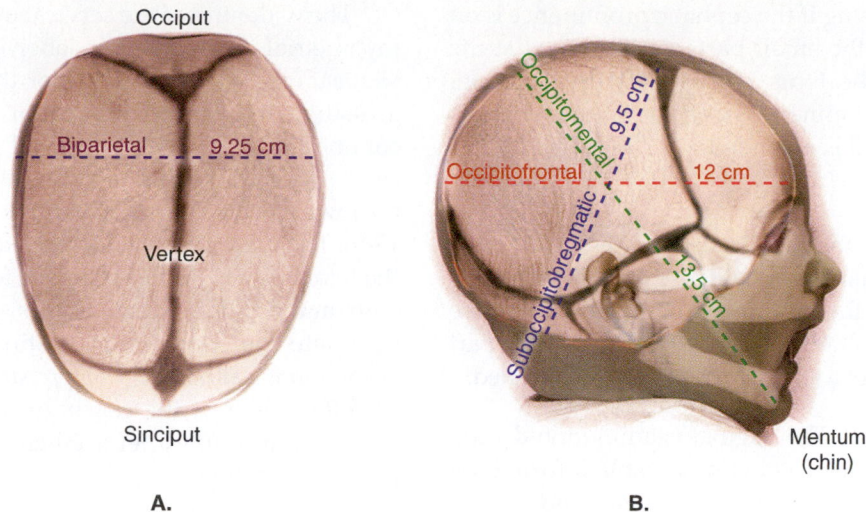

Figure 13-6   Fetal head measurements. A. Biparietal diameter. B. Cephalic diameters.

extremities. Both increased amniotic fluid and maternal obesity will make feeling the individual extremities more difficult, and in some cases only the back may be palpated. Determining the location of the back more anteriorly or transversely will give the examiner a more accurate idea of the fetal lie and presentation.

Third Maneuver

The third maneuver will help determine whether the previously detected presenting part is *engaged* (deep in the pelvis), and the attitude of the fetal head is in a cephalic

presentation. With the thumb and fingers of one hand, the examiner attempts to grasp the lower portion of the client's abdomen, just above the symphysis pubis. If a body part moves easily, the presenting part is not engaged. The fetal attitude can be determined in a cephalic

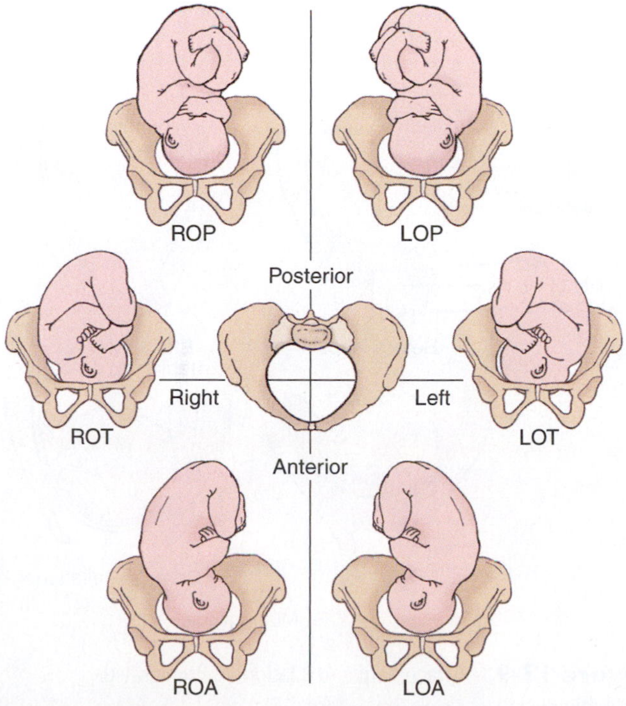

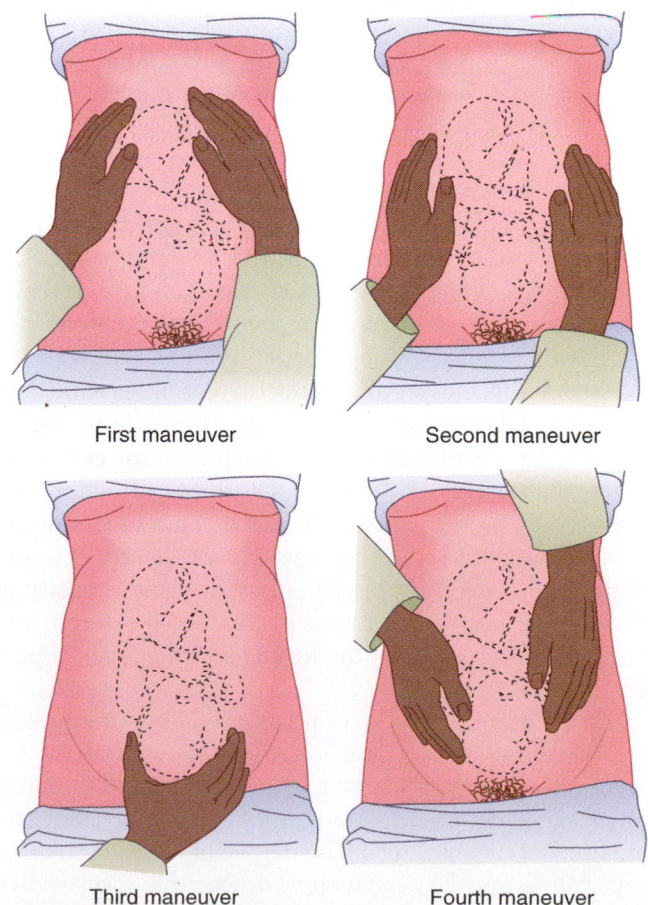

Figure 13-7   Positions of a vertex presentation.

Figure 13-8   Leopold's maneuvers.

presentation by assessing if the cephalic prominence is on the same side as are the small parts, indicating that the head is flexed and the fetus is in vertex presentation. When the cephalic prominence is on the same side as is the back, the fetal head is extended.

Fourth Maneuver

The examiner will face the client's feet to assess further the fetal attitude. This maneuver will use the fingertips of the palmar surface of the examiner's hands to outline the cephalic prominence of the fetus. When the presenting part is deeply engaged, only a small portion may be outlined.

Vaginal Examination. The vaginal examination during the labor process is done to obtain valuable information about the mother's progression during labor and the position of the fetus. Vaginal examination often can determine the fetal station and presenting part. The mother's cervix also can be assessed vaginally for how open, thin, and short it is and for the amount of dilation and effacement. Vaginal examination can help determine the adequacy of the pelvic size and shape for a vaginal delivery.

Powers

Two important types of powers are involved in the labor process, which are characterized as primary and secondary powers. The **primary powers** are the involuntary uterine contractions. The **secondary powers** are the mother's intentional efforts to push out the fetus.

Primary Powers

Uterine contractions are involuntary and generally are independent of extrauterine control. During labor, the uterus forms what is called the physiologic retraction ring, dividing itself into two portions. The upper contractile segments become thicker as labor advances. The passive lower uterine segment and the cervix expand and thin out as labor progresses. Uterine contractions are responsible for the effacement and dilation of the cervix, allowing the descent of the fetus. Uterine contractions are measured by their frequency, from the beginning of one to the beginning of the next contraction. The length of a contraction is how long it lasts in seconds. The intensity or strength of a contraction also is evaluated by external palpation of the firmness of the uterus and the level of pain perceived by the client.

As the uterine muscle contracts, the upper uterine segment shortens and causes longitudinal traction on the cervix. This leads to **effacement**, or shortening and thinning, of the cervix. Before labor, the cervix generally is 2 to 3 cm long and about 1 cm thick. The degree of effacement is described in terms of a percentage. For example, a cervix that is halfway effaced would be described as being 50% effaced.

The widening of the cervical opening that occurs from myometrial contractions in labor is referred to as **cervical dilation**. In general, before labor the cervix is closed, progressing to 10 cm open as labor advances. Dilation accommodates passage of the fetal head through the birth canal. When the cervix is fully dilated and retracted into the lower uterine segment, it is no longer palpable (Figure 13-9). The uterus elongates with each contraction, causing the fetal body to straighten. This fetal change exerts pressure on the fundus of the uterus, pushing the presenting part onto the cervix and assisting in dilation; this phenomenon is called *fetal axis pressure*. In the primigravida, the effacement of the cervix usually begins before dilation. In a multipara, effacement and dilation generally progress together.

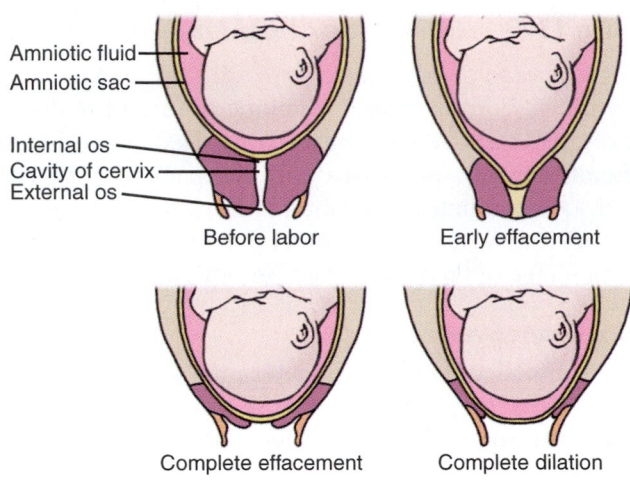

A. Primigravida

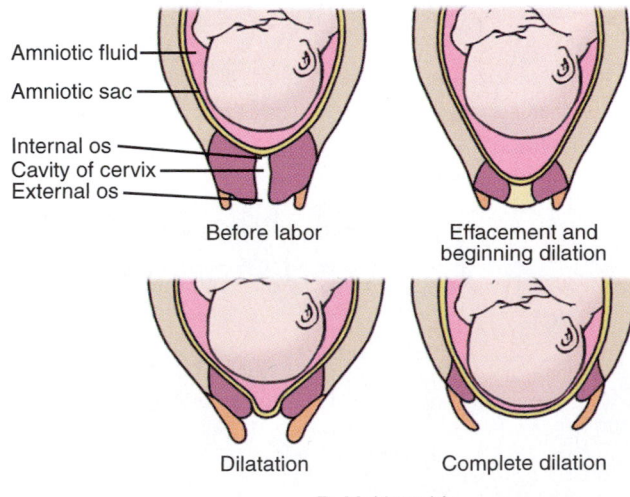

B. Multigravida

Figure 13-9   Effacement and dilation. A. Primigravida. B. Multigravida.

Secondary Powers

After the woman is fully dilated and effaced, the presenting part of the fetus descends to the pelvic floor. The uterine contractions begin to change and become more expulsive. The laboring woman begins to feel an involuntary urge to bear down or push. This begins the use of secondary, more voluntary efforts of labor. With each uterine contraction, the woman contracts her abdominal muscles to compress all sides of the uterus to aid in expelling the fetus. The woman's ability to push has an important role in the progression of the vaginal birth of the fetus.

Position

Maternal position in labor can have an effect on both the mother and fetus. Much disagreement exists regarding the influence of maternal position on labor progress, pain perception, and fetal well-being. During the first stage of labor, it may be psychologically beneficial for the mother not to be confined to lying supine in bed. If a client has an intravenous line in place, a movable pole should be used to allow ambulation. If a mother chooses to remain in bed, she should be encouraged to find her most comfortable position. A lateral recumbent position often is the most comfortable one and best for fetal well-being, particularly during the first stage of labor. The optimal position for an individual client, however, may range from sitting in a rocking chair to using a labor ball or being in a semi-reclined position. All positions have advantages and disadvantages. For example, although the squatting position may increase the size of the pelvic outlet, it may be difficult for a woman with an epidural to assume this position. In the absence of a clear-cut "best" position during labor, it is important to consider maternal needs, both physical and psychologic, as well as fetal well-being.

Psychologic Response of the Mother

Few reports exist in the nursing literature about the psychologic response to labor. Clark and Affonso (1978) identified some factors that make labor a meaningful positive event or the antithesis, a negative event for the mother. The first factor is the role of one's culture, that is, how a particular society views childbirth, which incorporates the woman's attitudes toward the labor process. Another factor that can negatively or positively affect the childbirth experience is the expectation and goals for the labor process. If the expectations about labor are realistic and can be met, the outcome is more likely to be positive; in contrast, if the expectations are unrealistic and unattainable, the experience is more likely to be negative. Finally, feedback from other people participating in the labor and birth process can add positive or negative aspects to the experience.

It is important for the nurse to assess these factors as soon as the client arrives in the labor suite. The nurse should communicate with the client and significant others involved in the labor experience and explore cultural ideas, attitudes, expectations, and goals. For example, a specific cultural need of the client that could be explored is the role of labor coach being taken on by the laboring woman's mother instead of the husband. Doulas, women who support laboring women, are sometimes used for added support during labor. These needs should be met when possible, even if the nurse providing care has different cultural attitudes.

A positive labor and birth experience can help the woman more easily transition into the maternal role. **Maternal role attainment** as defined by Rubin (1984) is the process by which a woman acquires knowledge of maternal behavior that aids in transforming her maternal identity. The first developmental stage of maternal role attainment is for the mother to seek a safe passage for herself and her child during pregnancy, labor, and delivery. Many factors contribute to maternal role attainment such as age, culture, support system, childbirth preparation, and previous birth experiences. Williams, Kramma, and O'Brian (1997) describe proper childbirth preparation as a valuable tranquilizer during the birth process that can lead to decreased need for analgesics to be administered during labor.

The labor and delivery nurse should provide a supportive and caring environment for the client and should respect the client's and family's needs and attitudes. Delivery of such care is attained through therapeutic communication and assessment of client needs.

Cultural Perceptions of Childbirth

Leininger (1985) defines *culture* as a "particular group's values, beliefs, norms and practices that are learned and shared and that guide thinking, decisions and actions in a patterned way." In examining this definition and relating it to childbirth, culture is one of the biggest influences on childbirth perceptions and the role of motherhood. A study by Callister, Vehvilainen-Julkunen, and Lauri (1996) compared childbirth perceptions among women who were American Mormon, Canadian Orthodox Jew, and Finnish Lutheran. The results showed that Finnish Lutheran women felt that motherhood was one of many roles women would encounter in life. In contrast, Canadian Jewish women and American Mormon women felt that motherhood was their purpose in life. The author points out that family structures are different in that husbands in Finland take a more active role in parenting. In contrast, American and Canadian fathers of these religious affiliations believe the mother's role is paramount and thus are less involved.

SIGNS AND SYMPTOMS OF IMPENDING LABOR

The signs and symptoms of impending labor are different for every woman, and an individual woman may experience all, some, or none of them. Some of the premonitory signs and symptoms of labor may include lightening, cervical changes, Braxton Hicks contractions, bloody show, an energy spurt, and gastrointestinal (GI) upset. Education of the woman and assessment of these signs and symptoms can help the nurse to provide anticipatory guidance for the onset of labor and delivery.

Lightening

Lightening is the movement of the presenting part of the fetus into the true pelvis. In primigravidas, lightening usually occurs about 2 weeks before the onset of labor. Clients often will describe a feeling of being able to breathe more easily because of less pressure on the diaphragm from the gravid uterus. Other discomforts however may become more apparent:

- Increased pelvic pressure and congestion, resulting in increased vaginal secretions and pelvic discomfort
- Increased urinary frequency from extrinsic pressure on the bladder
- Neuropathic pain related to the pressure of the presenting part on the nerves in the pelvis, particularly in the obturator foramen
- Edema of the lower extremities and increased venous stasis from inhibition of blood return by the pelvic pressure of the presenting part

Cervical Changes

As a pregnant woman approaches term, her cervix changes from being long and closed with a firm consistency to shortened (or effaced), thinned, dilated, and soft. The cervix of a multipara normally can be dilated 2 cm or more before the onset of labor. Primigravidas often will experience effacement before dilation, whereas multiparas will have concurrent effacement and dilation (Seidel et al., 2003). Effacement, however, is a subjective assessment.

Cervical changes are thought to occur from the remodeling of connective tissue secondary to the effects of prostaglandins. Because cervical ripeness varies at the onset of labor, it does not predict when the woman will go into labor. However, cervical ripeness can help predict that a client will go into labor when contractions begin and can help in deciding who is ready for induction of labor (Burst, Kriebs, Gegor, & Varney, 2004).

Braxton Hicks Contractions

Throughout the pregnancy a woman may experience painless irregular contractions called Braxton Hicks contractions or false labor. These often are felt in the front of the abdomen, whereas early labor is more commonly felt in the lower back. As true labor approaches, Braxton Hicks contractions may become more noticeable, frequent, painful, and difficult to differentiate from true labor without cervical examination. These contractions may be annoying and confusing to the pregnant woman, who often will come to the physician's office or hospital for evaluation. A woman experiencing false labor needs reassurance that true labor will eventually ensue.

Bloody Show

Soon after conception, thick tenacious mucus forms inside the cervical canal to act as a protective barrier. Before the onset of labor, as the cervix begins to soften and dilate, this mucous plug often is expelled. These blood-tinged secretions are referred to as bloody show. Labor usually ensues within 24 to 48 hours of expelling the mucous plug.

Energy Spurt

Although no physiologic basis is known for this, many women experience a burst of energy, known as nesting, 24 to 48 hours before going into labor. Many women report having the energy to do things that they recently have not had the ability to do because of the fatigue of pregnancy, for example, cleaning the house or washing windows. In providing anticipatory guidance, the nurse should warn clients of the possible energy spurt and how they need to conserve their energy for labor.

Gastrointestinal Disturbances

Diarrhea, indigestion, nausea, and vomiting sometimes are reported just before the onset of labor. There is no known physiologic explanation for these symptoms.

STAGES OF LABOR

There are four stages of the labor process. The first and longest stage of labor occurs between the onset of true labor and the point of complete cervical dilation and effacement. The second stage of labor is expulsion of the fetus, and the third stage of labor is delivery of the placenta. The fourth stage is the first 4 hours after delivery of the placenta.

First Stage

The **first stage of labor** begins with regular contractions and ends when the cervix is completely dilated. This stage is divided into three phases: latent, active, and transition phases.

Latent Phase

The **latent phase** of labor begins with the onset of regular contractions, which usually are mild. During this phase, contractions may be 15 to 20 minutes apart, lasting 20 to 30 seconds. As this phase progresses, however, the contractions will occur every 5 to 7 minutes and the duration will lengthen to 30 to 40 seconds. Many women remain at home during the early parts of the latent phase. This phase usually begins with little or no cervical dilation and ends when the cervix is 3 to 4 cm dilated. For the primigravida, the latent phase lasts an average of 9 hours; whereas in the multigravida, the latent phase generally lasts an average of 6 hours. Although the woman may exhibit some anxiety during this phase, she often is comfortable enough to verbalize her concerns. This is an excellent time for the nurse to establish rapport with the client and family. It is also an opportunity to assess the client's learning needs and provide teaching.

Active Phase

The **active phase** of labor begins when the woman is 3 to 4 cm dilated and ends when she is 8 cm dilated. During this phase, contractions occur every 2 to 3 minutes and last up to 60 seconds. The intensity of each contraction begins as moderate and continues to increase as the woman gets closer to the transition phase. The average length of the active phase in the primigravida is 6 hours and in the multigravida is 4.5 hours. Dilation rates should be at least 1.2 to 1.5 cm/h (Troyer & Parisi, 1993).

Transition Phase

The last and shortest part of the first phase of labor is **transition**, which typically is the most intense phase for the laboring woman. In transition, contractions occur every 1.5 to 2 minutes, with a duration of 60 to 90 seconds. The intensity of the contractions is very strong in the transition phase. The woman often becomes very restless and agitated and may have difficulty focusing during contrac-

tions. Many women exhibit anger at the coach, voice a desire to leave the hospital, request a cesarean section, hyperventilate, complain of nausea and vomiting, tremble, and experience rectal pressure. The nurse plays an important role for the client and her coach because the laboring woman often begins to withdraw from her coach's support. The coach may feel useless, and both the client and her partner will look to the nurse for reassurance and support. During this time the nurse will need to prepare the woman for the second stage of labor.

Second Stage

The **second stage of labor** begins when the cervix is completely dilated and effaced and ends when the fetus is expelled; it also is known as the **pushing stage**. The average length of the second stage of labor in a primigravida is 1.1 hours and 24 minutes in the multigravida. Many factors influence the length of the second stage of labor, including maternal parity, fetal size, uterine contractile force, presentation, position, pelvic size, method of anesthesia, and magnitude of maternal expulsive effort.

During contractions, the woman will bear down, causing the abdominal muscles to contract and helping the fetal head to descend through the birth canal. As the fetal head continues into the birth canal, the perineum begins to bulge. **Crowning** is defined as the point at which the fetal head is visible at the vulvar opening. When crowning occurs, birth is imminent.

Many women feel relief at the developing urge to push, partly because it signifies that the birth is very close. Other women, particularly those without support or child preparation classes, feel overwhelmed when it is time to push. Some women describe intense pain and burning of the perineum as the pressure increases on the vulva. Women are in various positions during the second stage of labor; the lithotomy position is the most common in the United States. Epidural anesthesia may interfere with the woman's perception of pushing and her ability to push forcefully. Nurses need to be aware of prolonged second stages of labor (Table 13-1) because intervention may be required.

Cardinal Movements or Mechanism of Labor

During the birthing process, the position of the fetal head and body must change to accommodate the maternal pelvis. These changes in fetal position are called *cardinal movements* or *mechanism of labor* (Figure 13-10). The cardinal movements are descent, flexion, internal rotation, extension, restitution, external rotation, and expulsion.

Table 13-1   Average Length of Labor Stages 1 and 2

CHARACTERISTIC	FIRST STAGE			SECOND STAGE
	LATENT PHASE	ACTIVE PHASE	TRANSITION PHASE	
Primigravida	8–10 h	6 h	2 h	1 h
Multigravida	5 h	4 h	1 h	15 min
Cervical dilation	0–4 cm	4–8 cm	8–10 cm	
Contractions				
Frequency	10–20 progressing to 5–7 min	3–5 min	2–3 min	2–3 min
Duration	15–20 progressing to 30–40 sec	40–60 sec	60–90 sec	60–90 sec
Intensity	Mild progressing to moderate	Moderate progressing to strong	Strong	Strong

Descent

Descent is the progression of the fetal head into the pelvis, which occurs because of three forces: the pressure of the amniotic fluid, direct pressure of the contracting uterus, and effects of the contractions on the maternal diaphragm and abdominal muscles. The head generally enters the pelvis in the transverse and oblique position. The degree of descent is measured by stations.

Flexion

Flexion occurs when the fetal head meets resistance from the pelvic floor and walls as well as the cervix, causing the head to flex with the chin against the fetal chest. This position achieves the smallest fetal diameters coming into the maternal pelvis.

Internal Rotation

The widest part of the maternal pelvis is the anteroposterior diameter because the fetal head must rotate to accommodate the pelvis. The pelvic muscles cause resistance to the fetal head, forcing it to rotate from left to right and aligning the fetal head with the long axis of the maternal pelvis. This occurs mainly during the second stage of labor.

Extension

As resistance is met by the pelvic floor, the fetal head pivots beneath the symphysis pubis. The head emerges through extension, led by the occiput, then the face, and finally the chin.

Restitution

Internal rotation causes the shoulders of the fetus to enter the pelvis in an oblique position. When the head is delivered in the extended position, the neck is twisted and the head realigns with the long axis of the fetus.

External Rotation

As a continuation of the restitution, the shoulders align in the anteroposterior diameter, causing the head to continue to rotate. The trunk navigates though the pelvis with the anterior shoulders descending first.

Expulsion

As the shoulders extend under the symphysis pubis, the anterior followed by the posterior shoulders are delivered by the woman's pushing effort. Once the shoulders are delivered, the trunk easily follows.

Reflections from a Laboring Mother

During my pregnancy, my labor lasted almost 48 hours. I had an epidural and felt pretty good but was getting more and more tired. The nurses couldn't believe how long I was taking to dilate (since they saw me—unusually—on more than one rotation). Finally, after about 40 hours, a new nurse came in and reviewed my chart. She introduced herself and said, "You are going to have this baby on my shift." She instructed me to turn every half hour, and she came into my room to make sure I did it. She was calm yet in control. I *did* have my baby on her shift and I whole-heartedly believe it was because she worked *with me* to make it happen.

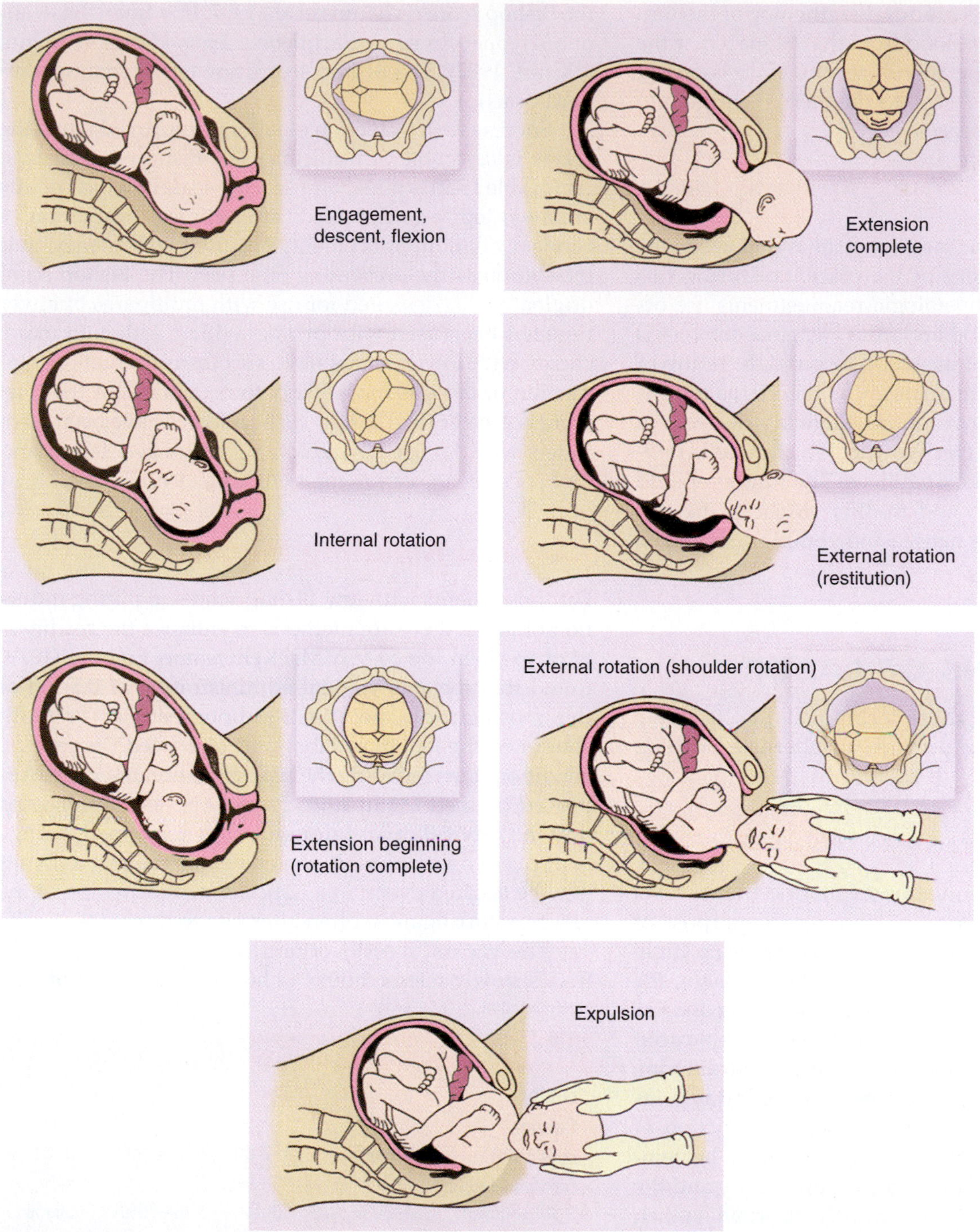

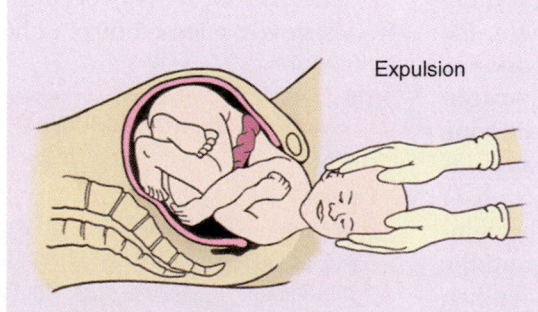

Figure 13-10 Mechanisms of labor.

Third Stage

The **third stage of labor** or **placental stage** begins as soon as the fetus is delivered and lasts until the placenta is delivered. The mechanism of placental separation is a combination of uterine contractions and involution. After expulsion of the fetus, the uterus continues to contract every 3 to 4 minutes. As the uterus contracts and begins the process of involution, shrinkage of the site of implantation of the placenta occurs. Within 10 to 15 minutes after delivery of the infant, most of the placenta has detached from the uterine wall. At this point, vaginal bleeding from the uncovered implantation site increases, and delivery of the placenta generally soon follows. The classic signs of placental separation are rounding up of the uterus, upward movement of the fundus, lengthening of the umbilical cord, and a rush of blood from the vagina. Once the placenta is delivered, the uterus continues to contract, closing off the spiral arterioles. As the uterus continues to shrink, the bleeding decreases.

Fourth Stage

The **fourth stage of labor** or **recovery stage** is defined as the first 4 hours after delivery of the placenta. During this time, many maternal physiologic readjustments are occurring. The average blood loss from a vaginal delivery is 250 to 500 mL. Because of the blood loss and the return of a more normal abdominal anatomy as the uterus returns to a more normal size (involution), there is a decrease in blood pressure and slight tachycardia. The fundus is midline and at the level of the umbilicus. The fundus should remain firm, contracted, and midline. Most of the discomforts of labor, such as nausea and vomiting, should be gone or clearly subsiding.

INTERVENTIONS OF LABOR

Interventions of labor are those techniques that facilitate the progress of labor or provide an alternate birthing mechanism.

Labor Induction

Labor induction is the stimulation of uterine contractions before the spontaneous onset of labor for the purpose of accomplishing delivery (ACOG, 1995). There are multiple medical and obstetric reasons for induction of labor, the most common being postterm gestation. Other indications for induction of labor include pregnancy-induced hypertension (PIH), diabetes mellitus, intrauterine growth restriction, intrauterine fetal demise, and various other maternal-fetal complications. Before induction of labor is performed, the benefit of delivery must be compared with the risks of continuing the pregnancy and the induction process itself (Bernstein, 2000). Certain women choose induction for convenience. Some of the contraindications to labor induction include placenta previa, transverse fetal lie, prolapsed umbilical cord, a previous classical uterine incision scar, and active genital herpes virus infection (ACOG, 1995).

In attempting to ensure the safety and ease of labor induction, Bishop (1964) established a cervical scoring system based on the clinical assessment of the cervix. Developed in the 1950s, the Bishop score has been studied extensively and compared with other methods of evaluation. Some authors have reported that cervical examination alone proves to be a more predictive value than does the Bishop score (Williams et al., 1997; Friedman, Niswander, Bayonet-Rivera & Sachtleben, 1966; Harrison, Flynn, & Craft, 1977). The Bishop score, however, remains standard practice.

Success with induction of labor is improved when the cervix is favorable or inducible. The Bishop scoring system (Table 13-2) is a 13-point scoring scale in which points are awarded (or subtracted) after clinical evaluation of cervical dilation, effacement, position, consistency, and the station of the presenting fetal part. The Bishop score originally was designed for use with multiparas but over time has been used with primigravidas. Although many clients with lower scores have successful inductions, induction of labor is more likely to be attained if the total score is greater than 8. Low Bishop scores have been associated with failure of induction, prolonged labor, and higher cesarean section rates (ACOG, 1995).

Cervical Ripening Methods

For those clients with low Bishop scores requiring induction of labor, there are methods to enhance the readiness of or to ripen the cervix. MacKenzie and Embrey (1979) found that the intravaginal administration of 0.5 mg of the prostaglandin gel (PGE$_2$) dinoprostone (Prepidil) shortened the length of labor and improved the cervical condition, thus reducing the risk for cesarean section. Approved by the FDA in 1992, Prepidil gel is administered into the cervical canal through a catheter-tipped syringe or applied to a diaphragm placed next to the cervix. Doses may be applied every 6 to 12 hours, with ripening of the cervix occurring most often after two to three doses.

The vaginal insert Cervidil contains 10 mg of PGE$_2$ that is slowly released over 12 hours. One benefit of Cer-

Table 13-2	Bishop Scoring System			
Factor	0	1	2	3
Cervical dilation	Closed	1–2 cm	3–4 cm	5–6 cm
Cervical effacement	1–30%	40–50%	60–70%	80+%
Fetal station	–3	–2	–1	+1, +2
Cervical consistency	Firm	Med	Soft	+
Cervical position	Posterior	Mid	Anterior	+

Predictive value:
Score: 0–4   45–50% induction failure rate
         5–9   10% induction failure rate
         10–13   0% failure rate

Note. From "Pelvic Scoring for Elective Inductions" by E. H. Bishop, 1964, *Obstetrics and Gynecology, 24,* p. 266.

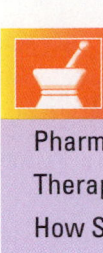

Oxytocin (Pitocin)

Pharmacologic Class	Pregnancy category X
Therapeutic Class	Oxytocic agent
How Supplied	Injection IM or IV; or given IV via piggyback into a mainline IV and controlled by an infusion pump. After delivery it is usually given IV but can be given IM.
Indications for Use	To stimulate or augment uterine contractions during the labor process. After delivery, oxytocin promotes uterine contraction and the beginning of the involution process. It may also be used to control postpartum bleeding.
Chemical Effect	Causes selective potent stimulation of the smooth muscle of the uterus and mammary glands; metabolized by the liver and kidneys and has a half-life of approximately 5 minutes
Therapeutic Effect	Stimulates uterine contractions, induces labor, and reduces postpartum bleeding
Dosage	When used postpartum: IV, 10 to 40 μ, are added to 1,000 mL of D_5W, D_5LR, lactated Ringer's Solution, or 0.9% normal saline at a rate of 20–40 mμ/min or a rate necessary to control bleeding; IM, 10μ
Side Effects and Adverse Reactions	Uterine hyperstimulation leading to uterine rupture, cervical and vaginal lacerations, postpartum hemorrhage, or uterine hypoperfusion. Fetal effects related to uterine hypoperfusion include fetal hypoxia, hypercapnia, bradycardia, and death. Cardiovascular reactions, including PVCs or other cardiac arrhythmias, increased heart rate, hypertension, nausea, and vomiting Excessive maternal fluid retention
Contraindications	Known hypersensitivity to oxytocin, CPD, unfavorable fetal presentation, fetal distress, severe pre-eclampsia, renal disease, or hypertension
Nursing Considerations	Monitor BP, P, R, FHR, contraction pattern every 15 minutes and with each increase in dose. Monitor intake and output. Monitor for nausea, vomiting, headache, hypotension, nonreassuring FHR. Perform vaginal exams with changes in frequency, intensity.
Client Teaching	Manage discomfort of intense uterine contractions.
Laboratory Finding	None

vidil is that the insert may be removed if hyperstimulation or active labor begins. Hyperstimulation of the uterus can be described as an inadequate rest between contractions and is a potential hazardous side effect of using any kind of PGE_2 for induction of labor. Maternal side effects of PGE_2, including vomiting, diarrhea, and fever, are avoided with local vaginal applications.

Monitoring of the client after receiving PGE_2 includes 30 minutes to 2 hours of external fetal monitoring for uterine contractions and reassuring fetal heart tones. Bed rest should be maintained for 30 minutes to ensure proper placement of the medication. If regular uterine contractions persist, fetal heart rate (FHR) monitoring should be recorded hourly for at least the first 4 hours (ACOG, 1995).

Misoprostol (Cytotec) is a synthetic PGE_1 used for the treatment and prevention of peptic ulcer disease. Although its use for the induction of labor is not approved by the FDA, studies have been conducted using the drug intravaginally to soften the cervix. ACOG (1999) outlined strict guidelines for the use of Cytotec in labor induction stating that for cervical ripening, one quarter of a 100 µg tablet should be used for the initial dose; doses should not be given more frequently than every 3 to 4 hours; oxytocin should not be given within 4 hours of the last dose; and Cytotec should not be used in clients with a previous cesarean delivery or a previous uterine scar. Wing, Lovett, and Paul (1998) also discourage use in clients with a previous uterine scar owing to the increased incidence of uterine rupture in their randomized trial of labor.

Oxytocin (Pitocin) is a hormone used to help induce labor, continue labor, or control bleeding after delivery. Pitocin is produced naturally by the posterior pituitary gland and stimulates contraction of the uterus. For those clients with low Bishop scores, cervical ripening may be initiated before using Pitocin.

Nursing Alert

Oxytocin (Pitocin)

An accidental bolus of oxytocin can be life-threatening for both the mother and fetus. To avoid this potential hazard, oxytocin should always be administered through an infusion pump and inserted by piggyback through the main intravenous line at the port closest to the client.

Intervention for Uterine Hyperstimulation

- Turn off the pitocin.
- Change the client's position (lying on the left side is best).
- Administer oxygen.
- Notify the physician.

Nursing Tip *Stripping the Membranes*

Stripping of the membranes can assist the commencement of spontaneous labor. Performed during a sterile vaginal examination, the technique entails placing the examining finger through the cervical os and sweeping in a circular motion to separate the chorioamniotic membrane from the internal surface of the lower uterus. Risks associated with the procedure include infection, bleeding, and accidental rupture of membranes. This procedure is done by physicians.

Oxytocin usually is diluted with 10 U in 1 L of an isotonic electrolyte solution (ACOG, 1995), although many hospital protocols may call for 20 U of oxytocin in a 1-L bag. Regimens for the initial dose and dose increases vary according to hospital protocols. Starting dosages of 0.5 to 2 mU/min with increases in increments of 1 to 2 mU/min every 20 to 60 minutes are acceptable dosages (ACOG, 1995).

Oxytocin does not cross the placenta; therefore, no direct effects on the fetus are seen. FHR deceleration as a result of uterine hyperstimulation is the most common adverse effect (ACOG, 1995). Adverse effects for the mother include uterine rupture and hyperstimulation. Refer to the oxytocin drug box.

Amniotomy

Amniotomy (artificial rupture of membranes) can stimulate and reduce the duration of labor. Amniotomy may be performed early in labor for urgent inductions (e.g., for preeclampsia), or later once cervical dilation has advanced for routine inductions. The longer the membranes have been ruptured, the greater the possibility of infection; therefore, amniotomy often is used in conjunction with oxytocin.

Augmentation of Labor

Augmentation of labor is the stimulation of uterine contractions after labor has begun. Indications for augmentation include prolonged labor, failure of cervical dilation to progress, or dysfunctional labor. Procedures for the augmentation of labor are the same as those for induction. Nursing assessment and management of the client undergoing augmentation also are the same as those for induction.

Forceps-Assisted Birth

Forceps are metal instruments used on the fetal head to provide traction or to provide a method of rotating the fetal head to an occiput-anterior position. There are several types of forceps. Some forceps have fenestrated (open) blades and some solid blades (Figure 13-11). All forceps have a locking mechanism that prevents the blades from compressing the fetal skull.

Forceps may be applied as follows:

- *Outlet forceps*—when head is crowning (Figure 13-12).
- *Low forceps*—when head is at +2 station or lower but not yet crowning.

According to Cunningham et al (2001), the indications of forceps-assisted birth are classified as maternal

Client Education

Pitocin

Explain the following to the client:

- The medication and reasons for use: induction of labor and improvement of contractions
- The reactions to expect: increased intensity and frequency of contractions
- The route of administration and the rate
- The monitoring of the fetal heart rate and contractions, including frequency, intensity, and resting tone
- The monitoring of the maternal blood pressure, pulse, and temperature
- The expected outcome
- That expectations may vary according to the Bishop score and other maternal-fetal factors

Nursing Tip   ***Interventions during Amniotomy***

1. Explain the procedure to the client and family.
2. Note and document the fetal heart rate before and after the procedure.
3. Assess the fluid color, odor, and consistency.
4. Note the time of rupture.
5. Assess the client's temperature every 1 to 2 hours to check for infection.
6. Frequently assess the client's level of comfort and provide pericare.
7. Maintain adequate intake and output records.
8. Document maternal and fetal assessments in the medical record.

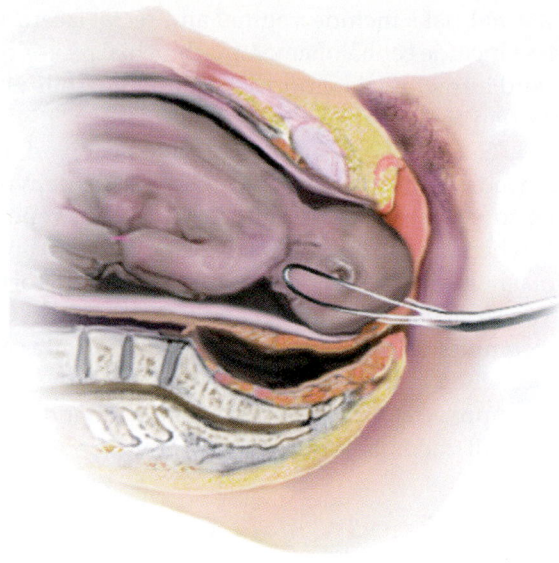

Figure 13-12   Forceps-assisted birth; traction is applied downward and outward during contractions.

and fetal. Maternal indications include heart disease, acute pulmonary edema, intrapartum infection, certain neurological conditions, exhaustion, or a prolonged second-stage labor. Fetal indications are prolapse of umbilical cord, premature separation of the placenta, and worrisome FHR patterns.

Before forceps are applied, the cervix must be completely dilated, membranes must be ruptured, and position and station of the fetal head must be known. The FHR must be checked, reported, and recorded *before* forceps are applied and again *after* forceps are applied to make sure the cord is not being compressed by the forceps. It may help the mother to understand about the forceps if it is explained that the forceps blades fit around the baby's head like two teaspoons fit around an egg (Lowdermilk & Perry, 2003). Traction is applied to the forceps only during contractions. Rotation is performed between contractions.

After the birth of the infant, the mother must be assessed for vaginal and cervical lacerations, hematoma, and bruising. The newborn infant may have facial bruising or edema.

Vacuum-Assisted Birth

A cup connected to suction is placed over the occiput on the fetal head. After the suction (negative pressure) is attained, traction downward and outward is applied during contractions (Figure 13-13). Indications are the same as for forceps-assisted birth.

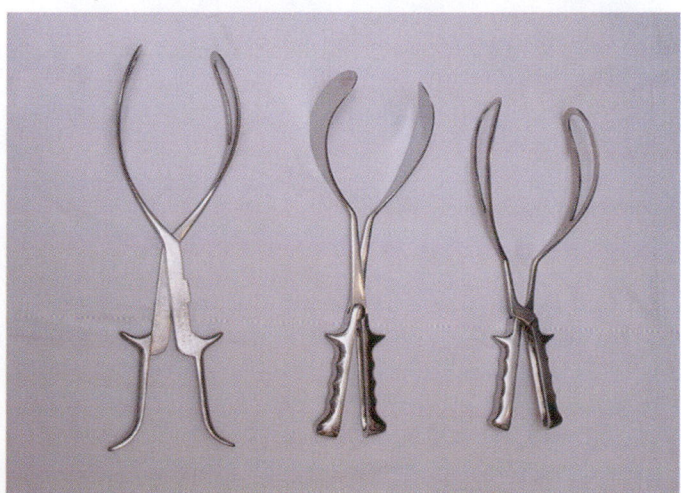

Figure 13-11   Types of forceps.

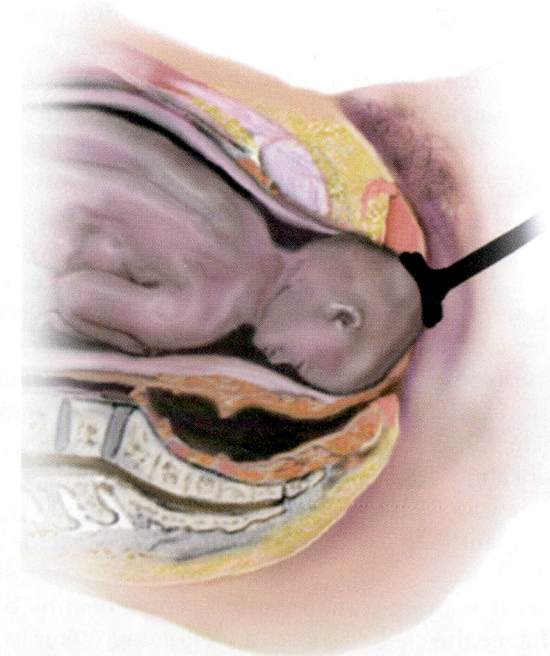

Figure 13-13   Vacuum-assisted birth.

Maternal risks include vaginal and rectal lacerations. Fetal risks include cephalohematoma, brachial plexus palsy, retinal and intracranial hemorrhage, and hyperbilirubinemia (O'Brian & Cefalo, 1996).

The U.S. FDA (1998) issued a public health advisory on the need for caution in vacuum-assisted deliveries. Two life-threatening complications have been reported: subgaleal hematoma (subaponeurotic hematoma) and intracranial hemorrhage. In response to the FDA report, the American College of Obstetrics and Gynecology (ACOG, 1998) recommends the continued use of vacuum-assisted deliveries when indicated. ACOG emphasizes the importance of appropriate training concerning the indications and use of all vacuum extraction devices.

Cesarean Section

Cesarean section, commonly called C-section, is the birth of the fetus through a surgical incision made in the mother's abdomen (Figure 13-14). The classical cesarean section involves a vertical incision through the skin and uterus and usually is performed only in cases of emergent delivery. The classical incision usually extends from the pubic hairline to the navel. The low transverse cesarean section is a horizontal (Pfannenstiel) incision of the skin and uterus. The incision scar from a low transverse cesarean section is a horizontal crease under the pubic hairline. Occasionally, the physician may perform a horizontal skin incision with a vertical uterine incision. Owing to the increased risk for uterine rupture in future pregnancies associated with a vertical uterine scar, it is important to maintain adequate documentation of both the skin and uterine incisions.

Indications for cesarean section are varied. **Dystocia** (failure of labor to progress), repeat cesarean section, breech presentation, and fetal distress are among the more common indications. Other indications for cesarean section include active genital herpes infection, placenta previa, placental abruption, prolapsed umbilical cord, PIH, and other maternal-fetal complications.

Cesarean section may be performed under regional (epidural or spinal) or general anesthesia. Because most surgeons use the low transverse cesarean section, vaginal birth after cesarean section is common practice. Risk for uterine rupture increases dramatically after a vertical uterine incision and therefore is a contraindication for vaginal delivery in subsequent pregnancies.

Counseling the client in preparation for cesarean section should include information about the surgery, anesthesia, and expected course of recovery. Clients undergoing cesarean section may express feelings of loss of a natural birth. Support and emphasis on a healthy baby may enhance the client's sense of well-being. Refer to the accompanying photo story on a cesarean delivery.

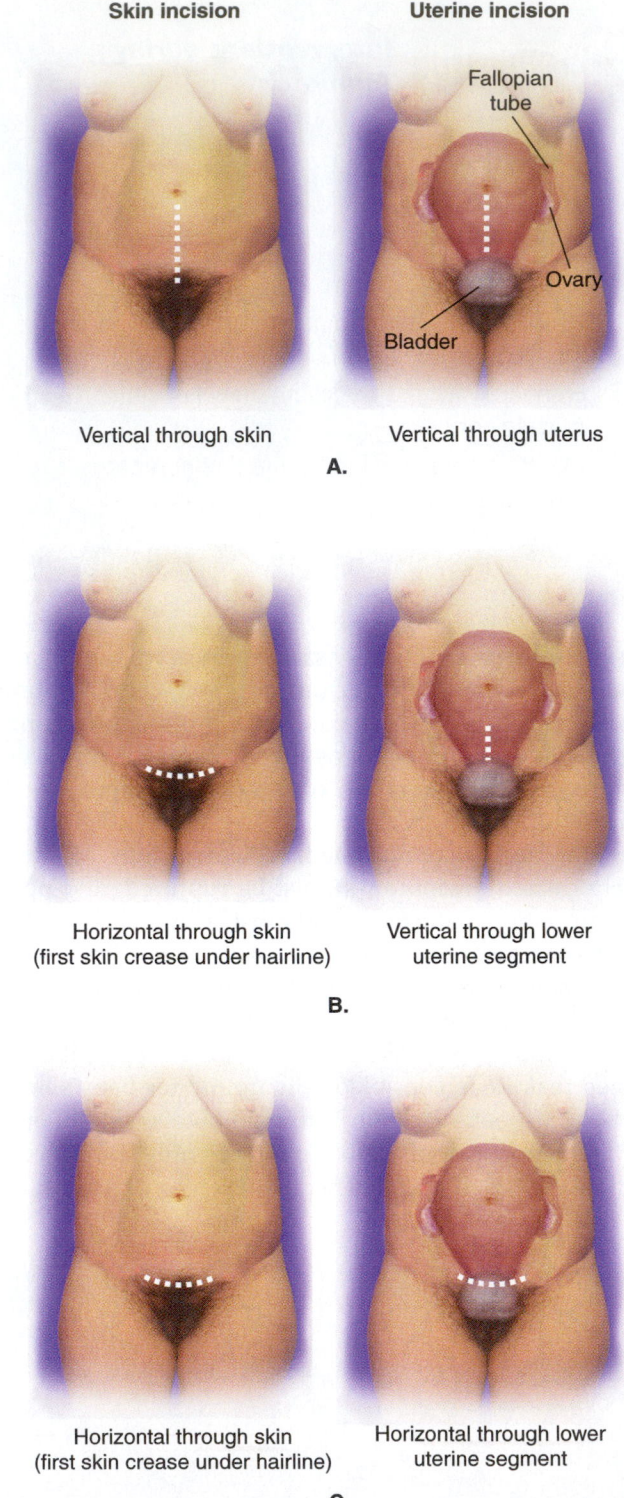

Skin incision   **Uterine incision**

Fallopian tube

Ovary

Bladder

Vertical through skin   Vertical through uterus

A.

Horizontal through skin (first skin crease under hairline)   Vertical through lower uterine segment

B.

Horizontal through skin (first skin crease under hairline)   Horizontal through lower uterine segment

C.

Figure 13-14   Cesarean incisions: A. Skin and uterine incisions classic, vertical skin incision with uterine incision; seldom used except in emergency situation; B. Horizontal skin incision with low vertical uterine incision; C. Horizontal skin incision with horizontal uterine incision.

One Couple's Cesarean Section Delivery and Tubal Ligation

When the operating room is set up and the client is secure on the table, anesthesia personnel monitor the client while the surgical team gathers.

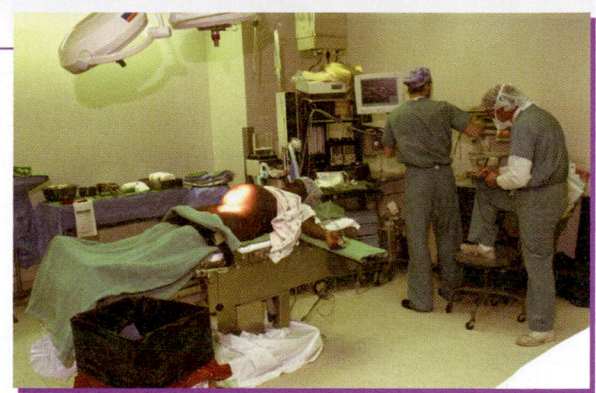

Nursery personnel arrive and check neonatal equipment and supplies in preparation to receive the newborn.

Identification bands are prepared for mother and infant.

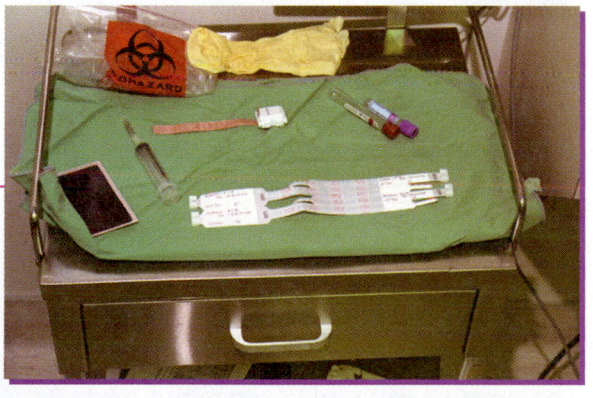

The circulating nurse performs a surgical scrub of the client's abdomen followed by a rinse with sterile water.

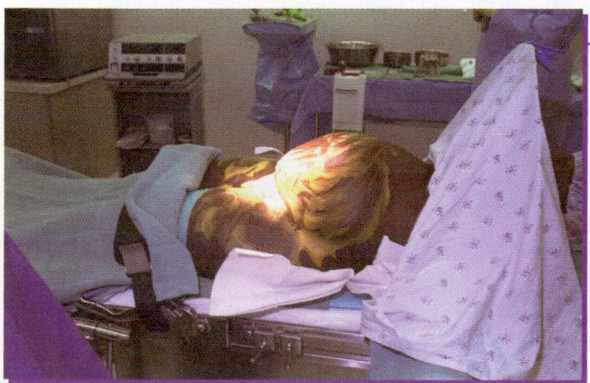

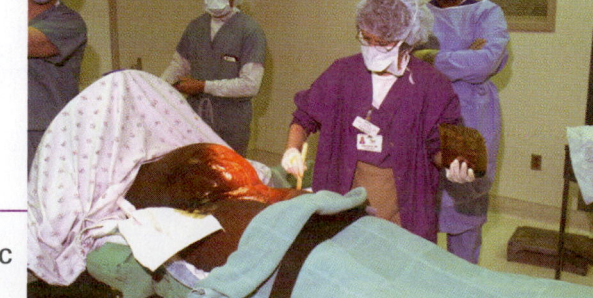

The client's abdomen is painted with an antiseptic solution to further reduce the risk of infection.

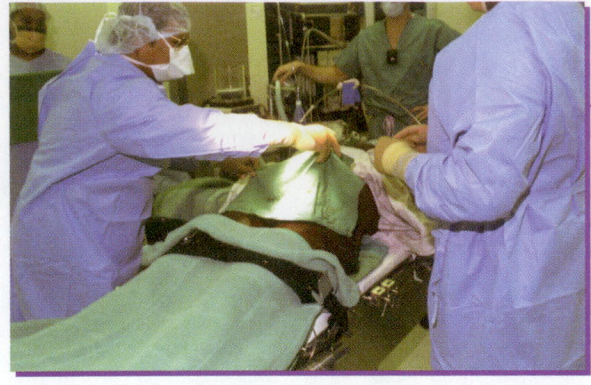

Sterile drapes are applied to provide a sterile field for the surgery.

The surgeon marks the targeted incision line along the previous C-section scar.

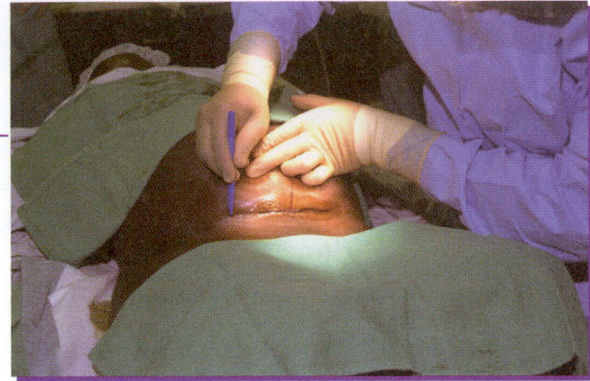

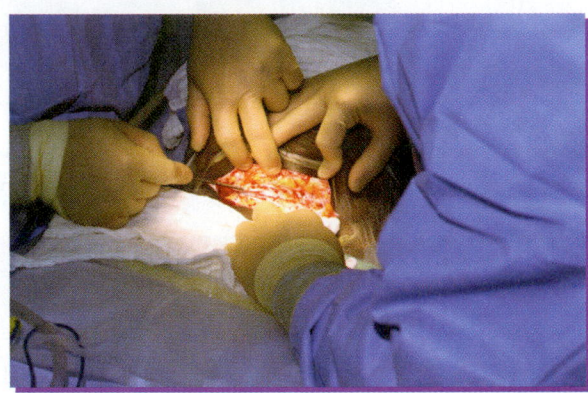

A Pfannenstiel incision is made.

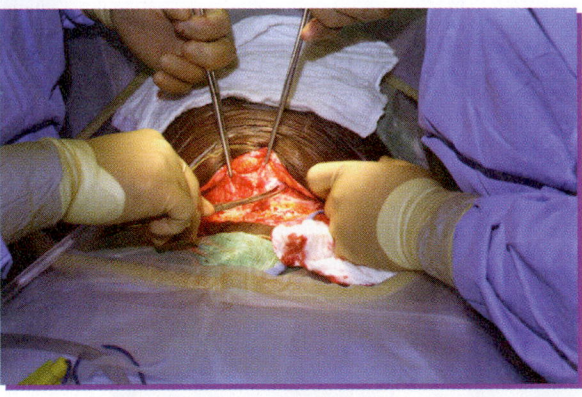

The central muscle is retracted and dissected to access the fascia.

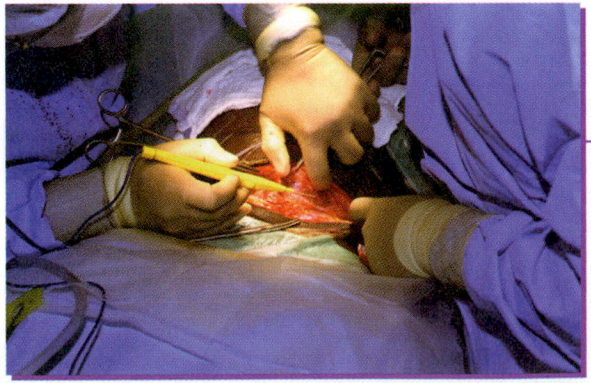

With routine C-sections, an attempt is made to control bleeding through cauterization.

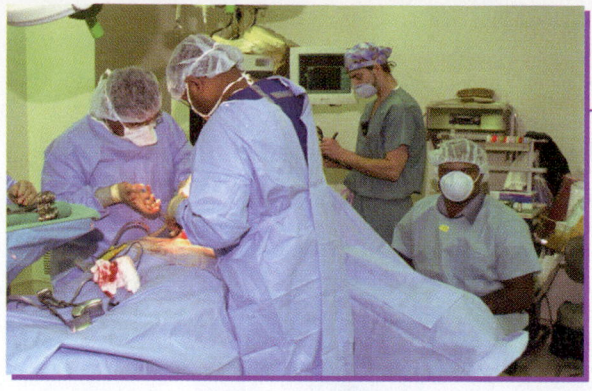

The father supports his partner and observes as the surgical team works.

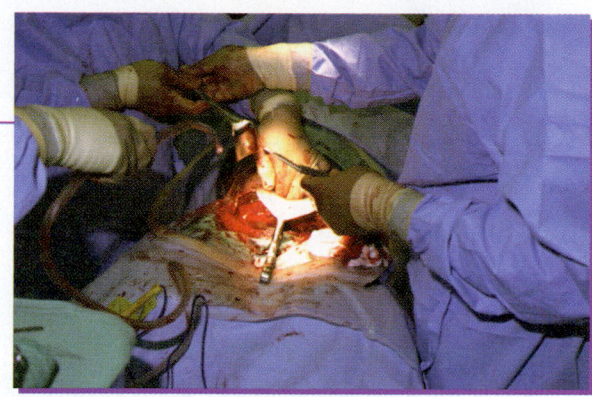

Prior to incision into the uterus, the bladder must be dissected away; a bladder blade is inserted into the abdominal cavity to retract the bladder.

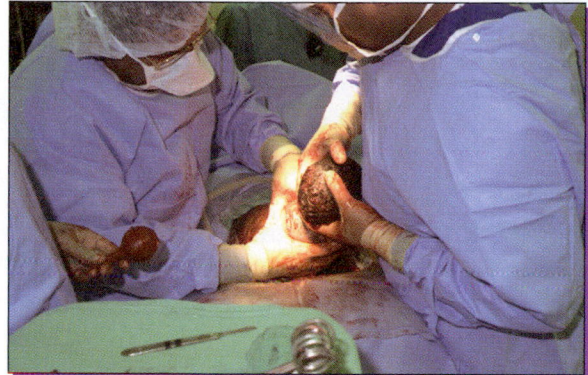

The infant's head is delivered through the incision, followed by the remainder of his body.

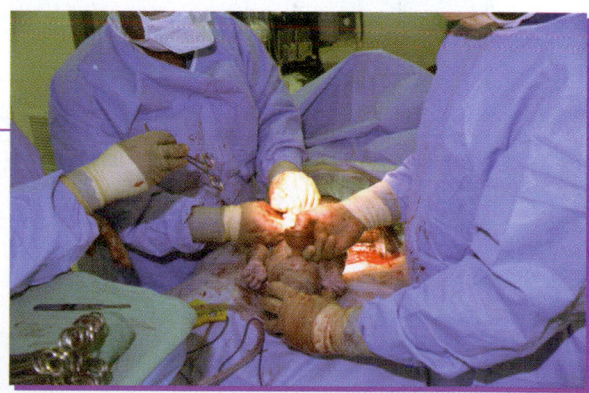

The infant's mouth and nose are suctioned immediately to remove amniotic fluid from the airway.

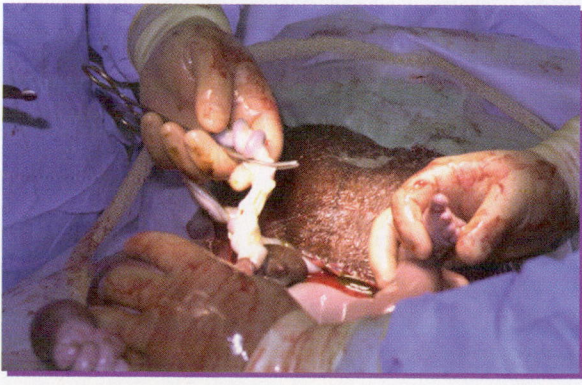

The infant's umbilical cord is cut and clamped.

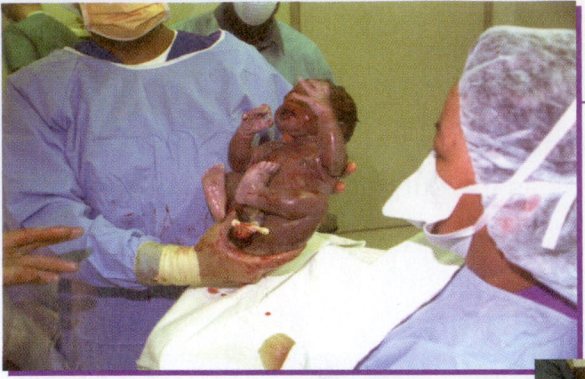

The infant is handed to the nursery personnel, who receive him in a sterile blanket.

Nursery personnel place the infant in a warmer and dry him to prevent heat loss by evaporation.

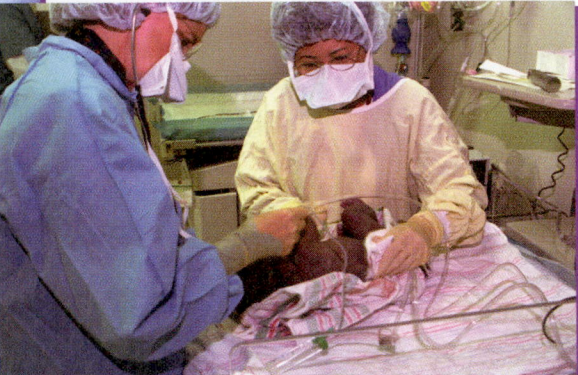

Cord blood samples are obtained.

The placenta is removed and the uterine cavity is examined for fragments of retained membranes.

The fundus of the uterus is removed from the abdominal cavity to assist the surgeon in visualizing the lower uterine segment for closure.

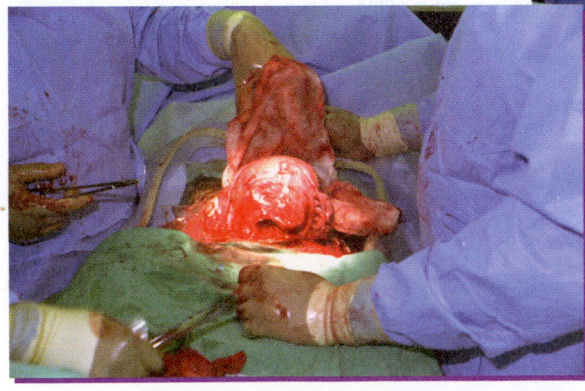

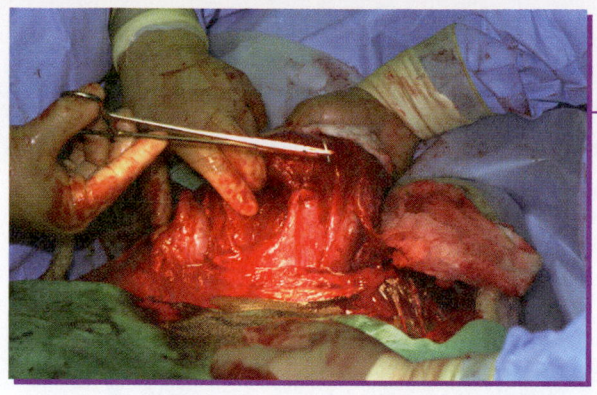

The surgeon sutures the lower uterine cavity to close the incision and control the bleeding.

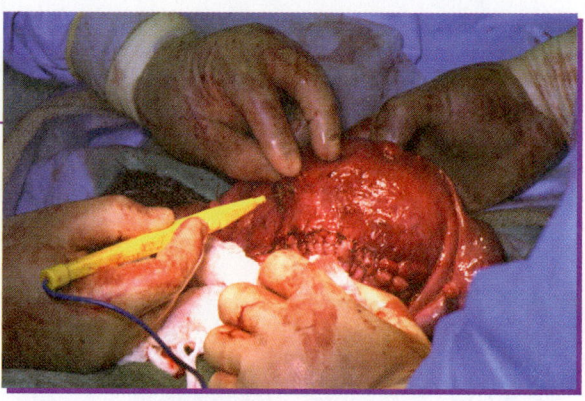

Once the major bleeding has been controlled, the smaller vessels are cauterized.

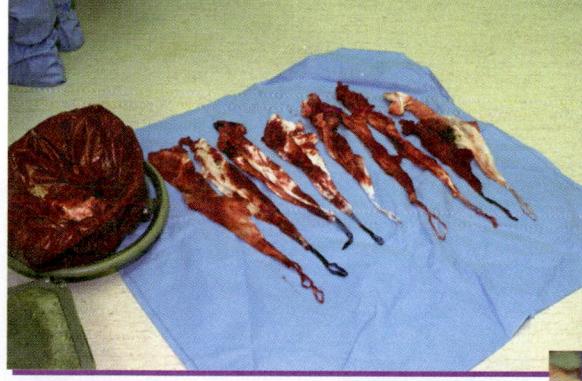

The circulating nurse and scrub nurse count lap sponges as the uterus is closed. A second sponge count occurs later, prior to closure of the peritoneum.

The bladder flap is repaired.

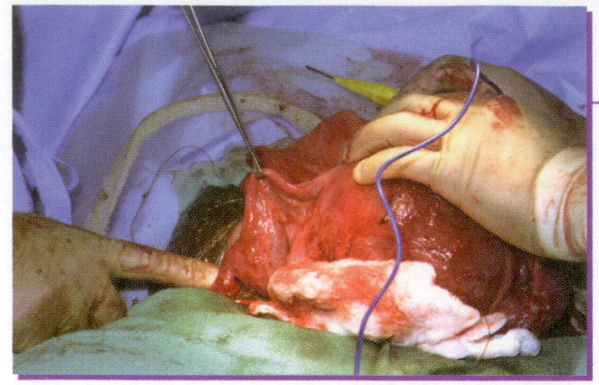

To begin the tubal ligation, the right fallopian tube is grasped with a Babcock clamp near the middle of the tube.

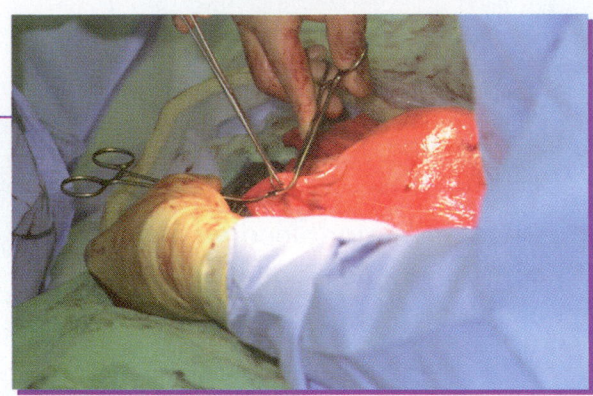

Kelley clamps are placed on each side of the Babcock.

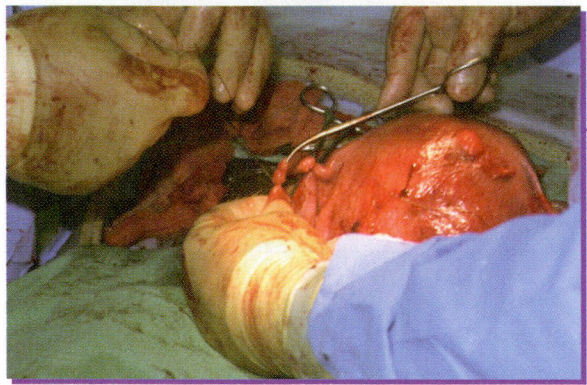

A suture is placed and tied to occlude the tube proximally and distally.

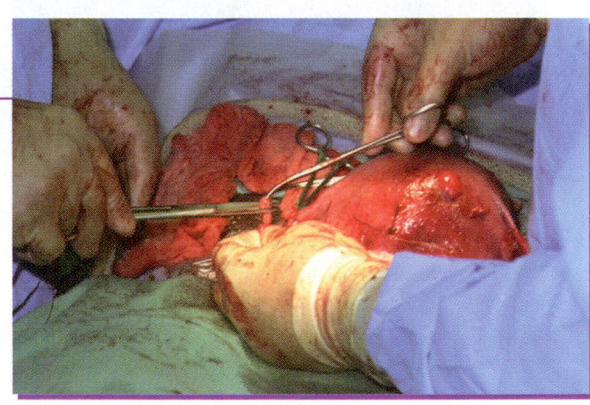

A segment of the tube between the two ligatures is removed.

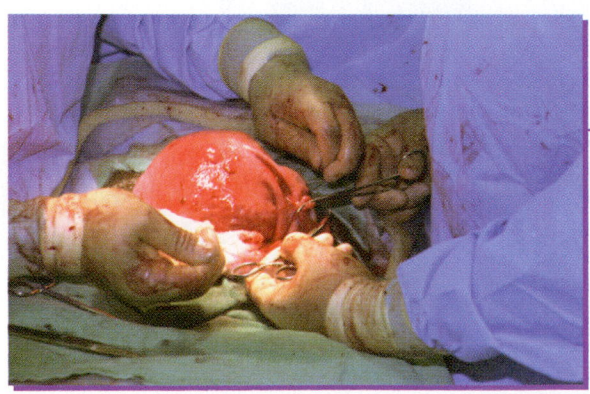

After the segment of tube is removed and the ligature is placed, the proximal end of the tube may be buried as an extra precaution.

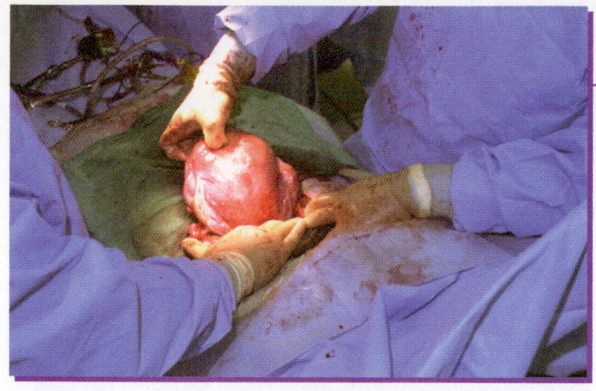

The contracted uterus is replaced into the abdominal cavity.

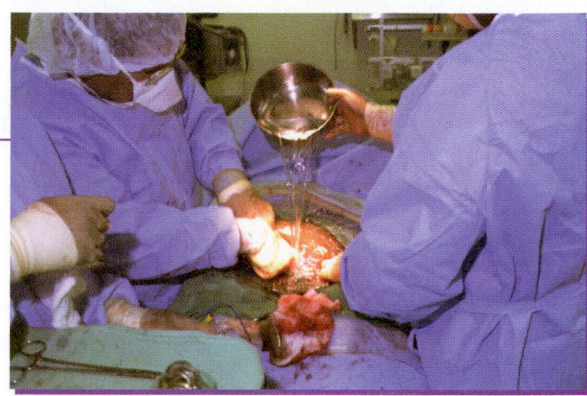

The abdominal cavity is irrigated to remove any blood clots and reduce infection.

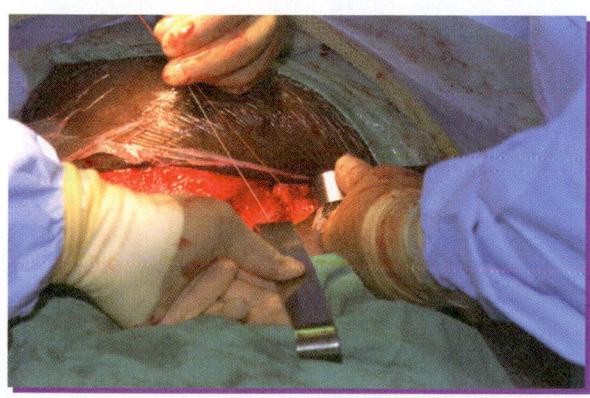

Each layer of tissue is reapproximated and sutured.

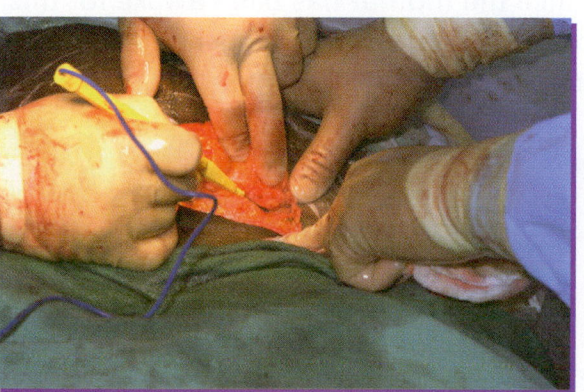

Care is taken to cauterize small bleeders during closure.

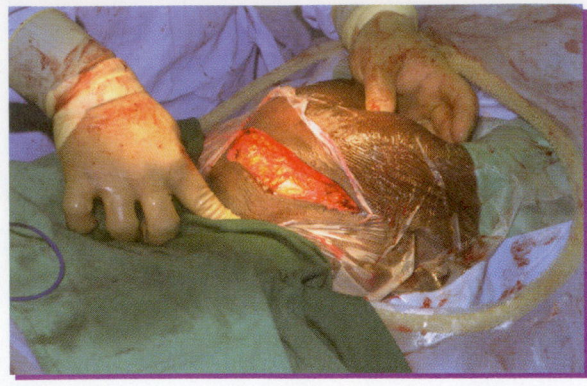

The abdominal opening is ready to be closed.

Skin staples are used to reapproximate the surface incision.

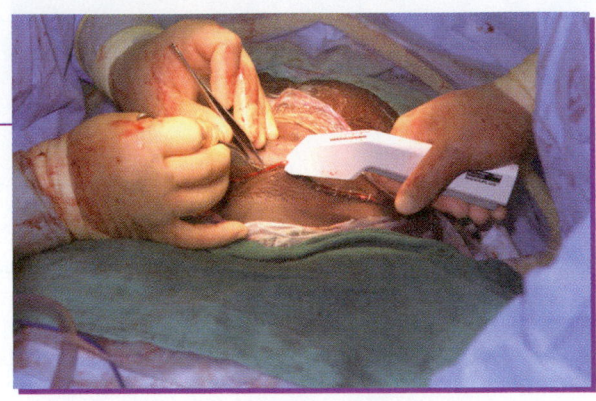

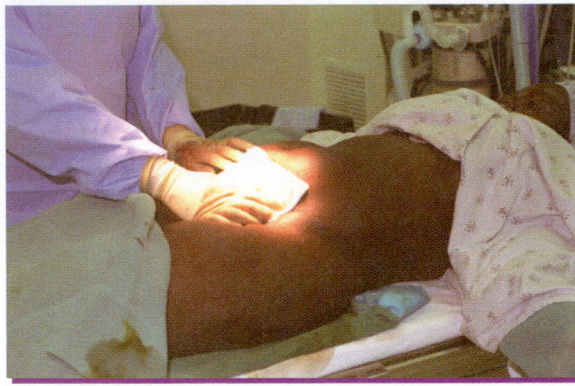

The lower abdomen is cleaned and a pressure dressing is applied.

Since the mother has been awake for this procedure, she and her husband have time to bond with their new son.

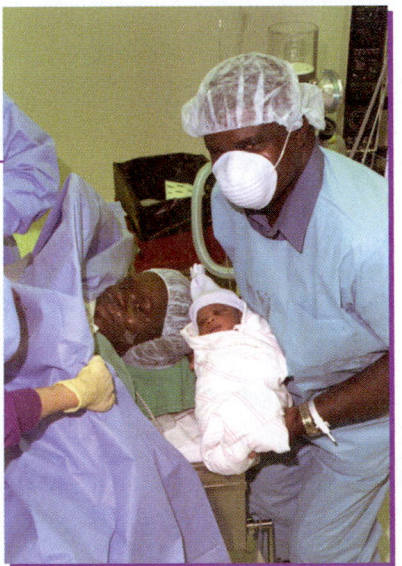

MATERNAL ADAPTATIONS TO LABOR

Maternal physiologic adaptations to the process of labor are complex and change rapidly throughout labor and delivery. To assess the client's status adequately, the nurse needs to understand the changes that occur during labor in the following systems: hematologic, cardiovascular, respiratory, renal, gastrointestinal, and endocrine systems.

Hematologic System

During labor, maternal hemoglobin levels increase slightly in response to the hemoconcentration. The increased hemoconcentration is related to the increases in erythropoiesis, muscular activity, and dehydration from blood and fluid loss. An increase in the leukocyte count is seen owing to an increase in neutrophils related to the stress response. It is not uncommon for a woman to have a leukocyte count from 25,000 to 30,000 mm^3 immediately after delivery, which often makes diagnosing an infection difficult.

The coagulation system is activated both before and after placental separation. The placenta and decidua are rich in thromboplastin, accounting for activation of the coagulation system. Because of all the changes in the coagulation system that occur during labor and immediately postpartum, the mother is in a hypercoaguable state. This is a compensatory mechanism to help protect the woman from postpartum hemorrhage (Blackburn & Loper, 2003).

Cardiovascular System

During labor a significant increase in maternal cardiac output occurs. Many factors contribute to this increase, including uterine contractions, pain, anxiety, and maternal position. During the first stage of labor, with each contraction approximately 400 mL of blood is emptied from the uterus into the maternal vascular system, increasing cardiac output by 10% to 15%. In the second stage of labor the increase in cardiac output is 30% to 50% (Blackburn & Loper, 2003).

An increase in blood pressure occurs during contractions, again related to the increase in blood flow to the maternal vascular system. An increase in systolic blood pressure of 10 mmHg can be expected with contractions in the first stage of labor. In the second stage of labor, systolic blood pressure may increase by 30 mmHg with each contraction. The diastolic pressure may increase by 25 mmHg with each contraction. It is important to carefully assess clients with underlying hypertension. Hypotension can occur in the supine position owing to compression of the ascending vena cava and descending aorta. In addition, medications used for anesthesia in labor sometimes can cause hypotension.

During the second stage of labor, the woman often is inclined to hold her breath and tighten her abdominal muscles, called the Valsalva maneuver, when pushing. The Valsalva maneuver can cause fetal hypoxia because the maternal pulse slows and cardiac output and blood pressure increase.

Respiratory System

An increase in oxygen consumption is associated with the increase in physical activity associated with labor. In addition, mild compensatory respiratory acidosis occurs to accommodate for mild metabolic alkalosis. By the end of the second stage of labor, the respiratory system can no longer fully compensate for the metabolic acidosis. Hyperventilation, which is common in labor, can cause respiratory acidosis, which can result in a decrease in the partial pressure of carbon dioxide in arterial blood. Symptoms of hyperventilation include dizziness and tingling. Nursing intervention includes counting the client's respirations aloud and informing her when a contraction is ending to help her relax. The acid-base disturbance quickly resolves after delivery because the respiratory rate returns to normal.

Renal System

During pregnancy the uterus displaces the bladder anteriorly, thus making it an abdominal organ, which causes a decrease in venous return, thus making it edematous. Edema and pressure placed on the bladder during labor can make voiding during labor very difficult and can cause overdistension of the bladder, often making urinary catheterization necessary.

Increased maternal and plasma renin levels as well as increased angiotensin levels are thought to be important in the control of uteroplacental blood flow (Blackburn & Loper, 2003).

Gastrointestinal System

During labor there are significant decreases in gastric emptying and gastric pH. The implication of these changes is the risk of vomiting with aspiration pneumonia. The use of narcotic pain medication can further decrease gastric emptying (Blackburn & Loper, 2003). Hyperventilation related to mouth breathing that occurs during labor can cause dehydration; however, because of the decreased gastric emptying it is important for the nurse to be cautious about the amount and type of oral fluids administered. With complete cervical dilation it is common for the client to experience nausea, belching, and sometimes vomiting. Diarrhea often is experienced at the onset of labor.

Endocrine System

As discussed previously, many changes occur within the endocrine system. In addition to the hormonal changes that occur during labor, metabolic change also occurs. An increase in the metabolic rate occurs related to the pain and work associated with labor, which is reflected by the decrease in glucose levels during labor.

FETAL ADAPTATIONS TO LABOR

Although the fetus experiences many mechanical and hemodynamic changes during parturition and birth, the full-term healthy infant can withstand these changes without adverse effects.

Fetal Heart Rate

Changes in the fetal heart rate (FHR) reflect fetal response to the labor process. Assessment of the FHR is an important nursing responsibility. During labor, the normal range for the FHR is 110 to 160 bpm (Feinstein & McCartney, 1997). Throughout labor, the nurse must record the FHR in terms of baseline, long-term variability, short-term variability, and the presence of periodic changes, that is,

accelerations and decelerations. Refer to the sections on assessment of fetal well-being for further discussion of these terms. For low-risk labors, FHR should be checked and recorded every 30 minutes for first stage of labor and every 15 minutes for second stage of labor.

Figure 13-15 illustrates areas for evaluating the FHR related to fetal position. The labor nurse must be knowledgeable about the effects of uterine activity, fetal movement, umbilical cord problems, vaginal exams, and medications on the FHR. In turn, the nurse must also know the appropriate responses and interventions to changes in the FHR that may indicate fetal intolerance of labor. Refer to the Nursing Alert regarding response to fetal intolerance of labor.

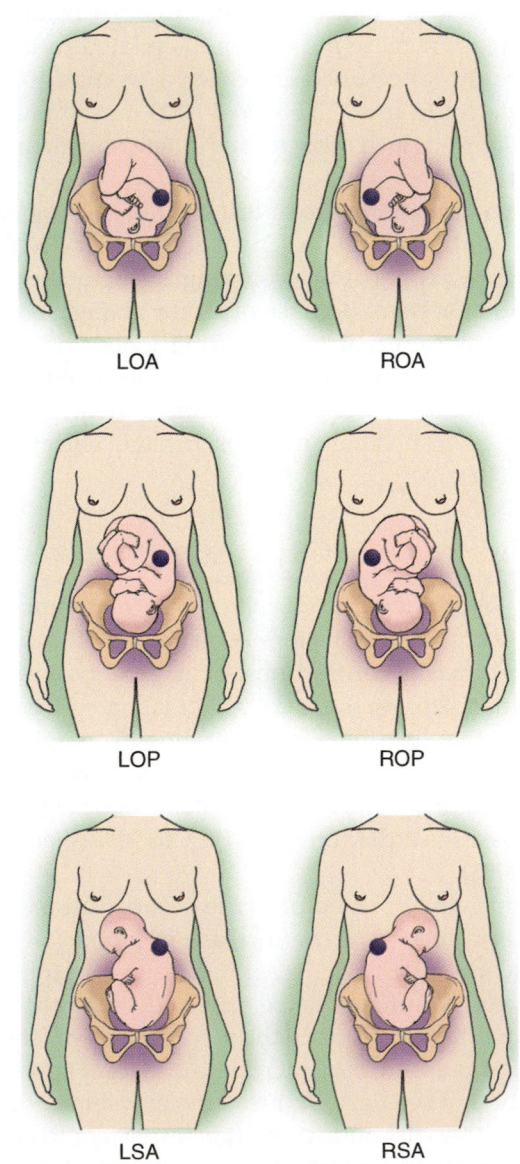

Figure 13-15   Based on Leopold's maneuvers, the fetal heart rate will best be heard in the marked areas for the various positions.

Nursing Alert

Management of Fetal Intolerance of Labor

The labor nurse must be prepared to respond to FHR changes such as bradycardia, decelerations, or changes in variability that may reflect fetal intolerance of labor. Interventions may include:

- Repositioning of the client to a side-lying position
- Turning off the oxytocin infusion
- Increasing the mainline IV
- Administering oxygen per facemask at 8 to 10 L/min
- Performing a vaginal exam to evaluate for umbilical cord prolapse
- Notifying the care provider
- Preparing to administer terbutaline (Brethine) 0.25 mg SQ if prescribed, to decrease uterine activity
- Continuously monitoring contractions and FHR

Fetal Respiratory System

The incidence of fetal breathing movements decreases before the onset of spontaneous labor. During active labor, fetal breathing movements continue to decrease. Fetal blood gases and pH change throughout the labor process. During early labor a gradual decrease in the capillary blood pH occurs; toward the end of labor this decrease is more rapid. The pH continues to decrease during the few minutes after birth. As the fetus passes through the birth canal, 7 to 42 mL of amniotic fluid is squeezed out of the fetal lungs. All of these changes help stimulate chemoreceptors in the aorta and carotids to prepare the fetus for spontaneous respirations after delivery (Manning, 1995).

Fetal Circulation

During the birth process the fetal circulation converts to that of an adult configuration within 60 seconds of the birth. The completion of this event may take up to 6 weeks. During this transition period the fetal oxygenation is transferred from the placenta to the lungs. As the placenta ceases to be the source of fetal circulation there is an increase in pulmonary blood flow and closure of the fetal cardiovascular shunts (Blackburn & Loper, 2003).

HISTORY OF ANALGESIA FOR CHILDBIRTH

The discomforts of childbirth have been acknowledged for thousands of years. For centuries it was thought that pain during childbirth was inevitable and to be endured. In comparison, the idea of pain relief during childbirth is a new concept (Morrision, Wildsmith, & Ostheimer, 1996). The advent of anesthesia in childbirth occurred in the mid-19th century in Great Britain and the United States. Dr. James Young Simpson, professor of midwifery at Edinburgh University is credited with being an early user of ether, and then chloroform, in obstetrical practice (Cohen, 1996). In 1849, the Committee on Obstetrics of the American Medical Association recommended the use of anesthesia in obstetrics, stating that pain relief in labor was justified (Morrison et al., 1996). After the early use of anesthesia in obstetrics, debate continued. Objections included medical concerns, need for physiologic pain during childbirth, and religious reasons. Medical concerns related to the newness of the field and safety of the mother and child. Some obstetricians regarded the mother's reaction to pain as a valuable guide to the progress of labor and, therefore, believed pain should not be relieved (Morrison et al., 1996). The religious objections were based on the interpretation of Genesis 3, verse 16, which was thought to imply that God had decreed that in pain would woman bring forth children (Cohen, 1996).

Rabbi Abraham De Sola, Canada's first rabbi, was asked to clarify the meaning of Genesis 3:16; in 1849, he published a three-part article detailing the interpretation. He concluded that the verse referred to the uterine contractions of labor and not the somatic sensation of pain, and, therefore, the use of anesthetics for pain relief in labor was not opposed by scripture (Cohen, 1996). The controversy died in Great Britain after Dr. John Snow administered chloroform to Queen Victoria, in 1853, for the birth of her ninth child, Prince Leopold (Morrison et al., 1996; Cohen, 1996; Kyle & Shampo, 1997; Ball, 1996). Because the queen was the head of the Church of England and defender of the faith, her use of anesthesia led to the end of the controversy on religious grounds, at least in Great Britain. Arguments continued over the safety of the practice (Connor & Connor, 1996). By 1862, however, chloroform and ether were in general use for anesthesia in obstetrics practice (Morrison et al., 1996).

During this same period, development proceeded in the use of parenteral opioids, first morphine and later meperidine (Demerol), and the use of both parenteral and inhalation anesthesia (Morrison et al., 1996). The early 20th century saw an increased use of twilight sleep, a result of the addition of scopolamine to morphine, with resultant analgesia, amnesia, and maternal restlessness. The high incidence of neonatal respiratory depression caused this technique to fall into disrepute (Morrison et al., 1996). Although a movement known as natural childbirth began in the 1940s and 1950s, it did not become prevalent in the United States until the 1960s when the Lamaze method of prepared childbirth was introduced (Sandelowski, 1984).

The technique of epidural anesthesia was known in the first half of the 20th century; however, its use in obstetrics was limited. Refinement of the technique and improvement in the available equipment and drugs led to an increased use of epidural anesthesia (Morrison et al., 1996). Research continues to make further refinements in techniques and medication combinations. Today, clients facing childbirth have a vast array of options for pain relief in labor and delivery.

THEORIES OF PAIN AND PAIN MANAGEMENT

Pain has been the subject of interest for centuries. In 1965, the gate-control theory of pain was proposed by Melzak and Wall (Morrison et al., 1996). The gate-control theory proposed that pain is a result of activity in several interacting neural systems. Each of these nervous systems, peripheral and central, has different functions. In the gate-control theory, sensory information can only pass from the peripheral nervous system to the central nervous

Nursing Alert

Over-the-Counter Medications

Remember to ask clients about over-the-counter medications and dietary supplements, including herbal preparations. Clients often do not volunteer this information unless specifically asked. Many of these preparations can interact with analgesic and anesthetic agents.

system (CNS) when the physiologic "gate" is open. When the gate is closed due to the release of inhibitory neurotransmitters, endogenous opioids, or lock, then sensory information is blocked. This mechanism explains the effectiveness of both physical (e.g., rubbing, massage, transcutaneous electrical nerve stimulation [TENS], and water therapy) and psychologic (e.g., focus points, breathing exercises, and encouragement) methods of pain relief (Nichols and Humenick, 2000).

Pain is an individual experience. It can be influenced by a number of factors such as cultural practices, anxiety, fear, previous experiences with pain, and psychologic support. These factors also are present during the experience of childbirth. It is useful for the nurse to identify in advance the most frequently seen client ethnic groups and develop profiles of culturally specific childbirth practices, including pain behaviors (Weber, 1996). However, the nurse should be concerned about stereotyping clients or failing to adapt to individual clients. The nurse must be aware of and sensitive to individual variations in a client's choices for dealing with pain in labor and delivery. The client may choose to use pharmacologic methods, nonpharmacologic methods, or both, to meet her needs. The nurse must be able to teach, review, and assist the client to implement a variety of pain relief methods. The nurse also must respect the client's prerogative to choose, as long as the method chosen is safe for the mother and child at that time.

ANALGESIA AND ANESTHESIA

It is important to have a clear understanding of the concepts of analgesia and anesthesia. **Analgesia** is the relief of pain. This can be complete relief or some lesser degree of relief. Analgesia can be provided by a variety of techniques, including administration of medications. **Anesthesia** is the absence of sensation. Whereas the absence of sensation could imply complete relief of pain, the opposite is not necessarily true. Anesthesia also can be provided by a variety of techniques.

Types of Anesthesia

Anesthesia techniques fall into three categories: local, regional, and general anesthesia. The different types of anesthesia have different applications, actions, effects, and requirements. Some types of anesthesia are instituted by the obstetrician or Certified Nurse Midwife (CNM); others require the assistance of a provider whose specialty is anesthesia.

Local Anesthesia

Local infiltration anesthesia refers to the loss of sensation from a small area of the body after infiltration with a local anesthetic. **Local anesthetic** refers to a class of drugs that produce reversible blockade of electrical impulses along nerve fibers (Williams, 1997). Blockade is produced by preventing sodium ions from passing through selective channels in the membrane of the nerve (Stoelting & Miller, 1994).

Regional Anesthesia

The second category of anesthesia techniques is **regional anesthesia**, which is the loss of sensation from a large area of the body owing to blockade of neural impulses. The most common regional anesthesia techniques in obstetrics are the subarachnoid block, or spinal, and the epidural. Pudendal nerve blockade is another form of regional anesthesia found in obstetrics and also is discussed subsequently.

General Anesthesia

The third category of anesthesia techniques is **general anesthesia**, which is the loss of sensation from the entire body secondary to the loss of consciousness produced by intravenous (IV) or inhalation anesthetic agents. Unconsciousness does not prevent the transmission of neural impulses of pain and other sensations; rather, it prevents the brain from interpreting the neural impulses into conscious awareness. Unconsciousness is not the only factor involved in general anesthesia. Other aspects—amnesia, analgesia, and muscle relaxation—also need to be provided through administration of other medications.

PAIN IN LABOR AND DELIVERY

In order to understand the requirements for analgesia or anesthesia, it is necessary to briefly review the nature and transmission of pain in the process of labor. Pain is a highly individualized experience with painful stimuli interpreted within the brain (Fiedler & Shaw, 1997). The philosophy behind prepared childbirth or psychoprophylaxis is that ignorance, misinformation, fear, and anxiety appear to intensify pain (Santos, Pederson, & Finster, 1997). Education of the client regarding expectations of labor increases her ability to deal with the stress of labor. The intermittent nature of pain in labor is a primary contributor to the challenge in providing analgesia through some options. These challenges include the contrast in pain levels between the peak of a contraction and the period between contractions. What would be an appropriate blood level of medication for pain relief at the peak of contractions would be too much for the periods between contractions.

Types of Pain

The pattern of pain in labor is fairly predictable (Nichols & Humenick, 2000) (Figure 13-16). During the first stage of labor, pain results from cervical dilation and uterine contractions. These pain impulses are carried via C-fibers through the lower thoracic dermatomes T-10 to L-1 (Fiedler & Shaw, 1997). A **dermatome** is an area of the body innervated through a specific spinal nerve (Figure 13-17). The degree of pain changes as dilation progresses, and

maternal tolerance of the changes varies but often is impacted by the duration of labor. Exhaustion from loss of sleep or prolonged labor contributes to increased pain perception (Youngstrom, Baker, & Miller, 1996; Morrision et al., 1996). When tired, a person may have less energy and a poor ability to deal with pain.

As labor progresses, with descent of the fetal head into the pelvis, another pathway appears to be the primary one (Fiedler & Shaw, 1997). The second stage of labor includes distention of the vagina and perineum by the fetal head, resulting in pain impulses being transmitted through the pudendal nerve. The pudendal nerve is composed of fibers that enter the spinal column through the sacral nerves S-2 to S-4 (Santos et al., 1997).

If the fetal head is descending in the occipitoposterior position, the force of contractions will push the fetal head into the client's sacrum and coccyx. The sacrum is in a relatively fixed position, and pressure exerted against it will result in the client perceiving pain to be in her lower back.

The stretching of the perineum just before delivery of the fetal head often is described by clients as an intense,

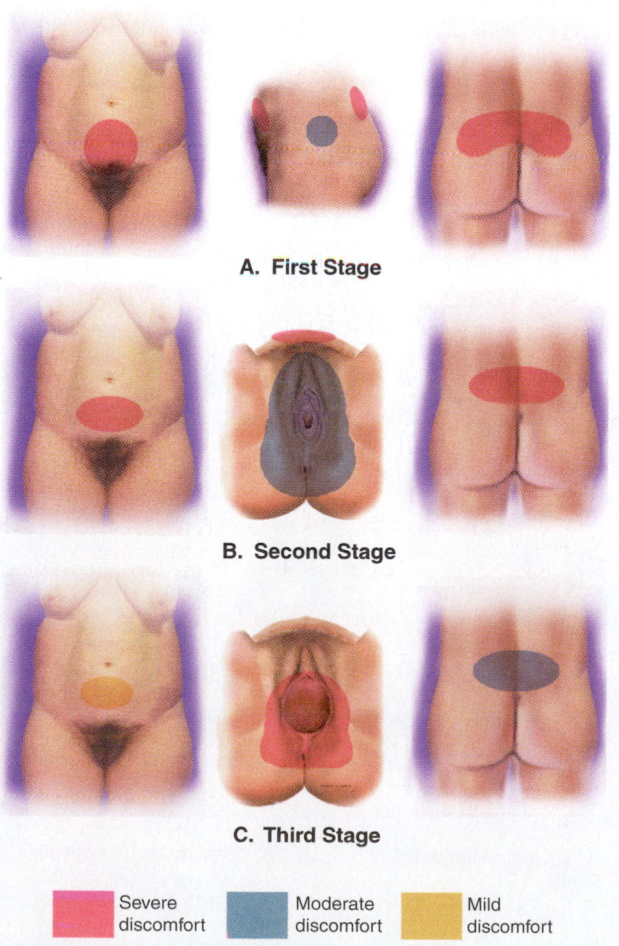

A. First Stage

B. Second Stage

C. Third Stage

| Severe discomfort | Moderate discomfort | Mild discomfort |

Figure 13-16   Intensity and distribution of labor discomfort.

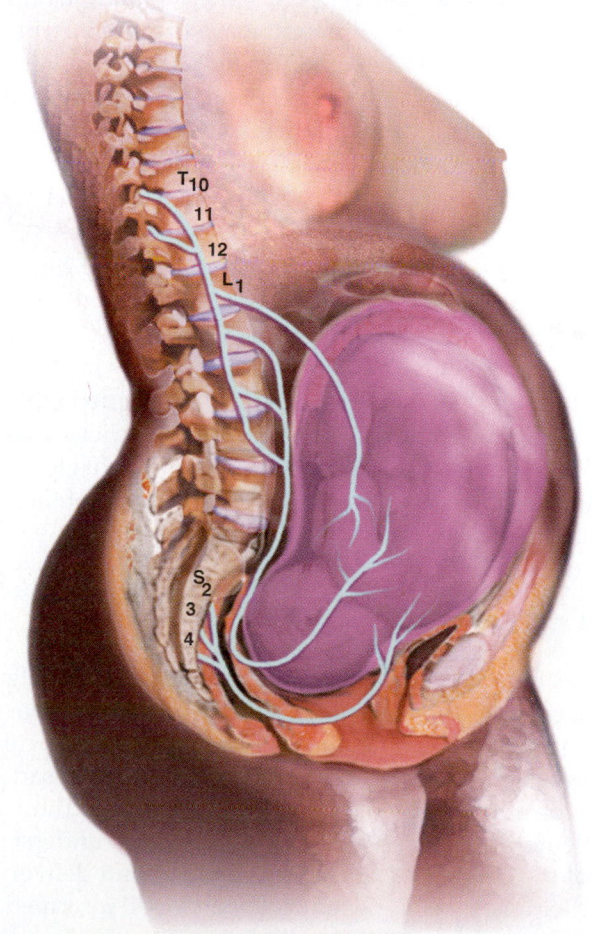

T10
11
12
L1

S2
3
4

Figure 13-17   Pain pathways.

burning sensation. Other specific pain sensations may be indicative of an abnormal presentation, such as an occipitoposterior position, or a different problem, such as uterine rupture (Fiedler & Shaw, 1997).

Considerations in Medication for Pain

Above all else, the first consideration regarding medication for pain in pregnancy, labor, and delivery is the safety of the mother and baby. The focal concern during labor is respiratory depression of either the mother or neonate and the possible complications as a result of maternal or neonatal depression. Therefore careful monitoring of clients choosing to use medications, including FHT and cervical dilation, is necessary. The nurse must be vigilant and knowledgeable about the medications being used and the individual nature of the response of the client to them.

Client Experience with Pain

The nurse must always recognize that pain is a very individual experience. It is subjective in nature and can only be defined by the client experiencing the pain, who may communicate in many different ways that are interpreted by the nurse. Misunderstandings may arise if the nurse is not aware of the personal beliefs and biases regarding pain and pain behaviors, particularly in clients from other cultural backgrounds (Weber, 1996).

Nursing Implications

Nurses and clients should discuss plans regarding pain relief early in labor. Assessment of the client's understanding of different methods of pain relief can illustrate educational needs. The nurse should convey information or act as the client's advocate to acquire needed information regarding pain relief methods. If the client asks for medication, the nurse should inform her of what to expect regarding the onset, duration, and side effects of the individual medication.

ANALGESIA IN LABOR

Clients currently have a number of options for analgesia during labor (Table 13-3). The nurse plays an important role in client education, that is, in conveying and confirming information regarding the advantages and disadvantages of many available options to the client. The client may enter the labor process with little or no understanding of the course or expectations of labor and delivery, or the client may be highly educated and well informed but seek the opinion of those she expects to have greater knowledge and experience. An understanding of the impact of parenteral and regional analgesia in labor will allow the nurse to anticipate problems that might, if undetected, jeopardize the safety of the mother and baby.

Parenteral Analgesia

Parenteral analgesia, administration of drugs by the IM or IV route, has a long history of use in obstetrics to provide some degree of analgesia for the client in labor. Refer to Table 13-3 for an explanation of this method of pain management in labor.

Regional Analgesia

Regional techniques, alone or in combination with other techniques, are commonly used to provide analgesia for labor pain (Ellis, 1997). Regional analgesia options for labor include the use of intrathecal opioids, epidural blocks, and spinal-epidural combination.

A review of the anatomy of the spinal column and epidural space is needed to fully understand the mechanism by which these techniques provide analgesia or anesthesia to the client (Figure 13-18). The spinal cord ends approximately at the level of the first or second lumbar vertebrae, L-1, L-2 (Ostheimer & Leavitt, 1996). It is

---

Reflections from a Nurse

Before epidurals were available I gave Demerol to clients in labor. There were some things that I could watch for because they happened a lot. I always put an emesis basin within reach because a fair number of the women would be nauseated or vomit. I had to really watch the multiparas when I gave them Demerol at 5 cm dilated, because after they threw up a couple of times they would look at you with eyes the size of dinner plates and say "The baby is coming." You had better believe them, because often they were right. The increased intra-abdominal pressure created by vomiting would push that baby down against the cervix, and they would go from 5 cm to complete in minutes. It didn't happen all the time but often enough to watch for it.

Table 13-3   Analgesia Options for Labor

TYPE OF ANALGESIA	MEDICATIONS USED	ROUTES OF ADMINISTRATION	ADVANTAGES	DISADVANTAGES	NURSING IMPLICATIONS
Parenteral Analgesia					
Opioids (also known as narcotics)	1. Demerol: appears to cause a lesser degree of neonatal respiratory depression than morphine 2. Fentanyl: useful in situations requiring rapid onset and short duration such as forceps application 3. Nubain (nalbuphine) and Stadol (butorpha-nol): can produce some maternal sedation, but have lower incidences of nausea and vomiting	These medications are generally administered IV at prescribed intervals. Demerol may also be administered via a patient-controlled intravenous infusion device (PCIA) or intramuscularly (IM).	Ease of administration Can be administered by a nurse	**Maternal:** Inadequate pain relief Nausea Vomiting Drowsiness Possible histamine release **Fetal:** Central nervous system depression Respiratory depression Decreased variability noted in the FHR tracing	Assess cervical dilation prior to administration. Provide client education about pain management in labor. Monitor maternal response. Monitor FHR. Prepare for possible neonatal respiratory depression at birth. This is especially important if opioids are administered within 4 hours of birth. Refer to the Nursing Tip on neonatal respiratory depression.
Regional Analgesia					
1. Intrathecal opioids	Morphine, fentanyl, or sufentanil (Sufenta)	Opioids, rather than local anesthetics, are injected just inside the dural sac. Medication is administered into the spinal fluid using a small-gauge spinal needle.	Rapid onset of pain relief No sympathetic block (no hypotension) No motor block (client is able to ambulate)	Labor may last longer than the duration of the analgesia. Maternal sedation Nausea Vomiting Itching Maternal respiratory depression is more common if morphine is used.	Provide client education regarding steps of the procedure and that the contractions will be perceived as pressure rather than pain. A consent must be obtained. Client must have IV access. Administer the prescribed bolus of IV fluid to counteract hypotensive effects. Assist the anesthesia provider with client positioning. Monitor maternal and fetal response.

(continues)

Table 13-3   Analgesia Options for Labor (continued)

TYPE OF ANALGESIA	MEDICATIONS USED	ROUTES OF ADMINISTRATION	ADVANTAGES	DISADVANTAGES	NURSING IMPLICATIONS
2. Epidural block	Dilute solution of a local anesthetic and an opioid	Medication is administered into the epidural space through a small catheter that is left in place.	Provides excellent analgesia Titratable when administered as a continuous infusion Indefinite duration	Client is confined to bed. Frequent vital signs are required. Hypotension is a possible side effect. May interfere with maternal pushing efforts Possible headache if the dura is punctured	In addition to all of the above: Frequently monitor vital signs. Instruct the client to remain in bed. Assess bladder filling, because client will not be aware of need to void.
3. Combined intrathecal-epidural block	An intrathecal opioid such as fentanyl or sufentanil followed by a continuous infusion of a local anesthetic and an opioid	First the dura is punctured using a spinal-epidural needle combination, and a small amount of fentanyl or sufentanil is injected. The spinal needle is withdrawn and a catheter is inserted through the epidural needle. This needle is withdrawn and the catheter is securely taped to the client's back.	Combines rapid pain relief with the ability to provide analgesia over an indeterminate amount of time After 30 minutes of monitoring for postural hypotension following administration of the intrathecal opioid, the client may ambulate. When the client becomes uncomfortable again, she returns to bed and the continuous epidural infusion is begun.	Accidental subarachnoid administration in the presence of a dural puncture	The same as for intrathecal opioids and then for an epidural block when that infusion is begun.
4. Paracervical block	Local anesthetic	Medication is injected into the vaginal wall near the cervix at 3 and 9 o'clock.	Good pain relief for the first stage of labor	Short acting and may need to be repeated Does not provide analgesia for second stage Associated with fetal bradycardia	Monitor maternal and fetal response. Be alert for fetal bradycardia.

Note. Adapted from *Maternal, Neonatal, and Women's Health Nursing* by L. Littleton and J. Engebretson, 2002, Clifton Park, NY: Delmar Learning.

Nursing Tip

Assessment and Treatment of the Neonate with Opioid-Induced Respiratory Depression

1. Place infant under warmer and dry thoroughly, removing wet linen.

2. Position and open airway, if needed.

3. Suction mouth and nose.

4. Evaluate respiratory efforts.

5. Provide tactile stimulation: rub back, flick the heel, or slap the foot briefly if infant does not have adequate respirations.

6. If neonate has no respirations or only gasping respirations, begin positive-pressure ventilation with a bag and mask to deliver 100% oxygen.

7. Evaluate heart rate.

8. If heart rate is below 60, continue ventilation and begin chest compressions.

9. If heart rate is 60 to 100 and increasing, continue ventilation.

10. If heart rate is below 80 and not increasing, continue ventilation and begin chest compressions.

11. If heart rate is above 100, watch for spontaneous respirations and discontinue ventilation.

12. If heart rate remains below 80 after 30 seconds of positive-pressure ventilation with 100% oxygen, medications may be needed and additional help should be summoned.

13. Evaluate color; if blue, continue to provide 100% oxygen.

14. If pink or there is peripheral cyanosis, observe and monitor.

15. Note: Careful observation of the neonate with suspected drug-induced respiratory depression continues after this period of stimulation because the decrease in stimulation may result in hypoventilation at this point.

16. If severe respiratory depression is present or maternal opioid has been administered in the past 4 hours, naloxone (Narcan) may be needed. The dosage is 0.1 mg/kg, preferably IV, or through an endotracheal tube. IM or SQ routes are acceptable but onset of action will be delayed.

17. Note: Duration of opioid may exceed duration of naloxone. Infant will need continued observation and assessment for return of respiratory depression. Notify nursery personnel of administration.

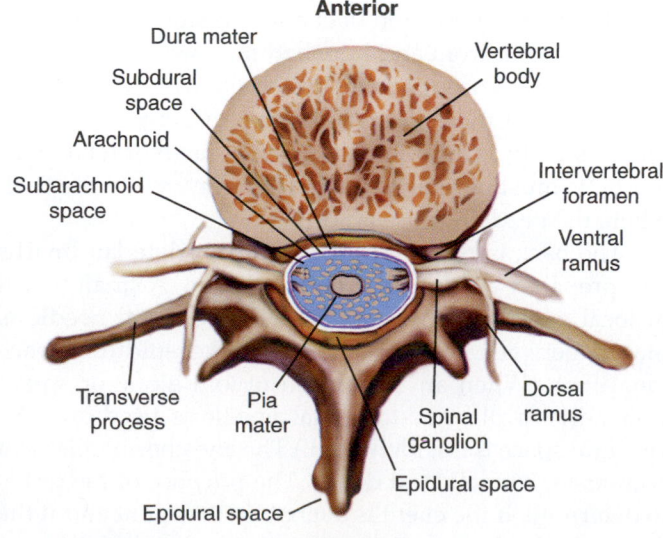

Figure 13-18   Cross-section of the spinal canal area.

protected by the dural sac and lies within the vertebrae. Below L-1, L-2 the dural sac contains spinal nerve roots. The epidural space lies between the dura and vertebral canal (Benards, 1997). Nerves and blood vessels travel through the epidural space, which is occupied by fat globules (Luyendijk, 1996).

The major factors involved in analgesia or anesthesia provided by regional techniques include the types of drugs used, dosages, anatomic level and area of placement, and client position. Individual differences in these factors impact the analgesia produced in a specific client. Refer to Table 13-3 for descriptions of regional techniques.

Preparation of the Client

The nursing actions to prepare the client and assist the anesthesia provider during initiation of intrathecal, epidural, or combined techniques are virtually identical.

Critical Thinking

Client and Partner Conflicts Regarding Analgesia and Anesthesia in Labor and Delivery

It is not unheard of for clients to change their minds regarding options for pain relief in labor and delivery, especially as pain intensifies.

- What will you do if the client requests medications or anesthesia and the partner disagrees?
- What if the client has had medications and now wants an epidural but her partner disagrees?
- Can the client give informed consent while under the influence of medication?
- What will you do?

Box 13-2

Contraindications to Regional Analgesia and Anesthesia

- Absolute
  - Client refusal
  - Severe hemorrhage
  - Significant coagulopathy
  - Infection at the site
- Relative
  - Sepsis
  - Neurologic disorder
  - Heparinization
  - Spinal deformity
  - Extensive spinal surgery or hardware
  - Metastatic disease in the lumbar spine

The client's desire for regional analgesia should be confirmed and the obstetrician notified before the procedure. IV access must be obtained, if not already available, and a bolus of fluid should be given just before the procedure. The CRNA or anesthesiologist must assess the client requesting regional analgesia. The client's medical history; physical status; understanding of the procedure, including risks and benefits; and consent for the procedure must be obtained (Fiedler & Shaw, 1997). It is very important to answer any questions the client may have regarding the risks and benefits of regional analgesia before the procedure is begun to create an atmosphere of trust and confidence and to fulfill conditions of informed consent. Box 13-2 lists the absolute and relative contraindications to regional analgesia and anesthesia.

After all questions of the client have been answered and informed consent has been obtained, the client is assisted to a sitting position (feet over the side of the bed, or cross-legged in front and hunched forward) or side-lying position (with knees and feet drawn up toward her chest), depending on the preference of the anesthesia provider (Figures 13-19 and 13-20). The client's gown or fetal monitor belts must be moved away from the area of the back where the needle will be placed.

The back is palpated for the appropriate landmarks and prepared with an antiseptic solution. A small wheal of local anesthetic is made, and the epidural needle is placed between the vertebrae and the epidural space identified. (When an intrathecal opioid alone or spinal anesthesia is planned, a spinal needle is used and the epidural space is not identified.) The anesthesiologist will administer a small "test dose." The purpose of the test is to determine if the client is allergic to the agent and if the catheter is in the correct position. Immediately following the procedure and each time a new dose is given, assess

---

Client Education

Important Information for the Anesthesia Provider

Before administration of medication, the anesthesia provider must ascertain the client's health history on the following:

- Drug or other allergies
- Smoking history
- Breathing problems
- Cardiac problems
- Other health problems
- Previous anesthetics
- Difficulties with nausea or vomiting with previous anesthetics
- CBC platelets

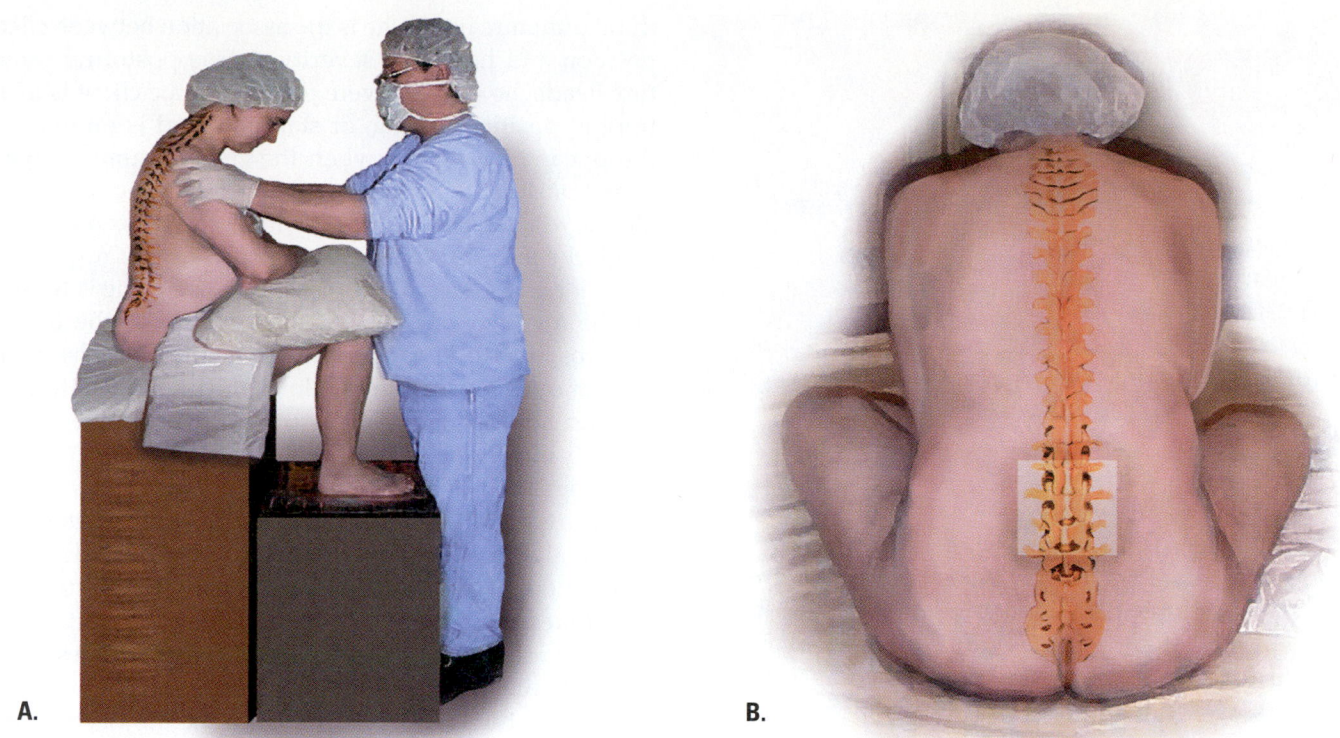

Figure 13-19   Sitting position for insertion of spinal or epidural anesthesia. A. Lateral view. B. Posterior view.

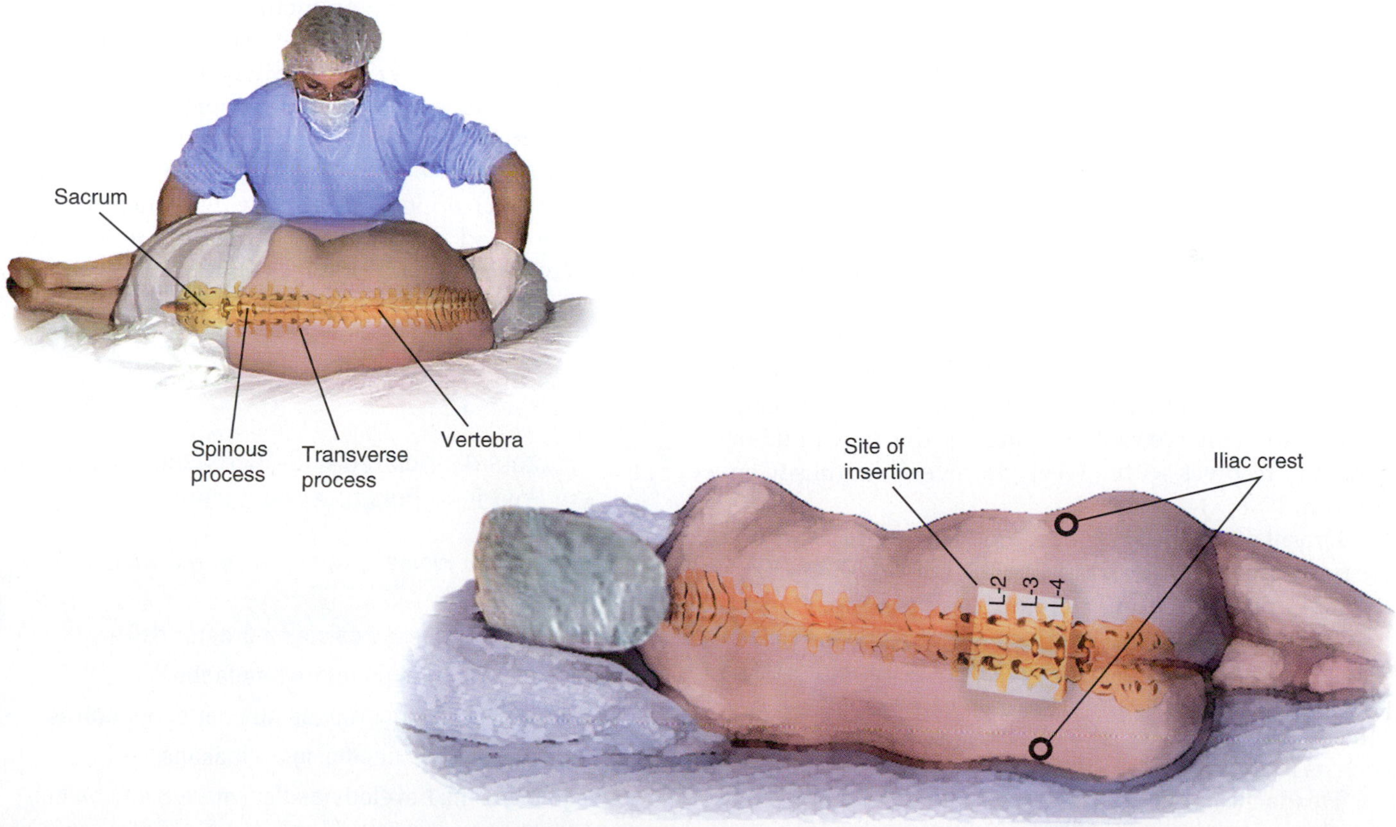

Sacrum

Spinous process

Transverse process

Vertebra

Site of insertion

Iliac crest

L-2

L-3

L-4

Figure 13-20   Side-lying position for insertion of spinal or epidural anesthesia.

Nursing Alert

Possible Side Effects and Complications of Epidural Analgesia

- Hypotension
- Urinary retention
- Total spinal anesthesia
- Neurologic injury
- Unsatisfactory block
- Unintentional subarachnoid (spinal) block

the fetal heart and the maternal blood pressure. A drop in blood pressure can be life threatening to the fetus. In addition, epidural anesthesia may cause a temporary rise in maternal temperature. This fact has led to an increase in unnecessary septic workups. The most important task of the nurse is to assist the client in not moving and remaining in an optimal position during the procedure. A knowledgeable nurse is a great asset to the anesthesia provider performing regional analgesia and anesthesia techniques (Fiedler & Shaw, 1997). The anesthesia provider will indicate when it is safe for the client to move.

Possible Complications with Regional Analgesia/Anesthesia

Numerous long-term complications from regional anesthesia are possible but very rare. Trauma to a nerve root or spinal cord is possible. Administration of lumbar puncture below the level of L-1, L-2 decreases the risk of spinal cord trauma because the spinal cord usually ends above this level. Trauma to the nerve root is possible but extremely rare (Concepcion, 1996). Paresthesias or hyperalgesia in the area innervated by that nerve root indicates damage to the nerve root. Fortunately, this type of injury generally resolves within weeks to several months (Concepcion, 1996).

Drasner and Swisher (1996) indicate that risk factors for postdural puncture headache include age, body habitus, specifics of the needle, and multiple insertion attempts (Box 13-3). Postdural puncture headache occurs when the dura mater of the spinal cord is punctured. The puncture can be deliberate, such as in administration of intrathecal opioids or spinal anesthesia, or accidental, such as in the case of epidural anesthesia.

Headaches after childbirth are not uncommon; they may be due to a number of causes other than regional anesthesia. The distinguishing characteristic of a post-dural puncture headache is the association between client position and headache severity. A true postdural puncture headache causes severe pain when the client is in an upright position, sitting, or standing, and is minimal or disappears completely when the client assumes a horizontal position (Chadwick & Ross, 1992). The onset usually is within the first 5 days after the procedure. The headache may last for days and usually is not responsive to minor analgesics. The cause of the headache is tension on the meninges of the brain as a result of the loss of cerebrospinal fluid through the puncture site. The lower level of cerebrospinal fluid allows the brain to shift more than usual when the client assumes the upright position, causing more severe pain when the client is sitting or standing. Treatment of postdural puncture headache includes hydration to assist the body in replacing the cerebrospinal fluid; analgesics, which may provide some relief; and oral or IV caffeine for cerebral vasoconstriction. When these treatments are unsuccessful, the next step is an "epidural blood patch." This technique is successful in over 95% of clients. It is an invasive technique, however, and carries the risks of additional puncture of the dura, which will result in worsening of headache, and arachnoiditis (if the blood is injected into the subarachnoid space). The technique involves placement of an epidural needle, preferably in the same vertebral interspace as the original puncture, and venipuncture and withdrawal of 20 mL of the client's blood by an assistant, often the nurse. The anesthesia provider then slowly injects the blood through the epidural needle into the epidural space. The client is instructed to lie quietly for the next 30 minutes and curtail activities over the next several hours. The epidural blood patch appears to work by two different mechanisms: the blood clots and plugs the hole in the dura; and the volume of blood in the epidural space increases

Box 13-3

Factors Associated with Increased Risk of Postdural Puncture Headache

- Age: younger women are at greater risk than are older women
- Body habitus: obesity carries a greater risk
- Previous postdural puncture headache
- Multiple attempts: increased number of punctures
- Needle size: large needle, more leakage
- Needle design: beveled needles, more than conical needles

Reflections from a Laboring Mother

When I got to the hospital I was 4 cm dilated. Although I had managed pretty well so far, I knew what was coming. With my first baby, once I got to be 6 cm the contractions started to hurt a lot worse and that's when I got the epidural. Talk about the difference between day and night! I felt the contractions as pressure, but they were not as painful as they had been before the epidural. With my second baby, I asked for the epidural as soon as I just got into the labor-delivery room. I didn't want to miss getting one because my labor was moving too fast.

the pressure within the spinal canal, which increases the cerebrospinal fluid level surrounding the brain (Fiedler & Shaw, 1997).

Hematoma in the spinal canal is a rare complication but one that can result in spinal cord compression or ischemia (Drasner & Swisher, 1996). The damage may range from sensory or motor weakness to quadriplegia and death. Presenting symptoms may include lower body muscle weakness, back pain, and sensory deficit. Delays in recognition, diagnosis, and treatment have been correlated with more severe damage (Drasner & Swisher, 1996). Concern about this complication is one of the reasons that spinal and epidural anesthesia methods are contraindicated in the presence of severe coagulopathies.

Epidural analgesia may contribute to some neurologic injuries. Because of the relaxation and decreased pain sensation provided by the epidural, it is possible to excessively flex the client's legs while positioning during pushing. Overstretching of the nerves passing through the pelvis may result. Clients may report parathesias or numbness in one foot or leg that can be severe or last long enough to require the use of a cane or walker for weeks to months. Any report of numbness, parathesisa, or weakness that lasts longer that the expected duration of the regional or epidural analgesia should be referred to the anesthesia provider for further evaluation.

The diminishment of uterine contractions after IV fluid boluses has been noted previously. Studies have indicated some diminishment in uterine activity in women receiving epidural analgesia with epinephrine-containing solutions (Chantigian & Chantigian, 1996).

An increased duration of the second stage of labor is common enough that the American College of Obstetricians and Gynecologists revised the guidelines for defining prolonged second stage of labor. In the presence of epidural analgesia, prolonged second stage of labor is defined as more than 3 hours in nulliparous women and more than 2 hours in parous women. These guidelines encourage careful assessment of the client's motor and sensory functions as she is preparing to start pushing. It has been recommended that pushing should be delayed if the client lacks motor or sensory function (Hawkins, Hess, Kubicek, Joyce, & Morrow, 1996).

The impact of epidural analgesia on the progress of labor and modes of delivery is a topic that has been studied by numerous researchers in the past and continues to be studied today. There are multiple studies with results that support both sides of the controversy. There is no definitive answer to the questions raised; however, research continues toward improving our understanding and refining techniques. The nurse should be aware of the ongoing research to further her own knowledge and assist the client in fully understanding the risks and benefits involved in the vast array of options currently available for pain relief in labor and delivery.

ANESTHESIA FOR DELIVERY

Anesthesia options for delivery include local anesthetic infiltration; regional techniques, such as a pudendal nerve block, a spinal, or an epidural; and general anesthesia. Without subjecting the client or fetus to unnecessary risks, the goal is to provide analgesia and anesthesia to meet the client's wishes and the requirements of the mode of delivery (Hawkins, Chestnut, & Gibbs, 1996). Modes of delivery include spontaneous vaginal, forceps (outlet, low, or mid), vacuum extraction, and cesarean section. Table 13-4 lists the specific modes of delivery and appropriate anesthesia techniques. The accompanying photo story highlights the technique of spinal anesthesia administration.

Local Infiltration

Infiltration of the perineal tissues with 10 to 20 mL of a local anesthetic (usually lidocaine) provides anesthesia during vaginal delivery to facilitate cutting or repair of the perineum and vagina. Episiotomy usually is performed by the obstetrician just before delivery of the fetal head (Hughes, Levinson, & Rosen, 2002). From a safety standpoint, local perineal infiltration has the least likelihood of complications (Hawkins et al., 1996).

Table 13-4	Modes of Delivery and Appropriate Anesthesia Techniques				
MODES	LOCAL INFILTRATION	PUDENDAL	SPINAL		EPIDURAL
Spontanous vaginal	X	X			X
Vacuum extraction	A	X			X
Outlet forceps		X	X		X
Low forceps		A	X		X
Cesearean section	B		X		X

A = Some clients may tolerate
B = Known technique but not used frequently

Regional Anesthesia

Regional anesthesia may be used for delivery as a continuation of the analgesia provided during labor or administered just before delivery, if required, for a specific mode of delivery.

Pudendal Block

A **pudendal block** is a minor regional block that is reasonably effective and also very safe owing to its lack of fetal effects (Hawkins et al., 1996). This block is administered by the obstetrician through the vagina by placing a local anesthetic in the area of the pudendal nerve, behind the sacrospinous ligament and near the right and left ischial spines (Cunningham et al., 2001; Hawkins et al., 1996; Hughes et al., 2002) (Figure 13-21). A pudendal nerve block can be used for spontaneous vaginal, outlet, and sometimes low forceps delivery. It also has been used effectively in some cases of vacuum extraction.

Spinal Anesthesia

Spinal anesthesia is rarely used for spontaneous vaginal delivery. It is likely to be used in low or midforceps deliv-ery and vacuum extraction. It is often used for cesarean delivery. A list of the advantages and disadvantages of spinal anesthesia is provided in Table 13-5. Differences in the levels of spinal anesthesia for vaginal and cesarean delivery are created by the dosage of medication administered and the position of the client after placement of the local anesthetic in the dural sac (Figure 13-22). For a vaginal delivery, the client will remain in a sitting position for a brief period (1 to 2 minutes) after the spinal anesthesia has been administered so that the local anesthetic solution will migrate downward toward the sacral area.

Cesarean section requires sensory blockade to at least the level of the xiphoid process, the T-8 dermatome (Cunningham et al., 2001). To obtain these levels a greater dosage of medication is required. The client is assisted immediately to a supine position, with left lateral tilt, after administration of the spinal anesthesia. The tilt causes a more cephalad spread of anesthesia, resulting in a higher level of sensory blockade. Hazards include maternal hypotension and the possibility of complete spinal anesthesia (Hawkins et al., 1996). Preloading with 1,500 to 2,000 mL of fluid may help decrease maternal hypotension (Ostheimer & Leavitt, 1996).

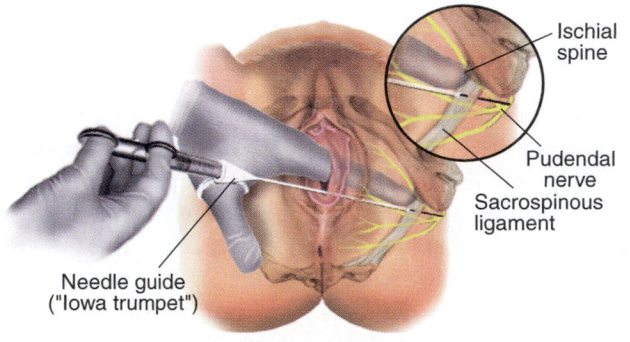

Figure 13-21 Pudendal block.

Table 13-5	Advantages and Disadvantages of Spinal Anesthesia
ADVANTAGES	**DISADVANTAGES**
Rapid onset	Finite duration
Dense block	Possible severe hypotension
Less shivering	Possible total spinal
Less systemic medication	
Little placental transfer	
Awake client	

Epidural Anesthesia

The epidural anesthesia technique provides the versatility required for all modes of delivery. This versatility is a result of differences in types, volumes, and concentrations of local anesthetics administered through a functioning epidural catheter (Figure 13-23). For a spontaneous vaginal delivery, additional local anesthesia can be administered just before delivery of the fetal head. Local anesthesia also may provide additional analgesia and anesthesia for episiotomy repair.

A slightly larger dose of local anesthetic can be administered for forceps or vacuum extraction delivery. The anesthetic should be administered 5 to 10 minutes before attempting forceps or vacuum extraction. It should be noted that the voluntary expulsive effort may be diminished with increased doses and longer elapsed time between administration and delivery. Two distinct advantages of epidural anesthesia are the ease and rapidity by which the anesthesia level can be increased to levels sufficient for cesarean delivery when forceps or vacuum extraction attempts are unsuccessful. The advantages and disadvantages of epidural anesthesia are summarized in Table 13-6.

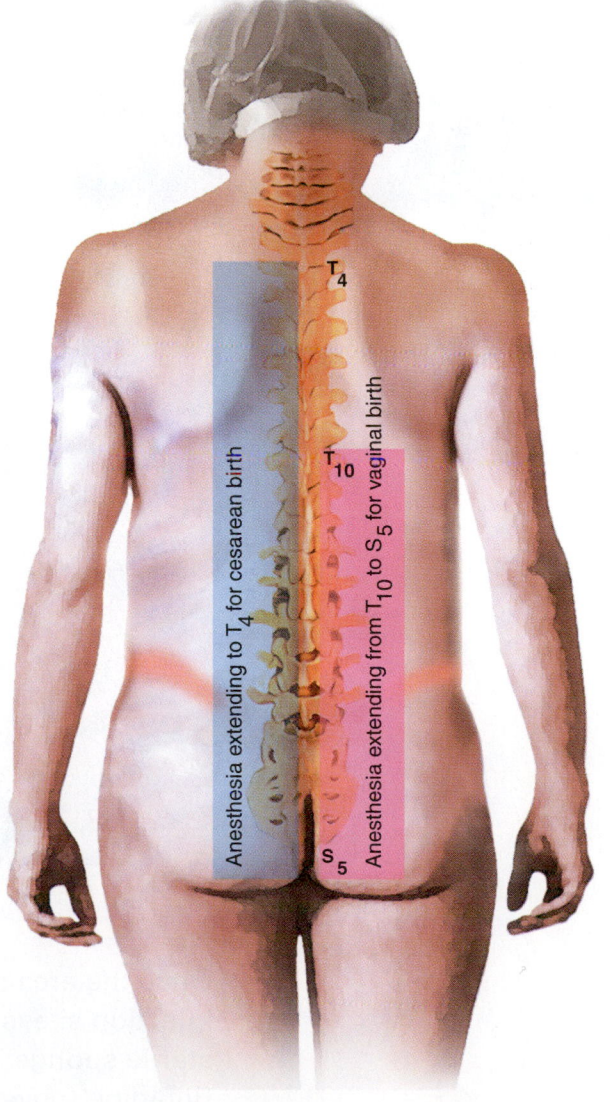

T_4

T_{10}

S_5

■ Anesthesia extending from T_{10} to S_5 dermatomes for vaginal birth

■ Anesthesia extending from T_4 to S_5 dermatomes for cesarean birth

A.

B.

Figure 13-22   Anesthesia levels for vaginal and cesarean births. A. Anterior view. B. Posterior view.

Administration of Spinal Anesthesia

This 29-year-old female is a gravida 4, para 3 who is being prepared for a repeat C-section. She will sit on the operating table with the nurse's assistance and support while the anesthesiologist assesses physical landmarks.

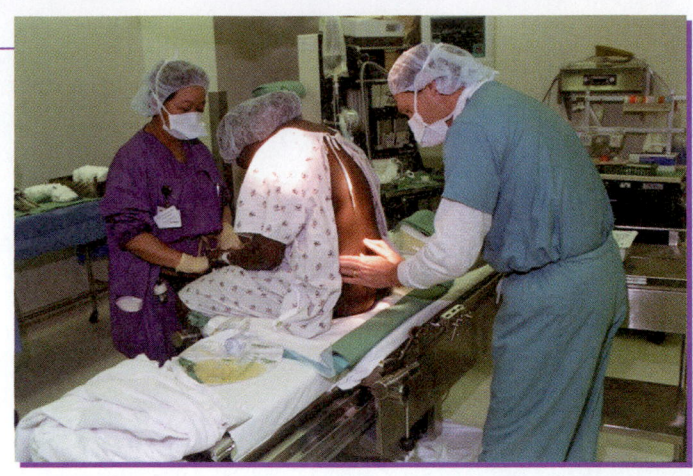

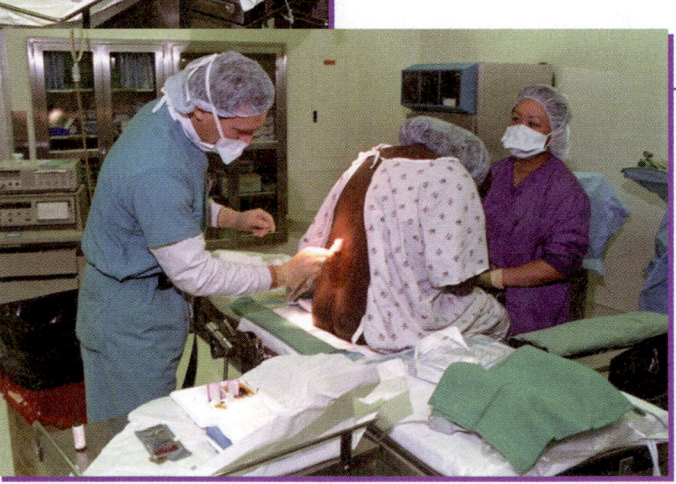

Upon identification of landmarks, preparations are made to cleanse the injection site.

The nurse has the responsibility to promote client comfort and limit motion during the procedure.

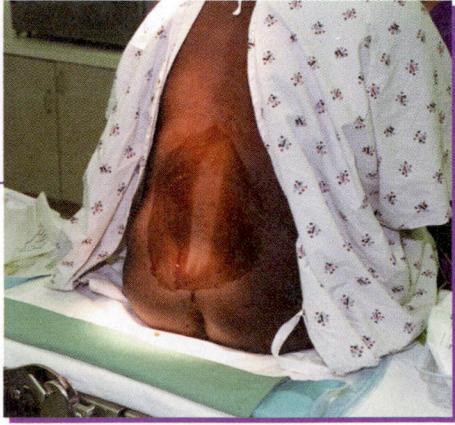

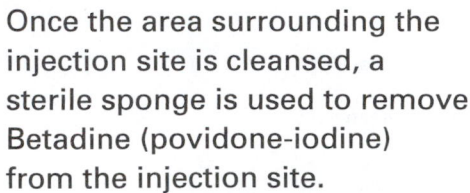

Once the area surrounding the injection site is cleansed, a sterile sponge is used to remove Betadine (povidone-iodine) from the injection site.

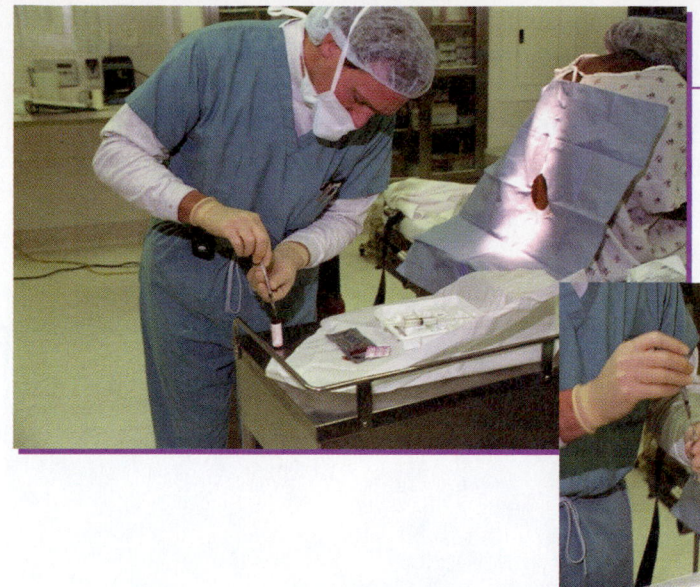

The anesthetic agent is prepared for injection using sterile technique.

Epinephrine is added to the anesthetic agent to produce local vasoconstriction and to prolong the action of the substance.

A local anesthetic is administered prior to the spinal to increase client comfort.

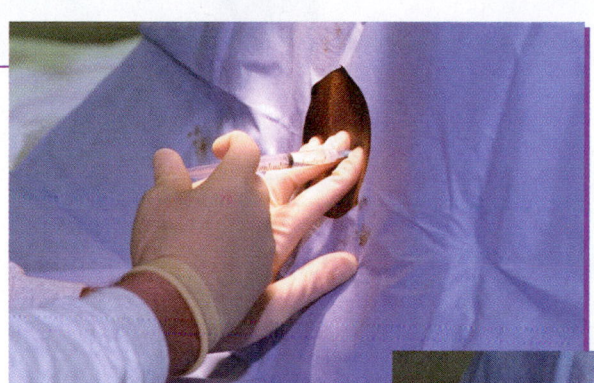

When the local anesthesia is completed, an 18-gauge introducer is inserted and the hub of the needle is left in place.

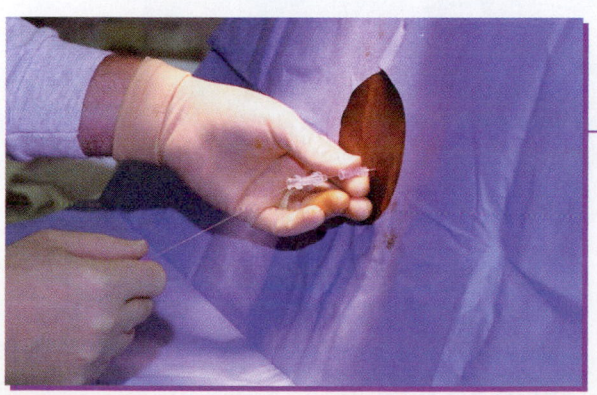

The stylus guide wire is removed from the hub of the needle and inspected for drops of spinal fluid.

495

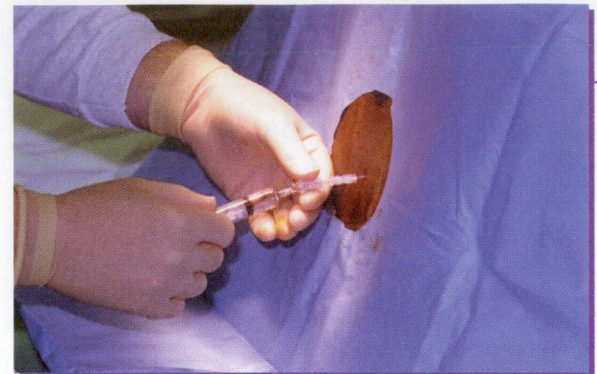

The syringe containing the anesthetic is connected to the hub of the needle.

The anesthetic agent is administered.

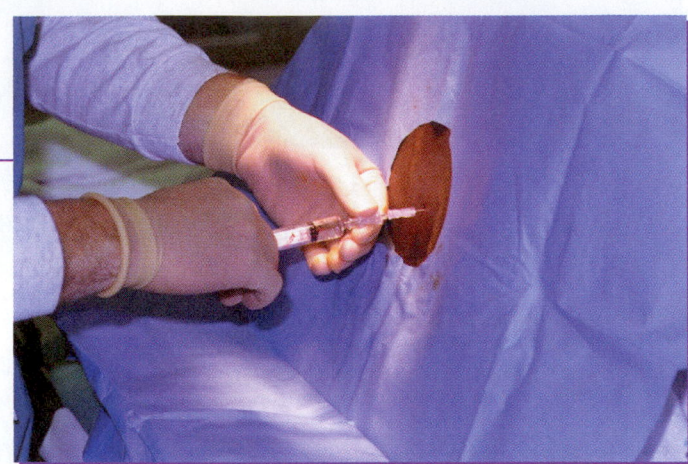

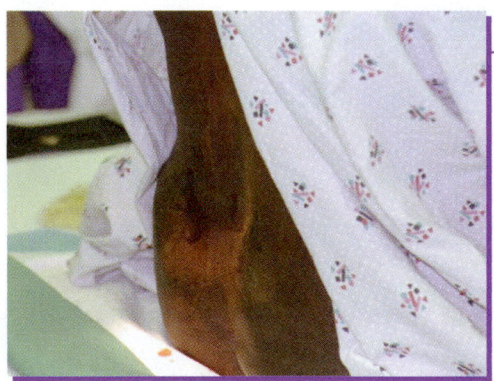

The anesthetic equipment is removed. The nurse assists the client in remaining seated until anesthesia personnel indicate the time is appropriate for the client to lie down. It is important to avoid vena cava syndrome by inserting a wedge or pillow under the right side of her back.

Anesthesia personnel will document the procedure and continue monitoring the client's condition.

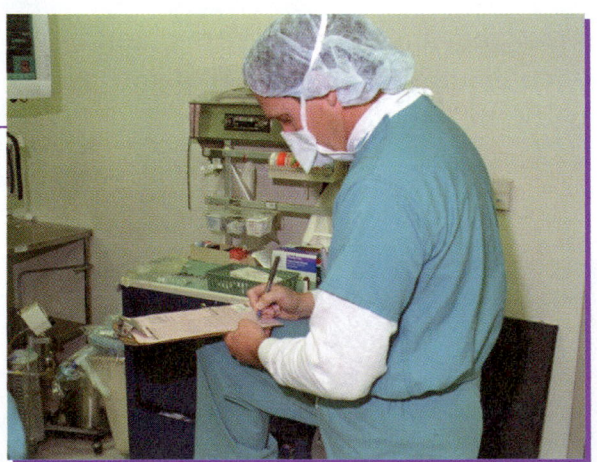

*T*he nurse's responsibility in assisting with an epidural is the same as assisting with a spinal. The difference is the epidural needle is inserted lower (L-4 to L-5), a larger needle is used, and a catheter remains in place for continuous dosing or reinjection.

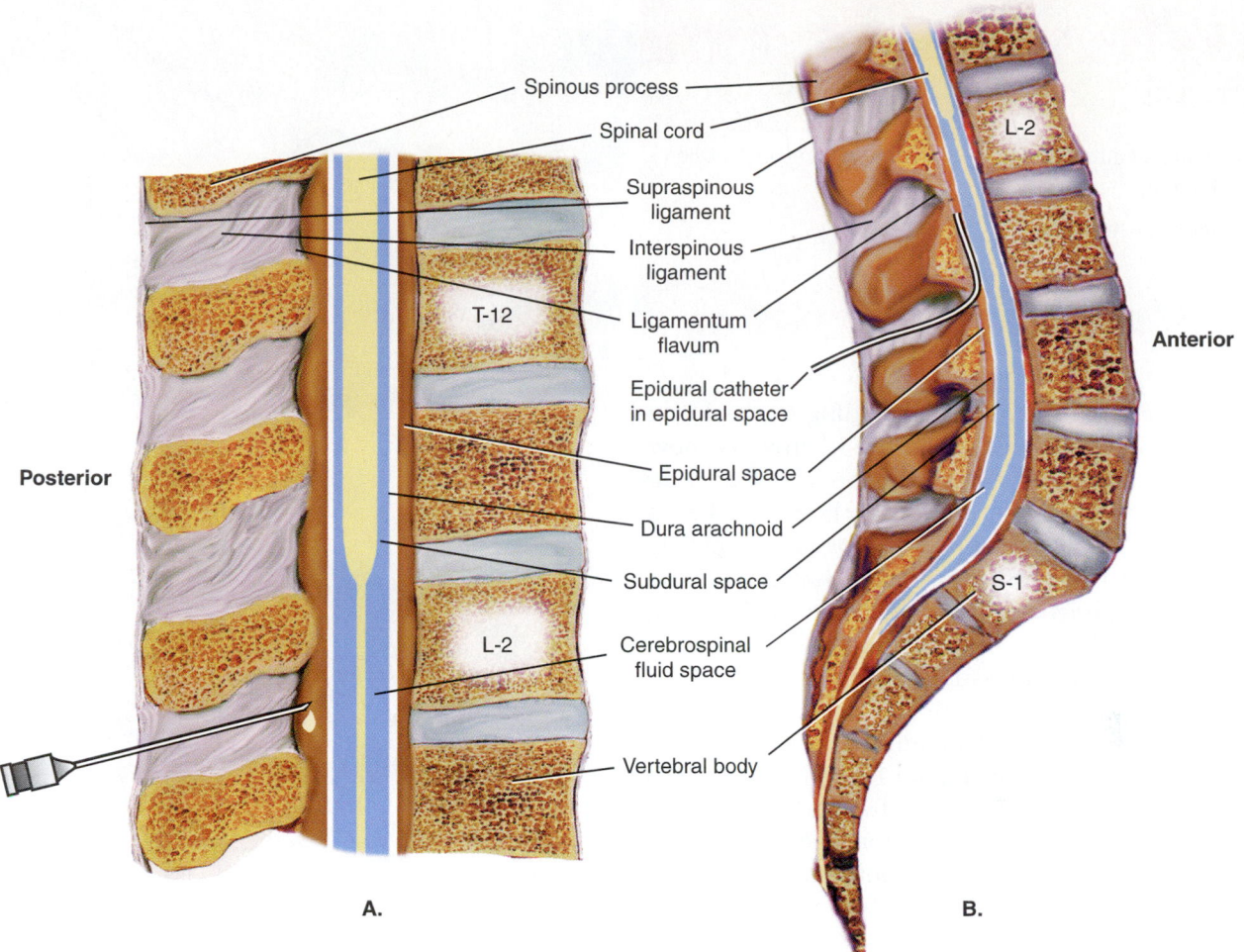

Figure 13-23   Side view of the anatomy of the spine. A. Epidural needle placed in the epidural space. B. Epidural catheter placed in the epidural space.

Except in the case of severe fetal distress, an epidural usually can be used to provide sufficient surgical levels of anesthesia in a short enough period of time for urgent cesarean section. General anesthesia is the technique of choice for true emergency cesarean sections such as in cases of severe fetal distress and substantial maternal hemorrhage (Santos et al., 1997).

Table 13-6	Advantages and Disadvantages of Epidural Anesthesia	
ADVANTAGES	**DISADVANTAGES**
Slower onset	Placement takes longer
Titratable level and duration	Possible systemic toxicity
Less hypotension	Larger placental transfer
Awake client	Higher incidence of inadequate block

General Anesthesia

General anesthesia for delivery involves rendering the client unconscious and intubation of the trachea with a cuffed endotracheal tube. Afterward, ventilation, oxygenation, unconsciousness, analgesia, and muscle relaxation are maintained. Emergence, or waking up the client, and extubation follow. The possible maternal and fetal complications of general anesthesia are listed in Table 13-7.

All anesthetic agents, whether given by IV or inhalation, cross the placenta and affect the infant. Muscle relaxants are the exception owing to their large molecular size. Resuscitation of an infant with respiratory depression should be anticipated, with adequate equipment and personnel present at delivery.

The two major causes of maternal morbidity and mortality from general anesthesia are failure to intubate and pulmonary aspiration (Hawkins et al., 1996). Pregnancy-induced changes such as engorgment of mucosa contribute to airway management problems.

Table 13-7	Possible Maternal and Fetal Complications of General Anesthesia
MATERNAL	**FETAL**
Hypertension at intubation	Drug-induced depression
Difficult or failed intubation	
Aspiration of gastric contents	
Awareness	
Uterine atony	

Management of the airway, including tracheal intubation, is in the hands of the anesthesia provider; however, the nurse should be aware of the possible difficulties in airway management. The nurse may be required to assist the anesthesia provider by calling for additional help, especially other anesthesia providers, if readily available, because extra experienced hands can be invaluable (Johnson, Lawlor, & Weiner, 1994). The nurse also may be needed to hold cricoid pressure or hand an endotracheal tube to a solitary anesthesia provider. To maintain cricoid pressure, use the thumb and forefinger to firmly compress the cricoid ring downward (Figure 13-24) (Chipas, 1997). The cricoid ring is the first and only tracheal cartilage ring that is a complete circle. Compression of this ring closes off the esophagus, helping to prevent passive regurgitation (Hughes et al., 2002). The most important part the nurse must remember is that *cricoid pressure is not released* until after the cuff of the endotracheal tube is inflated, with proper placement confirmed or the anesthesia provider indicating it can be released (Chipas, 1997).

Pulmonary aspiration of gastric contents can result in obstruction of lower airways, pneumonitis, pulmonary edema, and death (Cunningham et al., 2001). Two factors impact the severity of aspiration pneumonitis: volume

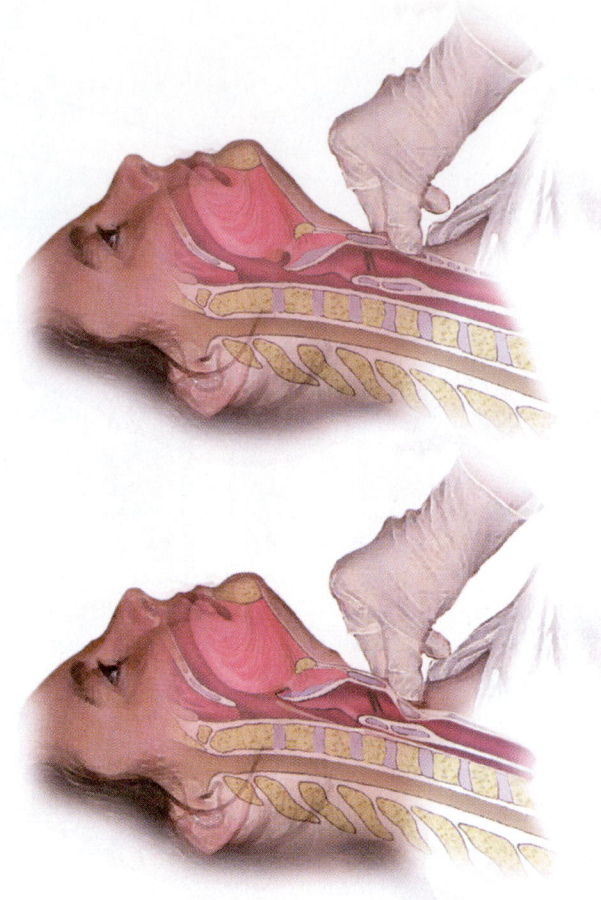

Figure 13-24   Downward force of the cricoid cartilage will compress the esophagus.

Nursing Alert

Cricoid Pressure
- The cricoid ring is located just below the thyroid bone.
- The cricoid ring is the only tracheal cartilage that forms a complete ring.
- With the client in the supine position, downward compression (with thumb and forefinger) will cause the cricoid cartilage to close off the esophagus and help protect the client against aspiration of gastric contents.

greater than 25 mL and pH less than 2.5 (Fiedler & Shaw, 1997). There are methods to decrease the risk of maternal aspiration or severity of a possible aspiration. The oral administration of a nonparticulate antacid (such as sodium citrate) just before induction of general anesthesia increases the gastric pH level and should be given routinely. Particulate antacids (such as Maalox) are not recommended because the particulate matter in the antacid can produce severe pulmonary reaction if aspirated (Fiedler & Shaw, 1997). Additional medications such as histamine blockers (cimetidine [Tagamet] or ranitidine [Zantac]) also may be administered to decrease the gastric pH level and volume.

Special Considerations for Cesarean Section

After securing of the airway, the obstetrician is directed to proceed with the cesarean section. Unconsciousness of the client is maintained through the use of a volatile anesthetic agent and oxygen. After delivery of the infant, nitrous oxide is often added to enhance the anesthesia. Additional doses of muscle relaxant are given as needed to maintain surgical conditions. After the procedure the client is awakened. Once she is responsive, is spontaneously breathing with sufficient rate and tidal volume, and has the protective airway reflexes, including swallowing, the oral cavity is suctioned, the cuff deflated, and the client extubated. At this time she is taken to the recovery room.

The two other complications listed in Table 13-7 are awareness during general anesthesia and uterine atony. It is possible for the client to have some degree of awareness under general anesthesia; this may be attributed to the attempt to minimize drug-induced depression of the neonate (Chadwick & Ross, 1992). Addition of nitrous oxide to the oxygen-volatile agent mixture can help decrease awareness but is not advocated by some practitioners until after the delivery of the fetus. Many anesthesia providers think that delivery of 100% oxygen until delivery of the infant is preferred because doing so should result in the highest level of oxygen available to the fetus. After delivery of the infant, additional doses of opioids and amnesics such as midazolam (Versed) as well as increased levels of volatile agents and use of nitrous oxide can help prevent maternal awareness. If the client describes incidences of awareness the nurse should take this seriously and notify the anesthesia providers so that the client can receive further assessment and explanation of the incident.

Uterine atony is possible in all deliveries regardless of the presence of anesthesia. The volatile agents used to maintain general anesthesia can produce a degree of dose-related decrease in uterine contractility and tone (Chadwick & Ross, 1992). At the level of volatile anesthetic agents and other drugs normally used, the uterus is responsive to the administration of oxytocin to induce contractions (Hughes et al., 2002).

POSTDELIVERY CARE FOR THE CLIENT RECEIVING ANESTHESIA

The care needed in the recovery period by the client who has received anesthesia varies greatly according to the type of anesthesia. The care related to the birth process itself is covered in Chapter 16. Care of the client related to analgesia and anesthesia in labor and delivery is discussed subsequently.

Local Anesthesia

The client with local infiltration anesthesia of the perineum requires little additional recovery care owing solely to the anesthetic. The nurse must be aware that the client may be unable to feel hot or cold in the area that has been anesthetized. She must ensure that ice or other sources of cold are not placed directly on the skin of the perineum because it is possible to cause cold thermal injury owing to impaired cold and pain perception in this area.

Regional Anesthesia

In the recovery of a client with regional anesthesia, the type and extent of the regional anesthesia will determine necessary care. The client with a pudendal nerve block requires the same care as does a client with local infiltration. One additional caution applies: the perineal area should be carefully assessed for swelling, which may indicate the development of vaginal wall or perineal hematoma. The impaired sensory perception may mask pain and delay the recognition of a developing hematoma.

The recovery of a client with spinal or epidural anesthesia requires careful attention to vital signs and the declining spinal level (sensory block). Monitoring of vital signs includes blood pressure, electrocardiogram, and pulse oximetry. Oxygen by nasal cannula may be needed if the client has received sedation or other depressive medications. A low spinal or saddle block has a lower sensory level and causes less maternal hypotension than does a spinal block for cesarean section. Positional changes from supine to semi-Fowler's to Fowler's position should be done incrementally, with assessment of the client for tolerance and hypotension. It is not necessary for the client to remain supine after regional anesthesia. The nurse should be aware that the sensory blockade recedes from the chest toward the feet. Analgesia for incision or episiotomy pain should be considered and administered before the block is completely gone. The client's ability to urinate may be impaired. The bladder should be assessed and catheterized if the client is unable to void.

The client with epidural anesthesia may need the care indicated above if epidural anesthesia has been used to provide sensory blockade for vaginal forceps or cesarean delivery. The type of local anesthetic used through the epidural greatly impacts the client's status in recovery. Bupivacaine (Lidocaine) is frequently used for its properties of sensory blockade with preservation of motor control. Clients who did not receive additional analgesia for delivery may not require specific care other than a warning that they will not have complete control of their legs for several hours and that full sensation does not mean full control. All clients should have assistance the first time they ambulate from the bed; however, the nurse should be even more cautious when helping to ambulate clients who have had regional anesthesia and should consider requesting additional help.

General Anesthesia

Recovery of the client from general anesthesia requires close observation and complete monitoring. Assessment of the client involves all major systems and preparations for immediate response to problems encountered. Respirations should be observed for rate and depth. Oxygen should be administered by nasal cannula or by mask (when higher concentrations are needed). Pulse oximetry should be employed to determine changes in oxygen saturation. Continuous electrocardiogram and frequent intermittent blood pressure monitoring are done. Suction equipment should be functioning and ready in case of vomiting. The nurse should be aware that the client should not be left alone at any time and that the most dangerous time in the recovery period can be those few minutes after the initial flurry of activity involved in admission to the recovery area. After the initial stimulation of monitor placement and assessment is over, the patient may drift back to sleep and hypoventilate. Vigilance is the key word for safe recovery of the client from general anesthesia.

WEB ACTIVITIES

- Search for obstetrics and gynecology client at Virtual Hospital, http://www.vh.org. Create a list of client teaching tips for the primipara and multipara.

- Visit the Web site of the National Library of Medicine at the National Institutes of Health at http://www.nlm.nih.gov. What time frames are outlined for the stages and phases of labor?

- Check out http://www.childbirth.org and the section Epidurals—Frequently Asked Questions.

- Type in the terms *childbirth* and *analgesia* in any Web search engine. You will get lists of thousands of Web sites. Check out a few just to see what is out there. Some information may be excellent and some may not be. Try to identify the information that is research-based.

Key Concepts

- There are many premonitory signs and symptoms of labor, which may include lightening, Braxton Hicks contractions, cervical change, bloody show, energy spurts, ruptured membranes, and GI disturbances.
- The five Ps of labor are important factors that may affect the labor process: passageway, passenger, powers, position of the mother, and psychologic response of the mother.
- The latent phase of the first stage of labor begins with the onset of labor and lasts until the woman's cervix is 3 to 4 cm dilated.
- The active phase of labor begins when the woman's cervix is 3 to 4 cm dilated and ends when it is 8 cm dilated.
- The transition phase of the first stage of labor begins when the woman's cervix is 8 cm dilated and ends when it is fully dilated.
- The second stage of labor begins when the cervix is completely dilated and effaced and ends when the fetus is expelled.
- The third stage of labor begins when the fetus is expelled and ends when the placenta is expelled.
- The fourth stage of labor lasts for 4 hours after the placenta is expelled.
- Theories of pain suggest that pain is a very individual experience influenced by cultural practices, previous experience with pain, and available support systems.
- Types of anesthesia include local (small area of the body), regional (large area of the body), and general (loss of consciousness).
- The primary consideration for use of pain medication during labor and delivery is always the health and well-being of the mother and baby.
- Sources of pain in labor and delivery include cervical dilation, uterine contractions, distension of the vagina and perineum, and pressure on the sacrum; perception of pain can be influenced by cultural expectations, exhaustion, loss of sleep, and duration of labor.
- Parenteral analgesia options during labor include a variety of opioids. Options for regional analgesia in labor include intrathecal opioids, epidural, combined intrathecal-epidural, and paracervical analgesia.
- During delivery, pudendal, spinal, and epidural blocks are the pain relief options of choice.

■ The nurse's role in caring for the client recovering from anesthesia emphasizes close observation, complete and frequent monitoring, and assessment; the nurse may also provide assistance to the client when ambulating.

Review Questions and Activities

1. How do hormones and prostaglandins affect the onset of labor?

2. Discuss the premonitory signs and symptoms of labor.

3. Name the five Ps of labor and explain how each affects the labor and delivery process.

4. Describe some aspects of the maternal attainment theory and how it is applied to labor.

5. Describe some of the maternal adaptations during the process of labor.

6. Name the different stages of labor, including the definition and the length of each.

7. Describe the fetal adaptations during the labor and delivery process.

8. Which of the following is not a process involved in nociception?
   a. Transduction
   b. Transmission
   c. Transudation
   d. Modulation

   The correct answer is c.

9. Which of the following types of anesthesia involves the loss of sensation from a large area of the body?
   a. General
   b. Regional
   c. Inhalation
   d. Local infiltration

   The correct answer is b.

10. Which of the following types of anesthesia does only a CRNA or anesthesiologist provide?
    a. General
    b. Regional
    c. Inhalation
    d. Local infiltration

    The correct answer is a.

11. In which stage of labor is the conduction of pain impulses through T-10 to L-1?
    a. Third stage
    b. Second stage
    c. First stage
    d. Fourth stage

    The correct answer is c.

12. In which stage of labor is the conduction of pain impulses through S-2 to S-4?
    a. Third stage
    b. Second stage
    c. First stage
    d. Fourth stage

    The correct answer is b.

13. Which of the following is one of the major causes of maternal morbidity and mortality from anesthesia?
    a. Emergency cesarean section
    b. Epidural catheter breakage
    c. Pulmonary aspiration
    d. Postdural puncture headache (spinal headache)

    The correct answer is c.

14. Which of the following is the most dangerous period for a client after general anesthesia?
    a. During transportation from the operating room to the recovery room
    b. After the initial flurry of activity on arrival to the recovery room
    c. Thirty minutes after arriving in the recovery room
    d. Just before transportation to the postpartum unit

    The correct answer is b.

References

American College of Obstetricians and Gynecologists (ACOG). (1995). *Induction of labor* (ACOG Tech. Bulletin #217). Washington, DC: Author.

American College of Obstetrics and Gynecologists (ACOG). (1998). *Delivery by vacuum extraction* (ACOG Committee on Obstetric Practice #208). Washington, DC: Author.

American College of Obstetricians and Gynecologists (ACOG). (1999). *Induction of labor with misoprostol* (ACOG Committee Opinion 228). Washington, DC: Author.

Ball, C. (1996). James Young Simpson, 1811–1870. *Anaesthesia & Intensive Care, 24,* 639.

Benards, C. M. (1997). Epidural and spinal anesthesia. In P. G. Barash, B. F. Cullen, & R. K. Stoelting (Eds.), *Clinical anesthesia* (3rd ed., pp. 645–680). Philadelphia: Lippincott-Raven.

Bernstein, P. S. (2000). Predicting successful induction of labor. *The American College of Obstetricians and Gynecologists 48th Annual Clinical Meeting.* Retrieved October 2000, from http://www.medscape.com/medscape/CNO/2000/ACOG-05.html

Bishop, E. H. (1964). Pelvic scoring for elective induction. *Obstetrics and Gynecology, 24,* 266.

Blackburn, S. T., & Loper, D. L. (2003). *Maternal, fetal, and neonatal physiology: A clinical perspective* (2nd ed.). Philadelphia, PA: W. B. Saunders.

Burst, H. V., Kriebs, J. M., Gegor, C. L., and Varney, H. (2004). *Varney's midwifery* (4th ed.). Boston: Blackwell Scientific Publications.

Callister, L. C., Vehvilainen-Julkunen, K., & Lauri, S. (1996). Cultural perceptions of childbirth: A cross-cultural comparison of childbearing women. *Journal of Holistic Nursing, 14*(1), 66–72.

Chadwick, H. S., & Ross, B. K. (1992). Causes and consequences of maternal-fetal perianesthetic complications. In J. L. Benumof & L. J. Saidman, *Anesthesia and perioperative complications* (pp. 520–547). St. Louis, MO: Mosby Year Book.

Chantigian, R. C., & Chantigian, P. D. M. (1996). Effect of lumbar epidural anesthesia on the progress of labor and the incidence of operative deliveries. In A. Van Zundert & G. W. Ostheimer (Eds.), *Pain relief and anesthesia in obstetrics* (pp. 943–954). New York: Churchill Livingstone.

Chipas, A. (1997). Airway management. In J. J. Nagelhout & K. L. Zaglaniczny (Eds.), *Nurse anesthesia* (pp. 708–725). Philadelphia: W. B. Saunders.

Clark, A. L., & Affonso, D. D. (1978). *Childbearing: A nursing perspective*. Philadelphia: F. A. Davis.

Cohen, J. (1996). Doctor James Young Simpson, Rabbi Abraham De Sola, and Genesis Chapter 3, verse 16. *Obstetrics & Gynecology, 88*(5), 895–898.

Concepcion, M. (1996). Acute complications and side effects of regional anesthesia. In D. L. Brown (Ed.), *Regional anesthesia and analgesia* (pp. 446–461). Philadelphia: W. B. Saunders.

Connor, H., & Connor, T. (1996). Did the use of chloroform by Queen Victoria influence its acceptance in obstetric practice? *Anaesthesia, 51,* 955–957.

Cunningham, F. G., Gant, N. F., Leveno, K. J., Gilstrap, L. C., Hauth, J. C., & Wenstrom, K. D. (2001). *Williams obstetrics* (21st ed.). New York: McGraw-Hill.

Drasner, K., & Swisher, J. L. (1996). Delayed complications and side effects of regional anesthesia. In D. L. Brown (Ed.), *Regional anesthesia and analgesia* (pp. 462–476). Philadelphia: W. B. Saunders.

Ellis, W. E. (1997). Regional anesthesia. In J. J. Nagelhout & K. L. Zaglaniczny (Eds.), *Nurse anesthesia* (pp. 1160–1197). Philadelphia: W. B. Saunders.

Feinstein, N., & McCartney, P. (1997). *Fetal heart rate monitoring: Principles and practice*. Washington, DC: Association of Women's Health, Obstetric and Neonatal Nurses.

Fiedler, M. A., & Shaw, B. (1997). Obstetric anesthesia. In J. J. Nagelhout & K. L. Zaglaniczny (Eds.), *Nurse anesthesia* (pp. 292–332). Philadelphia: W. B. Saunders.

Friedman, E. A., Niswander, K. R., Bayonet-Rivera, N. P., & Sachtleben, M. R. (1966). Relation of prelabor evaluation to inducibility and the course of labor. *Obstetrics and Gynecology, 28,* 495–501.

Harrison, R. F., Flynn, M., & Craft, I. (1977). Assessment of factors constituting an "inducibility profile." *Obstetrics and Gynecology, 49,* 270–274.

Hawkins, J. L., Chestnut, D. H., & Gibbs, C. P. (1996). Obstetric anesthesia. In S. G. Gabbe, J. R. Niebyl, & J. L. Simpson, *Obstetrics: Normal and problem pregnancies* (pp. 425–468). New York: Churchill Livingstone.

Hawkins, J. L., Hess, K. R., Kubicek, M. A., Joyce III, T. H., & Morrow, D. H. (1995). A reevaluation of the association between instrument delivery and epidural analgesia. *Regional Anesthesia, 20*(1), 50–56.

Hughes, S. C., Levinson, G., & Rosen, M. A. (2002). Schnider & Levinon's anesthesia for obstetrics (4th ed.). Philadephia: Lippincott Williams & Wilkins.

Johnson, C., Lawlor, M., & Weiner, M. (1994). The airway in the obstetrical patient. *AANA Journal, 62*(2), 149–159.

Kyle, R. A., & Shampo, M. A. (1997). James Young Simpson and the introduction of chloroform anesthesia in obstetric practice. *Mayo Clinic Proceedings, 72,* 372.

Leininger, M. (1985). Transcultural care diversity and universality: A theory of nursing. *Nursing and Health Care, 6*(4), 209–212.

Littleton, L., & Engebretson, J. (2002). *Maternal, neonatal, and women's health nursing*. Clifton Park, NY: Delmar Learning.

Lowdermilk, D., & Perry, S. (2003). *Maternity Nursing* (6th ed.). St. Louis, MO: Mosby Year Book.

Luyendijk, W. (1996). Anatomy of the lumbar and sacral spinal canal. In A. Van Zundert & G. W. Ostheimer (Eds.), *Pain relief and anesthesia in obstetrics* (pp. 167–182). New York: Churchill Livingstone.

MacKenzie, I. Z., & Embrey, M. P. (1979). A comparison of PGE_2 and $PGF_{2\alpha}$ vaginal gel for ripening the cervix before induction of labour. *British Journal of Obstetrics and Gynaecology, 86,* 167.

Manning, F. A. (1995). Fetal breathing movements. In F. Manning, *Fetal medicine: Principles and practices* (pp. 113–145). Norwalk, CT: Appleton and Lange.

Morrision, L. M. M., Wildsmith, J. A. W., & Ostheimer, G. W. (1996). History of pain relief in childbirth. In A. Van Zundert & G. W. Ostheimer (Eds.), *Pain relief and anesthesia in obstetrics* (pp. 3–19). New York: Churchill Livingstone.

Nichols, F. H., and Humenick, S. S. (2000) *Childbirth education: Practice, research and theory* (2nd ed.) Philadelphia: Saunders.

O'Brian, W. F., & Cefalo, R. C. (1996). Labor and delivery. In S. G. Gabbe, J. R. Niehyl, & J. L. Simpson (Eds.), *Obstetrics: Normal and problem pregnancies* (3rd ed.). New York: Churchill Livingstone.

Ostheimer, G. W., & Leavitt, K. A. (1996). Epidural anesthesia: Technique. In A. Van Zundert & G. W. Ostheimer (Eds.), *Pain relief and anesthesia in obstetrics* (pp. 288–295). New York: Churchill Livingstone.

Rubin, R. (1984). Maternal identity and the maternity experience. New York: Springer-Verlag.

Sandelowski, M. (1984). *Pain, pleasure, and American childbirth: From the twilight sleep to the Read method, 1914–1960*. Westport, CT: Greenwood Press.

Santos, A. C., Pederson, H., & Finster, M. (1997). Obstetric anesthesia. In P. G. Barash, B. F. Cullen, & R. K. Stoelting (Eds.), *Clinical anesthesia* (pp. 1061–1090). Philadelphia: Lippincot-Raven.

Seidel, H. M., Ball, J. W., Dains, J. E., & Benedict, G. W. (2003). *Mosby's guide to physical examination* (5th ed.). St. Louis, MO: Mosby.

Stoelting, R. K., & Miller, R. D. (1994). *Basics of anesthesia* (3rd ed.). New York: Churchill Livingstone.

Troyer, L. R., & Parisi, V. M. (1993). Management of labor. In T. R. Moore et al. (eds.). *Gynecology & obstetrics: A traditional approach* (pp. 575–588). New York: Churchill Livingstone.

Ulmsten, U. (1996). The onset of labor. *European Journal of Obstetrics, Gynecology and Reproductive Biology, 65,* 95–98.

U.S. Food & Drug Administration-Center for Devices and Radiological Health (1998). *FDA Public Health Advisory: Need for caution when using vacuum assisted devices*. Retrieved April 10, 2001, from http://www.fda.gov/cdrh/fetal598.html

Weber, S. E. (1996). Cultural aspects of pain in childbearing women. *Journal of Obstetric, Gynecologic, & Neonatal Nursing, 25*(1): 67–72.

Williams, J. R. (1997). Local anesthetics. In J. J. Nagelhout & K. L. Zaglaniczny (Eds.), *Nurse anesthesia*. Philadelphia: W. B. Saunders.

Williams, M. C., Krammer, J., & O'Brian, W. F. (1997). The value of the cervical score in predicting successful outcome of labor induction. *Obstetrics and Gynecology, 90*(5), 784–789.

Wing, D. A., Lovett, K., & Paul, R. H. (1998). Disruption of prior uterine incision following misoprostol for labor induction in women with previous cesarean delivery. *Obstetrics and Gynecology, 91*, 828.

Youngstrom, P. C., Baker, S. W., & Miller, J. L. (1996). Epidurals redefined in analgesia and anesthesia: A distinction with a difference. *Journal of Obstetric, Gynecologic, & Neonatal Nursing, 25*(4), 350–354.

Suggested Readings

American Academy of Pediatrics & American College of Obstetricians and Gynecologists. (1997). *Guidelines for perinatal care* (4th ed.). Washington, DC, Elk Grove, IL: Authors.

Cheek, T. G., & Gutsche, B. B. (1997). Analgesia for labor. In D. M. Dewan & D. D. Hood, *Practical obstetric anesthesia* (pp. 95–124). Philadelphia: W. B. Saunders.

Dewan, D. M., & Hood, D. D. (1997). *Practical obstetric anesthesia*. Philadelphia: W. B. Saunders.

Fine, P. G., & Ashburn, M. A. (1998). Functional neuroanatomy and nociception. In M. A. Ashburn & L. J. Rice (Eds.), *The management of pain* (pp. 1–16). Philadelphia: Churchill Livingstone.

Foster, S. D., & Jordan, L. M. (Eds.). (1994). *Professional aspects of nurse anesthesia practice*. Philadelphia: F. A. Davis.

Garde, J. F. (1997). Specialty practice of nurse anesthesia. In J. J. Nagelhout & K. L. Zaglaniczny (Eds.), *Nurse anesthesia* (pp. 23–27). Philadelphia: W. B. Saunders.

Jordan, L. M. (1994). Qualifications and capabilities of the Certified Registered Nurse Anesthetist. In S. D. Foster & L. M. Jordan (Eds.), *Professional aspects of nurse anesthesia practice* (pp. 3–10). Philadelphia: F. A. Davis.

Luxner, K. (2005). *Maternal infant nursing care plans*. Clifton Park, NY: Delmar Learning.

Moorhouse, M. F. (1999). *Maternal/newborn plans of care: Guidelines for individualizing care* (3rd ed.). Colorado Springs, CO: TNT-RN Enterprises.

Rawal, N. (1996). Combined spinal-epidural anesthesia. In A. Van Zundert & G. W. Ostheimer (Eds.), *Pain relief and anesthesia in obstetrics* (pp. 413–426). New York: Churchill Livingstone.

Rostant, D. M., Cady, R. F., & Miller, D. (1999). *Liability issues in perinatal nursing*. Philadelphia: J. B. Lippincott.

Vincent, R. D. Jr., & Chestnut, D. H. (1996). Analgesia during labor and delivery. In D. L. Brown (Ed.), *Regional anesthesia and analgesia* (pp. 587–608). Philadelphia: W. B. Saunders.

Resources

American Academy of Pediatrics, National Headquarters, 141 Northwest Point Boulevard, Elk Grove Village, IL 60007-1098, 847-434-4000, Fax: 847-434-8000, http://www.aap.org

American Association of Nurse Anesthetists (AANA), 222 South Prospect Avenue, Park Ridge, IL 60068, 847-692-7050, http://www.aana.com

American College of Nurse-Midwives, Suite 900, 818 Connecticut Avenue NW, Washington, D.C. 20006, 202-728-9860, Fax: 202-728-9897, http://www.midwife.org

American College of Obstetricians and Gynecologists, 409 12th Street, SW, P.O. Box 96920, Washington, DC 20090-6920, http://www.acog.com

American Society of Anesthesiologists (ASA), 520 N. Northwest Highway, Park Ridge, IL 60068-2573, 847-825-5586, http://www.asahq.org

Association of Women's Health, Obstetric and Neonatal Nurses, 2000 L Street, N.W., Suite 740, Washington, D.C. 20036, 800-673-8499 (U.S.), 800-245-0231 (Canada), Fax: 202-728-0575, http://www.awhonn.org

Lamaze International, Suite 800, 2025 M Street, NW, Washington, DC 20036-3309, 800-368-4404, http://lamaze-childbirth.com

March of Dimes, 233 Park Avenue South, New York, NY 10003, 212-353-8353, Fax: 212-254-3518, http://www.modimes.org

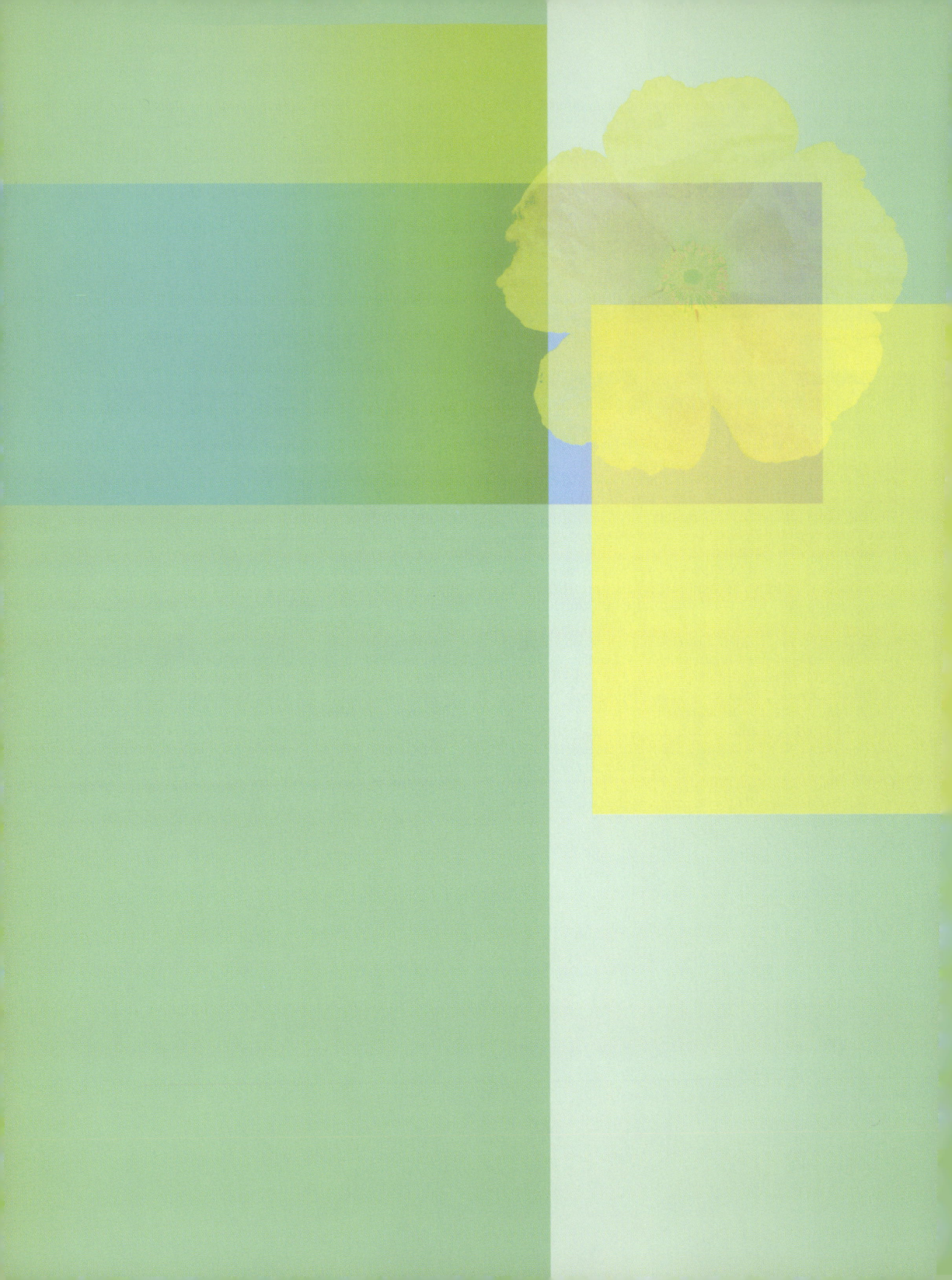

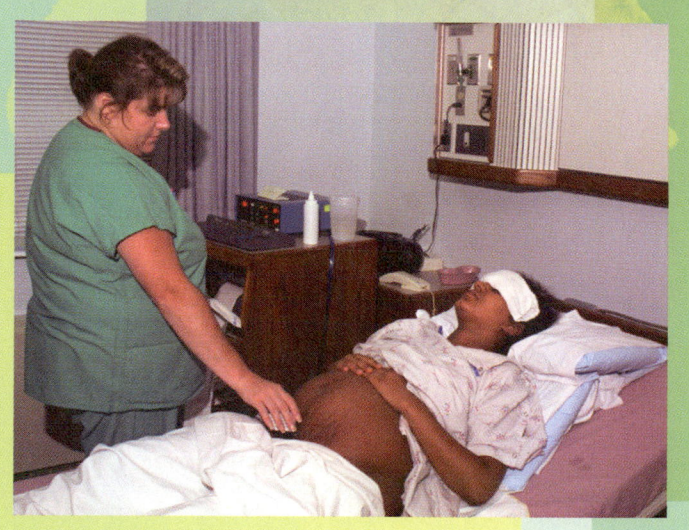

CHAPTER 14

NURSING CARE OF THE INTRAPARTAL FAMILY

Childbirth is one of the most meaningful, unique, and exciting times for the laboring woman and her partner, yet it also can be a time of stress and anxiety. Essential components of nursing care include a comprehensive knowledge of the processes of labor and delivery, competence in providing care that conforms with current standards, and provision of support for the childbearing family through this major event. Good interpersonal skills, including listening to the client, complement technical skills. A positive perception of the birthing experience and a feeling of empowerment are fostered by the nurse who gives sufficient information to the woman and her partner, in language they can understand, and who shows nonjudgmental support for their efforts.

An excellent intrapartum nurse is one who is skilled and knowledgeable and who deems it a privilege to provide care to a family during this momentous time. Many women remember every nuance of their labor and childbirth for many years afterward. These women especially remember the actions and demeanor of the major caregiver. Attentive and effective support, therefore, can make childbirth a satisfying experience for everyone involved and a treasured memory for the family.

Key Terms

Acceleration
Acme
Acrocyanosis
Active phase
Amniohook
Amnioinfusion
Amniotomy
Apgar score
Baseline fetal heart rate
Beat-to-beat variability
Bloody show
Chorioamnionitis
Contraction
Crowning
Deceleration
Dilation
Doula
Duration
Early onset deceleration
Effacement
Emergency childbirth
Episiotomy
Fern test
Fetal heart rate (FHR)
First stage of labor
Frequency
Gravidity
Hypertonic contractions
Hyperventilation
Intensity
Intrauterine pressure
   catheter (IUPC)
Inversion of the uterus
Labor
Laceration
Late onset deceleration
Latent phase
Long-term variability
Meconium

Montevideo units
Multipara
Nitrazine test
Nonperiodic fetal heart
   rate changes
Nuchal cord
Oligohydramnios
Overshoot
Parity
Parturient
Periodic fetal heart rate
   changes
Placenta previa
Polyhydramnios
Precipitous delivery
Premature rupture of
   membranes (PROM)
Presenting part
Preterm birth
Preterm premature
   rupture of membranes
   (PPROM)
Reactive nonstress test
Resting tone
Saltatory pattern
Second stage of labor
Short-term variability
Shoulder
Station
Striae gravidarum
Third stage of labor
Transition phase
True labor
Uterine atony
Uteroplacental
   insufficiency
Variability
Variable deceleration
Vertex

Competencies

Upon completion of this chapter, the reader should be able to:

1. Describe the initial assessment of the woman in labor.
2. Describe the subsequent maternal-fetal assessment during the four stages of labor.
3. Define the normal course of all four stages of labor.
4. Describe the primary nursing interventions in all four stages of labor.
5. Identify changes in client-fetal status that may alter the course of labor and delivery.
6. Discuss episiotomy use and subsequent nursing considerations.
7. Accurately document events and nursing interventions.

This chapter focuses on the nursing care of the woman experiencing an uncomplicated vaginal birth. All maternity clients have their individual expectations and reactions to labor and delivery. Emphasis on each of the varied roles of the nurse, as client advocate, support person, and expert caregiver, will depend on the client's particular circumstances and specific needs. For example, the young teenager who has received no childbirth preparation will need a greater amount of teaching than will the client who is giving birth to her fourth child, or a client who has attended childbirth classes. A woman with a planned pregnancy, good preparation, and a supportive family is more likely to find the experience joyful and rewarding than is the woman with an unplanned or unwanted pregnancy. The actions of the intrapartum nurse throughout the labor and delivery process are thoroughly described, beginning with the admission procedures and continuing with the ongoing observation and support of the client until completion of the fourth stage, or stabilization period. This is the sequence of events as the nurse encounters them. Although this chapter deals with uncomplicated vaginal delivery, every labor and delivery nurse must be able to recognize symptoms of complications that might develop and must know the appropriate nursing interventions.

Most women in the United States give birth in a hospital birthing room called a labor, delivery, and recovery room (LDR). In this setting, the woman is not transferred from a labor room to a delivery room, unless the need develops for operative intervention; she remains in the LDR for at least 1 hour after delivery. During this recovery period the infant remains with the woman, thus beginning the bonding process. After the recovery period, the woman is transferred to the postpartum unit. In some hospitals the woman remains in the same room (labor, delivery, recovery, and postpartum room [LDRP]) until discharge. With the introduction of LDRs, LDRPs, and birthing rooms, hospitals have attempted to create a family-centered approach that promotes an ambience of normalcy rather than a clinical atmosphere (Figure 14-1).

ASSESSMENT OF THE PHYSIOLOGIC PROCESS OF LABOR

Most women who arrive at the labor and delivery unit are excited about the birth of their baby but also anxious that everything should progress well. A woman often wonders whether she really is in labor, whether she will appear foolish if sent home, and if she is in true labor, how she will cope with the pain and stress of contractions and giving birth. The nurse can allay much of this anxiety by adopting a friendly and interested manner and keeping the woman and her support person fully informed. Teaching plays a major role in easing anxiety and includes events of labor and what to expect in the way of procedures. Care must be taken to maintain the client's privacy and confidentiality to promote trust and avoid undue

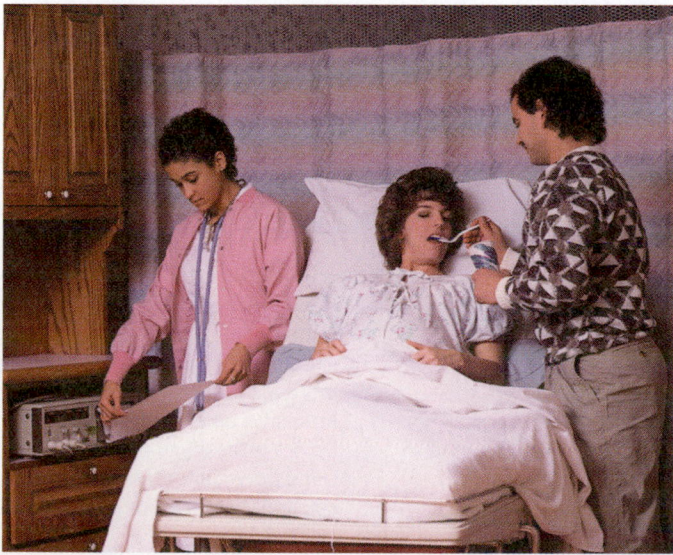

Figure 14-1   Many hospitals offer a pleasant, family-centered atmosphere for the birthing experience.

Critical Thinking

Who Delivers the Infant?

It is the woman who delivers the infant, not the physician or midwife. The laboring woman is the key player in this event. The health care team safeguards the mother and infant by providing a therapeutic environment, appropriate interventions, encouragement, reassurance, and feedback.

What do you believe is the most appropriate role for the professional nurse in providing care for the laboring woman and her fetus?

How do you think the nurse fits into the health care team?

stress. The woman in labor (the **parturient**), is the person of central importance in this situation, not the nurse, doctor, or nurse-midwife.

Maternal Status

Women arrive at the hospital or birthing center in different stages of labor and with different levels of wellness. Thorough initial and ongoing assessment by the nurse is critical to the well-being of mother and infant. Certain information is needed immediately for the nurse to establish appropriate priorities when developing the plan of care. Initial admission observations are aimed at establishing the fact that true labor has begun, ascertaining the imminence with which the birth might be expected, and alerting team members to existing or developing complications or risk factors. It is desirable for the prenatal care provider to transmit the client's health history, physical findings, and laboratory data to the hospital toward the end of the third trimester so that when the client is admitted to the labor and delivery unit her prenatal record can be reviewed and pertinent information recorded in the Admission Record.

Nursing Tip   *Introductions*

When meeting a client for the first time, it is wise to bear in mind that first impressions are lasting. The nurse should introduce herself, ask the names of the client and those accompanying her, and conduct them to the triage room or the assigned labor, delivery, and recovery room.

Labor Onset

One of the most critical diagnoses in obstetrics is the accurate diagnosis of labor status. The hallmark of true labor is cervical change; however, the woman at home has no way of knowing whether her cervix is dilating. Many women come to the hospital believing that they are in labor, only to be discharged home after a few hours, still pregnant. To conserve the use of LDRs, many hospitals have a triage unit in which the client's labor status is first evaluated before she is either discharged or moved to an LDR.

Although making a differential diagnosis between true and false labor sometimes is difficult, it usually can be done on the basis of certain very specific criteria (Table 14-1).

Initial Status Assessment

During the initial assessment the client is observed closely for clues to her status. Postures, facial expressions, and gestures can suggest tension, anxiety, or pain. Perspiration, varied breathing patterns, and frequent position changes also can indicate stress and discomfort. Grunting or breath-holding may signal the start of the second stage of labor. If the client is in active **labor** (the process by which the fetus is expelled from the uterus) the nurse may have to shorten the initial assessment and prioritize the questions (between contractions) to focus on her current labor status. Certain information is needed immediately to evaluate the extent of the woman's labor and to become alert to the woman with a history of rapid deliveries or problems indicating risk. The client should not have to guess the identifying information that is important for the nurse to know; therefore, skillful interviewing is essential. Questions that the nurse should ask include the following:

1. What is your reason for coming to the hospital?
   Information obtained: Presenting complaint (e.g., urge to push, back pain, "water" broke).

2. When is your baby due, and how many babies have you had?

COLLABORATIVE CARE

Communication for Intrapartal Team

When working as a member of a team, documentation is extremely important so that all members of the team have access to information they need to make appropriate decisions to develop a comprehensive plan of care.

Information obtained: Expected date of delivery and parity, possibility of a rapid labor if the woman is a **multipara**, that is, a woman who has had two or more pregnancies that reached viability.

3. When did your labor begin? How far apart are the **contractions** (tightening and shortening of the uterine muscles during labor)? Have they become stronger? Information obtained: The length of time the woman has been in labor, and the frequency and perceived **intensity** (strength of the contraction at its peak) of the contractions.

4. Has the bag of water (membranes) broken? At what time? What color was the fluid? Have you noticed any bleeding?
   Information obtained: Possible presence of abnormal bleeding (bloody discharge without mucus) or **bloody show** (a blood-tinged mucous discharge from the vagina that occurs as the cervix starts to dilate), whether membranes have ruptured, time of rupture of membranes, possible presence of meconium-stained amniotic fluid (**meconium** is fetal stool found in the bowel of a term neonate). Presence of meconium-stained amniotic fluid indicates that the fetus has experienced an episode of hypoxia.

5. How has your pregnancy been? Have you been hospitalized during this pregnancy? Is there anything

Table 14-1 True versus False Labor		
QUALIFIER	TRUE LABOR	FALSE LABOR
Contractions	Regular Intervals shorten Intensity increases Intensify with walking Lying down has no effect	Irregular Intervals do not shorten Intensity remains unchanged Do not intensify with walking Lying down lengthens interval
Cervix	Dilates and becomes effaced	Does not dilate or efface
Sedation	Does not stop true labor	Tends to stop false labor
Show (blood-tinged mucus from the cervical canal)	Often is present	Usually is absent

else about you or your pregnancy that I should know?

Information obtained: Any condition or information, especially medical, that may have an impact on labor, delivery, and the neonate.

6. Are you allergic to any foods or medicines that you know of? Are you allergic to latex? Have you ever had a bad reaction to a blood transfusion?

Information obtained: Any known allergies to medications, latex, or blood.

Other pertinent information can be outlined on the Obstetric Admitting Record (Figure 14-2).

Informed Consent

The fact that the woman comes to the birthing facility gives the implication of consent to treatment; nevertheless, informed consent should be obtained in the form of a signature before any invasive procedures are carried out. It is the physician's responsibility to give the client information and rationale for the type of interventions that may be performed, including benefits, possible risks, and available alternatives. Typically, however, it is the nurse who obtains and witnesses the client's signature on the consent form. An informed consent form should be signed before any treatment is carried out, particularly administration of medications that might impair the woman's ability to make decisions. Each hospital or birthing center may have its own variation of an informed consent form; however, all forms should cover delivery of the infant and include procedures that may be necessary in an emergency, for example, general anesthesia, cesarean delivery, blood transfusion, and hysterectomy.

Risk Factors

Often the physician or midwife on call will notify the labor and delivery unit of a client's pending arrival. If the prenatal record is available, it should be reviewed before the client arrives at the unit. The nurse reviews the medical history and antenatal care notes, and identified risk factors. Factors that put the woman or infant at high risk for morbidity must be recognized early so that appropriate and timely intervention can be made, including consultation with specialists in other medical departments. Early intervention can minimize fetal and maternal complications.

Many conditions in either the mother or fetus, some preexisting and others that have developed during the pregnancy, can result in a high-risk classification (Boxes 14-1 and 14-2). Cunningham (2001) listed three major categories that can be identified antepartum that put the client at increased risk: preexisting medical illness; previous poor pregnancy outcome, such as perinatal mortality,

Critical Thinking

Noncompliance

RL has phenylketonuria. Her doctor advised her to follow a diet low in phenylalanine before becoming pregnant and throughout the pregnancy to protect the fetus. RL refused to follow the low-phenylalanine diet and gave birth to a baby boy with severe neurologic damage. You overhear another nurse say, "People like her should be put in the hospital and obliged to follow the diet so that the baby would not be harmed."

What would be your response to this nurse?

preterm delivery, fetal growth retardation, malformations, placental accidents, and maternal hemorrhage; and inadequate maternal weight gain owing to malnutrition.

Expected Date of Delivery

The expected date of delivery (EDD) is noted in the Admission Record and the gestation calculated in weeks and days; for example, 38 weeks and 3 days would appear as 38 3/7 weeks. If the EDD is not known, the nurse may calculate the EDD from the date of the woman's last menstrual period using Naegele's rule (see Chapter 9). **Gravidity**, the number of times the woman has been pregnant, and **parity**, the number of pregnancies that have reached viability regardless of outcome, are noted.

Two methods are used to document gravidity and parity:

5-digit method:
a. Number of times the woman has been pregnant (gravidity)
b. Number of term births (parity)
c. Number of **preterm births**, that is, births after 20 weeks' gestation and before 37 weeks' gestation
d. Number of abortions (spontaneous or elective)
e. Number of living children

GTPAL: G6P4014 = 6 pregnancies, 4 to term, 0 premature, 1 abortion, 4 living

Nursing Tip *Parity*

Parity is determined by the number of pregnancies of viable duration, not the number of fetuses delivered. For example, a primigravida who previously delivered stillborn triplets at 29 weeks' gestation is a para 1.

Duplication of this form is strictly prohibited by law. © 2001 Briggs Corporation. All rights reserved.

Briggs CORPORATION

Obstetric Admitting Record
Maternal/Newborn Record System   Page 1 of 2
To order call: **1.800.245.4080**   Re-order No. **5710N**

Basic Admission Data
Date **6** / **23** / **04**   Time **1330**

☐ Ambulatory   ☐ Stretcher   ☑ Oriented to Unit
☑ Wheelchair   ☐ Transfer From _____   ☑ Safety/Security

| G. 111 | T. 11 | Pt. 0 | A. 0 | L. 11 | LMP | 9 / 28 / 03 | EDD 7 / 4 / 04 | Wks 38.5 |

EDD By Fetal Assessment **7 / 4 /04**

Race/Ethnicity **Caucasian**   Age **34**

Advance Directives ☑ **None** ☐ Living Will ☐ Medical Power of Attorney
Information Given ☑ Yes ☐ No (explain) _____
Organ Donor ☐ Yes ☑ No
Pain ☐ No ☑ Yes (site **abdomen/ lower back**)   Intensity 0 ___ **6-7** ___ 10
                                                                    none   highest

Type ☐ Aching ☐ Nagging ☐ Dull ☐ Heavy ☐ Crushing ☐ Sharp
☐ Stabbing ☐ Throbbing ☐ Radiating ☐ Burning ☐ Tingling
☑ Cramping ☐ Other: **squeezing**

Last Oral Intake
Fluids **orange juice /coffee** Time **0700**
Solids **toast** / ___ / ___ Time **0700**

Medications ☐ None

Type/Dose	Last Taken	With Patient No / Yes	Disposition
Prenatal vitamin	0700	☑ / ☐	at home
		☐ / ☐	
		☐ / ☐	

MD/CNM **Mark Brown**   Tel No **555-2300**   Support Person/Relationship **Frank/husband**   Tel No **555-9330**

Allergy/Sensitivity ☐ None   ☐ Latex
☑ Other **Demerol (severe nausea & vomiting)**

Reasons for Admission
☑ Onset of Labor
☐ Induction of Labor
☐ Spontaneous Abortion
☐ Cesarean Section
  ☐ Primary ☐ Repeat
  (reason for primary _____)
☐ Tubal Ligation
☐ Vaginal Bleeding
☑ ROM ☐ Premature ☐ Prolonged
☐ Preterm Labor

Detail Reasons for Admission **Contractions every 5-6 minutes since 1000. Spontaneous rupture of membranes at 1230.**

Observation Evaluation
☐ Fetal Status
☐ Ultrasound
☐ Amniocentesis
☐ NST ☐ CST
☐ Medical Complications
_____
☐ Obstetric Complications
_____

Personal Effects		Disposition		
Item	With Patient	With Support Person	Other (Describe)	
☑ Clothes		✓		
☑ Jewelry		✓	Gold metal watch	
	✓		Gold metal wedding band	

Patient Triage Data ☑ See Triage Record
Contractions ☐ **None** ☐ Palpation ☐ Tocotransducer
Frequency _____ Duration _____ Intensity _____
Began on ___ / ___ / ___ Time _____
Pain intensity 0 _____ 10
                      none   highest
Membranes ☐ Intact ☐ Bulging
☐ Ruptured (Date ___ / ___ / ___ Time _____)
☐ Nitrazine test (☐ pos ☐ neg) ☐ Sterile Speculum Exam
☐ Fern test   (☐ pos ☐ neg) (findings _____)

Fluid ☐ Clear ☐ Bloody ☐ Meconium Stained
      ☐ Foul Odor ☐ No Foul Odor ☐ None Observed
Vaginal Bleeding ☐ **None** ☐ Normal Show
      ☐ Bleeding (Describe _____)
Cervical Exam By _____
Station _____ Effacement _____ Dilatation ___ cms
Presentation ☐ Vertex   ☐ Transverse Lie
             ☐ Face/Brow   ☐ Compound
             ☐ Breech (type ___) ☐ Unknown

PRE-PROCEDURE CHECKLIST
(Check all that apply)
☑ History & Physical
☑ Prenatal Records
☑ X-rays and Ultrasounds
☑ Consents
☑ Patient ID
☐ Site ID / Verification
☐ Other _____
Timeout _____

Physical Assessment

Height 5 ft. 7 in.	Wt Pregrav/Grav 135 / 160	Temp 98⁸	Pulse 88	Resp 12	BP 128/88

Detail Abnormal Findings

System	Normal	Abnormal	
HEENT	☑	☐	
Neurologic	☑	☐	
Skin	☑	☐	
Breasts	☑	☐	(Pregnant)
Extremities	☑	☐	
Cardiovascular	☑	☐	
Respiratory	☑	☐	
Abdomen	☑	☐	(Pregnant)
Gastrointestinal	☑	☐	
Urinary	☑	☐	
Genitalia	☑	☐	

Initial Problems Identified ☑ None   Plan
1. _____
2. _____
3. _____

Fetal Evaluation Data   Multiple Gestation ☑ No ☐ Yes
Fundal Height **39** cms   Presentation   Position
Fetal Weight (est.) **8 lbs**   1. _____ _____
FHR **148**   2. _____ _____
☑ Fetoscope ☐ Fetal Monitor   3. _____ _____
☐ Doppler ☐ Other _____

Specimens Obtained (Check all that apply)

Urine Test	Time	Results	Blood Test	Time	Results
☑ Urinalysis	1400		☑ Hgb	1420	11.9
☐ C + S			☑ Hct	1420	35.2
☑ Glucose	1400	neg	☑ VDRL/RPR		
☑ Albumin	1400	trace	☐ Type/Screen		
☑ Ketones	1400	neg	☐		
☑ pH	1400	7.0	Cervical Culture		
☑ Blood	1400	neg	☐ GBS		
☐ Toxicology			☐		

Admitting Signature	Date/Time	Examiner Signature	Date/Time
Rae Baird RNC	6/23/04 1345	Mark Brown M.D.	6/23/04 1350

Form 5710N © 2001 Briggs Corporation, Des Moines, IA 50306
R404   To order, phone (800) 245-4080 www.BriggsCorp.com PRINTED IN U.S.A.

OBSTETRIC ADMITTING RECORD (Page 1 of 2)

Figure 14-2   Obstetric Admitting Record. (*Courtesy of Briggs Corporation.*)

Duplication of this form is strictly prohibited by law. © 2001 Briggs Corporation. All rights reserved.

Briggs
CORPORATION

Obstetric Admitting Record
Maternal/Newborn Record System   **Page 2 of 2**
To order call: **1.800.245.4080**   Re-order No. **5710N**

Significant Prenatal Data
Prenatal Records Available on Admission
☐ No ☑ Yes Source **Dr. Brown**
First Visit by 13 Wks ☑ Yes ☐ No
Regular Care ☑ Yes ☐ No
Prenatal Classes ☑ Yes ☐ No
Pediatric Provider
Michael Smith M.D.
General Health ☑ **Healthy**
☐ Functional Deficit (Type _____)
☐ Recent Exposure to Communicable Disease
  Type/Date _____ ___ /___ /___
  ☐ Illness (Less than or equal to 14 days prior to admission)
  Type/Treatment _____
  ☐ Chronic Condition
  Type _____
Immunizations ☑ Influenza ☐ Pneumonia ☑ Tetanus ☑ Hepatitis
  ☐ Other _____
Nutritional Status ☑ Well-nourished ☐ Malnourished ☐ Obese
Plan to Breast Feed ☑ Yes ☐ No
  ☐ Special Diet _____
Eating Disorder ☑ None ☐ Identify _____
Nutritional Problems ☑ None ☐ Identify _____

Lab Findings
☐ **None**
Blood Type & Rh **O+**
Rubella Titer **Immune**
Serology **Non-reactive**
HBsAg _____
HIV _____
GBS _____

Fetal Assessment Tests
☐ **None**

Date	Test	Result
2/14	Ultrasound	Normal 21 wk fetus
/		
/		
/		

Problems Identified ☐ **None**
	Active	Resolved
1. **Bicornate uterus**	☑	☐
2. _____	☐	☐
3. _____	☐	☐
4. _____	☐	☐

Hospitalizations ☐ **None**
1. ___ / ___ / **91** Reason **Tonsilectomy**
2. **8** / ___ / **00** Reason **Delivery**
   7 / **02** **Delivery**

Plans for Birth and Hospital Stay
☑ Birth Plan Attached
Support Person Present in L&D ☐ No ☑ Yes **Husband**
Other Family Members in L&D ☑ No ☐ Yes
Anesthesia ☐ **None** ☐ Local ☑ Epidural ☐ Spinal ☐ General
Delivery Site/Position **LDRP**
Personal Requests **None**

Adoption ☑ No ☐ Yes Contact with Infant ☐ No ☐ Yes
  Adoption Contact _____
Feeding Preference ☑ Breast ☐ Bottle
☐ Tubal Ligation Authorization Signed ☐ Yes ☐ No
☑ Circumcision Authorization Signed ☑ Yes ☐ No

Psychosocial Data ☐ See Prenatal Records
Emotional Status ☐ Happy ☐ Ambivalent ☐ Concerned
  ☐ Depressed ☐ Angry ☑ Other **Anxious**
Communication Barriers ☑ **None**
  ☐ Language ☐ Interpreter _____
  ☐ Vision ☐ Reading ☐ Writing ☐ Hearing
  ☐ Speech ☐ Other _____
Support System
  Marital Status: S ⓂSep D W Father involved ☑ Yes ☐ No
  Other Support ☐ None ☑ **mother and sister**
Occupation **RN** Education **BSN**
Religion ☐ N/A ☑ **Catholic**
Personal/Cultural/Religious Customs Affecting Care and/or Learning
  ☑ **None** ☐ Identify _____

Basic Needs Met Yes No If No, Explain
Food ☑ ☐
Clothing ☑ ☐
Housing ☑ ☐
Transportation ☑ ☐
Finances ☑ ☐
Life Stress No Yes If Yes, Explain
Physical Abuse ☑ ☐
Emotional Abuse ☑ ☐

Life Stress(Cont.)	No	Yes	If Yes, Explain
Major Change	☑	☐	
Self Care Needs	☑	☐	
Serious Illness	☑	☐	
Other	☐	☐	

Substance Use	No	Yes	If Yes, amt/day, last use
Tobacco	☑	☐	
Alcohol	☐	☑	1 glass wine – occasionally
Prescribed Drugs	☐	☑	Natabec 0700
Illicit Drugs	☑	☐	

Educational Needs	Mother	Support Person	Comments
Stages/Phases of Labor	☐	☐	
Coping Techniques	☐	☐	
Infant Feeding	☐	☐	
Infant Care	☐	☐	
_____	☐	☐	

Preferred Learning Methods	Yes	No
One-on-One Instruction	☐	☐
Group Instruction	☐	☐
Written Information	☑	☐
Audio/Visual Information	☐	☐
Demonstration/Practice	☐	☐
Other _____	☐	☐

Discharge Planning Data Planned Length of Stay **2** Days
Home Setting Yes No
Heat, running water, refrigeration ☑ ☐
Infant Care Supplies/Car Seat ☑ ☐
Phone in home ☑ ☐
Transportation available ☑ ☐
Adult assistance available ☑ ☐

Referrals
☐ RN Case Manager ☐ Utilization Review ☐ Other
☐ Home Care RN ☐ Social Service _____
☐ Nutritionist/Dietician ☑ Pediatric Provider

MD/CNM notified by **Rae Baird RNC** Date **6**/**23**/**04** Time **1355**
Admitting Signature **Mark Brown M.D.** Date **6**/**23**/**04** Time **1500**

Form 5710N © 2001 Briggs Corporation, Des Moines, IA 50306
R404 To order, phone (800) 245-4080 www.BriggsCorp.com PRINTED IN U.S.A.

OBSTETRIC ADMITTING RECORD (Page 2 of 2)

Figure 14-2 *(continued)*

Box 14-1

Pregnancy Risk Factors Identified from the Mother's Medical History

- Diabetes mellitus
- Sickle cell disease
- Prior cesarean delivery
- Chronic hypertension
- Heart disease
- Anemia
- Cigarette smoking, alcohol use, substance abuse
- Obesity
- Renal disease
- Infection, e.g., hepatitis B, syphilis, gonorrhea, chlamydia, human immunodeficiency virus, group B β hemolytic *Streptococcus*, active herpes virus
- Previous perinatal loss
- Age under 16 or over 35 years
- Seizure disorder

Box 14-2

Specific Risk Factors Developing during This Pregnancy

- Pregnancy-induced hypertension
- Polyhydramnios or oligohydramnios
- Preterm labor
- Bleeding in the third trimester
- Placenta abruption
- Prolonged or premature rupture of membranes
- Gestational diabetes mellitus
- Fetal congenital anomalies
- Gestational age 42 weeks or more
- Pre-eclampsia
- Multiple gestation
- Placenta previa
- Abnormal presentation
- Inadequate or no prenatal care
- Intrauterine growth restriction
- Isoimmunization (Rh or ABO)
- Drug exposure (OTC and Rx)

2-digit method:

a. Number of times the woman has been pregnant (gravidity)

b. Pregnancies that have reached a gestation of viability, regardless of outcome

G3P2: 2 pregnancies and 2 live births. G includes current pregnancy prior to delivery

Problems with Present Pregnancy

The client is asked about any problems she may have had, particularly those requiring hospitalization, pertaining to the current pregnancy. Problems such as preterm labor, vaginal infections, vaginal bleeding, gestational diabetes, and pregnancy-induced hypertension (PIH) are of particular importance. To make appropriate nursing diagnoses, a comprehensive nursing database must be compiled.

Findings of a preliminary history and screening serve to determine whether the woman is, in fact, in labor and whether there are any obvious problems. Relevant information includes but is not necessarily limited to the EDD; blood pressure; temperature; pulse; respirations; pattern and amount of weight gain and present nutritional status; symptoms experienced; deep tendon reflexes; edema; and urine screening for protein, glucose, and ketones.

Health History

The nurse obtains pertinent information from the prenatal record and by interviewing the client. Risk factors that may increase morbidity or mortality are evaluated. In order to make this evaluation, the nurse must possess a knowledge of perinatal factors and chronic physical conditions that might put the pregnancy into a high-risk category. Childhood diseases, emotional problems, and genetic defects are noted in the Admission Record. Chronic illnesses, such as hypertension, diabetes, positive human immunodeficiency virus (HIV) status, cardiac disease, phlebitis, renal disease, and seizure disorders, are conditions that place an additional burden on the body; therefore, these illnesses put the client and fetus at greater than normal risk for mortality or morbidity. Surgical operations are noted, particularly uterine surgeries (e.g., cesarean delivery, myomectomy) that would leave a weakened portion of the myometrium and thus a higher than normal risk of uterine rupture.

Demographic and Psychosocial History

Demographic and psychosocial information includes age; religious and cultural factors; and use of substances such as alcohol, tobacco, and illicit drugs. If the woman smokes cigarettes, she should be asked how many are smoked per day. If the woman admits to using illicit, so-called recreational, drugs she should be asked for details such as the

Critical Thinking

Cigarette Smoking during Pregnancy

Women who smoke cigarettes during pregnancy face serious health risks, including increased perinatal mortality, increased risk for placental abruption, low-birth-weight infants, small for gestational age infants, and preterm deliveries (ACOG, Sept. 1997).

If you were a nurse caring for a pregnant woman who smokes cigarettes, what would you tell her about cigarette smoking during pregnancy?

Would your advice differ if you were a cigarette smoker?

specific substance used and the amount taken. A drug screening should be done on any client who admits to or displays evidence that leads the caregiver to suspect substance abuse. Signs suggestive of substance abuse, such as needle marks or bruising, should be noted.

If the woman is admitted in an advanced stage of labor and is experiencing strong contractions, it may not be appropriate for the nurse to make an in-depth health history record. Priority assessments, however, include the following:

Is the woman able to ask for what she needs?

Is there a language barrier?

Does she talk freely with the nurse and her partner?

Does she avoid eye contact?

How much rest has she had lately?

The woman's culture and socialization as well as her perception of previous birth experiences are likely to influence her attitude toward her current situation and her postpartum emotional adjustment (Lowe, 1996).

The woman should be encouraged to ask about practices during labor and delivery that are important to her culture, and these requests must be entertained with respect and sensitivity. When a request is made that contradicts usual practice, nurses should ask themselves the following questions: How important is this to the client? Is it safe? Is it feasible to incorporate this request into the plan of care?

Safety Screening

Many studies report that violence may begin or escalate during pregnancy (Hilliard, 1985). Estimates of the prevalence of abuse during pregnancy, based on research studies or clinic-based statistics, range from 0.9% to 20.1%,

with the bulk of studies reporting a prevalence of 3.9% to 8.3% (Gazmararian et al., 1996). Thus, it is crucial for the nurse to inquire of all female clients as to the safety of their domestic situation, because hospitalization during childbirth may provide the only window of opportunity for an abused woman to seek assistance. Studies have revealed that women who are anxious or exposed to increased stress during pregnancy tend to have infants of lower birth weight than women without added stress; studies also have shown that women with high levels of stress hormones compared with those with low levels are more likely to deliver preterm (Teixeira, Fisk, & Glover, 1999; Wadhwa, Porto, Garite, Chicz-DeMet, & Sandman, 1998).

A client may not want to confide in the nurse about domestic violence until a relationship of trust has developed between the nurse and the client. Even then, the client may not volunteer information unless she is asked outright and is assured of confidentiality. Safety screening should always be performed in absolute privacy, when the client is alone with the nurse. Sometimes it is necessary for the nurse to ask the partner to step out into the waiting room. An Abuse Assessment Screen should be completed and placed in the client's medical record (Figure 14-3). If the client screens positive for abuse, the nurse must discuss possible options that are available, provide phone numbers of local shelters, and notify the hospital social worker. If there are overt signs of abuse, such as bruises or abrasions, the nurse should describe them and take photographs, which are then placed in the client's medical record.

Critical Thinking

Domestic Violence during Pregnancy

Complications of pregnancy, including low weight gain, anemia, infection, preterm labor, chorioamnionitis, and first and second trimester bleeding are significantly higher in women who are abused compared with women who are not abused (Parker, McFarlane, & Soeken, 1994; Berenson, Wiemann, Wilkinson, Jones, & Anderson, 1991). Also significantly higher are maternal rates of depression; suicide attempts; and use of tobacco, alcohol, and illicit drugs. Some studies report appreciably lower mean birth weights for infants born to women abused during pregnancy (McFarlane, Parker, & Soeken, 1996).

What responsibility does the nurse have in screening for domestic violence in pregnancy?

NAME _____

TODAY'S DATE _____

(Circle **YES** or **NO** for each question)

1. **IN THE YEAR BEFORE YOU WERE PREGNANT,** were you pushed, shoved, slapped, hit, kicked, or otherwise physically hurt by someone? . . . . . **YES   NO**

   If YES, by whom (Circle all that apply)

   Husband   Ex-husband   Boyfriend   Ex-boyfriend   Parent   Child   Friend

   Total number of times _____

2. **SINCE THE PREGNANCY BEGAN** have you been pushed, shoved, slapped, hit, kicked, or otherwise physically hurt by someone? . . . . . **YES   NO**

   If YES, by whom (Circle all that apply)

   Husband   Ex-husband   Boyfriend   Ex-boyfriend   Parent   Child   Friend

   DATE OF LAST INCIDENT _____, SCORE _____ (SEE BELOW)

   DATE OF WORST INCIDENT _____, SCORE _____ (SEE BELOW)

   → **MARK THE AREA OF INJURY ON THE BODY SCORE THE TWO INCIDENTS** according to the following scale:

   1 = Threats of abuse including use of a weapon

   2 = Slapping, pushing; no injuries and/or lasting pain

   3 = Punching, kicking bruises, cuts and/or continuing pain

   4 = Beating up, severe contusions, burns, broken bones

   5 = Head injury, internal injury, permanent injury

   6 = Use of weapon; wound from weapon

   (If any of the descriptions for the higher number apply, use the higher number)

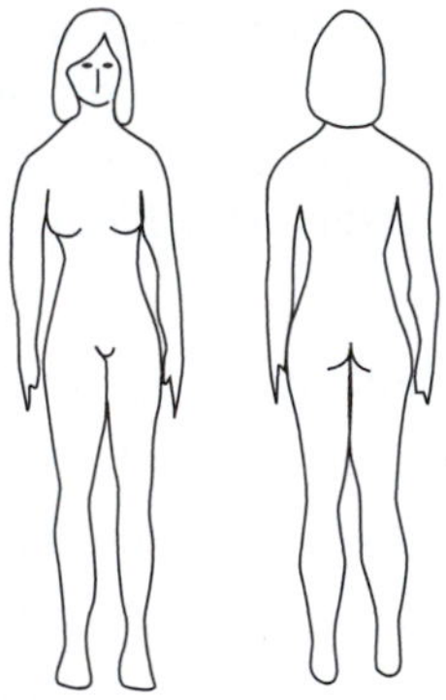

3. **IN THE YEAR BEFORE YOU WERE PREGNANT,** did anyone force you to have sexual activities? . . . . . **YES   NO**

   If YES by whom (Circle all that apply)

   Husband   Ex-husband   Boyfriend   Ex-boyfriend   Parent   Child   Friend

   Total number of times _____

4. **SINCE THE PREGNANCY BEGAN,** has anyone forced you to have sexual activities? . . . . . **YES   NO**

   If YES, by whom (Circle all that apply)

   Husband   Ex-husband   Boyfriend   Ex-boyfriend   Parent   Child   Friend

   Total number of times _____

Figure 14-3   Abuse Assessment Screen.

Obstetric History

When this is not the woman's first pregnancy, the characteristics of previous pregnancies and births are noted. Prenatal course, pregnancy outcomes, number of previous deliveries, and length of the client's last labor is information that might help to predict progress of the current labor. Useful details of the previous births would include gestation at delivery, birth weights, the type of anesthesia used, the kind of birth (spontaneous vaginal, forceps-assisted, vacuum-assisted, or cesarean birth), and whether there was postpartum hemorrhage.

Fetal Status

Initial assessment of the fetus gives reassurance of well-being and must be recorded appropriately. The fetal heart rate (FHR) may be evaluated by auscultation with a fetoscope or electronically by means of a Doppler or by electronic fetal monitoring (EFM). EFM has become routine in most labor and delivery units in the United States. The character of uterine activity and the response of the FHR to contractions provide considerable data. Leopold's maneuvers are performed by the nurse between contractions to assess fetal presentation, lie, and engagement, which aids in ascertaining the appropriate location for auscultating the FHR. Success of external fetal heart rate and maternal contraction monitoring depends largely on correct positioning of the ultrasound transducer and tocotransducer.

The **fetal heart rate (FHR)** is the number of times the fetal heart beats per minute (Cunningham, 2001). The Association of Women's Health, Obstetric and Neonatal Nurses (AWHONN) (1998) establishes guidelines for competency validation for FHR monitoring, and the American College of Obstetricians and Gynecologists (ACOG) publishes technical bulletins to guide clinical practice issues such as FHR monitoring (ACOG, July 1995).

Perinatal nurses are responsible for familiarizing themselves with practice guidelines regarding FHR monitoring. The FHR should be evaluated as soon as possible after the woman arrives at the labor and delivery unit

Nursing Tip *Confidentiality*

The client's partner may be unaware of past pregnancies, infants given up for adoption, abortions, or a positive human immunodeficiency virus status. A client's desire for confidentiality must be respected. Therefore, some questions are best asked when the partner, all family members, and all other support persons are out of the room.

Box 14-3

Nonstress Test

1. Place the fetal monitoring device on the client.
2. A **reactive nonstress test** is:

   2 accelerations of the fetal heart rate that are at least 15 beats above the baseline and last 15 seconds or more within 10 min.
3. If unable to obtain a reactive nonstress test within 30 min:

   Change the client's position.

   Administer oral or intravenous fluid.

   Use acoustic stimulation.
4. Continue to monitor for 30 more minutes.
5. If the fetal heart rate is not reactive after this time, inform the primary care giver.

(Box 14-3). The method and frequency of assessment will depend on risk factors and departmental policy. Monitoring can be continuous or intermittent.

Auscultation

Auscultation is an auditory method of monitoring the FHR. It is performed intermittently and usually with a DeLee-Hillis obstetric stethoscope or a Doppler device. Auscultation should be done during and immediately after a contraction. For the low-risk client in the active phase of the first stage of labor, auscultation should be performed at least every 30 minutes (ACOG, Dec. 1995). The Doppler ultrasound device is handheld and amplifies the sound of the FHR. The advantage of auscultation is that it allows for greater freedom of the client because she is not attached to a machine and does not have to wear belts to secure the ultrasound transducer and the tocotransducer. However, auscultation does not provide a printed record of the FHR for other medical professionals to see, nor does it provide an assessment of variability or other subtle changes in FHR.

Electronic Fetal Monitoring

Electronic fetal monitoring (EFM) is an auditory and visual monitoring method and provides a paper strip printout of FHR and variability, as well as a record of contraction frequency and duration (Figure 14-4, Box 14-4). EFM is used more frequently than is any other method; research has shown that EFM has increased the rate of surgical intervention and decreased perinatal mortality owing to fetal hypoxia (Vintzileos et al., 1995). Using EFM, the FHR can be assessed externally, or internally after the membranes have ruptured.

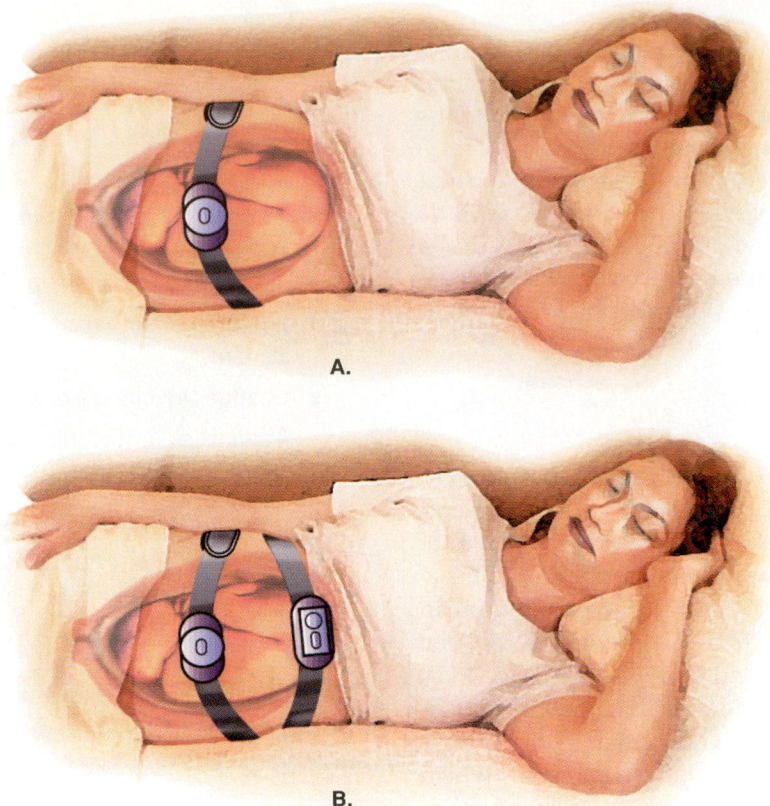

Figure 14-4 External fetal heart rate monitoring. A. Ultrasound transducer in place near the fetal heart. B. Tocotransducer in place over the uterine fundus. Tocotransducer placed over infant buttocks or lower back provides for better tracing of contraction pattern.

Box 14-4

General Approach to External Fetal Monitoring

1. Explain the procedure to the client.
2. Place the client in a position in which she feels comfortable and that is a semi-Fowler's, side-lying, or semi-recumbent position, with one hip tilted to the side.
   a. Turn monitor on.
   b. Press test button to ensure that monitor is functioning properly.
   c. Check date and time printed on strip.
   d. Mark the FHR monitor strip with the following information: client's name and medical record number, name of the physician or nurse-midwife, date, time, diagnosis, estimated date of delivery, and weeks of gestation.
3. Perform Leopold's maneuver to ascertain the position of the fetal back.
4. Apply water-soluble gel to the underside of the Doppler transducer for conduction of the fetal heart sounds.
5. Place the Doppler transducer on the maternal abdomen over the location of the upper portion of the fetal back (Figure 14-5).
6. Auscultate the fetal heart rate (FHR) while palpating the maternal pulse.
7. Place the uterine tocotransducer near the uterine fundus over the fetal buttocks (vertex presentation).
8. Check that the FHR tracing and contraction pattern are being printed and that the uterine reference has been zeroed.

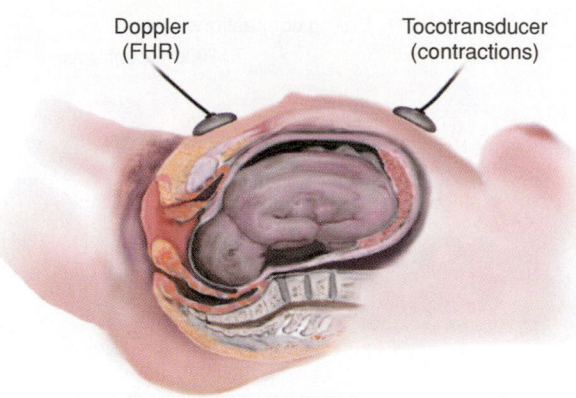

Figure 14-5   Lateral view of correct placement of Doppler and the tocotransducer on the maternal abdomen.

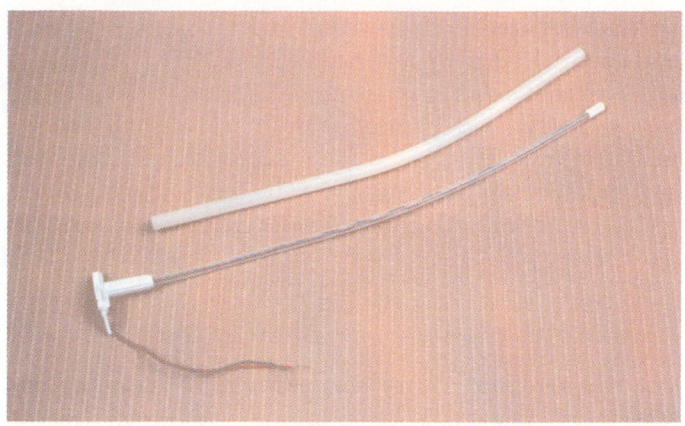

A.

In external electronic monitoring, the quality of the FHR strip depends on correct placement of the transducer (sometimes called a *Doppler*) on the maternal abdomen and the position of the fetus. The ultrasound waves strike the fetal heart, detecting the opening and closing of the valves, and direct a signal back to the transducer (ACOG, July 1995). The FHR can be observed from the bedside monitor or from a centrally located screen. Internal fetal heart rate monitoring requires a fetal scalp electrode (FSE) that attaches to the fetal scalp after rupture of the membranes (Figure 14-6). Internal uterine activity monitoring requires placement (by the physician or nurse-midwife) of an intrauterine pressure catheter (IUPC).

The frequency and method of fetal and contraction monitoring depend on institutional policy, maternal and

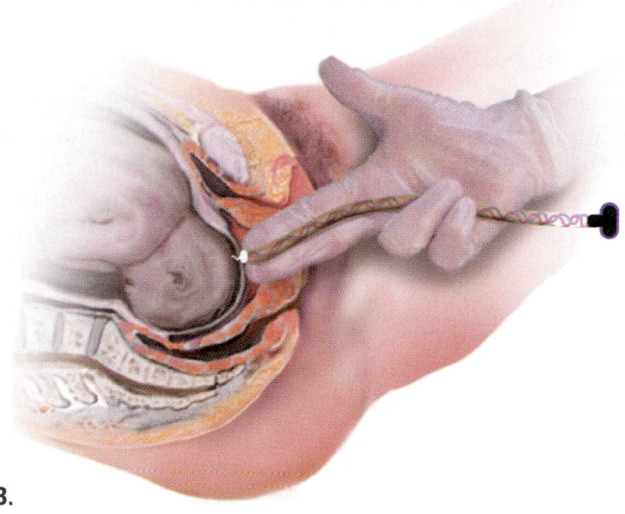

B.

Figure 14-6   A. Fetal scalp electrode. B. Placement of a fetal scalp electrode for fetal heart rate monitoring.

fetal risk factors, physician or nurse-midwife order, stage of labor, and client preference. When the electronic fetal monitor (EFM) is used intermittently, a 20-minute tracing is obtained on every woman on arrival to the labor and delivery unit (Table 14-2). The EFM is utilized periodically throughout the labor process based on the maternal and fetal status, stage of labor, and institutional policies. Auscultation of the FHR by Doppler and palpation of contractions are then performed by the nurse at intervals.

Critical Thinking

Fetal Monitoring Interpretation

Intrapartum nurses are legally responsible for interpreting the fetal heart rate (FHR) pattern and initiating appropriate nursing interventions. Timely notification of the primary caregiver in the event of a nonreassuring FHR pattern and documentation of all interventions and subsequent outcomes are nursing responsibilities. Should a difference of opinion arise between the intrapartum nurse and the physician or nurse-midwife regarding the appropriate intervention, the intrapartum nurse is responsible for initiating the institutional chain of command (AWHONN, 1998).

As a labor and delivery nurse, you have a client who has what you consider to be an ominous FHR pattern. You voice your concern to the physician several times, with no response. What is your duty as a nurse to provide for the safety of your client and her infant?

Table 14-2	Classification of Fetal Heart Rates	
Normal range		110–160 beats per minute (bpm)
Tachycardia	Mild	161–180 bpm
	Severe	>180 bpm
Bradycardia	Mild	100–110 bpm
	Moderate	80–100 bpm
	Severe	<80 bpm

When compared to intermittent auscultation of the FHR and manual palpation of contractions, EFM provides a more objective data-gathering tool. Electronic fetal monitoring provides a continuous graphical printout of the fetal heart rate and uterine contraction patterns. The labor and delivery nurse notes the FHR baseline, variability, and presence of accelerations or decelerations in the FHR pattern.

Labor Status

The client's labor status is assessed for uterine activity, fetal membrane status, cervical status, and fetal descent. Typically before assessing contractions, the nurse will perform Leopold's maneuvers to determine presenting part.

Uterine Activity

Assessment of uterine activity begins with the client's verbalization of when the contractions became regular and her perception of their strength. The nurse is able to confirm the intensity of the contractions by palpating the fundal area of the uterus. Assessment of uterine contractions by palpation requires no special equipment but, rather, nursing skill in touch and sensitivity. Evaluating the intensity via palpation is determined by the firmness of the fundal area noted by the nurse at the peak of the contraction. The nurse rests the palmar surface of the hand and fingertips on the fundus, where contractions start, and notes the changing firmness of the uterus as the contraction increases in intensity and then recedes. The firmness of the uterus at the **acme**, or peak, of the contraction is used to determine the intensity, which can be described as mild, moderate, or strong (Figure 14-7).

During mild contractions, the fundus can be indented easily by the fingertips. During moderate contractions, the fundus indents less easily and feels more rigid. During strong contractions, the fundus is firm and resists indenting by the slightly spread fingertips.

In addition to measuring the intensity of the contractions, their frequency and duration are also noted by the nurse. The **frequency** is measured from the beginning of one to the beginning of the next contraction. **Duration** of a contraction is the time from the start of a contraction to the end of the same contraction. The presence of uterine irritability or strong and prolonged contractions (**hypertonic contractions**) is noted by the nurse as well. It is also important for the nurse to evaluate the uterine resting tone. The **resting tone** is the firmness of the uterus between contractions and should be soft.

Electronically, contractions can be monitored by means of a tocotransducer, which is a pressure-sensing device placed on the fundus. The tocotransducer detects changes in the shape of the abdominal wall directly above the fundus as each contraction occurs. This noninvasive

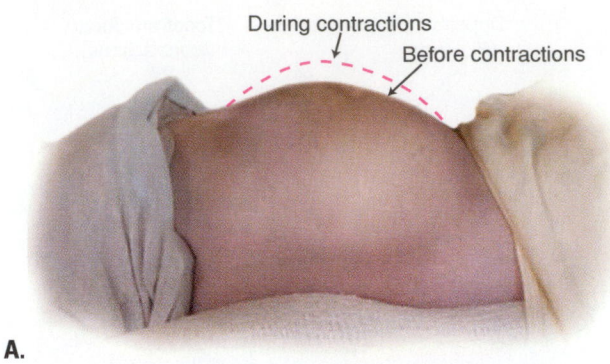

A.

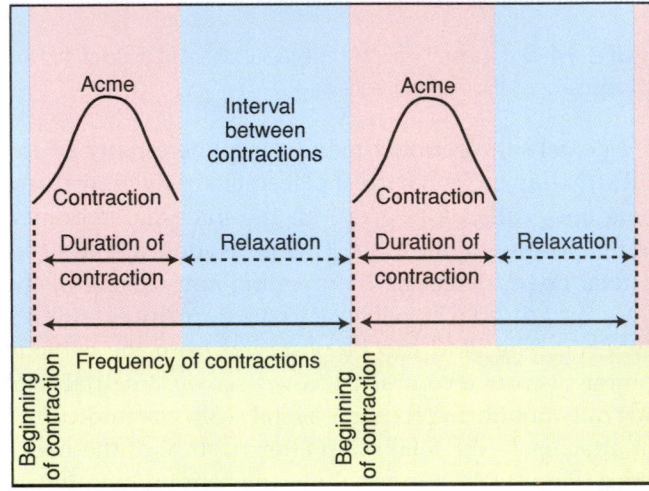

B.

Figure 14-7   A. Abdominal contour before and during a uterine contraction. B. Wavelike pattern of contractions on the fetal heart rate strip.

method gives the nurse information about the frequency and duration of the contractions but not the intensity. Because many women feel contraction pain in the lower back, or in the lower abdomen, they might question why the toco is placed over the fundus instead of where the pain is felt. The nurse should explain that the entire uterus contracts although the woman usually experiences pain mainly in the area of cervical stretching.

Accurate information concerning the intensity of contractions only can be obtained internally by means of the **intrauterine pressure catheter (IUPC)**. The IUPC is a fluid-filled catheter that is inserted directly into the uterine cavity through the cervix after the membranes have ruptured (Figure 14-8). In addition to the frequency and duration of contractions, the IUPC records contraction intensity by measuring the pressure of the amniotic fluid inside the uterus in millimeters of mercury (mmHg). Occasions that might necessitate the use of an IUPC include induction of labor, vaginal birth after cesarean section, failure to progress, and in the very obese client for whom attempts at external monitoring have been unsuccessful. Whether internal or external monitoring is used, it is important for

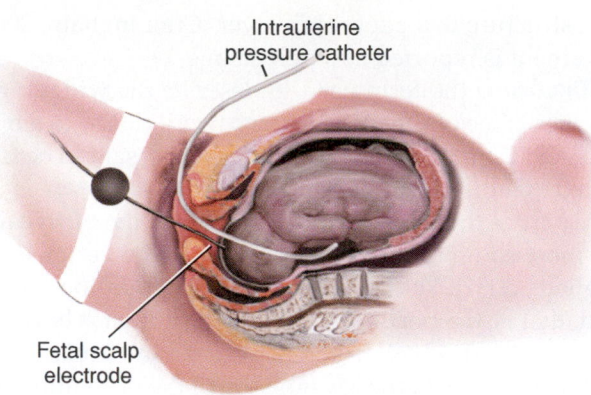

Figure 14-8   Placement of the intrauterine pressure catheter (IUPC) and fetal scalp electrode (FSE).

the nurse to remember to support the laboring woman based on her perception of the intensity of the contractions, not just the data detected by the electronic monitor.

Fetal Membrane Status

By the end of pregnancy the uterus contains about 1 L of amniotic fluid (Cunningham, 2001). In abnormal conditions the amount of fluid within the amniotic sac may vary from a few milliliters to several liters. The presence of more than 2 L of amniotic fluid is called **polyhydramnios** and less than 300 mL of fluid is referred to as **oligohydramnios** (Cunningham, 2001). Normal amniotic fluid is colorless and clear and contains particles of vernix. The odor is characteristic (not foul). As the nurse observes the perineum during physical examination, there may be pooling of amniotic fluid. It is important to establish the time of membrane rupture because a delay of 24 hours or more between membrane rupture and birth greatly increases the risk for intrauterine infection (Cunningham, 2001). Rupture of membranes may be confirmed by performing a **nitrazine test**, in which a dye-impregnated paper is dipped into a pool of suspected amniotic fluid or is touched to a cotton-tipped applicator soaked with vaginal secretions (Box 14-5). The color of the nitrazine paper is then compared with a color chart showing varying degrees of blue and the corresponding pH number (Table 14-3). Nitrazine paper that turns dark blue (pH 6.5) on contact with the alkaline amniotic fluid is consistent with ruptured membranes (Cunningham, 2001).

If a nitrazine test is not definitive and doubt still exists as to membrane status, a **fern test** may be done (Box 14-6).

The nitrazine test and the fern test may be done in conjunction with a vaginal examination. Most women will go into labor spontaneously within a few hours after membranes rupture. **Premature rupture of membranes (PROM)** is the term used to describe rupture of membranes before labor begins. **Preterm premature rupture of membranes**

Box 14-5

Procedure for Nitrazine Test for Presence of Amniotic Fluid

1. Explain the procedure to the woman and her partner.
2. Wash your hands, and put on sterile gloves. Do not use lubricating jelly.
3. Use a sterile cotton-tipped applicator to obtain fluid from the vagina. Touch the applicator to the test paper. Alternatively, a strip of nitrazine paper may be touched to the perineum when there is profuse drainage of clear fluid.
4. Compare the color of the nitrazine paper to the color chart.
5. Discard the gloves, and wash your hands.
6. Explain your findings and their implications to the client.
7. Document the numerical result.

Box 14-6

Procedure for Fern Test for Presence of Amniotic Fluid

1. Explain the procedure to the woman and her partner.
2. Wash your hands, and put on sterile gloves.
3. Use a sterile cotton-tipped applicator to obtain fluid from the vagina (usually done during a sterile speculum examination).
4. Draw the fluid-soaked applicator over a glass slide, and allow it to dry.
5. Examine the glass slide under a microscope and observe for the presence of a frondlike pattern, which indicates amniotic fluid.
6. Discard the gloves, and wash your hands.
7. Explain your findings and their implications to the client.
8. Document the result; that is, a positive or negative fern test.

Table 14-3   Findings on Nitrazine Paper

COLOR	PH	MEMBRANES
Yellow to olive green	5.0–6.0	Probably intact
Blue-green to deep blue	6.5–7.0	Probably ruptured

The pH values of blood, vaginal mucus, and secretions from some vaginal infections also are alkaline. Be aware of the possibility of false readings.

Nursing Tip — *Meconium Staining*

Presence of meconium in the amniotic fluid can be the result of vagal stimulation from transient umbilical cord compression or can be caused by fetal hypoxia. Fresh meconium staining in the presence of a nonreassuring fetal heart rate (FHR) pattern, such as severe variables or late FHR decelerations, is an ominous sign. The primary care provider should be notified immediately and requested to come to evaluate the client.

Nursing Tip — *Meconium Staining: Breech Presentation*

In a breech presentation, meconium frequently is passed because the fetal abdomen and buttocks are under pressure. This does not necessarily mean that the fetus is in distress.

(PPROM) describes rupture of membranes in a preterm pregnancy (less than 37 weeks' gestation) in the absence of contractions.

Abnormal findings upon or after rupture of membranes include meconium staining, foul odor, and dark-red fluid. Meconium, when present in the amniotic fluid in a cephalic presentation, often is an indication that the fetus has experienced an episode of hypoxia. Meconium turns the amniotic fluid to yellow or greenish-brown, depending on the amount of meconium present in the fluid. Meconium staining in the presence of a reassuring FHR pattern may indicate that the fetus is not currently in distress. Oligohydramnios, decreased amniotic fluid, reduces the cushioning effect of the fluid. As a result, the cord is more likely to become compressed. Cord compression, and consequent shutting off of the blood flow to and from the fetus, will result in a variable FHR deceleration.

The longer the fetal membranes have been ruptured, the greater the risk of **chorioamnionitis**, which is infection of the fetal membranes.

After taking the medical history, performing FHR monitoring, and assessing the labor status, a vaginal examination is performed to ascertain whether there has been cervical dilation; that is, whether the woman is in true labor.

Cervical Status and Fetal Descent

Vaginal examination is performed to determine the degree of cervical effacement and dilation, the fetal presenting part, and station. **Effacement** refers to the taking up of the cervical canal so that the cervix changes from a long thick structure to a paper-thin layer (Cunningham, 2001); effacement is reported as a percentage.

Dilation is the term used to describe the widening of the external os of the uterine cervix from closed to a maximum of 10 cm, at which time the cervix is said to be fully dilated (Cunningham, 2001). The **presenting part** is the body part of the fetus that is first to enter the birth canal. The most common presentation is cephalic vertex (Cunningham, 2001). **Vertex** refers to the crown of the infant's head, that is, the portion of the fetal head that is born first when the head is well flexed (Cunningham, 2001).

Station refers to the relationship of the presenting part to an imaginary line drawn between the ischial spines of the maternal pelvis (Figure 14-9), which is the narrowest diameter of the pelvis and designated as zero (0) station

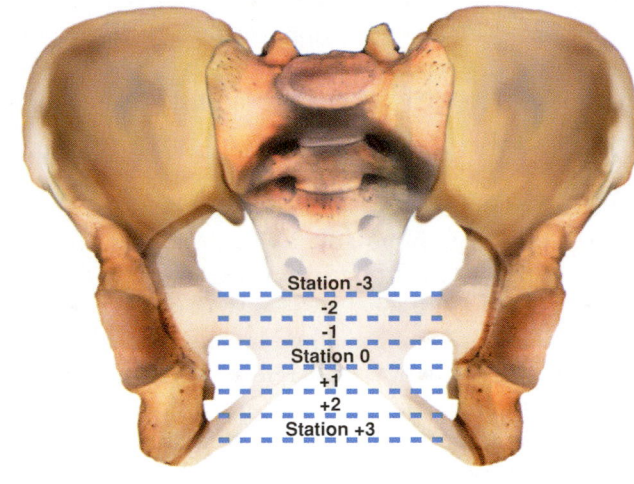

A.

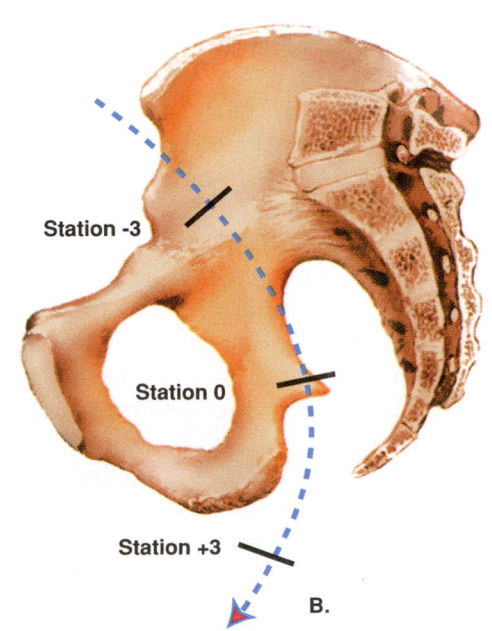

B.

Figure 14-9 Stations of the presenting part. A. Front view. B. Lateral view.

Nursing Tip *Effacement*

Effacement is a measurement of cervical thickness and is measured in percentages. The uneffaced cervix is about 1 inch thick (0% effaced). A cervix that is 2 inches thick is 50% effaced.

(Cunningham, 2001). The long axis between the pelvic inlet and the ischial spines can be divided into thirds, as described by Cunningham (2001), and labeled –3, –2, –1 accordingly; the axis between the ischial spines and the perineal outlet similarly can be divided into thirds and labeled +1, +2, and +3. When the presenting part can be seen at the woman's perineum it is said to be at +3 station.

Abdominal palpation for fetal lie and position, together with a check of fetal heart tones, should precede the initial vaginal examination. Situations such as PPROM or preterm labor contraindicate a digital vaginal examination, unless birth appears imminent, because of the infection risk. Vaginal examination should never be done by the nurse if the woman is experiencing significant vaginal bleeding or if placenta previa is known or suspected. Vaginal examination of a woman with placenta previa might cause severe bleeding.

Before vaginal examination the woman should empty her bladder; a full bladder will add to her discomfort. Vaginal examination can be performed between contractions or throughout a contraction. Examination during a contraction gives a much better picture of the fullest extent of dilation, effacement, and descent. Vaginal examination is an uncomfortable and stressful procedure for the woman. Efforts should be made to reduce stress by first giving a full explanation of the procedure and the information to be obtained from it in terms the woman can understand (Box 14-7). An informed woman is more likely to relax throughout the examination. Privacy must be maintained and modesty respected by closing the door or screening the room or triage

Box 14-7

Performing a Vaginal Examination on a Woman in Labor

1. Explain the procedure to the client in terms she can understand. Ensure privacy.
2. Position the client on the examination bed, semi-recumbent, with knees bent and legs apart and draped.
3. Wash your hands, and apply sterile gloves.
4. Apply sterile lubricating jelly to the index and second finger of the examining hand.
5. Inspect the general area of the introitus for presence and amount of bloody show, presence and color of amniotic fluid, malodorous discharge, and presence of blisters or ulcerated areas on the labia.
6. With the hand turned sideways and the thumb pointing upward, insert the first and second fingers of the examining hand gently into the vagina, keeping the fourth and fifth fingers bent inward to the palm of the hand. Insert the fingers the length of the vagina.

Membranes
7. Palpate for a soft, bulging membrane sac through the dilating cervix. Observe for running fluid during the examination, which would indicate that the membranes have ruptured.

Effacement
8. Palpate the thickness of the cervix and estimate the degree (0 to 100%) of thinning.

Dilation
9. Dilation of the cervix is measured in centimeters. One fingerbreadth is approximately 1.5 to 2 cm in width, although this measurement will vary among practitioners. Full cervical dilation is 10 cm in diameter.
10. Palpate for the presenting part.

Station
11. Determine the station by locating the lowest portion of the presenting part, then sweeping the fingers to one side of the pelvis to feel for the ischial spines.
12. Remove the fingers, and discard the gloves.
13. Wash your hands.

Nursing Alert

Vaginal Bleeding

If a client presents with bright-red vaginal bleeding, particularly if it is painless, you should suspect placenta previa, that is, implantation of the placenta near or over the cervical os.

1. Do *not* perform sterile vaginal examination.

2. Notify the primary care provider immediately.

3. Anticipate ultrasonography to rule out placenta previa.

4. Institute continuous electronic fetal monitoring.

Nursing Tip   Herpes Simplex Virus

When no lesions are visible at the onset of labor, vaginal delivery is acceptable. When primary or recurrent lesions are visible near the time of labor or when the membranes are ruptured or when there are prodromal symptoms of a recurrence (i.e., if the woman complains of herpeslike discomfort), cesarean delivery is performed (Roberts, Cox, Dax, Wendel, & Leveno, 1995).

Nursing Alert

Vaginal Examination

If raised vesicles or blisters are noted, the nurse should suspect active herpes viral infection. In the presence of active herpes infection, the examination is stopped and the primary care provider notified. Infants infected with the herpes virus during vaginal birth experience high morbidity (Kohl, 1997). Therefore, cesarean section is performed on all women who have herpes lesions at the time of delivery.

Nursing Tip   Station

Imagine a horizontal line from one ischial spine to the other. This line represents 0 station. Estimate how far (in centimeters) the tip of the presenting part is above or below the ischial spine. If the station is judged to be beyond 0, the pelvis probably is adequate for vaginal delivery.

area and asking the client whether she would like any family members present to step into the waiting room for a few minutes. Vaginal examination should be performed without delay if the woman complains of a desire to bear down or a perception of perineal pressure (Figure 14-10).

The woman is asked to lie down on the hospital bed, with legs bent and apart. Her legs are draped to avoid unnecessary exposure. If the woman knows a relaxation technique, such as slow deep breathing, she should be asked to use it and to try to relax. If it is not certain whether the membranes have ruptured, sterile lubricating jelly is not used because it can sometimes give a false-positive result on a nitrazine test. There may be sufficient vaginal mucus or bloody show to prevent dryness, or sterile water can be used instead of lubricating jelly. Presence of a large amount of bloody show indicates that labor is advanced.

Findings of the examination are communicated to the woman and related to her progress in labor. Information about the labor status may be reassuring to the woman and her partner.

Determine the onset of true labor (i.e., regular, strong contractions accompanied by cervical change). When doubt exists as to whether the woman is in labor, she may be advised to ambulate for several hours, taking frequent rest periods. Walking often helps to establish a good contraction pattern. The woman should be instructed to return to her room for FHR monitoring at 30- to 40-minute intervals, or to return immediately if any of the following occur:

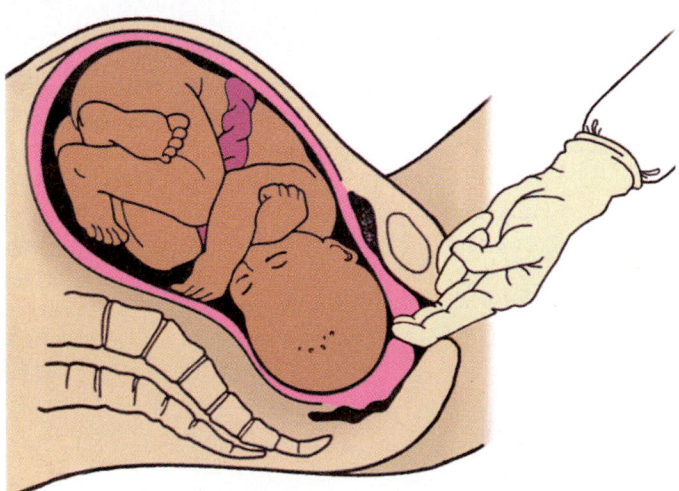

Figure 14-10 Vaginal examination to determine effacement, dilation, and fetal descent.

- Membranes rupture.
- Contractions become more frequent than 5 minutes apart.
- Bloody show increases.
- Nausea or vomiting occurs.
- An urge to push is felt.
- She requires analgesia or finds walking too tiring.

GENERAL SYSTEMS ASSESSMENT

The physical examination of the laboring woman is not as extensive as is that performed at the first prenatal visit. The initial assessment is carried out immediately to identify potential problems. Findings of the initial examination will provide a baseline for evaluation and comparison with future clinical findings. The general appearance of the woman is noted, particularly presence of edema in the face, hands, and feet as well as skin color, speech, manner, mood, state of awareness, gait, and personal hygiene. Initial information usually is recorded in the Admission Record; many facilities now have computer systems into which client information is entered directly from the bedside.

Vital Signs

Temperature, pulse, respirations, and blood pressure are assessed on admission and recorded in the Admission Record and nursing flowchart. Frequency of monitoring will depend on the risk status of the maternal-fetal dyad. Infection or dehydration will cause the client's body temperature to increase. The normal range is 97.4°F to 99.6°F, orally or tympanically. Normal heart rate range is 60 to 90 bpm. When auscultating the heart, the nurse will note that the point of maximal impulse is slightly more to the left than usual owing to displacement of the heart by the enlarged uterus. Increased heart rate may be due to excitement, anxiety, or contraction pain. Other possible causes of increased heart rate are cardiac problems or dehydration. Carefully taking the medical history should reveal preexisting medical problems. Dehydration should be considered as a possible reason for a rapid heart rate, in the absence of other causes, and the primary provider may require the administration of a 500 mL bolus of intravenous (IV) lactated Ringer's solution. The respiration rate will vary considerably, depending largely on the amount of pain being experienced. Counting of respirations should be done between contractions when the woman is not practicing a breathing technique.

Blood pressure is taken with the woman in a side-lying position, using the uppermost arm; the findings are compared with those on the prenatal record. A measurement showing an elevated systolic but normal diastolic blood pressure may indicate anxiety and should be repeated after the woman has had time to relax. To prevent supine hypotension and fetal distress caused by vena caval compression by the heavy uterus, the woman should be encouraged to lie on her side, or on her back with the uterus tilted to one side (Figure 14-11).

Abdomen

Inspect the abdomen for **striae gravidarum**, which are shiny, dark or reddish lines that appear as a result of stretching of the skin and underlying tissue, and for rashes, lesions, and scars. An abnormal shape of the abdomen should alert the nurse to a possible transverse lie, which would require cesarean delivery. Previous abdominal surgery will have been noted when the medical history was taken, and scarring may be evident. The history of the uterine incision must be obtained. If the uterine scar is classical (not low cervical), the primary care provider should be notified immediately. If a classical incisional scar is seen on the abdomen of a woman in active labor, the primary care provider should be notified immediately because a repeat cesarean delivery will be required and the woman, therefore, should not be left to labor. Although uterine rupture occurs in only 1 of every 2,000 deliveries (ACOG, 1998), it is more of a risk for women who have had a previous transfundal cesarean delivery and can be catastrophic for both mother and fetus. Palpate the uterus using Leopold's maneuvers to determine fetal lie.

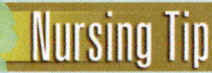

Nursing Tip *Presenting Part*

If you feel:

- The hard skull with the sagittal suture, it is a cephalic presentation.
- The softer buttock, it is a breech presentation.
- Irregular parts such as facial features, it is a face presentation.

Nursing Tip *Hypertension*

Compare blood pressure readings with those on the prenatal record. The client has hypertension if any of the following is noted:

- Blood pressure value of 140/90 mmHg or higher
- A systolic increase of 30 mmHg or higher
- A diastolic increase of 15 mmHg or higher

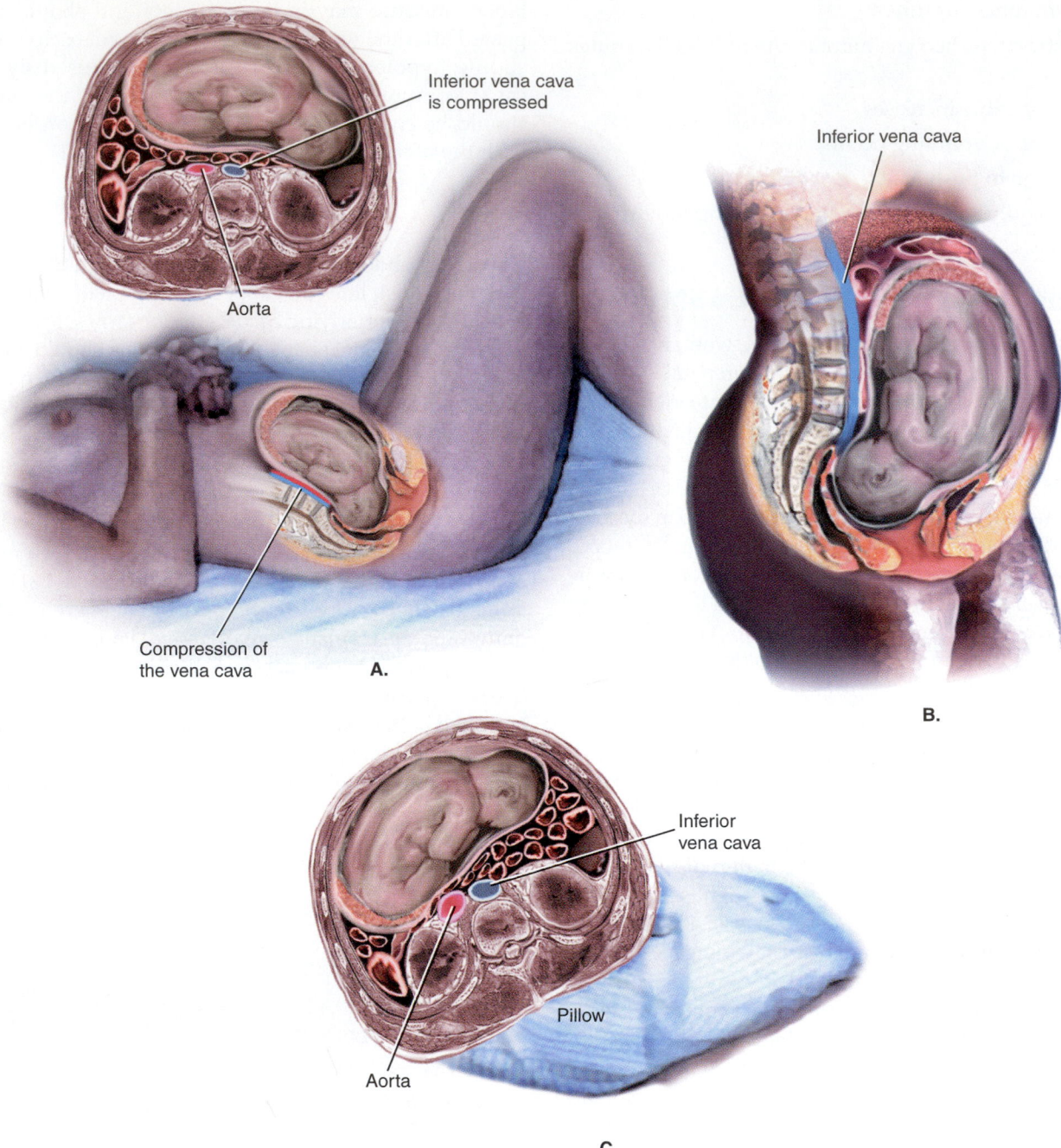

Figure 14-11 Vena caval compression (A) can be avoided by upright positioning (B) or by tilting to the side while lying supine (C).

Bladder

Gently palpate above the symphysis pubis to determine bladder fullness or suprapubic tenderness. Urinary frequency is common in late pregnancy; however, when the woman also complains of burning on urination, the nurse should suspect urinary infection. The nurse should send a catheter specimen or a clean-catch urine specimen for laboratory analysis.

Lower Extremities

Inspect the legs for varicosities and palpate with both hands for tenderness or areas of particular warmth, which might indicate thrombophlebitis. Other frequent physical findings in deep venous thrombosis are swelling, redness, and a positive Homan's sign (ACOG, March 1997).

Edema

Many women experience some dependent edema of the feet during late pregnancy from constriction of blood vessels by the pressure of the pregnant uterus (Box 14-8). Dependent edema usually is less evident when the woman is in bed. Pretibial edema, however, is an abnormal finding as are edema of the hands and edema around the eyes (periorbital edema), and is one of the signs of PIH. Findings of more than 2+ edema or periorbital edema should be reported to the primary care giver along with blood pressure readings and results of dipstick analysis of urine for albumin. The three cardinal signs of PIH are edema, hypertension, and albuminuria.

Deep Tendon Reflexes

Deep tendon reflexes (DTRs) are assessed by supporting the knee in a slightly flexed and quite relaxed position. The patellar tendon is briskly tapped just below the knee cap; responses are graded as per Table 14-4.

Nursing Tip *Positioning*

Ask the client to assume a side-tilt or side-lying position. These positions allow the heavy uterus to be displaced off the ascending vena cava and descending aorta, thus preventing a decrease in cardiac output that may lead to a decrease in maternal blood pressure and subsequent fetal bradycardia.

Table 14-4	Quantifying Deep Tendon Reflexes
RESPONSE	**GRADING**
More than normal (brisk)	3+
Normal	2+
Low or sluggish	1+
No response	0

Box 14-8

Procedure for Assessing Edema

Press firmly with the thumb for about 5 seconds over the pretibial area on both legs. Pretibial edema is assessed as follows:

1+ Small suggestion of fullness is felt.

2+ Sense of fullness.

3+ Blanching of the skin and depression seen as the thumb presses down.

4+ Indentation made by the pressure of the thumb remains for several seconds and gradually recedes.

Clonus

When the DTR is 3+ or greater (hyperactive), the nurse should be alert to the possibility of clonus, which is associated with pre-eclampsia. To test for clonus, the knee is supported in a partially flexed position while the nurse applies sharp dorsiflexion to the foot (Figure 14-12). As the foot is maintained in dorsiflexion it will oscillate rhythmically if clonus is present. An abnormal (positive clonus) is recorded as two or more "beats" clonus and indicates irritability of the central nervous system (CNS). The woman should be questioned about other possible indicators of pre-eclampsia such as nausea, dizziness, visual disturbances such as "halos" around the lights, epigastric pain, and headache.

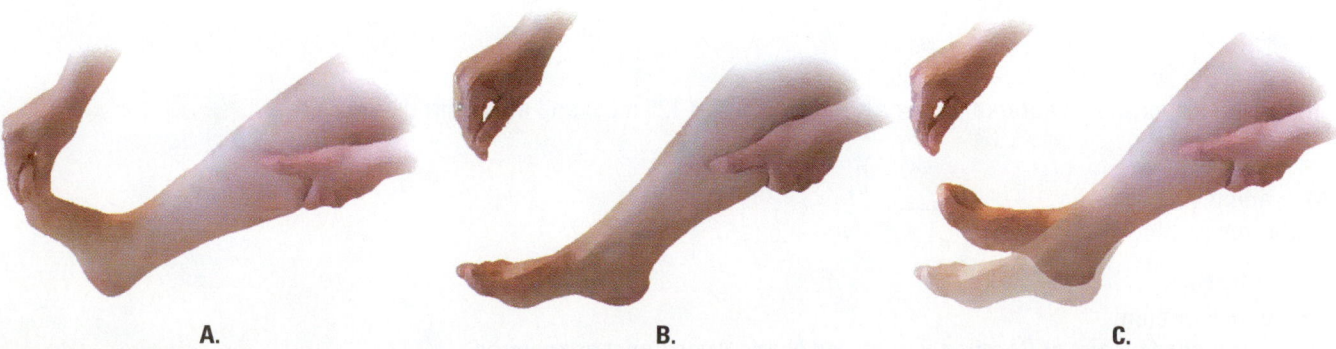

A.   **B.**   **C.**

Figure 14-12 Assessment for clonus. A. Dorsiflexion is applied to the foot. B. Foot returns to neutral position without pulsation. C. Foot oscillates, indicating clonus.

SETTING PRIORITIES AND MAKING DECISIONS

Care is prioritized and based on information obtained from the initial prenatal record, physical assessment, and medical history. Care of the laboring woman includes early identification and communication of conditions that might place the client in a high-risk category, educational needs, and discharge needs. A system of care is planned for the achievement of goals that are acceptable to both the client and nurse. A critical pathway of care that might be used is shown in Box 14-9. As labor progresses the plan of care is modified according to the ongoing maternal and fetal assessments as well as labor progress. Those women with critical care or high-risk conditions, or who are likely to give birth to an infant requiring neonatal intensive care, may require consultation with or transportation to a medical center with a neonatal intensive care unit.

Nursing Alert

C-Section Incisions

In assessing a woman with a history of C-section, the nurse needs to differentiate between the incision on the skin and the second incision on the uterus. The uterine incision is the determinant for repeat C-sections.

MATERNAL-FAMILY SUPPORT AND INTERACTIONS

A woman is more likely to have positive memories of her childbirth experience when she receives kind, sensitive care. Her partner, a significant family member, or friend should be encouraged to stay at the bedside and support

---

Box 14-9

Critical Pathway for a Client During Low-Risk Labor

Assessment

Monitor fetal heart rate and contractions as per protocol: Continuous _____   Intermittent _____
Sterile vaginal examination.
Blood pressure and pulse every hour.
Temperature every 4 h; every hour after rupture of membranes (ROM).
Laboratory tests: Typing, Rh status, complete blood count (CBC), rapid plasma reagin (RPR), hepatitis B surface antigen (HbsAg) (unless on prenatal record); HIV test is offered; Group B Beta Strep (GBBS); rubella status.
Input and output.
Cord gases: Yes _____   No _____
Cord blood sent to laboratory if Rh-negative or blood group type O.
Placenta sent to laboratory: Yes _____   No _____
Consent form signed.

Interventions

Oxygen per non-rebreather face mask at 8–10 L/min as required.
Straight catheter as required if unable to void. If receiving epidural, may insert Foley catheter as required.
Perineal preparation and stirrups at delivery.

Nutrition

Sips of water, ice chips, or clear liquids.
Intravenous hydration: Lactated Ringer's solution of 1 L at 125 mL/h and as required afterward.

Activity

May ambulate: Yes _____   No _____
Bathroom privileges (BRP):   Yes _____   No _____

Consultation

Notify pediatrician.
Notify anesthesiologist or Certified Registered Nurse Anesthetist as required.
Notify neonatologist as required.

Nursing Alert

Homan's Sign

Apply dorsiflexion to the client's foot, and ask her whether this action causes calf pain. Calf pain on dorsiflexion of the foot is a positive Homan's sign and must be investigated further for deep vein thrombosis.

Critical Thinking

Prioritize!

A client is rushed to labor and delivery in a wheelchair. She says she feels like pushing.

What would be your initial response?

How would you set your priorities?

the woman in labor. The support person also will need attention and should be provided with a comfortable chair and offered opportunities to take meal breaks. The nurse can show the family member how to provide comfort to the woman and should include the support person in discussions about the plan of care. Family interaction and the support system are evaluated as labor progresses, always taking cultural beliefs into consideration. When the woman does not have a support person with her, the nurse becomes the support person.

Many women attend childbirth preparation classes and develop expectations in the form of an individualized birth plan. When presented with a birth plan the nurse should consider the safety of the plan, importance of the plan to the client, and feasibility of incorporating some or all of the woman's wishes into the nursing process. It is important for the nurse to be respectful and flexible.

PSYCHOLOGIC CONSIDERATIONS DURING THE LATENT PHASE OF LABOR

The woman who comes to the hospital in the latent phase of labor often is mildly anxious both about her well-being and that of the baby, and also about how she will react to the pain of contractions. The hospital is an unfamiliar environment, and the nurse is a stranger to her. The nursing

Nursing Alert

Epigastric Pain

The presence of epigastric or right upper quadrant pain is a serious finding of possible severe preeclampsia. The pain is secondary to obstructed hepatic blood flow caused by fibrin deposits (Queenan & Hobbins, 1996) and the primary caregiver should be called immediately to assess the woman.

interview and interventions must be performed in a competent and respectful manner that promotes trust and facilitates relaxation. One of the most important nurse behaviors, as perceived by the client, is that the nursing staff know what they are doing (Manogin, Bechtel, & Rami, 2000). The approach of the nurse should be accepting and supportive of the woman as an individual. Cultural practices related to childbirth also need to be considered.

To provide appropriate teaching to the client, the nurse must first evaluate the amount of preparation for childbirth she has had. Other factors to consider are the stage of labor, maturity of the client, previous experience of childbirth, and educational level. During the initial orientation to the labor and delivery or triage room and the primary assessment, the nurse can make inquiries as to any childbirth classes the woman may have attended or books she has read. This also is a good time to ask whether the woman has specific concerns that may be causing anxiety. Family members also should be included in any teaching. Client teaching is an ongoing process, and it is important for the nurse to explain what is happening to the woman during each stage of labor. Examination findings also should be fully explained; some labor rooms have a chart depicting cervical dilation to which the nurse might refer.

The client participates in the plan of care. The rationale for recommended interventions, as well as risks, should be explained fully. Frequent reinforcement usually is necessary. Teaching includes an explanation of the purpose of equipment that is likely to be used, such as the electronic fetal monitor, the correct method of timing contractions, and activity that will be helpful to the woman. Many primary caregivers allow the woman to have sips of clear liquid and ice chips during normal labor. Some women prefer to ambulate during the early phase of labor, returning to the labor and delivery room for intermittent FHR monitoring. The woman and her support person should be shown the correct method of timing contractions.

Explanations are given about the current stage of labor and available options for pain management, when and how they can be administered, and the effect they are likely to have. Although the woman may have received previous instruction about breathing and relaxation techniques, these may need to be reviewed and reinforced. Teaching and the client's response should be recorded in the flowchart.

DOCUMENTATION AND COMMUNICATION

Admission data are documented in the medical chart and nursing flowchart and communicated to the appropriate health care team members such as the physician or nurse-midwife, social worker, pediatrician, or neonatologist. Charting of all interventions, medications, and clinical findings is done according to the accepted procedure of the facility and may involve flowcharts or computer-generated charting.

LABORATORY TESTS

After the initial assessment of the client, the nurse should anticipate the need for laboratory tests according to the hospital protocol.

Urine Specimen Analysis

Urinalysis can be done by the nurse, using a dipstick, to examine for the presence of protein, glucose, blood, and ketones. Urinalysis can be done using a voided specimen, as free as possible from debris. Urinalysis can alert the nurse to possible complications such as PIH (albuminuria), diabetes mellitus (glucose), or inadequate nutrition (ketones). Laboratory urinalysis can provide additional information about hydration status (specific gravity) and infection (presence of leukocytes).

Blood Tests

Blood tests vary with the hospital protocol and risk factors. Information that usually can be obtained from the prenatal record includes results of tests for the following: blood type, Rh factor, atypical antibodies, rubella, syphilis (rapid plasma reagin [RPR], or VDRL test), hepatitis B, glucose levels, HIV, and Groub B Beta Strep (GBBS).

Although sufficient information may be available from prenatal records, on hospital admission the hematocrit and hemoglobin levels should be rechecked and an RPR test performed. Many hospitals require a complete blood cell count (CBC), and confirmation of blood type and Rh factor. Platelets and clotting factors within CBC should be noted, as a change in these values could be an early warning for PIH, HELLP, and DIC. Blood may be saved in the laboratory for use in cross-matching should the client require a blood transfusion. A screening test for HIV is offered. The role of the nurse is to explain the purpose of drawing blood and often to draw blood and order the tests according to the hospital protocol. Only when all examinations, including laboratory review, are completed can a decision be reached about the normalcy of the pregnancy.

NURSING RESPONSIBILITIES DURING LABOR

Labor progresses through four stages, as outlined in Box 14-10. Nursing responsibilities to the laboring woman and family are tied to the stage of labor and the woman's changing needs.

First Stage

The **first stage of labor** begins with the initiation of regular contractions that produce cervical dilation and continues through complete dilation. The first stage is the longest one and is composed of three phases. The latent phase is followed by the active phase and then the transition phase. Nursing assessment of the mother and fetus is ongoing.

Maternal Assessment

Assessment of the woman in the first stage of labor includes evaluation of vital signs, hydration status, and elimination.

Box 14-10

Stages and Phases of Labor

First Stage (0–10 cm dilated)

Latent phase: 0–3 cm; contractions are mild every 15–30 min and last for 30 s

Active phase: 4–7 cm; contractions are moderate every 3–5 min and last for 40 s

Transition phase: 8–10 cm; contractions are strong every 2–3 min and last for 60 s

Second Stage (10 cm dilated to birth)

Contractions: Every 2–3 min

Duration of contractions: 60–90 s

Duration of second stage: 5 min–2 h

Third Stage (birth to delivery of placenta)

Duration: 5–45 min

Fourth Stage (recovery)

Duration: 1–4 h

Vital Signs

Vital signs of the mother include blood pressure, temperature, pulse, and respiration. Frequency of assessment is determined by the phase of labor and risk status of the maternal-fetal dyad. Monitoring will be more frequent in high-risk situations. Vital signs are monitored between contractions and recorded on the FHR strip and the nursing flowchart.

Blood pressure is measured between contractions every hour during active labor, if normal. During a uterine contraction approximately 500 mL of blood is shunted into the central circulation, elevating the maternal blood pressure. The normal range of blood pressure is 100 to 120 mmHg systolic and 60 to 80 mmHg diastolic. Hypertension is defined as a sustained blood pressure of 140 mmHg systolic or 90 mmHg diastolic, and the risk of developing PIH is increased in women with preexisting chronic hypertension (ACOG, 1996).

Temperature is an important indicator of hydration and infection and may be slightly elevated throughout labor. Temperature is taken on admission and every 4 hours until the membranes rupture, after which it is recorded every 1 to 2 hours. Once the fetal membranes are ruptured, there is an increased risk of ascending infection. For this reason all invasive procedures, such as vaginal examinations, are kept to a minimum. If the membranes are ruptured an elevated temperature could indicate chorioamnionitis, particularly if they have been ruptured for more than 12 hours. An increasing temperature should be reported to the primary caregiver. Foul odor of the amniotic fluid is a late sign of chorioamnionitis.

Meconium may support bacterial growth. For this reason, there is also a potential for chorioamnionitis when there is meconium staining.

Heart rate and respirations vary according to maternal exertion during labor, hydration, infection, and anxiety level. Respirations also are affected by the level of pain and breathing techniques used to cope with labor. **Hyperventilation**, a change in the oxygen-carbon dioxide exchange, is a consequence of breathing too rapidly and too deeply. If the woman complains of tingling sensations in the palms of her hands, she may be hyperventilating and should be urged to slow her breathing. This condition also can be corrected by having the woman rebreathe her exhaled air by breathing into a paper bag or oxygen mask with rebreather bag attached.

Hydration and Nutrition

Gastric emptying time is prolonged during active labor, so that ingested food remains in the stomach and may be vomited. Oral fluids usually are well tolerated throughout labor but should be limited to ice chips or sips of water or clear fluids, as tolerated. The various breathing techniques used by laboring women to cope with painful contractions usually result in a dry mouth and craving for sips of water or ice chips.

The woman is asked when she last had something to eat or drink, and the times are noted in the medical record. When general anesthesia is a possibility, the woman receives nothing by mouth to prevent vomiting. Aspiration of acidic gastric contents into the lungs is life-threatening to the woman and fetus. When the primary caregiver requires the woman to be NPO, the nurse provides mouthwashes and applies petroleum jelly to the lips to alleviate dryness.

Intravenous fluids provide calories and prevent dehydration in the laboring woman. Many facilities, particularly in physician-assisted deliveries, require IV hydration as part of the routine orders for the laboring woman. Starting an IV may be delayed for the woman in early labor who is ambulating. For hydration, an 18-gauge or 20-gauge cannula is inserted into a vein of the hand or forearm and connected to tubing attached to a 1 L bag of lactated Ringer's solution or dextrose 5% lactated Ringer's solution infusing at 125 mL/h. This constitutes the main IV line and facilitates administration of analgesics or other appropriate medications into one of the access ports. Antibiotics, oxytocics, or tocolytics can be diluted and inserted by piggyback into the main line. An accurate record of fluid intake and output should be maintained.

Elimination

Voiding every 2 hours is encouraged because a full bladder can impede descent of the presenting part. The nurse should palpate the suprapubic region to detect a distended bladder. When the bladder is readily palpated and the woman is unable to void, catheterization is indicated. If the woman wishes to get up to walk to the bathroom the nurse should assist her in doing so by lowering the bed, unplugging the FHR monitoring cables, and moving the IV pole. Urinary output is measured and dipstick testing for glucose, albumin, and ketones performed upon admission. In some institutions, dipstick testing is no longer a nursing function due to CLIA standards for laboratory quality assurance. All urine specimens are sent to the laboratory for analysis. The woman who is receiving epidural anesthesia should not be permitted to get out of bed to walk to the bathroom because partial loss of muscle strength in the legs is common. A Foley catheter, attached to bedside drainage, frequently is inserted if the woman is receiving epidural anesthesia because urinary retention is a very frequent side effect of this regional anesthesia.

The use of enemas is infrequent. As the fetal head descends, it exerts pressure on the lower bowel and any stool that is present will be expelled during the second stage of labor. Passage of fecal matter during the birth may be

Nursing Tip — *Elimination*

If the woman in active labor expresses the need to have a bowel movement, the nurse should perform a vaginal examination to assess cervical dilation and station. Examination may reveal significant descent of the presenting part.

Nursing Tip — *Fetal Bradycardia or Maternal Heart Rate?*

Always make certain that the rate you are recording using the external fetal heart rate monitor is not the same rate as the woman's radical or apical pulse. When the fetus changes position, the transducer may start picking up the maternal heart rate.

embarrassing for the client and also increases the risk for infection. Cleansing the perineal area throughout the second stage decreases this risk. As the fetal head descends, the woman will experience increased pressure in the rectal area.

Fetal Assessment

The FHR is assessed as per the hospital policy, taking into consideration the phase and stage of labor and maternal and fetal risk factors. Certain abbreviations are commonly used by labor and delivery personnel when documenting baseline, variability, and periodic changes in FHR (Box 14-11).

Baseline Fetal Heart Rate

In order to determine a **baseline fetal heart rate**, that is, the FHR between contractions and accelerations, the FHR must be observed *between* contractions. Because the FHR is an inherently irregular rate, accuracy will be improved by charting it as a *range*, for example, 130 to 140 bpm. The FHR baseline during the third trimester ranges from 110 to 160 bpm, and two FHR strips of at least 10 minutes each should be taken and compared before a baseline is established (ACOG, July 1995).

Fetal Heart Rate Variability

Fetal heart rate **variability** (fluctuations in the FHR) has two components: **long-term variability** (the slow rhythmic fluctuations above and below an average baseline rate, producing a wavelike pattern) and **short-term** (or **beat-to-beat**) **variability**, which are instantaneous fluctuations in the FHR. The combination of these two types of variability reflects the interaction between parasympathetic (which slows the heart) and sympathetic (which accelerates the heart) branches of the CNS.

The criteria for long-term variability (LTV) does not include accelerations or decelerations. Evaluation of the LTV helps identify changes in the fetal behavioral state and the response to labor. Absent LTV might also be described as a "flat" FHR. Marked LTV, or **saltatory pattern**, is

Box 14-11	
Common Abbreviations in Fetal Monitoring	
bpm	Beats per minute
EFM	Electronic fetal monitoring
FHR	Fetal heart rate
FSE	Fetal scalp electrode
UC	Uterine contraction
IUPC	Intrauterine pressure catheter
LTV	Long-term variability
STV	Short-term variability
TOCO	Tocodynamometer (external)
US	Ultrasonography

Nursing Alert

Causes and Physiology of Absent Long-Term Variability

- Fetal quiescent state that may last 90 min
- Medications, for example, central nervous system depressants
- Hypoxia owing to placental insufficiency
- Severe fetal anemia, for example, as a result of a fetal viral infection
- Arrhythmia such as a supraventricular tachycardia or complete heart block
- Fetal brain death or decerebration
- Congenital brain anomaly, for example, anencephaly or a heart anomaly or conduction defect
- Late sign of deterioration of the fetus having intrauterine growth retardation
- Terminal bradycardia (low baseline and absent LTV, not related to an arrhythmia, suggesting impending intrauterine death)

a term that describes a baseline that is chaotic and jumps up and down multiple times each minute. The presence of two spontaneous accelerations of greater than 15 bpm for at least 15 seconds' duration in 20 minutes is a reassuring sign. When LTV is present, STV also is almost always present.

Short-term variability (STV) or beat-to-beat variability can only be realistically visualized with internal FHR monitoring and is documented as minimal, moderate, or marked. STV variability can be present in the absence of LTV.

Periodic and Nonperiodic Fetal Heart Rate Changes

Periodic fetal heart rate changes are transient changes in FHR in association with contractions (Cunningham, 2001). **Nonperiodic fetal heart rate changes** are transient changes in FHR not associated with contractions, although they can occur during contractions. Specific classifications are defined by ACOG (July 1995) as follows:

1. **Acceleration:** An increase in FHR above the baseline level, with a return to baseline within 10 minutes. An increase in FHR lasting longer than 10 minutes is classified as an increase in FHR baseline.

2. **Deceleration:** A distinct decrease below the baseline, with a return to the baseline within 10 minutes. Decelerations are classified by their shape and timing in relation to uterine contractions as follows:

   Early—U-shaped deceleration that begins and ends with the contraction. The heart rate reaches its nadir at the peak of the contraction.

Variable—May have a V or W shape. May occur during or between contractions, onset is usually abrupt.

Late—Usually has a gradual onset. Nadir of the deceleration usually occurs after the peak of the contraction.

Accelerations

Accelerations are the most common type of FHR change (Figure 14-13). Periodic accelerations are not a sign of fetal distress; they are a reassuring sign that the fetus is able to increase his or her heart rate to compensate for the stress of contractions. Periodic accelerations begin with the onset of the contraction and return to the baseline at the end of the contraction. Nonperiodic accelerations are not associated with contractions. Nonperiodic accelerations most often are seen with fetal activity and during pelvic examination; they are reassuring of fetal well-being. Nonperiodic accelerations have no regular pattern. The presence of spontaneous accelerations of at least 15 bpm lasting at least 15 seconds is almost always an indication of the absence of fetal acidosis (ACOG, July 1995).

Early Onset Decelerations

Early onset decelerations involve a transitory decrease in FHR caused by fetal head compression, which stimulates the vagus nerve to decrease the heart rate. Early decelerations during the second stage of labor, in the presence of adequate descent of the presenting part, usually are benign and reflect compression of the fetal head as it enters the birth canal.

An early deceleration is characterized by a gradual onset at the beginning of a contraction and a slow return

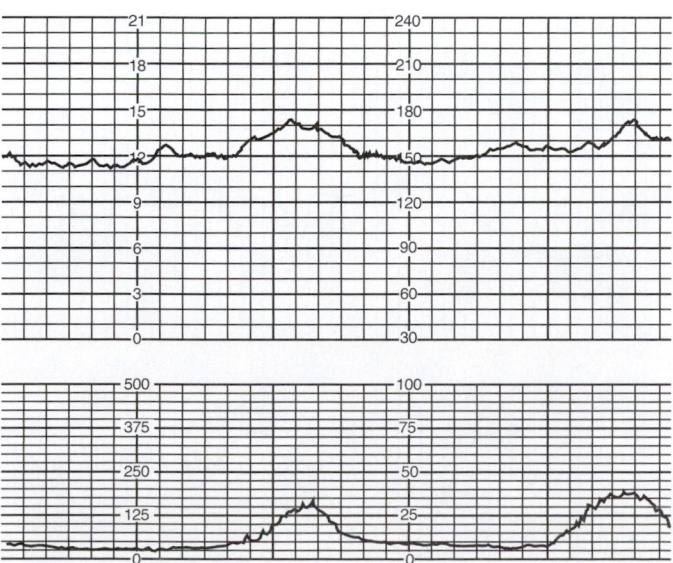

A.

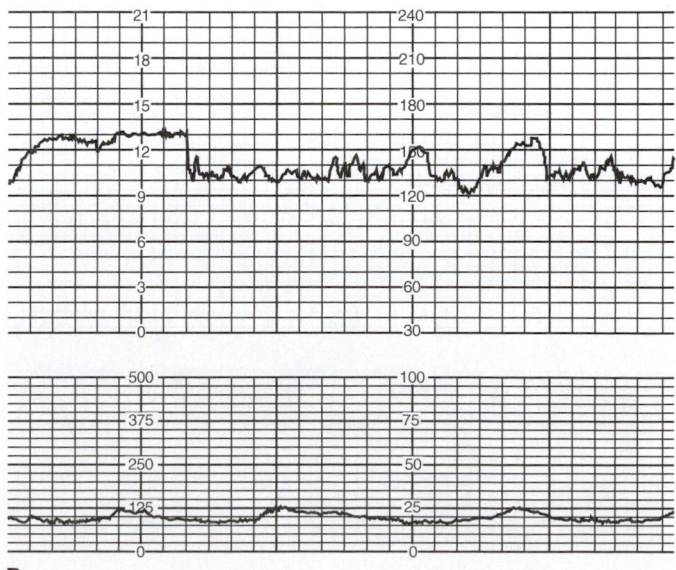

B.

Figure 14-13   A. Periodic accelerations. B. Nonperiodic accelerations.

Nursing Tip *Faster Baseline Heart Rate in the Premature Fetus*

The normal baseline fetal heart rate (FHR) ranges from 110 to 160 bpm. In early fetal life the sympathetic branch of the autonomic nervous system (ANS) establishes and maintains the baseline FHR, which tends to be in the upper range (150 to 160 bpm). As the fetus matures, the parasympathetic branch of the ANS exerts a slowing effect, bringing the baseline into the lower range (110 to 140 bpm) by term.

to the baseline soon after the contraction ends, like a mirror image of the contraction (Figure 14-14). The slope is gradual and the depth of the deceleration reflects the intensity of the contraction. Early decelerations occur most frequently with vertex presentations in the second stage of labor, during pushing.

No treatment is necessary for early decelerations that occur in the transition phase of the first stage of labor or during pushing in the second stage, provided the vertex is descending and the FHR recovers. If, during the second stage of labor, it becomes difficult to determine the baseline owing to the frequency of early decelerations, the woman should be instructed to stop pushing until the fetus has recovered and the FHR has returned to baseline. If early decelerations are observed while the presenting part is still above the level of the ischial spines, cephalopelvic disproportion should be ruled out.

Variable Decelerations

Variable decelerations are transitory decreases in FHR most often caused by umbilical cord compression, fetal movement, or head compression. Variable decelerations are characterized by rapid onset, rapid return to baseline, and a variable relationship to the contraction (Cunningham, 2001). As long as the baseline rate remains stable and the variability is good, variable decelerations are not associated with poor fetal outcome. Variable decelerations have no consistent shape and may appear V-shaped, W-shaped, or U-shaped; they may begin or end at any time in relation to the contraction curve (Figure 14-15).

Variable decelerations occur most frequently after rupture of membranes, when there is less amniotic fluid to provide a protective cushion around the cord. Other circumstances that could result in compression or stretching of the cord causing variable decelerations are the following: loops of the umbilical cord around the fetal neck or shoulder, a true knot in the cord, or prolapsed cord. Variable decelerations are defined according to their depth and duration (Table 14-5). Many variable decelerations are so brief that no treatment is necessary. When decelerations last longer than 30 seconds or when the recovery to the baseline is slow, treatment should be given to alleviate the cause of the compression.

Variable decelerations may be preceded or followed by acceleratory phases or shoulders. A **shoulder** is not an acceleration but is an acceleratory phase of a deceleration pattern. It is a compensatory sign of an intact fetal CNS. Appropriate descriptive documentation in the medical record should read as follows: "Variable decelerations with shoulders."

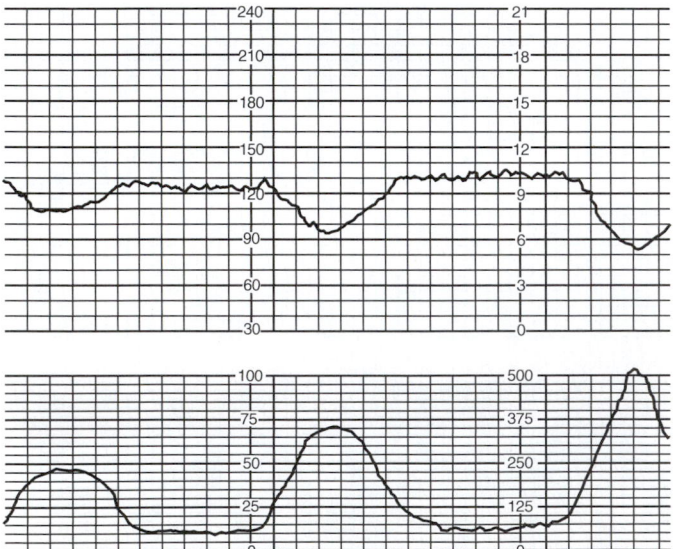

Figure 14-14 Early decelerations.

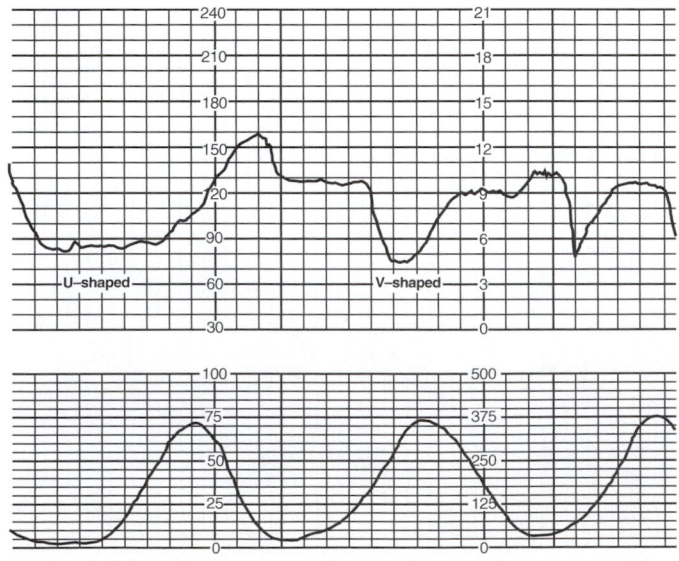

Figure 14-15 Variable decelerations.

Table 14-5	Variable Decelerations Defined
Mild	Any depth; duration, <30 s 70–80 bpm; duration, <60 s 80 bpm; duration, any
Moderate	<70 bpm; duration, 30–60 s 70–80 bpm; duration, <60 s
Severe	<70 bpm; duration, >60 s
Prolonged	Isolated deceleration; duration, >60–90 s

Occasionally, a rebound increase in the FHR occurs after a variable deceleration. This is called an **overshoot** and consists of an increase of 20 or more bpm above the baseline or an increase above the baseline for more than 20 seconds. An overshoot is not an acceleration but is part of a variable deceleration pattern (Murray, 1997). An overshoot is a nonreassuring sign and could indicate significant hypoxemia or hypoxia. The primary caregiver should be notified immediately of such a FHR pattern, particularly if there is absent STV or an increasing baseline (Murray, 1997).

Late Onset Decelerations

Late onset decelerations are transitory decreases in the FHR caused by **uteroplacental insufficiency**, which is compromised blood flow from the placenta to the fetus (ACOG, July 1995). Late decelerations have the following characteristics: uniform shape similar to early onset decelerations, smooth, and U-shaped (Figure 14-16). The late deceleration, however, starts at about the time the contraction is at its height and does not return to baseline until after the contraction has ended (ACOG, July 1995). When a pattern of late FHR deceleration occurs, the primary caregiver should be requested to review the FHR strip and assess the client without delay.

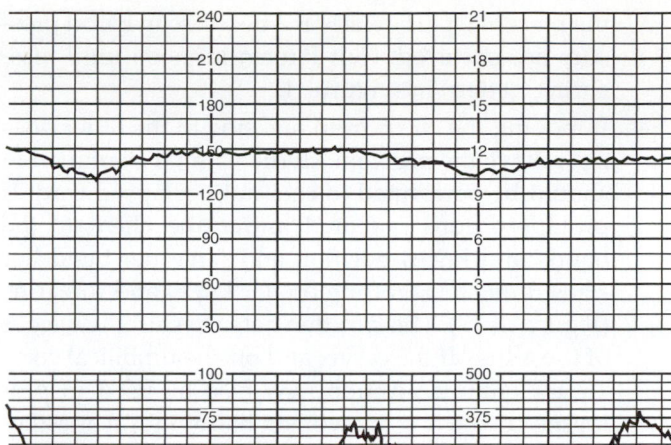

Figure 14-16   Late decelerations.

Interventions for Nonreassuring Fetal Heart Rate Pattern

Nursing interventions that should be initiated for a nonreassuring FHR pattern depend on the signs and probable cause, and include the following:

1. Change the maternal position from one side to the other side, particularly if umbilical cord compression is suspected. Changing the maternal position is almost always the first nursing intervention to consider and may be the only intervention necessary.

2. Oxygen therapy by non-rebreather face mask at 8 to 10 L/min. The theory is that oxygen therapy will saturate the mother's blood with oxygen so that when the cord compression is relieved, the fetus will have a good supply of oxygen to use in recovering a normal heart rate.

3. Increase the rate of the main IV fluid line (usually lactated Ringer's solution) to increase perfusion of

Critical Thinking

Early Decelerations

Your client has had an epidural and denies feeling pain with contractions. You note that with each contraction the fetal heart rate (FHR) decelerates so that the pattern looks like a mirror image of the contraction. What action should you take?

Perform a sterile vaginal examination to assess dilation of the cervix and descent of the presenting part.

The appearance of early FHR decelerations is an indication that labor may have progressed to the second stage; therefore, the cervix should be assessed.

Nursing Alert

Late Decelerations

Late decelerations are caused by uteroplacental insufficiency (low oxygen delivery) and are nonreassuring. The primary caregiver must be notified without delay of the appearance of late decelerations on the fetal heart rate monitor strip and should come to assess the client immediately.

the placenta, particularly if a decrease in blood pressure has occurred. Halt Pitocin infusion until reassuring pattern has returned.

4. If moving the client from one side to the other does not relieve the problem, sterile vaginal examination should be performed to rule out prolapsed cord. If prolapsed cord is feared, move the client to the hands and knees position and have her bend her arms until she is resting on her knees and forearms (Figure 14-17). This position helps to shift the weight of the fetus off the cervix and off the umbilical cord. Trendelenburg position may also be used in prolapsed cord when the woman has epidural anesthesia for pain relief.

5. Notify the primary care provider the time of occurrence, duration, severity, and frequency of decelerations and of nursing interventions given. The nurse also should document the rationale behind interventions provided.

6. Anticipate administration of a tocolytic such as terbutaline (Brethine), 0.25 mg subcutaneously or 0.125 to 0.25 mg IV (ACOG, Dec. 1995), if the woman is experiencing hypertonic contractions, resulting in inadequate resting tone between contractions.

7. Anticipate starting an **amnioinfusion**, which is instillation of an isotonic glucose-free solution (such as normal saline or lactated Ringer's solution) into the uterus to cushion the umbilical cord or to thin out meconium.

8. Chart all information, including the time the primary care giver was notified, the specific information given, and the response. It is acceptable to write, "No new orders received."

When interventions do not improve the FHR pattern, and depending on the seriousness of the deceleration and the stage of labor, the nurse should be prepared to move the client into the operating room for emergency cesarean delivery.

Labor Progress

The nurse assesses the woman throughout labor to establish normal progress during each stage and phase. The primiparous client may be expected to experience a longer labor than would the multiparous woman.

Uterine Assessment

Contraction patterns are monitored carefully, as discussed in the section on Admission Procedures. As the contractions intensify, the nurse continues to assess their frequency, duration, and intensity, and the adequacy of the resting tone. The minimal contractile pattern of 95% of women in spontaneous labor consists of three to five contractions in a 10-minute window. When the woman is having internal uterine monitoring, **Montevideo units**, or MVU (a numerical method of calculating adequacy of contraction strength), can be calculated. MVU equals the total strength of contractions, in mmHg, in a 10-minute window. The equation is as follows:

Total strength of all contractions in a 10-minute window

– Total resting tone of all contractions in a 10-minute

window = MVU

For example, if the woman has three contractions in 10 minutes of 90, 75, and 85 mmHg and the resting tone is 20 mmHg, then the MVU equals 190 mmHg:

$$(90 + 75 + 85 \text{ mmHg}) - (20 \text{ mmHg} \times 3)$$

$$= 250 \text{ mmHg} - 60 \text{ mmHg}$$

$$= 190 \text{ mmHg}$$

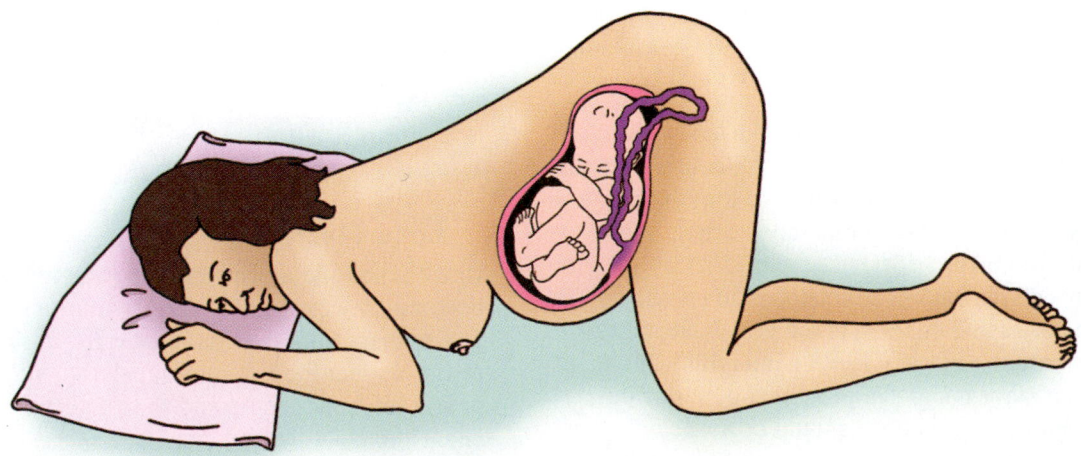

Figure 14-17   Elbows and knees position to relieve pressure on a prolapsed umbilical cord in a woman without an epidural.

Most women achieve 200 to 225 MVU, and some achieve 300 MVU. A woman is considered to have arrested labor when she exceeds a rate of 200 MVU for 2 hours without cervical change.

Rupture of Fetal Membranes

If the fetal membranes were still intact when the woman arrived at the hospital, they may rupture spontaneously during labor. If the woman states either that she has felt a sudden gush of fluid or has inadvertently urinated in the bed, the nurse should check the bed linen beneath the woman for pooling of amniotic fluid. When membranes rupture spontaneously, the first nursing responsibility is to check the FHR, because the gush of amniotic fluid could possibly cause a segment of umbilical cord to prolapse or become pinched between the fetal head and the cervix. The first indication of such an emergency would be a variable FHR deceleration.

If fetal membranes do not spontaneously rupture, the primary caregiver may perform **amniotomy**, artificial rupture of membranes (AROM). The rationale for AROM is to slightly shorten the length of labor, although there is no research to suggest that this is beneficial to either the mother or fetus.

One benefit of AROM is the earlier detection of meconium staining of amniotic fluid. Once the membranes are ruptured, a FSE can be applied for more accurate monitoring of the FHR. Amniotomy usually is done by the use of an **amniohook**, which is a plastic implement with a blunt hook at the distal end (Figure 14-18). AROM also can be effected by applying a FSE directly through the membranes, especially if there is no bulging forebag.

Nursing responsibilities during AROM are to assess the FHR both before and after amniotomy. The client usually is receiving continuous EFM. After AROM, the characteristics of the amniotic fluid are assessed and documented: color—clear, bloody, or meconium stained; odor; and amount—copious or scant. Notify the appropriate health care team members of the rupture of membranes and abnormal findings as per the hospital policy, procedure, and protocol. The primary caregiver should be

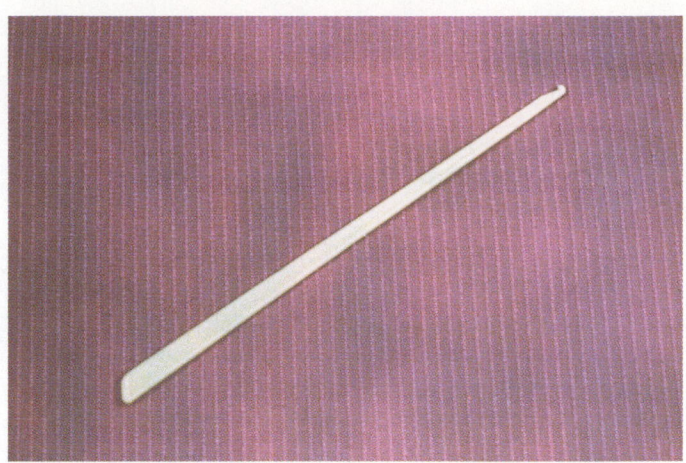

Figure 14-18   Amniohook.

notified immediately when meconium-stained amniotic fluid is first observed.

Documentation and Communication

Documentation of nursing care is made on a flowchart or entered directly into a bedside computer according to the hospital policy, procedure, and protocol and the client's clinical status communicated to other members of the health care team as appropriate (Figure 14-19). Although physicians and nurse-midwives make the obstetric management decisions, they cannot be in constant attendance at the bedside. It is the intrapartum nurse who alerts the physician or nurse-midwife when a change in the plan of care becomes necessary. Failure of the nurse to correctly interpret assessment findings is below the standard of care. Failure to communicate and document clinical findings are two reasons that the intrapartum nurse might be named as a defendant in a malpractice claim. The Board of Nurse Examiners Rules and Regulations, Standards of Professional Practice, require nurses to "accurately and completely report and document" (Rule 217.11 [4]).

Activity

When the woman is in bed, frequent position changes allow for better comfort. During normal labor, however, the woman does not need to be confined to bed, unless analgesics are being used. Many women prefer to walk, accompanied by a support person, and return to the LDR every 30 to 45 minutes for FHR assessment according to ACOG standards (July 1995). A comfortable chair may be beneficial, allowing the woman to maintain a more upright position than being semi-recumbent in bed. Many women use a rocking chair, preferring to rock through each contraction. Continuous EFM can continue with the woman sitting in a chair at the bedside. While in bed, the laboring woman should be allowed to assume the position that affords her the most comfort; additional

Nursing Alert

Prolapsed Cord

If spontaneous rupture of membranes is accompanied by a decrease in the fetal heart rate, the nurse should suspect umbilical cord prolapse and perform an immediate sterile vaginal examination to confirm or rule out this emergency.

Duplication of this form is strictly prohibited by law. © 2001 Briggs Corporation. All rights reserved.

Briggs CORPORATION

Labor Progress Chart
Maternal/Newborn Record System
To order call: **1.800.245.4080**   Re-order No. **5711N**

Admit Date	Admit Time	Blood Type and Rh	Age	G	T	Pt	A	L	EDD	Membranes		
6 / 23 / 04	1330	O+	34	III	II	O	O	II	7 / 4 / 04	☐ Intact ☑ Ruptured (SROM) AROM		
									LMP 9 / 28 / 03	☐ Bulging Date 6 / 23 / 04 Time 1230		

Current Date 6 / 23 / 04 Time →

		1335		1400		1430		1500		1530		1600		1630		1700		1730	
Vital Signs	Temperature	98⁸				98⁶				99				98⁸				98⁸	
	Pulse	88		80		82		84		86		86		88		86		84	
	Respiration / O₂ Saturation	12		18		18		16		16		14		16		18		18	
	Blood Pressure	128/88		130/86		128/86		130/88		128/88		130/86		130/86		130/84		128/86	
Maternal	Deep Tendon Reflexes (L/R)	2+/2+	/	/	/	/	/	/	/	/	/	/	/	/	/			2+/2+	/
	Urine (Protein/Sugar)	N/N	/	/	/	/	/	N/N	/	/	/	N/N		/	/	
	Vaginal Bleeding	NS				NS													
	Pain	6-7		6-7		7		7-8		8-9		9	9-10	10		10		10	
	Edema (site, extent)	O						O						O					
Uterine Activity	Monitor Mode	E		E		E		I		I		I		I		I	P	P	
	Frequency minutes	5 min	5 min			4 min	4 min			3 min	3 min			2 min	2 min	2 min	3 min	3 min	3 min
	Duration seconds	40 sec	40 sec			45 sec	45 sec					55 sec	55 sec	60	60	60	50-60	60	60
	Peak IUP	50	50	50-60	50-60	60	60	60	60	60	60	60-70	60-70	70	70	80	80	–	–
	Resting Tone	10	10	10	10	10	10	10	10	10	10	10	10	10	10	10	10	–	–
	Intensity	30-40	30-40	30-40	30-40	30-40	30-40	30-40	30-40	30-60	30-60	40-60	40-60	50-70	50-70	60-70	80	–	–
	MVUs	40	40	40-50	40-50	50	50	50	50	50	50	50-60	60	60	60	70	70	–	–
Fetal Assessment	Monitor Mode (Strip #_239_)	E	E	E	E	E	E	I		I		I		I		I		I	
	Baseline (FHR)	138	136	134	140	140	138	138	136	134	136	134	134	132	130	128	126	124	122
	STV	O	O	O	O	O	O	O	O	O	O	O	O	O	O	O	O	+	+
	LTV	O	O	1	1	+	+	+	+	+	+	+	+	+	+	+	+	+	+
	Accelerations	+	+	+	+	+	+	+	+	+	+	+	+	+	+	+	+	+	+
	Decelerations	N	N	N	N	N	N	N	N	N	N	N	N	N	N	N	N	N	N
	Membranes/Fluid	R/C/NF		R/C		R/C		R/C		R/C		R/C		R/C		R/C		R/C	
	Scalp pH							7.25		7.25		7.35		7.35		7.30		7.25	
Intake/Output (mL's/Hr)	IV	Begun				100				100				125				125	
	PO																		
	Urine	200						150								250			
	Emesis	–								100									
Cont Meds	Pitocin mU/min	–																	
	Magnesium sulfate gms/hr	–																	
Intervention	Treatments																		
	Teaching/Support			BRT		F		BRT						F					
	Touch							BR		E		E		BR	M	CP			
	Position/Activity	W		C		LS		RS		LS		RS		LS		RS		KC	
	Physical Care	PC												MC		BP	PC		
Initials		RB	RB	RB	RB	RB	RB	RB	RB	RB	RB	RB	RB	RB	RB	RB	RB	RB	RB

Abbreviations/Key

Deep Tendon Reflexes
0 = No Response
+1 = Sluggish
+2 = Normal
+3 = Hyperactive
+4 = Brisk + Hyperactive
C = Clonus

Vaginal Bleeding
NS = Normal Show
ABN = Frank Vaginal Bleeding

Pain
0 = No Pain
5 = Distressing Pain
10 = Highest Intensity

Uterine Activity Monitor Mode
P = Palpation
E = External
I = Internal

MVUs Montevideo Units
The sum of the peak of each uterine contraction minus its resting tone, in a 10 minute period.

Fetal Monitor Mode
A = Auscultation (Fetoscope)
D = Doppler
E = External
I = Internal

STV Short Term Variability
+ = Present (Roughness of Tracing Line Present)
ø = Absent (Tracing Line is Smooth)
LTV Long Term Variability
ø = 0- 2 BPM = Absent
↓ = 3- 5 BPM = Minimal
+ = 6-25 BPM = Average
↑ = greater than 25 BPM = Marked

Form 5711N © 2001 Briggs Corporation, Des Moines, IA 50306
R304 To order, phone (800) 245-4080 www.BriggsCorp.com PRINTED IN U.S.A.

LABOR PROGRESS CHART

Figure 14-19 Labor Progress Chart. (*Courtesy of Briggs Corporation.*)

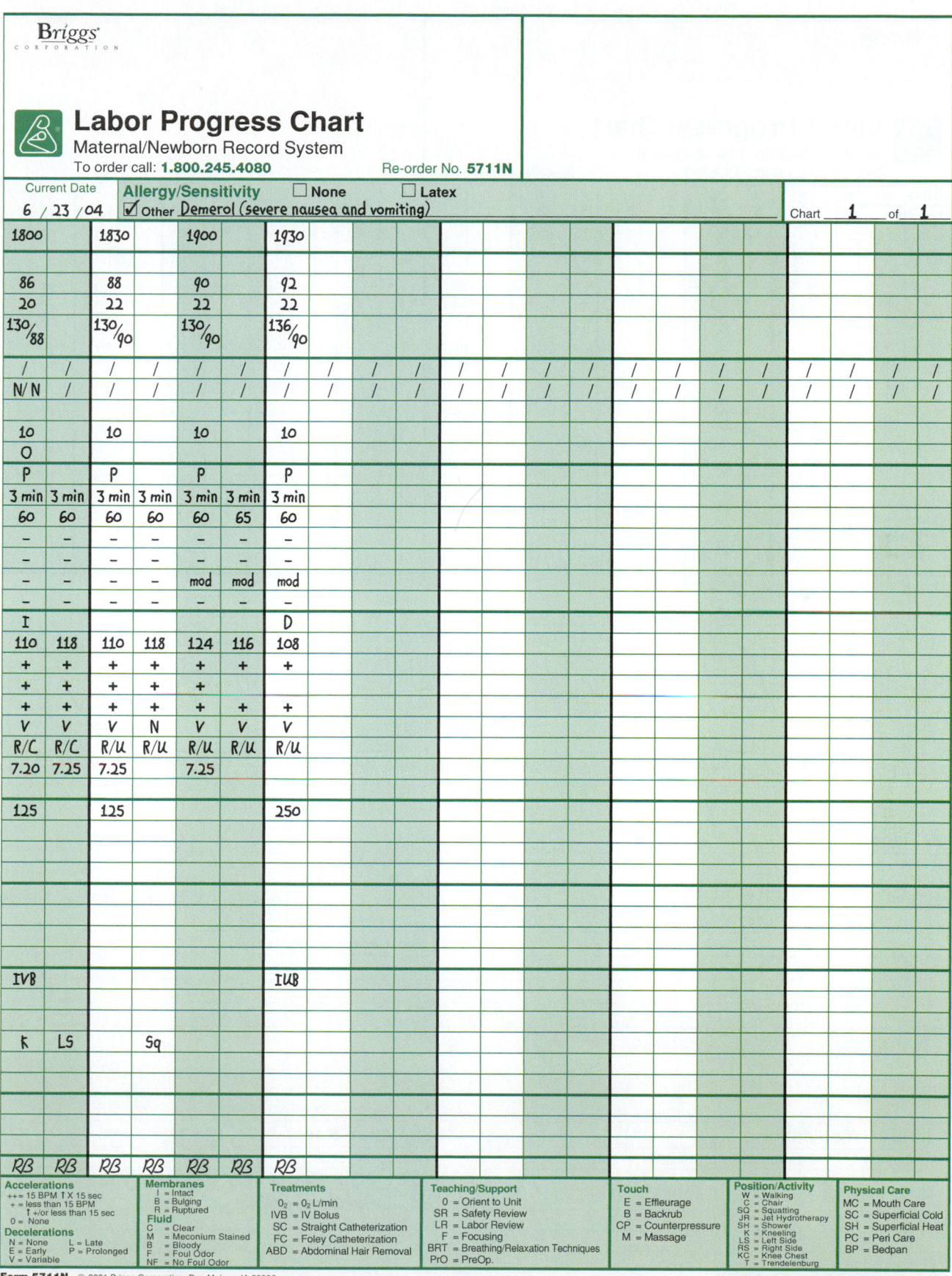

Briggs CORPORATION

Labor Progress Chart
Maternal/Newborn Record System
To order call: **1.800.245.4080**   Re-order No. **5711N**

Current Date	Allergy/Sensitivity	☐ None ☐ Latex	Chart
6 / 23 / 04	☑ Other Demerol (severe nausea and vomiting)		Chart __1__ of __1__

1800		1830		1900		1930															

86		88		90		92
20		22		22		22
130/88		130/90		130/90		136/90

| / | | / | | / | / | / | | / | | / | | / | / | | / | | / | | / | / | / |
| N/N | / | | / | | / | / | / | | / | | / | | / | / | | / | | / | | / | / | / |

| 10 | | 10 | | 10 | | 10 |
| O |
P		P		P		P
3 min	3 min	3 min	3 min	3 min	3 min	3 min
60	60	60	60	60	65	60
–	–	–	–	–	–	–
–	–	–	–	–	–	–
–	–	–	–	mod	mod	mod
–	–	–	–	–	–	–

I						D
110	118	110	118	124	116	108
+	+	+	+	+	+	+
+	+	+	+	+
+	+	+	+	+	+	+
V	V	V	N	V	V	V
R/C	R/C	R/U	R/U	R/U	R/U	R/U
7.20	7.25	7.25		7.25

| 125 | | 125 | | | | 250 |

| IVB | | | | | | IUB |

| K | LS | | Sq |

| RB | RB | RB | RB | RB | RB | RB |

Accelerations ++ = 15 BPM ↑ X 15 sec + = less than 15 BPM ↑ +/or less than 15 sec 0 = None **Decelerations** N = None L = Late E = Early P = Prolonged V = Variable	**Membranes** I = Intact B = Bulging R = Ruptured **Fluid** C = Clear M = Meconium Stained B = Bloody F = Foul Odor NF = No Foul Odor	**Treatments** O₂ = O₂ L/min IVB = IV Bolus SC = Straight Catheterization FC = Foley Catheterization ABD = Abdominal Hair Removal	**Teaching/Support** O = Orient to Unit SR = Safety Review LR = Labor Review F = Focusing BRT = Breathing/Relaxation Techniques PrO = PreOp.	**Touch** E = Effleurage B = Backrub CP = Counterpressure M = Massage	**Position/Activity** W = Walking C = Chair SQ = Squatting JR = Jet Hydrotherapy SH = Shower K = Kneeling LS = Left Side RS = Right Side KC = Knee Chest T = Trendelenburg	**Physical Care** MC = Mouth Care SC = Superficial Cold SH = Superficial Heat PC = Peri Care BP = Bedpan

Form 5711N © 2001 Briggs Corporation, Des Moines, IA 50306
R304   To order, phone (800) 245-4080 www.BriggsCorp.com PRINTED IN U.S.A.

LABOR PROGRESS CHART

Figure 14-19   *(continued)*

Duplication of this form is strictly prohibited by law. © 2001 Briggs Corporation. All rights reserved.

Briggs CORPORATION

Labor Progress Chart
Maternal/Newborn Record System
To order call: **1.800.245.4080**   Re-order No. **5711N**

TIME →	1335	1400	1430	1500	1530	1600	1630	1700								

Mark X ●

Station / Dilatation chart (values -4 to +3 / 2 to 10)

| Effacement % and/or position | 90% | | 100% | | ROP | | | ROA | | | | | | | | |
| Examined by: | MB | | RB | | RB | | RB | RB | | | | | | | | |

COMPOSITE NORMAL DILATATION CURVES

MULTIPAROUS (composite)   NULLIPAROUS (composite)

COMPOSITE CURVES OF ABNORMAL LABOR PROGRESS—MULTIPAROUS

Normal Dilatation curve   Prolonged deceleration curve   Protracted active phase   Secondary arrest of dilatation   Prolonged latent phase

Labor Progress Curves derived from the work of Emanuel A. Friedman, M.D.

IV Record

Start Date	Time	Site	Solution	Amount (mL's)	Medication/Dose Added	Initials	Infused Date	Time	Amount Infused
6/23/04	1345	left hand	#1 Ringer's lactate	1000mL	–	RB	6/23/04	1800	1000mL
	1950		#2 DSW	1000mL	–	RB			
			(#2 continued for recovery care)						

Interval Medications

Date Time	Medication/Dose	Route	Site	Initials

Signature Key

Initials	Signature
MB	Mark Brown MD
RB	Rae Baird RNC

Form 5711N © 2001 Briggs Corporation, Des Moines, IA 50306
R304   To order, phone (800) 245-4080 www.BriggsCorp.com PRINTED IN U.S.A.

LABOR PROGRESS CHART

Figure 14-19   (continued)

Briggs
CORPORATION

Labor Progress Chart
Maternal/Newborn Record System
To order call: **1.800.245.4080**   Re-order No. **5711N**

Progress Notes

Date	Time	Year 2004
6/23	1335	Gravida $\overline{\overline{\overline{\text{III}}}}$ Para $\overline{\overline{\text{II}}}$ admitted to LDRP 3. Temp 98⁸ P88 R12 B.P. 128/88. External monitor placed. Having moderate contractions every 5 minutes lasting 40 seconds. Describes pain as 6-7 on scale of 10. FHT regular at 138 per minute. Mother reports membranes ruptured at 1230 today. Nitrazine positive. Fern test pending ; fluid clear. Moderate amount of show. I.V. of 1000mL Ringer's Lactate started via #18 angiocath in left hand running at 100mL's per hour. Husband present. Admission physical per Dr. Brown. 2-3cm dilated, 90% effaced, vertex, 0 station. Refer to Labor Progress Chart. *Rae Baird RNC*
6/23	1400	Admission blood work drawn by lab tech. Ice chips. Encouraged to walk. Fern positive. *Rae Baird RNC*
6/23	1500	B.P. 130/88. Internal monitor placed. Contractions now every 3-4 minutes lasting 45-50 seconds. Intensity remains moderate at 30-40. FHT regular at 138. Scalp pH 7.25. Voided 150cc light yellow urine. Encouraged to focus. *Rae Baird RNC*
6/23	1600	Contractions now every 2-3 minutes lasting 55 seconds. Mother complaining of more discomfort but requests no pain medication at this time. B.P. 130/86. Complaining of nausea. Voided 100cc yellow urine at 1545. *Rae Baird RNC*
6/23	1630	8-9cm dilated. Contractions strong every two minutes, lasting 60 seconds. FHT stable at 132. I.V. increased to 125cc per hour. *Rae Baird RNC*
6/23	1715	Urge to push. Internal monitor discontinued. Fetal scalp monitor remains in place. Dr. Brown notified. FHT at 126. *Rae Baird RNC*
6/23	1800	Continue to push with each contraction. FHT 110, deceleration to 104 with receiving to 118. Patient most comfortable kneeling. O₂ begun at 6L 125mL I.V. bolus. *Rae Baird RNC*
6/23	1815	Baseline FHT's 118. O₂ maintained. Patient pushing while on L side. Dr. Brown present. ROP *Rae Baird RNC*
6/23	1830	Baseline FHT 120, occasional decelerations to 110 with recovery in 15-20 seconds. *Rae Baird RNC*
6/23	1845	Baseline FHT now 128. Mother squatting to improve force of pushing. *Rae Baird RNC*
6/23	1900	Patient continues to push. FHT's at 124. *Rae Baird RNC*
6/23	1915	FHT's baseline at 116. O₂ maintained at 6L per minute. Anesthetist alerted. Patient continues to push. *Rae Baird RNC*
6/23	1930	FHT 108, deceleration to 102 with recovery to 114 at 15 seconds. O₂ continues. Lying on left side. I.V. 250mL bolus. *Rae Baird RNC*
6/23	1940	Patient in semi-Fowlers position, slightly tilted to left. Pushing, beginning to crown. *Rae Baird RNC*
6/23	1946	Male infant delivered by Dr. Brown. Dr. Smith received infant. *Rae Baird RNC*
6/23	1947	Apgar 5 - bulb suctioned - O₂ per mask. *Rae Baird RNC*
6/23	1948	Placenta delivered. B.P. 112/76 P 78. *Rae Baird RNC*
6/23	1949	1% Xylocaine administered for episiotomy repair. *Rae Baird RNC*
6/23	1952	Apgar 9 - infant given to mother and father. Infant awake and alert. Band number 4515 applied to mother and infant. Mother attempting to nurse infant. Aquamephyton 1.0mg. I.M. right thigh given to infant. *Rae Baird RNC*

PRE-PROCEDURE CHECKLIST
(Check all that apply)
☐ History & Physical
☐ Prenatal Records
☐ X-rays and Ultrasounds
☐ Consents
☐ Patient ID
☐ Site ID / Verification
☐ Other_____
_____
Timeout_____

Form 5711N   © 2001 Briggs Corporation, Des Moines, IA 50306
R304   To order, phone (800) 245-4080 www.BriggsCorp.com PRINTED IN U.S.A.

LABOR PROGRESS CHART

Figure 14-19   *(continued)*

pillows can be provided to help in positioning. The supine position should be avoided because of the danger of vena caval compression.

Comfort Measures

Anxiety levels and coping mechanisms of the client, partner, and family are assessed continually as labor progresses. Anxiety and fear tend to lower a woman's pain threshold. The nurse should try to remain with the woman in active labor (client load permitting) to give encouragement and reassurance that normal progress is being made. Ignorance of the process and mechanism of labor can result in anxiety and fear of childbirth. Fear causes catecholamine secretion, which has the effect of decreasing peripheral blood flow. Adrenaline has a terbutaline-like effect in that it can cause labor to be prolonged as uterine contractions become less effective. The biggest factor in management of labor is nursing support and coaching. The value of having a caring skilled professional at the bedside cannot be overestimated.

A calm, competent, and gentle manner on the part of the nurse promotes trust and goes a long way toward alleviating client anxiety. Frequent feedback should be given and the findings of each test explained in language the client can understand. It also is important to take care of the woman's partner, and this can be done by providing a comfortable chair and including the person in discussions and explanations. Support for the laboring family is individualized according to the specific needs and expectations of those concerned as well as respectfully taking into account the cultural background.

Pain Management

A common concern of the pregnant woman is whether she will be able to cope with the pain of contractions, or whether she will lose control. There are a variety of measures that will promote relaxation and assist the woman in coping as contractions intensify.

The nurse may need to instruct the woman in breathing techniques or reinforce those already learned. Some women find counterpressure massage of the sacral area helpful during contractions, particularly when contraction pain is being experienced mostly in the lower back. Some

childbirth classes advise clients to bring a tennis ball to the hospital to roll in a circular fashion against the woman's lower back, while applying gentle pressure during a contraction. If the fetus is in an occipitoposterior position, the pressure of the fetal occiput on maternal spinal nerves will cause the woman to experience contraction pain mostly in the lower back. Counterpressure is helpful in lifting the occiput off these nerves, to some extent, thus providing pain relief. Changing positions frequently is helpful.

The comforting effects of a warm shower during the first stage of labor should not be underestimated. Some facilities feature a bathtub with whirlpool jets, such as a Jacuzzi, as a comfort measure to decrease muscle tension and promote relaxation (Figure 14-20). Having the client relax in a whirlpool, however, does not relieve the nurse of the responsibility of appropriate fetal assessment. Bathing during labor is associated with decreased pain and increased speed of cervical dilation (Lowe, 1996).

A **doula** is a woman who is employed by the pregnant woman to assist her through labor, delivery, and sometimes the first two weeks postpartum. The doula may be trained and certified, or may have no clinical training but be able to reinforce breathing techniques, massage, and sometimes provide ice packs or warm packs. The labor partner or nurse usually is more than able to provide physical and emotional support; however, when the nurse is assigned to more than one client or if the client has no family member with her, the services of a doula are particularly valuable.

The birthing ball is available in some labor and delivery suites. The ball provides a soft yet firm place to sit while promoting a desirable upright posture and allowing for decreased straining of the muscles. The birthing ball also is used to lie on.

Table 13-3 in Chapter 13 summarizes various methods of analgesia and anesthesia for labor and delivery.

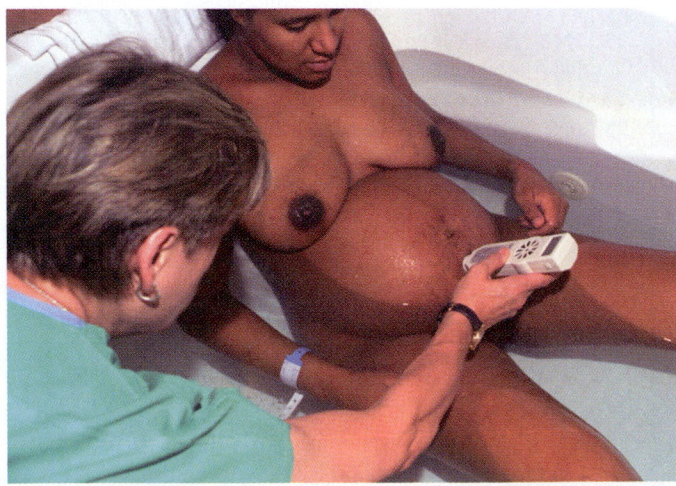

Figure 14-20 The nurse continues to monitor fetal status while the laboring woman relaxes in a whirlpool.

Nursing Tip

The Board of Nurse Examiners

If you are named as a defendant in a malpractice suit, bear in mind that the Board of Nurse Examiners is not there to protect nurses. Its sole concern is to protect the public from incompetent nurses. It does provide the guidelines that set standards of care.

Psychologic Considerations

As labor advances, anxiety levels secondary to pain increase in the woman who has not received epidural analgesia. It is important for the nurse to be present with the woman who is in active labor and to continue to offer encouragement and reassurance to the woman and family. As the transition phase approaches, the woman experiences stronger contractions while feeling tired, irritable, and less able to cope after all the hours of labor. She may feel trapped and apprehensive because of the increasing pain and vaginal pressure and will be less interested in her appearance and outside activities. To minimize environmental change, it is advisable for the same nurse, who already has developed a trusting rapport with the laboring woman, to continue care until she gives birth. Emphasis is on enhancing coping by assuring the client that all is going well, staying with her, and coaching her as necessary with her breathing techniques through each contraction. The client needs constant support during these phases of labor.

Labor Curve

Labor progress may be plotted by use of the labor curve, which was developed by Friedman (1970) as a method of graphically plotting the relationship of time to dilation of the cervix and station of the presenting part. When preparing to plot the labor curve, the number of hours the woman labors is written across the top of the graph, the dilation in centimeters up one vertical side, and the station (in descending order) down the opposite vertical side. The first time interval entered on the graph is the time the woman reported that regular contractions began.

Role of the Support Person

The friend or relative who provides companionship and encouragement to the laboring woman may be male or female; often is the husband or father of the infant who gives emotional support at this time. Some expectant fathers see their role as coach and will actively help the woman focus on breathing through her contractions. Partners who have not attended prepared childbirth classes with their mate, though not familiar with breathing techniques, often are quite willing to give physical comfort such as sips of water and back rubs. The nurse can fill in any knowledge gaps that the support person might have.

Some expectant fathers adopt a more passive role and are content to merely be present and to witness the birth. While being available to guide and encourage the man in taking an active part in the process, the nurse should in no way impose on him any personal philosophy of what his function should be. The laboring woman may be content that her partner is present and may not require him to do more than sit in a chair and read a newspaper while she is in labor. The woman is the one who knows her partner

Nursing Tip — *Nursing Diagnoses in the Second Stage of Labor*

Nursing diagnoses that apply to a woman during the second stage of labor might include the following:

- Risk for injury
- Disturbed sleep pattern related to the length of labor
- Deficient knowledge related to normal labor and delivery as evidenced by client's inexperience and lack of preparation
- Pain related to uterine contractions
- Fear or anxiety

best and probably has a fairly accurate idea of how much he will participate in the birth experience.

Second Stage

The **second stage of labor** begins when the cervix is fully dilated (10 cm), and ends with delivery of the baby. Inability to feel the cervix during vaginal examination confirms that the second stage has begun (Figure 14-21). When a woman has received epidural analgesia, she may not be aware that the contractions have become stronger. She will feel vaginal pressure with each contraction during the second stage of labor. Premonitory indicators that should alert the nurse that the client may have entered the second stage of labor include the following (Scott, DiSaia, Hammond, & Spellocy, 1994):

- Bearing down of her own accord
- Complaints that her contractions have become stronger and more painful
- Complaints of pressure on her rectum
- Increased amount of bloody show
- Increasing irritability and tearfulness, together with a decreased coping ability
- Nausea or vomiting
- Trembling limbs

The physician or nurse-midwife should be notified when the woman has begun the second stage of labor so

Nursing Tip — *Premature Pushing*

If the cervix is not fully dilated, pushing will not only tire the woman unnecessarily but will cause the cervix to become swollen and thus prolong labor. Repeated blowing or panting helps to counteract the tendency to push prematurely.

that he or she can be available to come to the LDR as soon as birth is imminent. The duration of the second stage varies greatly from woman to woman. A duration of more than 2 hours in a first pregnancy is considered prolonged, unless the woman is receiving epidural or other regional analgesia. In the multiparous woman, a second stage of more than 1 hour for a woman whose previous infant weighed over 6 pounds might be considered prolonged. The nurse notifies the appropriate health care provider of progress or lack of progress.

During the second stage of labor contractions usually occur every 2 to 3 minutes, with a duration of 60 to 90 seconds, and intensity is strong by palpation or 80 to 100 mmHg by IUPC. Uterine tone should palpate soft between contractions. Amniotic fluid is assessed for the presence of meconium, and bloody show is monitored for excessive bleeding. The FHR is assessed in accordance with institutional policy. During the second stage of labor the usual protocol requires FHR and uterine activity evaluation every 15 minutes for low-risk clients and every 5 minutes for high-risk clients (ACOG, July 1995).

Refer to the accompanying photo story for a complete account of one couple's birth story.

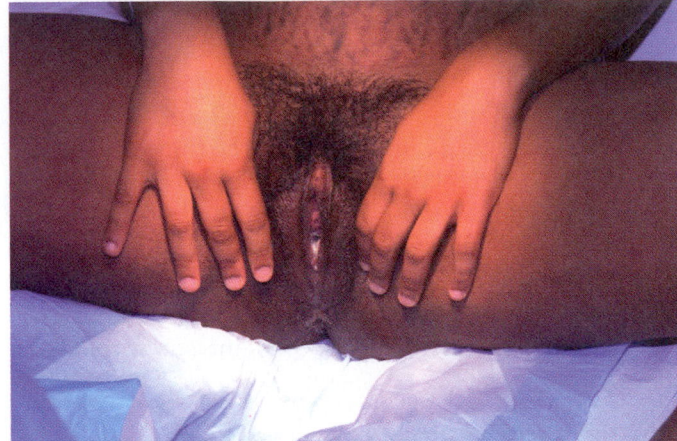

B.

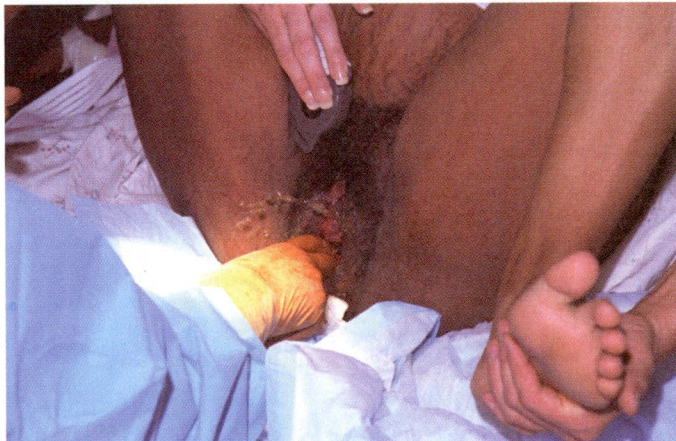

C.

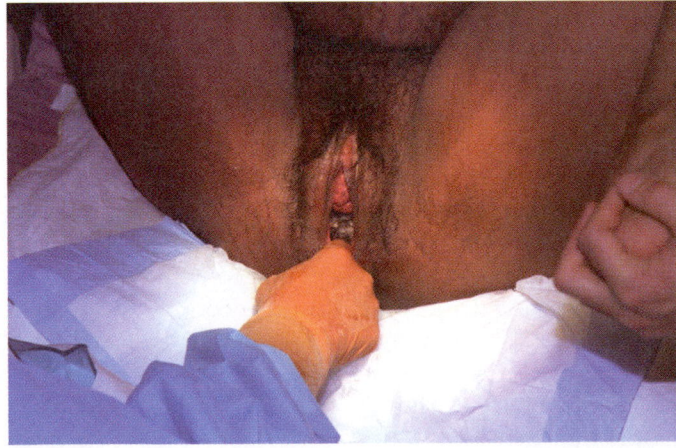

D.

Figure 14-21 A. Dilation of the cervix is assessed while the woman briefly bears down. B. Many women will want to feel the perineal bulge with their fingers to be assured that labor is progressing. C. Spontaneous urination occurs during a vaginal check. D. The infant's head is clearly visible, meaning that birth is imminent.

A.

One Couple's Birth Story

When the couple arrives at the hospital and labor is confirmed, the woman is admitted to Labor and Delivery. Certain admission procedures must be completed, including gathering baseline data and lab work.

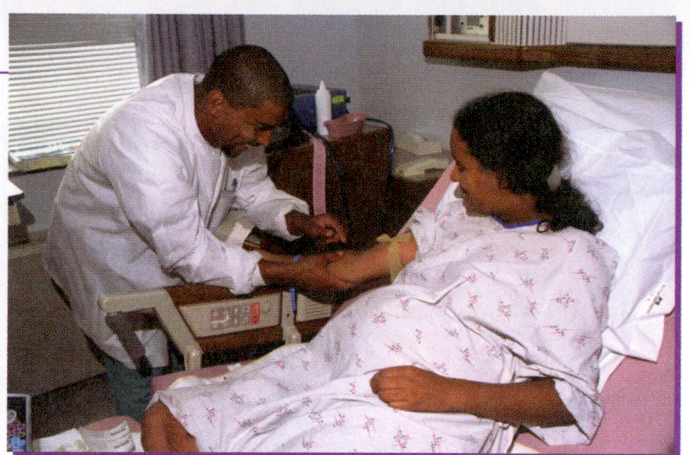

In the past, women were expected to remain NPO throughout their labor. This policy has been relaxed in most institutions and liquids are encouraged.

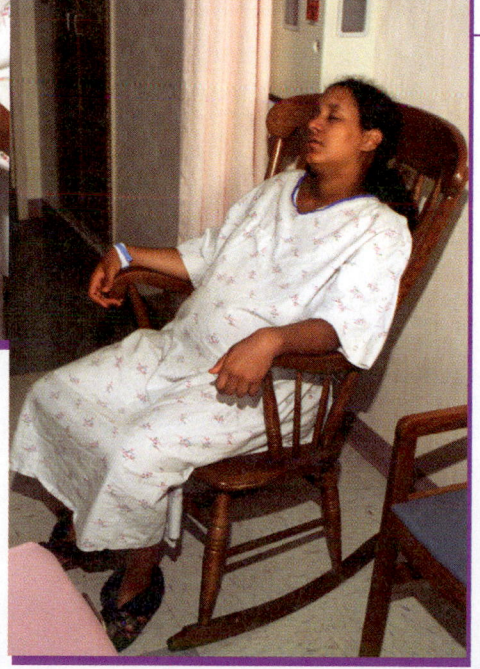

Many women find it more comfortable to ambulate or sit in a chair during early labor.

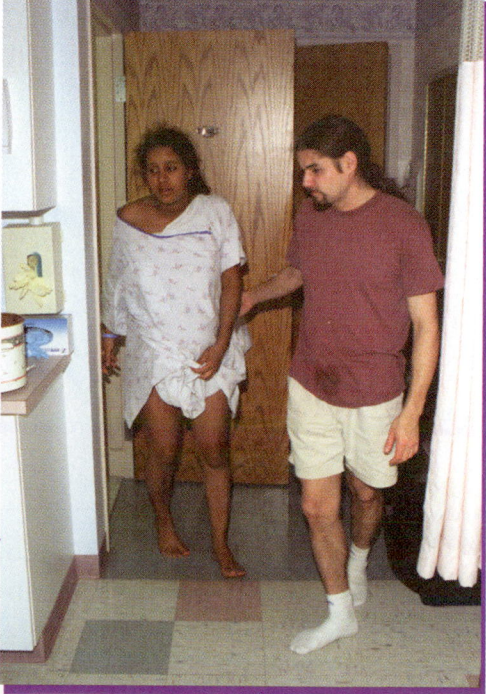

As labor progresses, the woman may want to rest in bed with the exception of trips to the bathroom.

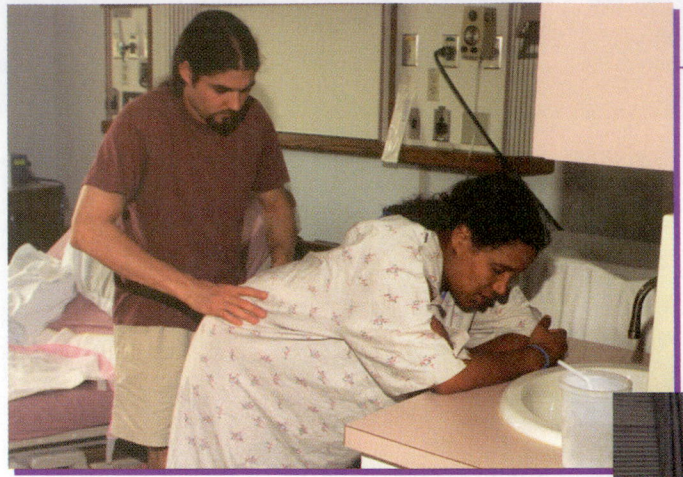

Some women find that a change of position and a backrub assists them in achieving comfort.

Most women try to rest between contractions to conserve energy.

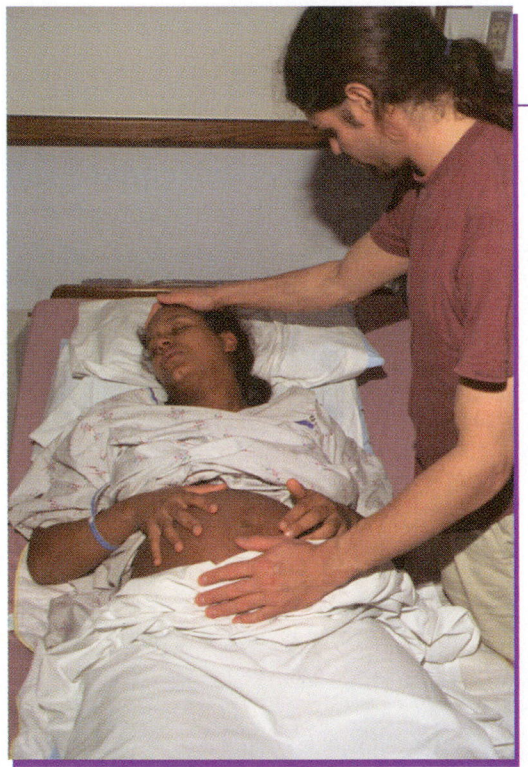

As contractions increase in frequency, duration, and intensity, the woman is less likely to be able to rest.

When the client becomes completely dilated, she feels an urge to push with her contractions. Her significant other is assisting her to assume a position conducive to pushing.

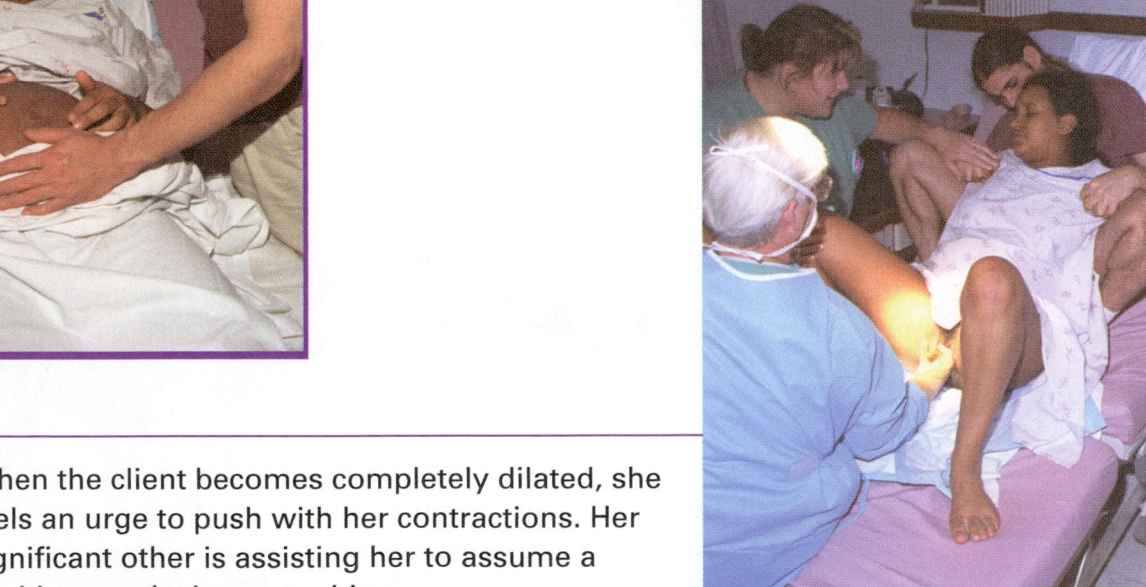

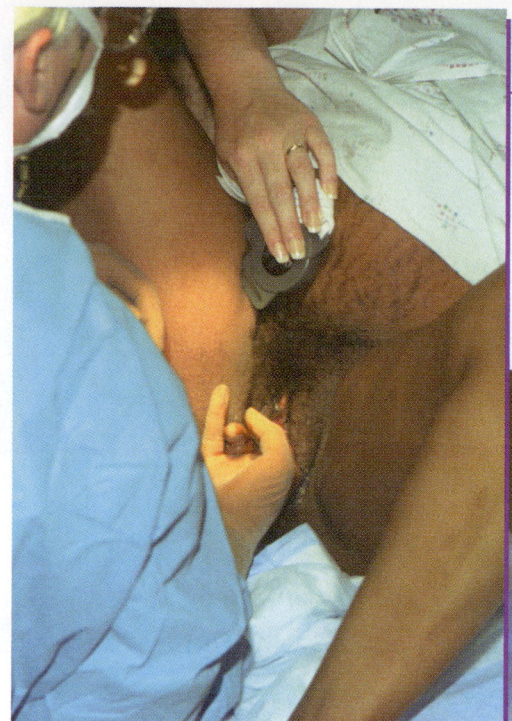

As the fetus descends through the pelvis, the nurse must monitor the fetal heart tones more frequently as well as the station of the presenting part.

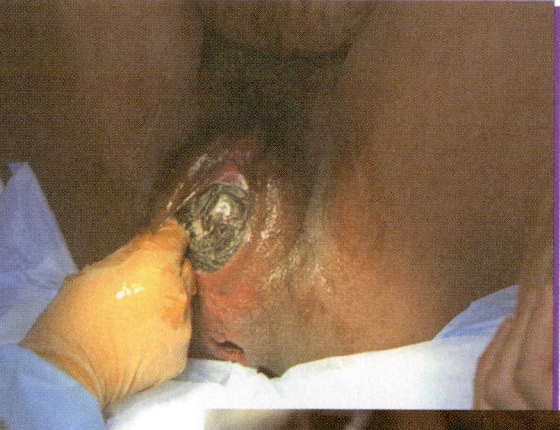

As the fetal head crowns, there is much thinning and pressure of the tissue. This pressure also involves the anus.

Finally, the baby's head is delivered between contractions to avoid perineal injury.

The midwife supports the head as external rotation occurs.

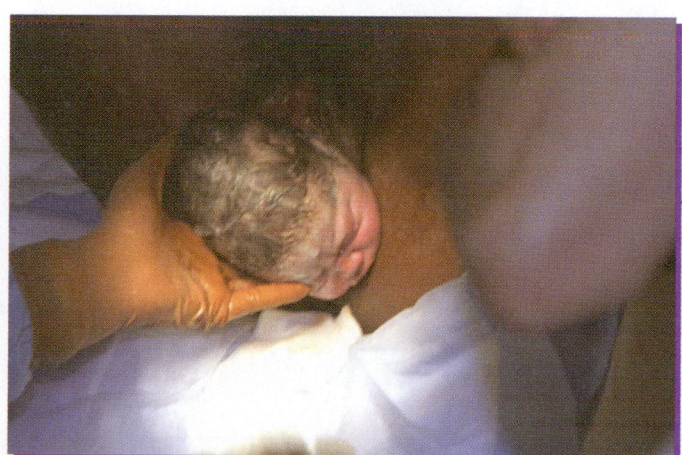

The baby's mouth and nose are suctioned immediately so the airway will be clear of amniotic fluid.

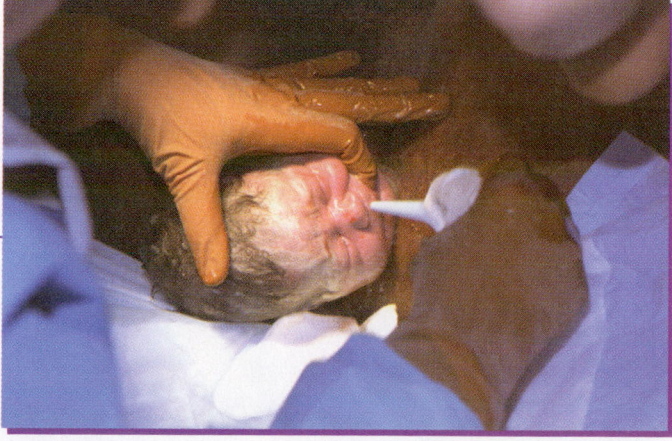

As restitution occurs, the midwife makes sure the baby's umbilical cord is not around its neck.

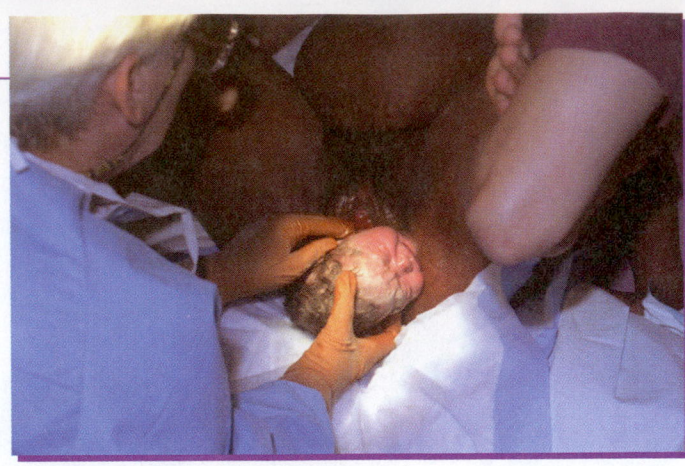

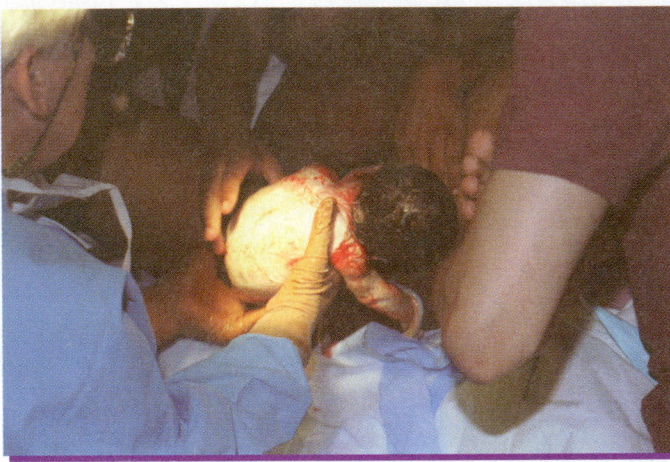

After the next contraction, the remainder of the body is delivered.

The baby is placed on the mother's abdomen while the midwife finishes the delivery.

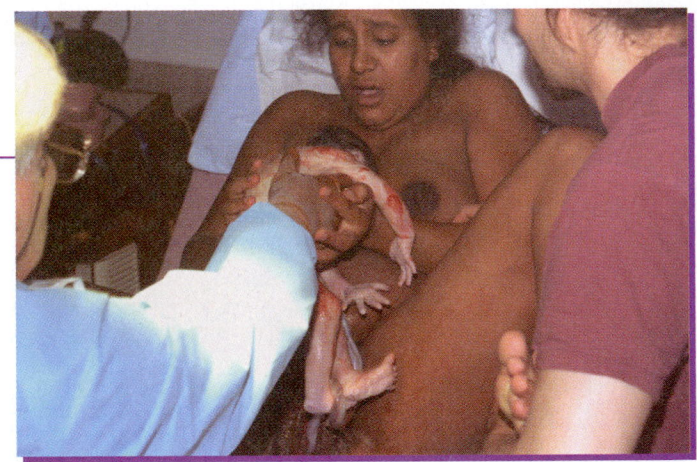

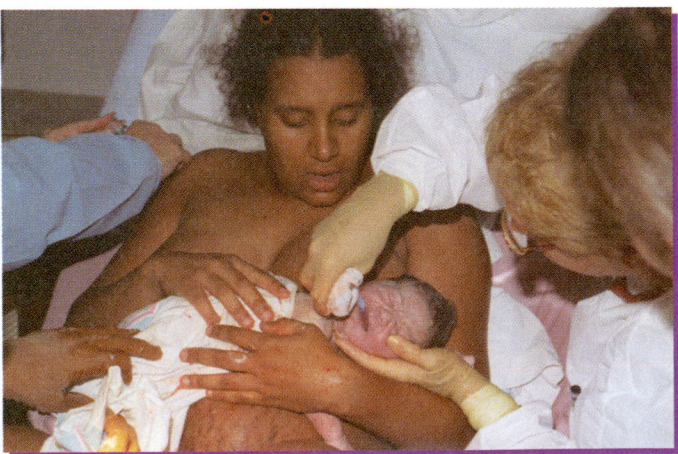

The infant is covered with a blanket and placed next to the mother's skin to prevent loss of body heat. The nurse suctions the baby's mouth again to ensure adequate air transport.

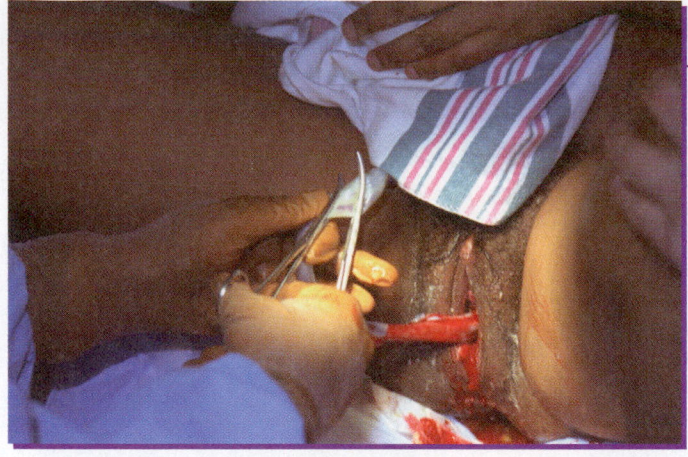

The midwife places two clamps on the umbilical cord.

The cord is cut between the two clamps by the baby's father.

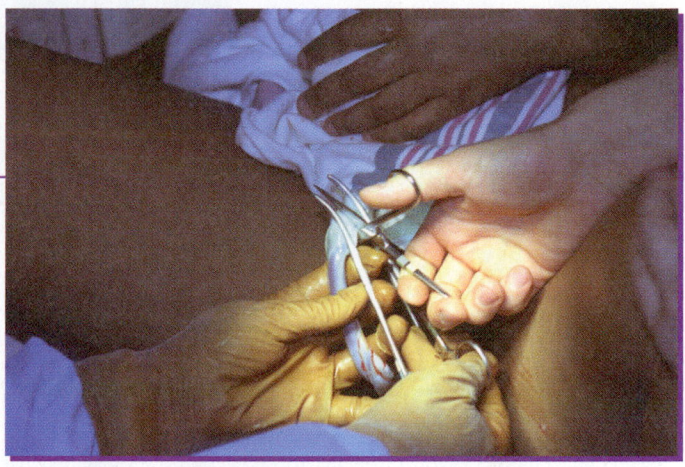

Waiting for the placenta to deliver. This usually occurs within a few minutes.

As the placenta separates, there is usually a gush of blood.

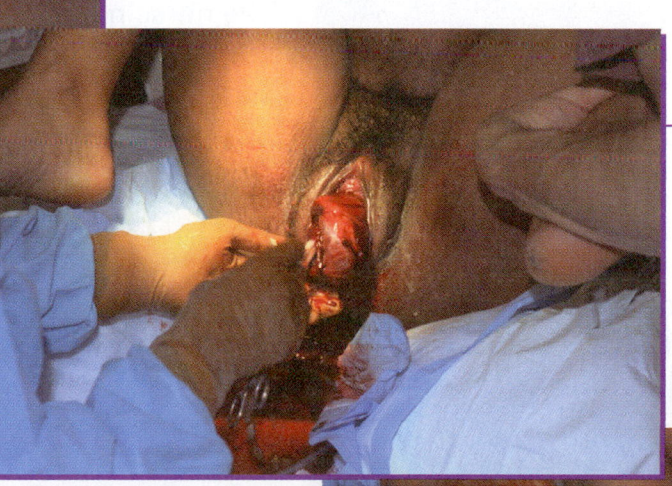

When the placenta has been delivered, it is inspected to ascertain that it is intact.

Many times women deliver without an episiotomy but may have small lacerations that need repair.

If the infant is placed at the mother's breast and sucks immediately following the delivery of the placenta, this assists in uterine involution through the release of maternal oxytocin.

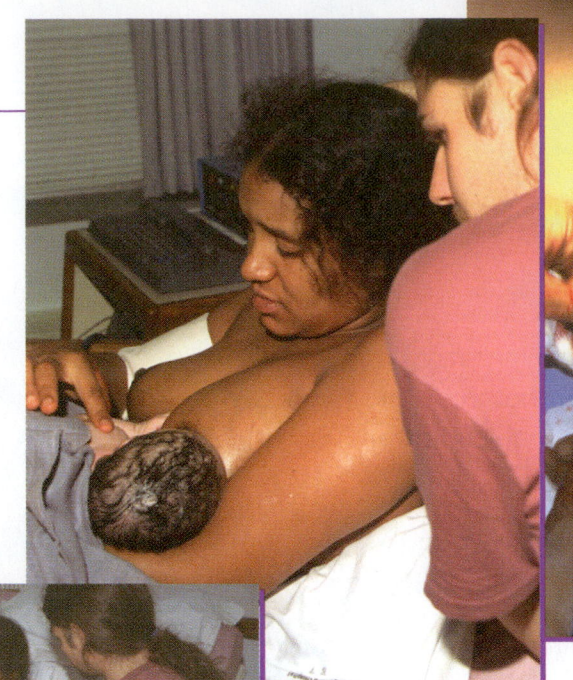

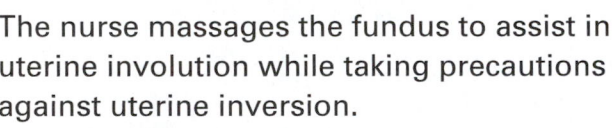

The nurse massages the fundus to assist in uterine involution while taking precautions against uterine inversion.

The baby's umbilical cord was intentionally left long at delivery. Now it is time to place a cord clamp and shorten the cord.

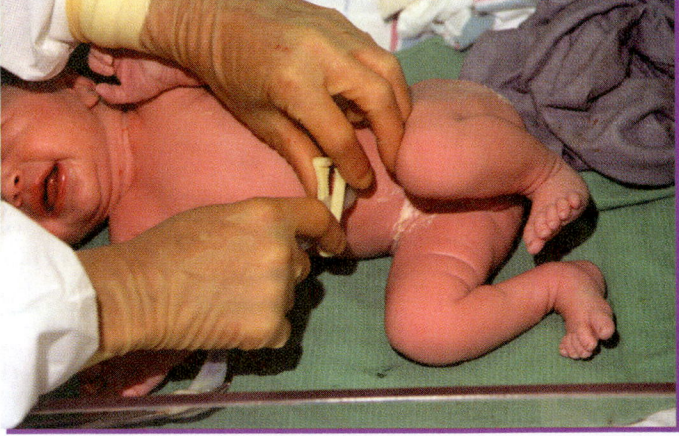

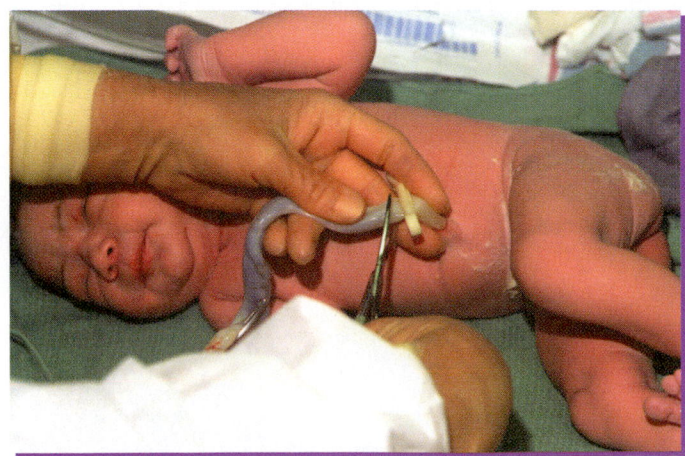

The cord is trimmed with sterile scissors.

The baby has a strong, lusty cry.

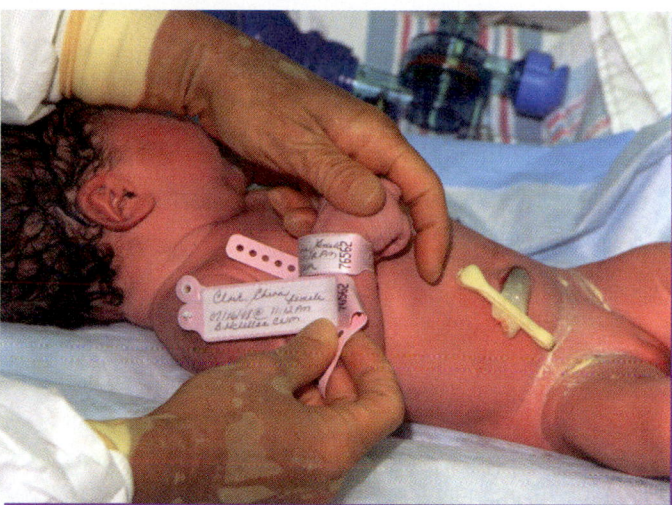

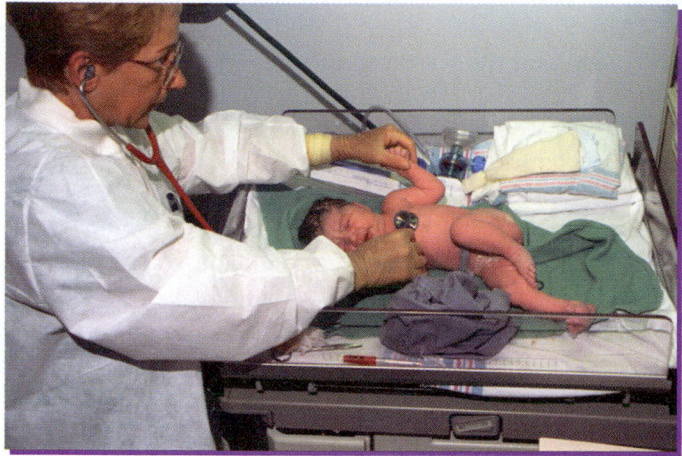

The nurse completes an assessment of the heart rate.

Matching arm bracelets are placed on the mother and infant for identification.

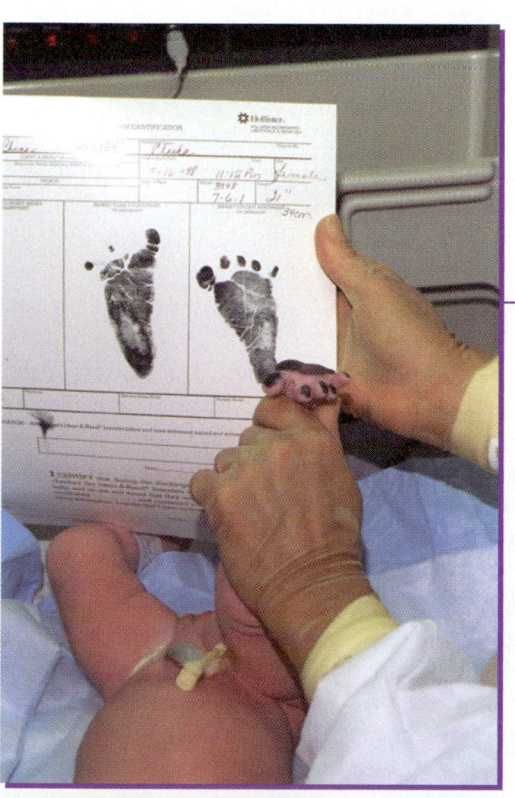

Infant footprints or cord blood DNA are obtained as a secondary means of identification.

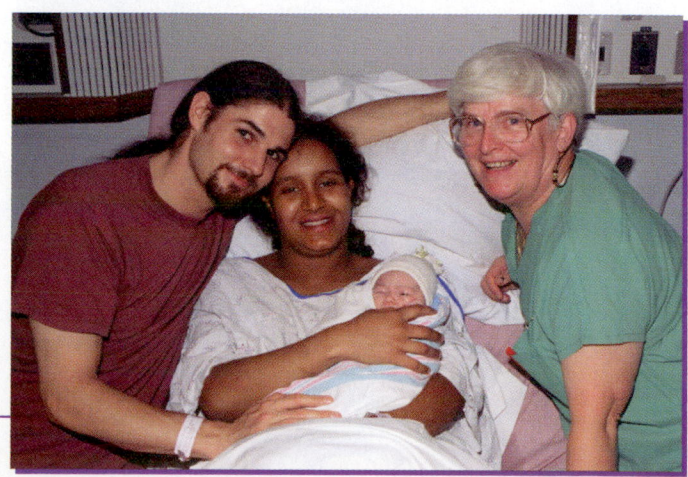

The happy family begins its life together.

Fetal Descent Assessment

Full dilation of the cervix is a function of descent; therefore, the continuing presence of a cervical lip indicates that the baby is not descending. Fetal descent is evaluated by performing a vaginal examination, or visually when the presenting part is at the perineum. When the cervix is fully dilated while the presenting part is still relatively high (0 to +1 station), the woman may wish to defer pushing efforts until after the fetal head has descended further.

The second stage can be divided into a passive phase and an active phase. In the passive phase of the second stage, the woman does not yet have any urge to push. Descent does not require pushing. During this phase, the fetal head should be allowed to descend by means of involuntary uterine contractions (primary powers). This action is called *laboring down*, and it helps to prevent stress on the fetus and exhaustion of the mother from extended pushing time. In the active phase of the second stage, pressure on S-2 to S-4 and stretch receptors in the vagina create the urge to push; therefore, the woman should begin her expulsive efforts (secondary powers). There are no benefits to pushing before the active phase of the second stage of labor. Visible signs of descent include bulging of the perineum and crowning (Figure 14-22).

Psychologic Considerations

The start of the second stage often is a relief for the laboring woman because she can now take a more active part in delivering her baby by augmenting the involuntary primary powers (uterine contractions) with secondary powers (pushing). Instead of panting through each contraction and fighting the almost uncontrollable urge to push, she can concentrate all her energies on pushing out the infant. Being able to push gives the woman a feeling

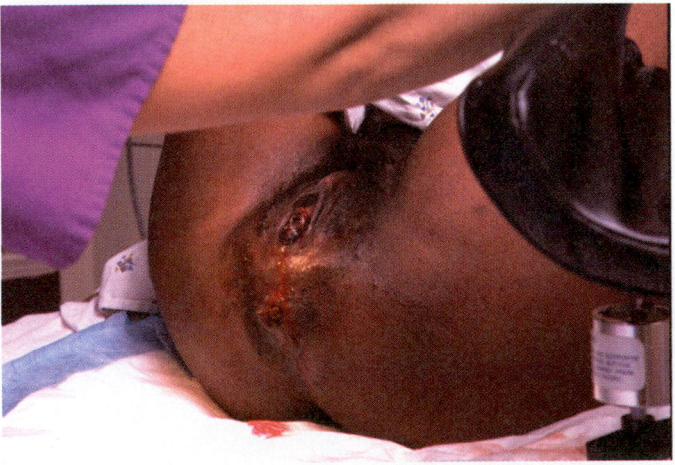

Figure 14-22 A bulging perineum is a visible sign of fetal descent.

of having some control over her labor (Box 14-12). The woman's perceptions are narrowed to the extent that she is all absorbed in the effort of pushing with contractions. Between contractions she should be encouraged to close her eyes take a deep cleansing breath and completely relax to conserve her strength for the next expulsive effort. The woman may experience nausea and may perspire with the effort of pushing.

The number of visitors permitted in a hospital room will vary and, as the time of delivery approaches, the nurse should ask the woman whom she would like to attend the delivery. This can best be done when visitors have temporarily stepped out of the room, so that the woman does not feel obliged to allow someone to see the delivery if she really does not want them there. The nurse can be an advocate for the woman by being the gatekeeper and ensuring that the woman's wishes in this regard are met.

Maternal Positioning

The nurse assists with maternal positioning to facilitate fetal descent and promote comfort. Several position options are available during pushing. The most commonly used position in the United States is the semi-Fowler's position in which the head of the bed is elevated about 45 degrees and the woman grasps her flexed knees or ankles. Epidural anesthesia has probably contributed to this semi-recumbent positioning. Women can benefit from pushing in a more upright position, which can be accomplished by leaning forward on a supported bedside table, a squat bar, or a birthing ball. Repeated studies have shown that upright positions, such as walking or standing, benefit both mother and fetus. These positions have a favorable effect on uterine contractility and reduce pain and perineal trauma (Mayberry et al., 1999). A lateral position also can be used for pushing and delivery. The pushing position used depends on the desires of the client and also requires flexibility on the part of the nurse and physician or nurse-midwife. Arbitrary limits on the second stage of labor should be abandoned if both the mother and fetus are doing well and progress is being made.

To assist with effective breathing and pushing, the nurse can ascertain which techniques the woman has learned in her prenatal classes and reinforce them. The woman is urged to listen to her body and bear down when she feels the urge to do so. The desire to bear down is an involuntary response to the pressure of the presenting part on the stretch receptors of the pelvic muscles. One drawback to this urge-to-push method is that the woman who has received epidural anesthesia may never feel the need to push. If the woman is not aware of contractions because of epidural analgesia, she needs to

Box 14-12

Pushing Technique

1. Encourage spontaneous bearing down. Allow the mother to rest until the fetal head has descended low enough in the pelvis to stimulate Ferguson's reflex (a reflex stimulated by stretch receptors in the pelvic floor, which usually occurs at a +1 station that stimulate in the mother an involuntary urge to push).

2. Consider fetal station, and position in addition to dilation in determining a woman's readiness for pushing.

3. Discourage prolonged maternal breath-holding (more than 6 seconds) during pushing.

4. Encourage four or more pushes per contraction.

5. Support rather than direct the woman's involuntary pushing efforts, whether they include grunting, groaning, exhaling, or breath-holding for less than 6 seconds (Figure 14-23).

6. Validate the normalcy of sensations and maternal sounds.

7. The woman who has received epidural anesthesia may require more directed support for her expulsive efforts during the second stage.

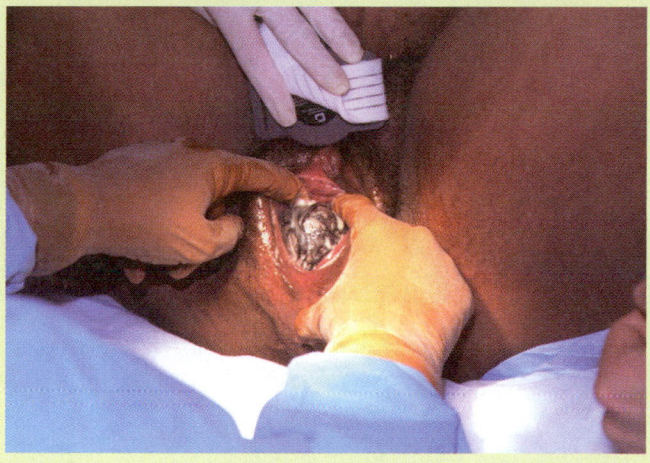
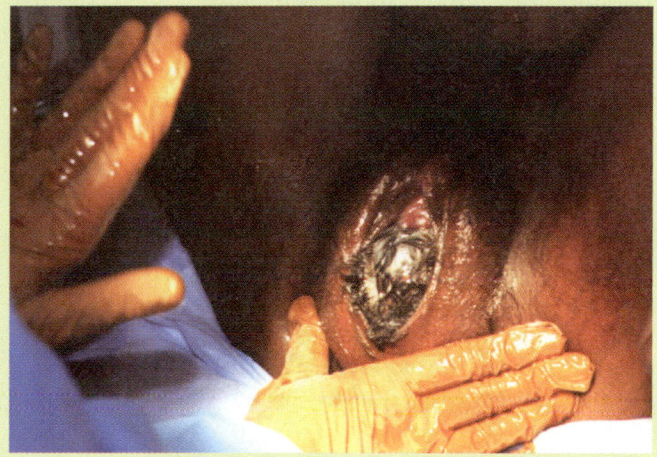

A.   **B.**

Figure 14-23   A. The perineum is stretched as the infant's head crowns. B. The health care provider supports the woman's efforts by encouraging her to stop pushing between contractions.

be coached to push during each contraction. Her partner may help by supporting the woman's head or shoulders during pushing, wiping her brow with a cool damp cloth, and offering words of encouragement. The nurse and partner need to understand that because of the stress of labor, pain, and exhaustion, it is not uncommon for the woman to say things that she would not otherwise say. The primary care provider is kept apprised of progress or lack of progress, as indicated. The woman, her partner, and family are kept informed of her progress, the expected sequence of events, and the delivery routine.

As the fetal head descends, bulging of the perineum occurs and rectal mucosa is exposed. Any stool in the rectum will be expelled. The fetal head passes under the pubic arch, and the vertex is visible as it pushes open the vaginal introitus, which is known as **crowning**.

Other Team Members

Other personnel required to be present during delivery will depend on the needs of the mother and infant as well as the protocol of the facility. If the woman is receiving epidural anesthesia, some facilities require a Certified Registered Nurse Anesthetist (CRNA) to be present during the delivery. The CRNA is there in case a bolus of analgesia is needed and to remove the epidural cannula immediately after the third stage is over and perineal repairs are completed.

If the amniotic fluid is meconium-stained, some facilities require that a neonatologist or a neonatal clinical nurse specialist be at the delivery to provide endotracheal suction to the newborn and ascertain whether meconium was aspirated by the baby. Many institutions now have neonatal resuscitation teams for at-risk deliveries. This team is often composed of an NICU nurse and a respiratory therapist with Neonatal Resuscitation Provider (NRP) certification. Other personnel that may be required, depending on the particular protocol are a surgical technician to assist with the instrument table and a second nurse to care for the baby. It is the primary nurse's responsibility to ensure that the primary caregiver and other health care team members as appropriate are notified of the impending delivery and are called in time.

Nursing Responsibilities in Preparing for Delivery

The client is never left alone during the second stage of labor; therefore, the nurse must anticipate the need for equipment and supplies. An instrument table is prepared and the individual requirements of the physician or nurse-midwife are considered (Figure 14-24). Other necessary items include a table containing sterile delivery instruments and an antiseptic such as Betadine (povidone-iodine), adequate lighting, personal protective equipment (PPE) such as gloves, masks, and eyewear, and oxygen and suction equipment for both mother and newborn. The radiant warmer or incubator should be prewarmed and spread with warmed baby blankets and a knit cap. Identification labels are prepared according to hospital protocol. Four identical identification bracelets usually are used for labeling the baby (two), mother, and partner. Two vials of oxytocin (Pitocin), 10 U, should be on hand for administration to the mother after the placenta has been delivered.

The nurse adjusts the birthing bed, delivery table, or operating table to accommodate the client and health care provider (who also may require a stool). In a physician-assisted delivery the client's legs often are supported in stirrups and the lower section of the delivery bed removed (Figure 14-25). A woman who has received epidural analgesia may have difficulty moving her legs;

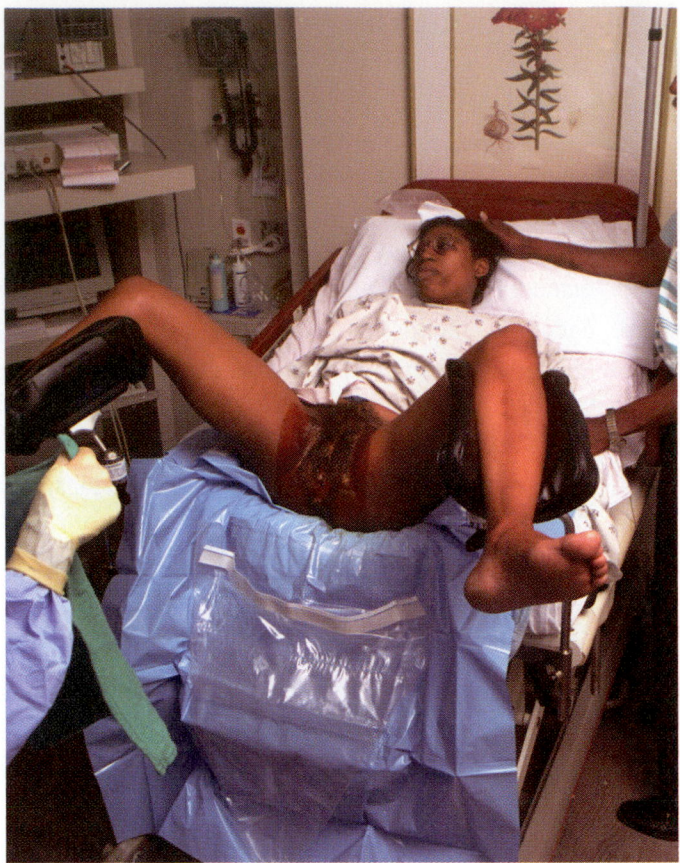

Figure 14-25   This woman is ready to deliver, with her legs supported in stirrups, the perineal area cleansed, and the foot of the bed removed.

therefore, the nurse must ensure that the woman's legs are completely secure in the stirrups. It is not advisable for the client's legs to be placed in stirrups until the baby's head is almost crowning and the primary caregiver is present in the delivery room, at which time the woman's legs are secured in the stirrups and the lower part of the delivery bed is removed. In a nurse-midwife-assisted birth, the bed is often not broken down and stirrups are not commonly used.

For the birth, the nurse wears personal protective equipment, a waterproof gown, and a mask with an eyeshield. Just before the birth, the nurse dons gloves and cleanses the maternal perineum, using technique as per the hospital policy and procedure (Figure 14-26). Some institutions no longer do a sterile scrub but rather a sanitary cleansing with the Betadine or Hibiclens (chlorhexidine gluconate) soap.

The nurse and client's partner continue to support and encourage the woman in her expulsive efforts, instructing her to modify her breathing and pushing technique as indicated. Xylocaine 1% (lidocaine HCl) local anesthetic should be available in case the primary caregiver decides that an **episiotomy**, an incision into the per-

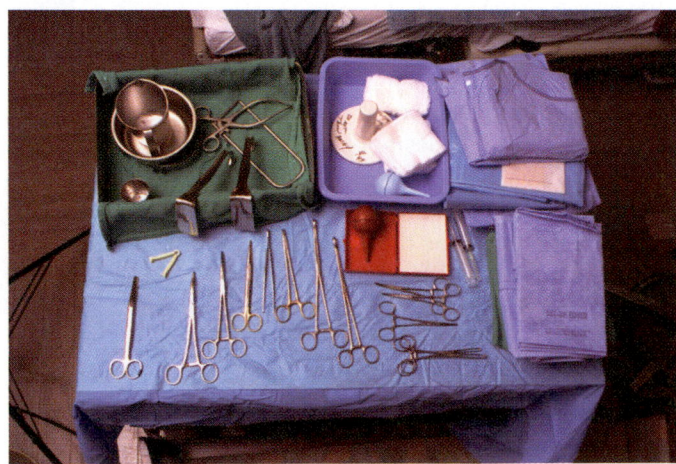

Figure 14-24   Delivery instrument table.

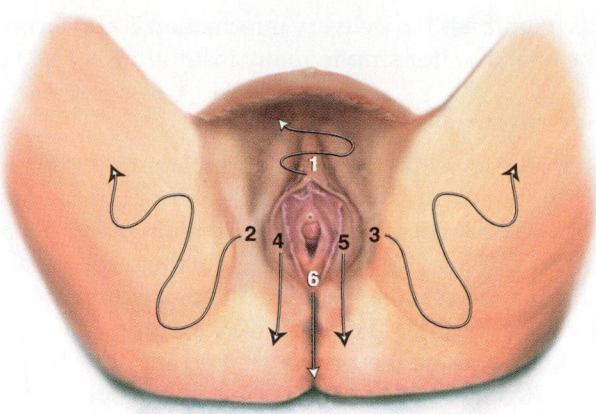

Figure 14-26   Perineal scrub; clean from the vagina outward, that is, from 1 to 6, moving bacteria away from and not toward the vagina.

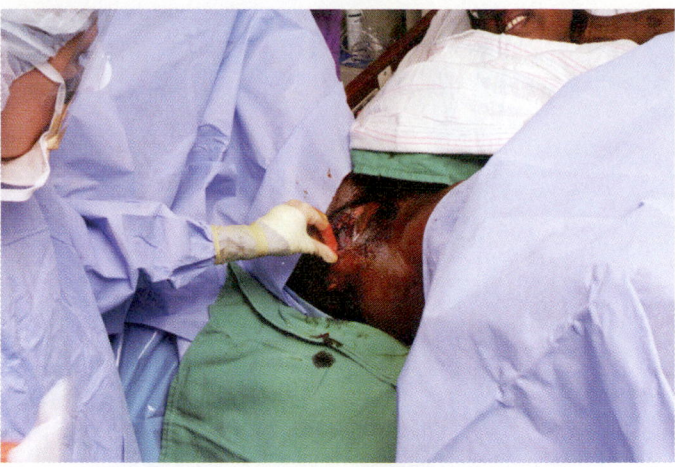

A.

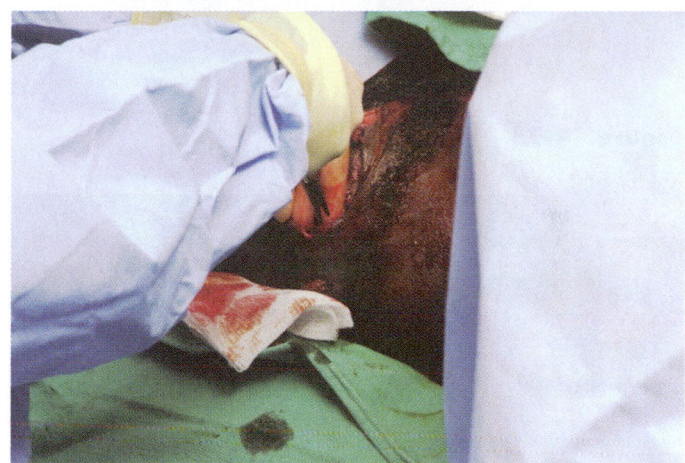

B.

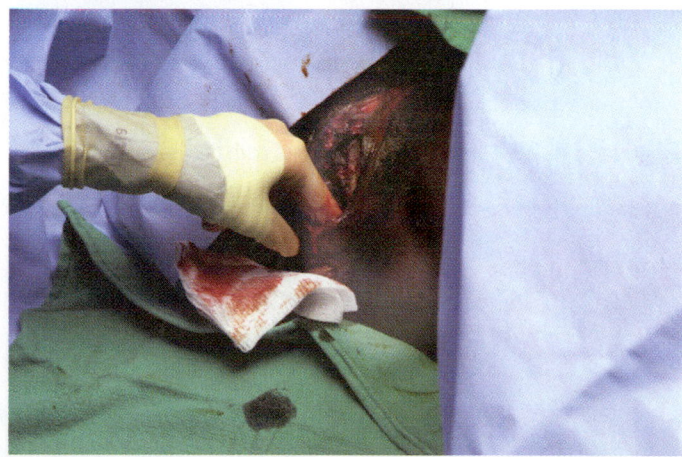

C.

Figure 14-27   Episiotomy procedure: A. Stretching of the perineum is assessed; B. Median incision is made; C. Some bleeding occurs.

ineum, is necessary, or to repair any lacerations that occur during the birth process.

Episiotomy and Nuchal Cord

At the time of crowning, when the largest diameter of the fetal head first becomes visible, the perineum is stretched extremely thin and may tear, particularly in the case of a nulliparous woman. The need to perform an episiotomy is determined by the primary caregiver's assessment of the perineum (Figure 14-27). Local anesthesia can be injected before the episiotomy.

The episiotomy incision is made in the midline downward (median or midline episiotomy), or it begins in the midline and is directed laterally and downward away from the rectum (mediolateral episiotomy) (Figure 14-28). An episiotomy incision is easier for the primary caregiver to repair than is a ragged **laceration**; however, research has shown that liberal use of episiotomy is not associated with a lower frequency of severe perineal tears (Anthony, Buitendijk, Zondervan, van Rijssel, & Verkerk, 1994).

After episiotomy has been performed, the fetal head often is delivered with the next contraction. The infant's head is born by extension and the primary caregiver feels around the infant's neck for **nuchal cord**, which is umbilical cord that has become wound once or more times around the infant's neck (Figure 14-29). If the cord can be felt around the neck, it often is loose enough to be pulled over the infant's head before delivery of the body. During the brief pause for restitution of the fetal head to take place, the primary caregiver may suction the mouth and nares of the infant before the infant's first breath. If the amniotic fluid has been stained by meconium, the infant's mouth and nares should be suctioned using a suction catheter to ensure that any meconium in the mouth or nose will not be aspirated (Figure 14-30). If the nuchal cord is tightly wound around the infant's neck the physician or nurse-midwife may need to double clamp and cut the cord to allow the infant to be delivered. Once the infant is born, the delivery time, date, and sex of the infant are noted on the mother's chart and on the infant identification

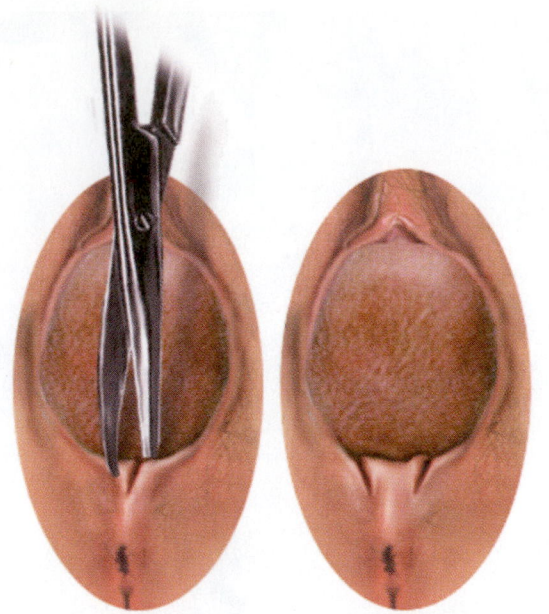

Figure 14-28   Episiotomy.

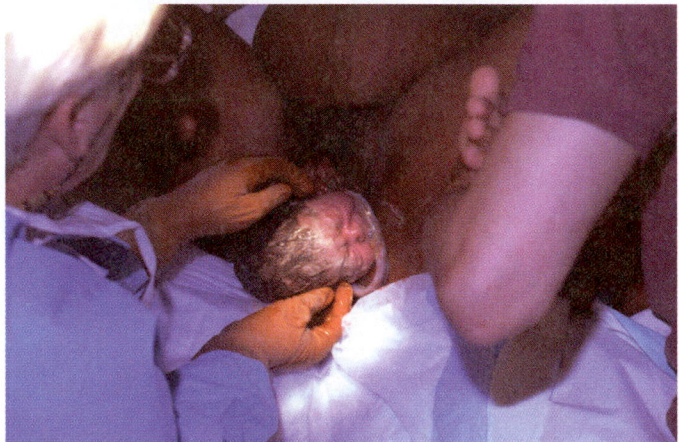

Figure 14-29   Birth of the fetal head with nuchal cord.

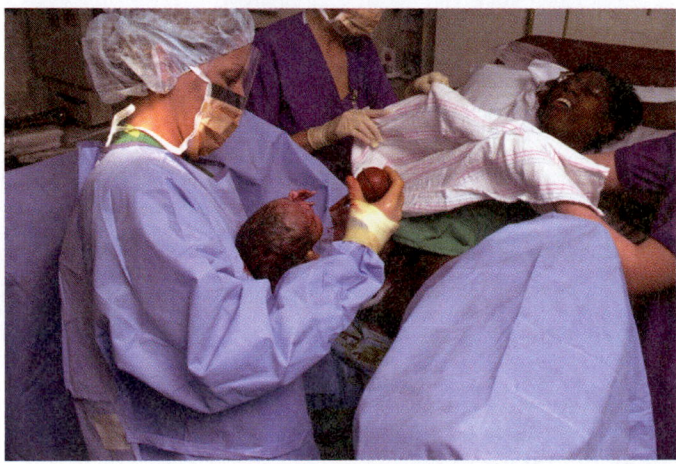

Figure 14-30   This infant was born so rapidly that there was no time to suction the mouth and nares until after the delivery was completed.

bands (Figure 14-31). Delivery information is also recorded on the fetal monitor strip in many institutions.

Meconium Aspiration

In utero, the fetus has two normal "breathing" patterns by which it moves amniotic fluid into and out of the lungs: shallow regular breathing (90% of the time) and deep irregular breathing (10% of the time). In the presence of hypoxia, the fetus may be stimulated to make compensatory gasping respirations. Hypoxia may result in passage of meconium, and the meconium-stained amniotic fluid can be aspirated into the fetal lungs if gasping respirations are stimulated by asphyxia.

When there is thick meconium in the amniotic fluid, the primary caregiver may order an amnioinfusion, introduction of warm normal saline or lactated Ringer's solution into the uterus by way of an IUPC, in an attempt to thin out the meconium and prevent meconium aspiration by the fetus.

At delivery, the neonatal resuscitation team should be present to provide prompt resuscitation and oxygenation as necessary. As the fetal head appears, the woman should be asked to refrain from pushing so that the primary caregiver can clear the airway, using a DeLee suction catheter, before the infant takes his or her first breath.

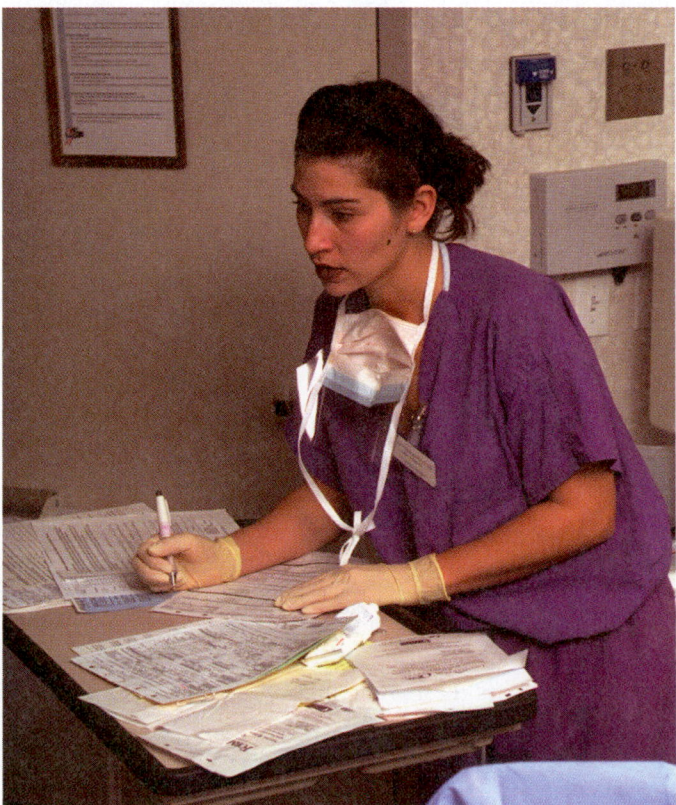

Figure 14-31   The nurse documents the delivery date, time, and the infant's gender on the mother's chart.

The neonatal resuscitation team may need to intubate the infant to clear the airway of meconium by way of an endotracheal tube. The decision to suction by way of intubation is based on infant activity and respiratory effort at birth, and consistency of the meconium.

Third Stage

The **third stage of labor** begins with delivery of the infant and ends with delivery of the placenta. This process may take up to 20 minutes. The nurse's attention at this time is divided between newborn and maternal care. In order to be prepared for complications, most institutions require two licensed nurses to be present in the delivery suite. One is assigned to the infant, while the other is assigned to the mother.

Newborn Care

The time of birth is noted in the delivery record, the fetal monitor strip, and the newborn's chart. When indicated, oral, pharyngeal, or endotracheal suctioning is performed according to the hospital policy, procedure, and protocol. Ideally, the infant is laid on the mother's abdomen and quickly covered with warm blankets to prevent heat loss by evaporation. The primary caregiver hands the infant directly to the nurse, who (wearing PPE), receives the infant into a baby blanket or towel. The nurse places the infant into a radiant warmer to prevent loss of body heat by evaporation while the infant is being dried. When necessary, the mouth and nares are again cleared by use of a suction bulb. While under the radiant warmer, the infant is dried thoroughly and a cap placed on the infant's head for extra warmth. As the nurse dries the infant, respiratory effort, color, and muscle tone can be observed. The

> ### Nursing Tip *Checking Newborn Heart Rate*
>
> Place a finger and thumb at the base of the umbilical cord. Count the pulsations for 6 seconds and multiply by 10 to calculate the infant's heart rate.

action of drying the infant with warm baby blankets acts to stimulate the baby to breathe deeply and cry. Lightly flicking the soles of an infant's feet also will stimulate an infant to cry.

While drying the infant the nurse notices any rib, sternal retractions, "grunting" sounds or nasal flaring, which indicate respiratory compromise. Heart rate is checked by placing the thumb and two fingers over the base of the umbilical cord and counting the pulsations, which should be within the range of 110 to 160 bpm. Skin temperature should be 97.8°F (36.5°C). While assessing respirations and heart rate, the nurse conducts a gross physical examination (Table 14-6). The infant should be crying and becoming pink. The infant's hands and feet usually are still slightly blue. This condition is known as **acrocyanosis** and may persist for 7 to 10 days. Respiratory support is initiated, if required, according to the hospital policy, procedure, and protocol. Respiratory support includes administration of oxygen or ventilation by bag or mask. Obvious abnormalities, such as spina bifida, cleft palate, and extra digits, are documented. The number of vessels in the umbilical cord also are noted; the umbilical cord should have two arteries and one vein.

The **Apgar score** (Apgar, 1966), a numerical expression of the newborn's well-being, is assigned at 1 and 5 minutes after birth as the neonate's immediate adaptation to extrauterine life is monitored (Table 14-7). A 10-minute Apgar is performed when the 5-minute score is under 7. The newborn is given a score of 0 to 2 in each of the fol-

> ### Nursing Alert
>
> #### "Floppy" Infant, Not Breathing
>
> When receiving an infant from the delivering primary caregiver: if the infant is "floppy" (lacking muscle tone) and is making no respiratory effort, it is wise to assume that the infant is already experiencing secondary apnea and, therefore, will be unresponsive to stimulation. Artificial ventilation with positive-pressure oxygen must be initiated at once. The nurse should not waste time by trying to stimulate the infant to cry but should call immediately for the neonatal resuscitation team and nursing assistance, while administering bag and mask ventilation with 100% oxygen.

Table 14-6	Newborn Evaluation at Delivery
ASSESS	**NORMAL FINDINGS**
Respirations	Rate 30–60 bpm, irregular No retractions No grunting
Apical pulse	Rate 120–160 bpm
Temperature	97.5°F (36.5°C)
Skin color	Body pink, with bluish extremities
Umbilical cord	Two arteries and one vein
Gestational age	Should be >37 weeks to remain with the parents for an extended time

Table 14-7   Apgar Scoring System

	SCORE		
SIGN	0	1	2
Respiratory effort	Absent	Slow, irregular	Good crying
Heart rate	Absent	Slow, below 100 bpm	Above 100 bpm
Muscle tone	Flaccid	Some flexion of extremities	Active motion
Reflex irritability	None	Grimace	Vigorous cry
Color	Pale blue	Body pink, blue extremities	Completely pink

Critical Thinking

What Is This Infant's Apgar Score?

The infant has just been delivered, and the physician hands the infant to you. You immediately lay the infant beneath the radiant heat lamp and begin your initial assessment as you dry the infant. The infant is breathing but not crying and the hands and feet are blue. The heart rate is 120 bpm, and the respirations are 30 breaths per minute and irregular. The infant's arms and legs are floppy. When you suction the mouth, the infant begins to cry more vigorously.

What is the 1-minute Apgar score that you will assign to this baby?

Answer: 6 (respiratory effort, 1; heart rate, 2; muscle tone, 0; reflex irritability, 2; skin color, 1).

lowing five categories: respiratory effort, heart rate, muscle tone, reflex irritability, and skin color.

Newborn laboratory studies vary according to the hospital protocol but might include cord blood samples if the mother is Rh-negative or has type O blood group. Cord blood for neonatal blood type and Rh factor is obtained by the birth attendant while awaiting placental separation (Box 14-13). Cord blood gas analysis to evaluate biochemical status may be requested if the infant has a low Apgar score (Figure 14-32).

If the Apgar is less than 9 at 5 minutes, the infant should be stabilized rather than remaining with the mother in the LDR. Other situations that would require stabilization by the neonatal personnel include the following: "Grunting" respirations or rib retractions, nasal flaring, heart rate below 120 bpm or above 160 bpm, pallor, serious congenital anomalies such as spina bifida, a mother who is insulin-dependent, less than 38 weeks' gestational age, or small for gestational age appearance.

After the Apgar evaluation, identification procedures are completed according to the hospital policy and proto-

Box 14-13

Procedure for Collection of Umbilical Cord Blood for Blood Gases

1. Before delivery, request that a 6- to 8-inch segment of umbilical cord be clamped, cut, and passed off the surgical field as soon as possible after delivery.

2. One person is needed to attend the delivery and care for the neonate; another is needed to collect the blood samples.

3. Prepare a cup or Ziploc bag of crushed ice, two 1 mL insulin syringes with 23-gauge needles and rubber stoppers, two laboratory slips, and two specimen labels.

4. Don gloves and goggles.

5. Using a bevel-down approach, aspirate 1 mL of blood from one of the umbilical arteries first.

6. Remove air bubbles: Air contamination has no effect on pH, partial pressure of carbon dioxide, or bicarbonate but may increase the partial pressure of oxygen (Gaskins & Goldkrand, 1994).

7. Remove the needle from the syringe with a hemostat, and cap the syringe with the rubber stopper.

8. Repeat the process with the umbilical vein (see Figure 14-32). Compare the color of the blood in the syringes. The pinker blood is venous, and the darker blood is arterial.

9. Label each syringe with name, identification number, source, and time; place both syringes in the bag of ice.

10. Expedite delivery of the blood samples to the laboratory for blood gas analysis.

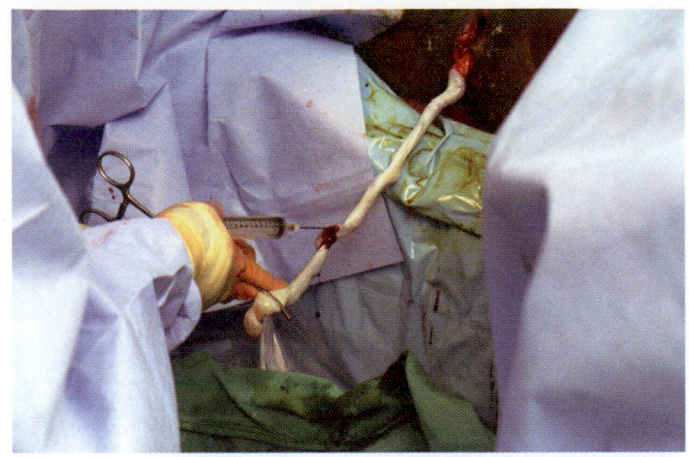

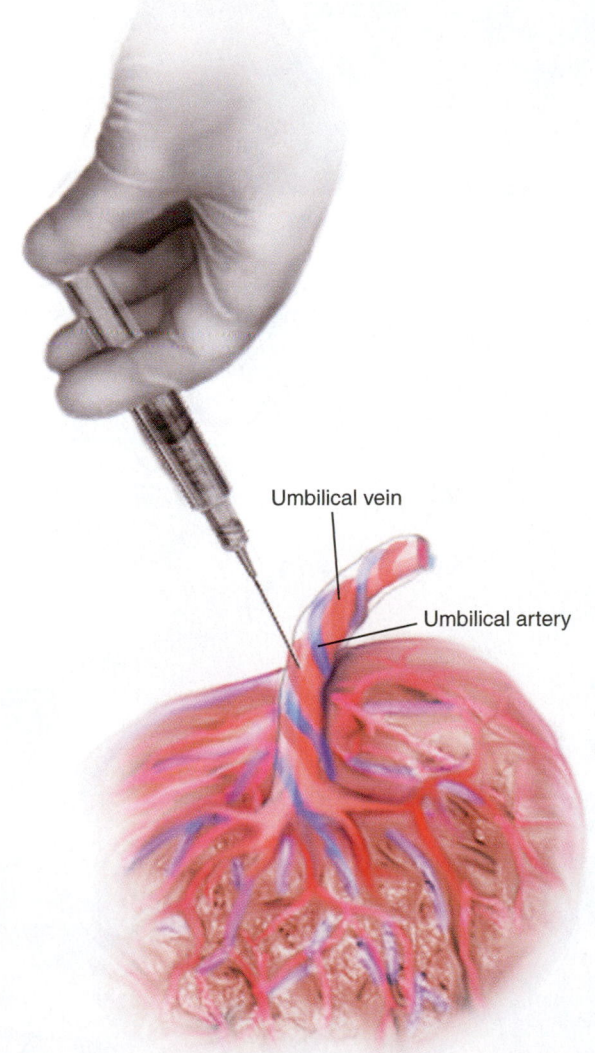

Umbilical vein

Umbilical artery

Figure 14-32   Aspiration of umbilical cord blood.

col (Figure 14-33). Identification may include taking the footprints of the infant and a fingerprint or thumbprint of the mother, and labeling. A common labeling protocol involves preparation of a set of four identically numbered waterproof bracelets with the mother's name, sex of the baby, physician or nurse-midwife of record, and the date and time of delivery. The baby wears two bands and the mother and her partner wear the others.

Delivery of the Placenta

The third stage of labor begins after the birth of the newborn and ends with delivery of the placenta. The priority at this time is the complete separation and expulsion of the placenta and prevention of hemorrhage from **uterine atony**, which is inability of the uterus to contract. After the baby is born, the height of the fundus is ascertained by palpating the abdomen. As long as the uterus remains contracted and there is no bleeding, the policy is one of watchful waiting for signs of placental separation. Separation of the placenta may take as long as 20 minutes but more often takes place within 1 to 10 minutes of the birth. During the waiting time the physician or nurse-midwife may examine the cervix and vagina and perform any necessary perineal repairs; however, repairs usually are undertaken after the third stage is complete. Contractions during the third stage of labor are of much less intensity than are those experienced during the second stage.

The placenta is attached to the endometrium by numerous fibrous villi, which break when uterine contractions cause the placental site to shrink. If the uterus remains flaccid, the placental site does not contract and thus the placenta cannot detach from the endometrium. Attempts to deliver the placenta, before it detaches from the uterus, by using cord traction or fundal pressure can result in tearing of the cord or membranes or inversion of the uterus. **Inversion of the uterus**, turning the uterus inside out, results in serious hemorrhage and shock. Indications that the placenta has separated from the uterine endometrium are the following (Cunningham, 2001):

- A firmly contracting fundus
- Globular shape of the uterus as the separated placenta descends into the lower uterine segment
- A small spurt of blood from the vagina
- Apparent lengthening of the umbilical cord at the introitus as the placenta descends into the lower uterine segment

When signs of placental separation are evident, the mother should be asked to bear down for the final time (Figure 14-34). Whether the shiny fetal surface of the placenta appears first (Schultze mechanism) or the dark roughened

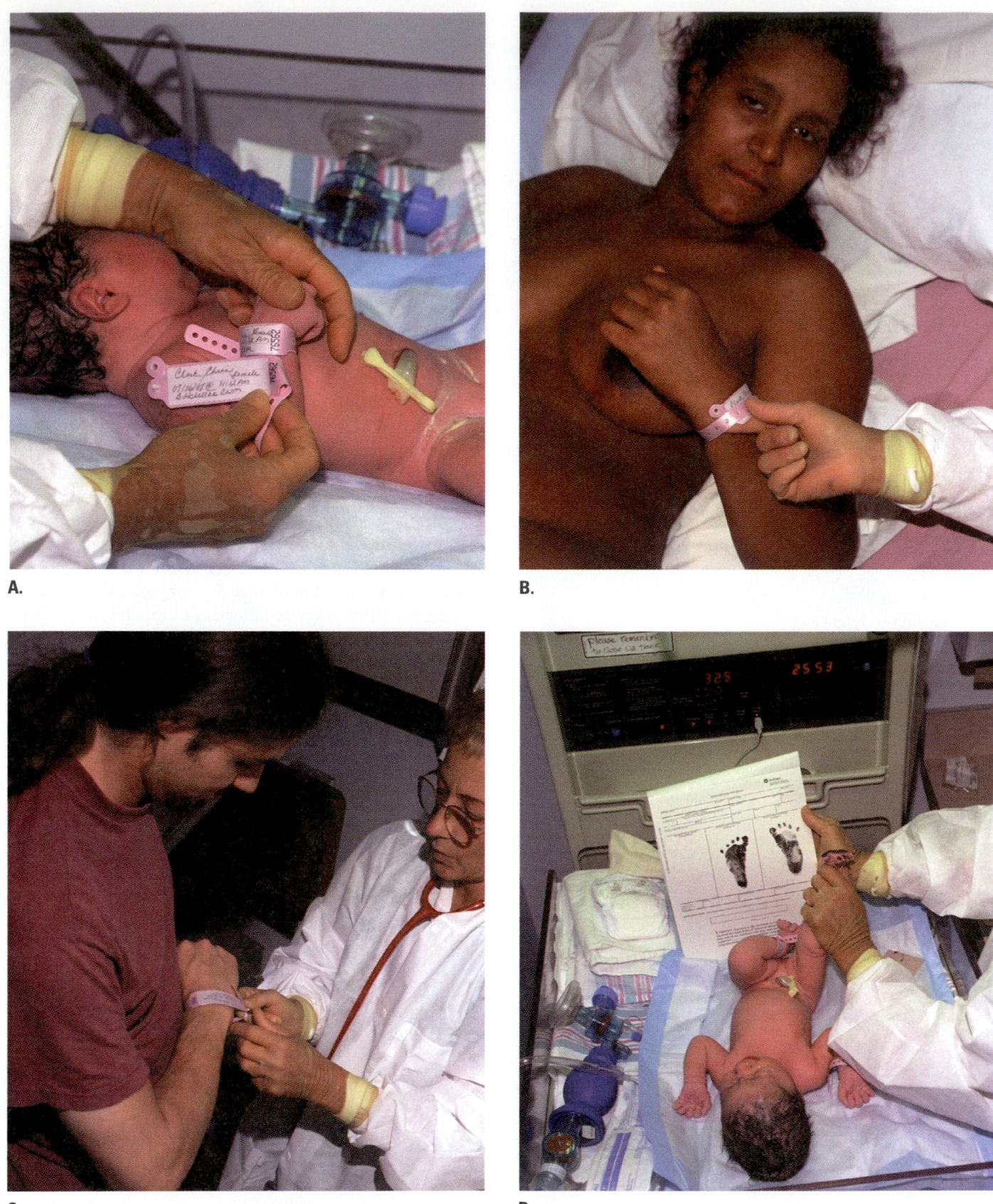

Figure 14-33   Matching identification bands are placed on the (A) infant, (B) mother, and (C) father; (D) the infant's footprints are taken.

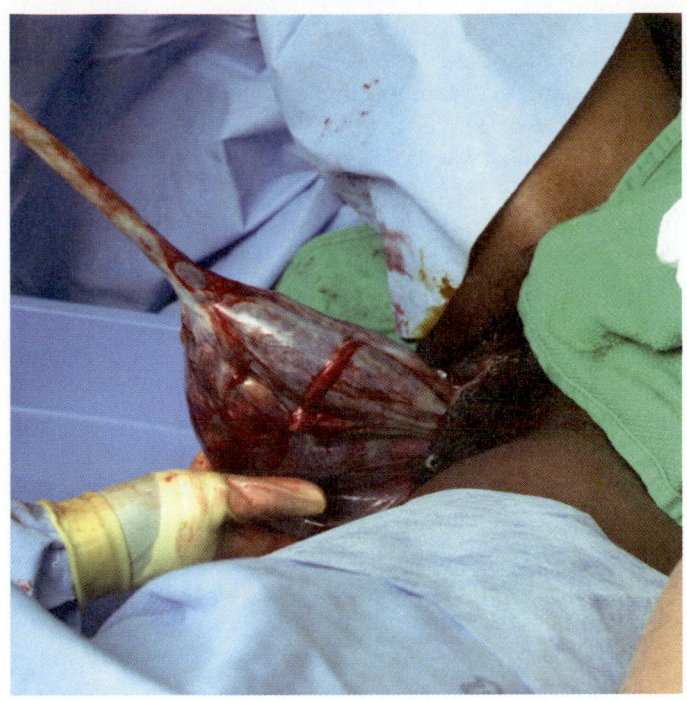

A.

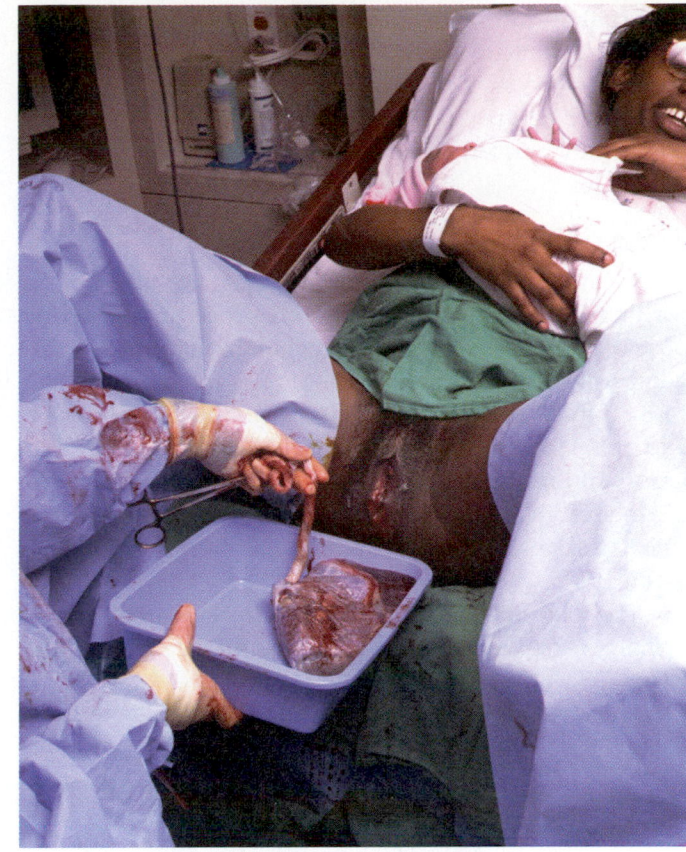

B.

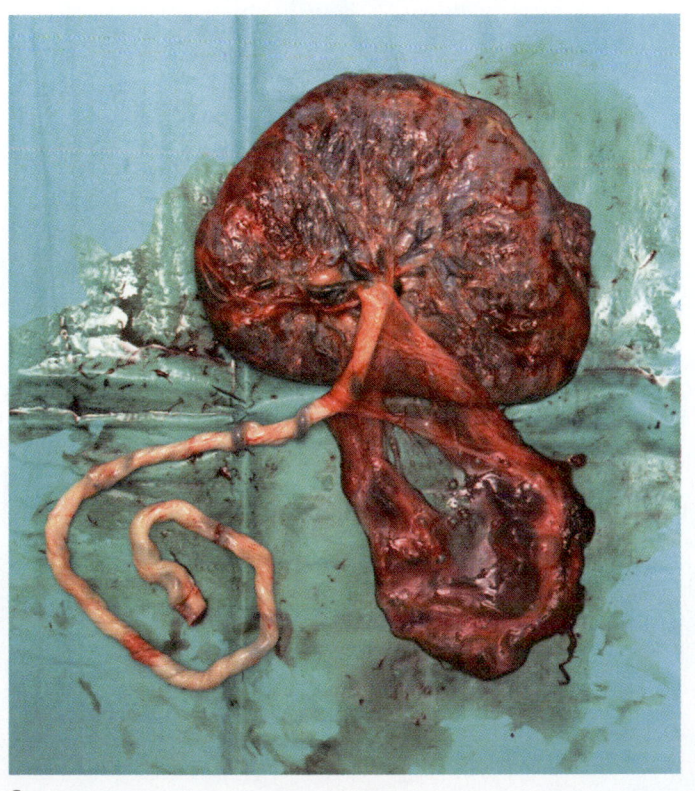

C.

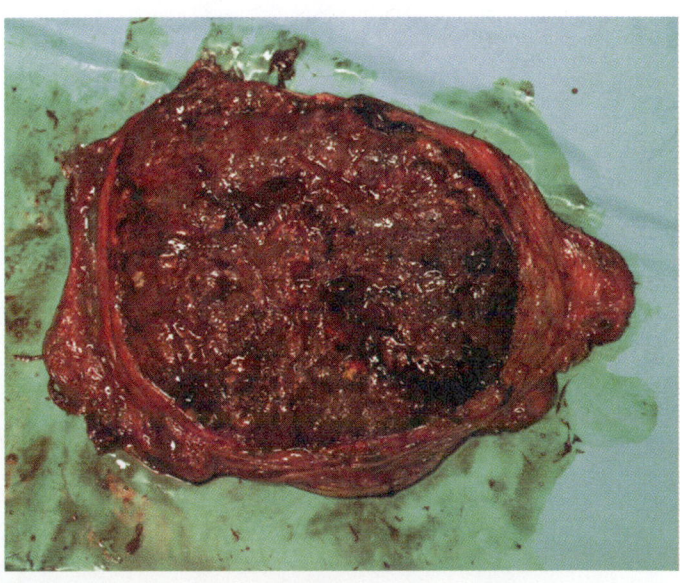

D.

Figure 14-34 A. Delivery of the placenta. B. Inspection of the placenta. C. Fetal side (note empty amniotic sac). D. Maternal side.

maternal surface shows first (Duncan mechanism) is of no consequence (Cunningham, 2001) (Figure 14-35). Perineal repairs for laceration (tear in the perineum, vagina, or cervix caused by childbirth) and episiotomy are usually performed after the birth of the placenta (Figure 14-36).

Oxytocin Administration

Oxytocin is given at the end of the third stage of labor, according to the hospital policy and procedure. The purpose of oxytocin administration is to prevent postpartum hemorrhage by stimulating the uterus to contract (Table 14-8). If the woman has an IV line, a frequent protocol is to add of oxytocin (Pitocin), 20 U, to 1 L lactated Ringer's solution and infuse over 40 to 60 minutes. A second liter of oxytocin (Pitocin), 20 U, in 1 L lactated Ringer's solution or 5% dextrose lactated Ringer's solution is sometimes given at a rate of 125 mL/h.

The placenta and membranes are examined by the primary caregiver for completeness, and the placenta may be sent for pathological examination. Cultures or tissue specimens are obtained as per the request of the primary caregiver and according to the hospital protocol.

The time of delivery of the placenta, its condition, and any abnormal characteristics are recorded in the Delivery Record. The amount of blood loss during delivery is estimated by the physician or nurse-midwife and noted in the Delivery Record by the nurse. The average blood loss at vaginal delivery is up to 500 mL (ACOG, 1998). The degree and type of episiotomy or laceration is recorded in the Delivery Record (Table 14-9). The mother's perineum is cleansed gently and a peripad applied. An ice pack should be applied to the perineum to prevent swelling and pain, particularly if there are lacerations or an episiotomy. The lower portion of the delivery bed is replaced, and the woman's legs are carefully and slowly removed from the stirrups and placed back on the bed. If the woman has received continuous epidural analgesia, it is discontinued and the cannula removed by the CRNA. The nurse who circulates the delivery is often institutionally

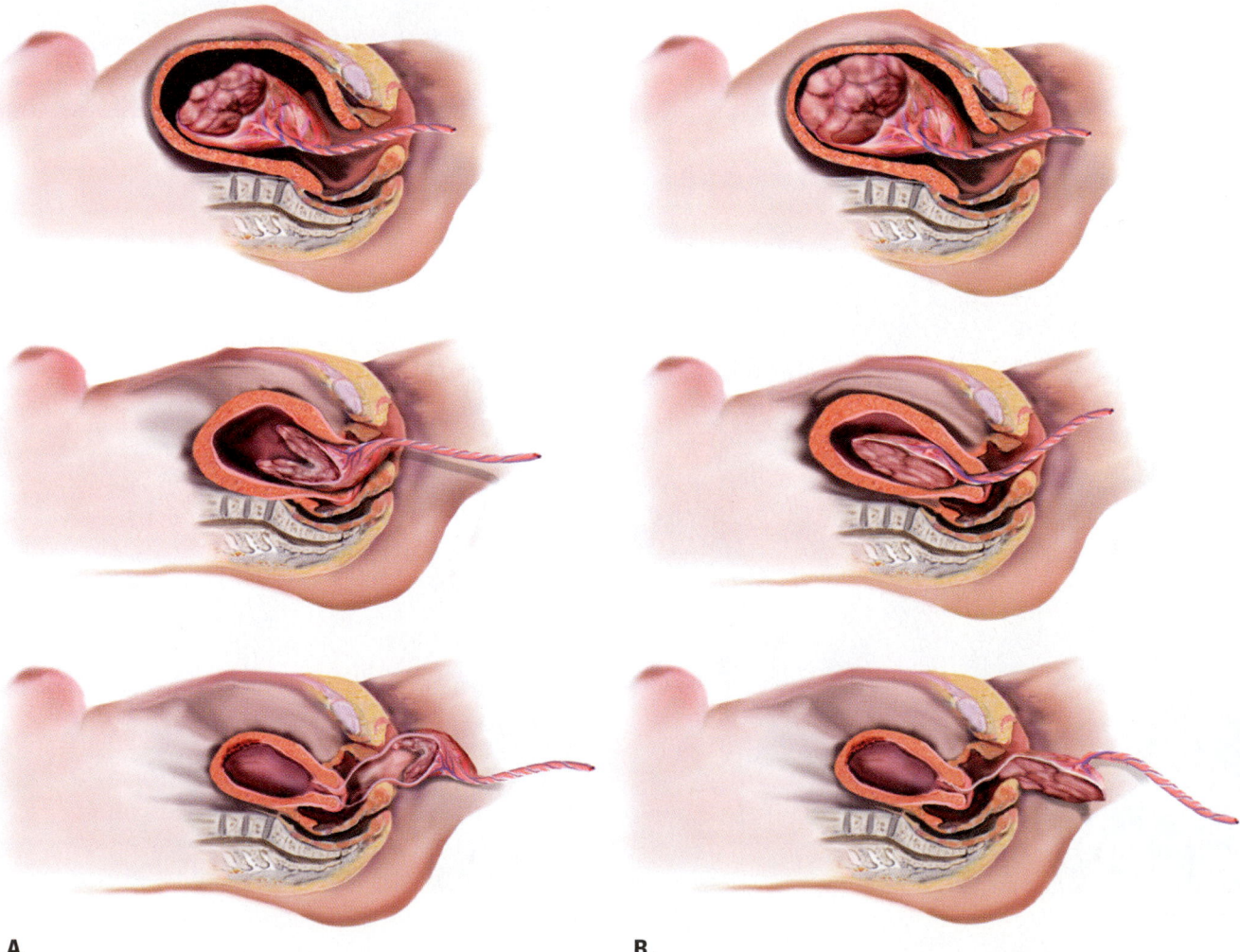

A.

B.

Figure 14-35 Placental separation. A. Schultze mechanism. B. Duncan mechanism.

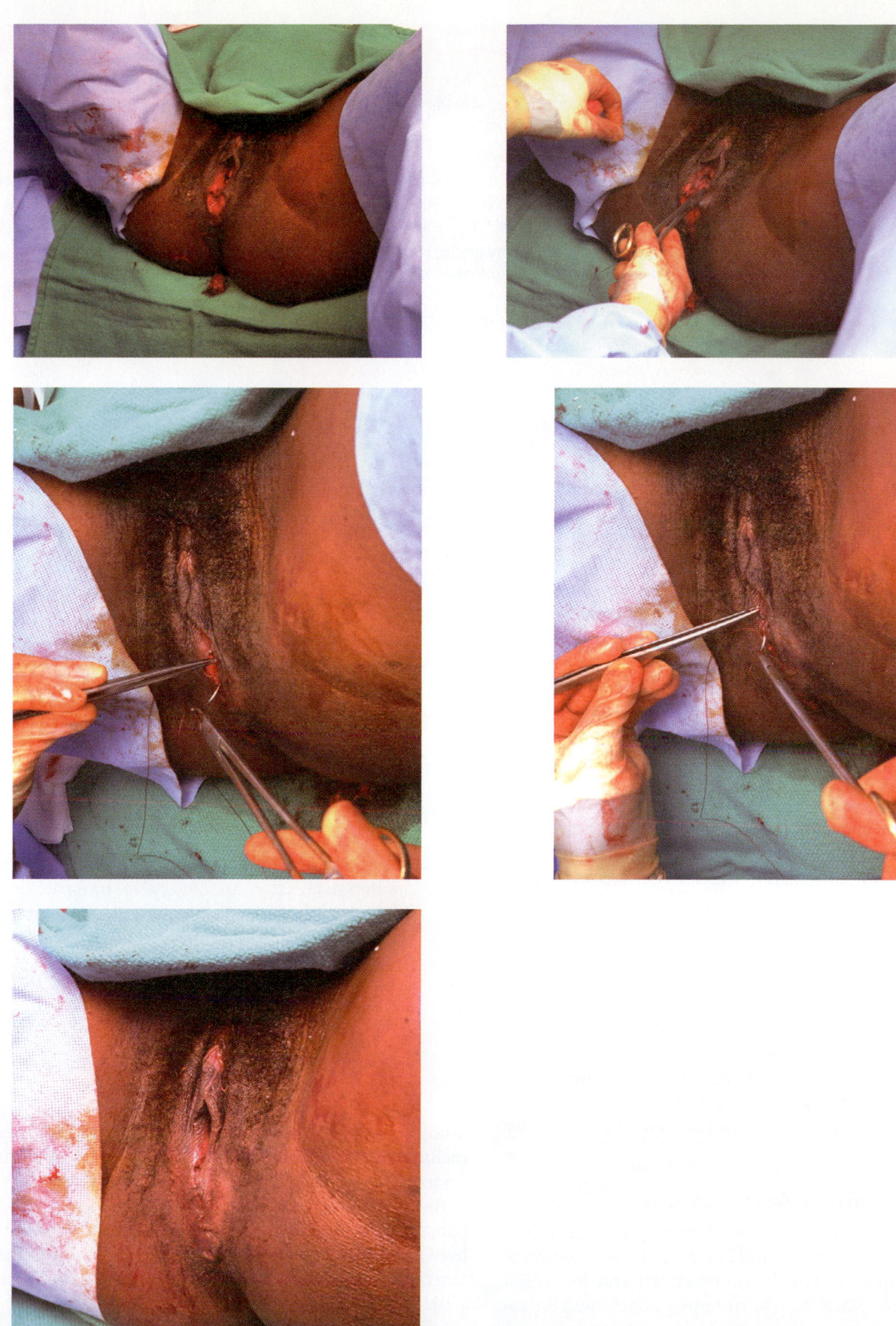

Figure 14-36   Perineal repair for laceration and episiotomy.

Table 14-8	Oxytocin Administration after Delivery of Placenta
Oxytocin (Pitocin)	Polypeptide hormone.
Action	Increases myometrial contraction by increasing the availability of intracellular calcium. Binds to oxytocin receptors in the decidua and myometrium.
Indication	Delivery of the placenta.
Dosage and route	Oxytocin, 20 U (range 10 U to 40 U), in 1 L lactated Ringer's solution or dextrose 5% lactated Ringer's solution. Administer the first liter at a rapid rate. When a second liter of solution is ordered, administer at 125 mL/h. Oxytocin for control of postpartum bleeding may be diluted and administered by IV, or 10–20 U IM.
Adverse effects	With too rapid an infusion, tachycardia may occur; hypotension or hypertension also may occur. The antidiuretic effect may cause oliguria, fluid overload, arrhythmia, water intoxication, nausea, vomiting, or headache.
Nursing considerations	Assess the fundus for contraction. Assess the amount of lochia. Monitor vital signs, record intake and output, and assess the bladder.

Table 14-9	Lacerations of the Birth Canal
DEGREE	**INVOLVEMENT**
First	Fourchette, perineal skin, and vaginal mucous membrane
Second	Fourchette, perineal skin, vaginal mucous membrane, and fascia and muscles of the perineal body
Third	A second-degree tear involving the anal sphincter
Fourth	A third-degree tear extending through the rectal mucosa to expose the lumen of the rectum

certified to remove the epidural catheter after delivery. It is important for the nurse to document that the tip was intact at removal. Warm blankets can be provided for comfort. All care is documented in the delivery record (Figure 14-37).

Fourth Stage (Recovery)

The recovery phase immediately after delivery of the placenta often is referred to as the fourth stage of labor. This is a misnomer because labor and delivery are completed with the expulsion of the placenta. The fourth stage is the critical time that begins after delivery of the placenta and ends when the mother's systems have stabilized, usually 1 to 4 hours later.

Newborn-Family Attachment

The recovery period is a time of relative peace after the exertion and activity of labor and delivery. It also is a time of becoming acquainted with the newborn and for initial bonding to take place. Newborn-family attachment is promoted by encouraging touch and eye contact as soon as possible after delivery and by giving the family time to

Nursing Tip

Nursing Diagnoses, Postpartum

Appropriate nursing diagnoses during this stage are the following:

- Deficient fluid volume related to hemorrhage as evidenced by blood loss secondary to uterine atony or perineal trauma
- Impaired skin integrity secondary to median episiotomy or lacerations
- Interrupted family process related to addition of a new member
- Grieving related to the birth experience not being as was expected, or the newborn not being the desired sex, as evidenced by the mother refusing to hold the newborn
- Risk of uterine and perineal infection related to bacterial invasion secondary to trauma during labor and delivery, episiotomy, and extended time with ruptured membranes
- Health-seeking behaviors related to newborn care, self-care, normal postpartum physiologic occurrences as evidenced by the client asking questions
- Pain related to uterine cramping

hold and admire the baby. Maternal bonding behaviors include smiling and talking softly to the baby, holding it up to her face and making eye contact, and breastfeeding. If the mother displays a negative behavior toward the baby, such as refusing to hold the baby or look at him or her, further exploration and supportive follow-up are warranted as are documentation and communication with the other nurses caring for the family.

Some women wish to breastfeed immediately after the baby is born. At this time, the newborn usually is quite

Duplication of this form is strictly prohibited by law. © 2001 Briggs Corporation. All rights reserved.

Briggs
CORPORATION

Labor and Delivery Summary
Maternal/Newborn Record System   Page 1 of 2
To order call: **1.800.245.4080**   Re-order No. **5712N**

Labor Summary

G	T	Pt	A	L	Type and Rh	EDD
⊹⊹⊹	⊹⊹	ŏ	ŏ	⊹⊹	O pos	7 / 4 / 04

Prenatal Events   ☑ None
☐ No Prenatal Care
☐ Preterm Labor (less than or equal to 37 Weeks)
☐ Postterm Labor (greater than or equal to 42 Weeks)
☐ Previous Cesarean
☐ Prenatal Complications

Intrapartal Events
Maternal
☐ Febrile (greater than or equal to 100.4°F/38°C)
☐ Bleeding—Site Undetermined
☐ Preeclampsia (mild) (severe)
☐ Seizure Activity
☐ Medications   ☑ None

Date	Time	Medication	Dose	Route

☐ Transfusion _____ units
  Blood Component _____
☐ _____

Amniotic Fluid
☑ SROM ☐ AROM Date 6/23/04 Time 1230
☐ Premature ROM ☐ Prolonged ROM
☑ Clear
☐ Meconium-Stained (describe) _____
☐ Bloody
☐ Foul Odor
  ☐ Cultures Sent _____ Time _____
☐ Polyhydramnios
☐ Oligohydramnios
☐ _____

Placenta
☐ Placenta Previa
☐ Abruptio Placenta
☐ _____

Labor
☐ Precipitous Labor (less than 3 hrs)
☐ Prolonged Labor (greater than or equal to 20 hrs)
☐ Prolonged Latent Phase
☐ Prolonged Active Phase
☑ Prolonged 2nd Stage (greater than 2.5 hrs)
☐ Secondary Arrest of Dilatation
☐ Induction   ☑ None
  ☐ AROM   ☐ Oxytocin ☐ _____
☐ Augmentation ☑ None
  ☐ AROM   ☐ Oxytocin ☐ _____

Labor Summary (Cont'd.)
Fetus
Gestational Age (Wks) __38.5__ By Dates
                      __38.5__ By Ultrasound

Presentation   **Position**
☑ Vertex | L | O | A |
☐ Face/Brow
☐ Breech   ☐ Frank   ☐ Complete
              ☐ Single Footling
              ☐ Double Footling
☐ Transverse Lie ☐ Back-up ☐ Back-Down
☐ Compound
☐ Unknown
☐ Cephalopelvic Disproportion (CPD)
☐ Cord Prolapse
☐ Dystocia _____

Monitor ☐ None   FHR   UC
          External   ☑   ☑
          Internal   ☑   ☑
☑ STV   ☑ Present ☐ Absent
☑ LTV greater than 25 BPM last 20
☐ Fetal Bradycardia   minutes of labor
☐ Fetal Tachycardia
☐ Sinusoidal Pattern
☐ Accelerations ☐ Spont. ☐ Uniform
☑ Decelerations ☐ Early   ☐ Late
              ☑ Variable ☐ Prolonged
☑ Scalp pH less than or equal to 7.2
☐ _____
FM Discontinued 6/23/04 Time 1930
FHR Prior to Delivery 108 bpm Time 1930

Delivery Data
Support Person Present ☑ Yes ☐ No
Delivery Location
  ☐ LDR ☑ LDRP ☐ DR ☐ OR
  ☐ Birthing Center ☐ _____

Method of Delivery
☑ Vaginal ☐ VBAC
        Number Previous Cesareans _____
☑ Vertex
  ☑ Spontaneous
  ☐ Assisted [|] to [|]
    ☐ Manual Rotation
    ☐ Forceps (type _____)
      ☐ Outlet ☐ Low ☐ Mid
  ☐ Vacuum Extraction Duration _____ Min.
    Degree of suction _____ kg/cm²
☐ Breech (type _____)
  ☐ Spontaneous
  ☐ Partial Extraction (assisted)
  ☐ Total Extraction
  ☐ Forceps Assist
    ☐ Piper ☐ _____

Method of Delivery (Cont'd.)
☐ Cesarean
  ☐ Scheduled   ☐ Emergency
  ☐ Primary   ☐ Repeat (x_____)
  ☐ Other
Operative Indication
  ☐ Previous Uterine Surgery
  ☐ Failure to Progress
  ☐ Placenta Previa
  ☐ Abruptio Placenta
  ☐ Fetal Malpresentation _____
  ☐ Non reassuring FHR Pattern _____
  ☐ Other _____
Uterine Incision
  ☐ Low Cervical, Transverse
  ☐ Low Cervical, Vertical
  ☐ Classical
  Hysterectomy   ☐ No ☐ Yes
  Tubal Ligation ☐ No ☐ Yes
  Skin Incision
  ☐ Vertical
  ☐ Pfannenstiel

Episiotomy   ☐ None
☑ Midline
☐ Mediolateral L R
Laceration/Episiotomy Extension ☑ None
☐ Periurethral
☐ Vaginal
☐ Cervical
☐ Uterine
☐ Perineal ☐ 1° ☐ 2° ☐ 3° ☐ 4°
Repair Agent Used 000 chromic
☑ Vagina free of sponges

Placenta
☑ Spontaneous
☐ Expressed
☐ Manual Removal
☐ Adherent (type _____)
☐ Uterine Exploration
☐ Curettage
Configuration
☐ Normal
☐ Abnormal
Weight __580__ gms
Disposition to lab

Cord
☐ Nuchal Cord (x_____)
☐ True Knot   Length _____ cms
☐ 2 Vessels
☑ 3 Vessels
Cord Blood ☑ To Lab ☐ Refrig ☐ Discard
Lab ☑ Type + Rh ☐ Cultures ☐ Coombs
    ☐ pH   ☐ _____

Surgical Data
Sponge Counts Correct
☐ N/A ☐ Yes ☐ No _____
Needle Counts Correct
☐ N/A ☐ Yes ☐ No _____

                              Date
Rae Baird RNC   Completed 6 /23 /04
(Signature)

Figure 14-37   Labor and Delivery Summary. (*Courtesy of Briggs Corporation*)

Duplication of this form is strictly prohibited by law. © 2001 Briggs Corporation. All rights reserved.

Briggs CORPORATION

Labor and Delivery Summary
Maternal/Newborn Record System — Page 2 of 2
To order call: 1.800.245.4080   Re-order No. 5712N

Delivery Data (Cont'd.)

Surgical Data (Cont'd.)
Vaginal Pack Count Correct
☐ N/A ☑ Yes ☐ No _____
Estimated Blood Loss **less than 250** ccs

Delivery Anesthesia ☐ **None**
☑ Local ☐ Pudendal ☐ General
☐ Epidural ☐ Spinal

Date	Time	Medication	Dose	Effect
6/23/04	1949	1% Xylocaine		

Complications ☑ **None**

Delivery Medications ☑ **None**

Date	Time	Medication	Dose	Route Site	Init

Chronology Date

	Date	Time		
EDD	7/4/04			
Admit to Hospital	6/23/04	1335		
Membranes Ruptured	6/23/04	1230		
Onset of Labor	6/23/04	1000	Total Time Hrs/Min	
Complete Cervical Dilatation	6/23/04	1715	7	15	I
Delivery of Infant	6/23/04	1946	2	31	II
Delivery of Placenta	6/23/04	1948		02	III
			9	48	Total Labor

Infant Data ☑ Male ☐ Female
ID/Band No. **8163**
Condition ☑ Alive
☐ Stillbirth ☐ Antepartum
☐ Intrapartum
☐ Neonatal Death
Birth Order **3** of 1 2 ③ 4
Repeat Apgar every 5 min until score greater than or equal to 7

Apgar Score	1 min	5 min	10 min
Heart Rate	1	2	
Respiratory Effort	1	2	
Muscle Tone	1	2	
Reflex Irritability	1	2	
Color	1	1	
Total	5	9	

Scored by **Rae Baird RNC**

Infant Data (Cont'd.)
Airway
☑ Bulb Suction
☐ Suction Catheter Size ____ Fr
  ☐ Mouth Pressure ____ mm Hg
  ☐ Nose ☐ At Delivery
  ☐ Pharynx
☐ Endotracheal Tube Size ____ Fr
  ☐ Meconium Below Cords Times ____

Breathing
☑ Spontaneous
☐ O₂ **2** # Liters
  ☐ Free Flow Time Init. ____
  ☐ PPV
    ☑ Bag/Mask Time Init. ____
    ☐ ET Tube Size ____ Fr Time Init. ____
    ☐ CPAP ____ mm
less than one minutes to First Gasp
2 minutes to Sustained Respiration

Circulation
☑ Spontaneous
☐ External Cardiac Massage
  Time Initiated ____ Time Completed ____
  ____ minutes for HR greater than 100
  Heart Rate (bpm)
  ____ Time ____
  ____ Time ____
  ____ Time ____

IV Access
☐ Umbilical Catheter
☐ Peripheral Line
Person Managing Resuscitation:
Michael Smith M.D.

Neonatal Medications ☐ **None**

Date	Time	Medication	Dose	Route Site	Init
6/23/04	1951	Aquamephyton	1.0 mg	Inj. right thigh	RB

Lab Data ☑ **None**   Time ____

Blood Gases	Sent	Umb Art	Umb Vein
pH			
pO₂			
pCO₂			
HCO₃			

Test	Result
Dextrostix	

Initial Newborn Exam
Weight **3789** gms **8** lbs **5.5** ozs ☐ Deferred
Length ____ cms **20.5** ins ☐ Deferred
Head **34.7** cms **13.5** ins ☐ Deferred
Chest **32.6** cms **12.7** ins ☐ Deferred
Abdomen **32** cms **12.5** ins ☐ Deferred
Temp **98** ☐ Rectal ☑ Axillary
AP **144** Resp **42** BP **not done**
☑ No Observed Abnormalities

Initial Newborn Exam (Cont'd.)
☐ Abnormalities Noted
☐ Meconium Staining ☐ Cephalhematoma
☐ Petechiae ☐ Other
Describe ____

Intake ☐ **None**
  Breast Fed ☑ Yes ☐ No
Output ☐ **None**
  ☑ Urine ☐ Stool (type ____)
  ☐ Gastric Aspirate ____ cc or ml/hr
Examined By **Michael Smith M.D.**
Transfer ☐ With Mother
  ☐ To Newborn Nursery
  ☐ To NICU
  ☑ Remains in LDRP
Date __/__/__ Time ____
Mode of Transport ____

Delivery Personnel
RN (1) **Rae Baird RNC**
   (2) **Kathleen Ammon RN**
Anesthesiologist/CRNA **Jeff SaHoy CRNA**
CNM ____
Physician—Attending **Mark Brown M.D.**
Physician—Assist (1) ____
   (2) ____
Pediatric Provider **Michael Smith M.D.**
☐ Notified ☑ Present at Birth
Remarks **Prolonged second stage of labor. Apgar at one minute 5, 9 at 5 minutes. Spontaneous respirations. Variable decelerations with recovery last 1.75 hrs. of labor.**

Rae Baird RNC
(Signature)   Date Completed **6/23/04**

Figure 14-37 (continued)

alert and amenable to breastfeeding. Suckling the baby as soon as possible after the birth is desirable from the mother's viewpoint because it stimulates the release of oxytocin, which helps the uterus to contract and thereby prevents hemorrhage.

After the excitement and stress of labor and delivery, the recovery time is an appropriate time to review events with the parents and give positive reinforcement. The nurse encourages verbalization of the birth experience and provides explanations so that the client and family can better incorporate these events into their life experience. During this time it is not unusual for the mother to apologize to the nurse for making "too much" noise or for being irritable during labor. The nurse can promote positive recall of the birth experience by commending the woman for her efforts and reassuring her that she fulfilled her part well. The objective is for the woman to remember her childbirth experience as an empowering and satisfying event.

Maternal Status

As the mother's organs begin the task of readjusting to the nonpregnant state, careful observations are recorded by the nurse. The priority of care during the recovery period is prevention of hemorrhage from the placental site.

In LDR settings, the woman remains in the labor and delivery area for 1 to 2 hours of intense observation. Findings during these first 2 hours are charted in the Obstetric Recovery Record according to the hospital protocol (Figure 14-38). Handwashing precedes assessment. Nonsterile latex gloves are worn when the perineum is inspected or when there is a possibility of contact with mucous membranes, skin that is not intact, blood, or other body fluids. Hands are washed again after removal of gloves.

Uterus

The uterus is assessed every 15 minutes for the first hour. The woman is positioned with knees flexed and head flat. The nurse uses one hand to stabilize the uterus just above the symphysis pubis and the outer edge of the other hand to locate the fundus. Position of the fundus is noted in relation to the umbilicus and recorded as centimeters above or below the umbilicus. During the fourth stage, the fundal height usually is at the level of the umbilicus. Placement of the uterus also is noted in relation to midline. Consistency is noted: If the uterus is not firm, it is referred to as *boggy*, and the fundus is massaged gently in a circular motion until the uterus contracts and becomes firm (Figure 14-39).

Clots are expelled at this time by the nurse placing both hands on the mother as if for measuring fundal height and applying gentle but firm pressure downward with the upper hand while observing the perineum for amount and size of expelled clots. The nurse must be careful to avoid exerting too strong a pressure, as this may cause the uterus to invert. Once the fundus is palpated firm, the nurse should not continue to massage because overmassaging is unnecessary and painful for the woman. A full bladder should be suspected when the uterus requires repeated massage to contract, remaining at the level of the umbilicus or above and being displaced to one side.

Lochia

Lochia is monitored every 15 minutes for the first hour, and the findings are recorded. The nurse notes the amount, color, and presence of clots. The red lochia encountered during this stage is known as lochia *rubra*. A standardized method for estimating the amount of lochia after delivery was devised by Jacobson (1985):

- Scant: Blood on tissue only when wiped or less than a 2-inch stain
- Light: Less than a 4-inch stain on the peripad
- Moderate: Less than a 6-inch stain on the peripad
- Heavy: A saturated peripad within 1 hour

A perineal pad that is completely soaked with blood contains about 68 to 80 mL of blood (Lugenbiehl, Brophy, Artigue, Phillips, & Flak, 1990). When lochia is heavy, pads and linens should be saved for inspection by the physician or nurse-midwife. Continuous bleeding in the presence of a well-contracted uterus indicates soft tissue damage or retained products of conception such as placental tissue or membranes.

Prevention of Hemorrhage

Hemorrhage from the placental site is controlled by contraction of the uterus. Anything that impedes contraction of the uterus may result in postpartum hemorrhage. Assessments are designed to identify events that presage postpartum hemorrhage. The loss of at least 500 mL of blood is considered postpartum hemorrhage. The uterus is palpated at 15-minute intervals to ensure it is firm. A well-contracted uterus will not fill with blood. The peripad is

Nursing Alert

Checking for Hemorrhage

When assessing a newly delivered woman for bleeding, always look beneath her buttocks. Sometimes the perineal pad is barely soiled because blood is running down and pooling beneath the mother. The client may be completely unaware that she is hemorrhaging.

Duplication of this form is strictly prohibited by law. © 2001 Briggs Corporation. All rights reserved.

Briggs CORPORATION

Recovery Flow Record

Maternal/Newborn Record System

To order call: 1.800.245.4080 Re-order No. 5713N

Maternal Data Admitted 6 / 23 / 04 Time 2000 | G iii | T iii | Pt o | A o | L iii

Pain: 0-10 2 Site: Lower abdomen and perineum

Type: ☐ Aching ☐ Nagging ☐ Dull ☐ Heavy ☐ Crushing ☐ Sharp ☐ Stabbing ☐ Throbbing ☐ Radiating ☑ Burning ☐ Tingling ☑ Cramping ☐ Other:

Delivered 6 / 23 / 04 Time 2000 Age 34

☑ Vaginal ☐ VBAC ☐ Cesarean (☐ Scheduled ☐ Emergency)

☐ Tubal Ligation ☐ Preanesthesia T 98.8 P 84 R 18 BP 128/86

Episiotomy ☐ None ☑ Midline ☐ LML ☐ RML

Perineal Laceration/Extension ☑ None ☐ 1° ☐ 2° ☐ 3° ☐ 4°

Abdominal Incision ☑ No ☐ Yes

Anesthesia Local

Complications Prolonged second stage labor

Mother's Physician Mark Brown M.D. Planned LOS 2 days

Allergy / Sensitivity ☐ None ☐ Latex

☑ Other Demerol (severe nausea and vomiting)

Infant Data ☑ Male ☐ Female

ID/Band No. 4515 Name Bradley Michael

Condition ☑ Live/Normal ☐ Live/Abnormalities Noted ☐ Fetal/Neonatal Death

Feeding ☑ Breast ☐ Bottle

Location ☑ With Mother ☐ Nursery ☐

Adoption ☑ No ☐ Yes

Problems Identified ☑ None ☐ Yes

Visitors Present ☐ None ☑ Husband, mother, sister

Maternal Assess — (PAR Score) Admission 10, Transfer Remains in LDRP, 10 at 2145

Time	Temperature	Pulse	Respirations/O₂Sat.	Blood Pressure	Level of Consciousness	Activity	Color	Fundus	Bladder	Abdomen	Lochia	Perineum	Pain	Intake (PO mL's)	Output (Urine mL's)	Response to Infant	Comments	Init
2000	99	88	22	128/88	2	2	2	Firm at U	F	–	Mod	WA	2	ice chips	–	3	Passed 2 clots, I.V. to 150ml/hr	KA
2015		80	18	126/86	2	2	2	Firm at U	F	–	Mod	WA	1+2	–	–	3	Talking, pleased with son	KA
2030		76	18	124/80	2	2	2	Firm 1UU	E	–	Mod	WA	2	–	500	3	Voided on bed pan; ice to perineum	KA
2045		78	20	120/78	2	2	2	Firm 2FU	E	–	Mod	WA	1	100ml	–	3	Nursing infant – cradling	KA
2115		70	16	120/80	2	2	2	Firm 2FU	F	–	Mod	WA	1	–	–	3	To bathroom. Instructed in pericare	KA
2145	98.8	68	18	122/82	2	2	2	Firm 1FU	E	–	Sm	Ec	1	100ml	–		Light lunch. I.V. discontinued	KA

Intake (IV)

Start Date	Time	Solution	Amount mL's	Medication/Dose Added	Initials	Infused Date/Time	Amount
6/23	1345	#1 Lactated Ringers	1000	–	KA	6/23/04 1800	1000
6/23	1950	#2 D5W	1000	–	KA	6/23/04 2145	175

Medication

Time	Medication	Dose	Route/Site	Initials

Released By ______ Date __/__/__ Time ____

Transferred To ______ via ______ Time ____

Report To ______ Time ____

Remains in LDRP 2150

Kathleen Ammon RN Signature

Infant Assess

Time	Temperature	Pulse	Respirations	Skin Color	Muscle Tone	Behavior State	Feeding	Urine	Stool	Gastric	Comments	Init
2000	98	150	56	pink	++	QA					In bed with mother – wrapped – side lying	KA
2015		152	42	pink	++	QA		✓			Side rails up	KA
2030		144	50	pink	++	C					Parents talking – attempting to quiet infant	KA
2045	98.6	146	48	pink	++	S	✓		Mec		Nursing – poor grasp at areola, proper technique	
2115				pink	++						demonstrated	KA
2145		140	42	pink	++	S					Sleeping	
2215		138	40	pink		S					Sleeping	
						S					To nursery	

Transferred To Nursery via crib Time 2215

Report To Bev Lee RN Time 2215

Signature

Initials	Signature	Initials	Signature
KA	Kathleen Ammon RN		
Initials	Signature	Initials	Signature

Form 5713N R404 © 2001 Briggs Corporation, Des Moines, IA 50306 To order, phone (800) 245-4080 www.BriggsCorp.com PRINTED IN U.S.A.

RECOVERY FLOW RECORD

Duplication of this form is strictly prohibited by law. © 2001 Briggs Corporation. All rights reserved.

Assessment Key

Post Anesthesia Recovery (PAR) Score Worksheet *(circle one in each category upon admission and transfer)*

Respiration		Admission	Transfer
Able to breathe and cough	=	2	2
Dyspnea or limited breathing	=	1	1
Apnea	=	0	0
Blood Pressure			
Less than 20% of preanesthetic level	=	2	2
Plus or minus 20-50% of preanesthetic level	=	1	1
Greater than 50% of preanesthetic level	=	0	0
Level of Consciousness			
Fully awake	=	2	2
Arousable	=	1	1
Not responsive	=	0	0

Activity		Admission	Transfer
Able to move 4 extremities	=	2	2
Able to move 2 extremities	=	1	1
Able to move 0 extremities	=	0	0
Color			
Normal / pink	=	2	2
Pale, dusky, blotchy, jaundiced	=	1	1
Cyanotic	=	0	0

Maternal Assessment

Bladder
E = Empty
F = Filling
D = Distended

Perineum
R = Red
Ec = Ecchymotic
Ed = Edematous
NA = Not Approximated
WA = Well Approximated

Pain
0 = None
10 = Highest Intensity

Abdomen (Dressing/Incision)
D/I = Dry/Intact
Dr = Drainage
S&C = Saturated and Changed
NA = Not Approximated
WA = Well Approximated

Lochia
Sc = Scant 0-25% pad saturation
Sm = Small 25-50% pad saturation
Mod = Moderate 50-75% pad saturation
Lg = Large 75-100% pad saturation

Response to Infant
0 = No visual contact. No verbal response, demanding or rejecting tone. No attempt to touch infant, rough handling.
1 = Occasional glances. Single words, no inflection. Minimal touch, holding baby away from body.
2 = Looks at infant at intervals. Short phrases, average tone. Holds infant, explores with fingertips.
3 = Seeks en face with infant, smiles at infant. Long phrases, soft, soothing tone. Comments on infant appearance. Enfolds infant, explores with hands.
4 = Maintains en face with infant. Speaks in rhythmic pattern, loving tone. Uses infant name or "pet" name. Enfolds infant, cuddles, strokes, rocks.

Infant Assessment

Skin Color
P = Pink
R = Ruddy
PL = Pale
M = Mottled
C = Cyanotic

Muscle Tone
+ or 1+ Hypotonic (Floppy; poor head control; limp extremities)
++ or 2+ Normal (Flexed; resistant to opposing flexion)
+++ or 3+ Hypertonic (Tightly flexed or stiffly extended extremities; easy startle)
++++ or 4+ Jittery (Persistent tremors, twitches; myoclonic jerks)

Behavior State
S = Asleep or drowsy
QA = Quiet, alert
C = Crying

Form 5713N R404 © 2001 Briggs Corporation, Des Moines, IA 50306 To order, phone (800) 245-4080 www.BriggsCorp.com PRINTED IN U.S.A.

RECOVERY FLOW RECORD

Figure 14-38 Recovery Flow Record. (*Courtesy of Briggs Corporation*)

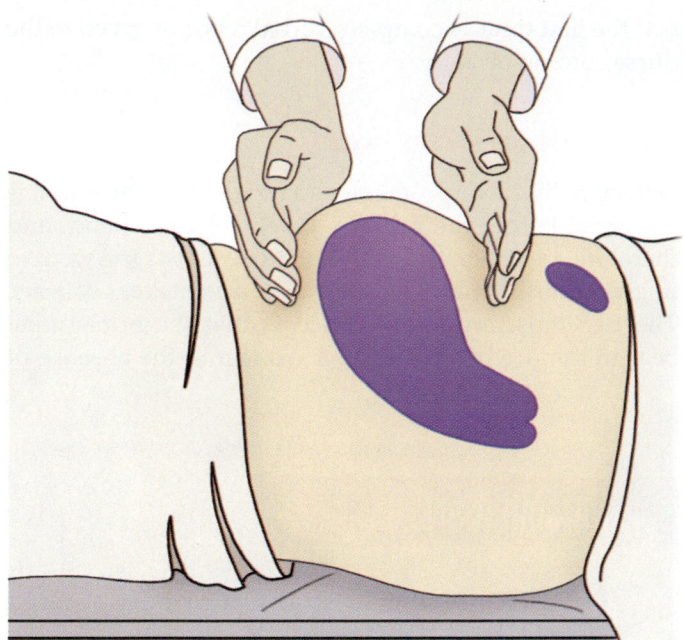

Figure 14-39   Recovery assessment of the fundus.

Nursing Tip   **Make Sure the Bladder is Empty**

When your client is to be transferred after the recovery hour from an LDR room to a busy postpartum unit (with a higher nurse-client ratio), it is prudent to have the woman empty her bladder before she is transferred. A client who has not voided after delivery is at risk for hemorrhage secondary to uterine displacement by a full bladder.

checked every 15 minutes to monitor lochia. The fundus normally is firm or can become firm after gentle massage and expulsion of any clots that have accumulated within the uterus. Certain factors are associated with postpartum uterine atony:

- Rapid labor
- Prolonged first and second stages of labor
- Overdistention of the uterus (owing to hydramnios, multiple gestation, or large fetus)
- Previous postpartum hemorrhage
- Advanced maternal age
- Parity of four or more
- Abruptio placentae or placenta previa
- Induced labor
- Pre-eclampsia and eclampsia
- Use of tocolytics

Perineum

The perineum is observed every 15 minutes for the first hour to assess the episiotomy site or laceration repair to ensure it is intact and for edema, bleeding, and hematoma. Ice packs provide comfort and prevent swelling. In some cultures, such as Southeast Asian and Hispanic, women may prefer warmth to the perineum following delivery, to draw out the pain.

Bladder

The woman may have difficulty voiding spontaneously owing to bruising of the meatus or the effects of epidural anesthesia. The nurse should palpate the bladder for filling every 15 minutes during the first hour. When the mother's vital signs are stable and she is not suffering the effects of sedation or anesthesia, she may be assisted to the bathroom to void. Alternatively, a bedpan may be offered. Urine is measured and the time of voiding recorded. A full bladder usually causes the uterus to become boggy and be displaced to the right, and may lead to increased bleeding. When the woman is unable to void even though the bladder is palpable, or the uterus is displaced, catheterization is necessary.

Blood Pressure

Recording of blood pressure provides a database for possible diagnosis of complications such as hypertension and hypovolemia. Under normal circumstances, few alterations in blood pressure are seen and pressure readings should return to prelabor levels within the first hour of vaginal delivery. Blood pressure is monitored every 15 minutes for the first hour, or more frequently if the client's condition warrants (AAP & ACOG, 1997).

Heart Rate

Pulse readings are recorded every 15 minutes for the first hour, and rhythm and regularity are assessed. The pulse usually returns to the prelabor rate within the first hour after vaginal delivery. If the nurse detects tachycardia, dehydration, hypovolemia, or infection should be ruled out.

Temperature

A temperature reading is taken during the first hour. It is not unusual for the woman's temperature to increase to at least 100.4°F (38°C) owing to the dehydrating effects of labor; however a higher temperature than this should be reported to the primary caregiver.

Psychosocial Status

The mother may be emotionally and physically exhausted but at the same time elated. She may be talkative and eager to phone friends and relatives with news of the newborn. Women often feel hungry immediately after delivery; however, food usually is withheld until after the recovery hour because of possible nausea. The intestinal tract is still slowed from the hormones of labor.

Pain

The mother may experience abdominal cramping commonly referred to as afterpains as the uterus contracts. Uterine contractions are necessary to prevent abnormal blood loss. Oxytocin administration after delivery of the placenta also will stimulate uterine contractions, and the nurse can explain to the woman the rationale for oxytocin administration and how this may cause some cramping. Analgesics should be administered according to the hospital policy, procedure, and protocol. NSAIDS are particularly effective for uterine afterpains.

Maternal Teaching

The mother should be instructed in palpating her own uterus and how to massage it when necessary. The nurse can guide the woman's hand so that she can feel the firm contracted uterus (about the size of a grapefruit). It often is less uncomfortable for the mother to massage her own fundus than for this to be done by the nurse; however, teaching the mother in no way relieves the nurse of the responsibility of checking the fundus for firmness every 15 minutes during the recovery hour. It should be stressed that neither the woman nor the nurse should massage the fundus if it already is firm.

Transfer to the Postpartum Unit

In some hospitals the mother remains in the same room for labor, delivery, recovery, and the postpartum period and the same nurse may care for the mother and infant. At other institutions the care may be handed over to a postpartum nurse. Many hospitals take the newborn to a nursery for 2 to 4-hours' transition time, during which the infant is observed closely. If the baby is to go to the nursery, the LDR nurse should encourage the partner to accompany it. When the father goes with the infant to the nursery, the mother may feel more at ease because she knows a family member is in attendance.

Recovery from Anesthesia

If the woman is to be transferred from the LDR to the postpartum unit, she should not be discharged from the LDR until her vital signs are stable. If she received epidural analgesia, she should be sufficiently recovered from its effects to be able to move both legs and raise her hips in order to move from the delivery bed to a wheelchair. Effects of an epidural may take several hours to completely dissipate; therefore, the mother should be instructed to call for nursing assistance before getting out of bed the first time. A complete verbal report is given to the nurse coming on duty.

Precipitous Delivery

Occasionally, labor progresses so rapidly that the infant is delivered before the primary caregiver can attend, and therefore, the labor and delivery nurse assists the woman in giving birth. This is referred to as a **precipitous delivery**. The two most important concepts that the nurse must bear in mind when assisting a woman in the absence of

Nursing Alert

Nursing Interventions During Precipitous Delivery

1. Instruct the woman to pant with contractions if the fetal head is crowning.

2. With a gloved hand, apply gentle pressure against the fetal head occiput or vertex to maintain flexion and prevent it from popping out quickly. Support the perineum with the other hand.

3. When the fetal head is born, instruct the woman to pant and not to push. Suction the fetal mouth and nares with a bulb syringe.

4. Insert two fingers along the back of the fetal neck to check for a nuchal cord. If present, pull it over the infant's head. If the cord is too tight to pull over the infant's head, clamp it twice and cut between the clamps. Unwind the cord from around the neck.

5. While requesting the woman to push gently, place one hand on each side of the infant's head over the ears and exert gentle downward pressure on the head to assist in the birth of the anterior shoulder. Then exert gentle upward pressure to assist with the posterior shoulder. Support the rest of the infant's body as he or she is born.

6. Place the newborn on the maternal abdomen, and dry the infant with warm blankets. Keep the newborn covered. Use the bulb syringe to suction the mouth and nares as needed.

7. Check the firmness of the fundus and observe for vaginal bleeding.

8. Watch for signs of placental separation (change in shape of placenta, lengthening of umbilical cord, spurt of dark red blood).

the primary caregiver, is to support the fetal head as it descends, preventing it from popping out quickly, and to ensure that the newborn has a patent airway.

Delivery in a Nonhospital Setting

Childbirth that occurs too rapidly for the mother to get to the hospital is referred to as **emergency childbirth**. Because there may be a certain amount of panic on the part of the mother and those with her, it is important that the person helping the mother remain calm and reassuring. Someone should call 911 as soon as possible so that help will be on the way. Most infants born under such nonconventional circumstances do very well, although they are at risk for cold stress. If there are other persons willing to give assistance, here are some main points to keep in mind.

1. Someone must be designated to take notes as the events unfold. The primary helper can dictate as the events unfold so that times will be accurate. Important information to record during emergency birth includes:
   a. Time the membranes ruptured, color of the amniotic fluid, and any unusual odor
   b. Fetal position and presentation
   c. Time of delivery
   d. Presence or absence of the nuchal cord and the number of loops
   e. Apgar scores at 1 and 5 minutes after birth
   f. Resuscitation efforts, if needed
   g. Condition of the infant
   h. Sex of the newborn
   i. Time of delivery of the placenta and its appearance
   j. Amount of bleeding
   k. Woman's condition: interventions to control bleeding and condition of the perineum
2. Try to ensure some privacy.
3. If the mother is lying on the floor, put something beneath her such as towels, a blanket, or layers of newspaper.
4. Help her to remove her clothing as necessary.
5. If you have a few minutes and the head of the infant is presenting, it is best to have the mother push between contractions rather than at the height of the contraction. This will help to prevent tearing. Positioning the mother on her side also will lessen the intensity of the contractions and lessen the pressure, which, in turn, will help prevent the infant's head from popping our precipitously. A lateral position and pushing between contractions also will lessen the risk for perineal tearing.

6. Place your hand against the infant's head to provide support and to prevent it from popping out precipitously.
7. Check whether the amniotic sac is intact. If it is, then try to tear the sac so the newborn will not breathe in amniotic fluid with the first breath. Sometimes the fetal membranes are covering the infant's face and are too slippery to be grasped. If this is the case, break the membranes when the head is out by inserting a finger into the infant's mouth. When the infant is born encased in the amniotic sac, this is referred to as being born "in the caul."
8. When the infant's head is out, have the mother relax and stop pushing while external restitution takes place. Watch as the infant's face turns toward the mother's inner thigh.
9. While restitution is taking place, feel around the infant's neck for a possible nuchal cord. If you feel the cord, and it is loose, slip it over the infant's head.
10. After restitution there is no need for manipulation of the shoulders unless more than 3 or 4 minutes has passed since the birth of the head. Placing your hands on each side of the infant's head, covering the ears, and pushing gently down on the head toward the floor may help free the anterior shoulder, and then lifting up the infant may facilitate birth of the lower shoulder.
11. The infant must be supported as it emerges. Hold the newborn at the level of the uterus to facilitate blood flow through the umbilical cord. Bring the infant up onto the mother's abdomen and cover it with whatever is available, preferably a clean cloth or towel. Wipe the infant's nose and mouth with a cloth or towel.
12. It is essential to keep the infant warm at all times. The best way to do this is to lay the infant skin to skin on the mother and cover them both. While the mother is holding the infant close to her body, stimulate the infant to cry by gently drying the skin with the cloth. Assign an Apgar score without exposing the infant to cold air. There is no need to tie or cut the umbilical cord. It will stop pulsating within a few minutes.
13. If the infant is showing no signs of spontaneous respiration, rescue breathing must begin (adult mouth over infant's nose and mouth).
14. To facilitate separation of the placenta and membranes, by contraction of the uterus, the mother should be encouraged to put the infant to her breast at this time. Suckling of the infant stimulates uterine contractions through release on oxytocin from the pituitary gland.

15. Watch for signs of placental separation. When the placenta has separated, have the woman give one slow steady push and catch the placenta in your hands. Gently twist the placenta so that the trailing membranes will twist to form a rope as they slowly separate from the uterus. Try not to let the membranes tear away from the placenta.

16. Wrap the placenta and place it together with the infant; it will provide some warmth.

17. Check the firmness of the uterus. The fundus may be massaged to stimulate contractions and decrease bleeding.

18. Clean the area under the mother, and inspect the perineum for lacerations. Bleeding from lacerations may be controlled by pressing a clean peripad against the perineum and instructing the woman to keep her thighs together.

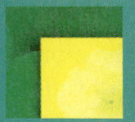

CASE STUDY/CARE PLAN
THE CLIENT WITH PAIN DURING A VAGINAL DELIVERY

Maria Brown, a 26-year-old gravida 3, para 2, is admitted to the labor and delivery unit at 41 weeks' gestation. Maria says that she thinks her "bag of waters" has broken. The nurse orients Ms. Brown and her boyfriend to the labor, delivery, and recovery room (LDR). After Ms. Brown has undressed and put on a hospital gown, external fetal heart rate (FHR) monitoring is begun. The FHR has a baseline of 140 bpm and good variability.

The nurse has Maria sign a consent form and proceeds with the interview and assessment. No risk factors are identified from the prenatal record and the nursing assessment. A vaginal examination indicates Maria's cervix is 80% effaced and 3 cm dilated. The presenting part is vertex at −1 station. No amniotic sac is palpated, and there is clear fluid draining from the vagina and pooling in the bed. Nitrazine paper, when touched to the wet bed linen, turns deep blue, indicating the presence of amniotic fluid. When asked the time the membranes ruptured, Maria indicates that they have been ruptured for 2 hours. The nurse-midwife is notified and states that she is en route to the hospital.

Maria's labor continues uneventfully. Blood is drawn for routine laboratory tests. Maria's temperature is taken every 2 hours. Various measures are employed to ensure her comfort during the first few hours. She ambulates up and down the hall with her boyfriend, and he brings her back to the LDR every 30 minutes for intermittent fetal monitoring. After 3 hours of labor, Maria says that she would like to rest in bed. The nurse and Maria's boyfriend help her into a comfortable lateral position and support her with extra pillows.

At 5 cm dilation, Maria becomes increasingly uncomfortable and requests epidural anesthesia. The nurse starts IV lactated Ringer's solution, 1 L, to infuse over the next 30 minutes. The anesthesiologist briefly interviews Maria as the nurse positions her to receive the epidural anesthesia. The boyfriend helps to support Maria in the required position.

Thirty minutes after the epidural is placed and Maria is feeling comfortable once more, vaginal examination reveals the cervix to be 8 cm dilated, 100% effaced, and the vertex at 0 station. At this time, the FHR decelerates from the 140 bpm baseline to 90 bpm, and then to 60 bpm. Maria's blood pressure is 94/44 mmHg. The nurse quickly turns Maria on her side and opens the IV to give a rapid bolus of fluid. Oxygen is started by way of a non-rebreather mask, at 10 L/min. After 2 minutes, Maria's blood pressure is 100/54 mmHg, and the FHR has returned to baseline. After a 500 mL bolus of IV fluid has been infused, the nurse slows the rate to 125 mL/h. Vaginal examination reveals the cervix still 8 cm dilated, 100% effaced, but the vertex is at +1 station. A fetal scalp electrode is placed for internal FHR monitoring. The amniotic fluid remains clear, and Maria is afebrile. A Foley catheter is inserted and attached to bedside drainage. Intake and output are recorded carefully.

Labor continues uneventfully for the next 3 hours, when Maria is fully dilated and the presenting part is at +2. Because of the effects of the epidural, Maria does not have an urge to push. The nurse instructs Maria how to support her knees, and to push when there is a contraction. After 1 hour of pushing, a viable male is delivered and placed skin to skin on the mother's abdomen. Maria's boyfriend, the baby's father, is able to cut the umbilical cord. The Apgar scores are 8 and 9. The placenta and membranes are delivered 5 minutes later and inspected by the midwife. Total blood loss is 250 mL; the perineum is intact although swollen. An ice pack is applied. Maria and her boyfriend are jubilant as she prepares to breastfeed their new son.

(continues)

Assessment

MB is 26 years old and in labor with her third baby. External fetal monitoring is in progress and the FHR shows average variability, with a baseline of 140 bpm. Vaginal examination reveals MB's cervix is 3 cm dilated, 80% effaced, and vertex presentation at −1 station. Membranes are ruptured, and the amniotic fluid is clear. Contractions are moderate in intensity. MB is gasping with each contraction and sometimes verbalizing pain.

☐ Nursing Diagnosis

Pain related to uterine contractions and cervical dilation as evidenced by MB's facial contortion and gasping when uterine contractions occur and her statement: "I am really hurting now."

Expected Outcome	Maria will verbalize decreased discomfort with uterine contractions and experience a degree of relaxation.
Planning	The nurse must take into account the length of time Maria's labor is likely to endure (she is only 3 cm dilated), and structure care to help Maria cope with labor progress.
NOC	Pain control
NIC	Pain management

Nursing Interventions	Rationales
1. Assess MB's preparation for labor.	1. Clients who have attended childbirth preparation classes often use psychoprophylactic methods to reduce pain.
2. Teach MB breathing techniques during early labor.	2. Controlled thought and focused breathing will increase relaxation. Clients are more receptive to teaching during early labor.
3. Encourage MB's boyfriend in methods that may help to reduce her discomfort: offering fluids, ice chips as ordered, back rubs; assisting MB into comfortable position, giving praise.	3. Measures are often more effective when delivered by a familiar person. Studies have shown that a support person helps to reduce the length of labor.
4. Provide comfort measures.	4. Ambulation, back rubs, change of position, extra pillows, warm shower, and other comfort measures help to reduce the discomfort of labor.
5. Explain what analgesics and anesthesia are available for use during labor and mode of administration.	5. Explanation of pharmacological methods of pain control will provide knowledge to help MB make decisions about analgesia and anesthesia.
6. Assist in the placement of an epidural catheter, if ordered.	6. Regional anesthesia provides analgesia and anesthesia during labor and delivery.
7. Keep MB aware of her progress and review the process of labor.	7. Knowledge that she is making expected progress will allay anxiety and increase coping.
8. Encourage regular voiding to decrease the chance of distention.	8. Bladder distention can increase discomfort during contractions and impede the progress of labor.
9. Encourage conscious relaxation between contractions.	9. Fatigue contributes to increased pain perception and inability to cope with pain.

Evaluation	MB verbalizes decreased discomfort with her contractions during early labor with the assistance of her boyfriend and the nurse, who supplied back rubs, extra pillows, encouragement, information, assistance in positioning, and ambulation. As labor progressed, and after receiving information about analgesia and anesthesia, MB made the decision to have epidural analgesia. After the epidural was placed, MB was able to rest peacefully and stated: "I can no longer feel any pain with my contractions."

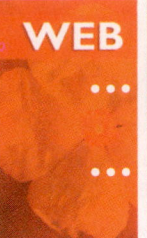

WEB | ACTIVITIES

••• What information can you find on the Doulas Web site?

••• Outline client teaching tips drawn from the Lamaze Internet offerings.

Key Concepts

■ Nursing care of the laboring woman is very complex because the nurse must ensure the well-being of the mother and fetus throughout the labor process.

■ Although labor and delivery are normal physiologic events, there is a great potential for negative outcomes.

■ In many birthing units, the nurse is the sole health care provider with which the client interacts throughout labor.

■ The nurse who provides intrapartum care must have a thorough understanding of the labor process as well as signs of fetal status to identify actual or potential labor complications.

■ Initial and ongoing assessment for risks and changes in condition are of paramount importance.

■ Every woman deserves to have the most positive birth experience possible considering her condition.

■ Interventions that provide relaxation and comfort to the laboring woman facilitate the birth process.

■ Every woman deserves to know her birth experience was special.

Review Questions and Activities

1. When a client arrives at the L & D unit, what should the nurse ask first if the woman states her bag of waters broke?
   a. Presence of bloody show
   b. Time the membranes ruptured
   c. Frequency of contractions
   d. Appearance of the fluid

   The correct answer is d.

2. Which maternal position should be strongly discouraged during labor?
   a. Lateral position
   b. Squatting position
   c. Standing position
   d. Supine position

   The correct answer is d.

3. Which of the following anatomical structures is involved when an episiotomy is performed?
   a. Glans clitoris
   b. Labia minora
   c. Levator ani muscle
   d. Labia majora

   The correct answer is c.

4. Which of the following is an expected characteristic of amniotic fluid?
   a. Deep yellow color
   b. Clear, with small white particles
   c. Nitrazine test shows acidic result
   d. Absence of ferning

   The correct answer is b.

5. A woman whose membranes have ruptured prior to the onset of or early in labor is at increased risk for:
   a. Hemorrhage
   b. Precipitous labor
   c. Supine hypotension
   d. Intrauterine infection

   The correct answer is d.

6. When assessing a woman in the first stage of labor, the nurse recognizes that the most conclusive sign that uterine contractions are effective would be:
   a. Progressive dilation of the cervix
   b. Presence of caput succedaneum on the vertex
   c. Rupture of amniotic membranes
   d. Increase in bloody show

   The correct answer is a.

7. The nurse who performs vaginal examinations to assess a woman's progress in labor should:
   a. Perform an examination at least once every hour during the active phase
   b. Perform the examination more frequently if vaginal bleeding is present
   c. Wear two clean gloves for each examination
   d. Discuss the findings with the woman and her labor partner

   The correct answer is d.

8. The second stage of labor begins when the:
   a. Amniotic membranes rupture
   b. Cervix cannot be felt during a vaginal examination
   c. Woman experiences a strong urge to bear down
   d. Presenting part has descended below the ischial spines

   The correct answer is c.

9. The most critical nursing action when caring for the newborn immediately after birth is:
   a. Keeping the newborn's airway clear
   b. Fostering parent-newborn attachment
   c. Drying and wrapping the newborn in a blanket
   d. Recording the time of birth and Apgar score

   The correct answer is a.

10. The nurse prepares to administer oxytocin to a woman, after expulsion of the placenta, to:

a. Relieve pain

b. Stimulate uterine contraction

c. Prevent infection

d. Facilitate rest and relaxation

The correct answer is b.

References

American Academy of Pediatrics & American College of Obstetricians & Gynecologists. (1997). *Guidelines for perinatal care* (4th ed.). Elk Grove Village, IL: Authors.

American College of Obstetricians and Gynecologists (ACOG). (1995, July). *Fetal heart rate patterns: Monitoring, interpretation, and management* (ACOG Tech. Bulletin No. 207). Washington, DC: Author.

American College of Obstetricians and Gynecologists (ACOG). (1995, December). *Dystocia and the augmentation of labor* (ACOG Tech. Bulletin No. 218). Washington, DC: Author.

American College of Obstetricians and Gynecologists (ACOG). (1996). *Hypertension in pregnancy* (ACOG Tech. Bulletin No. 219). Washington, DC: Author.

American College of Obstetricians and Gynecologists (ACOG). (1997, March). *Thromboembolism in pregnancy* (ACOG Educational Bulletin No. 234). Washington, DC: Author.

American College of Obstetricians and Gynecologists (ACOG). (1997, September). *Smoking and women's health* (ACOG Educational Bulletin No. 240). Washington, DC: Author.

American College of Obstetricians and Gynecologists (ACOG). (1998). *Postpartum hemorrhage* (ACOG Educational Bulletin No. 243). Washington, DC: Author.

Anthony, S., Buitendijk, S. E., Zondervan, K. T., van Rijssel, E. J., & Verkerk, P. H. (1994). Episiotomies and the occurrence of severe perineal lacerations. *British Journal of Obstetrics & Gynaecology, 101*(12), 1064–1067.

Apgar, V. (1966). The newborn (Apgar) scoring system: Reflections and advice. *Pediatric Clinics of North America, 13*, 645.

Association of Women's Health, Obstetric and Neonatal Nurses (AWHONN). (1998). *Standards and guidelines* (5th ed.). Washington, DC: Author.

Berenson, A. B., Wiemann, C. M., Wilkinson, G. S., Jones, W. A., & Anderson, G. D. (1994). Perinatal morbidity associated with violence experienced by pregnant women. *American Journal of Obstetrics and Gynecology, 170*(6), 1760–1766.

Cunningham, F. G., Gant, N., Gilstrap, L., Hauth, J., Leveno, K., & Wenstrom, K. (2001). *Williams obstetrics* (21st ed.). New York: McGraw-Hill.

Friedman, E. A. (1970). An objective method of evaluating labor. *Hospital Practice, 5*(7), 83.

Gaskins, J. E., & Goldkrand, J. W. (1994). Air contamination in umbilical cord blood sampling. *American Journal of Obstetrics & Gynecology, 171*(6), 1546–1549.

Gazmararian, J. A., Lazorick, S., Spitz, A. M., Ballard, T. J., Saltzman, L. E., & Marks, J. S. (1996). Prevalence of violence against pregnant women. *Journal of the American Medical Association, 275*(24), 1915–1920.

Hilliard, P. J. (1985). Physical abuse in pregnancy. *Obstetrics & Gynecology, 66*, 185–190.

Jacobson, H. (1985). A standard for assessing lochia volume. *Maternal-Child Nursing, 10*(3), 174–175.

Kohl, S. (1997). Neonatal herpes virus infection. *Clinics in Perinatology, 24*(1), 129–150.

Lowe, N. K. (1996). The pain and discomfort of labor and birth. *Journal of Obstetric, Gynecologic, and Neonatal Nursing, 25*(1), 82–92.

Lugenbiehl, D. L., Brophy, G. H., Artigue, G. S., Phillips, K. E., & Flak, R. J. (1990). Standardized assessment of blood loss. *Maternal Child Nursing, 15*, 241.

Manogin, T. W., Bechtel, G. A., & Rami, J. S. (2000). Caring behaviors by nurses: Women's perceptions during childbirth. *Journal of Obstetric, Gynecologic, and Neonatal Nursing, 29*(2), 137–168.

Mayberry, L. J., Wood, S. H., Strange, L. B., Lee, L., Heisler, D. R., & Nielson-Smith, K. (1999). Managing second-stage labor. *Lifelines, 3*(6), 28–34.

McFarlane, J., Parker, B., & Soeke, K. (1996). Physical abuse, smoking, and substance abuse during pregnancy: Prevalence, interrelationships, and effects on birth weight. *Journal of Obstetric, Gynecologic & Neonatal Nursing, 25*(4), 313–320.

Murray, M. (1997). *Autopartal and intrapartal fetal monitoring* (2nd ed.). Albuquerque, NM: Learning Resources International.

Parker, B., McFarlane, J., & Soeke, K. (1994). Abuse during pregnancy: Effects on maternal complications and birth weight in adult and teenage women. *Obstetrics and Gynecology, 84*(3), 323–328.

Queenan, J., & Hobbins, J. (Eds.). (1996). *Protocols for high-risk pregnancies* (3rd ed.). Cambridge, England: Blackwell Science.

Roberts, S. W., Cox, S. M., Dax, J., Wendel, G. D., & Leveno, K. J. (1995). Genital herpes during pregnancy: No lesions, no cesarean. *Obstetrics & Gynecology, 85*(2), 261–264.

Scott, J., DiSaia, P., Hammond, C., & Spellocy, W. (Eds.). (1994). *Danforth's obstetrics and gynecology* (7th ed.). Philadelphia: J. B. Lippincott.

Teixeira, M., Fisk, N. M., & Glover, V. (1999). Association between maternal anxiety in pregnancy and increased uterine artery resistance index: Cohort based study. *British Medical Journal, 318*, 153–157.

Vintzileos, A. M., Nochimson, D. J., Guzman, E. R., Knuppel, R. A., Lake, M., & Schifrin, B. S. (1995). Intrapartum electronic fetal heart rate monitoring versus intermittent auscultation: A meta-analysis. *Obstetrics & Gynecology, 85*(1), 149–155.

Wadhwa, P. D., Porto, M., Garite, T. J., Chicz-DeMet, A., & Sandman, C. A. (1998). Maternal corticotropin-releasing hormone levels in the early trimester predict length of gestation in human pregnancy. *American Journal of Obstetrics and Gynecology, 179*, 1079–1085.

Suggested Readings

Carroli, G., & Belizan, J. (2000). Episiotomy for vaginal birth (Cochrane Review). In *The Cochrane Library Issue 1*. Oxford: Updated Software.

Fraser, W. D., Turcot, L., Krauss, I., & Brisson-Carrol, G. (2000). Amniotomy for shortening spontaneous labour (Cochrane Review). In *The Cochrane Library, Issue 1*. Oxford: Updated Software.

Hall, S. (1997). The nurse's role in the identification of risks and treatment of shoulder dystocia. *Journal of Obstetrics, Gynecology, and Neonatal Nursing, 26*(1), 25–32.

Hodnett, E. D. (2000). Caregiver support for women during childbirth (Cochrane Review). In *The Cochrane Library, Issue 1.* Oxford: Updated Software.

Horger, E. (1995). Shoulder dystocia. *Female Patient, 20*(12), 12–58.

Salamalekis, E., Loghis, C., Panayotopoulos, N., Vitoratos, N., Giannake, G., & Christodoulacos, G. (1997). Non-stress test: A fifteen-year clinical appraisal. *Clinical & Experimental Obstetrics & Gynecology, 21*(2), 79–81.

Tucker, S. M. (1996). *Pocket guide to fetal monitoring assessment* (3rd ed.). St. Louis, MO: Mosby.

Resources

American Academy of Husband-Coached Childbirth, P.O. Box 5224, Sherman Oaks, CA 91413, (800) 422-4784, http://www.bradleybirth.com

American College of Nurse-Midwives, 8403 Colesville Rd., Suite 1550, Silver Spring, MD 20910, (240) 485-1800, http://www.midwife.org

American College of Obstetricians and Gynecologists (ACOG), 409 12th Street, SW, P.O. Box 96920, Washington, DC 20090, 800-762-2264, http://www.acog.org

American Society for Reproductive Medicine, 1209 Montgomery Highway, Birmingham, AL 35216, 205-978-5000, http://www.asrm.org

Association of Nurse Advocates for Childbirth Solutions, http://www.anacs.org

Doulas of North America, P.O. Box 626, Jasper, IN 47547, (888) 788-DONA, http://www.dona.org

International Childbirth Education Association, P.O. Box 20048, Minneapolis, MN 55420, (952) 854-8660, http://www.icea.org

March of Dimes Birth Defects Foundation, National Foundation/March of Dimes, 1275 Mamaroneck Avenue, White Plains, NY 10605, 914-428-7100, 888-663-4637, http://www.modimes.org

Maternity Center Association, Inc., 281 Park Avenue South, 5th Floor, New York, NY 10010, 212-777-5000, http://www.maternitywise.org

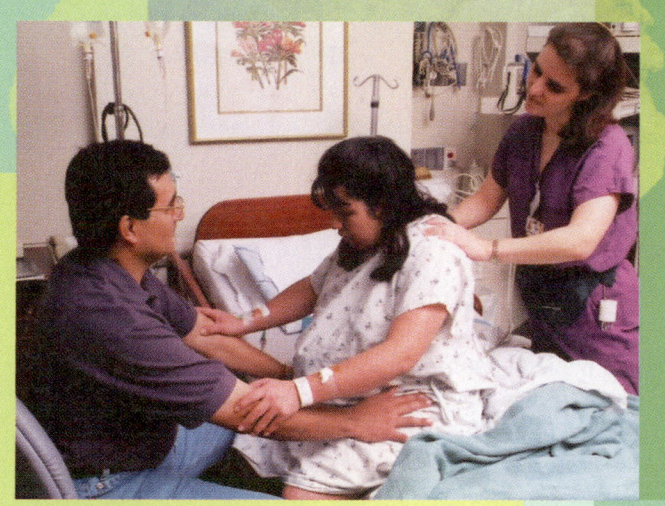

CHAPTER 15

HIGH-RISK BIRTHS AND OBSTETRIC EMERGENCIES

Complications arise suddenly and often quite dramatically in obstetrics. Complications can transform a routine antepartum or intrapartum experience into an emergent situation, with both maternal and fetal well-being at stake. Because of the ever-present potential for complications, the obstetric nurse should possess strong critical thinking skills coupled with anticipatory preparations that allow immediate intervention. The nurse must incorporate these skills and preparations without compromising the birthing environment in which the client and her family are seeking to participate. Balancing the goals of positive birth experiences with acute and intensive support of maternal and fetal status can be quite a challenge for the professional nurse. As you review the following questions, reflect on your own personal views, experiences, and coping mechanisms:

- How do I feel about being responsible for the fetus whose status may be difficult to assess because of limited available assessment data?
- How do I react in emergency situations?
- Have I ever been present during a cesarean section? How did I feel?
- Have I ever been present at a delivery where complications occurred? How did I respond?
- Have I or has anyone close to me experienced a perinatal loss, had a baby born with a birth defect, or had an infant injured at birth? How do I feel about that experience now?
- How do I feel about comforting a client who will have or has had a baby requiring intensive care, or who has had an infant who will not or did not survive?

Key Terms

Abruptio placentae
Amniotic fluid embolism
Amniotomy
Anencephaly
Breech presentation
Brow presentation
Cephalopelvic
    disproportion (CPD)
Contracted maternal
    pelvis
Dysfunctional labor
    pattern
External cephalic version
Face presentation
Fetal distress
Hydrocephalus
Hypertonic labor
Hypotonic labor
Intrauterine pressure
    catheter (IUPC)
Kleihauer-Betke test
Labor augmentation
Long-term variability
    (LTV)

Malposition
Malpresentation
Multiple gestation
Oligohydramnios
Placenta percreta
Placenta previa
Polyhydramnios
Precipitate labor
Short-term variability
    (STV)
Shoulder dystocia
Shoulder presentation
Transverse lie
Turtle sign
Umbilical cord
    compression
Umbilical cord prolapse
Undulating variability
Uterine rupture
Vasa previa
Velamentous insertion of
    the cord

Competencies

Upon completion of this chapter, the reader should be able to:

1. Identify selected dysfunctional labor patterns and the nursing interventions to enhance maternal and fetal well-being.

2. Identify and differentiate the common fetal malpositions and malpresentations. Discuss the assessment data relative to confirming the fetal position. Explain the delivery concerns for each of the malpositions and malpresentations.

3. When fetal distress occurs, integrate the nursing process by focusing on assessment, diagnoses, and implementation of appropriate interventions to achieve the desired outcomes. Describe the evaluation parameters that will verify successful implementation.

4. Discuss the assessment data found in clients who have experienced uterine rupture and the plan for implementing care and evaluation of outcomes.

5. Compare and contrast the assessment parameters found with placenta previa and abruptio placentae. Differentiate the plans of care and evaluations of outcomes.

6. Discuss the assessment findings that indicate a prolapsed umbilical cord and the emergent implementation of required interventions.

7. Identify the hemorrhagic conditions that predispose obstetric clients to coagulopathies, such as disseminated intravascular coagulation, or DIC.

8. Discuss the maternal and fetal implications when a diagnosis of oligohydramnios or polyhydramnios has been confirmed, and identify the contributing causes of these conditions.

9. Describe the assessment data indicative of amniotic fluid embolism and two critical factors impeding maternal survival.

Pregnant clients at risk for or who incur obstetric emergencies are dependent on the entire health care system to support their needs during pregnancy, labor, and delivery. Because of the constant interaction with the professional nurse during the labor and delivery process, clients and their support persons anticipate and trust that the nurse will be ready to identify problems that develop and intervene immediately. The goal is clear: a positive outcome for both mother and child. That goal, however, is not always easily achieved.

Integration of the nursing process into the high-risk obstetric setting can be challenging. Assessment of clients includes reviewing historical and prenatal data; completing a maternal physical assessment; assessing fetal status; and obtaining pertinent emotional, cultural, developmental, and educational data. The development of outcomes or goals must be done with regard to the current plan of medical management. Nursing plans and interventions may combine one-on-one interactions, such as massaging and positioning clients, with highly technical skills, such as maternal-fetal monitoring and management of multiple medications to augment labor. Evaluation of the process depends on the confirmation of assessment data, success of the nursing interventions, and comparison of the actual with the desired maternal-fetal outcomes.

The obstetric nurse working in labor and delivery often provides care in an atmosphere of a relaxed home environment. The nurse's initial interactions with the client and her significant others include acknowledging their hopes and dreams for their expected baby. The expectations of the client and her support persons for the pregnancy, labor, and delivery are affected by various factors: family structure; cultural aspects, including language barriers; educational levels; and religious beliefs. The relationship that develops between the nurse and client often is a personal one that may last throughout the labor and delivery experience. The nurse must take the time to establish rapport and trust with the client. Rapport may enable the nurse to accomplish necessary interventions quickly and efficiently, while minimizing the client's fear and anxiety (Manogin, Bechtel, & Rami, 2000). The nurse also must be able to recognize the many feelings that the woman may experience as an obstetric client at high risk. These feelings vary with the person and the chronicity of the problem but may include a sense of entrapment or being held prisoner, boredom, loss of control, reversal of the role of caregiver to one of being cared for, and frustration with the limitations imposed by bed rest and hospitalization. The nurse is challenged to incorporate interventions that minimize negative feelings and support optimal coping (Gupton, Heaman, & Ashcroft, 1997). Establishing a strong relationship between the nurse and client, and the client's support persons, confirms the nurse's role as a client advocate during the course of care.

Assessment of maternal-fetal status is critical. The total clinical picture should incorporate data from both the mother and fetus that offer reassurances of maternal stability and fetal well-being. The assessment process is very dynamic in the intrapartum period because changes that compromise the maternal-fetal status may occur in minutes. Interventions also are completed quickly and often have results requiring immediate evaluation. Quick interventions, however, should not be the result of an incomplete assessment.

Reflections from a Nurse

The miracle of birth is an awesome experience. To participate and support a client throughout the course of her labor and delivery is rewarding. Encountering and overcoming the challenges of high-risk situations, complications, and obstetric emergencies to achieve a positive birth outcome truly result in a victory for the obstetric health care team! Regardless of the outcome, providing professional, supportive, and compassionate care is equally challenging.

Complete assessment of critical information best enables the nurse to formulate diagnoses, intervene appropriately, and achieve successful and timely outcomes.

The intensity and speed of the labor and delivery process may at times produce a feeling of being overwhelmed in clients, support persons, and even the nurse. These feelings become more intense as high-risk situations, complications, or emergent situations arise. It is important for the nurse to remain calm, use critical thinking skills, communicate clearly, and intervene appropriately. To help increase the efficiency of interventions during an emergent situation, the nurse should anticipate client needs; ready equipment and other personnel; and put in place well-established lines of communication with the physician or Certified Nurse Midwife (CNM), nursery, anesthesia services, and additional team members.

Several conditions make the intrapartum period one of high risk. Conditions that will be addressed in this chapter include dysfunctional labor patterns, fetal malpresentation, maternal and fetal structural anomalies, multiple gestation, fetal distress, uterine rupture, placental anomalies, umbilical cord anomalies, and amniotic fluid anomalies. Each condition requires astute nursing care to ensure positive maternal and fetal outcomes.

DYSFUNCTIONAL LABOR PATTERN

A **dysfunctional labor pattern** is a labor process that does not proceed normally. Normal labor is characterized by uterine activity that causes cervical change in effacement and dilation, and fetal descent, resulting in a vaginal delivery (Cunningham et al., 2001). Dysfunctional labor patterns often are medically classified as labor dystocias (Bashore, 1992). Labor dystocias are ranked as the leading cause of primary cesarean sections at approximately 43% (Cunningham et al., 2001). Labor dystocias during the first stage of labor occur in 8% to 11% of vertex presentations. They occur at approximately the same rate during the second stage of labor (Wiznitzer, 1995). Hypertonic labor, hypotonic labor, and precipitate labor are three types of dysfunctional labor patterns, or dystocias, attributed to uterine dysfunction.

Hypertonic Labor

Hypertonic labor is classified as an "abnormality of the expulsive forces" of the uterus in *Williams Obstetrics* (Cunningham et al., 2001). The pattern of uterine activity includes uterine irritability, poor resting tone, and contractions occurring at a frequency of closer than every 2 minutes. Whereas this pattern of uterine activity is painful to the pregnant client, it usually is not effective in causing the cervical changes necessary for labor to progress and the fetus to descend. Maternal and fetal factors that contribute to hypertonic labor include primiparous labor, fetal presentation other than cephalic, persistent occipitoposterior position (Joshi & Bharadwaj, 2000), flexion of the fetal head, and increased fetal size. Up to 50% of the time, however, no attributable cause for the dysfunction can be clearly identified (Cunningham et al., 2001).

The consequences of a hypertonic uterine pattern may include maternal exhaustion and inadequate pain relief from prolonged uterine activity, a prolonged latent or active phase of labor, increased risk for maternal or fetal infection when the membranes have ruptured, and increased risk for maternal or fetal injury.

Medical management of hypertonic labor patterns may be approached in more than one way. The physician or CNM may choose to allow the client to rest using hydration and sedation, which also will reduce uterine irritability and allow reevaluation of uterine activity (Cunningham et al., 2001). When the membranes have already ruptured, resting the client is not an option. The physician or CNM also may choose to use oxytocin to stimulate a more effective contraction pattern (Bashore, 1992). When oxytocin is used to enhance ineffective uterine activity, the procedure is called **labor augmentation** (Payton & Brucker, 1999).

The nursing process begins with thorough maternal and fetal assessments. Data that will assist in confirming a hypertonic uterine pattern focus first on assessment of uterine activity. Manual palpation of uterine activity and the uterine activity recording found on the external fetal monitor tracing provide valuable information to the

Critical Thinking

Oxytocin (Pitocin) and Propranolol (Inderal)

A 1996 study reported the comparison of oxytocin augmentation alone with oxytocin augmentation accompanied by the additional administration of intravenous (IV) push doses of propranolol in the treatment of dysfunctional labor. The study results were favorable, with the group receiving both oxytocin and IV propranolol having fewer cesarean sections. In addition, no increase in poor maternal or fetal delivery outcomes were reported. The outcomes of this study will change the management of dysfunctional labor patterns. What is your opinion of the value of the oxytocin-propranolol combination?

Note. From "Randomized Trial of Oxytocin Alone and with Propranolol in the Management of Dysfunctional Labor," by L. Sanchez-Ramos, M. J. Quillen, and A. Kaunitz, 1996, *Obstetrics and Gynecology, 88*(4), pp. 517–520.

nurse. Contraction activity may occur closer than every 2 minutes, with poor uterine relaxation between contractions. Contractions that are occurring closer than every 2 minutes or lasting longer than 90 seconds can lead to fetal hypoxia. The contractions usually will not feel firm even at peak intensity, although the client may voice variable levels of discomfort. The pelvic examination should include assessment of cervical dilation and effacement and fetal station, presentation, and position. Failure to observe changes in the cervix or fetal descent in the presence of irritable uterine activity indicates an ineffective pattern of labor. Membrane status must be assessed. When the membranes have ruptured, the risk for infection becomes a consideration in the client's medical management. Augmentation is the primary medical management of a hypertonic pattern of labor when the membranes have ruptured.

Fetal tolerance to the contraction pattern also must be assessed (Box 15-1). Assessment is accomplished through auscultation or, better, intermittent or continuous external fetal monitoring. When fetal monitoring is employed, data used to make the assessment include fetal heart rate baseline, the presence of heart rate variability, the presence and type of periodic changes, and any nonperiodic changes (Feinstein & McCartney, 1997). Maternal vital signs, including temperature and input and output status, may offer information about her physical tolerance of the labor pattern. The assessment also should indicate the client's level of knowledge, particularly of the labor expe-

> **Box 15-1**
>
> Fetal Monitoring Terms and Parameters
>
> **Baseline Data**
> **Rate:** Maintained for a minimum of 10 minutes.
> > **Normal:** 120–160
> >
> > **Tachycardia:** >160
> >
> > **Bradycardia:** <110
>
> **Fetal Heart Rate Variability:** The heart rate changes from beat to beat or over an extended period of time measured in 1-minute intervals that indicate central nervous system status.
> > **Short-term variability (STV):** Measured in beat-to-beat changes in the baseline as either present or absent. Only measurable with internal mode of fetal monitoring.
> >
> > **Long-term variability (LTV):** Measured in minute intervals from the baseline and rated as follows: decreased, 0–5 bpm; average, 6–25 bpm; or marked, >25 bpm (on a 3-point scale).
> >
> > **Undulating variability:** Waveform variation that is repetitive and almost uniform in appearance, including sinusoidal and pseudosinusoidal patterns.
>
> **Rhythm**
> > **Regular**
> >
> > **Irregular**
>
> **Periodic Changes:** Heart rate changes in response and relation to the occurrence of uterine activity.
> **Accelerations*:** Variations upward from baseline. Presence, frequency, peak, and duration of accelerations are assessed.
> **Decelerations*:** Variations downward from baseline. Presence, frequency, shape, type classification, depth, and durations are assessed.
> > **Variable:** Frequency and timing in relation to contractions, shape, and duration vary.
> >
> > **Early:** Shape and occurrence are more uniform before or with contractions; "mirroring."
> >
> > **Late:** Shape and occurrence also are uniform but begin during or after contractions.
> >
> > **Prolonged:** >2 minutes but <10 minutes in duration.
>
> ---
>
> *Accelerations and decelerations also may occur without a defined relationship to the contraction and are then termed nonperiodic or spontaneous in occurrence.
>
> *Note.* Adapted from *Fetal Heart Monitoring Principles and Practices*, 2nd ed., by N. Feinstein, P. McCartney, and AWHONN, 1997, Dubuque, IA: Kendall/Hunt.

rience, and the cultural and religious considerations that may affect her response to the labor process.

Nursing diagnoses for a client experiencing a hypertonic labor pattern may include the following:

1. Risk for infection (maternal or fetal) related to prolonged latent labor process, as evidenced by maternal fever of 100.4°F, maternal tachycardia, fetal tachycardia, or a combination of these (Feinstein & McCartney, 1997).

2. Acute pain (maternal) related to uterine irritability and prolonged labor, as evidenced by frequent or persistent maternal requests for pain relief, frequent uterine contractions, poor uterine resting tone, and failure of the cervix to dilate 1 to 2 cm/h on cervical assessment.

3. Deficient knowledge of labor processes and variations related to inexperience and unfamiliarity with intervention options, as evidenced by client questions and an inability to cooperate with requested interventions.

4. Fatigue (maternal) related to a prolonged labor process, as evidenced by an inability to rest between contractions, inadequate pain relief, client statements of exhaustion, and client inability to cooperate with requested interventions.

5. Impaired gas exchange (fetoplacental) related to hyperstimulation of the uterus with oxytocin augmentation, as evidenced by nonreassuring fetal tracing inclusive of severe variable decelerations; late decelerations; bradycardia; or loss of long-term or short-term variability, or both. Inadequate fetoplacental oxygenation as a result of uterine hyperstimulation can adversely affect the fetus (Feinstein & McCartney, 1997).

6. Anxiety related to unfamiliar experiences, surroundings, and unexpected medical interventions, as evidenced by client verbal and nonverbal behaviors.

Desired outcomes are based on the nursing diagnoses developed for the client. Prevention of risks for problems or resolution of actual problems are addressed in the following outcome statements:

1. Client and fetus will not experience infection related to a prolonged labor process.

2. Client will verbalize effective pain relief without demonstrating adverse maternal or fetal response to the selected interventions.

3. Client and support persons will verbalize an understanding of the uterine pattern; plan of care to address it; and expected outcomes, including the projected mode of delivery. The client also will be able to participate in and cooperate with requests from the nurse.

4. Client will not experience exhaustion related to prolonged fatigue during a hypertonic labor pattern.

5. Fetus will not exhibit **fetal distress**, a nonreassuring fetal heart rate response to the intrauterine environment as a result of the hypertonic labor pattern or oxytocin augmentation of labor.

6. Client will demonstrate effective coping behaviors in response to heightened anxiety.

Achieving the above outcomes requires ongoing assessment with 80% of occurrences and support of the client by the professional nurse. The nurse must assess maternal-fetal status and relay the pertinent information to the attending physician or CNM. Critical elements include monitoring of uterine activity, results of the pelvic examination (changes in cervical dilation or fetal descent), maternal vital signs, and fetal heart rate data. Changes in maternal-fetal status may alter the current medical plan of management. For instance, if the initial medical plan was to rest the client and on reassessment the fetal heart rate data are of concern, the physician or CNM may decide to augment the labor pattern and move toward delivery.

Assessment data should include ongoing monitoring for signs of infection. The fetal heart rate and the maternal temperature, heart rate, and respirations may increase with the onset of infection. Fetal tachycardia is most frequently the result of maternal fever or maternal or fetal infection (Feinstein & McCartney, 1997). Monitoring maternal input and output reduces the likelihood of dehydration being a cause of maternal fever and maternal or fetal tachycardia. Monitoring of the input and output also is critical when oxytocin is administered because of its antidiuretic effect and the potential for water intoxication (Payton & Brucker, 1999; Cunningham et al., 2001). Ongoing maternal-fetal assessments become even more imperative once the membranes rupture and this barrier of defense is no longer intact.

Anxiety can increase catecholamine secretion and thus lead to a dysfunctional labor process (Feinstein & McCartney, 1997). Aside from the physiologic effects, anxiety impacts the client's perception of the birth experience and can further impact the resolution or successful integration of the events into her adaptation from pregnancy to parenthood. Lack of knowledge can increase the anxiety levels of both the client and her support persons. Thus, all interventions should be explained in a manner best understood by the client and questions should be encouraged and answered. Initially establishing rapport with the client and her support persons is fundamental in developing trust. In turn, trust can allay fears and reduce anxiety. A trusting relationship also makes it easier for the client to follow instructions and better participate in the labor process. When the client and her support persons feel the nurse is aware and respectful of their level of knowledge and any cultural or religious considerations, they are more likely to cooperate and actively participate in the plan of care. Finally, when they believe the nurse is knowledgeable and capable of managing the client's care, the labor experience is more likely to be perceived as being positive, regardless of the need for technical intervention (Manogin, Bechtel, & Rami, 2000).

The nurse can help provide pain relief by using physical comfort measures such as position changes, lower back rubs, counterpressure at the lower back during a contraction (pressing the fist firmly into the identified pressure point low on the back), and administration of analgesic medications. The physical presence of the nurse along with sincere encouragement may further alleviate anxiety that may enhance pain perception (Manogin, Bechtel, & Rami, 2000). An explanation about the medications and the likely responses after administration may further reassure the client regarding pain relief. Ensuring that the environment is conducive to rest by reducing external stimuli (e.g., lowering lighting levels, reducing the volume on noise-producing equipment, and turning off televisions) is another intervention the nurse can use. Although the nurse does not insert or administer epidural anesthesia, assisting with adequate hydration, assessing baseline vital signs, positioning the client, and evaluating maternal-fetal responses to the effects of the epidural anesthesia are all within the nursing role. Finally, the nurse can help the client achieve adequate pain relief and reduce fatigue by evaluating her responses to the medications, regional anesthesia, and physical comfort measures taken, and by promoting rest opportunities between contractions.

When the physician orders oxytocin to augment labor, the nurse should ensure that the orders and protocols for administration are observed. Adding the correct amount of oxytocin to the IV solution and administering it to the client by IV pump through a piggyback approach to the main IV line are all important steps in this process. Monitoring the maternal-fetal responses to the augmentation process is critical because the increase in dosage is titrated to these responses. Some protocols require dosage increases of a set amount of milliunits every 15 to 30 minutes until an effective labor pattern is achieved. The parameters may be established by the individual physician after a low-dosage regimen or may follow a high-dosage regimen. The administration rate of a low-dosage regimen is 0.5 to 2 mU/min and is increased by the nurse every 15 to 40 minutes, with a maximum dosage limit between 20 and 40 mU/min. When a high-dosage protocol is ordered, the starting rate may be 6 mU/minute, with increases every 20 to 40 minutes and a maximum dosage of 40 mU/min (Payton & Brucker, 1999). Regardless of the protocol, the nurse should try to ensure the occurrence of regular contractions of moderate to firm intensity that last 30 to 60 seconds every 2 to 5 minutes, without causing maternal or fetal compromise.

Once an effective labor pattern is established and cervical change occurs, the physician may choose to perform an **amniotomy**, which is artificial rupture of the membranes to further augment the labor process (Figure 15-1). When assisting with the amniotomy, the nurse should ensure that the fetal heart tracing remains stable and note the color, amount, particulate matter in, and odor of the fluid. At that time, fetal monitoring options may include internal monitoring modes to increase the accuracy of uterine activity assessment (**intrauterine pressure catheter [IUPC]**), fetal heart rate assessment (fetal spiral electrode [FSE]), or both. Having the amniotomy hook, internal monitoring devices, sterile gloves, appropriate monitor cables, towels, and fresh hip pads readily available will enhance the efficiency of the procedure. Although the modes of data attainment may have changed, the nurse is still responsible for ongoing maternal-fetal assessments as the client progresses through labor.

Evaluation of maternal-fetal status ensures that the interventions employed have been effective. Medical man-

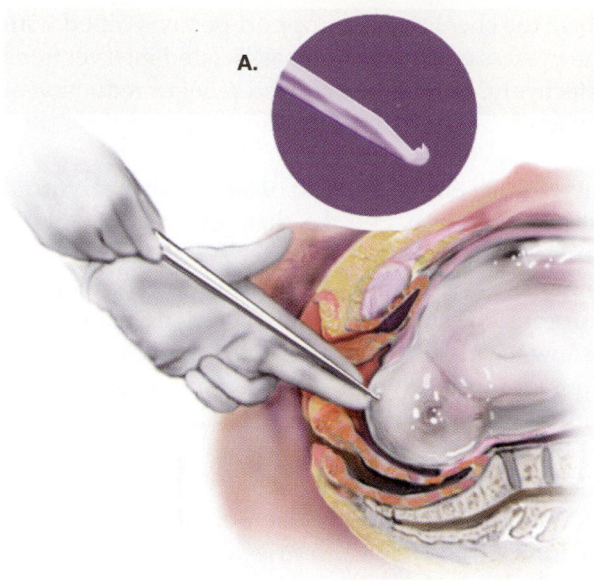

Figure 15-1   A. Disposable amniohook to rupture membranes. B. Technique for amniotomy.

agement and nursing interventions may need to be altered or continued based on the findings of the evaluation.

1. Are signs of infection present? Are maternal and fetal vital signs stable? Is the fetal heart rate tracing reassuring, with long-term variability and accelerations present?

2. Is the client's pain relieved? Does she state there is less pain? Does she appear less distressed? Is there less uterine irritability, or is there better uterine relaxation between contractions? Are the contractions less frequent? If an epidural is in place, is it intact? Has the client stated she has adequate pain relief from the epidural without demonstrating hypotensive responses, fetal bradycardia, or prolonged decelerations?

3. Does the client understand what is happening? Does she ask appropriate questions? Is she cooperative? Does she verbalize understanding? Do her support persons verbalize an understanding of the process? Do they express confidence in the management of care?

4. Does the client rest between contractions? Does she verbalize resting between contractions? Does she participate in her care?

5. Does the client's labor pattern become effective? Is there cervical change? Is there fetal descent? Are the maternal-fetal responses to the augmentation of labor reassuring or stable?

6. Have the client and her support persons coped with the process of labor and the associated interventions effectively? Has she verbalized relief or reduction of anxiety?

A hypertonic uterine pattern of labor may evolve into a normal labor pattern, and the client eventually will deliver vaginally. In contrast, an ineffective pattern of labor may continue, necessitating a cesarean section either as a result of arrested labor or because the maternal or fetal status shows evidence of compromise. The professional nurse must continuously assess maternal-fetal status and communicate this information to all health care providers to optimize outcomes. Readiness to initiate alternative interventions in the event the desired outcomes are not achieved is essential. The physician or CNM, anesthesia services, nursery, and all health care personnel required at the delivery should be kept abreast of the client's changing status. Finally, the nurse is responsible for recording the following: assessment data, interventions employed, maternal-fetal responses, and evaluations of outcomes.

Hypotonic Labor

Hypotonic labor refers to uterine contractions that are inadequate in terms of frequency, intensity, or duration. Hypotonic labor tends to occur during the latent or active phase of labor. The client experiences contractions that are ineffective in causing cervical dilation or effacement, or fetal descent. Risk factors that contribute to the occurrence of a hypotonic labor pattern include large fetal size, fetal malpresentation, and early or repeated maternal sedation in labor. Recent concerns have been voiced regarding epidural administration as a contributing cause of hypotonic labor patterns. Current studies do not support the claim that epidural anesthesia negatively impacts labor, although it is frequently used for pain management in clients with ineffective labor patterns because of increased need for adequate pain relief (Thompson, Thorp, Mayer, Kuller & Bowes, 1998). In another study, Clark, Carr, Loyd, Cook, and Spinnato (1998) further found that epidural anesthesia did not increase the rate of cesarean sections in women with dystocia managed actively with oxytocin. Similar findings were the result of a study by Bofill et al. (1997). The significance of these studies impacts the nurse in two ways. Epidural anesthesia is a viable pain relief intervention that is monitored throughout its duration of action by the nurse. In addition, each study acknowledges the need for strict active management of the labor method that employs the high-dosage oxytocin protocol. This method requires the nurse to intensively monitor maternal-fetal responses and oxytocin titration based on uterine activity. The results of a hypotonic labor include prolonged latent labor, prolonged active labor, or

both; increased risk for maternal or fetal infection; increased risk for fetal compromise from insufficient reserve; maternal fatigue and exhaustion; and the need for additional medical, technical, and nursing interventions, including altering the client's desired birth plan.

Medical management of the hypotonic labor pattern is similar to that used for the hypertonic labor pattern. The physician or CNM may choose to allow the client to rest by administering hydration and sedation and then reevaluate her later for cervical changes, fetal descent, and improved uterine contraction activity. The other management option is to augment the labor with IV piggyback administration of oxytocin or amniotomy, or both.

Nursing considerations for the client with hypotonic labor include assessment information obtained from the monitoring of uterine activity and the pelvic examination. Maternal vital signs and fetal status must be assessed and monitored closely for changes that may indicate either complications or progression of labor. The nursing assessment should explore the client's level of formal or experiential knowledge, cultural and religious considerations, influence of support persons, and her perceived fear and anxiety level.

As with the hypertonic labor pattern, the nursing diagnoses for hypotonic labor address the risk for maternal and fetal infection. Prolonged labor processes related to hypotonic labor patterns also can impair fetoplacental gas exchange relative to the sheer duration of the labor process and the lack of further fetal reserve (Feinstein & McCartney, 1997). Maternal pain and fatigue and knowledge deficit of the client and her support persons also are risk factors in hypotonic labor. The client may incur heightened anxiety, particularly when it seems as if little to no progress is being made. The desired outcomes for these diagnoses also will be similar to those for hypertonic contraction patterns. The ultimate outcome is for the client to deliver vaginally, without evidence of maternal or fetal compromise.

The nursing plan and interventions employed also are similar to those used for hypertonic labor patterns. Continuous monitoring for signs of maternal or fetal infection and fetal intolerance to oxytocin augmentation is imperative. Implementation of client comfort measures, use of labor pain relief methods, emotional support of the client and her support persons, and ongoing client teaching are instrumental throughout the labor process. The nurse must always anticipate alternative outcomes that require rapid intervention. Communication and documentation of assessment data, interventions, and evaluations also are necessary. Communication and documentation cannot be overstressed in an area where dramatic changes may occur very rapidly.

In evaluating outcomes the nurse should ask pertinent questions of the situation.

- Is the maternal-fetal status stable?
- Have the outcomes been achieved or are further interventions required?
- Is the medical management of the client changing?
- Will the nursing interventions need to change to support the medical management?
- Is the client coping effectively?
- Are her support persons able to support her and participate in her care?
- What is the delivery outcome?
- Is the neonate stabilized easily at birth?
- Is the mother able to initiate bonding interactions with her newborn?

Precipitate Labor

Precipitate labor refers to a labor pattern that progresses rapidly and ends with delivery occurring less than 3 hours after the onset of uterine activity. Maternal and fetal contributory factors for precipitate labor include maternal multiparous status, small fetus, relaxed pelvic and vaginal musculature, and a history of rapid labors with previous deliveries. Maternal and fetal risks include a delivery out of asepsis, maternal soft tissue injuries, and fetal injuries from rapid expulsion at delivery. Medical diagnosis and management include a readiness on the part of the entire health team for the delivery, particularly when the client has a history of rapid labor. The American College of Obstetricians and Gynecologists (ACOG) acknowledges that a history of rapid or precipitous labors is a reason for medical induction to ensure a hospital delivery and increase the likelihood for a controlled delivery that minimizes the potential for maternal and fetal injuries.

The nursing assessment of the client should include a thorough history of gravidity, length of previous labors, and delivery outcomes. Uterine activity should be assessed by palpation or fetal monitoring, or both. Precipitate delivery may occur as a result of pelvic relaxation; however, intense and frequent contractions may contribute to rapid progression of labor. When uterine relaxation is inadequate, fetoplacental gas exchange may be compromised. Assessment of fetal position using Leopold's maneuvers, review of ultrasonography information for position, and estimation of fetal weight may provide information regarding the likelihood of rapid delivery. The pelvic examination will reveal information on cervical status, fetal station, and adequacy of pelvic outlet. Subsequent examinations will denote changes, and a rapid or significant change may be a predictor of a short labor process. Assessment of client responses, such as intensity of behavior, bearing down, and increased anxiety, may reveal a need for the nurse to reevaluate the progression of labor. Fetal tolerance to labor should be assessed continuously. Maternal vital signs are significant for baseline information because women who experience particularly intense, precipitous labor and deliveries are at a higher risk for amniotic fluid embolism and uterine atony after delivery than are women who do not (Cunningham et al., 2001).

Nursing diagnoses for the client experiencing precipitous labor and delivery include a recognition of risks for the following: maternal or fetal soft tissue injury related to rapid descent and expulsion, maternal or fetal infection if delivery occurs outside of aseptic surroundings, and maternal hemorrhage if atony results after delivery. The nurse also must consider maternal pain and anxiety. The goals of these client outcomes are to avoid the risks of soft tissue injury, infection, and hemorrhage, while reinforcing maternal comfort and attempting to reduce or limit anxiety.

Nursing care involves vigilant attendance, client safety, preparations for delivery in advance, client comfort measures, and education and emotional support for the client and her support persons. The onset of rapid labor can be frightening and overwhelming. When uterine relaxation is minimal, little reprieve between contractions is provided. Thus, the opportunity of resting, refocusing, and preparing for the next contraction is limited. Communication with the physician or CNM and all other team members anticipated at delivery must be clear, concise, and timely to avoid the lack of critical support personnel during delivery.

The nursing plan of care and interventions should include continuous reassessment of maternal-fetal status. Any change in status, maternal or fetal tolerance, or sign of impending problems must be communicated in a timely manner to the physician or CNM and all other required health care providers. The nurse should inform the client of any change in the plan of care. As changes are made, the nurse should explain all procedures and offer reassurance to the client of the readiness of the health care team for delivery. Visually seeing the nurse set up for the anticipated delivery may reassure the client and her support persons that the nurse trusts their concerns and is responding by preparing for the birth of their baby. Teaching or reinforcing relaxation techniques may assist the client in optimizing rest periods between contractions. Rapid labor may prevent the client from obtaining regional anesthesia; however, small IV dosages of pain medication may be ordered when cervical dilation has not progressed to the second stage of labor or immediately preceding this stage. When medication is administered, maternal responses and vital signs and fetal heart rate responses should be evaluated. The nurse also should anticipate successful relaxation and a resulting rapid delivery when providing pharmacologic interventions. When labor progresses too rapidly for even small amounts of pain medication, the nurse can support the client by staying with her and encouraging and assisting her into a comfortable position. After delivery, monitoring maternal vital signs, assessing the uterine fundus for uterine atony, and observation for signs of soft tissue hematoma or increased vaginal bleeding that may indicate a hidden laceration should be done at frequent intervals (every 15 minutes, if stable; more frequently, if there are concerns). The nurse should assess the neonate for soft tissue injuries and monitor vital signs to ensure stability after delivery.

Evaluation of client outcomes involves answering the questions that recognize the success of the established outcomes.

- Did the neonate have bruising, swelling, or signs of injury after delivery?

- Is the mother demonstrating signs of hematoma, lacerations, or increased bleeding?

- If lacerations were present, are the repairs intact with heavy bleeding evident?

- Are maternal vital signs stable?

- Is the mother or neonate demonstrating signs of infection?

- Did the delivery occur in an appropriate setting?

- Are temperatures and respiratory efforts within normal limits?

- Are there signs of maternal hemorrhage after delivery?

- Is the fundus firm and at the umbilicus?

- Is excessive fundal massage required to increase fundal tone?

- Did the client demonstrate reduced anxiety with the nursing support interventions?

- Did the client verbalize enhanced relaxation or reassurance with the nursing interventions?

- Did the client verbalize or demonstrate reduced pain?

- Were pharmacologic interventions helpful?

- Were the maternal-fetal responses reassuring, without evidence of vital sign or fetal heart rate compromise?

- Were nonpharmacologic comfort interventions helpful to the client?

FETAL MALPRESENTATION AND MALPOSITION

Fetal malpresentation and malposition may interfere with the progression of labor and fetal descent. **Malpresentation** refers to a fetal presenting part other than the vertex and includes breech, transverse, compound, shoulder, face, and brow presentations. Malpresentations may be identified late in pregnancy or may not be discovered until the initial assessment during labor. Fetal **malposition** refers to a position other than an occipitoanterior position. Malpositions include occipitotransverse, occipitoposterior, and oblique, or acynclytic, positions of the fetal head in relation to the maternal pelvis. Fetal malpositions are assessed during labor. Fetal malpresentation or malposition may pose risks to maternal-fetal well-being and may necessitate operative vaginal delivery, cesarean section, or other interventions to accomplish delivery.

Breech Presentation

Breech presentation occurs when the fetal buttocks, legs, feet, or a combination of these parts presents first into the maternal pelvis. Classifications of breech presentation include complete, frank, and footling (double or single) (Figure 15-2). The complete breech presentation is best described as when the thighs are flexed on the abdomen and the legs are upon the thighs. In the frank breech presentation the fetus appears as if it is folded in half, with its feet in its face and the buttocks presenting. The fetal legs are extended in the frank breech presentation, unlike the crossed legs found in the complete breech presentation. The fetus in the footling breech presentation has one or both feet presenting first in the maternal pelvis followed by the buttocks. Breech presentation is frequently found

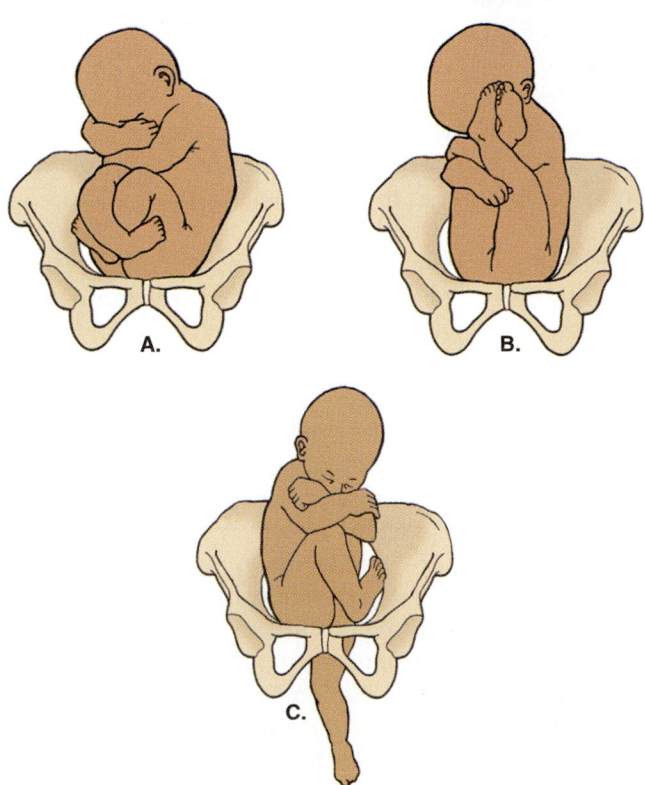

Figure 15-2   Breech presentations. A. Complete. B. Frank. C. Footling.

in pregnancies of 28 weeks' gestation and less; however, it is documented in approximately 3% to 4% of term pregnancies (Toth & Jothivijayrani, 1999; Acien, 1995; Albrechtsen, Rasmussen, Dalaker, & Irgens, 1998). Of breech presentations, 65% are frank, 25% are footling, and the remaining 10% are complete breech presentations.

The most common contributing factors to malpresentation and malposition include prematurity; fetal anomalies, such as **hydrocephalus** (increased circulating cerebrospinal fluid, resulting in an increase in the size of the fetal head) and **anencephaly** (failure of the fetal brain, skull, and head to fully develop; this condition is incompatible with life); multiple gestation; placental placement abnormalities; maternal uterine or pelvic abnormalities; and **polyhydramnios**, a condition in which the amount of amniotic fluid in the uterus is increased to two or more liters within the third trimester (Toth & Jothivijayrani, 1999). Advanced maternal age also has been associated with an increased incidence of breech birth (Acien, 1995; Rayl, Gibson, & Hickok, 1996).

Maternal risks from breech labor and delivery include prolonged difficult labor, potential for soft tissue injury, lacerations, and need for cesarean section. Fetal risks from breech delivery exceed maternal risks for injury. Even without fetal anomalies present that can be exacerbated by a vaginal delivery, risks to the fetus include umbilical cord prolapse, with compression and resultant hypoxia; brachial plexus injuries; and fetal head and neck injuries from entrapment.

Medical management of the client with a suspected breech presentation includes plans to confirm the fetal presentation. Sonography also is used to screen for apparent anomalies and obtain an estimate of the fetal weight. The physician or CNM will find these data to be instrumental in determining the best plan of care for the client. The physician or CNM will determine whether a vaginal trial of labor or cesarean section is in the best interests of both the mother and fetus. In some cases, there is an attempt to perform **external cephalic version**, which is a procedure by which the physician manipulates the fetus externally through the maternal abdomen to turn the fetus from the abnormal presentation to a cephalic presentation. This procedure is successful roughly 15% to 30% of the time. The ideal time to perform a version is 37 weeks' gestation. The use of tocolytics has added to the success rate. Most importantly there is a risk of fetal distress and maternal complications so the client may have to have an emergency Cesarean birth. Repeated studies have documented the danger of a vaginal birth for a breech presentation. With a cephalic presentation the head molds over several hours and this is not possible in breech presentation. There is an increase in the risk of severe fetal distress with intracranial hemorrhage, cord compression, and tentorial tears, which result in gross

motor and mental incapacity. This is why there are few doctors trained in vaginal breech delivery. Most breech presentations are delivered by cesarean section due to the dwindling number of skilled physicians able to safely deliver breech babies (Cunningham et al., 2001).

Cesarean delivery is commonly used in the following circumstances: (1) a large fetus; (2) any unfavorable shape of the maternal pelvis; (3) a hyperextended fetal head; (4) maternal indications for delivery including pregnancy-induced hypertension (PIH) or ruptured membranes for 12 hours or more without labor; (5) uterine dysfunction; (6) footling presentation; (7) a healthy, viable preterm fetus of 25 to 26 weeks or more with the mother in active labor or in need of delivery; (8) severe fetal growth restriction; (9) previous perinatal death or children suffering from birth trauma; and (10) a request for sterilization (Cunningham et al., 2001). Trial of labor may be attempted when estimated fetal weight is equal to or less than previous delivery weights (2,500 to 3,800 g), pelvic assessment reveals adequacy of the outlet, the position is frank breech, the fetal head is flexed, and the gestational age of the fetus is 36 weeks or more (Toth & Jothivijayrani, 1999).

During the initial assessment the nurse should take into account the gestational age of the fetus, keeping in mind that breech presentations are more frequently found in premature gestations. The nurse should review the client's prenatal history and inquire if a breech presentation has already been suspected or diagnosed, if there is a multiple gestation, or if there has been a prenatal diagnosis of fetal or maternal anomalies. Initial assessment of the gravid abdomen with Leopold's maneuvers may reveal a suspicion of breech presentation. Auscultation of the fetal heart rate at or above the umbilicus may increase this suspicion of a noncephalic presentation. Finally, pelvic assessment may further increase or confirm a breech presentation by palpation of feet, buttocks, or genitalia. Confirmation of presentation with a limited sonographic scan may be permitted as an institutional protocol. Suspicion of breech presentation during the initial maternal assessment should be relayed to the physician or CNM. Care should be taken to avoid rupturing the membranes because there is an increased risk of prolapsed umbilical cord with a noncephalic presentation.

Nursing diagnoses in the management of breech presentation include the risk for fetal injury related to hypoxia from cord prolapse, and injury to the fetal head, neck, soft tissue, and nerves related to traumatic delivery. Potential maternal problems include the risk for hemorrhage and infection related to soft tissue injury or lacerations from operative vaginal or cesarean delivery. Maternal pain, anxiety, and knowledge level are actual diagnoses routinely addressed in all laboring clients.

Maternal and fetal outcomes evolve from both medical and nursing management. The medical plan of care and nursing interventions strive to prevent fetal hypoxia, fetal injury, and maternal hemorrhage and infection. These critical interventions are provided concurrently while promoting physical comfort, ensuring adequate pain management, and offering both emotional and educational support for each obstetric client at high risk.

In order to achieve these outcomes, the professional nurse must continuously monitor and update the maternal-fetal assessment and relay the information to the physician. To prevent injury from cord compression related to prolapse and avoid artificially rupturing the membranes, pelvic examinations should be conducted with care. The nurse also should instruct the client to report suspicion of her membranes rupturing. When membranes rupture spontaneously, the nurse should assess for the presence of the umbilical cord in the vaginal vault. The fetal heart rate should also be assessed to ensure it is stable and within normal range. When the medical plan includes a cesarean section, all health team members required at the surgery should be notified. When a vaginal trial of labor is the plan, the nurse should have a double delivery setup available. A double setup consists of a vaginal delivery table setup and a cesarean section instrument table ready to be opened in the surgical suite. Special instruments such as Piper forceps should be in the room, if not open on the instrument table. The nursery personnel should be made aware of any complicating factors, such as prematurity or fetal anomalies.

Pain interventions should be implemented according to the client's assessed needs. Position changes, back massage, IV medication per physician orders, and regional anesthesia may be used to relieve maternal pain during labor. Labor support, reassurance, client education, and validation of client response to the comfort interventions are all interventions the nurse may employ for pain relief. For cesarean section, regional anesthesia is used when possible to minimize fetal anesthetic effects that could occur with a general anesthetic. The nurse's role may include assisting with client positioning for insertion of the regional anesthetic. Although the client is monitored by the anesthesiologist throughout the cesarean section, monitoring during recovery is within the scope of the nurse's role.

Client anxiety may be heightened by the discomfort of the labor and threat of the unknown. Assessment of baseline knowledge, feelings, and perceptions helps the nurse reassure and educate the client to reduce anxiety. Validating information with the client provides appropriate feedback to promote her emotional and physical support during breech labor or a cesarean section. Manogin, Bechtel, and Rami (2000) reported that providing the laboring client with information about her status and the plan of care for delivery enables her to incorporate the information into her experience and develop a healthier, positive perception of the delivery process.

The nurse caring for the client with breech presentation may be required to function in the role of a circulating nurse during the cesarean section. This role includes preparing the client for the operative procedure (shaving when ordered, insertion of a Foley catheter, and preanesthesia fluid loading) and transporting her, as necessary. The circulating nurse supports the needs of the anesthesiologist and obstetrician during the delivery, records sponge and instrument counts, documents occurrences during the procedure, and ensures both equipment and team readiness to receive the neonate. A cesarean section performed for breech presentation may require additional supplies. Obtaining verification of special requests for supplies from the obstetrician promotes readiness. These supplies may be present in the operative suite unopened, unless needed. After the case is completed, the nurse also may be required to monitor the client during the recovery period.

When a client undergoes a trial of labor for vaginal breech delivery, similar preparations should be anticipated. The physician may request additional personnel to assist with delivery or additional supplies. The labor process may be prolonged related to lack of a firm presenting part to enhance dilatory processes. Augmentation may be required to avoid dystocia, which can result in heightened discomfort and anxiety. The nurse's meticulous attention to client responses to labor discomfort will not only promote client support and better meet pain needs but also should reduce anxiety. At delivery, the physician may request administration of amyl nitrite or nitroglycerin to obtain rapid uterine relaxation should head entrapment become apparent. Having the requested medication readily available reduces delays at a critical time in the delivery.

After delivery, vaginal or operative, rapid feedback to the mother regarding the status of the neonate offers reassurance and reduces additional anxiety. Neonatal assessment for soft tissue injuries, swelling, lack of mobility, and lack of flexion of the extremities is critical once respiratory support and thermoregulation are established. Any deviation from normal neonatal assessment should be reported to the nursery or neonatal staff receiving the infant.

Evaluations of the maternal-fetal outcomes answer several questions.

- Did the fetal heart monitoring provide reassuring rates, accelerations, and variability?
- Did the client experience frank or occult prolapse and compression of the umbilical cord?
- Did the neonate demonstrate effective respirations or require minimal support at delivery?
- Did the neonate experience injury at delivery?
- Was assessment rapid, and were interventions initiated immediately?

- Did the client express adequate pain relief verbally or nonverbally?
- Did maternal-fetal status remain stable throughout pharmacologic interventions?
- Did the client express comfort with the plan of care?
- Were questions by the client asked and answered?
- Did the client verbalize reduced anxiety?
- Did maternal vital signs remain stable?
- Did fluid balance remain stable?
- Did the client experience hemorrhage?
- Did the client experience laceration or hematoma?
- Was aseptic technique observed?
- Did the client or fetus demonstrate signs of infection?

Shoulder Presentation

Transverse lie involves the fetus assuming a more horizontal position in the uterus. This type of lie results in a **shoulder presentation** in which the presenting part of the fetus is the shoulder or combination of shoulder, arm, and hand (Figure 15-3). When the fetal back faces the maternal abdomen, it is referred to an acromiodorsoanterior position. When the fetal back faces the maternal back, it is referred to as an acromiodorsoposterior position. Cunningham et al. (2001) has identified the incidence of transverse lie with shoulder presentation as 1 in 420 singleton deliveries. Common contributing factors for transverse lie and shoulder malpresentation include grand multiparity (as a result of relaxed abdominal musculature), prematurity, multiple gestation, placenta previa, polyhydramnios, and abnormalities of the maternal pelvic structure. When this presentation is identified antenatally, external cephalic version may be attempted to reposition the fetus into cephalic or even breech presentation. Risks to the client include uterine rupture, a high probability of cesarean section, and sepsis if the fetal arm prolapses after membrane rupture and returns through the uterus during cesarean section. Fetal risks include umbilical cord prolapse and fetal injury from attempted and failed version. Medical management is aimed at confirming the transverse lie and shoulder presentation. The usual plan of care is cesarean section once the malpresentation is confirmed.

The nursing assessment is instrumental as a first indicator of malpresentation. A review of maternal prenatal history may promote identification of risk factors. Initial abdominal assessment with Leopold's maneuvers often will identify the transverse or oblique lie. Pelvic assessment may reveal a very high presenting part or no presenting part at all. Care should be exercised to prevent accidental rupture of membranes because this malpresentation also carries a high risk of umbilical cord prolapse. Fetal heart rate assessment should be performed, and the nurse may locate the fetal heart rate at the umbilicus or laterally to it.

From the data obtained in the nursing assessment, the nursing diagnoses should address the risk for the following: fetal injury related to hypoxia from prolapsed umbilical cord or uterine rupture; maternal injury related to hemorrhage from uterine rupture; infection from prolonged labor, with eventual chorioamnionitis; and postoperative infection.

Once malpresentation has been confirmed the nursing plan of care is based on the medical plan of management. Preparation for cesarean section must be completed before the physician attempts external version because the potential for injury exists. Otherwise, the nurse will repeat the interventions for the breech malpresentation in preparing, accompanying, assisting, and monitoring the operative recovery of the client.

Outcome evaluation validates the following: neonatal physical stability at delivery, maternal physical stability during and after cesarean section, maternal coping with and understanding of procedure, and the absence of signs of infections postoperatively.

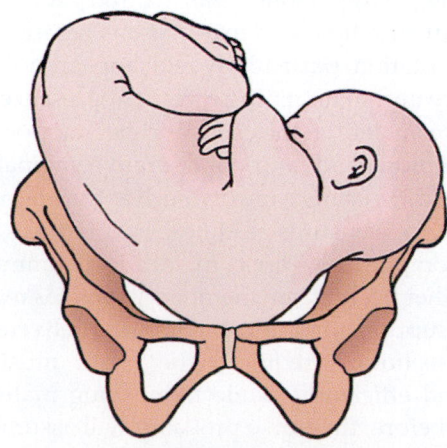

Shoulder presentation
(transverse lie)

Figure 15-3   Shoulder presentation.

Face Presentation

Face presentation occurs when the fetal head is hyperextended and the fetal face descends into the pelvis, as opposed to the flexed position, resulting in fetal vertex presentation. **Brow presentation** occurs when the area between the anterior fontanelle and the fetal eyes descends first (Figure 15-4). *Williams Obstetrics* (Cunningham et al., 2001) reports the incidence of face presentation as 1 in 600,

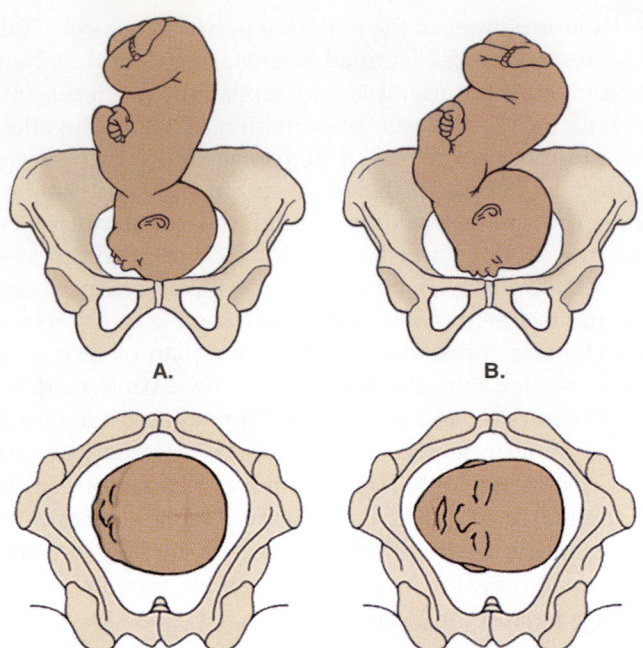

Figure 15-4   A. Brow presentation. B. Face presentation.

or 0.17%. Brow presentation is described as occurring less frequently than does face presentation at a rate of 0.02%, or 1 in 4,470 births. Contributing causes are less clearly defined for face and brow presentations but do include maternal multiparity, fetal macrosomia, fetal anencephaly, and abnormalities of the maternal pelvis. Brow presentation is presumed rare because of its expected conversion to face or occiput presentation to allow vaginal delivery. Unless the maternal pelvis is generously adequate or the fetus is small, persistent brow presentation is not a viable presentation for vaginal birth (Cunningham et al., 2001). This fact may increase the likelihood of prolonged or difficult labor, and failed vaginal delivery, and increases the potential for surgical delivery. Fetal risks for both of these presentations include significant facial edema and bruising and the potential for aggressive interventions at the time of vaginal delivery.

Medical management is expectant in nature, meaning that the client is allowed to labor and her progress is evaluated (Shields & Medearis, 1992a). As stated previously, the brow presentation usually will convert to face or vertex presentation so the fetus can pass through the pelvis. Oxytocin augmentation may be employed for dystocia. When arrested dilation or descent occurs, medical management may then be operative delivery. Aggressive interventions involving midpelvic manipulation are not currently recommended because they increase fetal morbidity and mortality (Shields & Medearis, 1992a).

The nursing assessment should include client history, including perinatal diagnosis of any anomalies or multi-

ple gestation. Estimated gestational age should be documented and verified. Auscultation or fetal monitoring indicates fetal well-being. The pelvic assessment is the one most likely to reveal a nonvertex presentation by palpation of the soft facial features or anterior fontanel to brow. Sonography may be performed to confirm position, flexion, hyperextension, and fetal size.

The nursing diagnoses for the face or brow presentation are similar for all cephalic labors, plus the risk for fetal injury related to the difficult delivery and the potential for infection should operative vaginal or cesarean delivery become necessary. The outcome for the client based on the first additional diagnosis is that the fetus will not incur permanent injury. Realistically, little can be done to avoid the facial edema associated with a face delivery. The other specific diagnosis addresses maternal well-being and absence of postdelivery infection.

The nursing plan should address both vaginal and cesarean delivery potentials. The nurse must continuously monitor maternal labor progress, fetal well-being, and maternal pain and coping behaviors. Ongoing labor assessment allows early identification of abnormal labor processes so that the physician or CNM may intervene with orders for augmentation when deemed appropriate. When augmentation is ordered, nursing actions include careful IV medication administration and monitoring of uterine activity to prevent hyperstimulation, while promoting an effective labor pattern. The nurse also must continuously reassess the fetal response through fetal heart rate monitoring. Communication with the physician or CNM by the nurse is instrumental to being a client advocate. The nurse must assess client pain responses, offer comfort interventions, administer pain medications as ordered, assist with regional anesthesia, and monitor the client after administration of anesthesia. In order to educate and reduce anxiety, the nurse may offer explanations to the client and support persons regarding the plan of care; reason for augmentation; and expectations regarding face or brow presentation, particularly fetal appearance. Offering reassurance and maintaining a vigilant presence also will help reduce anxiety in the client and her support persons.

Preparation in advance for operative vaginal delivery with any additional instruments, such as forceps or vacumn suction devices, ensures readiness and reduces potential delays if complications arise. In addition, communication with the other health team members promotes ready availability of support for the neonate once delivered. When cesarean section is required the nurse must prepare quickly and efficiently, while monitoring maternal-fetal status. As before, the nurse probably will assume the role of circulating nurse during the cesarean section or operative vaginal delivery, and possibly will assume the role of recovery nurse after the procedure. The continuity of the nurse's attendance should reassure the client and limit anxiety throughout the delivery process.

Evaluation of the outcomes unique to face and brow presentations addresses the neonate's stability and presence or absence of injury. Evaluation of maternal pain management and anxiety requires obtaining feedback verbally and observing behavioral responses. Periodic evaluation throughout labor and delivery allows for revision or reinforcement of the nursing interventions to better meet the emotional and educational needs as well as the physical care of the client and her fetus.

Malpositions

Malpositions include persistent occipitoposterior and persistent occipitotransverse positions, which result from fetal rotation as the fetus descends through the pelvis. When the extension process is incomplete, the rotational process also may be incomplete. Fetal and maternal contributing factors include macrosomia and pelvic abnormalities, respectively. A malposition may result in increased discomfort during labor, particularly back pain; prolonged, abnormal labor; soft tissue injury; lacerations; or an extensive episiotomy incision. The fetus in a malposition may experience extensive caput and molding from the sustained occipitotransverse or occipitoposterior position. Caput succedaneum is swelling of a portion of the fetal head most commonly occurring when the head is in the lower portion of the birth canal after the resistance of a rigid vaginal outlet is encountered (Cunningham et al., 2001).

Molding refers to the movement of the bones in the skull of the neonate to fit through the maternal pelvis. The degree to which the neonate's head is capable of molding may make the difference between successful vaginal delivery and cesarean section (Cunningham et al., 2001). When the fetus has macrosomia, the potential exists for shoulder dystocia. **Shoulder dystocia** is a condition in which the fetal shoulders are large and cannot be delivered spontaneously by the maternal pelvis (Figure 15-5). Most cases of malposition resolve spontaneously, and less than 10% fail to resolve (Cunningham et al., 2001). Those cases that do not resolve may be managed with operative vaginal delivery, including outlet forceps to assist delivery in the occipitoposterior position, forceps rotation of the fetal head to an occipitoanterior position, and manual rotation of the fetal head for subsequent delivery (Thompson, 1995; Hankins & Rowe, 1996). When arrest of descent occurs and macrosomia or abnormal pelvic outlet is suspected, the physician may choose delivery by cesarean section.

The nursing assessment should include the historical, physical, emotional, and educational information necessary to plan for the holistic support of the client, her fetus, and her support persons. The history should include information that may indicate macrosomia, such as maternal diabetes, excessive weight gain, results from sonography showing large for gestational age status, and a history of an infant with macrosomia. A history that includes prolonged labor or operative vaginal delivery also may indicate the potential for a malposition to occur. The experienced obstetric nurse may be able to assess malposition during the pelvic examination by denoting fetal suture line and fontanel position in relation to the maternal pelvis. However, assessment becomes much more difficult once significant caput is present. Fetal heart rate monitoring for well-being and labor tolerance should be performed. Uterine activity assessment is necessary to ensure adequacy of contractions and early identification of signs of abnormal labor. Client complaints of pain may be focused on her back when the fetal position is occipitoposterior. Assessing the location of pain allows better intervention and provides indications of fetal position. Client level of knowledge, fear, and anxiety also should be assessed.

The nursing diagnoses address fetal injury, maternal injury, maternal pain, anxiety, and knowledge deficits. The outcomes seek prevention and resolution of these potential or actual problems. Nursing interventions include ongoing assessment of maternal-fetal status and the progression of labor. Particularly useful in converting malpositions in labor are maternal position change laterally or onto her hands and knees in the form of a knee-chest position (Ou, Chen, & Su, 1997). In addition, nursing support for pain management, containment or reduction of anxiety, and client education are essential interventions. Because of the likelihood and intensity of back labor, nursing support should include a variety of comfort measures, including position changes; low back counterpressure during contractions; and the use of, if permitted and

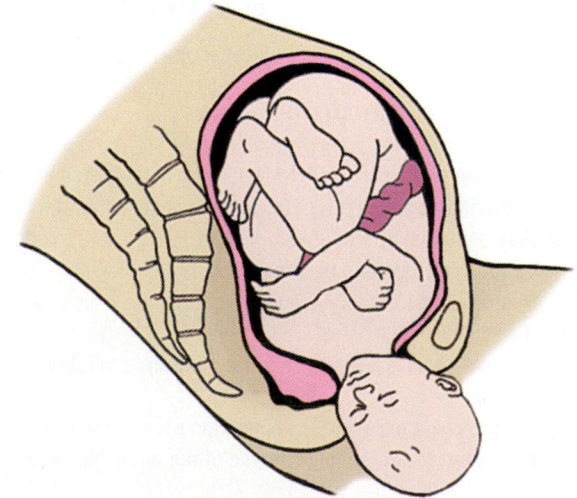

Figure 15-5   Shoulder dystocia.

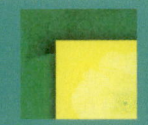

CASE STUDY/CARE PLAN
CLIENT WITH FETAL MALPRESENTATION

Linda is a 29-year-old gravida 2, para 1001 at 39 5/7 weeks' estimated gestational age. She arrives in labor and delivery with her partner, Tim. She states that she is having contractions every 5 minutes and denies that her membranes have ruptured. Her first baby weighed 6 pounds, 7 ounces and was born after 14 hours of labor. Her physician has voiced concern that this baby appears much bigger than that based on ultrasonography, Leopold's maneuvers, and fundal height measurements. After orientation to her room and the unit, Linda is assessed for labor status. External fetal monitoring is applied. Fetal heart tones are located at the maternal umbilicus and are in the 130s. Accelerations are present. Maternal vital signs are the following: temperature, 98°F; pulse, 88; respirations, 18; and blood pressure, 120/72. Pelvic examination reveals cervical dilation of 4 cm, 80% effaced, and −2 station with palpable intact membranes. The presenting part feels softer than a vertex (fetal skull), raising the suspicion of a breech presentation; Linda states she is uncertain what this means for her delivery status.

The nurse finds that critical elements of the assessment are suspicions of a larger baby than the first, who weighed 6 pounds, 7 ounces. In addition, fetal heart tones are located around the maternal umbilicus. Finally, the presenting part seems more like a breech presentation, which is a malpresentation. The cervical dilation of 4 cm may play a role in the face of spontaneous rupture of membranes. In such a case, if the breech presentation is not well applied to the cervix, prolapse of the umbilical cord could occur.

Assessment

- 39 5/7 weeks
- P 88
- BP 120/72
- T 98°F
- R 18
- 4 cm dilated
- −2 station
- FH status

Nursing Diagnosis

Risk for injury (fetal) related to possible umbilical cord prolapse with spontaneous rupture of membranes, soft tissue injury, or nerve compression from macrosomia or a complex delivery owing to malpresentation, as evidenced by signs of acute fetal cord compression or fetal trauma after operative or cesarean birth.

Expected Outcome	Fetus will not incur injury from cord prolapse or complex delivery maneuvers.
Planning	Alert care team to potential risks and prepare for emergency procedures.
NOC	Risk detection
NIC	Electronic fetal monitoring: Intrapartum

Nursing Interventions	Rationales
1. Report to the physician or CNM suspicion of malpresentation. Supplemental confirmation of large baby is also important because a vaginal breech delivery is probably not the option of choice for this client due to large fetal size.	1. Medical management is necessary to carefully assess fetal presentation, fetal size, maternal pelvic size, and mode of delivery.
2. Order and report ultrasonography results to the physician or CNM.	2. Information about presentation and fetal weight is critical to determining course of action.
3. Monitor maternal vital signs and fetal tolerance to labor.	3. Constant monitoring of maternal and fetal well-being is most important in fetal malpresentation.
4. Instruct the client to report any sensation of ruptured membranes and to be alert for potential prolapse of the umbilical cord.	4. With a breech presentation, a significant fetal risk includes umbilical cord prolapse.

(continues)

Evaluation	Fetal vital signs are stable and cord did not prolapse before delivery. Fetal tracing showed no cord compression. No fetal injuries, bruising, brachial nerve compression, or hip problems were noted.

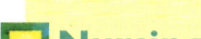 Nursing Diagnosis

Risk for injury (maternal) related to operative procedure, as evidenced by postoperative infection, hemorrhage, or hematuria.

Expected Outcome	Client will not experience postoperative infection or injury from operative delivery.
Planning	Prepare client for postdelivery care procedures so that she may anticipate and accept nursing care measures.
NOC	Risk control
NIC	Risk identification

Nursing Interventions	**Rationales**
1. Preoperative procedures to minimize the risk for infection and operative injury may include abdominal shaving and preparation and insertion of an in-dwelling Foley catheter.	1. These steps will reduce the risk of infection.
2. Give Tim appropriate scrubs and position for procedure to support Linda without contaminating surgical setup.	2. Partner participation in the birth process must be in line with the need to maintain a sterile environment.
3. After surgery, carefully monitor the client according to postanesthesia unit standards to minimize the risk of postoperative complications.	3. Febrile morbidity is rather frequent after cesarean deliveries because of postpartum infection.

Evaluation	Maternal vital signs are stable and there is no maternal fever or signs of infection, hemorrhage, or shock.

Nursing Diagnosis

Anxiety (maternal and family) related to altered plans for childbirth experience and unfamiliarity with the management of breech presentation, as evidenced by client verbalization and nonverbal behaviors.

Expected Outcome	Client and support persons will verbalize concerns regarding birth plans, alterations, and possible management, while demonstrating effective mechanisms for coping with the stress of the labor and delivery process.
Planning	Work with client and partner so they understand and accept the delivery options that are now likely.
NOC	Anxiety level
NIC	Anxiety reduction

Nursing Interventions	**Rationales**
1. Remain in the room with the client while the attending physician or CNM visits with the client and family, and listen to the plan of care and how it is presented.	1. This enables the nurse to reinforce the plan of care with the client and family.
2. Answer client questions regarding the attendance of her partner, Tim, at the scheduled cesarean section and access to infant after delivery.	2. Client education and support reduces anxiety and stress.

(continues)

Evaluation	Client and family verbalized and demonstrated effective coping with the altered plan of a cesarean section.

Nursing Diagnosis

Acute pain (maternal) related to an active labor pattern, as evidenced by verbalization and nonverbal behaviors.

Expected Outcome	Client will verbalize effective pain relief from pharmacologic and nonpharmacologic interventions.
Planning	Help client to mentally prepare for the impending labor and delivery.
NOC	Pain control
NIC	Pain management

Nursing Interventions	Rationales
1. Use positional comfort interventions along with lower back counterpressure to assist the client. Reassess labor progress and FHR.	1. Comfort measures, including frequent position changes, low back counterpressure, and appropriate pain control are all nursing support measures aimed at reducing client anxiety and facilitating labor progression.
2. Consult the anesthesia service for consideration of regional anesthesia and analgesia for vaginal or cesarean delivery.	2. Imminent cesarean delivery will require appropriate preparation.
3. Assess FHR and cervical dilation. Administer pharmacologic agents as ordered after informed consent is obtained for both treatment and anesthesia.	3. Pharmacologic and nonpharmacologic measures combined will provide the greatest measure of client relief.

Evaluation	Client verbalizes effective pain relief.

requested, epidural anesthesia. IV anesthesia also is helpful but should not be used late in labor to avoid fetal sedation and fetal respiratory depression at delivery. Additional needs for vaginal delivery, such as forceps or vacumn suction devices, should be anticipated and equipment made available. Evaluations should obtain the objective and subjective feedback necessary to determine whether interventions have been successful or require revision. Interventions are successful when no fetal or maternal trauma occurs, pain is adequately managed, and the clients' anxiety and educational needs are met.

MATERNAL AND FETAL STRUCTURAL ABNORMALITIES

Variations in maternal and fetal structural proportions that may result in high-risk deliveries include cephalopelvic disproportion and macrosomia.

Cephalopelvic Disproportion

Cephalopelvic disproportion (CPD) exists when the maternal pelvis cannot accommodate the fetal head as it descends. A contracted maternal pelvis and fetal macrosomia con-

tribute to CPD (Bashore, 1992). A **contracted maternal pelvis** refers to abnormalities in measurements that fall short of those required for an average delivery. Congenital or acquired (from trauma) pelvic deviations may exist. Relative CPD is said to exist when the fetus is larger than the maternal pelvic inlet-outlet or when the fetal position places the head at an angle that is larger than the size the pelvis can facilitate. Relative CPD is particularly important when considering the mode of delivery for subsequent pregnancies. A 1998 study that reviewed cesarean deliveries for CPD showed that 68% of the women successfully delivered their subsequent neonate vaginally and 47% had larger babies (Impey & O'Herlihy, 1998). These data should encourage practitioners, including nurses, not to predetermine the mode of delivery for clients attempting trial of labor who have a history of cesarean section for CPD. Contracted maternal pelvic outlets are reported in less than 1% of the delivering population. The reported incidence of macrosomia using 4,000 g as the weight index is 5.1%. Using 4,500 g as the weight index, the incidence is 0.4% (Cunningham et al., 2001).

Contributing factors for CPD include congenital nongynecoid pelvic (flattened, narrow, or irregular) shape or post-traumatic contractures as a result of a crushed or fractured pelvis. The risks to the laboring client are a prolonged and painful labor and failure of the cervix to dilate or the fetus to descend, with resultant need for operative delivery. The potential also exists for maternal uterine rupture from prolonged thinning of the lower uterine segment during a nonprogressive but active labor process. Fetal risks include extensive caput and molding from the prolonged labor; fetal intolerance, with resultant hypoxia from the prolonged labor; and the potential for birth injury related to a difficult and traumatic delivery.

Medical management will carefully assess pelvic and fetal sizes. Sonography may be beneficial, although estimates of fetal weight with very large fetuses are not very reliable. X-ray pelvimetry measures were more commonly used several years ago but offer true pelvic measures. The management of labor may be expectant when labor activity is adequate, or augmentation may be attempted when the contraction pattern is not regular or firm. At the point of delivery in CPD, the physician may attempt outlet forceps delivery or vacuum suction to assist in delivering the fetus vaginally. When measurements or these interventions are not satisfactory, or the fetal heart rate demonstrates intolerance of the delivery process, the physician may order preparations for cesarean delivery.

The nursing assessment history may help identify a pelvic adequacy problem. Risk factors are maternal diabetes, previous prolonged labor, previous fetal or maternal trauma at delivery, previous need for operative vaginal delivery (extensive episiotomy, use of forceps or vacuum extraction), and previous cesarean delivery. Leopold's maneuvers may reveal a fetus that is not well descended into the maternal pelvis. Pelvic examination that identifies caput or molding, particularly while the fetus remains at station 0 or higher, may indicate a problem. Pelvic examination by the nurse that fails to reveal cervical change hourly despite regular contractions that are moderate to firm in intensity also may be significant in identifying CPD. These assessment variables help to indicate potential CPD; however, they do not preclude the initial thorough and complete assessment of maternal-fetal status or the dynamic elements that are reassessed every 5, 15, 30, or 60 minutes, depending on the stage of labor, client risk status, and fetal tolerance (Feinstein & McCartney, 1997).

Nursing diagnoses address the risks for maternal and fetal injury and infection and the concerns for maternal pain, anxiety, and lack of knowledge during labor and delivery. Desired outcomes designate that no fetal or maternal injury or infection will occur, and adequate pain and anxiety management and appropriate education will be achieved.

While the nursing interventions to meet the above outcomes may seem routine, the dynamics of the potential problem require the nurse to be alert for changes that are either reassuring or nonreassuring in nature. The in-dividualization of the emotional and educational support as well as the unique interaction between the nurse and each client prevent the experience from being routine or less than challenging. The client experiencing CPD or relative CPD may experience a prolonged labor process and require extensive medical intervention for an operative vaginal delivery, or she may need to undergo a cesarean section. The nurse does not control the medical management of labor and eventual delivery; however, assisting the client to achieve optimal delivery outcomes with a minimum of negative occurrences is a nursing role. Evaluation of successful or less than successful outcomes provides the nurse with feedback from which new interventions or further support can be applied.

Macrosomia

Macrosomia is a cause of relative cephalopelvic disproportion. The increased size of the fetus can make passage through an adequate-sized pelvis difficult or impossible. As stated previously, macrosomia is more common than are contracted maternal pelvic disorders, with a 5.1% incidence (Cunningham et al., 2001). When the fetus does descend, the passage may be further complicated by delivery of the fetal head but then halted abruptly because of shoulder dystocia. Shoulder dystocia occurs when the fetal shoulder width is so large that it is not deliverable beneath the maternal symphysis pubis without additional delivery intervention or fetal injury. Shoulder dystocia occurs when the anterior shoulder of the fetus is aligned with the anteroposterior line of the pelvis and becomes lodged behind the symphysis pubis; the alignment is appropriate but the size of the shoulders prevents anterior shoulder progression toward delivery; or the posterior shoulder becomes lodged behind the sacral promontory (Hall, 1997). The delivery of the shoulders can be extremely difficult for the mother to experience, and fetal injury may be impossible to prevent regardless of the skill and experience of the physician or CNM. Shoulder dystocia is considered an obstetric emergency (Hall, 1997; Wagner, Nielsen, & Gonik, 1999). The reported incidence of shoulder dystocia varies from 0.2% to 2% because of variable definitions of true shoulder dystocia. Within this range, the low percentages are attributable to those cases requiring classic delivery maneuvers and the high percentages are based on fetal weights with documentation of shoulder dystocia (Cunningham et al., 2001; Hall, 1997).

The literature shows that the most frequent risk factor leading to shoulder dystocia is macrosomia (Cunningham et al., 2001; Hall, 1997; Lewis et al., 1998; Wagner et al., 1999). Other risk factors include concurrent maternal diabetes, a history of a previous large infant, prolonged second stage of labor, and excessive weight gain during pregnancy (Toohey et al., 1995; Lewis et al., 1998). Less

Reflections from a Mother

I was feeling very alone as I neared my due date. I had friends, but the father of my baby was not involved. My parents tried to be supportive. However, they were not pleased with my status as a single pregnant woman. When I arrived in labor and delivery in active labor, I was scared and hurting terribly from my contractions. When the nurses saw the heart beat on the monitor everything began to happen very fast. I had three people working on me at the same time. I had an oxygen mask on my face, and the smell of plastic was awful. My parents' faces had looks of concern and fear. They stood away from me while everyone was busy working on me. I was so scared!

Then I saw Marta. She is a nurse who was called into my room when the other nurses saw my baby's heart beat recording. She calmed everyone down, and they worked fast without panic. She explained what was happening and why. She assured me my doctor was aware of what was happening and was coming immediately. She asked me if I had questions, and then she asked my parents. She brought my mother to one side and let her hold my hand. Up until then, my mother and I had said little to each other because of her disappointment in me. Now, however, we just held hands and prayed my baby would be okay.

Marta seemed to calm everyone. When my baby did not respond to the oxygen, IV fluids, and all the different positions they had me move to, she appeared concerned but did not panic. My doctor came in and confirmed her expectations for a cesarean section. Even though everything happened very fast, I trusted Marta. She stayed with me and encouraged me throughout my surgery. She showed me my baby as soon as he was ok. She explained to me the things that were around me. I wasn't scared with everyone working around me, because she told me they would help my baby adjust to being outside. I have a healthy son, Aaron, because the labor and delivery team worked so hard and fast. I have a good memory of my experience because of Marta.

clear as risks but still frequently believed to be contributory are advanced maternal age, previous history of gestational diabetes, multiparity, short maternal stature, and maternal obesity (Hall, 1997; Lewis et al., 1998). Two acronyms summarize the risk factors that should be assessed routinely: Diabetes Obesity Postterm Excessive (DOPE) fetal or maternal weight gain, and Age + DOPE (ADOPE) (Cunningham et al., 2001; Hall, 1997).

Risks to the client that are related to shoulder dystocia include soft tissue injury; bladder injury; cervical, vaginal, or perineal lacerations; separation of the symphysis pubis; uterine rupture; postpartum hemorrhage; and cesarean section (Hall, 1997). Risks to the fetus include fractures of the clavicle and humerus and nerve damage, resulting in Erb's or Klumpke's palsy. Erb's palsy affects mobility of the upper arm; Klumpke's palsy affects mobility of the lower arm and hand and tone. The fetus also may experience increased intracranial pressure, hypoxia, acidosis, and asphyxia (Cunningham et al., 2001).

Medical management is determined by early identification of risk factors and consideration of delivery op-

tions. Both early elective induction and scheduled cesarean section have been evaluated for delivery of infants with macrosomia whose mothers have diabetes, with variable results (Gonen et al., 1998; Conway & Langer, 1998; Wagner et al., 1999). These measures are anticipatory in nature. Many times, however, shoulder dystocia must be dealt with at the time of occurrence.

Nursing considerations are significant in the recognition of and intervention for shoulder dystocia. The nurse's initial and ongoing assessments during labor may be the first data indicating shoulder dystocia. Labor delays, particularly with fetal descent, should be communicated to the physician or CNM. Pronounced caput or molding even at a relatively high station (above zero) may also be indicative of impending shoulder dystocia. Observation during maternal pushing may allow recognition of the turtle sign. The **turtle sign** occurs when the fetal head pulls back instead of completing the external rotation process and progressing forward into the maternal perineum. The appearance is as if the head is retracting back into the shell of the pelvis. Once the head is delivered, the inability to deliver the anterior shoulder beneath the symphysis pubis with gentle traction is diagnostic of shoulder dystocia (Hall, 1997; Cunningham et al., 2001).

The nurse should remain with the physician or CNM and call from the room for assistance. Once shoulder dystocia is recognized, constant monitoring of fetal status at 1-minute intervals is essential. Fetal acidosis can begin after 5 minutes. The fetus may experience low Apgar scores or signs of asphyxia after only 7 to 10 minutes (Hall, 1997). Several maneuvers may be used by the physician or CNM to complete the delivery process. It is essential that the nurse remain calm to assist in delivery, reduce the client's anxiety, and facilitate client cooperation while these maneuvers are being attempted (Hall, 1997; Simpson, 1999).

The McRoberts maneuver requires maternal position changes in which the client's legs are bent at the knees and hyperflexed against her abdomen to straighten the sacrum and alter the angle, allowing for the anterior shoulder to be dislodged (Figure 15-6). Preferably two nurses assist the mother, with one nurse supporting each leg in the hyperflexed position while the physician or CNM attempts to complete the delivery. When reviewed as a first procedure used for reducing shoulder dystocia, the McRoberts maneuver was successful in 47% of cases. The remaining deliveries reviewed required additional interventions (Gherman et al., 1997).

Suprapubic pressure is another procedure that the nurse may be requested to perform. By applying suprapubic pressure either in an oblique or lateral approach (Rubin technique) or posteriorly and laterally (Mazzanti technique), the anterior shoulder may be compressed and slip beneath the symphysis pubis (Figure 15-7). These techniques may be combined with maternal pushing, or the client may be requested not to push and rely only on the traction of the physician or CNM. The client's bladder should be empty to prevent trauma. The nurse may have already emptied the bladder before delivery, or the physician or CNM may do so before performing these maneuvers.

The other maneuvers employed for shoulder dystocia are more invasive in nature. They include the Woods corkscrew maneuver in which the physician or CNM places his or her fingers within the vagina against the anterior chest wall of the fetus to push the posterior shoulder back and rotate it 180 degrees. Either shoulder may deliver as a result of this maneuver. The physician may request that the nurse apply suprapubic pressure to keep the anterior shoulder in an adducted position. The Rubin maneuver requires the physician or CNM to place his or her fingers within the vagina against the scapula of the anterior shoulder and rotate it forward 180 degrees. This maneuver also may be used to rotate the posterior shoulder anteriorly. Once again, the nurse may be requested to provide suprapubic pressure. When the rotational maneuvers are unsuccessful in dislodging the shoulders and delivering the fetus, the physician may then attempt to deliver the posterior arm. In this procedure, a hand is inserted into the vagina to the posterior arm to trace the path to the elbow, allowing flexion, retrieval, and delivery of the arm. This procedure allows for room to dislodge the anterior shoulder. This maneuver may result in fracture of the fetal humerus. When these maneuvers fail, the fetal head may be rotated to direct occipitoanterior position and pressure applied to replace the head within the pelvis

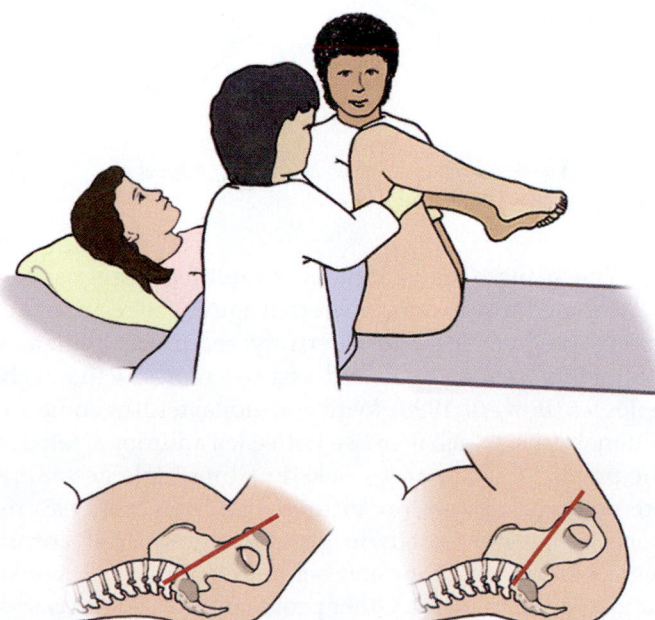

Figure 15-6   In the McRoberts maneuver, the client's legs are bent at the knees and hyperflexed against her abdomen. The result is straightening of the sacrum and altering of the angle, allowing the shoulder to dislodge.

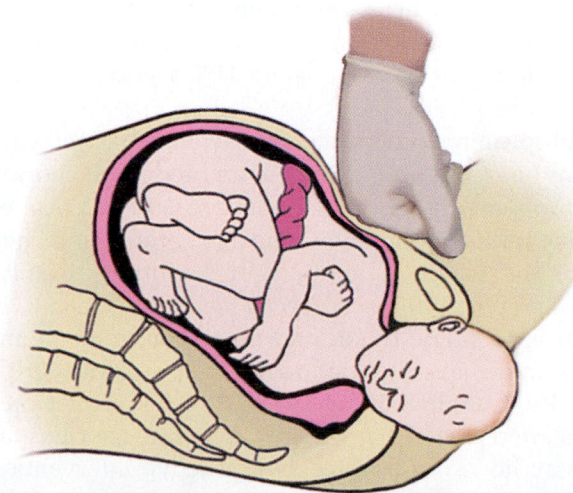

Figure 15-7   Suprapubic pressure may release shoulder dystocia.

for retrieval through emergent cesarean section. The person supporting the head will remain in that position until the cesarean is complete and the fetus delivered. The morbidity is much higher with this procedure; however, the alternative may be stillbirth when the shoulders cannot be delivered vaginally (Hall, 1997; Cunningham et al., 2001).

Nursing diagnoses for macrosomia include risks of fetal injury and fetal hypoxia, risks of maternal injury and infection, as well as the usual nursing diagnoses. The outcomes seek to prevent negative outcomes from occurring. Interventions during the labor process focus on the ongoing assessment that indicates possible shoulder dystocia, communicating concerns effectively, remaining with the physician or CNM, calling for help, remaining calm, offering reassurance and information to the client and support persons, assisting with maneuvers, notifying nursery personnel, and documenting the events that transpired as accurately and systematically as possible (Hall, 1997; Simpson, 1999).

MULTIPLE GESTATION

Multiple gestation refers to the carrying of more than one fetus during the same pregnancy (Figure 15-8). With the increase in infertility management and assisted reproductive technology, such as in vitro and gamete transfer technology, the incidence of twins, triplets, and higher-order gestations (quadruplets, quintuplets, and so on) has increased significantly. Bowers (1998) reviewed the 1995 U.S. statistics and found there were 96,736 neonates born alive as twins, 4,551 as triplets, 365 as quadruplets, and 57 as quintuplets or higher-order multiple births. In 1990, the reported incidence of twins was 1 in 43 live births and that of triplets was 1 in 1,341 live births. Ovulation induction and assisted reproductive technology are identified as the causes of 83% of triplet pregnancies and 95% of quadruplet pregnancies (Eganhouse & Petersen, 1998). Higher-order pregnancies, inclusive of triplets, have increased rapidly at approximately 11% a year since 1997 (Bowers, 1998).

Multiple fetus pregnancies are evaluated for separate amnions and chorions. Shared amnion and chorions allow for shared placental circulations and physical entanglement issues. Shared placentas, amnions, and chorions are the result of monozygotic splitting. *Williams Obstetrics* reports that *monozygotic twinning*, (when twins occur from a single ovum and may share a single placenta, amnion, and chorion) occurs in approximately 1 in 250 births (Cunningham et al., 2001). Most triplet pregnancies are reported as trizygotic (separate chorions and amnions); however, assisted reproductive interventions have increased the likelihood of monozygotic triplets (Eganhouse & Petersen, 1998).

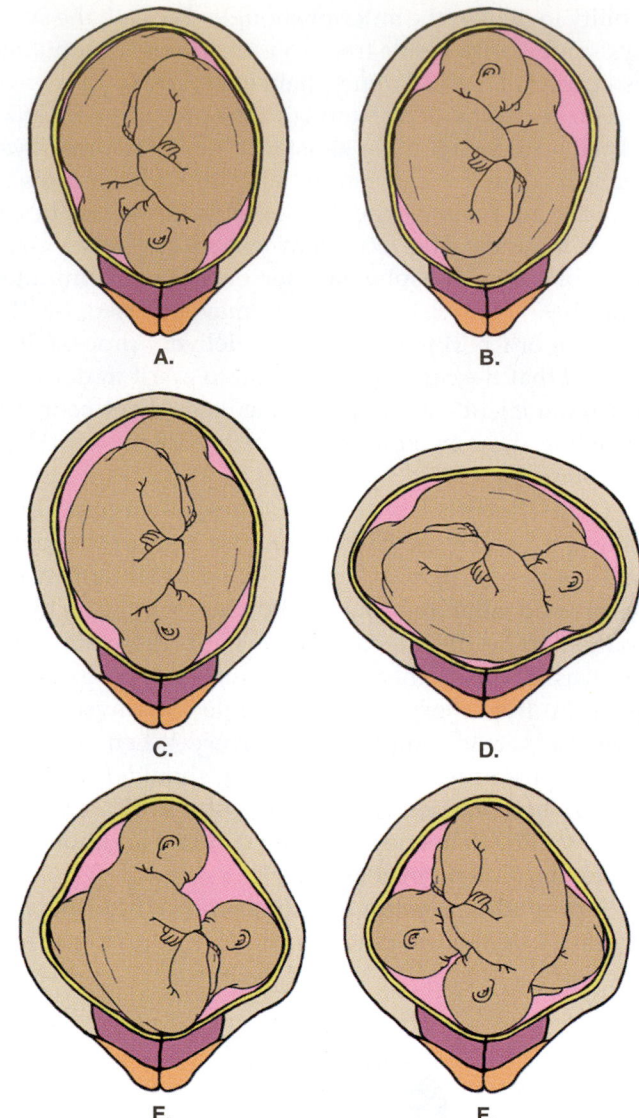

Figure 15-8   Twin fetuses can assume any number of presentations.

The increase in the number of multifetus pregnancies is attributed to advanced maternal age as the result of delaying pregnancies and infertility requiring ovulatory stimulation medications and assisted reproductive technologies (Bowers, 1998). With additional fetuses come additional risks, which increase with each additional fetus in the pregnancy. The major risks in all multiple gestations are prematurity and low birth weight. Bowers (1998) reported that 47.9% of twin gestations and 87.8% of all higher-order gestations end before the 37th week, unlike singleton pregnancies. Other problems are also increased, with twin gestations experiencing an overall complication rate at least twice that of singleton pregnancies. Triplets and higher-order multiples experience much higher complication rates than do twins. Over 92% of higher-order multiples fall into the low-birth-weight category, and 35%

are reported as having very low birth weights (Bowers, 1998). In addition, the infant death rate for higher-order multiples exceeds that of singleton gestations by 12 times.

Among the fetal risks are *conjoining abnormalities* (when twins have incomplete separation and demonstrate a common organ or portion of the body), placental abnormalities, twin-to-twin transfusions, and discordant fetal growth (when the growth of one twin exceeds that of the other(s) by at least 25%). Cerebral palsy and other neurologic impairments, stillbirth, glucose instability at birth, and birth injuries also occur more frequently (Cunningham et al., 2001). Fetal mortality ranges from 9.8% to 13.6% (Eganhouse & Petersen, 1998). Perinatal mortality is described as being five times higher for twin gestations than for singleton pregnancies (Ellings, Newman, & Bowers, 1998).

Maternal complications of multiple gestations also increase with the number of fetuses carried. All of the physiologic changes that occur to the client carrying a singleton gestation are increased to the extreme with multiple gestations. These include cardiac output, diastolic blood pressure, plasma volume, and venous distention. In contrast, maternal cardiac reserve, pulmonary residual volumes, and even gastrointestinal tone and motility are decreased (Bowers, 1998). Problems that can occur with pregnancy, such as anemia, pyelonephritis, cholelithiasis and cholestasis, peripartum cardiomyopathy, and fatty liver disease, are more likely to occur in women with multiple gestations; and preexisting chronic problems affecting any organ system are likely to be exacerbated (Bowers, 1998). Maternal challenges also include increased nutritional demands, increased discomforts and compromises from uterine distention, and the risk for preterm labor. The complications that result from treating these problems also are challenges for the client. Pre-eclampsia, uterine atony after delivery, and postpartum hemorrhage are also risks the client with multiple gestation faces (Shields & Medearis, 1992b; Ellings et al., 1998). Psychosocial risks for the client and support persons include the incorporation of the multiple fetuses into the client's and the family's pregnancy plan and adaptation; acceptance as a high-risk obstetric client; altered activities, including prolonged hospitalizations; financial concerns related to the loss of income and hospital costs; and the overriding fear of potential fetal loss (Bowers, 1998; Sather & Zwelling, 1998). The potential for anxiety and depression related to all of the concerns listed is well documented in families of multiple gestations (Leonard, 1998).

Medical management of the multiple gestation surrounds early diagnosis, monitoring of maternal and fetal well-being, and interventions as indicated in the face of complications. Medical surveillance may rely on laboratory values (for anemia), sonogram data (to assess fetal growth, chorionicity, and complications such as entanglement of cords) (Aisenbrey et al., 1995), fetal viability, and cervical assessment (for stable labor status). Intrapartum management of multiple gestations may consider vaginal delivery for twins; however, many twins and all higher-order gestations are delivered by cesarean section.

Nursing considerations for the client and her support persons experiencing a multiple gestation are numerous. Whether the client is receiving nursing care in a high-risk antepartum hospitalization, is trying to halt the threat of preterm labor, or is in labor and delivery for her high-risk delivery, the nurse will be an integral part of a multidisciplinary team. The focus of care is to minimize or prevent antepartal and intrapartum complications (Bowers, 1998). The need for emotional support also is tremendous (Sather & Zwelling, 1998). The thoroughness of the nursing assessment is critical to identify even subtle concerns or changes in maternal-fetal status. The assessment should focus on maternal stability, fetal well-being with serial nonstress testing, and the absence or presence of uterine activity recorded on the fetal monitor. Psychosocial assessment should address the client's adaptation to the multiple pregnancy, the current situation, anticipatory grief processes, basic knowledge, coping skills, the ability to cooperate with the plan of care, and her support system (Bowers, 1998; Sather & Zwelling, 1998). An awareness of the potential for peripartum depression is particularly important. The nurse may facilitate the client in seeking additional support that may reduce the likelihood of impaired maternal-infant attachment or even neglect or abuse (Leonard, 1998). The nurse may become the hub of the team by communicating needs, problems, plans, and readiness to other team members, such as the physician, the neonatal nursery team, social services, pastoral care, lactation support persons, and postpartum caregivers. An additional benefit to the client is provided through the nurse's consistent presence in an organized and calm environment (Bowers, 1998). Readiness for delivery and the necessary fetal and neonatal support are essential to prevent delay in resuscitative efforts or stabilization of all neonates. Perioperative procedures should be strictly observed to reduce the potential for infection. Provision of information and answering of questions should be done to meet the client's and support person's educational needs and reduce anxiety.

Evaluations of outcomes for the client and her neonates in a multiple gestation require review of the events.

- Was preterm labor halted long enough to achieve fetal viability, growth, and optimal survival?
- Did the delivery result in minimal problems for the fetuses and mother?
- Were the emotional needs of the client and her family met?

- Were resources consulted to assist with social and economic challenges?
- Were spiritual needs, inclusive of grief, addressed and supported?

The challenge of providing care for the client with multiple gestation is becoming more frequent and requires that the nurse provide highly technical care coupled with careful attention to the emotional well-being of the whole family.

FETAL DISTRESS

Nonreassuring fetal status, inclusive of the term **fetal distress**, refers to the response of the fetus to the antepartum or intrapartum uterine environment. Distress refers to the lack of fetal reserve or presence of fetal hypoxia, acidosis, or asphyxia. The fetal monitor tracing may demonstrate repetitive late decelerations; loss of variability; increasing baseline; or deep prolonged decelerations, with failure to return to baseline. A low scalp pH may indicate distress. A poor biophysical profile score also may indicate fetal compromise.

Any pregnant client may demonstrate a nonreassuring fetal status. It is safe to assume, however, that obstetric clients with high-risk conditions, such as prematurity, postmaturity, infectious processes, hemorrhagic conditions, and pre-eclampsia, are more likely to experience problems. Fetal risk factors include permanent injury or death as a result of sustained hypoxia, with resultant acidosis and asphyxia. Maternal risks include the potential for operative vaginal or cesarean section, once the condition is diagnosed, and the resultant complications.

Concurrent medical management depends on whether the client is antepartal or intrapartal and the extent of the nonreassuring data. For example, when a client who is antepartal undergoes a fetal nonstress test that is nonreactive, despite adequate maternal hydration and various fetal stimulation interventions, the physician or CNM may choose to obtain a biophysical profile or other evaluation of the fetus. In contrast, when a client who is antepartal demonstrates **oligohydramnios** (less than 5 cm total of four quadrant measurements) on a biophysical profile along with a nonreactive stress test, the physician or CNM may choose to deliver. A client who is intrapartal and demonstrates deep variables in labor may respond to interventions and continue without additional problems. In contrast, the client who is intrapartal and demonstrates deep variables, decreasing variability, lack of accelerations, and delayed return to the baseline may require immediate delivery.

Nursing assessment of fetal status is critical. Fetal heart rate baseline, variability, the presence of periodic or nonperiodic accelerations, the presence of periodic or

Nursing Tip — *Amnioinfusion*

Amnioinfusion may be ordered to be performed at a bolus rate (up to 800 mL at one instillation); continuous flow rate (3 mL/min); or combination of an initial bolus (600 to 800 mL at 10 to 15 mL/min followed by continuation at 3 mL/min), with a subsequent continuous flow rate. Amnioinfusion requires ruptured membranes and an intact intrauterine pressure catheter (IUPC), preferably a double-lumen one. You must:

1. Check the functioning of the IUPC.
2. Connect the primed tubing by way of the controller pump to the instillation port of the IUPC. Set the rate for bolus or continuous flow.
3. Use warmed solution, which is standard practice; some policies require a warmer to maintain temperature.
4. Monitor the maternal abdomen for tension, the perineum for outflow of fluid on the hip pad, and the fetal tracing for symptomatic relief of cord compression.
5. Discontinue as per orders or if complications arise (e.g., no fluid return and fetal intolerance).
6. Document preinfusion data, amount, maternal fetal response, and tolerance to amnioinfusion.

Note. Adapted from a protocol in "Fluid Check: Making the Case for Intrapartum Amnioinfusion," by J. Schmidt, 1997, AWHONN Lifelines, 1(7), pp. 47–51.

nonperiodic decelerations, depth, and duration should all be assessed in detail. Maternal status that can affect fetal response, including position, maternal infection, hydration, uterine activity, blood pressure, and medication, also must be assessed. Psychosocial elements, such as anxiety, pain, and lack of knowledge, also may affect maternal tolerance and thus fetal oxygenation.

The nursing plan is based on the initial and ongoing maternal-fetal assessment. Nursing interventions specifically used to increase fetal oxygenation may include use of maternal position changes to either side or even a modified knee-chest position to relieve pressure on the umbilical cord in utero. The nurse may apply supplemental oxygen by face mask at 8 to 10 L/min to enhance maternal-fetal oxygenation; increase IV fluid hydration to correct dehydration or dilute oxytocin stimulatory effects; and reduce or discontinue oxytocin uterine stimulation, particularly in the face of hyperstimulation. The nurse may be able to increase the accuracy of fetal monitoring by applying an internal fetal electrode for direct electrocardiogram monitoring or inserting an intrauterine pressure catheter (IUPC) to accurately assess intrauterine pressure during contractions and at rest. Application of these devices may be done by individual order, standing order, or critical pathway orders. Application should be done by the physician, CNM, or a nurse with additional expertise and experience. Each institution has policy parameters for performing these procedures based on the nursing practice act of the state and community norms. The nurse may be requested to start, maintain, and monitor an *amnioinfusion*, which is an invasive procedure that instills warm fluid into the uterine cavity by infusion pump to increase fluid volume and relieve pressure on the umbilical cord. This procedure also serves to dilute thick meconium and, therefore, may reduce the likelihood of meconium aspiration syndrome (Schmidt, 1997). Finally, in the face of nonreassuring responses, the nurse needs to make preparations for an emergent delivery.

Although not specific for fetal distress, the nurse also must incorporate general nursing monitoring and support interventions for client well-being. It is critical that the nurse maintain excellent channels of communication with the physician or CNM to discuss maternal-fetal status, interventions, and results. The intervention process should be calmly explained to reassure the client and support persons, convey concern and confidence in the interventions, and help reduce the overall level of anxiety. Finally, communication with the neonatal team is also important so that the members can prepare for any neonatal resuscitative efforts.

UTERINE RUPTURE

Uterine rupture involves a separation of the uterine wall that may allow protrusion of fetal parts into the maternal abdomen. A longitudinal rupture, sometimes referred to as a classic rupture, occurs over the body of the uterus and is an acute emergent situation. Maternal shock and fetal distress may quickly become apparent to the nurse providing care. Uterine rupture of a low transverse segment over a scar from a previous low transverse cesarean section may have less acute symptoms; however, all ruptures place the mother and fetus at risk. Ruptures are classified as complete and incomplete. A complete rupture extends into the peritoneal cavity; an incomplete rupture maintains peritoneal integrity. Dehiscence refers to the separation of the old scar line and does not result in protrusion of fetal parts into the peritoneal cavity (Cunningham et al., 2001).

The rate of uterine rupture varies by institution, with reported incidences ranging from 1 in 1,280 to 1 in 3,000 deliveries (Cunningham et al., 2001). One 10-year review from Singapore has revealed an incidence of 1 in 6,331 de-

liveries, with a ratio of three previous cesarean scarred uteri to one unscarred uterus (Chen, Tan, & Yeo, 1995). The incidence of rupture in an unscarred uterus is even less common and has been reported in one study as 1 in 16,849 deliveries (Miller, Goodwin, Gherman, & Paul, 1997). Contributing factors to uterine rupture include a previous cesarean scar, major surgery involving the uterus, such as a myomectomy; congenital abnormality of the uterus; grand multiparity; and use of oxytocin or prostaglandins (Al Sakka, Dauleh, & Al Hassani, 1999; Caughey et al., 1999; Kirkendall, Jauregui, Kim, & Phelan, 2000; Cunningham et al., 2001; Miller et al., 1997). Rupture also has been reported when forceps were used (Miller et al., 1997). Blunt trauma also has been associated with spontaneous uterine rupture (Cunningham et al., 2001). There have been reports, although rare, of spontaneous rupture of the unscarred primigravid uterus in the absence of uterine trauma or an infectious process. The second such case ever recorded was associated with an abnormally implanted placenta (**placenta percreta**; abnormal placental attachment that completely penetrates the uterine myometrium) in the second trimester and occurred as a spontaneous acute event (Imseis, Murtha, Alexander, & Barnett, 1998).

Maternal consequences of rupture include hypovolemic shock, bladder injury, anemia, emergent hysterectomy, anemia, transfusion, bowel injury, and death; fetal and neonatal outcomes include low Apgar scores, brain damage, intrapartal death, and neonatal or infant death (Kirkendall et al., 2000). Admissions to the neonatal intensive care unit and increased neonatal acidosis at delivery also have been associated with uterine rupture (Menihan, 1998).

Medical management of uterine rupture includes identification of risk factors, such as the client being a candidate for vaginal birth after cesarian section; careful management of all intrapartum clients; and surgical intervention and repair, as indicated. Clients who have had previous cesarean sections are evaluated carefully, including previous scar documentation, before undergoing a trial of labor after cesarean (TOLAC) section. Clients with longitudinal uterine scars usually are not considered candidates for TOLAC. Clients with low transverse uterine scars, an adequate pelvis, and an appropriate-sized fetus without indication of malposition or malpresentation may be considered candidates for TOLAC. Management of prostaglandins and oxytocin should follow accepted medical standards of care. Many institutions require the ready availability of the physician or CNM when oxytocin is being administered during labor. Medical awareness of signs and indications of possible uterine rupture and ready availability for surgical intervention are necessary to ensure optimal maternal-fetal outcomes. Finally, repair of any sustained injuries and possible hysterectomy coupled with appropriate volume and blood replacement are part of the medical management of the client experiencing uterine rupture.

Nursing considerations for providing care for the client with potential uterine rupture are to identify risk factors with a thorough nursing assessment. Maternal history should be reviewed for previous cesarean section and type of uterine scar (longitudinal or low transverse), previous uterine surgery (such as a myomectomy in which uterine fibroids were removed), and trauma. Nursing assessment should focus on maternal uterine activity, especially contraction frequency, intensity, duration, and resting phases. When oxytocin is being administered, care should be taken to avoid hyperstimulation of the uterus. The client's abdomen also should be assessed for signs of abdominal trauma, bruising, tenderness, pain, and rigidity. Maternal vital signs may indicate shock with an elevated pulse, shallow respirations, and decreasing blood pressure. Maternal complaints of acute pain without interruption or evidence of fetal distress may support suspicion of uterine rupture.

Nursing diagnoses specific for uterine rupture identify the risks for injury to both mother and fetus from hemorrhage, shock, sustained hypoxia, hypovolemia, and acidosis. Nursing diagnoses also should address the emotional and educational needs of the client and family. Grief challenges should be included among the nursing diagnoses.

Nursing interventions center around prevention of uterine rupture induced by aggressive use of oxytocin, immediate recognition and stabilization of the client experiencing this obstetric emergency, and notification of the physician or CNM (and team members) to perform an emergency cesarean and possibly a hysterectomy. During this urgent situation the nurse should remain calm, offering explanations and reassurances to the client and informing the family of the status of the mother and fetus. Specific interventions to stabilize the client include monitoring maternal vital signs, ensuring IV access with fluid volume replacement, discontinuation of oxytocin, placement of an oxygen face mask at 10 L/min, and monitoring fetal status. Immediate laboratory tests should include, at minimum, a complete blood count (CBC), platelet count, typing, and crossmatching. Operative preparations, including insertion of a Foley catheter, are managed urgently. The nurse also may need to assist in obtaining and administering blood products as ordered.

PLACENTAL ABNORMALITIES

Placental abnormalities also may contribute to a high-risk delivery or obstetric emergency. Placental abnormalities may be related to the implantation depth or site in the uterus; early separation from the uterine wall; or developmental problems, such as poor attachment of the cord, veins, or arteries to the body of the placenta. All of these placental abnormalities place the client and fetus at risk for hemorrhage, hypoxia, and even death. The incidence of hemorrhage related to placental abnormalities varies related to differing definitions but ranges somewhere between 3% and 7% (Cunningham et al., 2001).

Placenta Previa

Placenta previa is a condition in which the placenta implants low in the uterus (Figure 15-9). It is referred to as a *complete placenta previa* when the cervical os is completely covered by the placenta. When the cervical os is only partially covered, it is called a *partial previa*. When the placenta borders on the edge of the cervical os, it is referred to as a *marginal previa*. A placenta that implants very close to the edge is called a *low-lying placenta* (Cunningham et al., 2001; Schmidt, 1998). The incidence of placenta previa is reported to be between 0.33% and 0.5% (Crane, van de Hof, Dodds, Armson, & Liston, 1999; Cunningham et al., 2001). The problem with such low implantation is that as the uterus contracts or the cervix dilates, the placenta is separated from the cervix and bleeding occurs. Acute or chronic bleeding may adversely affect the mother and fetus. Acute, dramatic bleeding places the mother and fetus at risk for hypovolemia, shock, and diminished perfusion. Chronic bleeding over the second and third trimester may result in impaired fetal perfusion and growth. Ultrasonography may identify placenta previa in the second trimester before the first episode of antepartum or intrapartum bleeding. As the gestation advances, however, as many as 90% of marginal and low-lying placentas resolve (Ricci, 1992). Placenta previa demonstrates a higher rate of abnormal implantation in the uterus. *Placenta acreta* refers to abnormal implantation to the myometrium. *Placenta increta* extends into the myometrium. *Placenta percreta* implants through the myometrium. These conditions further increase the risk for hemorrhage, uterine injury, and infection (Cunningham et al., 2001). With the exception of low-lying placentas and some marginal presentations, cesarean section is the mode of delivery for clients with placenta previa.

Contributing factors to placenta previa include previous placenta previa, advanced maternal age, multiple gestations, multiparity, uterine scars from previous cesarean sections, abortions, and endometriosis (Cunningham et al., 2001). Smoking also has been associated with increased risk for placenta previa (Cunningham et al., 2001; Andres, 1996). Consequences for the pregnant client include acute or chronic hemorrhage accompanied by resultant anemia and coagulopathies, including disseminated intravascular coagulopathy (DIC). Additional ma-

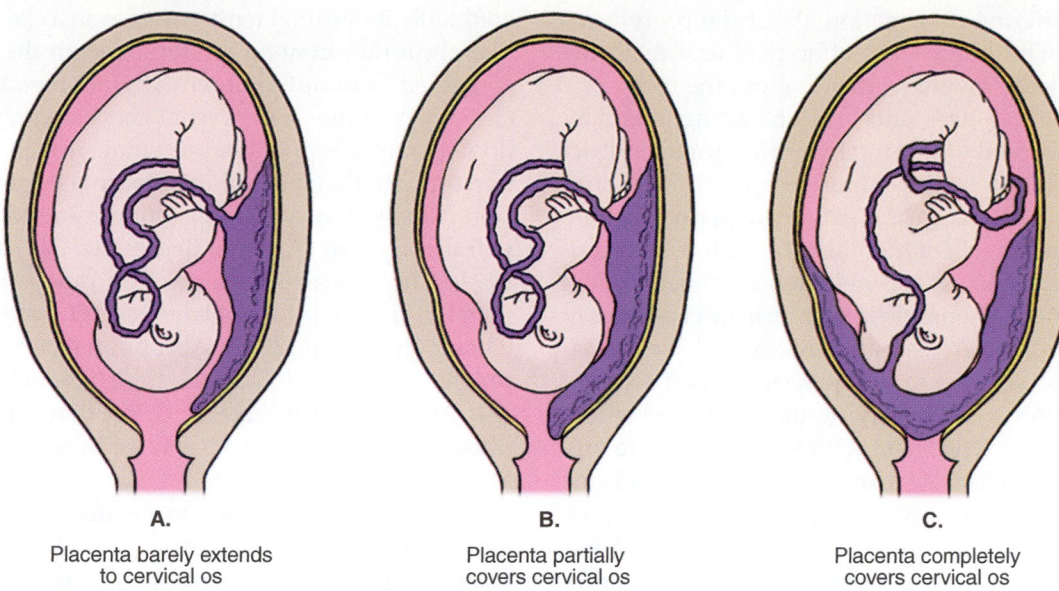

A.
Placenta barely extends
to cervical os

B.
Placenta partially
covers cervical os

C.
Placenta completely
covers cervical os

Figure 15-9   Placenta previa. A. Low implantation (marginal). B. Partial placenta previa. C. Total placenta previa.

ternal risks include the potential that the previa has abnormally implanted as a placenta acreta, increta, or percreta. These conditions not only necessitate emergent cesarean delivery but require hysterectomy (Cunningham et al., 2001; Lin, Adamczyk, Montag, Zelop, & Snow, 1998). Fetal risks include impaired placental perfusion that may inhibit growth and survival. Complications reported by Crane et al. (1999) include preterm delivery, respiratory compromise, anemia, and a higher rate of congenital defects.

Medical management strives to identify placenta previa before the onset of bleeding; however, this is not always successful. Even when placenta previa is identified, the onset of bleeding is not always predictable. Close monitoring of maternal-fetal status with blood tests to evaluate hemodynamic stability is necessary for maternal and fetal well-being, regardless of whether the client is hospitalized or is managed on an outpatient basis. Outpatient management requires frequent office visits and concurrent home health care. When maternal-fetal status is nonreassuring or the client is approaching term, cesarean delivery is performed.

Nursing considerations when managing an obstetric client who is bleeding include identification of the source or cause of the hemorrhage and stabilization of the client and fetus until cesarean section can be performed. Assessment data should include review of prenatal history, predisposing risk factors to suggest previa, other antepartum bleeding events, maternal Rh-factor status, and whether Rho(D) immune globulin (RhoGAM) was received if indicated. The current assessment should include when the bleeding began, the amount, the duration, whether or not the bleeding was associated with pain,

and the presence or absence of fetal movement. Vaginal bleeding should be assessed for color, amount, and presence of clots. The assessing nurse should not perform a vaginal examination in the presence of bleeding. Fetal monitoring should be performed to assess for signs of fetal well-being or nonreassuring fetal status. Blood for initial laboratory testing should be drawn to evaluate hemodynamic stability. The nurse may anticipate orders for a complete blood count, typing, and crossmatching. Clotting studies, such as prothrombin time (PT), partial thromboplastin time (PTT), fibrinogen, fibrin split products, and fibrin degradation products also may be performed. A **Kleihauer-Betke test** may be performed to denote evidence of fetal cells in the maternal circulation, which is significant for clients who are Rh negative. The nurse should be aware of the acute onset of abdominal or referred pain that may indicate a placental abruption coexisting with or instead of placenta previa. Unit-based ultrasonography may allow confirmation of the placental abnormality and provide better information with which to plan care.

Nursing interventions include ongoing maternal-fetal assessment, establishment of IV access with a large-bore cannula in anticipation of transfusions, continuous monitoring of maternal vital signs, maternal pulse oximetry, oxygen supplied by face mask at 10 L/min, and insertion of an in-dwelling Foley catheter for strict intake and output measures. Assessment of bleeding can be obtained by weighing the hip pads before and after use and by counting the total number of saturated pads. As a rule, 1 g is equivalent to 1 mL. Positioning the client laterally to increase good circulatory return is useful. The nurse should perform these interventions while explaining the reasons for them and offering information about the procedures as they occur. The nurse may offer reassurance to the client and family by giving feedback about the fetus.

If the client stabilizes and stops bleeding, she may remain in the hospital or eventually return home on strict bed rest, with home health nursing support. Maintaining a client on bed rest for an extended period of time causes challenges for client mobility, strength, loss of control, coping mechanisms, and heightened anxiety. When the client with placenta previa is near term or continues to bleed, preparations for cesarean delivery and the associated communications, setup, and preparations are carried out while informing and involving the client and family as much as possible. The client with known placenta previa who has been bleeding chronically may actually be quite relieved at the prospect of impending delivery; the client with newly diagnosed placenta previa who has acute bleeding may be highly anxious and frightened. These differences should be assessed by the nurse to individualize client and family support. Finally, nursing considerations should include spiritual and grief support, as indicated, keeping in mind that uncontrolled acute hemorrhage may result in maternal or fetal illness, permanent injury, and even death.

Abruptio Placentae

Abruptio placentae is a condition in which the placenta separates prematurely from the uterine wall (Figure 15-10). Partial abruption involves a portion of the placenta and may be very small or nearly completely separate. In complete abruption, the entire placenta separates from the uterus. When complete placental separation occurs, fetal demise is certain and maternal morbidity is high. Hemorrhage is the chief characteristic of placental abruption. The bleeding may be frank, bright red, and associated with abdominal tenderness, as in a classic abruption. The abruption may be hidden beneath the placenta and concealed, without apparent vaginal bleeding. Pregnancies can continue with partial concealed abruptions that do not exceed 50% of the placental surface. When abruption of more than 50% of the placenta occurs, fetal perfusion usually is very severely compromised and the fetus will die in utero (Ananth, Berkowitz, Savitz, & Lapinski, 1999). The incidence of abruption ranges from approximately 1 in 100 to 1 in 200 deliveries (Ananth et al., 1999; Cunningham et al., 2001). Abruption recurs in subsequent pregnancies up to 16% of the time (Schmidt, 1998). Misra and Ananth (1999) have reported that initial abruption rates average 1.7%, whereas rates in second pregnancies average 2.2%.

Factors that contribute to the development of abruption include advanced maternal age, advanced parity, and crack-cocaine use. Abruption also occurs more frequently in Black women than it does in Caucasian or Hispanic women. The most significant contributing factor, however, is maternal hypertension (Cunningham et al.,2001; Schmidt, 1998). There seems to be no difference in potential for abruption based on whether maternal hypertension is chronic and preexisting or acute, as in pre-eclampsia. Other risk factors for abruption include smoking, preterm premature rupture of membranes, external trauma from motor vehicle accidents, internal trauma from insertion of an IUPC, maternal cocaine use, uterine leiomyomas beneath placental implantation, and a short umbilical cord (Andres, 1996; Misra & Ananth, 1999; Reis, Sander, & Pearlman, 2000; Handwerker & Selick, 1995; Cunningham et al., 2001; Schmidt, 1998). Maternal risks include shock, severe anemia related to hemorrhage, hypovolemia, risk for DIC, risk for embolism during the placental separation process, and death. Fetal risks include fetal growth impairment when the abruption is small and chronic; prematurity; severe hypoxic insults resulting in permanent neurologic damage; and intrauterine fetal demise (Ananth et al., 1999).

Medical management centers around the earliest possible identification of abruption, emergent cesarean delivery when the fetus is still alive, and maternal hemodynamic stabilization. When the abruption is minimal and maternal-fetal status is stable, an attempt at expectant management to allow fetal maturing may be considered cautiously, with emergent cesarean delivery an ever-present probability (Cunningham et al., 2001). Tocolysis may be provided to control uterine irritability and contractility that may increase the process of placental separation (Cunningham et al., 2001; Towers, Pircon, & Heppard, 1999). When the fetus is no longer alive in utero, vaginal delivery may be attempted with regard to maternal coagulopathy (DIC) that predisposes her to significant hemorrhage (Corbett & Fonteyn, 1995). Hypovolemia is

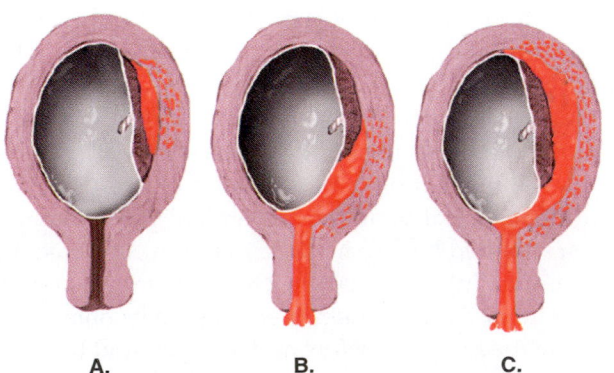

Figure 15-10 Abruptio placentae. A. Central abruption, concealed hemorrhage. B. Marginal abruption, external hemorrhage. C. Complete abruption, external hemorrhage (could also be concealed).

treated with IV fluids and blood product replacement (cryoprecipitate, packed erythrocytes, and platelets), as indicated.

Nursing considerations in the care of the client experiencing an abruption depend on a thorough but efficient nursing assessment, keying in on risk factors that may signal this potential emergency. The nurse should also explore habits and events leading up to the point of maternal symptoms, such as abdominal trauma, cocaine use, or a history of heavy smoking. During the physical assessment the nurse should pay special attention to maternal vital signs, especially in the face of hypertension or shock indices (hypotension, tachycardia, and tachypnea); vaginal bleeding; and uterine tenderness, rigidity, or hypertonic response. Noting an increase in abdominal girth may alert the nurse that the client is bleeding into the uterine muscle, resulting in a Couvelaire uterine hematoma. Vaginal bleeding should be assessed with a hip pad count, with before and after weights of the pads being documented. Monitoring the fetal status is critical to establishing fetal well-being or identifying fetal distress as close as feasible to the onset of compromise. Particular attention should be paid to the presence of tachycardia, bradycardia, late decelerations, sinusoidal pattern, and loss of variability. IV access with a large-bore catheter is essential for delivery of lactated Ringer's solution and blood products. Necessary laboratory tests include a CBC, a platelet count, clotting studies, typing, crossmatching, baseline electrolyte and chemistry studies, and liver and renal functions studies. An in-dwelling Foley catheter should be inserted, with strict measurement of intake and output. Pulse oximetry monitoring should be used, if available, and supplemental oxygen delivered by face mask. When the maternal hemodynamic status is not stable or oliguria is not corrected with administered fluids and blood products, the client may require hemodynamic monitoring with a central venous line or pulmonary catheter. The mode of delivery depends on maternal-fetal status and maternal clotting status.

If the fetus is alive, the nurse may anticipate an emergent cesarean. If the fetus is not alive, a vaginal delivery may be in order, with oxytocin stimulation required. When oxytocin is ordered, careful titration must be observed to prevent further uterine trauma (Cunningham et al., 2001). In the midst of rapid medical and nursing interventions employed to stabilize the client and her fetus, the nurse must also provide the vital information necessary to quickly educate and reassure the client and her family. In the event of fetal demise, grief and spiritual support also must be considered. This aspect of care is particularly challenging because the family may have numerous unanswered questions as they try to cope with overwhelming grief related to the loss of their baby and uncertainty regarding maternal survival.

Other Placental Anomalies

Other placental abnormalities may contribute to poor fetal outcome, because maternal hemorrhage may go undetected until it is discovered at or after delivery. These abnormalities may be developmental or the result of superimposed trauma, such as from hypertensive episodes. Hypertension, either chronic or pregnancy-induced, may cause placental injuries called *infarcts*. These areas of tissue injury are no longer able to facilitate placental circulation. When these areas of damaged placental tissue are large or numerous, perfusion to the fetus may be compromised. Fetal growth may be affected over an extended period of time. Fetal heart tracings on the monitor may be nonreassuring, particularly during the stress of labor. Such fetal intolerance may result in fetal distress and necessitate cesarean section.

UMBILICAL CORD ANOMALIES

Developmental errors may occur as the umbilical cord joins into the placenta. **Velamentous insertion of the cord** refers to the junction of the cord at the edge of the placenta. The vessels separate into the membranes before reaching the insertion site. This abnormality can result in chronic altered fetal perfusion. More significantly, this abnormality can undergo trauma and compression during labor and delivery, resulting in rupture and hemorrhage. **Vasa previa** involves the cord vessels crossing the cervical os and results in significant compression and possible rupture from the pressure of the fetal head during descent. Fetal compromise may include hypoxic injury, hemorrhage, hypovolemia, and death. Before the ability to diagnose vasa previa in the antepartum period, the mortality rate was 33% to 100% (Oyelese et al., 1998). Both velamentous insertion and vasa previa tend to accompany other placental abnormalities, such as placenta previa and bilobed or irregularly developed placentas. These abnormalities also occur more frequently in multiple pregnancies and pregnancies that result from in vitro fertilization. With the advent of more detailed ultrasonography, vasa previa and cord abnormalities may now be detected before labor, allowing for an alternative form of delivery in highly suspicious cases (Oyelese et al., 1998; Lee et al., 2000).

Umbilical cord events and abnormalities may occur that result in a high-risk pregnancy or emergent status. Problems may be developmental, as in an umbilical cord having only two vessels instead of three. The absence of one of the umbilical cord arteries occurs in 0.72% to 0.85% of delivered infants, and it occurs more frequently in Caucasian women and even more frequently in women who have diabetes (Cunningham et al., 2001). Labor and delivery may proceed without any indication of problems until the neonate's cord stump is assessed at delivery and found to have only two vessels. Antenatally, sonography currently can screen for the presence of a three-vessel cord at the anatomic scan performed during the second trimester. Although this abnormality is not a problem during labor and delivery, neonates with only two vessels in the cord have been found to have a higher incidence of multisystem abnormalities (spinal, gastrointestinal, renal, and cardiac). Other cord problems may become evident during labor, such as cord length. Whereas *Williams Obstetrics* (Cunningham et al., 2001) identifies the average cord length as 55 cm, the variances range from 0 to 300 cm. Higher risks of rupture, abruption, and inversion of the uterus are associated with a short umbilical cord. An exceptionally long umbilical cord may result in fetal entanglement, with an intrauterine fetal demise being the result.

Umbilical cord compression involves pressure applied to the umbilical cord. Compression can occur as the presenting part presses against the cord on descent or from entanglement or looping around a body part, such as the neck or shoulder, or from the existence of a true knot. Fetal perfusion is interrupted as cord compression increases or persists. Cord compression has been associated with nonreassuring fetal tracings, low Apgar scores, meconium-stained fluid, emergent cesarean section or operative vaginal delivery, neonatal resuscitation, and admission to the neonatal intensive care unit (Jauniaux, Ramsay, Peellaerts, & Scholler, 1995; Larson, Rayburn, Crosby, & Thurnau, 1995). Longer cords also may incur a true knot (occurring in 1.1% of cords) or prolapse during labor once the membranes rupture.

Umbilical cord prolapse occurs when the cord precedes the presenting part into the birth canal (Figure 15-11). Fetal position, multiple fetuses, artificial rupture of the membranes, and fetal activity may contribute to the likelihood of a prolapsed cord. Maternal risks include hemorrhage, uterine inversion accompanied by profound shock, and trauma from emergent interventions. Fetal risks include decreased or obliterated perfusion, hypoxic injury, and death. The incidence of umbilical cord prolapse has been reported to be as frequent as 1 in 426 births or 0.4% to 0.5% (Murphy & MacKenzie, 1995; Cunningham et al., 2001). The prolapse may be either frank, with obvious fetal response and the umbilical cord found in the vagina or protruding from the introitus vaginae, or the prolapse may be occult, compressed between the presenting part and the cervix and not discovered until the time of delivery. Time is essential once a prolapse is suspected or confirmed. Delays in intervention for a prolapsed cord can result in fetal injury or death. Prabulos and Philipson (1998) reported that in a review of 26,545 cases of cord prolapse, a significant percentage of negative fetal outcomes still occurred despite diagnosis-to-delivery times averaging 11 minutes, 9 minutes less than the average vaginal delivery time of 20 minutes from diagnosis of cord prolapse to delivery of the baby. This study emphasized the need to deliver emergently once a diagnosis of prolapse has been made and also raised questions about the possibility of other variables contributing to negative neonatal outcomes.

Medical management of cord compression and prolapse involves early recognition, intervention, and delivery to avoid fetal compromise or death. Medical management of prolapse is an obstetric emergency. Umbilical cord compression can be managed conservatively as long as the fetal tracing is reassuring. When fetal intolerance becomes evident, alternative medical management may become necessary, including emergent cesarean section.

Nursing considerations focus on assessment of risk factors and evidence to support concerns about fetal perfusion. Most significant will be the fetal response recorded on the monitor tracing. Cord compression may be accompanied by variable decelerations that become deeper, wider, or return slowly to the baseline. Loss of variability or increasing baseline may signify loss of fetal reserve and indicate fetal compromise. In a frank cord prolapse, an acute and sustained bradycardia, decreasing fetal base-

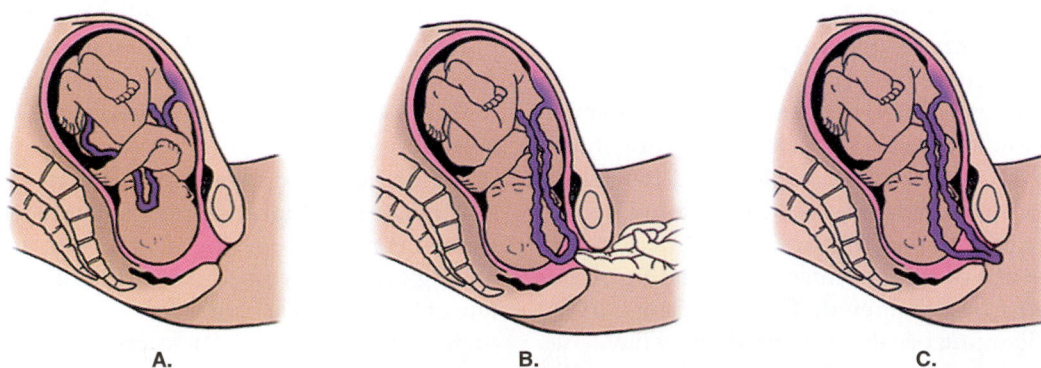

A.   **B.**   **C.**

Figure 15-11   Prolapsed cord. A. Occult (hidden, cannot be seen or felt). B. Complete (cannot be seen but may be felt). C. Visible (can be seen protruding from vagina).

line, or prolonged deceleration lasting more than 60 seconds may be observed on the tracing. The pelvic examination also may assist the nurse to identify risk factors. When the presenting part is not well applied to the cervix or when a malposition or malpresentation (e.g., in breech and transverse lie presentations) is present, the client is at high risk for prolapse of the umbilical cord. Cord compression may be more apparent in the client with oligohydramnios, a condition in which the amniotic fluid volume equals 5 cm or less of the estimated total volume at or near term. A client with ruptured membranes also may experience more frequent compression because limited fluid is available to prevent pressure on the cord in utero. When the nurse suspects a prolapse, a pelvic examination should be performed. When the umbilical cord is palpated, the nurse can attempt to gently lift the presenting part away from it, thus permitting cord perfusion to resume. Once this is done, the examiner should not remove the examining hand. Fetal monitoring should continue, and the client either may be positioned with her head slightly downward or assume a modified knee-chest position to further remove the presenting part off the cord. The nurse should call for assistance while remaining with the client. It is important to explain to the client what is happening and why the interventions are being performed. Supplemental oxygen with a face mask should be added to enhance placental fetal perfusion. Frank cord prolapse is an emergent condition. An emergent cesarean section is needed to deliver the fetus before significant circulation is interrupted and fetal hypoxia and acidosis occur.

Vaginal deliveries sometimes occur when the prolapse is occult, or hidden. In these cases, deep, broad variables may be observed on the fetal tracing. Maternal position changes and supplemental oxygenation with a face mask may provide some relief of the cord compression and enhance circulating oxygen until delivery occurs. If the fetal tracing becomes nonreassuring or demonstrates loss of fetal well-being, the physician may choose to perform operative vaginal delivery with low outlet forceps or vacuum suction if delivery is imminent. A cesarean section may be necessary if labor is early. Having supplies available for these options is a part of the anticipatory preparations the nurse can make once the fetal monitor tracing becomes suspicious for problems.

The nurse providing care for the client experiencing cord compression may employ similar interventions, with maternal position changes from side to side or even a modified knee-chest position. The client may benefit from oxygen supplementation by face mask. The nurse may be asked to start and maintain an amnioinfusion to instill fluid within the uterus to replace the cushioning effect of amniotic fluid and relieve cord compression. The nurse should carefully monitor labor progression. When labor is progressing rapidly, the fetus may better tolerate the effects of cord compression. When cord compression is significant in early labor or during a sluggish labor, the fetal tracing may become nonreassuring before vaginal delivery is feasible. It is particularly important that the nurse complete preparations for delivery, including notifying the nursery personnel and having resuscitation supplies available in the event the fetus has respiratory depression from chronic cord compression. Emotional support and educational information are helpful to reduce or alleviate client anxiety that accompanies high-risk situations.

AMNIOTIC FLUID ABNORMALITIES

Problems with amniotic fluid also can make a pregnancy and delivery high risk. Amniotic fluid amounts that deviate from normal can result in complications for the client and her developing fetus. Abnormal amounts of amniotic fluid are referred to as polyhydramnios (or hydramnios) and oligohydramnios. Amniotic fluid embolism is a critical event with an unclear cause. These three amniotic fluid aberrations can result in significant maternal and fetal complications.

Polyhydramnios

Polyhydramnios refers to an increased amount of amniotic fluid within the uterus. An amount of 2 L at term is considered to be polyhydramnios (Cunningham et al., 2001). This measurement is often based on clinical assessment of uterine size and perceived amount of fluid using Leopold's maneuvers. Another way of measuring polyhydramnios is to calculate the amniotic fluid index, which measures a pocket of amniotic fluid in each of the four quadrants using sonography. If the sum of the measures in the four quadrants exceeds 24 cm, the client is diagnosed with polyhydramnios. The advent of routine sonography has offered a more objective way to evaluate amniotic fluid volume. The reported incidence of occurrence is approximately 0.9%, with most cases identified as mild hydramnios (Cunningham et al., 2001).

The occurrence of polyhydramnios has been associated with maternal diabetes; multiple gestations; and maternal isoimmunization, with resultant fetal hydrops (Kellogg, 1998). Polyhydramnios is also found in the fetus with neural tube malformations such as spina bifida or anencephaly, with increased fluid loss through meningeal membranes, gastrointestinal problems that interfere with the normal swallowing, and absorption of amniotic fluid (Cunningham et al., 2001). Maternal effects of polyhydramnios include general discomfort from overexpansion of the uterus, respiratory compromise, uterine irritability from overdistention, premature labor, and uterine rupture.

Fetal risks include premature delivery, cord prolapse, malpresentation, macrosomia, and cesarean delivery (Kellogg, 1998; Panting-Kemp, Nguyen, Chang, Quillen, & Castro, 1999). An earlier study had concluded similar findings in hydramnios when the condition was persistent throughout the second and third trimesters. When hydramnios resolved in the third trimester, the incidence of negative outcomes decreased significantly (Golan, Wolman, Sagi, Yovel, & David, 1994b).

Medical management of the client with polyhydramnios is related both to an identified cause and symptomatic complaints. When hydramnios is severe, amniocentesis to remove fluid is performed. The procedure is carried out with ultrasound guidance, and the amount of fluid is measured and recorded. Otherwise, medical management addresses the client and fetus at the time of labor (i.e., prematurity, maternal diabetes, fetal anomalies, and so on).

Nursing considerations also depend on the contributing causes and maternal symptoms. For instance, when the client is admitted in preterm labor, the nursing care focuses on tocolysis, fetal and maternal monitoring, and prevention of therapy side effects. In addition to the cause of hydramnios, if known, client comfort is a particularly important nursing issue. Maternal comfort in late pregnancy is always challenging, and the addition of more amniotic fluid that causes further uterine distention and dyspnea is even more so. Elevation of the head of bed, pulse oximetry, and humidified oxygen supplementation by nasal cannula may be beneficial in late antepartal care. Oxygen by face mask is still preferred in labor. Fetal monitoring may be difficult related to the additional uterine expansion and bulk. Leopold's maneuvers also may be more difficult because of the taut abdominal skin and the large volume of fluid to try and "feel through." Once delivery is inevitable, the neonatal team should be notified of the premature labor and anticipated fetal anomalies. The client experiencing hydramnios has the additional challenges of coping with increased physical discomforts; causative factors, such as diabetes; and the overriding concern for the well-being of the infant. The chronicity of the condition may be extremely fatiguing and become comparable to the client on extended bed rest for multiple gestation or preterm labor. Diligent client education, emotional support, and encouragement are nursing interventions that may assist the client to better cope with her situation.

Oligohydramnios

Oligohydramnios refers to the amniotic fluid being significantly less than expected for pregnancy. The volume measurement is 500 mL or less between 32 and 36 weeks' gestation, or an amniotic fluid index of 5 cm or less (Kellogg, 1998; Cunningham et al., 2001). Sonography has allowed early identification of oligohydramnios along with follow-up surveillance of the client with persistent oligohydramnios. Oligohydramnios identified early in the pregnancy has a more negative prognosis relative to the cause and chronicity of the condition (Cunningham et al., 2001). The incidence varies with the associated cause; however, a 1994 study found a rate of 0.58% in a review of 25,000 obstetric clients (Golan et al., 1994b). A more recent study of 6,423 pregnancies found an occurrence rate of 2.3% (Casey et al., 2000).

Contributing causes toward the development of oligohydramnios include fetal anomalies, especially of the renal system. Fetal anomalies were identifed as being the cause in over 50% of cases of oligohydramnios in the second trimester of pregnancy and almost 25% of cases in the third trimester (Shipp, Bromley, Pauker, Frigoletto, & Benacerraf, 1996). Fetal renal agenesis (known as Potter's syndrome), or the failure of the fetal kidneys to develop, is associated with severe chronic oligohydramnios. The renal agenesis is accompanied by pulmonary hypoplasia. The fetal renal and pulmonary systems are significant in maintaining and rebuilding amniotic fluid volumes (Cunningham et al., 2001). Without their existence or development, the fetus is compressed within the uterus. Renal agenesis is an anomalous condition that is incompatible with life outside the uterus. Other fetal problems that contribute to oligohydramnios include renal system obstruction and polycystic kidneys. Maternal factors that contribute to oligohydramnios are hypertension; leaking or premature rupture of membranes; and most frequently, gestations that continue beyond 41 weeks (Cunningham et al., 2001).

Perinatal outcomes reported in a study examining the various complications included increased rate and need for labor induction, increased stillbirths, nonreassuring fetal heart rate tracings, neonatal intensive care unit admissions, meconium aspiration, and neonatal death (Casey et al., 2000). Cesarean section and an Apgar score of less than 7 at 5 minutes were found more frequently in clients with oligohydramnios (Chauhan, Sanderson, Hendrix, Magann, & Devoe, 1999). Increased rates of maternal hypertension, second trimester bleeding, fetal intrauterine growth retardation, fetal skeletal and renal system anomalies, and perinatal mortality were reported in a 1994 study (Golan et al., 1994a). Even borderline amniotic fluid levels ranging between 5 and 10 cm on the amniotic fluid index have been associated with increased intrauterine growth problems and perinatal complications (Banks & Miller, 1999). *Idiopathic* (meaning unknown cause) oligohydramnios without associated fetal growth problems as followed on surveillance sonography did not demonstrate a higher incidence of fetal complications other than premature delivery in a 1997 study reported by Garmel, Chelmow, Sha, Roan, and D'Alton.

Medical management of the client with oligohydramnios includes early diagnosis with anatomy surveillance for anomalies. When maternal conditions such as hypertension and postdate gestation are contributory, evaluation for delivery must be considered. Use of the biophysical profile may augment the practitioner's plan of care by providing feedback on fetal well-being. When oligohydramnios results from premature leaking or rupture of membranes, medical care may be expectant. That is, maternal-fetal status is monitored for stability and infection while the opportunity is provided for amniotic fluid to accumulate. When signs of infection are apparent, delivery plans replace expectant management to minimize the risk of sepsis. When oligohydramnios is severe or associated with fetal anomalies, the client and family must be informed and prepared for the likely outcomes.

Nursing considerations in the care of the client with oligohydramnios are determined by assessment data related to the cause of the oligohydramnios and the medical plan of care. When expectant management is the plan, nursing considerations include thorough maternal-fetal assessment, with the fetal tracing providing critical information on fetal status. Monitoring for signs of infection in the event the membranes are leaking or ruptured also is a nursing concern. The client with hypertension may be on strict bed rest and required to undergo repeated surveillance sonograms and nonstress tests. Anticipatory grief support may be the most important support offered to the client with a fetus that has significant anomalies. When delivery is planned, the nurse can anticipate orders for an amnioinfusion to relieve cord and fetal compression and thus reduce overall stress during labor. Ongoing fetal monitoring may reveal deep variables and prolonged decelerations related to severe umbilical cord compression. Maternal position changes may be futile relative to the uterine compression of the fetus in severe cases of oligohydramnios but should be attempted to achieve optimal fetal response. Supplemental oxygenation may benefit fetal perfusion and can be administered by face mask. IV hydration should be maintained to avoid perfusion complications that increase fetal stress. As in all high-risk delivery settings, the neonatal team should be ready in the event neonatal resuscitation is required.

Acknowledging parental grief and acceptance of their loss in the event the fetus or neonate does not survive is a critical nursing concern. The nurse should assess the parental needs and readiness for grieving and provide adequate time for the parents to see, hold, and bond with their infant with privacy, respect, and any requested spiritual support. Many facilities have protocols for perinatal loss support that include photographs, time together, burial layettes, and memory books with a lock of hair and handprints and footprints of their baby. Recognizing that all persons grieve differently should provide insight into how to implement and observe such a protocol without offending or upsetting the mother and family if they are not ready or are unable to participate in such a personal farewell. In some cases, the memorabilia is collected and saved in a labeled envelope in case the parents desire it at a later time.

Amniotic Fluid Embolism

Amniotic fluid embolism is a very rare but life-threatening condition. Amniotic fluid embolism involves the presence of an embolus composed of amniotic fluid along with particulate matter (such as vernix caseosa, lanugo, meconium, and other fetal cells) that enters the maternal circulation and causes acute respiratory distress, cardiovascular collapse, severe coagulopathy, shock, and death (Austin, 1998). The reported occurrence is 1 in 65,000 deliveries, and the maternal mortality rate is up to 80%. A 1995 review of national registry records reported a maternal mortality rate of 61% (Clark, Hankins, Dudley, Dildy, & Porter, 1995). A more recent study in 1999 reviewed approximately 1.1 million deliveries and identified an incidence of 1 per 20,646 deliveries and an associated maternal mortality rate of 26.4% (Gilbert & Danielsen, 1999). Half of all maternal survivors of amniotic fluid embolism have significant neurologic sequelae (Locksmith, 1999). The embolic event occurs during or immediately after delivery when the placenta separates from the uterine wall and maternal veins are open for transport of the embolus. Intrauterine pressures are favorable for transport of the embolus, especially when there is aggressive uterine stimulation; tumultuous, hypertonic labor; or placental abruption. Amniotic fluid embolism is more common when the labor has been precipitous or strong; when premature placental separation makes maternal access available sooner; and when more particulate matter, such as meconium, is available to compose the embolus (Cunningham et al., 2001). Studies repeatedly have reported classic responses of maternal respiratory distress, cardiovascular collapse, shock, and coagulopathy; however, the similarities between amniotic fluid embolism and anaphylaxis or septic shock are identified as possible potentiators that increase the mortality rate (Clark et al., 1995; Locksmith, 1999; Weiwen, Ningyu, Lanxiang, & Yu, 2000).

Clinical presentation of an amniotic fluid embolism is abrupt and spontaneous and includes complaints of respiratory difficulty and pain, cyanosis, and chest pain, with rapid onset of shock and cardiovascular collapse (Weiwen et al., 2000). In the previously cited study, the time of onset of symptoms to the time of death was reviewed. Thirty-nine percent of mothers died within 1 hour of onset of symptoms, and one-third died within the first 30 minutes. Women who survive are at significant risk of neurologic impairment from severe hypoxemia. If

Reflections from a Nurse

Labor and delivery was my passion! I had just attained a level of clinical comfort as an experienced labor and delivery nurse. I had participated in numerous high-risk deliveries, started IVs in almost nonexistent veins, protected seizing clients from self-injury, managed Pitocin and magnesium sulfate, transfused blood, and raced my clients to the OR like lightning in an emergent situation. I prided myself on bonding with the clients, their families, and even their newborns.

Then entered our newest admission. Kate was 31 and in labor with her first child. She and her husband, Scott, were so excited about their baby. They worked together in labor, and her labor was tough. Strong contractions were exhausting but she coped well with minimal pharmacologic intervention. She pushed hard to deliver a strong, loud, healthy boy weighing in at 9 pounds. They were oblivious to the repair as it was in progress. Within 10 minutes of the placental delivery, she began complaining of chest pain and acting so anxious. Her color paled and she became diaphoretic. We had to initiate resuscitation in another few minutes. Minutes felt like hours. The ABCs of CPR rang in my ears. The response of everyone was admirable and quick, but futile. Later as I would clean and prepare Kate for her return to her horrified husband, I reviewed the process and wondered what else could have been done. I hugged him, cried with him, and told him how sorry I was.

Still later as I reviewed my chart and followed the process for closing a chart that would undergo immediate risk review, I tried to retrace the events to explore one more time what could have been done. Nothing. How humbling that thought. We are but human. We did all that could be done. Alone, on my way home, I cried for us all; Kate, Scott, their newborn son, my colleagues, and myself.

---

delivery has not been completed, the fetus is at the same risk of hypoxemia and subsequent damage or death.

Medical management depends on recognition of the clinical symptoms and is supportive in nature because there is no known curative protocol (Locksmith, 1999). Rapid intervention involves immediate and aggressive resuscitation to maintain oxygenation; volume replacement; monitoring of cardiac output and vital signs; and transfusions of cryoprecipitate, fresh frozen plasma, and packed erythrocytes and platelets to control the coagulopathy (Cunningham et al., 2001). When delivery has not occurred, it must be performed surgically and immediately if the fetus is to survive.

Nursing considerations include astute assessment of maternal-fetal status throughout the third and fourth stages of delivery. Attention should be focused on vital sign stability and any maternal complaints of shortness of breath, chest pain, heightened anxiety, and sensation of impending doom. Other assessment data include listening to breath sounds, observing for increased bleeding from the perineum or incision, and monitoring the level of maternal consciousness. The nurse should never leave an unstable or deteriorating client unattended. Calling for assistance and emergency supplies such as the crash cart should be done immediately on identification of maternal problems. The first interventions are based on the classic

ABCs of resuscitation: airway, breathing, and circulation. Maintaining or reestablishing an airway is first and foremost, and may be as simple as initially applying an oxygen face mask at a rate of 10 L/min. However, maintaining the client's airway may progress rapidly from oxygen supplementation to manual ventilation with a self-inflating resuscitation bag, and finally to assisting with intubation and support by ventilator. Circulation and perfusion are maintained with IV fluids, chest compressions if cardiac arrest occurs, and assisting with defibrillation as necessary. Multiple pressor drugs may be ordered to help maintain blood pressure and promote adequate perfusion. Continuous monitoring of maternal vital signs is critical. Pulse oximetry should be used until a pulmonary catheter and an adjunctive arterial line are put in place for accurate cardiac output assessment and monitoring of blood gases. The nurse can anticipate orders for various laboratory tests, including CBC, platelet count, typing, crossmatching, a clotting panel (PT, PTT, fibrinogen, fibrinogen split products, and fibrin degradation products), and chemistry panels to assess electrolyte stability and renal function. An in-dwelling Foley should be inserted, with strict intake and output monitored hourly. Receiving and following through with orders for the various blood products and strict compliance with administration procedures also are nursing responsibilities.

Monitoring ongoing blood loss and recording of amounts are important factors in estimating replacement needs.

The resuscitative process can be overwhelming to the health care team. The process certainly will be a terrifying experience for the family and support persons who witness a cardiovascular arrest, significant hemorrhage, and the incredibly aggressive response. Because such events are unexpected, the scene can appear chaotic as supplies and team members are rapidly assembled and participate in the resuscitative efforts. Quick explanations about the situation to the family and support persons should be provided. They may be asked to move to an area in the room where they can remain close or to wait outside the room. Available space in the room or hospital policies may determine where the family and support persons will be asked to stay. Whenever possible, a social worker or spiritual counselor should remain with the family to provide support while resuscitative efforts continue. If the client is stabilized and placed on ventilatory support, the family should be allowed to see her before she is transferred to the intensive care unit. If the client does not survive, the family should receive grief support and be allowed to spend time saying farewell. If the fetus does not survive, the family's grief will be further increased. If the neonate survives, support will be needed to enable a healthy adaptation with the surviving family.

Most of the time, obstetrics is a happy nursing specialty area. In the event of maternal or fetal death, the health care team must deal with their own personal feelings of loss and possibly failure. It may be helpful for a grief or spiritual counselor to meet with the team that was involved to assist them with coping, both personally and professionally. Review of all resuscitations can be expected as a part of risk management and quality improvement requirements. Careful review of the chart documentation, including entering of any late entries, should also be done after a resuscitation.

WEB | ACTIVITIES

••• Visit ACOG's and AWHONN's Web sites. Do they include information specific to some of the dysfunctional labor patterns discussed in this chapter? Compare information regarding the nurse's role versus the physician's role.

••• Search the Internet for information for parents of multiples. Are there chat rooms? Support groups? Toll-free numbers? Resource materials, such as books and videos?

Key Concepts

- Dysfunctional labor patterns include hypertonic, hypotonic, and precipitate labor patterns. Oxytocin may be used to regulate and normalize a dysfunctional labor pattern.

- Malpositions include occipitotransverse and occipitoposterior. Malpresentations include breech, acromion, face, brow, and transverse presentations. Persistent malpositions and malpresentations place mother and fetus at risk for cesarean section or operative vaginal delivery.

- Fetal distress indicates fetal intolerance to the intrauterine environment or labor, or both. When left untreated, the fetus can experience hypoxic injury, acidosis, and death. Nursing interventions focus on increasing fetal oxygenation and perfusion.

- Uterine rupture is more likely to occur in a scarred uterus and may result in fetal death and maternal shock and hemorrhage. Uterine hyperstimulation may contribute to rupture.

- Placenta previa and abruptio placentae are hemorrhagic conditions of pregnancy. Placenta previa frequently presents as silent, nonpainful bleeding that may initially occur in the second and third trimesters. Abruptio placentae is more frequently acute and associated with abdominal pain. Complete placenta previa necessitates cesarean section, as does acute abruption. Abruption of over 50% is incompatible with fetal survival. Two consequences of abruption include DIC and a higher risk of amniotic fluid embolism.

- Prolapsed umbilical cord is an obstetric emergency. When unrelieved, the cord compression may result in fetal death.

- Abruption, uterine rupture, and amniotic fluid embolism predispose the obstetric client to DIC.

- Oligohydramnios refers to less than normal amniotic fluid volume in the second and third trimesters. Fetal cord compression, intolerance to labor, and negative fetal outcomes are increased in clients with oligohydramnios. This abnormality is frequently found in pregnancies with fetal anomalies. Maternal factors include hypertension and postdatism.

- Polyhydramnios refers to a greater than normal amniotic fluid volume and can result in maternal respiratory compromise, fetal malpresentation, and cord prolapse. Polyhydramnios is frequently found in pregnancies with maternal diabetes, multiple gestation, and isoimmunization.

- Amniotic fluid embolism is a rare event with a high maternal mortality rate as a result of obstetric shock from cardiopulmonary collapse and hemorrhagic coagulopathy. The physiologic response is comparable to anaphylactic and septic shock.

Review Questions and Activities

1. Ms. J. is an obstetric client who is in observation status in labor and delivery. Her contractions are occurring irregularly every 2 to 10 minutes. She states that she has had contractions like these for 9 hours. She is afebrile, and her vital signs are stable: pulse, 90; respirations, 18, and blood pressure, 114/72. The fetal heart rate is in the 140s, the baseline tracing demonstrates several accelerations, and no decelerations are noted. What other assessment information should you gather to assist in formulating diagnoses and a plan of care for Ms. J?

2. Ms. P. is a 32-year-old gravida, para 2002. She arrives in labor and delivery breathing, panting, and holding her abdomen near the suprapubic region. She tells you her membranes ruptured 10 minutes ago and that she now feels the urge to push. As you take her to a bed, you continue to gather additional information and discover she had her last baby en route to the hospital after a 30-minute labor. Without a pelvic examination performed, what action might you take?

3. Ms. R. is a gravida 2, para 1001. She has been completely dilated and at +1 station for 2 hours. She had an epidural and was unable to push well with contractions. She has begun to feel the pressure sensation and believes she can push better now. The fetal heart rate is in the 130s with long-term variability present, no decelerations noted, and an occasional acceleration observed. Ms. R.'s vital signs are stable. What interventions might you try to enhance her pushing efforts? What signs might you observe that may indicate a problem with fetal descent?

4. Ms. B. is a gravida 3, para 1011. She is 36 5/7 estimated gestational age with a twin gestation and presents with contractions that are 3 minutes apart, lasting 45 seconds, and moderate to firm in intensity. The twins' heart rates are identified at the right lower quadrant and left upper quadrant and range in the 130s and 150s, respectively. Discuss the assessment information you require for a safe labor and delivery process for this client. What factors may affect her mode of delivery and outcomes?

5. Ms. K. is a gravida 2, para 1001, and is attempting a trial of labor after having a cesarean section. Her original cesarean was 4 years ago for arrested descent. She complains of intense burning pain over the parapubic region. What other assessment para-

meters must you evaluate to identify a uterine rupture? What preparations have you already completed knowing this client has had a previous cesarean section and is undergoing trial of labor?

6. Ms. T. arrives in the labor and delivery unit by stretcher from an ambulance. Her vital signs follow: pulse, 120; respirations, 24 and shallow; blood pressure, 84/50 and faint. She complains of acute abdominal pain that began abruptly 1.5 hours ago. She has a very scant amount of bright red bleeding. Fetal heart tones are auscultated in the 90s. What do you suspect has occurred? Formulate a priority-based plan to ensure the best outcome for Ms. T. and her fetus.

7. As you begin your shift you receive a report on Ms. A. She is a gravida 4, para 0030, at 37 2/7 estimated gestational age, with a history of late pregnancy losses for unknown reasons. She is currently in a low Fowler's position, on continuous fetal monitoring, and having contractions of moderate intensity that are 4 minutes apart and last for 45 seconds. While you review her fetal monitor tracing, you note that the baseline is in the 120s. You do not note any accelerations and, in fact, notice late decelerations occurring after each contraction for the last 15 minutes. Identify interventions to attempt to alleviate this nonreassuring pattern. Are there other tests to reinforce your concerns or establish a sense of well-being in the client?

8. Ms. F. presents to labor and delivery in active labor. Examination finds that she is 4 cm dilated, has 80% effacement with bulging membranes, and the presenting part is at –3 station. Fetal heart tones are reactive in the 130s to 140s, with accelerations present. As you enter laboratory requisitions at the desk, you note on the central monitor that the fetal heart rate is now in the 90s. You return to find Ms. F. saying she just was going to call you because her membranes have ruptured. What are your next actions in a prioritized order?

9. Ms. Y. is a 26-year-old gravida 3, para 3003, who just delivered 15 minutes ago. You are assessing her vital signs and talking with her about her baby while the physician repairs her perineal laceration when she suddenly looks worried and tells you she cannot breathe well. You note that she has become pale and clammy in this few moments. Her vital signs are reflecting changes with a pulse that is increasing and at 106, a blood pressure that is decreasing and at 88/56, and respirations that are shallow and rapid at 28. She is gasping and looks panicky. What do you suspect is occurring? Discuss the prioritized interventions and complications that may arise secondary to her immediate diagnosis.

References

Acien, P. (1995). Breech presentation in Spain, 1992: A collaborative study. *European Journal of Obstetrics, Gynecology and Reproductive Biology, 62*(1), 19–24.

Aisenbrey, G., Catanzarite, V., Hurley, T., Spiegel, J., Schrimmer, D., & Mendoza, A. (1995). Monoamniotic and pseudomonoamniotic twins: Sonographic diagnosis, detection of cord entanglement, and obstetric management. *Obstetrics and Gynecology, 86*(2), 218–222.

Albrechtsen, S., Rasmussen, S., Dalaker, K., & Irgens, L. (1998). The occurrence of breech presentation in Norway 1967–1994. *Acta Obstetrics and Gynecology Scandinavia, 77*(4), 410–415.

Al Sakka, M., Dauleh, W., & Al Hassani, S. (1999). Case series of uterine rupture and subsequent pregnancy outcome. *International Journal of Fertility and Women's Medicine, 44*(6), 297–300.

Ananth, C., Berkowitz, G., Savitz, D., & Lapinski, R. (1999). Placental abruption and adverse perinatal outcomes. *Journal of the American Medical Association, 282*(17), 1646–1651.

Andres, R. (1996). The association of cigarette smoking with placenta previa and abruptio placenta. *Seminars in Perinatology, 20*(2), 154–159.

Austin, D. (1998). Labor and delivery at risk. In S. Mattson & J. Smith (Eds.), *AWHONN: Core curriculum for maternal newborn nursing* (Chap. 34). Philadelphia: W. B. Saunders.

Banks, E., & Miller, D. (1999). Perinatal risks associated with borderline amniotic fluid index. *American Journal of Obstetrics and Gynecology, 180*(6, P. 1), 1461–1463.

Bashore, R. (1992). Dystocia. In N. Hacker & J. Moore (Eds.), *Essentials of obstetrics and gynecology* (2nd ed., Chap. 23). Philadelphia: W. B. Saunders.

Bofill, J., Vincent, R., Ross, E., Martin, R., Norman, P., Werhan, C., & Morrison, J. (1997). Nulliparous active labor, epidural analgesia and cesarean delivery for dystocia. *American Journal of Obstetrics and Gynecology, 177*(6), 1465–1470.

Bowers, N. (1998). The multiple birth explosion: Implications for nursing practice. *Journal of Obstetric, Gynecologic and Neonatal Nursing, 27*(3), 302–310.

Casey, B., McIntire, D., Bloom, S., Lucas, M., Santos, R., Twickler, D., et al. (2000). Pregnancy outcomes after antepartum diagnosis of oligohydramnios at or beyond 34 weeks' gestation. *American Journal of Obstetrics and Gynecology, 182*(4), 909–912.

Caughey, A., Shipp, T., Repke, J., Zelop, C., Cohen, A., & Lieberman, E. (1999). Rate of uterine rupture during a trial of labor in women with one or two prior cesarean deliveries. *American Journal of Obstetrics and Gynecology, 181*(4), 872–876.

Chauhan, S., Sanderson, M., Hendrix, N., Magann, E., & Devoe, L. (1999). Perinatal outcome and amniotic fluid index in the antepartum and intrapartum periods: A meta-analysis. *American Journal of Obstetrics and Gynecology, 181*(6), 1473–1478.

Chen, L., Tan, K., & Yeo, G. (1995). A ten year review of uterine rupture in modern obstetric practice. *Annals Academy of Medicine in Singapore, 24*(6), 830–835.

Clark, A., Carr, D., Loyd, G., Cook, V., & Spinnato, J. (1998). The influence of epidural analgesia on cesarean delivery rates: A randomized, prospective clinical trial. *American Journal of Obstetrics and Gynecology, 179*(6, P. 1), 1527–1533.

Clark, S., Hankins, G., Dudley, D., Dildy, G., & Porter, T. (1995). Amniotic fluid embolism: Analysis of the national registry. *American Journal of Obstetrics and Gynecology, 172*(4, P. 1), 1158–1167.

Conway, D., & Langer, O. (1998). Elective delivery of infants with macrosomia in diabetic women: Reduced shoulder dystocia versus increased cesarean deliveries. *American Journal of Obstetrics and Gynecology, 178*(5), 922–925.

Corbett, J., & Fonteyn, M. (1995). Treating disseminated intravascular coagulation. *American Journal of Maternal Child Nursing, 20*(5), 290.

Crane, J., van de Hof, M., Dodds, L., Armson, B., & Liston, R. (1999). Neonatal outcomes with placenta previa. *Obstetrics and Gynecology, 93*(4), 541–544.

Cunningham, F., Gant, N., Leveno, K., Gilstrap III, L., Hauth, J., & Wenstrom, K. (2001). *Williams obstetrics* (21st ed.). New York: McGraw-Hill.

Eganhouse, D., & Petersen, L. (1998). Fetal surveillance in multifetal pregnancy. *Journal of Obstetric, Gynecologic and Neonatal Nursing, 27*(3), 312–321.

Ellings, J., Newman, R., & Bowers, N., (1998). Prenatal care and multiple pregnancy. *Journal of Obstetric, Gynecologic and Neonatal Nursing, 27*(4), 457–465.

Feinstein, N., McCartney, P., & AWHONN. (1997). *Fetal heart monitoring principles and practices* (2nd ed.). Dubuque, IA: Kendall/Hunt.

Garmel, S., Chelmow, D., Sha, S., Roan, J., & D'Alton, M. (1997). Oligohydramnios and the appropriately grown fetus. *American Journal Perinatology, 14*(6), 359–363.

Gherman, R., Goodwin, T., Souter, I., Neumann, K., Ouzounian, J., & Paul, R. (1997). The McRobert's maneuver for the alleviation of shoulder dystocia: How successful is it? *American Journal of Obstetrics and Gynecology, 176*(3), 656–661.

Gilbert, W., & Danielsen, B. (1999). Amniotic fluid embolism: Decreased mortality in a population-based study. *Obstetrics and Gynecology, 93*(6), 973–977.

Golan, A., Lin, G., Evron, S., Arieli, S., Niv, D., & David, M. (1994a). Oligohydramnios: Maternal complications and fetal outcome in 145 cases. *Gynecologic and Obstetric Investigation, 37*(2), 91–95.

Golan, A., Wolman, I., Sagi, J., Yovel, I., & David, M. (1994b). Persistence of polyhydramnios during pregnancy: Its significance and correlation with maternal and fetal complications. *Gynecology and Obstetric Investigation, 37*(1), 18–20.

Gonen, O., Rosen, D., Dolfin, Z., Tepper, R., Markov, S., & Fejgin, M. (1998). Induction of labor versus expectant management in macrosomia: A randomized study. *Obstetrics and Gynecology, 89*(6), 913–917.

Gupton, A., Heaman, M., & Ashcroft, T. (1997). Bed rest from the perspective of the high-risk pregnant woman. *Journal of Obstetric, Gynecologic and Neonatal Nursing, 26*(4), 423–430.

Hall, S. (1997). The nurse's role in the identification of risks and treatment of shoulder dystocia. *Journal of Obstetric, Gynecologic and Neonatal Nursing, 26*(1), 25–32.

Handwerker, S., & Selick, A. (1995). Placental abruption after insertion of catheter tip intrauterine pressure transducers: A report of four cases. *Journal of Reproductive Medicine, 40*(12), 845–849.

Hankins, G., & Rowe, T. (1996). Operative vaginal delivery: Year 2000. *American Journal of Obstetrics and Gynecology, 175*(2), 275–282.

Impey, L., & O'Herlihy, C. (1998). First delivery after cesarean delivery for strictly defined cephalopelvic disproportion. *Obstetrics and Gynecology, 92*(5), 799–803.

Imseis, H., Murtha, A., Alexander, K., & Barnett, B. (1998). Spontaneous rupture of a primigravid uterus secondary to placenta percreta. *Journal of Reproductive Medicine, 43*(3), 233–236.

Joshi, R., & Bharadwaj, A. (2000). Occiputposterior vertex in labor, an under recognized cause of dystocia. *Obstetrics and Gynecology, 95*(4, Suppl. 1), S40.

Jauniaux, E., Ramsay, B., Peellaerts, C., & Scholler, Y. (1995). Perinatal features of pregnancies complicated by nuchal cord. *American Journal of Perinatology, 12*(4), 255–258.

Kellogg, B. (1998). Placental development and functioning. In S. Mattson & J. Smith (Eds.), *AWHONN: Core curriculum for maternal newborn nursing* (Chap. 5). Philadelphia: W. B. Saunders.

Kirkendall, C., Jauregui, I., Kim, J., & Phelan, J. (2000). Catastrophic uterine rupture: Maternal and fetal characteristics. *Obstetrics and Gynecology, 95*(4, Suppl. 1), 74.

Larson, J., Rayburn, W., Crosby, S., & Thurnau, G. (1995). Multiple nuchal cord entanglements and intrapartum complications. *American Journal of Obstetrics and Gynecology, 173*(4), 1228–1231.

Lee, W., Lee, V., Kirk, J., Sloan, C., Smith, R., & Comstock, C. (2000). Vasa previa: Prenatal diagnosis, natural evolution and clinical outcome. *Obstetrics and Gynecology, 95*(4), 572–577.

Leonard, L. (1998). Depression and anxiety disorders during multiple pregnancy and parenthood. *Journal of Obstetric, Gynecologic and Neonatal Nursing, 27*(3), 329–337.

Lewis, D., Edwards, M., Asrat, T., Adair, C., Brooks, G., & London, S. (1998). Can shoulder dystocia be predicted? Preconceptive and prenatal factors. *Journal of Reproductive Medicine, 43*(8), 654–658.

Lin, C., Adamczyk, C., Montag, A., Zelop, C., & Snow, J. (1998). Placenta previa percreta involving the left broad ligament and cervix. A case report. *Journal of Reproductive Medicine, 43*(9), 839–843.

Locksmith, G. (1999). Amniotic fluid embolism. *Obstetric and Gynecologic Clinics of North America, 26*(3), 435–444.

Manogin, T., Bechtel, G., & Rami, J. (2000). Caring behaviors by nurses: Women's perceptions during childbirth. *Journal of Obstetric, Gynecologic and Neonatal Nursing, 29*(2), 153–157.

Menihan, C. (1998). Uterine rupture in women attempting a vaginal birth following prior cesarean birth. *Journal of Perinatology, 18*(6, P. 1), 440–443.

Miller, D., Goodwin, T., Gherman, R., & Paul, R. (1997). Intrapartum rupture of the unscarred uterus. *Obstetrics and Gynecology, 89*(5, P. 1), 671–673.

Misra, D., & Ananth, C. (1999). Risk factor profiles of placental abruption in first and second pregnancies: Heterogenous etiologies. *Journal of Clinical Epidemiology, 52*(5), 453–461.

Murphy, D., & MacKenzie, I. (1995). The mortality and morbidity associated with umbilical cord prolapse. *British Journal of Obstetrics and Gynaecology, 102*(10), 826–830.

Ou, X., Chen, X., & Su, J. (1997). Correction of occipito-posterior position by maternal posture during the process of labor. *Zhonghua Fu Chan Ke Za Zhi* [article in Chinese], *32*(6), 329–332.

Oyelese, K., Schwarzler, P., Coates, S., Sanusi, F., Hamid, R., & Campbell, S. (1998). A strategy for reducing the mortality rate from vasa previa using transvaginal sonography with color Doppler. *Ultrasound Obstetrics and Gynecology, 12*(6), 434–438.

Panting-Kemp, A., Nguyen, T., Chang, E., Quillen, E., & Castro, L. (1999). Idiopathic polyhydramnios and perinatal outcome. *American Journal of Obstetrics and Gynecology, 181*(5, P. 1), 1079–1082.

Payton, R., & Brucker, M. (1999). Drugs and uterine motility. *Journal of Obstetric, Gynecologic and Neonatal Nursing, 28*(6), 628–638.

Prabulos, A., & Philipson, E. (1998). Umbilical cord prolapse: Is the time from diagnosis to delivery critical? *Journal of Reproductive Medicine, 43*(2), 129–132.

Rayl, J., Gibson, P., & Hickok, D. (1996). A population-based case-control study of risk factors for breech presentation. *American Journal of Obstetrics and Gynecology, 174*(1, P. 1), 28–32.

Reis, P., Sander, C., & Pearlman, M. (2000). Abruptio placentae after auto accidents. A case control study. *Journal of Reproductive Medicine, 45*(1), 6–10.

Ricci, J. (1992). Antepartum hemorrhage. In N. Hacker & J. Moore (Eds.), *Essentials of obstetrics and gynecology* (2nd ed., Chap. 14). Philadelphia: W. B. Saunders.

Sanchez-Ramos, L., Quillen, M., & Kaunitz, A. (1996). Randomized trial of oxytocin alone and with propranolol in the management of dysfunctional labor. *Obstetrics and Gynecology, 88*(4), 517–520.

Sather, S., & Zwelling, E. (1998). A view from the other side of the bed. *Journal of Obstetric, Gynecologic and Neonatal Nursing, 27*(3), 322–328.

Schmidt, J. (199). Fluid check: Making the case for intrapartum amnioinfusion. *AWHONN: Lifelines, 1*(7), 47–51.

Schmidt, J. (1998). Hemorrhagic disorders. In S. Mattson & J. Smith (Eds.), *AWHONN: Core curriculum for maternal newborn nursing* (Chap. 28). Philadelphia: W. B. Saunders.

Shields, J., & Medearis, A. (1992a). Fetal malpresentations. In N. Hacker & J. Moore (Eds.). *Essentials of obstetrics and gynecology* (2nd ed., Chap. 20). Philadelphia: W. B. Saunders.

Shields, J., & Medearis, A. (1992b). Multiple gestation. In N. Hacker & J. Moore (Eds.). *Essentials of obstetrics and gynecology* (2nd ed., Chap. 21). Philadelphia: W. B. Saunders.

Shipp, T., Bromley, B., Pauker, S., Frigoletto, F., & Benacerraf, B. (1996). Outcome of singleton pregnancies with severe oligohydramnios in the second and third trimesters. *Ultrasound Obstetrics and Gynecology, 7*(2), 108–113.

Simpson, K. (1999). Shoulder dystocia. Nursing interventions and risk management strategies. *MCN American Journal of Maternal Child Nursing, 24*(6), 305–310.

Thompson, J. (1995). Forcep deliveries. *Clinical Perinatology, 22*(4), 953–972.

Thompson, T., Thorp, J., Mayer, D., Kuller, J., & Bowes, W. (1998). Does epidural analgesia cause dystocia? *Journal of Clinical Anesthesia, 10*(1), 58–65.

Toohey, J., Keegan, K., Morgan, M., Francis, J., Task, S., & deVeciana, M. (1995). The "dangerous multipara": Fact or fiction? *American Journal of Obstetrics and Gynecology, 172*(2, P. 1), 683–686.

Towers, C., Pircon., R., & Heppard, M. (1999). Is tocolysis safe in the management of third trimester bleeding? *American Journal of Obstetrics and Gynecology, 180*(6, P. 1), 1572–1578.

Wagner, R., Nielsen, P., & Gonik, B. (1999). Shoulder dystocia. *Obstetric and Gynecologic Clinics of North America, 26*(2), 371–383.

Weiwen, Y., Ningyu, Z., Lanxiang, Z., & Yu, L. (2000). Study of the diagnosis and management of amniotic fluid embolism: 38 cases of analysis. *Obstetrics and Gynecology, 95*(4, Suppl. 1), S38.

Wiznitzer, A. (1995). Obstructed labor and shoulder dystocia. *Current Opinions in Obstetrics and Gynecology, 7*(6), 486–491.

Suggested Readings

Abitbol, M., Bowen-Ericksen, M., Castillo, I., & Pushchin, A. (1999). Prediction of difficult vaginal birth and of cesarean section for cephalopelvic disproportion in early labor. *Journal of Maternal Fetal Medicine, 8*(2), 51–56.

Halle, J. (1998). Diagnostic evaluation of high-risk pregnancies. In S. Mattson & J. Smith (Eds.), *AWHONN: Core curriculum for maternal newborn nursing* (Chapt. 11). Philadelphia: W. B. Saunders.

Love, C., & Wallace, E. (1996). Pregnancies complicated by placenta previa: What is appropriate management? *British Journal of Obstetrics and Gynecology, 103*(9), 864–867.

Maymon, E., Ghezzi, F., Shoham-Vardi, I., Silberstein, T., Wiznitzer, A., & Mazor, M. (1998). Isolated hydramnios at term gestation and the occurrence of peripartum complications. *European Journal of Obstetrics, Gynecology and Reproductive Biology, 77*(2), 157–161.

McDougall, R., & Duke, G. (1995). Amniotic fluid embolism syndrome: A case report and review. *Anaesthesia Intensive Care, 23*(6), 735–740.

Richey, M., Gilstrap, L., III, & Ramin, S. (1995). Management of disseminated intravascular coagulation. *Clinics in Obstetrics and Gynecology, 38*(3), 514–520.

Turley, G. (1998). Essential forces and factors in labor. In S. Mattson & J. Smith (Eds.), *AWHONN: Core curriculum for maternal newborn nursing* (Chap. 14). Philadelphia: W. B. Saunders.

Resources

American College of Obstetricians and Gynecologists (ACOG), 409 12th Street, P.O. Box 96920, Washington, DC 20090-6920, http://www.acog.com

Association of Women's Health, Obstetric and Neonatal Nurses (AWHONN), Suite 740, 2000 L Street, NW, Washington, DC 20036, U.S.: 800-673-8499, Fax: 202-728-0575, Canada: 800-245-0231, http://www.awhonn.org

National Association of Neonatal Nurses (NANN), 4700 W. Lake Avenue, Glenview, IL 60025-1485, 800-451-3795, http://www.nann.org

National Organization of Mothers of Twins Clubs, Inc., P.O. Box 438, Thompson Station, TN 37179-0438, 615-595-0936, 877-540-2200, http://www.nomotc.org

Resolve Through Sharing, 812-353-8506

Sidelines National Support Network, P.O. Box 1808, Laguna Beach, CA 92652, 888-447-4754, http://www.sidelines.org

TWINS Magazine, 11211 E. Arapahoe Rd., Suite 101, Centennial, CO 80112-3851, 888-55-TWINS, http://www.twinsmagazine.com

UNIT 6

Postpartum Nursing Care

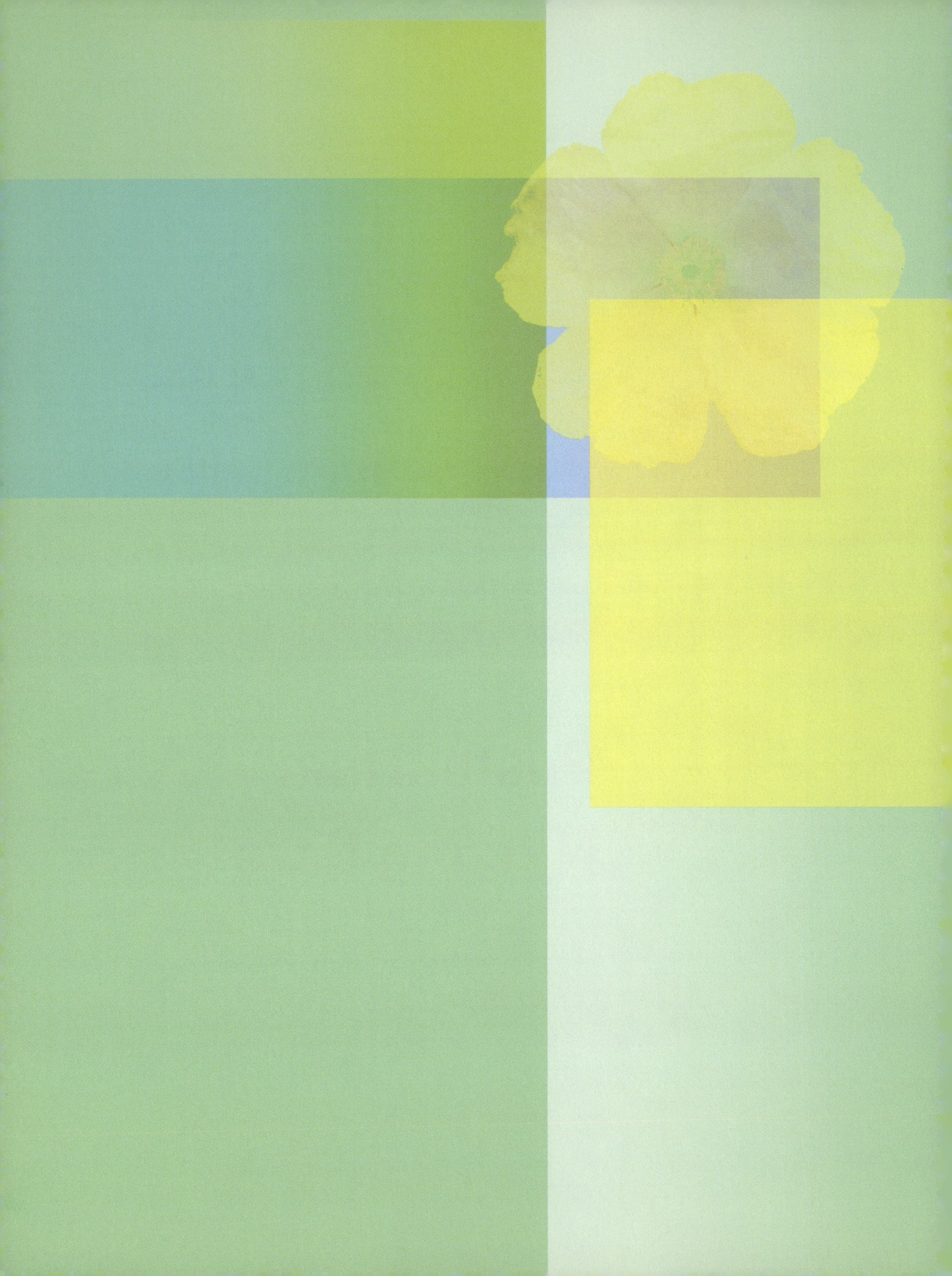

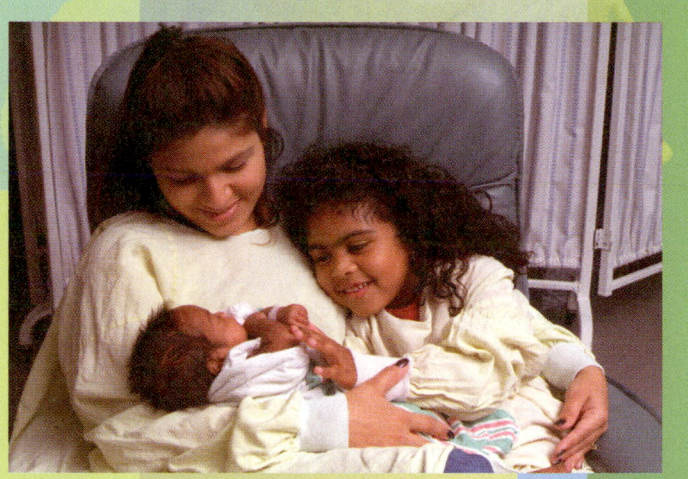

CHAPTER 16

NURSING CARE OF THE LOW-RISK POSTPARTUM FAMILY

After delivery, the new mother's body undergoes many changes as the process of involution takes place. In addition to the physical changes, the new mother and her family begin to adapt to the new roles of parenting and incorporating a new family member into their lives. To increase your awareness of the needs of new mothers and their families during the postpartum period, ask yourself the following questions:

- Reflect on the physiological changes that occur in the woman during pregnancy. What do you think happens as the body returns to a nonpregnant state?
- What would it be like to have another member in your family?
- If you have had a baby, recall what it was initially like to be totally responsible for an infant.
- If you have not had a baby, what do you think it would be like to be totally responsible for an infant?
- How would a baby change your life and that of your family on a day-to-day basis?

Key Terms

Afterpains
Atony
Attachment
Boggy
Diastasis recti
Endometritis
Engorgement
Episiotomy
Fundus
Involution
Letting-go phase

Lochia
Maternal-infant bonding
Puerperium
Residual urine
Role attainment
Role transition
Sleep-wake cycle
Striae
Subinvolution
Taking-hold phase
Taking-in phase

Competencies

Upon completion of this chapter, the reader should be able to:

1. Describe a systematic, logical approach to postpartum assessment.
2. Identify the expected values and clinical assessments to be evaluated in the care of the woman postpartally.
3. Summarize the systemic physiologic changes women experience after childbirth.
4. Describe infant behaviors facilitating or inhibiting the attachment process.
5. Outline three phases of maternal role adjustment.
6. Assess maternal and paternal role adjustment.
7. Identify and describe appropriate nursing interventions for the postpartum woman.

The postpartum period, or **puerperium**, lasts from delivery of the placenta to approximately 6 weeks afterward. The immediate postpartum period consists of the first 24 hours after delivery. The early postpartum period lasts from the second day after birth to the end of the first week. The postpartum period, also known as the fourth trimester, continues until 6 weeks postpartum.

The obstetric nurse will see the pregnant client experience various physiologic and psychosocial changes when she makes the transition from a pregnant woman to a mother. Postpartum nursing should include specific nursing responses based on appropriate assessments to the entire postpartum family. Assessments should be based on a complete understanding of the physiological and psychological processes to both the mother and the neonate during the puerperium.

The needs of the client and her family in the postpartum period can best be met through coordinated multidisciplinary care. Physicians, midwives, nurses, social workers, lactation consultants, and others must ensure that clients receive the services they need. The responsibilities of the obstetric nurse in caring for the client postpartally include being able to make relevant assessments, plan and implement a family-centered plan of care, and evaluate the effectiveness of her care. The nurse also has the potential to significantly affect the client's postpartum health by presenting self-care and infant care education, preparing for hospital discharge, and providing follow-up for the mother and infant.

POSTPARTUM CARE

The birth of a child most often is a joyous occasion for the family. The initial family-infant interaction in the first hours of the postpartal period begins the bonding process. Unless complications occur, the father, significant

COLLABORATIVE CARE

Postpartum care can involve many disciplines and resources in the care of the mother, infant, and family. This care extends from the hospital into the community. Even if nurses are based in the hospital setting, there are many opportunities to refer the postpartum family to other professional resources, such as:

- Physicians: obstetricians, pediatricians, neonatologists
- Advanced practice nurses: Certified Nurse Midwives, nurse practitioners, clinical nurse specialists
- Social workers
- Lactation consultants (many are board certified)
- Nutritionists
- Community health nurses
- Health educators
- Doulas

other, or other supportive family members and friends should remain with the mother and infant after birth. Encouraging family members to hold the infant and point out special physical characteristics promotes family-infant interaction and bonding in this initial introductory period.

Mother-Baby Nursing

The postpartum nurse may need to be prepared to care for both the mother and her infant. Some hospitals continue to offer a traditional postpartum unit and separate nursery. In this type of setting the postpartum nurse is responsible for caring for the mother, whereas another nurse cares for the infant. Most facilities (i.e., birth centers) have now transitioned to family-centered maternity care (FCMC) in which the nursing philosophy is based on the concept of mother-baby nursing or couplet care (Phillips, 1997). The approach to care in this nursing strategy is based on the family being the primary caregivers. The mother's well-being is interdependent with that of her newborn as they adjust to multiple physical, congnitive, and psychosocial changes during the postpartum period (Box 16-1). One team of health care providers (e.g., a nurse and technician or aide) cares for both the mother and her newborn as a unit, viewing them as an interdependent couplet.

A gradual shift has occurred from the nurse providing all the newborn care while the mother watches, to the mother independently caring for her newborn. Education about self-care and newborn care is integrated during the nurse's daily physical care for the couplet. The expanded role of the "mother-baby nurse" involves early parent-infant interaction, demand feeding, flexible care schedules, personalized parenting education, and family visitation.

In addition to mother-baby care, there is a separate concept of rooming-in, where the infant remains in the mother's room at her bedside (Figure 16-1). The infant rooms in with the mother unless medically contraindicated

---

Box 16-1

Practicing Mother-Baby Nursing

The benefits of mother-baby nursing for the family and newborn include the following:

- Facilitating earlier establishment of biologic rhythms with flexible feeding and sleeping cycles
- Fostering breastfeeding
- Decreasing the incidence of cross-infection
- Providing individualized, one-on-one care
- Promoting the mother's role and attachment
- Increasing educational opportunities
- Fostering continuity of care and reduction of confusion of messages between caregivers
- Promoting the mother's learning about her newborn and self-care capabilities
- Increasing maternal self-confidence in caring for her newborn
- Eliminating anxiety about whether the newborn is properly cared for

The benefits of mother-baby nursing for the nursing staff include the following:

- Streamlining responsibilities of care and teaching
- Increasing nursing involvement and responsibility for client care and learning
- Increasing accountability
- Improving communication between the family and caregivers
- Replacing fragmented care with continuity of care
- Eliminating duplication of services
- Facilitating discharge planning
- Increasing efficiency and productivity
- Improving teamwork and interdisciplinary communication
- Increasing job satisfaction through the provision of individualized care, a more stimulating work environment, and positive feedback from families

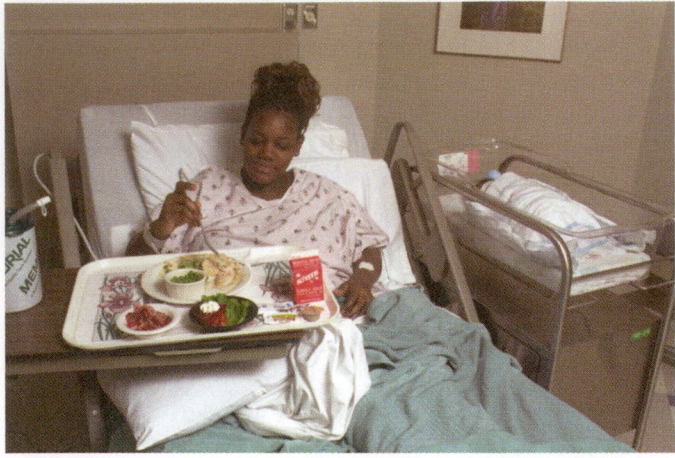

Figure 16-1 The practice of rooming-in allows mother and baby to be together throughout the day.

or the mother is unable to care for her infant owing to medical problems or emotional difficulties. This facilitates the mother-infant attachment process and allows the mother to adapt to caring for the newborn.

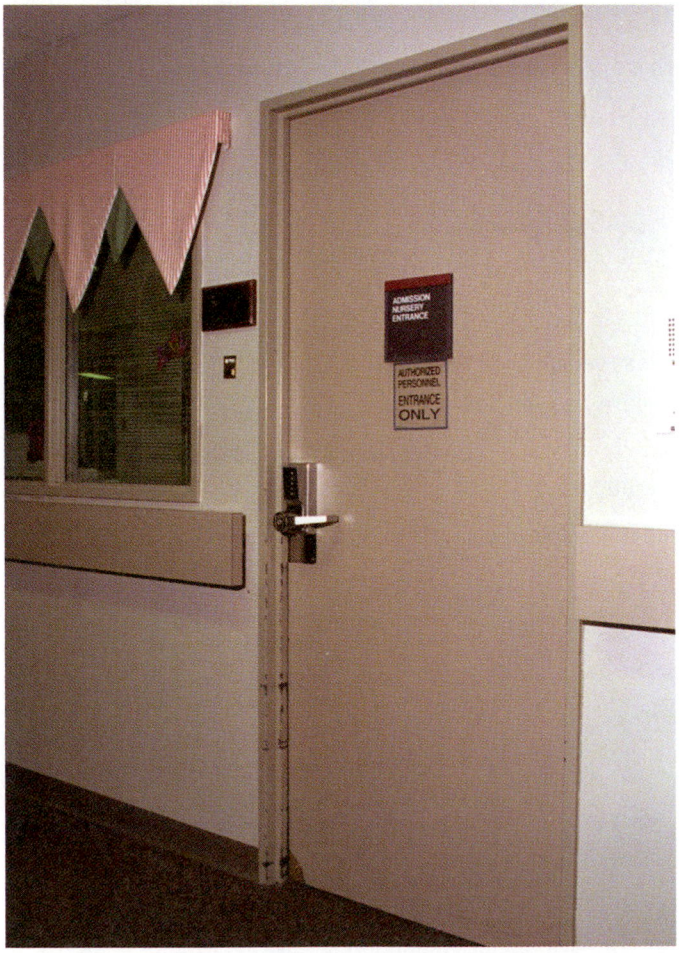

Figure 16-2 Security measures in the postpartum unit and nursery always are in force.

Infant Security

An important aspect of postpartum care is infant security. Cases of infant abduction have directed hospitals to institute infant safety and security systems. The nursing staff must be alert and educate mothers and families about proper security and identification processes (Figure 16-2). The nurse should always check the identification bands on both the mother and infant when providing care. This also ensures appropriate mother-infant match. Many hospitals are applying additional security measures related to visitors.

Hospital Length of Stay

Historically, routine hospital stays after uncomplicated vaginal delivery had ranged from 12 hours to one week. The current hospital length of stay for mothers having normal vaginal delivery is 24 to 48 hours. Today, federal law dictates that third-party insurance companies cannot restrict benefits for hospital stays in connection with childbirth to less than 48 hours after a vaginal delivery and 96 hours after a cesarean delivery. The attending provider is permitted to discharge the client earlier if the client agrees.

Mothers now have less time to recover from the birth process while under professional supervision than in the past. Nurses, in turn, have less time to ensure that new

Critical Thinking

Practicing Family-Centered Maternity Care

Progressive new hospitals have transitioned obstetric services to offering family-centered maternity care (FCMC) (Phillips, 1997). This style of care includes not only physical dimensions but social, spiritual, psychological, and economic dimensions as well.

The elements of FCMC are based on principles designed to promote greater family self-determination, decision-making capabilities, and control. The families are empowered to be responsible for their own care. The family is recognized as a whole unit and care is not necessarily limited to the nuclear family.

- How can you collaborate with families while providing appropriate care and education with respect to their structure, cultural background, and racial and ethnic group?

- How can you be flexible, accessible, and responsive to the needs of families while also respecting their privacy?

mothers are physiologically stable, able to safely provide care for themselves and their new infants, and able to assume the responsibilities of motherhood. Because the purposes of hospitalization after birth are to (1) identify maternal and neonatal complications and (2) provide professional assistance at a time when the mother is likely to need supportive care (American Academy of Pediatrics [AAP] & American College of Obstetricians and Gynecologists [ACOG], 1997), it is essential that the postpartum nurse effectively complete the nursing process to successfully attain an optimal outcome.

CLINICAL ASSESSMENT

Before providing care for the postpartum client, the nurse should review the medical record for the antepartum and intrapartum histories. A nursing report from the labor and delivery nurse should communicate pertinent information regarding the intrapartum course. Information such as length of labor, estimated blood loss, and the presence of episiotomy will alert the postpartum nurse to potential complications.

The nurse should be prepared to provide physical and psychosocial nursing care. The new mother may want to discuss the events of her child's birth in the immediate postpartum period. Retelling what happened during birth validates the events for her and gives the nurse an idea of the mother's state of mind. Active listening by the nurse may elicit potential problems that may occur later in the postpartum period (e.g., "I pushed for 3 hours. I am so tired, and now my bottom really hurts").

During the entire hospital stay, the nurse must incorporate client teaching in all aspects of nursing care. Although the new mother may be emotionally and physically overwhelmed after birth, she must be provided with baby care, self-care, nutrition, and activity information. The nurse can instruct the mother with each step and will explain the reasoning for doing it. (For example, the nurse might say, "I am checking your lochia. It should normally be bright red for the first 3 days.") Client education after birth is important and should be provided at the same time the nursing care is being performed. Ensuring privacy before examining the client will convey respect and may help ease the new mother's fears.

The nurse also should remember to approach the client with sensitivity, taking cultural and religious practices into consideration. For example, some clients may have deep beliefs regarding personal hygiene and modesty or foods to eat (e.g., hot versus cold). The nurse should consult a reference guide, such as *Cultural Assessment* by Geissler (1998), that addresses cultural considerations for the type of client population she serves in her community. This guide annotates health care beliefs, predominant sick care practices,

health team relationships, food practices and intolerances, birth and death rites, infant feeding practices, and child-rearing practices for many nationalities.

In addition to cultural differences, the nurse may find herself unable to communicate to her client if the woman speaks a different language. A family member or professional interpreter may assist in relaying important information to the client.

The nurse assesses the postpartum woman closely. The physiological changes occur rapidly and during these changes, the mother is at risk for complications. A focused clinical assessment used in the postpartum period is an abbreviated form of a full assessment that allows the nurse to monitor closely the postpartum course. In interpreting the assessment data, the nurse must always keep in mind the process of involution and the potential for hemorrhage, infection, and other common complications of the puerperium. The nurse can also use assessment to teach the new mother measures to reduce discomfort and prevent complications, as well as what to expect in the physiological process. This teaching is extended to instructing the new mother in what to expect after she leaves the hospital, self-care, newborn care, and family adjustment.

Vital Signs

The recovery period normally lasts for the first few hours after delivery and until the client is stable. Depending on the protocol of the particular unit, the nurse should assess vital signs, fundus, and lochia every 15 minutes for the first hour, every 30 minutes for the second hour, at the third and fourth hour, and then every 8 hours thereafter (Association of Women's Health, Obstetric and Neonatal Nurses [AWHONN], 1996). Close monitoring assists in identifying potential complications such as hemorrhage and infection. Clients who received some type of conductive anesthesia (e.g., an epidural or spinal) should be monitored during recovery by trained staff in an area with appropriate resuscitative equipment.

Blood Pressure

The client's blood pressure usually changes minimally in the postpartum period. Within the first 6 hours, the blood pressure should stabilize to or remain consistent with the client's baseline before delivery. Blood pressure may be lowered due to the effects of analgesia or anesthesia. Hypotension may result from administration of epidural anesthesia or hemorrhage. Signs of orthostatic hypotension may include dizziness or faintness immediately after sitting or standing. Hemorrhange in the postpartum client may be difficult to identify because the blood pressure may be within normal limits. Blood volume increases 30% during pregnancy, and, therefore, time is needed for it to return to prepregnancy volumes. The postpartal client may

Critical Thinking

Cultural Differences in Postpartum Care

Soon after childbirth, American women are encouraged to get out of bed, ambulate, and care for themselves. Other cultures treat new mothers differently.

A new mother on the Japanese island of Goto Archipelago will stay in bed for 1 month after delivering her baby (Epstein, 2000). It is normal in this culture to have an extended postpartum recovery period. Female relatives, such as grandmothers, aunts, and others, take turns "mothering" the mother and her infant until she feels ready to care for her baby herself.

Based on anthropologic research, historical tribes also mothered new mothers for the first year postpartum (Griffin, 2000). They treated the mothers with massage to help them relax and to restore normal circulation. Massage also was thought to facilitate musculoskeletal healing. Some mothers were treated to a daily full-body massage for the first 3 months after birth.

The balance of opposites such as hot and cold is part of a belief system in many cultural groups, such as Chinese, Filipinos, and Hispanics. They believe there are natural external factors that must be kept in balance to maintain health. To restore a disrupted balance, for example, the treatment is to apply the use of opposites. To treat a so-called hot condition, such as a fever, the person should eat cold foods, such as fresh vegetables, dairy products, and meats. To treat a so-called cold condition, such as a headache, the person should consume hot foods, such as eggs, cheese, chocolate, and aromatic beverages.

How would you incorporate these beliefs and practices into your nursing care to ensure that your practice embodied cultural sensitivity?

Nursing Tip
Vital Signs

Despite a stable blood pressure, the presence of both tachycardia and tachypnea may suggest hypovolemia secondary to early hemorrhage. In a client with hypertension, it may be difficult to determine hemorrhage because blood pressure may appear normal when she actually may have hypovolemia.

Pulse

Due to epinephrine from stress of childbirth, pulse may be increased immediately after birth. A heart rate greater than 100 bpm may indicate pain, fever, anxiety, dehydration, infection, or hypovolemia (Figure 16-3).

Respiratory Rate

Without the presence of respiratory disease or medications, such as an epidural narcotic, the normal respiratory rate should be 16 to 24 breaths per minute. Epidural narcotics include fentanyl and morphine, both of which have the potential to depress the respiratory rate to less than 12 breaths per minute. The nurse should carefully monitor the respiratory rate and have a narcotic antagonist (e.g., naloxone [Narcan]) readily available.

Temperature

The client's oral temperature should range from 36.2°C to 38°C (98°F to 100°F). A temperature greater than 100.4°F in the first 24 hours after delivery may indicate dehydration (Figure 16-4). A temperature greater than 38°C (100.4°F)

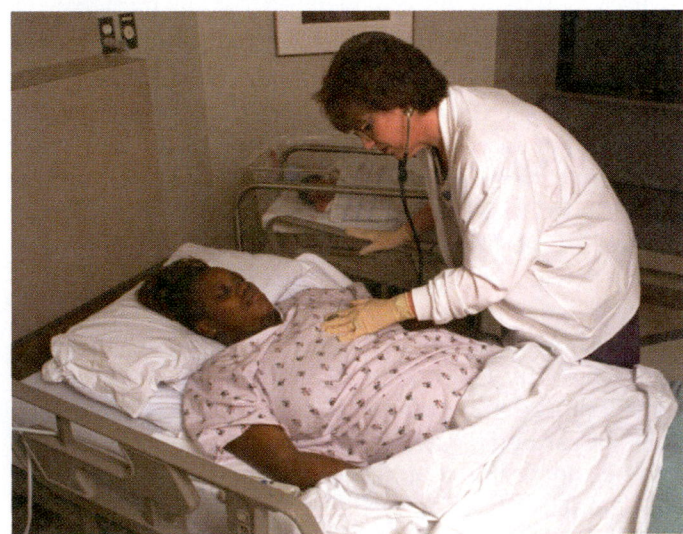

Figure 16-3 The nurse assesses the apical pulse of the postpartum mother.

be in moderate shock before blood pressure changes occur; thus, a decrease in blood pressure may be a late sign of hemorrhage.

Blood pressure elevation may be related to oxytocin administration or excessive use of medications (AWHONN, 1996). Hypertension may be the result of pregnancy-induced hypertension (PIH), anxiety, or essential hypertension. When a client has PIH, her blood pressure values may remain elevated 5% above the norm until 4 days postpartum (AWHONN, 1996). Clients with pregnancy-induced hypertension (PIH) should be monitored more frequently, measuring blood pressure every 4 hours for the next 48 hours because the risk for seizures may continue into the postpartum period.

Nursing Tip *Postpartum Shivers*

Shivering immediately after delivery may be caused by chills or an infection. Many women experience tremors or shaking, sometimes uncontrollably. Changes in hormones, adrenaline, and the physiology of the body cause shivering. You should assess the client's vital signs and risk factors for infection. Once infection has been ruled out, reassure the client that the tremors are normal and soon will pass. Placing a warm blanket over her can reduce the shivering.

6 hours apart after the first 24 hours after delivery for 2 consecutive days may indicate a postpartum infection (AWHONN, 1996). Unless proved otherwise, fever in the postpartum period suggests the presence of an infectious process, usually somewhere in the genitourinary tract (Williams & Cooper, 1993).

Physical Assessment

The nurse should follow an organized method when examining the postpartum client. This manner provides a consistent, quality approach to nursing care. The acronym BUBBLE-HE can serve as a helpful reminder of the elements in a postpartum assessment. BUBBLE-HE stands for:

- Breasts
- Uterus
- Bladder
- Bowel
- Lochia
- Episiotomy
- Homan's sign
- Emotional status

The nurse should assess these elements every 8 hours, along with vital signs (AWHONN, 1996).

Nursing Tip *Discharge Planning for the Low-Risk Postpartum Client*

Preparation for discharge of the postpartum client begins with periodic assessments and includes evaluation of the mother's status and comfort level, self-care education, and resource referral as needed.

Assessment

Monitor vital signs, fundus, and lochia every 15 minutes for first hour, every 30 minutes for second hour, each hour for third and fourth hours, then every 8 hours. Check breasts, uterus, bladder, bowel, lochia, episiotomy, Homan's sign, and emotional status every 8 hours (BUBBLE-HE).

Interventions

Mother should be encouraged to ambulate often and care for the newborn. Ice packs and sitz baths may be used for comfort.

Client Teaching

Self-care preparation for discharge includes perineal care and hygiene, breast care, activity, nutrition, and sleep. Postpartum exercises can help restore muscle tone, especially in abdomen and perineum. New mothers can be counseled about sexuality and contraception. Care and feeding of the infant, including breastfeeding if that is the family's choice, parenting, and family adaptation should be included. Warning signs of postpartum and neonatal complications, including postpartum depression, need to be incorporated.

Referrals

The family should have identified a pediatrician and have a follow-up appointment, along with a follow-up obstetrical appointment. Lactation consultants and other community resources may be included to support family adjustment.

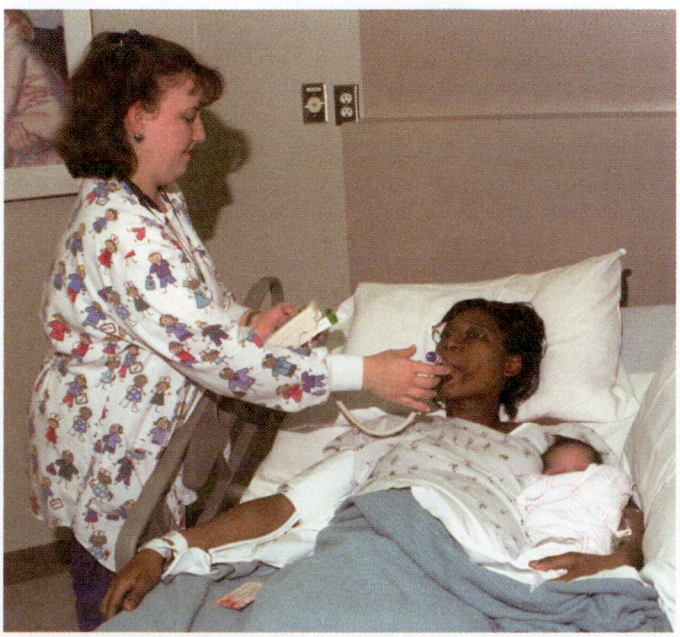

Figure 16-4   The nurse should assess the new mother's temperature regularly in the early postpartum period because fever may suggest an infectious process.

Breasts

On palpation after delivery, breasts usually are enlarged, soft, warm, and contain only a small amount of colostrum, the precursor of milk. The nipples should be intact without redness, tenderness, cracks, or blisters. Colostrum may be expressed. If the mother is not breast-feeding, the breast changes as a result of pregnancy regress after 1 to 2 weeks postpartum.

The mother may experience breast **engorgement** (enlargement and filling of the breasts with milk), which may begin as a tingling sensation in her breasts, 2 to 4 days after delivery. The breasts feel very full, tender, and uncomfortable until the milk is either released through infant sucking, manual expression, or pumping. The discomfort from engorged breasts normally subsides once stimulation to produce milk is decreased. The nursing mother's breasts should be inspected for the presence of inverted nipples, cracks, blisters, fissures, and palpated for fullness and tenderness (Figure 16-5). Some women

Client Education

Breast Care in Nonlactating Women

For the nonlactating client to successfully care for her breasts, you should teach her the following:

- Do not manually express milk from the breasts.

- Do not stimulate the nipples.

- Wear a tight-fitting bra.

- Use ice packs to constrict the superficial blood vessels.

- Take analgesics to minimize discomfort.

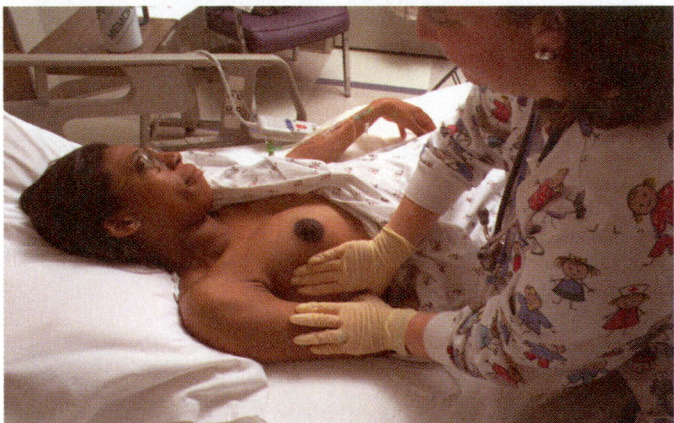

A.

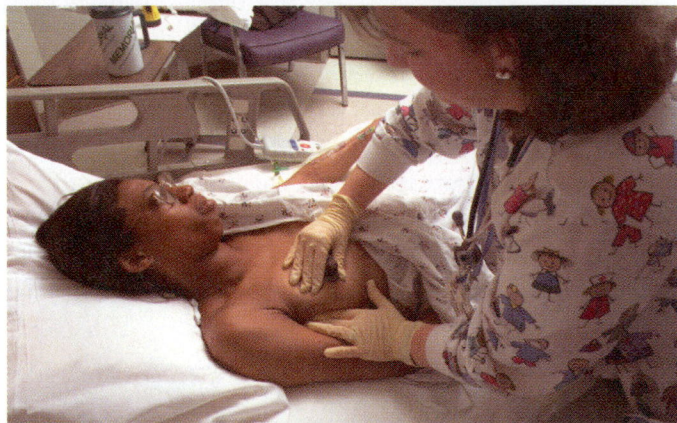

B.

C.

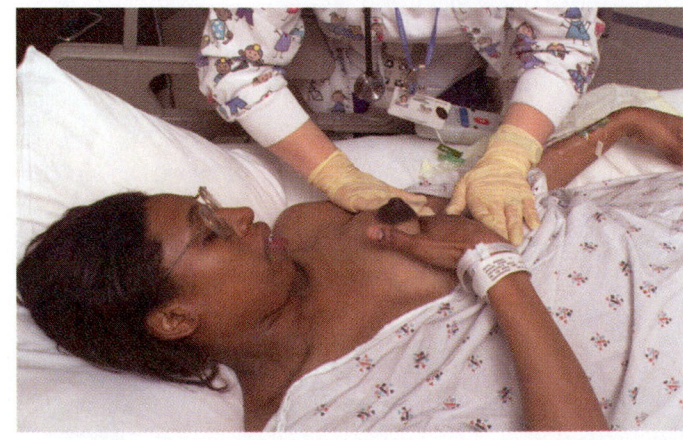

D.

Figure 16-5   Postpartum breast assessment. A. The nurse palpates the breast for tenderness and lumps, which may indicate a plugged milk duct. B. The nipples are assessed for inversion, cracks, blisters, and tenderness; colostrum may be expressed during compression of the areola. C. Showing the new mother how to assess her breasts is an important element of postpartum teaching. D. After assessing the first breast, the nurse examines the second breast.

may have cultural implications of touching breasts or being examined by males. Nurses need to be sensitive when approaching the examination.

When a client chooses to bottle-feed her infant, it is essential to teach the client about lactation suppression. Suppression can be achieved through a variety of methods: decreasing stimulation to the breasts (e.g., securely binding the breasts with a snug support bra and with an ace bandage if more support is needed), avoiding warmth (e.g., hot shower water) on the breasts, and applying ice packs to the breasts. The mother can take acetaminophen (Tylenol) for breast discomfort. These methods can be used until milk production stops.

Uterus

Immediately after delivery the uterus begins the process of **involution** or reduction in size. It generally takes 6 weeks for complete physiologic involution and for the reproductive system to be restored to its nonpregnant state, except for the nursing mother's breasts. **Subinvolution**, or the failure of the uterus to return to a nonpregnant state, occurs when the process of involution is prolonged or stopped as a result of hemorrhage, infection, or retained placental parts.

Uterine involution involves the return of the uterus to a nonpregnant condition—diminishing in size and weight—and anatomic location back into the pelvis (Figure 16-6). The endometrial decidua is shed, as noted by the lochial vaginal bleeding. By the end of the 3 weeks postpartum, the endometrial lining and site of the placental attachment should have returned to a nonpregnant state. The placental site usually is completely healed without scarring by 6 weeks postpartum.

Immediately after delivery, the uterus weighs about 1,000 g (2 lb, 4 oz), measuring 14 by 12 by 8–10 cm, which is two to three times the nonpregnant size (Table 16-1). At the end of 6 weeks postpartum, the uterus weighs 50 to 100 g (2 oz) (AWHONN, 1996). Breastfeeding or breast

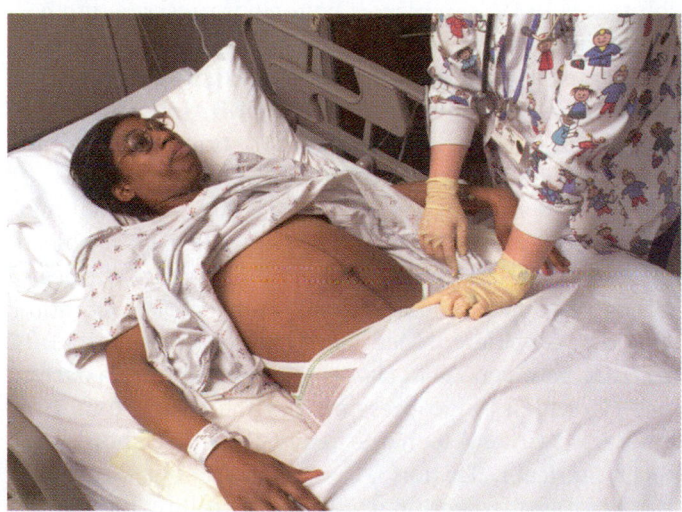

A. Primipara (top and bottom photo)

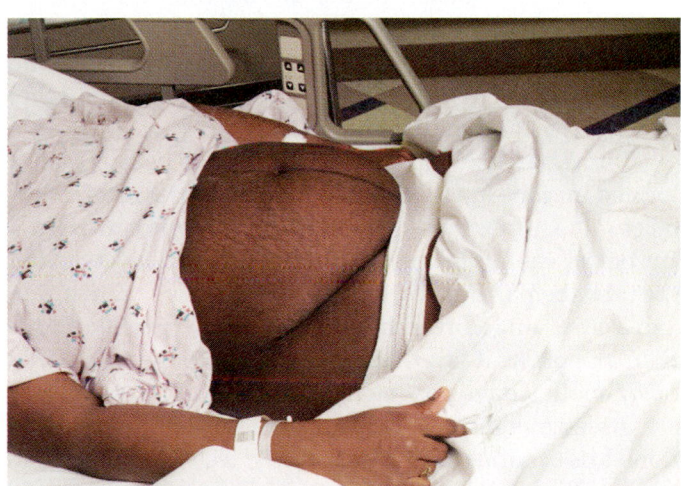

B. Multipara (top and bottom photo)

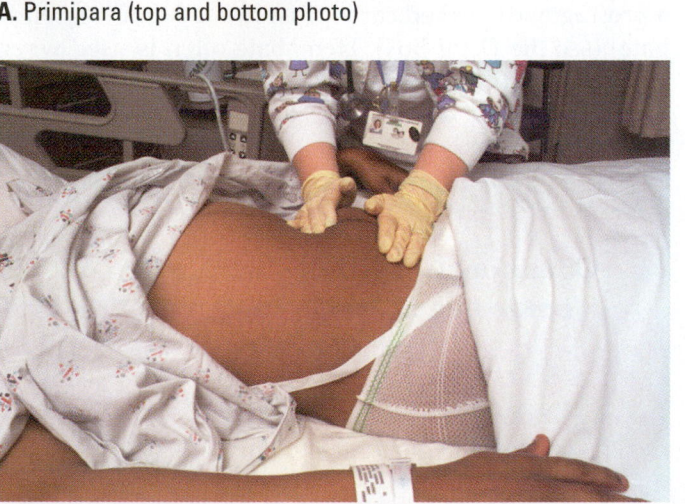

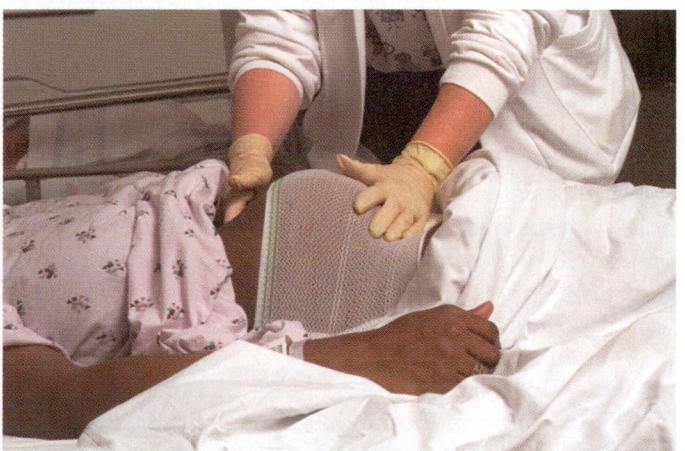

Figure 16-6   Uterine involution 4 hours after delivery in the primipara (A) and the multipara (B). Note the size and shape of the abdomen (top), and the size of the palpated uterus (bottom).

Table 16-1	Weight of Uterus after Delivery
TIME	SIZE (g)
After delivery	1,000
End of first week	300–350
End of second week	100
End of sixth week	50

Nursing Tip   *Assessing Bleeding*

Postpartum hemorrhage should be considered if a pad is saturated with blood within 15 minutes or two pads within 30 minutes (AWHONN, 1996). A slow, steady seepage of blood also may lead to postpartum hemorrhage.

stimulation assists in hastening the speed of uterine involution. There generally is no difference between primiparas and multiparas regarding healing time. Multiparas may have less abdominal muscle tone, however, and the cervix does not completely return to its closed nonpregnant appearance. The parous cervix is easily distensible and appears as a slit.

Assessment of the Fundus

When assessing the location and firmness of the uterine **fundus**, the top portion of the uterus, the nurse should place the client in a supine position with the bed flat. Using a two-handed approach, the nurse places one hand beneath the uterus to support it, while using the other hand to cup the fundus (Figure 16-7).

Immediately after delivery, the fundus usually can be located midline at the level of or one to two fingerbreadths below the umbilicus. The fundus is approximately 1 cm below the umbilicus at 12 hours after delivery. After the first postpartum day the fundus descends or involutes 1 to 2 cm (1 fingerbreadth) each day. Finally, the fundus is nonpalpable as it gradually descends into the true pelvis on or about 9 days postpartum (Figure 16-8).

Assessments may be documented using the abbreviations ML (midline) at "U + 2, U + 1, @U, U-1, U-2" from the umbilicus, or u/1, 1/u.

The fundus should be massaged to firmness (Procedure 16-1) Fundal massage provides the opportunity to maintain contraction of the uterine blood vessels where the placenta was once attached, preventing potential hemorrhage and expelling placental fragments and blood clots (Figure 16-9). Immediately after delivery of the placenta, the fundus should be firm upon palpation. If it is not firm or palpable, the fundus may feel soft or **boggy**. A boggy uterus may be related to an overdistended uterus or structural anomalies (e.g., fibroids). A fundus that remains boggy is a warning sign of uterine **atony** and potential postpartal hemorrhage. Assessment will also include monitoring for risk factors for hemorrhage such as tocolytics, high parity, and prolonged labor.

The position of the fundus also should be noted. Because the broad and round ligaments were greatly stretched during pregnancy and become very lax after the loss of the enlarged uterus after delivery, the uterus is easily displaced (usually above the umbilicus and deviated to the right) by an overfilled bladder. This displacement interferes with the uterus' ability to contract after delivery, resulting in uterine atony and hemorrhage. Women who have had several pregnancies or large babies may have a large uterus that is palpated higher than is normally expected.

Management of Bleeding

After delivery of the placenta, 20 to 40 U of oxytocin (Pitocin) often are added to the mainline intravenous (IV) solution if an IV is in place. Oxytocin is prescribed to hasten uterine contractility and control bleeding. When IV access is not present, other options include administering oxytocin (10 U) intramuscularly (IM), initiating early breastfeeding, or performing nipple stimulation (see the Drug Box on Oxytocin in Chapter 13).

When the uterus remains boggy despite fundal massage and oxytocin administration, other reasons for bleeding must be determined. When bleeding continues, a second pharmacologic agent, such as an ergot preparation, should be considered. Methylergonovine (Methergine), 0.2 mg, may be given IM to clients who do not have a current history of high blood pressure (see the Drug Box). If the fundus is firm and lochia is heavy, the nurse should suspect a cervical laceration.

Another medication useful in controlling bleeding is a prostaglandin called carboprost tromethamine (Hemabate) (see the Drug Box). Hemabate often is used when

Nursing Alert

Common Causes of Postpartum Hemorrhage

1. Uterine atony
2. Retained placenta
3. Cervical or perineal laceration
4. Subinvolution
5. Bleeding disorders

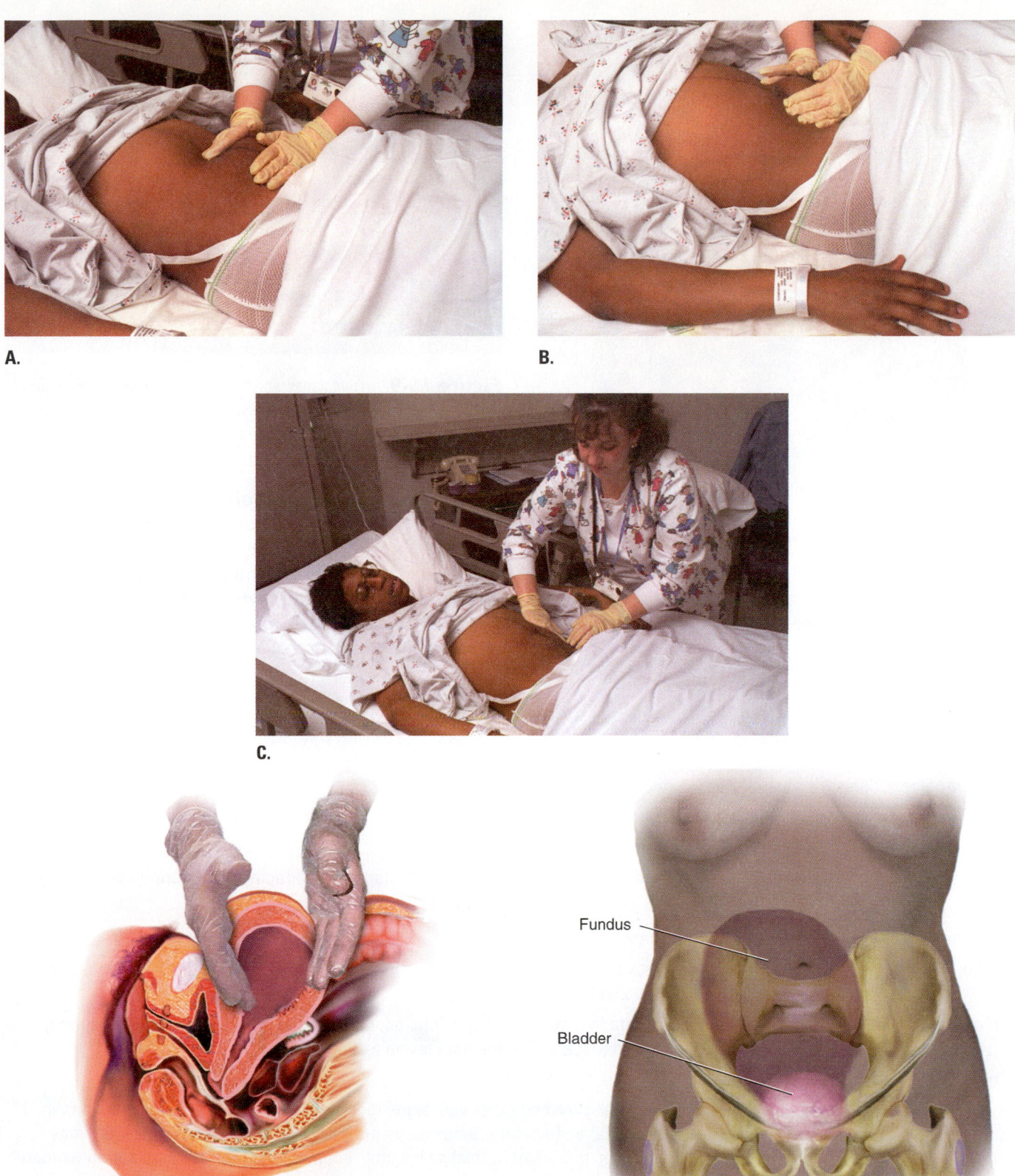

A.

B.

C.

D.

E.

Fundus

Bladder

Figure 16-7   Assessment of the fundus. A. The nurse supports the uterus with her left hand held beneath it while cupping the fundus (top of the uterus) in her right hand. B. The nurse palpates the uterus to determine if it is firm or boggy. C. The nurse assesses the position (midline or displaced to the left or right) of the uterus, which must be done at each fundal assessment. D. View of the uterus during fundal assessment. E. A full bladder displaces the uterus and prevents its contraction.

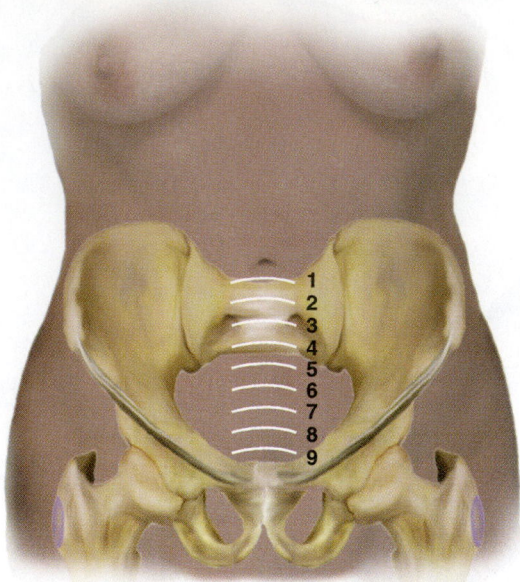

Figure 16-8 Height of the fundus after delivery; numbers indicate postpartum day and level of fundus, in fingerwidths, in relation to the umbilicus.

fundal massage and second-line medications such as methergine do not stop the hemorrhage, or when methergine is contraindicated.

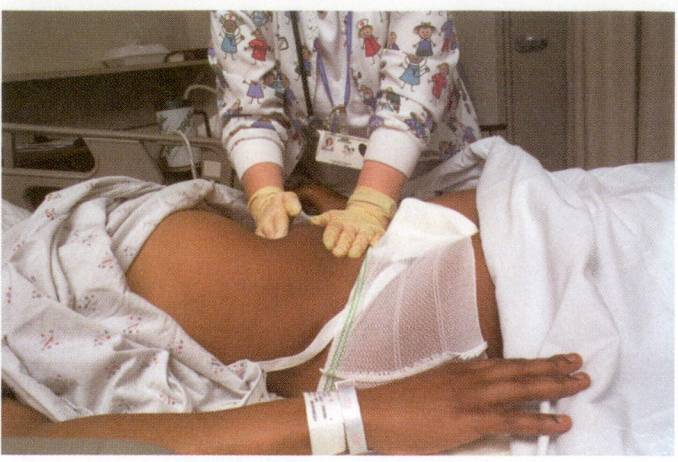

Figure 16-9 Fundal massage helps the uterus return more quickly to its prepregnancy state; massage also helps prevent hemorrhage and expel placental fragments and blood clots.

Assessment of Uterine Pain

Abdominal cramping or **afterpains** are caused by uterine tonic contractions, which are the efforts of the uterus to expel blood clots and placental fragments. The contractions are enhanced with oxytocin. A history of multiple gestation, multiparity, or uterine overdistention usually increases the perception of afterpains.

 **Methylergonovine (Methergine)**

Pharmacologic Class	Pregnancy category C
Therapeutic Class	Oxytocic agent
How Supplied	IM or IV, 0.2 mg/mL; PO, 0.2 mg
Indications for Use	Manages and prevents postpartum hemorrhage by producing firm uterine contractions
Chemical Effect	Stimulates rate, tone, and amplitude of uterine contractions
Therapeutic Effect	Stops postpartum hemorrhage
Dosage	IM, 0.2 mg, every 2 to 4 h; IV, 0.2 mg, slow IV push over 1 min; PO, 0.2 mg three to four times a day 2 to 7 d
Side Effects and Adverse Reactions	Dizziness, headache, seizures, hypertension, palpitations, thrombophlebitis, dyspnea, diaphoresis, nausea and vomiting, uterine tetany
Contraindications	Pregnancy, toxemia, hypertension
Nursing Considerations	Monitor blood pressure and other vital signs for evidence of shock or hypertension while administering IV; abdominal cramps may continue for 3 h after administration; may dilute IV dose up to 5 mL of normal saline; not recommended for use in lactating women
Client Teaching	Report signs and symptoms of ergotism, nausea and vomiting, headache, numbness of fingers and toes, chest pain, weakness; may have abdominal cramps
Laboratory Finding	None

Note. Data from *PDR Nurse's Drug Handbook,* by G. R. Spratto and A. L. Woods, 2004, Clifton Park, NY: Delmar Learning.

Nursing Alert

Precautions for Methylergonovine

Methylergonovine should only be given to clients who *do not* have high blood pressure. Take a blood pressure reading before administering the medication. If the client with hypertension or risk of hypertension has a blood pressure greater than normal parameters, do not give the medication, and notify the physician.

The uterus of the primipara woman tends to remain in a better or more prolonged state of contraction compared with that of a multipara woman. Thus, the multipara woman's afterpains will seem more intense, contracting vigorously at regular intervals. Afterpains usually become milder after 3 days. When abdominal pain becomes significantly more intense or the uterus is tender to palpation, the nurse should assess for further indications of problems, such as **endometritis**, an infection of the uterine lining. Severe pain that is not relieved by medications should be reported to the health care provider.

PROCEDURE 16-1

Postpartum Fundal Massage

Purpose

To promote uterine involution and expulsion of uterine contents

Equipment

Exam gloves

Peripads or Chux

Actions and Rationales

1. Ensure that your hands are warm and clean. *This procedure promotes client comfort and safety.*

2. Inform the client what you are going to do. *Client understanding of the reasoning for the procedure aids in cooperation and in the client's feeling involved in care.*

3. Determine if the client needs to empty her bladder. *A full bladder impedes uterine involution.*

4. Put the client in a supine position with her legs slightly flexed. *This position promotes client comfort and allows maximum access to abdominal area.*

5. Gently touch the client's abdomen to decrease tension on it. *Light touch gives client notice that you are about to begin and helps the client relax the muscles.*

6. Tell the client you are going to place (cup) one hand on top of the symphysis pubis to support and hold the lower part of the uterus. *Having the client understand your movements helps her relax and accept the procedure.*

7. Place (cup) the other free hand on the fundus. *Correct placement of the hands facilitates a successful massage.*

8. Gently palpate the fundus and massage with a downward, steady pressure. If you cannot locate the fundus, move your hand higher or lower as needed. The fingers should lay flat on top of the abdomen while massaging. Do not massage for more than a few minutes because overstimulation of the fundus may cause muscle fatigue and continued agony. *Gentle palpation and massage of the fundus facilitates contraction of the organ and expulsion of uterine contents.*

(continues)

PROCEDURE 16-1 *(continued)*

9. Note the consistency of the fundus, that is, whether it is soft and boggy or firm. The firm fundus will feel hard like a softball. *Firmness indicates that the uterus is naturally contracting and shrinking.*

10. If the fundus is soft, massage it until it contracts and becomes firm. *A soft, boggy fundus indicates that the uterus is not contracting.*

11. Teach the client how to massage the fundus. If the woman is breastfeeding, putting the infant on the breast will help the uterus contract. *These health promotion techniques involve the client actively in her postpartum care. Advise the client that the uterine contractions may be painful, especially during breastfeeding, and that this is normal.*

12. Note the location of the fundus. When the fundus is greater than the level of the umbilicus, the nurse should assess for the possibility of uterine filling with blood or blood clots and uterine displacement by a distended bladder. *Any condition other than normal uterine involution should be investigated further by the physician.*

13. It is best to observe the perineum at the same time you palpate the fundus to note the amount and color of lochia or clots that may be discharged during massage. The bleeding may increase during massage. *Expulsion of blood and clots is expected during massage; let the client know that this is normal.*

14. Replace the old peripad, as needed. *Promote client comfort and cleanliness by keeping the perineal area as clean as possible.*

15. Cover the client and reposition her in the bed, as needed. *Return the client to a state of privacy and comfort.*

16. Document findings in the client's medical record. *Note state and height of fundus, and results of massage, so involution can be monitored.*

Follow-up

Measuring postpartum bleeding and uterine descent is crucial to monitoring successful involution and the risk of hemorrhage or other untoward sequelae.

If the third stage of labor is mismanaged by pulling on the cord before readiness of the placenta to detach from the uterine wall, uterine inversion or prolapse may occur. Although rare, this is a life-threatening occurrence that requires emergency measures and immediate notification of the physician. The client may go into shock. The uterus must be reinserted immediately by returning it to a normal position in the pelvis, a procedure that must be performed by a physician.

Bladder

In the immediate postpartum period, the bladder is congested, edematous, and hypotonic from the effects of labor. Unless a urinary tract infection is present, these effects should resolve within 24 hours of delivery. Considerable diuresis—up to 3,000 mL per day—occurs in the first 2 to 3 days postpartum (AWHONN, 1996). The diuresis results from the decreasing production of aldos-terone hormone (sodium retention decreases and urine production increases) and the body's method of removing excess fluid. The renal pelvis and ureters, stretched and dilated during pregnancy, return to normal by the end of 4 weeks postpartum.

In the immediate postpartum period, urinary distention, incomplete emptying, and residual urine may occur. These complications are related to an edematous perineum, pain, reflex spasms, and bladder desensitization, and can lead to a full bladder. A full bladder interferes with uterine contractions and increases the risk for hemorrhage.

Risk factors for these problems include: episiotomy (surgical incision to enlarge the vaginal opening for delivery of the infant's head), perineal edema or tenderness, long labor, assisted vaginal delivery (forceps or trauma may cause neural blockage), lacerations, previous catheterization (secondary to pain and swelling associated with an episiotomy), and anesthesia (bladder tone may

Carboprost Tromethamine (Hemabate)	
Pharmacologic Class	Pregnancy category C
Therapeutic Class	Oxytocic; uterine stimulant
How Supplied	IM, 250 µg/mL
Indications for Use	Prevents and treats postpartum hemorrhage not managed by conventional methods
Chemical Effect	Produces immediate strong uterine contractions
Therapeutic Effect	Stops postpartum hemorrhage
Dosage	IM, 250 µg/mL, deep IM every 1.5 to 3.5 h, may increase to 500 µg if bleeding is not controlled; total dosage should not exceed 12 mg
Side Effects and Adverse Reactions	Nausea, vomiting, diarrhea, fever, chills
Contraindications	Uterine tetany
Nursing Considerations	Monitor drug's effectiveness by evaluating uterine contractions and cessation of bleeding; may prophylactically administer an antidiarrheal drug, such as diphenoxylate and atropine (Lomotil)
Client Teaching	Client will experience uterine contractions
Laboratory Finding	None

be temporarily lost, resulting in urinary retention and diminished perception of bladder fullness).

Nursing responsibilities include teaching the newly delivered mother to empty the bladder often after birth to assist in controlling pain and bleeding. Immediately after delivery, the client should be assisted to the bathroom the first two or three times to protect against falls; the nurse must monitor her for orthostatic hypotension and faintness (Figure 16-10). Early ambulation and comfort facilitate urination. After delivery the client should be able to urinate within 4 hours, at least 300 mL, with complete emptying of the bladder (AWHONN, 1996). The nurse should note complaints of urinary frequency, dysuria, and retention. The primary provider should be notified if the woman has not voided 6 to 8 hours after delivery, frequently covered in routine orders.

The nurse should closely observe for bladder distention and adequate emptying after urinary efforts. After urination, the fundus should be repalpated for location to ensure appropriate emptying of the bladder. The bladder normally should be nonpalpable. If the bladder remains distended, the client may be retaining residual urine. **Residual urine** is defined as urine remaining in the bladder after elimination. Residual urine can result in urinary tract infection.

The nurse may need to perform a straight catheterization when the client cannot urinate, the bladder remains distended, and the client is uncomfortable. The

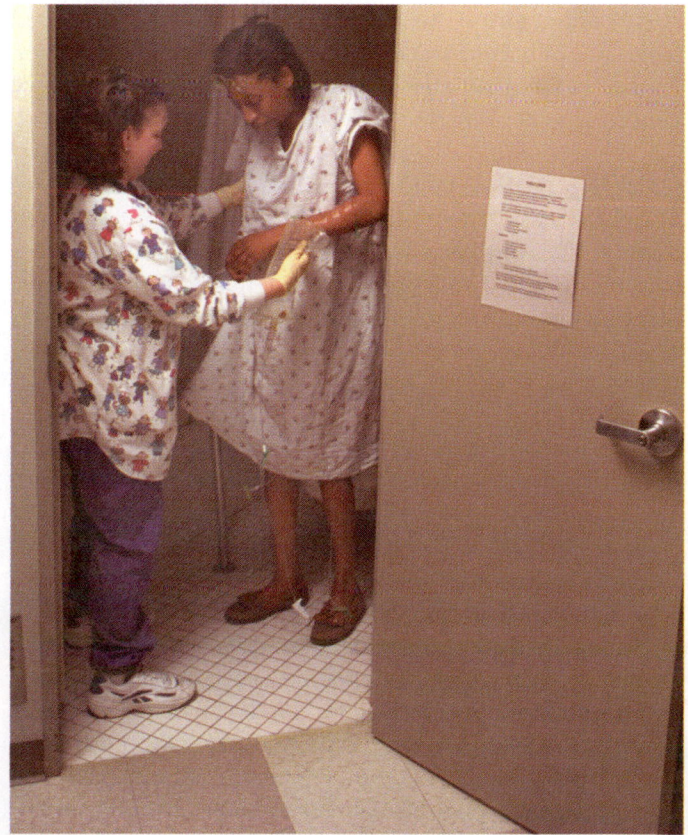

Figure 16-10   The nurse should assist the new mother the first few times she attempts to ambulate after delivery.

Nursing Tip   *Urination after Delivery*

The newly delivered client may need assistance in urinating. Therapeutic actions, such as mental relaxation, taking an analgesic before voiding, drinking fluids, running the tap water, blowing bubbles through a straw in a glass, pouring water over the perineum, concentrating on relaxing part of the perineum using pelvic tightening exercises (Kegel), or standing in the shower, may aid in stimulating urination. A few drops of peppermint oil in the toilet water also is helpful in stimulating the urge to urinate.

judgment to perform a straight catheterization depends on the client's circumstances: the degree of bladder distention, location of the displaced uterus, amount of bleeding, amount of fluid or IV intake since the last voiding, and the techniques used to encourage voiding. When all of these parameters are not extreme or have not been met, catheterization should be delayed an hour or so until further assessment.

An indwelling catheter should be inserted when the client cannot empty her bladder completely. An increased incidence of bacteriuria exists with an indwelling catheter. An indwelling catheter inserted before cesarean delivery generally is kept in place for 24 hours.

Bowels and Gastrointestinal System

The client's appetite typically will return to normal immediately after delivery, with the new mother usually becoming hungry 1 to 2 hours after delivery. If there are no complications from anesthesia, diet habits with regular

Nursing Alert

Detecting a Distended Bladder

When the bladder is full and distended, on palpation it will feel like a ballottable cystic mass or rounded bulge. The mound may fluctuate as does a water-filled balloon. Dull percussion may be heard over the symphysis pubis. A full bladder tends to displace the uterus up and to the right. Lochia may be more than normal because the uterus is unable to contract effectively. A distended bladder takes longer to regain its original tone because muscle tone may have been lost as a result of stretching.

Critical Thinking

Voiding after Delivery

Marissa, your newly delivered 30-year-old grava 2, para 2, mother, is unable to void 5 hours after delivery. She received an epidural when she was 5 cm dilated, and a Foley catheter was inserted after the epidural when she was unable to void. She quickly progressed through labor, delivering a 9 lb, 7 oz baby boy.

- Which methods would you use in assisting your client to urinate?
- Which nursing intervention must be performed if the client is unable to void spontaneously?
- Which other assessments should you monitor if the client has a distended bladder?

food may be resumed. The client who had vomited during labor may not have an appetite. The nurse should encourage her to increase her fluid intake and choose foods high in potassium and protein. Especially after a long and difficult labor, the new mother will be thirsty and will need nourishment with food and fluids to regain her strength.

A woman's nutrition continues to be important throughout the postpartum period, regardless of choice of infant feeding methods. The physical stresses of labor and delivery and the psychological demands of being a new mother take a toll on her body. The client may need a diet high in protein and iron if she has experienced heavy blood loss. Adequate dietary protein and iron facilitate tissue healing and restore iron levels from the normal hemoglobin hemodilution of pregnancy.

The client's bowel pattern should remain unchanged after a vaginal delivery, with a bowel movement normally occurring by 2 or 3 days postpartum. Often, a woman may defecate while pushing during the second stage of labor. When gastric motility does not return by 2 or 3 days after delivery, constipation may occur. The nurse should assess the client's abdomen for nondistention, softness, and bowel sounds.

Constipation in the early postpartum period may be the result of several factors. Due to the increases in progesterone toward the end of pregnancy, bowel tone is slowed. During labor, bowel motility and decreased fluid intake further slow bowel action. The side effects of medications and anesthesia and the self-restraint or hesitancy to defecate owing to perineal or rectal discomfort also lead to postpartum constipation. For women who have had an episiotomy, fear of tearing the stitches may lead to or exacerbate the occurrence of constipation.

Nursing Alert

Use of Enemas and Suppositories after Delivery

Do not administer enemas or suppositories to women who have experienced a fourth-degree laceration because they are at risk for dehiscense (breakdown) of their episiotomy.

The client's possible inhibition must be assessed because it may lead to fecal impaction. The nurse should explain that the stitches are inserted in layers and assure the client that the normal effort of bearing down with rectal pressure will not affect the episiotomy. The client should be encouraged to drink six to eight 8 ounce glasses of fluids daily and eat a high-fiber diet (e.g., whole grains, legumes, vegetables, and fruits). Warm sitz baths, topical anesthetics (e.g., chloroprocaine [nesacaine]), and stopping medications that cause constipation (e.g., Tylenol with Codeine) are helpful interventions to lower the chances of constipation.

When constipation is severe, administering an analgesic and a stool softener (e.g., docusate [Colace]) before ambulation may assist in facilitating a bowel movement. Many health care providers order a mild prophylactic laxative, such as magnesium hydroxide (Milk of Magnesia), 30 mL/day, for women who have had a fourth-degree laceration. If the client has not yet had a bowel movement by 2 to 3 days postpartum, mineral oil, bisacodyl suppository (Dulcolax), or Fleet enema may be prescribed to stimulate intestinal activity.

Hemorrhoids

Examination of the bowels includes assessment for the presence of hemorrhoids. Hemorrhoids present during pregnancy may enlarge during labor. If the hemorrhoids are too large, they may cause pain if they become thrombosed and may subsequently cause constipation. Treatments with witch hazel or a topical anesthetic spray may relieve discomfort.

Lochia

The usual uterine discharge of blood, mucus, and tissue after childbirth is called **lochia**. Lochia contains the sloughing of decidual tissues, including erythrocytes, epithelial cells, and bacteria. Lochia is assessed according to its amount, color, and change with activity and time. The duration of lochia is not affected by breastfeeding or the use of oral contraceptives (Bowes, 1996).

The descriptive name of lochia changes with the changes in color. *Lochia rubra* is the term given for the discharge in the first 3 days after delivery. Lochia rubra is small to moderate in amount and has a bright-red color, secondary mainly to decidual tissue and bloody content. The color becomes progressively paler. Small clots may be present.

Lochia serosa, which occurs 4 to 10 days after delivery, is a watery, pink, or brown-tinged color, which is lighter in amount than is lochia rubra. Lochia serosa primarily contains serous fluid, leukocytes, erythrocytes, and decidual tissue.

The lochia transitions into *lochia alba*, a whitish-yellow creamy discharge on days 10 to 17. Many women may have minimal discharge by day 14; however, it is not uncommon for lochia alba to last until 6 weeks postpartum (Bowes, 1996). Lochia alba consists of a mixture of leukocytes, decidual tissue, and decreasing fluid content. The nurse should inform the client that there likely will be an episode of heavy vaginal bleeding between days 7 to 14 when the placental eschar sloughs off (Bowes, 1996).

The flow of lochia rubra is evaluated by examining the blood saturation on a peripad that occurs in 1 hour or less. The nurse should document her assessment of lochia using the descriptive term and the amount of blood saturation. Descriptions of lochia can be scant (less than 2.5 cm, or 1 in), light/small (less than 10 cm, or 4 in), moderate (less than 15 cm, or 6 in), or heavy/large (one pad saturated within 15 to 30 min) (Figure 16-11).

Determining the exact amount of blood on a peripad can be a challenge. Health care providers often mistakenly underestimate blood loss. Quantifying blood loss is a learned skill that should be practiced to accurately assess blood loss.

Saturation of a pad within 15 to 30 minutes may indicate hemorrhage. When the client is bleeding heavily, the nurse needs to ensure that the blood is not coming from another source, such as a cervical or vaginal laceration. Lacerations are more highly suspected when heavy bleeding continues despite a firm uterus. The nurse also should check under the woman's buttocks for bleeding on the underpad and bed sheets.

The peripad, along with the Chux or pads used, may be weighed (1g = 1 mL fluid). Blood tests can be used as an indicator of blood loss. A complete blood count (CBC) may indicate a 1.0 to 1.5 g/dL decrease in hemoglobin and a 3% to 4% decrease in hematocrit, which is consistent with a loss of 500 mL of blood (AWHONN, 1996).

The amount of lochia varies with position changes but should continually decrease throughout the first 4 to 6 weeks postpartum. The blood pools in the vaginal vault when the client is recumbent and drains when standing up. Clot formation occurs as a result of the pooling in the uterus or vagina. An increase in bright-red bleeding and

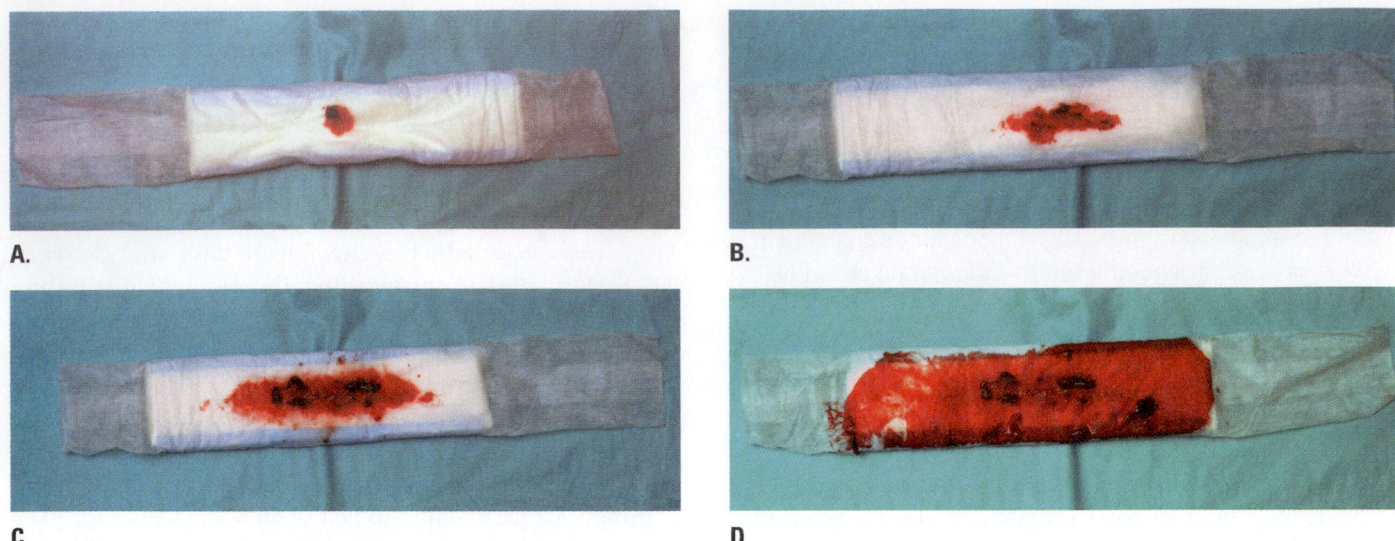

A.   **B.**

C.   **D.**

Figure 16-11   Assessment of lochia is based on the amount of blood saturation on a peripad. A. Scant. B. Light/small. C. Moderate. D. Heavy/large.

the passage of clots also may occur during physical activity or breastfeeding. Lochia with a reddish color that persists after 2 weeks of delivery may indicate subinvolution of the placental site or retained placental parts; this finding must be reported to the physician (Bowes, 1996).

The client should be instructed to notify the nurse if blood clots larger than 1 cm or roughly the size of a silver dollar are passed. Nursing actions include assessing the fundus for firmness and amount of lochia (Figure 6-12). When clots persist, the nurse should notify the health care provider because an examination may be required to evaluate for other sources of continued bleeding.

Lochia has a characteristic menstrual-like musky or fleshy smell. A foul-smelling discharge, along with other indicators, such as fever and uterine tenderness, may suggest an infection, such as endometritis. Lochia serosa

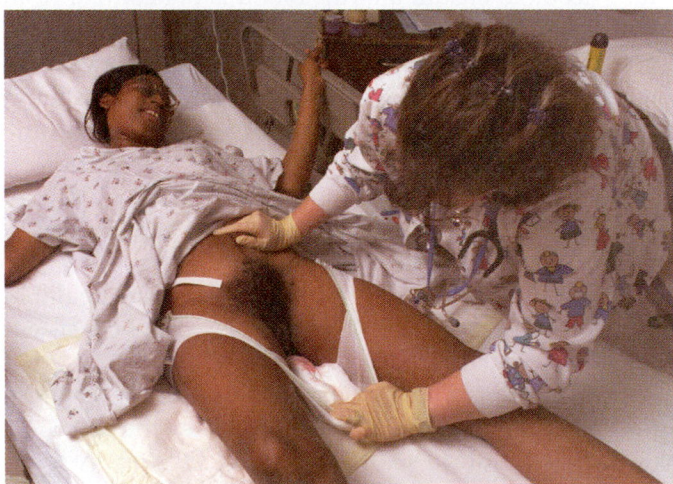

Figure 16-12   The nurse places a hand on the fundus while assessing the amount of lochia.

emits the strongest odor, which increases if mixed with perspiration. Because lochia is an excellent medium for bacterial growth, clients should be taught to change the peripad at every urination.

The first menstrual period usually begins within an average of 8 weeks after delivery for most nonlactating women. The timing may be delayed from 2 to 18 months in breast-feeding mothers; however, ovulation may occur without the onset of the first menstrual period (AWHONN, 1996). Thus, it is possible for a woman to become pregnant before the return of menses. Consistent, continuous breastfeeding increases prolactin levels, thus postponing the resumption of ovulation. Once breast stimulation decreases, prolactin levels decrease and FSH and LH hormone levels increase, inducing ovulation.

Client education includes teaching the client to report signs and symptoms of problems, such as foul-smelling lochia, heavy flow or change in normal flow, presence of large clots, and lochia rubra that continues past 4 days postpartum or that returns after initial cessation. Absence of lochia may indicate perineal infection.

Episiotomy

An **episiotomy** is the surgical incision made to enlarge the vaginal opening for delivery of the baby's head. Depending on client preference, situation, and provider preference and judgment, some women experience delivery with an episiotomy. The episiotomy may be incised midline down the center of the perineum, or mediolaterally, which extends in a diagonal angle to either the left or right side. With or without an episiotomy, the perineum may suffer from lacerations during childbirth. Lacerations are classified as first, second, third, or fourth degree (Table 16-2). Severe pain may indicate a hematoma.

Table 16-2	Classification of Perineal Lacerations
CLASSIFICATION	**DESCRIPTION**
First degree	Involves only the skin and superficial structures above the muscle
Second degree	Extends into the perineal muscles
Third degree	Reaches into the anal sphincter muscles
Fourth degree	Continues into the anterior rectal wall

Nursing Tip *Using Ice Packs*

Many commercially prepared ice packs are available; however, an inexpensive way to make an ice pack is right on your unit. A condom or latex glove filled with crushed ice and wrapped with a disposable paper towel can be used as an ice pack. Fresh ice will easily mold on the woman's body; however, frozen packs will last longer before they begin to melt. Caution should be used to not leave the ice pack on too long because it may cause tissue damage.

To assess an episiotomy and the condition of the perineum, it is best to have the client lie on her side, flexing her upper leg toward her hip. The nurse can then lift the buttocks to expose the perineum. Using a good light source, such as a gooseneck lamp or flashlight, facilitates visualization of the incision and repair (Figure 16-13). The REEDA (redness, edema, ecchymosis, discharge, and approximation) scoring scale can be used when assessing the episiotomy. At the client's request, the nurse can provide a mirror to show her the episiotomy to help dispel fears and misconceptions about healing of the perineum.

Care of the vulva includes applying ice packs to the perineum for the first 24 hours to help decrease edema and pain. Ice packs also assist in constricting blood vessels, minimize the risk of hematoma formation, and decrease muscle irritability and spasm (Bowes, 1996). Ice packs should not be applied directly to the skin; they should be wrapped with an absorbent disposable type of covering.

After the first 24 hours after delivery, a sitz bath with warm water or moist heat may be used to reduce the local discomfort caused by perineal trauma and an episiotomy. The change from cold to warm therapy enhances vascular circulation and healing. The sitz bath may be used until the episiotomy heals (Procedure 16-2). Use of a heat lamp two or three times a day also will assist in the healing process, although many institutions no longer support this practice.

The client should be taught perineal hygiene, including daily washing with warm water and mild soap. The perineum should be cleansed after each voiding and bowel movement. A squeeze-bottle filled with warm tap water may be used to clean the perineum. The water should be comfortably warm on the wrist (approximately 38°C, or 100°F). The nozzle should be directed toward the perineum. The perineum should be wiped from the anterior to the posterior, or in a front-to-back motion, to avoid contamination from the anal region. Practices such as changing the peripad frequently (after each voiding and bowel movement or at least four times a day, removing the pad from front to back, and hand washing will help decrease the risk for infection and promote wound healing for episiotomy and repaired lacerations. Soiled pads should be placed in an appropriate disposal container. Pain should be assessed and medication provided as needed.

Immediately after delivery, the vagina appears edematous, bruised, stretchable, and may gape at the introitus. By week 4, the vaginal ruggae return. Always remaining slightly larger than in the prepregnant state, the vagina returns to its prepregnant state by 6 to 8 weeks postpartum. The nurse should teach the client how to perform perineal exercises, such as Kegel exercises, to assist in

Nursing Tip *REEDA Scale*

Use the REEDA acronym as a nursing tool when evaluating an episiotomy (Davidson, 1974). REEDA stands for redness, edema, ecchymosis (purplish patch of blood flow), discharge, and approximation (closeness of the skin edges).

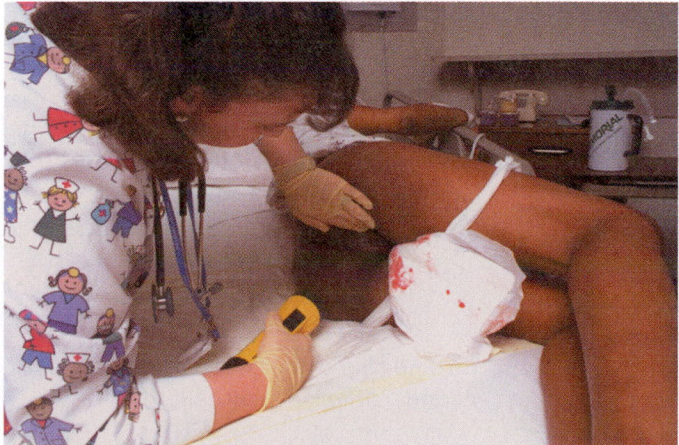

Figure 16-13   The nurse inspects the episiotomy site with the client lying on her side.

PROCEDURE 16-2

Sitz Bath

Purpose

To promote client comfort and perineal hygiene

Equipment

Sitz bath kit	Dry towels
Warm water	Peripads
Toilet	Exam gloves

Actions and Rationales

1. Inform the client about the rationale and process of using a sitz bath. *Client understanding of the reasoning for the procedure aids in cooperation and in the client's feeling involved in care.*

2. Remove the contents from the package. *This allows preparation of the materials for use.*

3. Clamp the tubing. *Clamping prevents water leakage prior to intended use.*

4. Fill the enclosed bag with warm water and hang the bag on a hook by the toilet. *Warm water is more comfortable for the client, and this position facilitates flow of water through the tubing.*

5. Fill the container halfway with warm water. *Warm water is more comfortable for the client.*

6. Lift the toilet seat and place the container on the toilet with the overflow opening facing toward the back. *Proper positioning of the basin ensures client safety and proper use.*

7. Attach the tube into the opening in the container. *Proper fitting prevents leakage.*

8. Position client on toilet seat and release clamp. *This allows the warm water to irrigate the perineum.*

9. Instruct the client to sit atop the container for 15 to 20 min. *This is the suggested time frame for a therapeutic bath.*

10. Adjust the water level and temperature of the water by opening the clamp and releasing more water into the container. *Client comfort is enhanced by ensuring that the water temperature and level are appropriate.*

11. Instruct the client to dry the perineum and apply a clean peripad when finished. *Removing excess moisture promotes healing of the site.*

12. Flush the water in the basin into the toilet and clean the basin. *A cleaned container can be reused.*

13. Teach client to use sitz bath at home. *Clients may find comfort in performing this procedure at home following discharge.*

14. Assess the perineum.

15. Document the use of a sitz bath and assessment of the episiotomy site.

Follow-up

Remind clients that a sitz bath can be performed at home to provide comfort and freshness, and to relieve perineal or episiotomy pain.

restoring vaginal and perineal tone and elasticity and to help reduce urinary incontinence. (See the Client Education box for instructions on performing Kegel exercises, on page 641.)

Extremities

Assessment of the extremities should include examination of varicosities, deep tendon reflexes (DTRs), tenderness, and presence of edema or nodular areas on the legs. DTRs should be no greater than +1 to +2. Brisk DTRs (+3 to +4) may present hyperactive reflexes suggestive of PIH. Pretibial or pedal edema may be present, especially in the client with PIH.

Preconditions of blood hypercoagulability, severe anemia, traumatic delivery, and obesity are risk factors for developing superficial or deep vein thrombosis. Pain, erythema, or local swelling on the legs, especially the calves, may signify thrombophlebitis. The nurse should assess for Homan's sign as a positive indicator of thrombophlebitis (Figure 16-14). Early ambulation in current practice reduces the incidence of developing thrombophlebitis.

In addition, the client's legs should be assessed for sensation and mobility when epidural or spinal anesthesia has been administered. The nurse may place a needle or sharp object on the client's torso to determine the level of tactile sensation, which should begin to approach T-11 or T-12 within the first hour of delivery. With appropriate return of mobility, the client should be able to move her toes and lift her buttocks off the bed within 2 to 4 hours after the discontinuation of the anesthesia.

Emotional Status

The immediate postpartum period is an emotional roller coaster, and almost any emotions may be observed. Nevertheless, the nurse should be continually assessing the parents for appropriate responses to their infant.

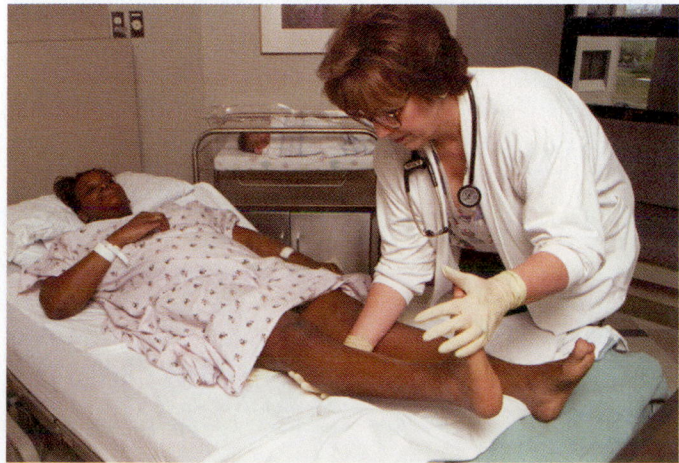

Figure 16-14   The nurse assesses for Homan's sign by checking for calf pain when the foot is flexed.

Nursing Tip   *Assessing Homan's Sign*

Homan's sign is assessed by straightening the client's leg flat on the bed. Place one hand on the knee, applying gentle pressure to keep the leg straight. Place the other hand on her foot, gently flexing the foot toward the body. The leg may be more easily examined when the woman slightly bends her knees and places the foot flat on the bed. The feeling of calf pain on flexion in either foot is a positive sign of thrombophlebitis. Use both hands on either side of the leg to palpate the calf for warmth and tenderness. Examine the calves for redness, hardness, or nodules along a vein. In addition, check the ankle and pretibial areas for edema (see Figure 16-14).

Many times the client experiences a sense of elation immediately after the birth of her baby. She is excited and relieved that labor is finally over. The mother may want to relive the experience by talking about the labor. If she went through a particularly long and painful labor and delivery, however, she also may be exhausted and need sleep and rest to restore her body to health. In this "taking-in phase," the mother wishes to meet her own rest and

Nursing Tip   *Prevention of Thrombophlebitis*

Clients who remain in bed up to 8 hours should perform leg exercises to prevent formation of clots (thrombus) in the legs, which can develop into thrombophlebitis or thromboembolism. Deep vein thrombosis (DVT) is a serious condition. A clot formed in the deep pelvis leg veins may fragment from the original clotted site and lodge into the lungs as pulmonary embolus. Superficial thrombophlebitis is noted as a hard, painful, warm, and red vein. Unlike DVT, there is little potential for pulmonary embolism with superficial thrombophlebitis.

Teach clients to flex and extend both feet and legs alternately while in bed. In a rhythmic motion, press then relax the backs of the knees into the mattress. Clients should also be taught other ways to prevent thrombus formation, such as keeping the legs uncrossed while seated, not flexing the legs at the groin, resting the legs without putting pressure on the back of the knees, wearing support hose or antiembolism stockings when varicosities are present, and padding pressure points during lithotomy positions.

Assess the client for signs of pulmonary embolism: dyspnea, coughing, and chest pain.

nutritional needs before focusing her energy on her new-born. The attainment of parental roles, infant care, and family adaptation should also be assessed.

OTHER ASSESSMENTS

In addition to the basic postpartum assessments addressed in the approach using the acronym BUBBLE-HE, other important body systems need to be examined.

Hemodynamic Status

Blood values return to normal within the first 6 weeks after delivery. A CBC may show marked leukocytosis, predominantly neutrophils, both during and after labor. The leukocyte count may increase during labor up to 25,000/mm^3, increase to as high as 30,000/mm^3 during a prolonged labor, and remain elevated for the first 2 days postpartum (AWHONN, 1996). The average leukocyte count is 14,000 to16,000/mm^3. A possible infectious process should be ruled out in the presence of such increased counts or an increase of more than 30% from baseline during the first 6 hours after delivery.

Hemoglobin, hematocrit, and erythrocyte levels may fluctuate during the first postpartum days. When considerable blood loss occurs, the levels may decrease below those measured before labor. Immediately after delivery the hematocrit begins to rise owing to hemodilution, increase in plasma volume, and dehydration. By 4 to 5 weeks, the hematocrit returns to normal values of 37% to 47% (AWHONN, 1996).

Blood coagulation normalizes a few days after delivery; profiles secondary to PIH remain elevated. Findings may include uterine clot formation at the placental attachment site or pooled blood in the uterine cavity. It takes 3 to 4 weeks for the blood volume to return to prepregnant levels, depending on the amount of blood lost during delivery. Cardiac output remains increased for at least 48 hours after delivery.

> ### Reflections from a Family
>
> The recovery period was difficult for me. I waited 9 months to be able to hold my baby for the first time, but I didn't get the chance to do it. I was bleeding a lot after the delivery so the doctor was rubbing real hard on my belly. I just couldn't deal with holding my baby when I was bleeding.

Integumentary System

The newly delivered client may wonder if the stretch marks or **striae** on her breasts, thighs, and abdomen will ever go away. The striae eventually fade to a pale color but may never completely disappear, especially in dark-skinned women (Figure 16-15). Skin discolorations that appeared during pregnancy (e.g., chloasma) usually disappear toward the end of pregnancy. However, hyper-pigmentation of the areolae and linea nigra may be permanent (Cashion, 1997).

After giving birth, the mother may complain of profuse perspiration, especially at night, which is normal during the first week as the body rids itself of excess fluid from pregnancy. The nurse should inform the mother that this is normal, and encourage her to change her gown as needed.

Some women may note an eruption of mild acne from hormonal changes (AWHONN, 1996). Women who suffered from pruritic urticarial papules and plaques of pregnancy (PUPPP) will note a rapid regression of this

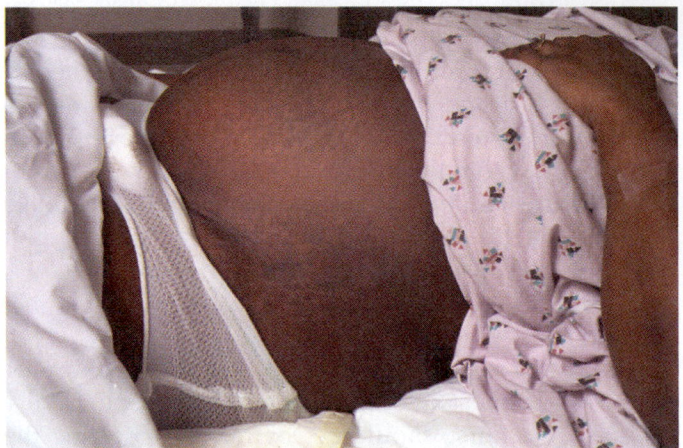

A.

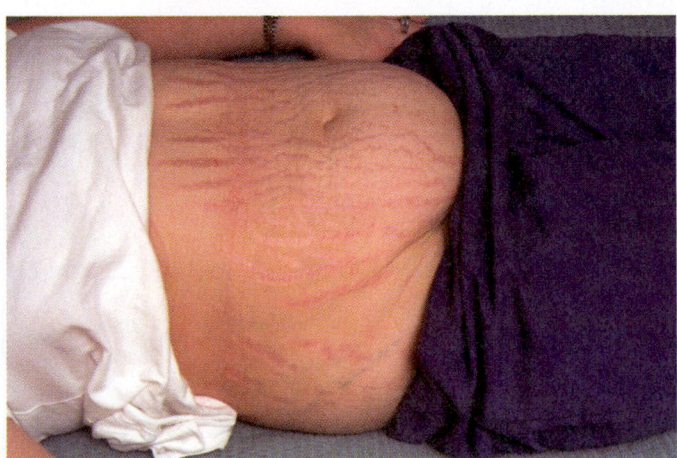

B.

Figure 16-15 Postpartum striae, or stretch marks, in (A) dark-skinned and (B) light-skinned clients.

uncommon pregnancy rash within 1 to 2 weeks after delivery (Gordon & Landon, 1996). Topical steroids are the standard treatment for controlling the intense pruritus.

Other changes include hair loss for the first 2 months after delivery. The mother may become concerned with the large amount of hair found at the bottom of the tub or shower; the nurse should reassure her that this is normal owing to hormonal changes. The increase in fine hair usually disappears; however, coarse or bristly hair may remain (Cashion, 1997). The rapid decrease in estrogen also induces the regression of vascular abnormalities, such as palmar erythema and spider angiomas.

Musculoskeletal System

Because the abdomen stretches during pregnancy, the mother's abdominal walls relax or become flaccid after delivery. When visually assessing and palpating the abdomen and fundus, the nurse may notice some degree of muscle separation, called **diastasis recti**, along the center of the abdomen. This separation is due to pressure from an enlarging uterus and may increase with each subsequent pregnancy. The severity depends on the client's general physical condition, muscle tone, timing between pregnancies, parity, and other circumstances that distend the uterus and abdomen. Multiple gestation, macrosomia, and hydramnios also distend the uterus to a larger than average size, making it difficult for the client to regain her prepregnant muscle tone.

Activity

Many mothers complain of fatigue after childbirth. They require time to recuperate and recover from the effects of labor and delivery. Once the postpartum woman is stable, the nurse should encourage her to ambulate often. The advantages of early ambulation are well established (Box 16-2)

Box 16-2

Advantages of Early Ambulation

In general, the client will feel better and stronger if she begins to ambulate early after delivery. The following are the specific medical advantages of early ambulation:

- Fewer bladder infections
- Less frequent constipation
- Decreased incidence of deep vein thrombosis
- Decreased incidence of pulmonary embolism

Women who deliver vaginally often are able to ambulate to the restroom within a few hours of delivery.

Although the nurse must be ready to assist a client out of bed, the client should be offered the use of a wheelchair, when necessary. Before rising from the bed, the client should be assessed for dizziness and motor weakness from weak knees or legs. Ask the client how she feels when she rises from a recumbent position and if she is able to stand straight without assistance. When the mother is very tired or has received an epidural or analgesics that may cause drowsiness, she may not have the ability to stand and walk independently. When assisting the client in getting up from bed for the first time, the nurse should accompany her because she may experience orthostatic hypotension and be at risk of falling.

The client should be encouraged to return to normal activities of daily living as soon as possible. She should be able to provide independent self-care before going home. Once home, depending on the physician's instructions, she may perform light household chores. Family members or friends can take on the primary responsibility for major household chores such as meal preparation. When episiotomy has been performed, the client should shower instead of using a tub until the incision has healed and the flow of lochia has diminished.

Exercise

Although vigorous exercise should be delayed until the client feels well-recovered, a woman who has had an uncomplicated vaginal delivery can begin moderate exercise soon afterward. The client may perform mild stretching and flexing of muscles, especially abdominal muscles, which may relieve tension and muscle strain (Figure 16-16). Care should be emphasized because joints do not stabilize until 6 to 8 weeks postpartum. Other safe exercises include Kegel exercises, deep breathing, and pelvic tilts. Exercising too much and too soon may result in an increase in bright-red vaginal blood flow. The client must not lift anything heavier than her baby for the first 2 weeks after childbirth. She should avoid climbing stairs for about 2 to 3 weeks.

A safe healthy exercise program should include 30 to 60 minutes of aerobic exercises that increase the heart rate at least four times a week. Even exercising 1 hour a day, such as taking a brisk walk while pushing the baby in a stroller or carrying the infant in a sling will burn off 400 calories. The exercises should include abdominal and back strengthening exercises to support the organs, protect the back, improve posture, and improve appearance.

The mother may not fit into the clothing she wore very early in her pregnancy. Although she may not relish the idea of wearing maternity clothes again, she can wear pants with an elastic waist and a loose top.

Nursing Tip *Pampering Yourself Postpartum*

Suggest to the new mother to prepare a "Personal Postpartum Pampering Plan Checklist" to follow once she returns home after childbirth. A sample plan follows:

- Ask friends and family to cook meals (double menus, and freeze half). Ask friends to bring food if they are coming to visit, or let them cook for you when they arrive.
- Wear a gorgeous bathrobe, or wear comfortable clothing.
- Take a warm, soothing bath. Have someone else watch your baby during this break.
- For routine household chores, hire cleaning help, ask friends or family, or hire a neighborhood teenager.
- Get out of the house. Go shopping. Take a walk in the park. Go to the local fitness club. Call other new mothers to accompany you, and take the babies together.
- Take frequent naps.
- Enjoy your baby.

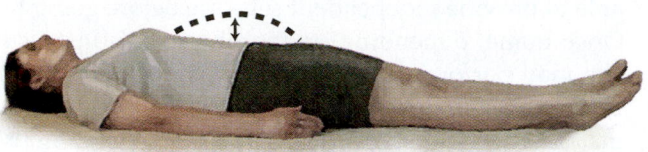

A. Deep breathing

Breathe deeply, expanding your abdominal muscles; then slowly exhale, tightening your abdominal muscles.

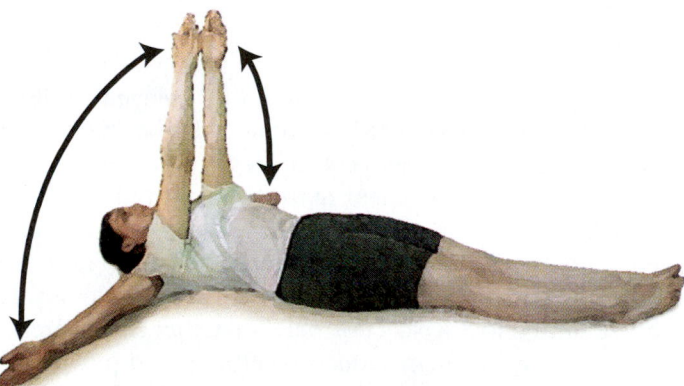

B. Arm raises

Place your arms at right angles to your body: slowly raise them, touch your hands together, then slowly lower your arms.

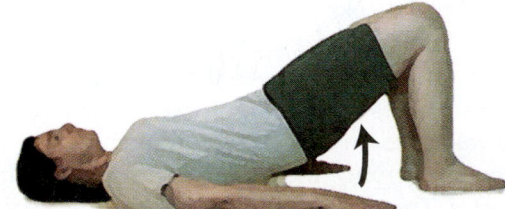

C. Pelvic tilt

Place your arms at your sides and your feet flat on the floor. Tighten abdominal and buttock muscles, press back into floor, then tilt pelvis toward ceiling.

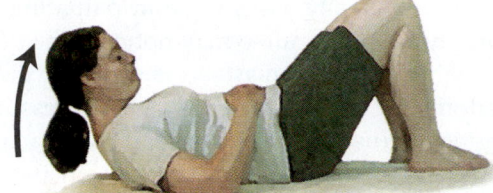

D. Head raises

Lie with your knees flexed, feet flat on the floor. Contract your buttocks, lift your head.

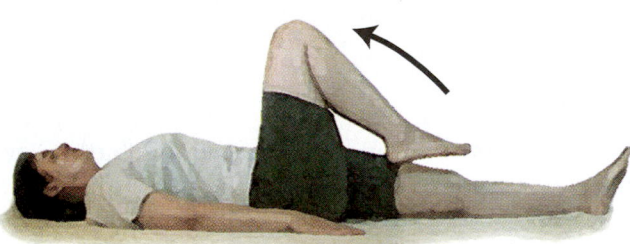

E. Knee flexes

Flex one knee toward your abdomen; lower your foot toward the floor, then straighten your leg.

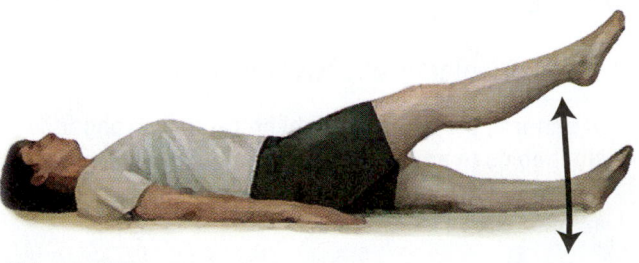

F. Leg raises

Straighten legs and point toes. Slowly raise then lower one leg and then the other using your abdominal muscles.

Figure 16-16 Postpartum exercises.

Weight Loss

Although the woman's figure does not immediately return to prepregnancy form, there is immediate loss of weight after delivery, representing the combined weights of the infant, placenta, and amniotic fluid. Average weight loss is 12 to 15 lb after delivery. An additional 5 lb is lost during the first week postpartum owing to extracellular fluid diuresis. Another 10 lb may be lost in the next 6 weeks.

Most women return to their prepregnancy weight 6 months after delivery; however, postpregnancy weight loss is difficult to achieve for some women. The client's ability to lose weight is related to the amount of weight gained during pregnancy, number of pregnancies, smoking, and the opportunity to return to work outside the home.

Exercises that flatten the stomach muscles and eating a healthy diet will help the woman return to her prepregnant size and weight. The woman should keep in mind that because the skin has been stretched greatly during pregnancy, the abdomen may not return to a totally flat appearance. The stretched muscles also may not return completely. First, the client should set goals and tailor her exercise and nutrition programs to her needs. She should include foods from the four basic food groups, increase her fluid intake, and avoid eating junk food.

The main approach to losing weight should be to adjust her metabolism gradually with a healthy diet. She should avoid fad and starvation diets that include in their regimens the practice of skipping meals. She should calculate her basic daily caloric needs, which is the number of calories of balanced nutrition she can consume to maintain a feeling of well-being without gaining weight. The diet should contain 1,500 calories or more, while the client simultaneously increases the intensity and duration of exercise (Sears & Sears, 2000). Breastfeeding mothers need at least 500 extra calories for lactation. Abstaining from only

Client Education

Performing Kegel Exercises

Pregnancy, childbirth, and being overweight can weaken the pelvic floor muscles and cause leaking of urine and stool. The muscles are weak if the client notes symptoms such as leaking urine when she sneezes, coughs, or lifts heavy objects. As with other muscles, exercises can make the pelvic floor muscles stronger. The pelvic floor muscles between the legs attach to the front, back, and sides of the pelvic bone. Two pelvic muscles do most of the work. The largest muscle stretches as does a hammock; the other is shaped like a triangle.

You should teach the client to perform Kegel exercises properly. The client should be instructed to find the muscles that are stretched using two methods:

1. She should try to stop and start the flow of urine when sitting on the toilet.

2. She should imagine she is trying to stop passing gas or complete a bowel movement. She should squeeze the rectal muscles she would use. She will feel a pulling sensation when she is using the correct muscles.

There are two types of Kegel exercises: quick and slow. In doing the quick ones, the client should tighten and relax the muscles rapidly. In doing the slow ones, she should tighten the muscles for 5 to 10 seconds and then relax.

The client should work up to doing 10 to 15 repetitions each time, three times a day. It is important to instruct the client about the following:

- She should not overdo exercising the muscles.

- She should not hold her breath.

- She should take care not to tighten other muscle groups, such as the stomach, buttocks, and legs. Squeezing the wrong muscles can put more pressure on the bladder control muscles.

Kegel exercises can be done anywhere: sitting in a chair while watching television, standing in the kitchen cooking, or sitting in a car while stopped at a red light. The client should do the exercises in three different positions: sitting, lying, and standing. Doing so makes the muscles the strongest.

The client should be advised to have patience in seeking results. Improvement in bladder control may not occur for 3 to 6 weeks but may occur earlier. The client should try to tighten her muscles before sneezing, lifting, or jumping to protect them from more damage.

> ### Nursing Tip
> ### *Tips for Making Sexual Intercourse after Birth Easier*
>
> You can give the client the following tips to educate her on how to make sexual intercourse easier after delivery:
>
> - Try positions that may be more comfortable for the newly delivered mother. The woman-on-top position gives her greater control over the depth of penetration and allows her to move in a way that is most pleasurable for her.
> - Use a water-based lubricant to ease vaginal dryness.
> - Try having sex at different times of the day if you are too tired when you go to bed at night.
> - Move your baby into another room to preserve the privacy and intimacy of your bedroom.
> - If sex is too painful, engage in noncoital sex as a safe and satisfying alternative.
> - Keep the lines of communication open by talking about and exploring new ways to satisfy each other physically.

one nonnutritious snack a day (e.g., one chocolate chip cookie contains about 100 calories) will reduce the daily caloric intake by 500 calories, or 3,500 calories a week, which is enough to lose 1 lb of weight. The mother can keep track of her success by monitoring her eating habits and weekly weight loss.

The client must approach losing weight in a positive way and try to do it slowly (about 1 lb a week). The slower the weight loss, the better she will feel and the more likely the weight will stay off. The exercise program will invigorate her physically and mentally. Although the changes will be gradual, she will feel satisfied with herself once she reaches her weight and fitness goals.

Sexuality

There is no prescribed time when to resume sexual intercourse after childbirth. Mothers are warned to avoid sexual activity until their episiotomy has healed, which can take 6 weeks or more, or until they are comfortable and desire to have sex. Some women feel like resuming sexual activity as early as 2 weeks after birth; others may wait for 5 or 6 months until they are ready physically and emotionally. Bleeding and infection are less likely to occur once 14 postpartum days have passed. Because of perineal discomfort or swelling, some mothers often wait to resume sexual intercourse until after the 6-week checkup.

Several factors affect a woman's desire for sexual activity after the birth of her child. The birth experience places incredible stress on the body. Episiotomy stitches (if present) will have tightened the vagina, making it less elastic at first so that intercourse may hurt the first time after delivery. Breastfeeding mothers may have decreased estrogen production, leading to vaginal atrophy and dryness, making sexual intercourse difficult and painful. The client should use a water-based lubricant, such as K-Y jelly, for vaginal dryness.

The physical demands of taking care of a newborn infant with frequent feedings often leave both parents deprived of sleep. The new father may feel some cautiousness because he may be afraid of hurting his partner during sexual activity. It is helpful if both partners communicate openly about their feelings and discuss what is compatible and what is painful. The breasts of the lactating mother also are more sensitive to stimulation and might be tender to touch. The milk might leak or letdown might occur during breast stimulation and orgasm; wearing a nursing bra or nightgown or having a towel nearby may help with this problem.

Contraception

Many women may not think about contraception immediately after birth, or they may be waiting for their 6-week checkup, or for the return of menses. However, many women resume sexual activity prior to the 6-week checkup and may get pregnant before return of menses. Therefore, it is important for the nurse to discuss contraception before discharge from the hospital.

The decision about contraception depends on many things: the client's and her partner's motivation, the number of children desired, the state of the client's health, whether she is breastfeeding, and the couple's religious beliefs.

The use of oral contraceptives while lactating is controversial (Bowes, 1996). When prescribed, providers often suggest starting contraceptives after breastfeeding has been firmly established. The mother who is not breastfeeding can begin to take oral contraceptives as early as 2 to 3 weeks after delivery. The mini pill has shown to be safe for breastfeeding women.

Other choices in steroid contraception include depot medroxyprogesterone acetate (DMPA), which is given IM every 3 months. The major advantages of this method are client convenience and easy administration.

If the client chooses to use a barrier method, such as a diaphragm, she will need to be fitted for the proper size at her 6-week postpartum checkup even if this method was used previously. The cervix will require time to return to the more normal nonpregnant size. The breastfeeding woman will experience vaginal dryness and tightness secondary to involution, which will make fitting more difficult. Use of the diaphragm also requires a spermicidal lubricant.

If an intrauterine device (IUD) is the method of choice, it usually is inserted after the 6-week postpartum checkup. Some providers may decide to insert it in the immediate postpartum period because fewer perforations occur when it is inserted between weeks 1 and 8; however, the risk of expulsion is higher, with rates from 10% to 21% (Bowes, 1996).

If the couple is undecided on the method of family planning or is postponing oral contraceptive therapy until 6 weeks, the use of condoms in combination with spermicides may be a good choice. If the couple is sure about permanent sterilization, this can often be accomplished during a cesarean delivery or 24 to 48 hours after delivery. The timing must be carefully planned. Immediate postpartum sterilization often is associated with guilt and regret (Bowes, 1996). If the couple decides to postpone the procedure until 6 to 8 weeks after delivery, it will provide them time to ensure their infant is healthy and to be sure they are making the correct decision.

Pain Management

After delivery, the mother is at risk for various types of discomfort. She may complain of perineal discomfort, uterine cramping, sore nipples, or a headache if she received incorrectly administered spinal anesthesia. The most common source of discomfort is from the afterpains related to uterine contractions.

Postpartum medications commonly given for episiotomy or uterine pain may be oral nonsteroidal anti-inflammatory drugs (NSAIDS), such as ibuprofen (Motrin), 400 to 800 mg orally every 4 to 6 hours as needed. Acetaminophen with codeine (Tylenol with Codeine) may be given for more severe cramping. Emptying the bladder every hour or so is an effective measure to reduce afterpains. Another useful method is for the client to lie on her abdomen with a pillow against her lower abdomen because this creates pressure that keeps the uterus contracted (Jordan, 1998).

Topical anesthetics (e.g., chloroprocaine [Nesacaine]) may provide temporary relief from episiotomy pain. The anesthetic spray should be used sparingly 3 to 4 times a day after voiding. Ice packs and sitz baths also may provide relief for the mother.

Immune System

Before discharge, the nurse should check the client's record for proper immunization status, particularly against rubella. If the mother is rubella nonimmune with a titer below 1:8, she should be vaccinated before leaving the hospital. The client may need to sign a consent form to receive the vaccine. Because the effects of congenital rubella syndrome (CRS) have devastating teratogenic effects on a fetus, it is important that the nurse counsel the client against becoming pregnant again before receiving the vaccine—if she has declined to receive it in the hospital—and for the next 28 days after receiving the vaccine (ACOG, 1992). The client should know that she may experience a brief period of rubella-like symptoms such as a rash, lymphadenopathy, joint symptoms, and a low-grade fever 5 to 21 days after the vaccination. The vaccine is safe to give to breastfeeding mothers.

Unsensitized mothers who are $RH_o(D)$-negative and have given birth to an infant who is Rh-positive also should receive 300µg of $RH_o(D)$ immune globulin (RhoGAM) within 72 hours of delivery (see the Drug box) (ACOG, 1990). RhoGAM is administered even if the mother received RhoGAM in the antepartum period. Depending on the extent of the hemorrhage and exchange of maternofetal blood, a larger dose of RhoGAM may be necessary.

Although standard precautions should be practiced with all clients, particular care must be taken with the postpartum client who has the human immunodeficiency virus (HIV) or acquired immunodeficiency syndrome (AIDS). Personal protective gear (e.g., latex gloves and safety glasses) should be worn to prevent the transmission

Nursing Tip   *Relieving Afterpains*

Suggest to the client an exercise called mini head lifts that can assist in managing afterpains. The client should be instructed to lie down with her knees bent. She should take a deep breath and as she exhales, lift her chin so it rests on her chest. She should perform the head lifts 5 to 10 times each time afterpains are felt, several times a day, to encourage uterine contraction.

Nursing Alert

Assessing Unrelieved Perineal Pain

When medications do not relieve complaints of perineal pain, you should assess the site more carefully. Pain unrelieved by other means may indicate a possible perineal hematoma. Episiotomy pain normally is relieved by 3 weeks after delivery. The postpartum client with a perineal hematoma will be in severe pain, often unable to sit comfortably.

Rh₀(D) Immune Globulin Vaccination (RhoGAM)

Pharmacologic Class	Immune serum, Pregnancy category C
Therapeutic Class	Anti-Rh₀(D)-positive prophylaxis agent
How Supplied	IM, 300 µcg vial (standard dose); 50 µg vial (microdose)
Indications for Use	Anti-Rh₀(D)-positive prophylaxis agent during situations such as abortion, miscarriage, ectopic pregnancy, postpartum
Chemical Effect	Suppresses active antibody response and formation of antibodies to antigens from Rh-positive fetal blood, which results in erythroblastosis fetalis
Therapeutic Effect	Blocks the adverse effects of Rh-positive exposure; prevents sensitization and subsequent development of antibodies to antigens from Rh-positive fetal blood, which results in erythroblastosis fetalis
Dosage	300 µg vial (standard dose) IM if fetal erythrocyte count <15 mL; provide more than one vial if fetomaternal hemorrhage is >15 mL
Side Effects and Adverse Reactions	Low fever, anaphylaxis, discomfort at injection site
Contraindications	History of anaphylactic or severe systemic reaction to human globulin; contraindicated in RH₀(D) antigen-negative or splenectomized individuals and in patients who are Rh immunized (Rh antibody positive)
Nursing Considerations	Must administer medication within 72 hours of delivery; obtain confirmation of fetal blood type from sample of cord blood and maternal blood type before administration
Client Teaching	Ensure client knows the reason for receiving RhoGAM. Carry card identifying dates RhoGAM was received.
Laboratory Finding	Rh₀D is negative and direct Coombs is negative test, give RhoGAM.

Client Education

Congenital Rubella

Although the incidence of congenital rubella has decreased over the years, about 10% to 20% of women are susceptible. Congenital rubella is a serious disease, with the fetus experiencing severe physical abnormalities.

You have the opportunity to teach the client that if she is not immunized, the rubella virus can cross the placental barrier. The frequency and intensity of infection depends on the timing of the infection. The more severe infections occur in the first 4 weeks of pregnancy, that is, at a time when she will not know she is pregnant. During this time, half of infants exposed to the virus will become infected. The rate decreases to less than 1% when the infection occurs after the first trimester.

Inform the client that a wide variety of severe abnormalities result from congenital rubella syndrome. The four most common problems are deafness, eye defects, central nervous system (brain) defects, and cardiac malformations (patent ductus arteriosus). Other abnormalities include a small head (microcephaly), mental retardation, susceptability to pneumonia, small size (intrauterine growth restriction), enlarged liver, and blood dyscrasias (hemolytic anemia and thrombocytopenia).

You can instruct the client about prevention. Prevention of congenital rubella can be obtained by receiving the rubella vaccine. About 95% of women who receive it become immunized. Inform the client that there are only a few rare side effects from the vaccine, for example, a low-grade fever, fatigue, and arthralgia. When the vaccine is given immediately after delivery the effects may be delayed for up to 21 days (Bowes, 1996). The vaccine is not contraindicated in women who are breastfeeding. She should also avoid getting pregnant for at least 1 month after the vaccination.

Nursing Alert

RhoGAM and Rubella Vaccine

RhoGAM and rubella vaccine should not be administered to the same woman prior to discharge. RhoGAM prevents antibody formation, whereas the rubella vaccine promotes antibody production. This prevents rubella immunity from being fully established.

of blood and other bodily fluids. The nurse should advise the mother to avoid contact of her bodily fluids with her infant's mucous membranes and open skin areas. The client also should be cautioned not to breastfeed and thus take the risk of transmitting HIV to her infant (Duff, 1996). Clients with HIV or AIDS may receive medications postpartally, such as zidovudine.

Client Education

Receiving RhoGAM After Delivery

You should educate the client by telling her that if she has Rh-negative blood, she may need to receive RhoGAM after delivery. If the father's blood is Rh-positive, the blood of the baby also may be Rh-positive. If the baby has Rh-positive blood, small amounts of the baby's blood may have escaped into the mother's bloodstream during delivery. Natural antibodies are then released into the bloodstream as the body tries to destroy the foreign Rh-positive cells from the baby. When this happens, the client will become permanently sensitized to Rh-positive blood cells. If she has an Rh-positive baby in a future pregnancy, her body will have sensitized antibodies that will attack her baby's blood cells during pregnancy. Her baby may then develop a disease called erythroblastosis fetalis.

Instruct the client that to avoid this potentially fatal disease in an unborn baby the immune globulin RhoGAM should be given after the first pregnancy. Once her body becomes sensitized, it can never be reversed, even if given RhoGAM. Once she receives RhoGAM, future pregnancies with Rh-positive babies will not be affected because her blood will be free from anti-Rh-positive antibodies.

Documentation

Daily care of the woman after delivery encompasses assessments of the same parameters, such as episiotomy, lochia, and breastfeeding. If written in narrative format, the nurse may use the acronym BUBBLE-HE to assist her in ensuring that all pertinent assessments are charted completely at least every shift or more frequently, depending on the client's acuity and the facility's policy on nursing documentation (Figure 16-17). In general, nursing documentation should follow the nursing process.

Flowcharts or clinical pathways facilitate the documentation process (Figure 16-18). The use of flowcharts and graphs provide the ability to quickly note trends and changes from one shift to another. Columns at the top of the flowchart provide ease in checking off a box, using the coded legend, or placing the nurse's initials, as appropriate.

FAMILY CONSIDERATIONS

The birth of a baby is one of life's most exciting and challenging events. Brazelton (1981) pointed out that parenthood is an opportunity for personal growth and maturity, because a baby presents parents with the task of becoming a family with all the feelings and responsibility that entails. Adapting to the role of parent can be challenging, because developmental tasks must be successfully accomplished to integrate the new role. **Role transition**, or the process of adopting new behaviors related to change and developmental tasks, involves not only the birth of a firstborn child for the new parents but also the expanding of the family. Since family adjustment and attainment of developmental milestones are complex, health care providers can be instrumental in helping families make these transitions.

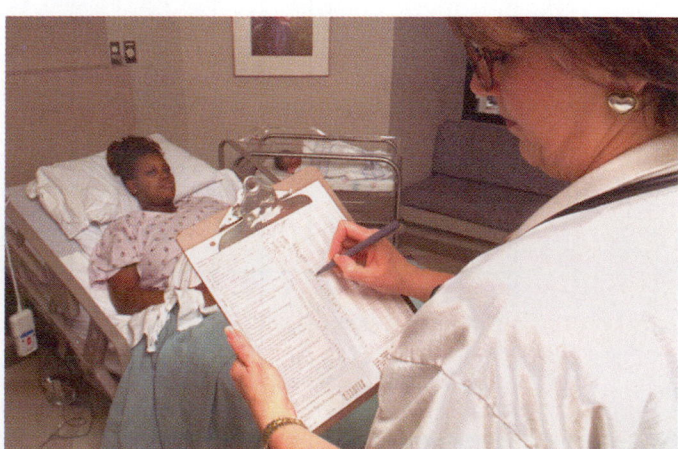

Figure 16-17   Careful documentation is the closing step of each assessment encounter.

Date											
Time											
Initials											
Breasts											
Fundus											
Lochia											
Perineum											
Diet											
Activity											
Bowels											
Bladder											
Homan's Sign											
Emotions											
IV											
Meds											

Legend:

Breasts
S=Soft
F=Filling
E=Engorged
NT=Nontender
T=Tender

Fundus
F=Firm
B=Boggy
at U +/−
ML=Midline

Lochia
Sc=Scant
Sm=Small
M=Moderate
L=Large
R=Rubra
S=Serosa
A=Alba

Perineum
N=Normal
E=Edematous
B=Bruised
H=Hemorrhoids
    present
IP=Icepack in use
S=Sitz bath in use

Diet
NPO
Reg=Regular
CL=Clear Liquid
ADA=Diabetic

Activity
AL=Up AdLib
BR=Bed rest

Bowels
BM=Bowel
    movement
F=Flatus

Bladder
QS=Voiding
    quantity
    sufficient
F=Foley catheter

Homan's Sign
−=Negative
+=Positive
BL=Bilaterally

Emotions
N=Normal
S=Sad
H=Happy
N=Neutral
O=Other

Figure 16-18 Sample Postpartum Assessment Flowchart. These may be incorporated into computerized charts.

Adaptation to parenthood is not an easy process. There has been a great deal of research about the developmental course of early attachment relationships (Waters, Posada, Crowell, & Lay 1994). **Attachment** is the process of connecting with another human being. Ideally, a mother's attachment to her offspring is a strong bond that lasts a lifetime. Attachment usually begins during pregnancy and intensifies as the pregnancy progresses and a fantasy child is perceived.

In the period after birth, or the postpartum period, the mother-infant acquaintance begins as the infant is compared to the child who was perceived in the womb. This "getting-to-know you" period is characterized by behaviors that initiate the attachment process. Researchers speak of this period as a time when parents begin to identify with their newborn. It is a time when parents begin to integrate the newborn into their lives as they reconcile the fantasy child with the real child and begin to view their role as parents.

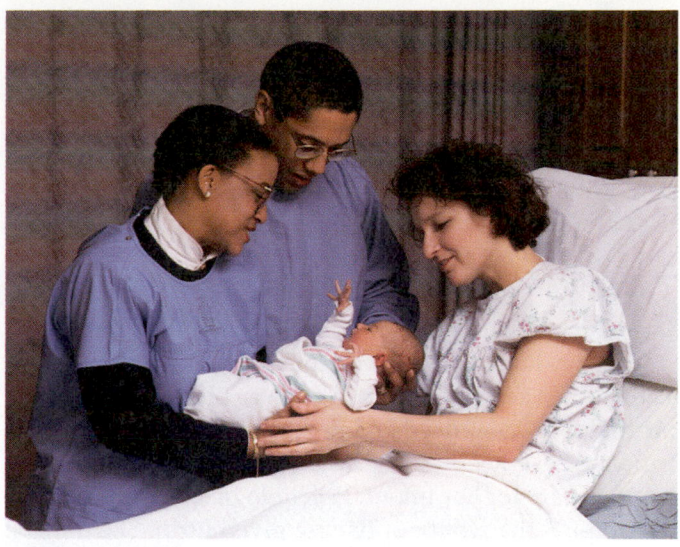

Figure 16-19   The nurse can help create an environment conducive to parental attachment behaviors by encouraging early parent-infant contact.

Maternal-Infant Attachment

The attachment process does not occur overnight. Brazelton (1981) reported that parents often believe in the romanticized version of parenthood characterized by instinctive, instantaneous attachment, which is not necessarily immediate, but often a continuing process. Early research conducted by Klaus and Kennel (1982) examined maternal attachment and found that the period when a mother falls in love with her baby was not easily identified. They reported it was common for mothers to experience distress and disappointment if they did not experience feelings of love for their infants in the first minutes or hours after birth. Many of the mothers studied developed an affection for their infant within the first week; however, the onset of maternal feelings of affection toward their infant was delayed if labor was painful, amniotic membranes were ruptured artificially, or the mother had received narcotic drugs for pain relief.

Klaus and Kennel (1982) referred to the first hour following birth of an infant as a period when maternal-infant attachment begins and labeled this attachment as **maternal-infant bonding**. Because a mother's physical and emotional state can be adversely affected by exhaustion, pain, anesthesia, the absence of support persons, or an unwanted outcome, a delay or block in the attachment process can occur. By encouraging early maternal-infant contact, nurses can provide an environment that fosters attachment behaviors (Figure 16-19). The close contact aids in thermoregulation of the infant. In addition, by encouraging attachment behaviors, such as early contact, suckling, and *rooming-in*, infant abandonment was reduced. Rooming-in involves the infant remaining in the mother's room throughout hospitalization.

Maternal Adjustment and Role Attainment

The postpartum period is a time for mothers to adjust to the new role of motherhood as the attachment process continues. Nurses can assist the mother and family with role transition by understanding maternal **role attainment**, which is the process of accomplishing the developmental tasks of a

Critical Thinking

Mother-Infant Attachment and Early Infant Contact

The concept of early contact immediately after birth has been discussed as a necessary experience for mother-infant attachment. However, some mothers are too exhausted during the first hour after a difficult labor and delivery or deliver a high-risk infant, who is immediately taken to the nursery. Do you think these mothers experience less attachment toward their infant? Do you think they feel a sense of loss, depression, and anxiety because they missed an experience that has been promoted as important to the mother-child relationship? Can maternal-infant attachment behaviors be postponed? Do you think the presence of a support person enhances the attachment process? How can nurses facilitate early maternal-infant contact? What nursing behaviors may interfere with early maternal-infant contact? What interventions can you suggest to help parents of high risk infants?

new social role. Classic research by Reva Rubin (1984) explored the process of maternal role attainment. According to Rubin, after the delivery, the mother shifts her attention from an inward focus that is characteristic of labor and delivery to focusing outward on her relationship with her infant. Rubin identified three adjustment phases involved in the process of assuming the maternal role (Table 16-3).

Taking-In Phase

The taking-in phase of maternal adjustment is characterized by basic maternal needs for food, care, and comfort. The mother's initial goal is to recover physically from the birth and to meet needs related to rest, comfort, and nutrition. These needs must be met before the mother can begin to care for her infant. Psychologically, the mother is "taking-in" the reality of having given birth. She may be content to be a passive observer of her infant's care. The nursing focus at this stage is to provide a quiet, restful environment to facilitate the mother's recovery and promote mother-child interaction.

Taking-Hold Phase

Following the initial phase of dependency, mothers move on to the taking-hold phase, which occurs after they have had a chance to rest and have received relief from discomfort. This phase may begin 24 to 48 hours after delivery. Characteristically, mothers in this phase begin to show an increased interest in participating in their infant's care.

Today, with early hospital discharge, this phase often occurs earlier or may occur after discharge. Nurses have a key role in assisting the mother to feel confident in her ability to care for herself and her newborn. It is important to assess learning needs and provide positive reinforcement during the teaching-learning process. By praising the mother's accomplishments, the nurse can foster maternal confidence in the mother's ability to care for herself and her infant (Figure 16-20).

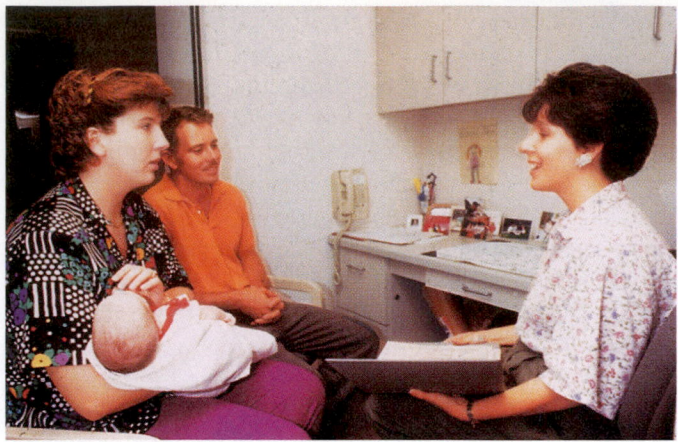

Figure 16-20 Including support persons in postpartum teaching encourages parental self-confidence.

Letting-Go Phase

Mothers move last to the letting-go phase. This phase is characterized by role attainment and relationship adjustments. It may take several weeks to reach and is influenced by cultural beliefs. Maternal role attainment often occurs slowly, as maternal self-confidence increases and maternal-child attachment strengthens. The goal of the letting-go stage is to achieve relationship and role stability.

Table 16-3	Rubin's Phases of Maternal Adjustment
PHASE	**MATERNAL CHARACTERISTICS**
Initial: *Taking-in*	Passivity and dependence Preoccupation with self Reviews the reality of giving birth Compares infant to her "fantasy child" Concerned with rest, food, and comfort
Second: *Taking-hold*	Resumes control over her life Concerned about self-care Interested in caring for her newborn Begins to gain self-confidence
Third: *Letting-go*	Maternal role attainment Relationship adjustments

Nursing Tip
Promoting Attachment Behaviors

Nurses have a special role in promoting maternal-infant attachment behaviors:

1. Always refer to the infant by name.
2. Unwrap the infant and initiate exploration of the infant's body.
3. Answer concerns that the parents may have (such as those regarding cord care or circumcision).
4. Encourage the mother to pick up and hold her infant.
5. Encourage the mother to hold her infant in an *enface* (face-to-face) position.
6. Talk directly to the infant in a calm, soothing voice.
7. Use the infant's grasp reflex to hold onto the mother's finger.
8. Demonstrate comforting techniques, such as gentle patting and rocking.
9. Assess the mother's readiness to learn infant care.
10. Point out the infant's response to maternal stimulation.

Reflections from a Mother

When I delivered my first baby at age 21, my husband was not able to attend the birth because of a military assignment. After the delivery of our son, the nurse gave him to me to hold and encouraged me to put the baby to breast. However, I really did not want to nurse at that time, because I was in too much pain from a difficult delivery and was upset about not having my husband with me. I felt so guilty about not having an immediate attachment to my baby; it felt like I was looking at someone else's baby. These feelings made me feel like crying; I thought I was being a bad mother. With extreme feelings of guilt, I asked the nurse to take the baby and give me some pain medication. She seemed to disapprove of my unwillingness to nurse my baby. It made me feel so sad and confused.

Role Attainment

Nurses can also facilitate maternal role attainment by carrying out a complete assessment of family interactions and available support systems. Mothers should be encouraged to verbalize concerns and identify stressors that

Client Education

Helping Parents Adjust to Parenthood

Adjusting to the birth of a baby involves many changes, both physiological and psychological. It is important that parents:

- Recognize that adjusting to parenthood takes time.
- Discuss feelings with support persons.
- Obtain adequate rest and nutrition.
- Use community resources.
- Seek out support from family and friends.
- Understand postpartum and newborn care.
- Refer to written plans of care for postpartum and newborn care.
- Keep postpartum and newborn followup appointments.

may impede maternal role attainment. By using therapeutic communication skills and active listening, nurses can develop a collaborative plan of care and initiate referrals to support services when indicated.

Paternal Adjustment

Initial research by Jordon (1990) examined paternal role attainment and found that a father's quest toward role identification and relevance involved three steps:

1. Initial acceptance of the reality of the pregnancy
2. Being recognized by his mate in the role of father
3. Becoming more involved as a father

Ferketich and Mercer (1995) reported that inexperienced, first-time fathers, at 4 and 8 months following birth of their child, had greater anxiety and depression than experienced fathers and that a sense of mastery and family functioning were predictors for paternal role competence. Nurses can facilitate paternal adjustment by encouraging fathers to participate in childbirth preparation classes, during which they are given an active supportive role. In years past, fathers assumed a passive role, sitting in a waiting area anxiously awaiting the birth. Today, their role as coaching partners allows them the opportunity to experience the birth process with the mother and be actively involved in attachment behaviors immediately after birth.

Similar to maternal attachment, paternal attachment is a gradual process that occurs over weeks or months. Participation in childbirth preparation classes facilitates paternal antenatal attachment behaviors and prepares the father for the birth process and the needs of the expanding family. Thus, it is important for nurses to help fathers adjust to their role by taking time to listen to their concerns, letting them know it is acceptable to express their emotions, and showing them how they can become involved in the care of the child. By slowly introducing fathers to the care needs of their child and assessing their

Reflections from a Father

When my daughter was born I was elated and very proud. In the early weeks, there was little chance for me to play with her because all she did was sleep and eat. Then one day, when I was changing her diaper, she looked directly at me and smiled. I felt extreme love and attachment. I was hooked for life.

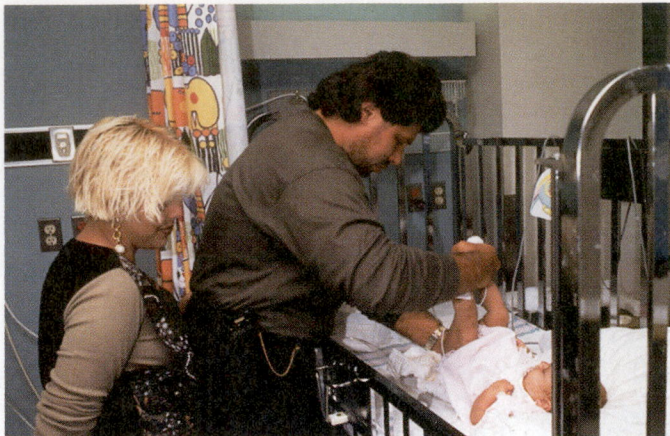

Figure 16-21 Most fathers are eager to learn how to care for their newborn.

readiness to participate, nurses can reduce role strain and enhance family adjustment (Figure 16-21).

Infant Behaviors Influencing Attachment

As a new mother begins to get acquainted with her new-born, infant behavioral cues can assist in facilitating maternal-child attachment. Nurses should be aware of infant behaviors to assist parents to understand their infant's cues and to recognize when their infant is most receptive to stimulation. Brazelton (1984) identified six stages in the infant's **sleep-wake cycle** that affect alertness and responsiveness: deep sleep, light sleep, drowsiness, quiet alertness, active alertness, and crying (Table 16-4). A mother must be able to identify an infant's state of quiet alertness when the baby is most responsive to stimulation. During this state, the infant responds to stimulation

Critical Thinking

Transition to Fatherhood

Male emotions are not well accepted in Western culture. Men are taught to be strong, and crying is thought to be a sign of weakness. Do you think that fathers experience strong emotional feelings at the birth of their child? How do you feel when you see a man cry? Are men conditioned to hold in their emotions? What is the result of emotional restraint? What do you think is the impact of the added responsibilities on the new father? How can the nurse help the father adjust? How does culture influence the father's response?

Nursing Tip — Assisting Parental Role Adjustment

1. Establish rapport early to promote effective communication and verbalization of positive and negative feelings.
2. Assess the goals of the parents and include them in the planning process.
3. Give parents a feeling of empowerment by giving them choices regarding participation in maternal and infant care.
4. Encourage alone time with the infant to explore and get acquainted.
5. Promote rooming-in for the infant and the mother's partner to foster knowledge of their infant's normal patterns and encourage touching and holding behaviors.
6. Assess readiness to learn and participate in providing care.
7. Identify support figures and encourage involvement.
8. Encourage sibling visitation where possible.
9. Refer to community classes for parenting, nutrition, new fathers, infant massage, or similar activities.

Table 16-4   Newborn Sleep-Wake States

STATE	OBSERVED ACTIVITY
Deep sleep	Very little movement Occasional startle motion Regular breathing
Light sleep	Some body movements Eye fluttering Smiles occasionally Irregular breathing
Drowsiness	Mild startle movements Intermittent eyelid opening Glazed eyes
Quiet alertness (most attentive state)	Some increase in activity Widening of the eyes More alert face
Active alertness	Increased motor activity Fussiness Decreased attention to stimulation Increased reaction to discomfort
Crying	Increased motor movement Extreme response to discomfort

Note. Data from *Neonatal Behavioral Assessment Scale* (2nd ed.), by T. B. Brazelton, 1984, London: Heineman.

with a widening of the eyes and increased alertness; this is an optimum time for maternal-infant interaction.

Nurses can assist parents to recognize infant behaviors to optimize parent-newborn interactions and facilitate the attachment process. Nurses can also teach parents infant cues of overstimulation, which are particularly helpful if the infant is sick or premature.

Sibling Adjustment

Another challenging aspect of adjustment for the growing family involves the adjustment of siblings. When a newborn is introduced into the family structure, siblings must adjust and assume the role of the older brother or sister. Anxiety and feelings of jealousy may occur as the sibling reorganizes his or her place in the family. It is not unusual to see regression to earlier behaviors, such as bed-wetting and thumb sucking. Jealousy may also be used to gain parental attention. Sibling adjustment can be made easier if the parents involve the older child in a sibling preparation class. Nurses have developed these classes to assist children in adjusting when they visit the hospital nursery and are addressed as the "big brother" or "big sister." In many areas, older children are permitted to attend the birth. The sooner older children are involved in the preparation for a new family member, the more positively involved they are likely to be (Brazelton, 1981). By allowing

visitation time for older children to greet their new sibling, nurses can foster behaviors that initiate a positive attachment (Figure 16-22). This attachment is further strengthened by finding ways in which the older child can carry out the role of "big brother" or "big sister" through participation in the infant's care. Older children can feel important when they help by retrieving supplies or carrying the diaper bag. Many parents find it helpful to set

---

Nursing Tip — Sibling Visitation Postpartum

Early inclusion of older siblings helps to facilitate adaptation of older children to their new role and promotes a sense of being a family.

1. Promote early contact with the newborn to facilitate integration into the family unit.

2. Enhance the older sibling's feeling of importance within the family as a "helper."

3. Include the sibling in a celebration party to promote a feeling of belonging.

4. Take precautions against cross-infection by questioning parents to see if their older child has been exposed to a communicable disease in recent weeks or presently has symptoms of an infection, such as vomiting, coughing, runny nose, fever, diarrhea, or rash.

5. Educate parents regarding sibling hand washing to promote safe sibling contact with the newborn and facilitate appropriate sibling attachment behavior.

Client Education

Strategies for Managing Sibling Rivalry

Observed Behavior: Regression

Regression is a coping mechanism whereby the child returns to a coping behavior of an earlier stage of development. This is a normal behavior for young children to exhibit in times of stress. Behaviors such as thumb sucking, temper tantrums, and increased dependency help the child cope with stress. Strategy: Be patient, don't scold, and use a calm, caring approach. With time, the behavior will pass.

Observed Behavior: Jealousy

This is a normal behavior when young children see a new baby taking most of the parents' time. Strategy: Set aside special times for outings with the older child. Don't address negative coping behaviors. Focus on encouraging the older child to express feelings through verbalization, drawings, or play. Listen attentively and help older children sort out their feelings. Most of all, older children need to feel important and loved.

Observed Behavior: Anger or Tantrums

Recognize this as attention-getting behavior. Strategy: Ignore the tantrum by avoiding eye contact and moving out of view, but nearby. Do not make statements such as, "Stop acting like a baby," or threaten to spank the child. If anger is directed toward harming the baby, set rules in a calm manner; "time out" may be enforced. Encourage positive interactions with supervision and give praise for positive behavior. Involve older children by asking them to get supplies and to help by carrying the diaper bag, and praise children for being a big helper (Figure 16-23). Never leave an angry child unattended near the newborn. With time, love, positive involvement, and rule setting, the problem behaviors will pass. Older children need praise, hugs, and a parent's undivided attention to help them adjust to the change.

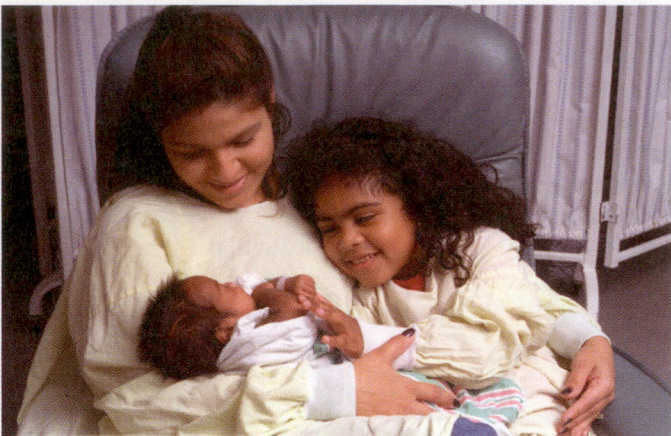

Figure 16-22 Encourage parents to introduce older siblings to the newborn as soon as feasible.

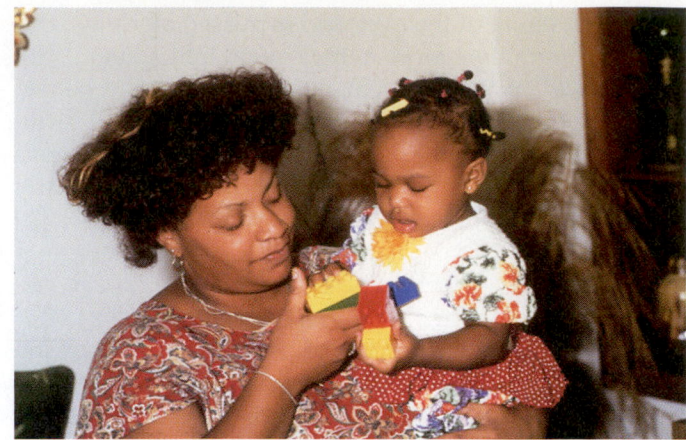

Figure 16-24 Grandparents can be a source of help and wisdom for new parents and sometimes may even take over the parenting role, if the new parents are unable to manage the responsibilities.

aside special time alone with the older child in a play activity. During this time, the older child should be encouraged to express feelings. Parents must understand that there will always be some level of sibling adjustment, and that they should not feel guilty or inadequate if difficulties arise.

Grandparent Adjustment

Grandparents can be a source of support for new parents. Grandparents are unique in that they have the experience to assist new parents as they adjust to the role of parent (Figure 16-24). A grandmother's expertise can be helpful to a new mother as she learns to care for her infant. Having someone who has raised children is a valuable source of information and support that can lessen the anxiety of new parents and give the mother a chance to rest and focus on her role.

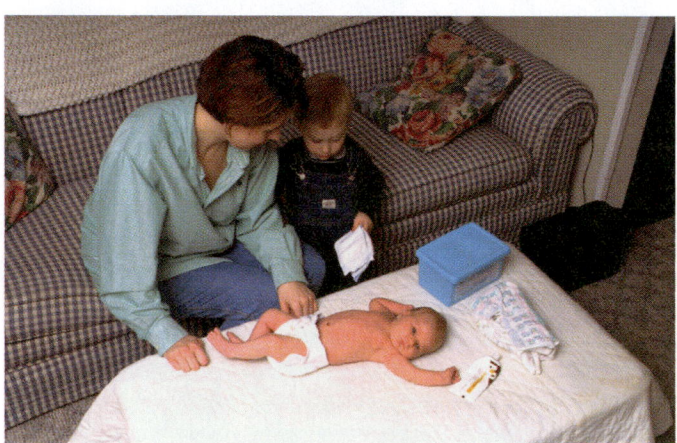

Figure 16-23 Older siblings feel important if they can help care for the new baby through simple tasks, such as retrieving a clean diaper.

However, the role change can be a stressful time for both the parents and grandparents. It is not unusual for grandparents to be unsure of how much involvement they should have. Many grandparents are still employed and unable to provide assistance, or they may give unsolicited advice and spoil the child with gifts. This can be a source of disagreement between the parents and grandparents.

The Postpartum Adolescent Mother

Adolescence is a time of great change as teens address developmental milestones of independence and strive to achieve self-identity. When developmental progress is interrupted, a situational crisis occurs that affects the entire family. An unplanned pregnancy during the teen years generally results in a major personal and family crisis. The pregnancy can block the adolescent's successful completion of developmental tasks. The pregnant adolescent has an increased dependence on others at a time when she is striving for independence. It is important to listen to the teen mother's concerns, include her in health care decisions, collaborate with her when planning interventions, and include support persons to assist the teen mother throughout the pregnancy, delivery, and postpartum period to facilitate positive adjustment. The adolescent's ability to adapt to the pregnancy and respond with realistic expectations depends on effective sources of support to assist her to clarify feelings and set realistic goals (Figure 16-25).

DISCHARGE PREPARATION

Hospital stays for new mothers have decreased to an average of 48 hours or less (based on client preferences). To qualify for early discharge, it must be determined that the mother is at low risk and has had an uncomplicated an-

Critical Thinking

The Impact of Adolescent Pregnancy

Adolescence is a time of change when many teens are trying to develop a sense of identity and begin to move toward independence. Do you think adolescent pregnancy impedes the developmental process? Do you think pregnant adolescents suffer from low self-esteem? Do you think adolescents can successfully attain the maternal role? Do you think single adolescent mothers are able to parent effectively? Do you think adolescent mothers can successfully adapt to the role of mother if they actively participate in planning interventions? Do you think adolescent mothers need close follow-up during the postpartum period? Do you think the unwed father should play an active supporting role throughout the pregnancy and after birth?

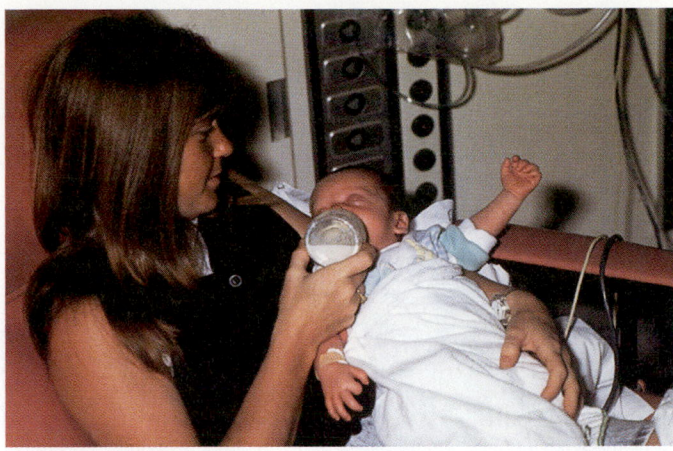

Figure 16-25   This teenage mother is accepting the responsibility of caring for her newborn.

tepartum and intrapartum course and a normal vaginal delivery. Guidelines for discharge vary with each hospital. Each facility should have policies in place that identify the circumstances and processes that must occur for the new mother and infant to be discharged early from the hospital. The *Guidelines for Perinatal Care* (AAP & ACOG, 1997) state specific criteria that must be met before a mother and her infant may qualify for early discharge from the hospital (Box 16-3).

Before the new mother's discharge, the postpartum nurse should include an assessment for adequate support at home. Does she have a designated support person available to help with the household duties, such as cleaning and preparing meals? The new mother may become overwhelmed with the responsibility of caring for herself and her new infant without adequate support.

NURSING IMPLICATIONS

Client education comprises much of the nurse's responsibilities throughout the postpartum stay. With shortened hospital stays, the nurse must streamline her teaching methods, assessing the new mother's and family's personal teaching needs. Client interactions should become more efficient, focusing on communicating knowledge to clients. The focused interactions should be directed toward desired client outcomes, empowering the woman and her family. Ideally, the nurse should assess the mother's current knowledge regarding self-care and infant care because the mother's prior experiences with pregnancy and infant care may change the direction of the nurse's teaching plans.

Box 16-3

Criteria for Early Discharge Mother (Within 48 Hours)

Mother

- Uncomplicated pregnancy, labor, birth, and postpartum course
- No evidence of premature rupture of membranes
- Stable blood pressure and no fever
- Ability to ambulate
- Ability to void without difficulty
- Intact perineum without third- or fourth-degree perineal laceration
- Hemoglobin level greater than 10 g/dl
- No significant vaginal bleeding (mild to moderate)

Infant

- Term infant (37-41 weeks) with birth weight of 2,500–4,500 g
- Normal findings on physical assessment
- Normal laboratory data, including negative results for Coombs test and normal hematocrit
- Stable vital signs
- Stable temperature
- Successful feeding (normal suckling and swallowing)
- Apgar score greater than 7 at 1 and 5 minutes
- Normal voiding and stooling
- Newborn screening test completed

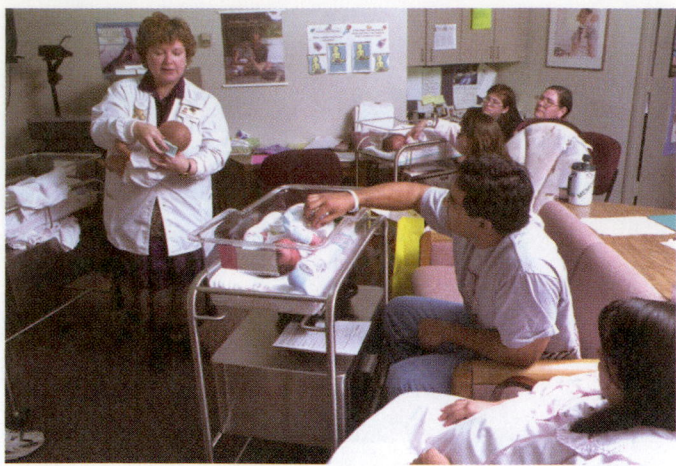

Figure 16-26 Infant care, self-care, and family adaptation are topics typically covered in postpartum education classes.

Before being discharged, the new mother must learn how to care for herself and her infant (Figure 16-26). Self-care topics include those activities that help her to manage, anticipate, and recognize health problems or danger signs. Infant care encompasses activities such as feeding, dressing, and recognition of health problems.

Client Education

General Discharge Instructions

You should provide these general discharge instructions to the new mother:

- Take it easy when you go home.
- Do not lift anything heavier than your baby. Do not move furniture or vacuum for the first few weeks.
- Get lots of rest. Sleep when the baby sleeps.
- Take advantage of offers of help from others.
- Ignore housework for the first few weeks. Enjoy your baby.
- If you have an episiotomy, avoid having sexual intercourse until it heals or until your bottom feels better. You may need to use a lubricant to help with dryness.
- Try to take older siblings' feelings into consideration.
- Take your medications as prescribed.
- Keep your postpartum follow-up appointment.
- Call your health care provider if you have any of the warning signs of sickness.

General instructions, in addition to other client education discussed throughout this chapter, should be given to the client. The nurse should also instruct the client on warning signs of complications after delivery.

As part of the discharge process, the nurse may use a facility-specific checklist to ensure all care has been provided (e.g., birth certificate completed, laboratory testing obtained, and teaching handouts and pertinent information received). The nurse should ensure the client is instructed on any discharge medications ordered and where to obtain them. Some women may continue to take their prenatal vitamins and iron until the postpartum checkup, especially if the hematocrit is low. If the woman experienced a third-or fourth-degree laceration, she may be prescribed a stool softener. The provider may order over-the-counter or prescription pain medication for home use.

A postpartum follow-up examination usually is scheduled for 6 weeks after delivery, or earlier depending on the primary provider. Before discharge the new mother should leave the hospital with a follow-up clinic appointment already in hand or with clear instructions on how to obtain one.

NURSING PROCESS

For the postpartum family, nursing care is an ongoing process that is used to develop an individualized plan of care. It involves careful collection of a database that supports a problem-solving approach to client care. The nursing process identifies areas in which the postpartum family requires nursing intervention.

Assessment

Postpartum assessment begins at delivery and the nurse monitors involution. Family assessment focuses primarily on maternal and father-partner assessment. When taking a history and observing family dynamics, nurses begin to identify problem areas for collaborative intervention.

Nursing Diagnoses

Identification of actual or potential problems early in the postpartum period is necessary for effective planning and intervention. On the basis of assessment data, cultural influences, spiritual needs, medical considerations, and family interactions, problem areas are analyzed and nursing diagnoses are developed.

Outcome Identification

Outcomes for nursing interventions lay the groundwork for nursing care. Goals are set through mutual determination of priorities between the nurse and the family. Identified outcome criteria act as a pathway for nursing interventions. An example would be: the nursing diagnosis of knowledge deficient related to inexperience with infants could have as one possible goal that the mother is able to demonstrate proper infant positioning during feeding.

Planning

Individualized nursing plans of care are established to include nursing actions, available resources, and client willingness to participate. For example, when developing a plan for a mother who is unsure about breastfeeding, the plan of care could include a referral to a resource, such as a lactation consultant.

Nursing Intervention

Identification of reasonable actions that can achieve desired outcomes is based on an individualized plan. These actions may be independent nursing actions or collaborative actions involving other health care team members. Actions are developed to resolve or lessen an identified problem and provide direction for nurses and other health care professionals.

Evaluation

Evaluation of goal achievement starts with assessment of the client and continues during data gathering to determine if the outcome has been reached or needs adjusting.

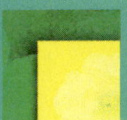

CASE STUDY/CARE PLAN
POSTPARTUM TEEN MOTHER

Megan is a 16-year-old primigravida who delivered an 8-lb girl by cesarean section. She is unwed and has no contact with the baby's father. She was in her junior year in high school, until her parents sent her to another state to live with an aunt for the last trimester and delivery. The parents are busy with their professional careers and have no interest in raising a grandchild. Because they are attorneys, they were able to arrange for adoption.

On the day following delivery, Megan was found crying. She told the nurse that she wanted to see her baby but was afraid to hold her. She expressed a desire to stay with her aunt and keep the baby. She also wanted to finish high school and get a job. Her aunt has been very loving and supportive, but she is raising three children alone as a divorced parent and cannot take on the added responsibility. Megan asked the nurse for pain medication while looking sadly at and holding her swollen abdomen. She tearfully said she would never get her figure back.

Assessment
Subjective data obtained through the interview process:

- Client was sent away to have her baby and give the baby up for adoption.
- Client is an unwed adolescent.
- Client desires to finish high school.
- Client has expressed a desire to keep her baby.
- Client desires to see her infant and is afraid to hold her.
- Client has no contact with the baby's father.
- Client has busy parents who give her monetary support and arranged the adoption.
- Client has an aunt who is supportive but unable to care for her niece and newborn.
- Client requested pain medication.
- Client states she will not get her figure back.

Objective data obtained through observation:

- Client is tearful and crying.
- Client looks anxious when talking about the baby.
- Client is holding her hands over incisional area.
- Client looks at the physical changes in her body.

(continues)

Nursing Diagnosis

Pain related to cesarean incision as evidenced by supporting the incisional area and requesting medication.

Expected Outcome   Client will have pain reduction by 3 points on a 10 point scale within 1 hour after medication administration.

Planning   Collaborating with client, determine how pain medication is to be administered and how often.

NOC   Pain control

NOC   Pain management

Nursing Interventions	Rationales
1. Assess need for pain medication using a scale from 1 to 10. Use guided imagery to refocus and enhance medication effectiveness.	1. Relief of pain is achieved with pharmacologic and nonpharmacologic means.

Evaluation   Pain medication schedule is effective in reducing client's pain within 1 hour after administration.

Nursing Diagnosis

Ineffective coping related to personal vulnerability in a crisis as evidenced by inability to manage situation and lack of support.

Expected Outcome   Client will be able to clarify feelings and improve coping skills by discharge.

Planning   By collaborating with client and support services, determine interventions to increase coping with situational crisis.

NOC   Coping

NIC   Coping enhancement

Nursing Interventions	Rationales
1. Take time to listen and assist to clarify feelings and improve coping skills. Address situational crisis via referral to a social worker.	1. Showing respect to client by listening and offering referrals will encourage confidence and realistic view of situation.

Evaluation   Client is able to collaborate with social worker through family counseling to clarify feelings, improve coping skills, and set realistic goals regarding situational crisis by discharge.

Nursing Diagnosis

Anxiety related to situational crisis as evidenced by conflict with adoption issue.

Expected Outcome   Client will demonstrate use of alternative relaxation techniques to reduce anxiety by discharge.

Planning   Collaborating with client, determine methods to reduce level of anxiety.

NOC   Anxiety control

NIC   Anxiety reduction

Nursing Interventions

1. Encourage ventilation of feelings; take time to listen. Incorporate alternative relaxation techniques, such as music, therapeutic touch, or focal breathing.

Rationales

1. Encouraging verbalization of feelings and relaxation exercises will help to lessen anxiety.

Evaluation Client is able to effectively carry out alternative relaxation techniques to reduce anxiety by discharge.

Nursing Diagnosis

Disturbed body image related to physical changes as evidenced by concern about appearance.

Expected Outcome Client will demonstrate an understanding of postpartum body changes and exercise and nutritional program by discharge.

Planning Collaborating with the client, determine actions to increase realistic perception of self through physical and nutritional interventions.

NOC Body image

NIC Body image enhancement

Nursing Interventions

1. Address concerns related to physical changes. Review postpartum exercise program, which may include yoga or walking. Refer to dietitian if calorie reduction is indicated.

Rationales

1. Realistic understanding of physical changes promotes acceptance of body image. Knowledge of available resources assists in maternal adjustment.

Evaluation Client is able to understand physical changes during postpartum and incorporate a progressive exercise program by discharge.

WEB ACTIVITIES

• • • Which online site provides information on recovering from labor and delivery?

• • • Which resources on the Internet can you find regarding general postpartum care?

• • • Where can you find information on how to perform Kegel exercises?

• • • Where can you find a sample postpartum exercise routine?

Key Concepts

- The parent-child attachment process occurs over a period of time.
- Parental adjustment takes time and is facilitated by nursing interventions.
- Siblings are affected by role change and seek nurturing by significant others.

- Nurses need to be aware of cultural influences that affect parental role adjustment.
- Postpartum adolescents require assistance in achieving role adjustment and meeting the developmental tasks of adolescence.
- Although pregnancy is considered to be wellness oriented, the postpartum nurse utilizes clinical decision-making and critical thinking skills to provide safe, high-quality nursing care.
- Vital signs indicative of problems, such as hemorrhage and infection, are important elements in the assessment of the client postpartally.
- A systematic evaluation of postpartum women consists of examining the breasts, uterus, bladder, bowels, lochia, episiotomy, Homan's sign, and emotional status.
- Uterine involution to nonprepregnant size and return of other pregnancy changes to normal functioning occur 4 to 6 weeks after delivery.
- Although eager to lose her pregnancy weight, the new mother must approach weight loss and exercise slowly and in a healthy manner.
- Various approaches to pain relief can include traditional pharmacologic interventions as well as holistic alternative treatments.

■ Before discharge the nurse must ascertain the client's immune status; the Rh-negative mother who delivered an infant who is Rh-positive should receive RhoGAM, and the mother who is rubella non-immune should be immunized with rubella vaccine before her next pregnancy.

■ Because of short hospitalizations, the postpartum nurse should try to identify key self-care and infant-care information that the new mother needs and wants to learn; the nurse should guide her teaching plan toward meeting these needs.

■ The nurse incorporates consideration of client and family needs into planning her nursing care, including being aware of cultural diversity.

■ Throughout the hospital stay, the nurse should educate and counsel the client (and family) as she encourages the client to progress toward confident, independent care of herself and her new baby.

Review Questions and Activities

1. Which of the concepts regarding assessment of vaginal bleeding are incorrect?
   a. Lochia rubra is a normal characteristic the first few days after delivery.
   b. The passage of a large amount of bright-red blood with multiple clots is a normal finding the first 24 hours after delivery.
   c. Blood may accumulate in the vaginal vault and gush out when the client moves from a horizontal to a vertical position.
   d. Bleeding usually is controlled with up to 40 U of oxytocin added to an IV bag of fluids.

   The correct answer is b.

2. Lochia undergoes changes over the course of a few weeks. What does lochia look like during the first 24 hours?
   a. Bright red in color owing to decidual tissue sloughing and blood components
   b. Pink or brown-tinged in color owing to its serous fluid, leukocyte, erythrocyte, and decidual tissue components
   c. Whitish-yellow in color and creamy in consistency owing to its leukocyte content and decreasing serous fluid content
   d. A large amount of dark-red blood owing to passing of multiple blood clots

   The correct answer is a.

3. What nursing actions facilitate parent-child attachment?

4. List infant behaviors that can facilitate the parent-child attachment process.

5. How can sibling adjustment be facilitated?

References

American Academy of Pediatrics (AAP) and American College of Obstetricians and Gynecologists (ACOG). (1997). *Guidelines for perinatal care* (4th ed.). Washington, DC, and Elk Grove, IL: Authors.

American College of Obstetrics and Gynecology (ACOG). (1990). *Prevention of D isoimmunization* (Tech. Bulletin, pp. 1–4).

American College of Obstetrics and Gynecology (ACOG). (1992). *Rubella and pregnancy.* (Tech. Bulletin, pp. 1–8).

Association of Women's Health, Obstetrics, and Neonatal Nurses (AWHONN). (1996). *Compendium of postpartum care.* Washington, DC: Author.

Bowes, W. A. (1996). Postpartum care. In S. G. Gabbe, J. R. Niebyl, & J. L. Simpson (Eds.), *Obstetrics: Normal and problem pregnancies* (pp. 692–713). New York: Churchill Livingston.

Brazelton, T. B. (1984). *Neonatal behavioral assessment scale* (2nd ed.). London: Heineman.

Brazelton, T. B. (1981). *On becoming a family: The growth of attachment.* New York: Dell.

Cashion, K. (1997). Normal postpartum. In D. L. Lowdermilk, S. E. Perry, & I. M. Bobak (Eds.), *Maternity and women's health care* (6th ed.). St. Louis, MO: Mosby.

Davidson, N. R. S. (1974). REEDA: Evaluating postpartum healing. *Journal of Nurse Midwifery, 19*(2), 6–8.

Duff, P. (1996). Maternal and perinatal infection. In S. G. Gabbe, J. R. Niebyl, & J. L. Simpson (Eds.), *Obstetrics: Normal and problem pregnancies* (pp. 692–713). New York: Churchill Livingston.

Epstein, B. A. (June 6, 2000). New baby, new stress. In *The doctor's office.* Retrieved from http://www.allkids.org/Epstein/Articles/New Baby Stress.html.

Ferketich, S. L., & Mercer, R. T. (1995). Predictors of role competence for experienced and inexperienced fathers. *Nursing Research, 44*(2), 88–95.

Geissler, E. M. (1998). *Cultural assessment.* St. Louis, MO: Mosby.

Gordon, M. C., & Landon, M. B. (1996). Dermatologic disorders. In S. G. Gabbe, J. R. Niebyl, & J. L. Simpson (Eds.), *Obstetrics: Normal and problem pregnancies* (pp. 1184–1187). New York: Churchill Livingston.

Griffin, N. (2000, June 25). *After-the-birth mother care.* Retrieved from http://wospace.cnation.com/Health/Hlth Mother-Care .html.

Jordan, P. (1998). *Losing belly after childbirth.* Retrieved from http://www.allhealth.com/health/followup/print/0,4197,6936 968,00.html.

Jordon, P. L. (1990). Laboring for relevance: Expectant and new fatherhood. *Nursing Research, 39,* 11–16.

Klaus, M. (1998). Mother and infant: Early emotional ties. *Pediatrics, 102*(5), 1244–1246.

Klaus, M. H., & Kennel, J. H. (1982). *Parent-infant bonding* (2nd ed.). St. Louis: C. V. Mosby.

Phillips, C. (1997). *Mother-baby nursing*. Washington, DC: Association of Women's Health, Obstetrics, and Neonatal Nurses.

Rubin, R. (1984). *Maternal identity and the maternal experience*. New York: Springer.

Sears, W., & Sears, M. (2000). *Postpartum basics: Getting your body back*. Retrieved from http://www.2.parentsoup.com/firstyear/articles/postpartum/body/0,5302,,00.html.

Spratto, G. R., & Woods, A. L. (2001). *PDR nurse's drug handbook*. Clifton Park, NY: Delmar Learning.

Water, M. A., & Lee, K. A. (1996). Difference between primigravidae and multigravidae mothers in sleep disturbance, fatigue, and functional status. *Journal of Nurse Midwifery, 41*(5), 364–367.

Waters, E., Posada, G., Crowell, J. A., & Lay, K. L. (1994). The development of attachment: From control system to working models. *Psychiatry, 57*(1), 32–42.

Williams, L. R. & Cooper, M. K. (1993). Nurse-managed postpartum home care. *Journal of Obstetrics, Gynecologic, and Neonatal Nurses, 22*(1), 25–31.

Suggested Readings

Association of Women's Health, Obstetrics and Neonatal Nurses (AWHONN). (1991). Postpartum nursing care: Vaginal delivery. *OGN nursing practice resource*. Washington, DC: Author.

Barclay, L., Everett, L., Rogan, F., Schmied, V., & Wyllie, A. (1997). Becoming a mother—an analysis of women's experience of early motherhood. *Journal of Advanced Nursing, 25* (4), 719–728.

Beger, D., & Loveland Cook, C. A. (1998). Postpartum teaching priorities. The viewpoints of nurses and mothers. *Journal of Obstetric, Gynecologic, and Neonatal Nurses, 27*(2), 161–168.

Freedman, L. H. (1999). *Birth as a healing experience. The emotional journey of pregnancy through postpartum*. Old Saybrook, CT: Harrington Park Press.

Health Care Financing Administration. (June 21, 2000). *The newborns' and mothers' health protection act of 1996*. Retrieved from http://my.webmd.com/content/dmk/dmk article 5462944.

Lewis-Copeland, C. (1997). *Mother's first year: A realistic guide to the changes and challenges of motherhood*. Berkeley, CA. Berkeley Publishing Group.

Mattson, S., & Smith, J. E. (Eds.). (1993). *Core curriculum for maternal-newborn nursing*. Philadelphia: W. B. Saunders.

Moran, C. F., Holt, V. L., & Martin, D. P. (1997). What do women want to know after childbirth? *Birth, 24*(1), 27–34.

Noble, E. (1995). *Essential exercises for the childbearing year: A guide to health and comfort before and after your baby is born* (4th ed.). Harwich, MA. New Life Images.

Placksin, S. (2000). *Mothering the new mother: Women's feelings and needs after childbirth a support and resource guide*. New York: Newmark Press.

Rogan, F., Schmeid, V., Barclay, L., Everitt, L., & Wyllie, A. (1997) Becoming a mother—developing a new theory of early motherhood. *Journal of Advanced Nursing, 25*(5), 877–885.

Roye, C. F., & Balk, S. J. (1997). Caring for pregnant teens and their mothers, too. *Maternal Child Nursing, 22*, 153–157.

Stern, D. (1998). Mothers' emotional needs. *Pediatrics, 102*(5), 1250–1252.

Wheeler, L (1997). *Nurse-midwifery handbook: A practical guide to prenatal and postpartum care*. Philadelphia: Lippincott, Williams & Wilkins.

Resources

About Busy Cooks: http://busycooks.about.com

About Pregnancy/Birth: http://pregnancy.about.com (search for "Postpartum Exercise Routine")

Alexian Brothers Medical Center: http://www.alexian.org

Baby Business: http://www.babybusiness.com

Baby Center: http://www.babycenter.com

Baby Workshop (Sesame Workshop): http://www.ctw.org/baby workshop

Bayfront Medical Center: http://www.bayfront.org

Child Care Experts National Network: http://www.childcare-experts.org

Depend Absorption Products: http://www.depend.com

EngenderHealth: http://www.engenderhealth.org

Family Education Network: http://www.familyeducation.com

Family Fun: http://familyfun.go.com

iVillage Parent Soup: http://www.parentsoup.com

iVillage Parents Place: http://www.parentsplace.com

Johnson & Johnson: http://www.jnj.com

National Center for Fathering: http://www.fathers.com

National Parenting Center: http://www.tnpc.com

NetWellness (University of Cincinnati): http://www.netwellness.org

Pampers Parenting Institute: http://www.pampers.com

Parenthood: http://www.parenthood.com

University of Nebraska Medical Center: http://www.unmc.edu

Very Best Baby (Nestle): http://www.verybestbaby.com

Welcome Addition (Abbott Laboratories): http://www.welcomeaddition.com

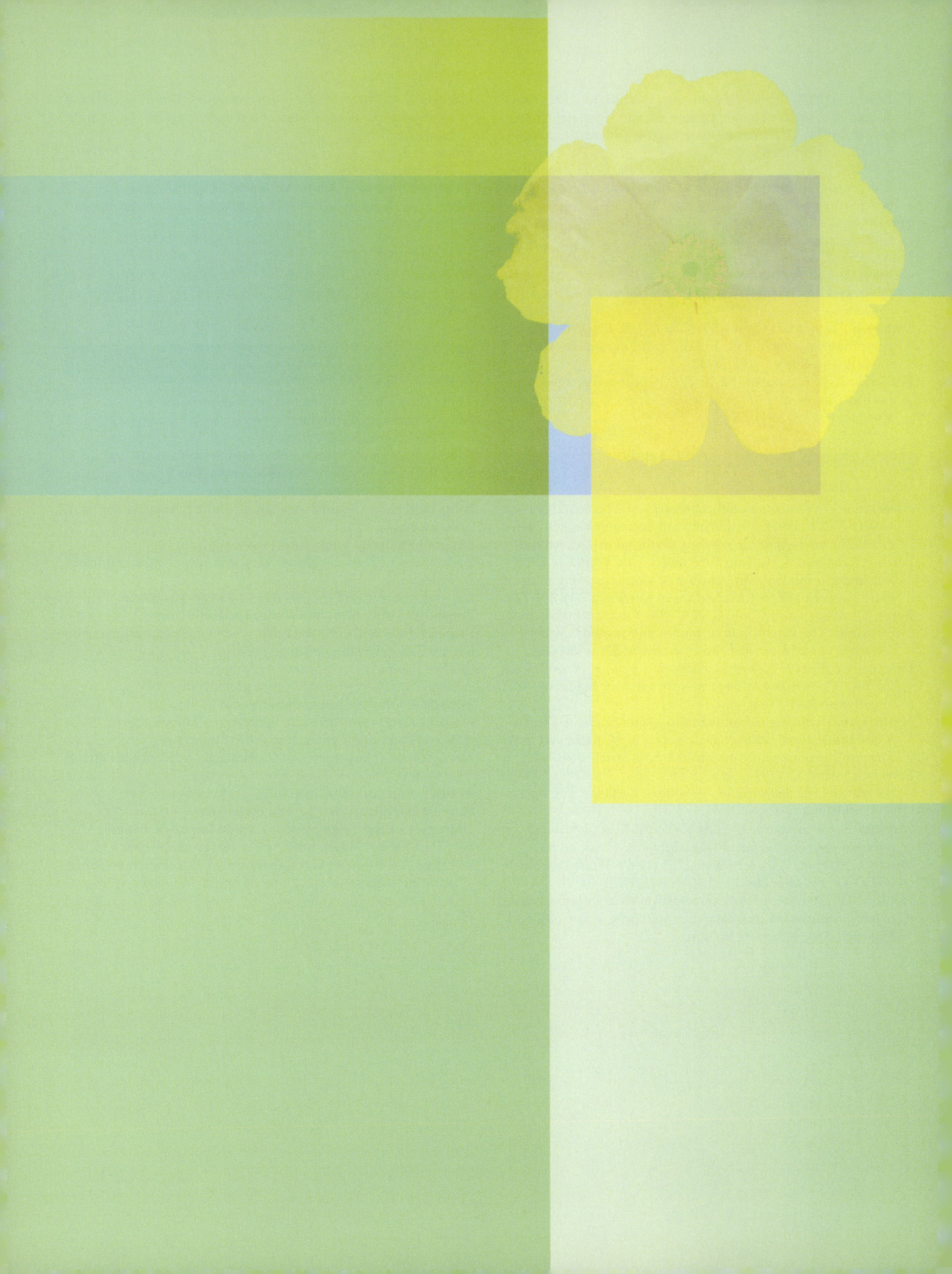

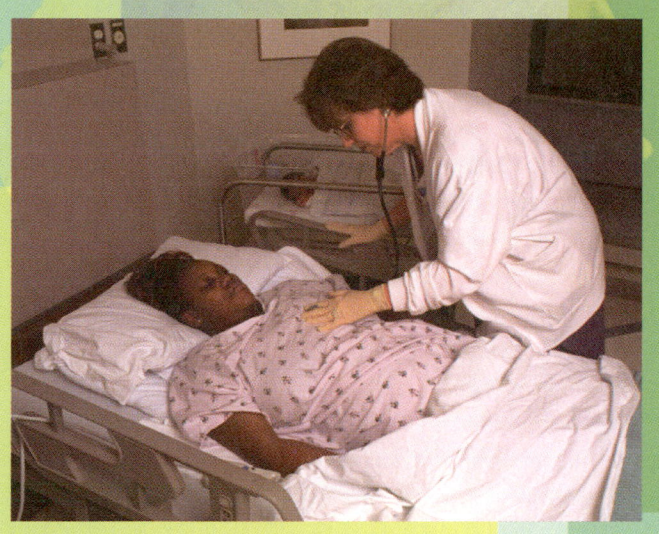

CHAPTER 17

COMPLICATIONS OF POSTPARTUM AND NEONATAL LOSS

Postpartum units are often oriented to happy, excited couples adjusting to a healthy newborn. Throughout the postpartum period, nurses are always alert for signs of complications. These may be physical or psychologic complications of the mother. Complications of the postpartum period may include the neonate with serious health problems, or a neonatal death. To prepare yourself for working with postpartal complications, ask yourself the following questions:

- What would happen if the nurse did not do periodic assessments to pick up early signs of complications?
- How do I feel about depressed mothers who are unable to care for their infants?
- What would it be like to be a newly delivered mother on a mother-baby unit and have just lost your newborn?

Key Terms

Anticipatory Grieving
Atony
Grief
Grief work
Mastitis
Pathologic grief

Puerperal sepsis
Relinquishment
Reproductive loss
Sudden infant death
    syndrome (SIDS)

Competencies

Upon completion of this chapter, the reader should be able to:

1. Describe the causes, classifications, and signs of postpartum hemorrhage.
2. Discuss the most common types of postpartum infection and the most common infectious agents.
3. Discuss nursing care of the client with postpartum complications.
4. Differentiate among postpartum blues, postpartum depression, and postpartum psychosis.
5. Discuss nursing care of the family dealing with loss from neonatal illness or neonatal death.
6. Develop a plan of care for a family experiencing maternal complications.

The majority of pregnancies end with a healthy neonate and a healthy mother who recovers to a nonpregnant state without complications. Complications can emerge during the physiologic process of involution, the psychologic process of adaptation, and from dealing with the health of the neonate. However, the process of involution is very comprehensive and numerous physiologic changes occur over a relatively short time. During these changes, the postpartum client is vulnerable to complications. The most common of these relate to hemorrhage and infection. The psychologic changes involve response to birth, adjusting to the newborn, emergence of parenting roles, and family adaptation. These psychologic changes are also influenced by the physiologic changes in hormonal levels and changes in sleep patterns. Parents who have neonates who are in intensive care, or who have been born with a serious health problem or defect, or whose infant has died will have psychologic grieving and coping with the loss in addition to all the other postpartum adjustments. This chapter covers the most common physiologic postpartum complications, postpartum depressions, and family issues related to neonatal losses.

POSTPARTUM PHYSICAL COMPLICATIONS

In caring for the low-risk healthy woman after delivery, the nurse must monitor and prevent the development of complications that may occur during the puerperium. The most common complications discussed in this section include hemorrhage, perineal hematoma, and infection.

Postpartum Hemorrhage

Maternal hemorrhage is the most frequent complication in the postpartum period. It is one of the three leading causes of maternal morbidity and mortality in the United States (ACOG, 1990). Normal blood loss during an uncomplicated vaginal delivery is 500 mL or less (Beneditti, 1996). Hemorrhage is defined as blood loss greater than 500 mL for a vaginal delivery. The diagnosis of postpartum hemorrhage is based on the clinician's judgment of the estimated blood loss (EBL); however, providers tend to underestimate blood loss.

Risk factors for postpartum hemorrhage include:

- Cesarean delivery
- Unusually large episiotomy
- Operative delivery (forceps or vacuum extractor)
- Precipitous labor
- Atypically attached placenta (accreta, previa, abruption)
- Fetal demise
- Previous uterine surgery

Hemorrhage can be classified as early or late. Early or acute hemorrhage occurs within the first 24 hours after delivery. The majority of early hemorrhages are manifested within the first 2 hours postdelivery. The most common cause (80% to 90%) of early postpartum hemorrhage is uterine **atony**, or lack of uterine muscle tone. Uterine atony is when the uterus fails to contract and becomes boggy, or soft. This failure to contract leads to continued bleeding from the site of placental insertion. Risk factors for uterine atony include:

- Overdistention of the uterus (polyhydramnios, multiple gestation, macrosomia)
- Uterine anomaly (bicornuate uterus, presence of fibroids)
- Poor uterine muscle tone (high parity, rapid or prolonged labor, induction/augmentation of labor, chorioamnionitis, magnesium sulfate, general anesthesia)

Retained placental fragments are the second leading cause of early postpartum hemorrhage. Risk factors for retained placental fragments include:

- Mismangement of third stage
- Second trimester delivery
- Abnormal uterine anatomy
- Abnormal placental implantation (accreta, previa, abruption)
- Placental malformation (succenturiate lobe)

Another frequent cause of early hemorrhage is tears or lacerations of the birth canal. Risks factors for lacerations include:

- Operative deliveries (forceps or vacuum extractor)
- Precipitous delivery
- Abnormal tissue scarring (conization, abnormal cervical cells, history of D&C or abortion, presence of HPV lesions)
- Extensions of episiotomy or perineal lacerations
- Varices
- Hematoma formation

Bleeding also may be related to systemic coagulopathies, such as disseminated intravascular coagulation (DIC). The risk of DIC is higher in women having PIH, abruptio placentae, clotting abnormalities, thrombocytopenia, fetal demise or retention of a dead fetus, amniotic fluid embolism, and infectious processes, and in whom anticoagulants have been used.

Postpartum hemorrhage can be very rapid, and often is very dramatic. Health care providers must be able to recognize the signs and symptoms early and respond immediately. During the immediate postpartum period the nurse bears great responsibility in assessing for potential hemorrhage. Knowledge of predisposing factors and careful examination of the client alert the nurse to the potential for hemorrhage and help anticipate it, thus preventing further complications. Many cases of postpartum shock are not recognized until the client is in moderate to severe shock, which requires more aggressive treatment to reverse. Table 17-1 lists the signs and symptoms seen in shock and the reasons for these conditions. Table 17-2 differentiates among mild, moderate, and severe shock.

Table 17-1	Signs and Symptoms of Shock
SIGNS AND SYMPTOMS	**CAUSES**
Hypotension	Stroke volume and cardiac output
Tachycardia, weak thready pulse	Symptomatic vasoconstriction; chemoreceptor stimulation, progressing to medullary respiratory stimulation secondary to metabolic acidosis
Decreased pulse pressure	Stroke volume
Cool, pale, clammy skin	Peripheral vasoconstriction
Cyanosis	Excessive vasoconstriction of reduced hemoglobin in blood
Oliguria or anuria	Renal perfusion
Extreme thirst	Extracellular fluid
Hypothermia	Metabolism
Apathy, lethargy, confusion, coma	Cerebral blood flow, acidosis
Irritability and anxiety	Epinephrine secretion; hypoxia

Nursing Alert

Signs of Disseminated Intravascular Coagulation

Bleeding from other nongenital sites in the body, such as venous puncture sites, may suggest the development of disseminated intravascular coagulation (DIC).

Nursing Tip *Uterine Atony*

Uterine atony is the most common cause of postpartum hemorrhage. When excessive postpartum bleeding is encountered the first intervention by the nurse is fundal massage. If the uterus is firm and bleeding remains heavy, inspection for placental fragments or lacerations is indicated. The physician or midwife should be called if heavy bleeding continues.

Table 17-2	Classifications of Hemorrhagic Shock					
SIGNS AND SYMPTOMS	BLOOD PRESSURE	PULSE	RESPIRATION	SKIN	URINARY OUTPUT	LEVEL OF CONSCIOUSNESS
Mild	Normal or hypertensive	Increased, tone becoming weaker	Increased, deep	Cool and pale	Normal (average 30 mL/h)	Alert, oriented, mildly anxious
Moderate	Systolic, 60–90 mmHg	Tachycardic, tone becoming irregular	Tachypneic, becoming shallow	Cool, pale, and moist	Decreased (10–22 mL/h)	Oriented, increasing anxiety and restlessness
Severe	Systolic, <60 mmHg	Tachycardic, thready and irregular	Tachypneic, irregular	Cool, clammy, central cyanosis	Oliguric (<10 mL/h)	Lethargic

Nursing Tip — Assessing for Decreased Perfusion

To subtly test for decreased perfusion in the extremities, squeeze the hypothenar area of the hand for 1 to 2 seconds and then release the pressure. If the client has a normal volume, the skin will initially blanch and then return to a normal color after 1 to 2 seconds. Circulatory refill in the blanched hand will be delayed in the client with a 15% to 25% volume deficit.

Classification of Postpartum Hemorrhage

Management of acute hemorrhage includes determining the cause of the bleeding, estimating blood loss, and trying to control the bleeding. Hemorrhage often occurs immediately before or after delivery of the placenta (Beneditti, 1996). Treatment of hemorrhage is based on identification of the classification and percentage of blood loss (Table 17-3).

Class 1 is often asymptomatic so careful monitoring of blood loss is important.

Table 17-3	Classifications of Hemorrhage	
CLASS	PERCENT OF BLOOD LOSS	ESTIMATED BLOOD LOSS (mL)
1	15	<900
2	20–25	1200–1500
3	30–35	1800–2100
4	40	>2400

Clients with Class 2 hemorrhage will begin to demonstrate clinical signs, such as tachycardia or tachypnea (Beneditti, 1996). Tachypnea is considered a nonspecific and early sign of mild volume deficit. Minute ventilation often is double its normal rate and should be interpreted as a sign of impending problems. Blood pressure changes include orthostatic hypotension and decreased perfusion to the extremities. The pulse pressure begins to narrow; when it decreases to 30 mmHg or less, the client may be experiencing further volume loss (Beneditti, 1996).

The postpartum client with a Class 3 hemorrhage will begin to exhibit marked tachycardia (120 to 160 bpm) and tachypnea (30 to 50 bpm). Overt hypotension is present, and the nurse may note cool, clammy skin. The client with a greater than 40% blood loss has a Class 4 hemorrhage. The nurse may not be able to detect a blood pressure in a client with profound shock. Pulses often are absent and urine output is minimal (oliguria) to none (anuria). Examination of the hematocrit may assist in estimating a large blood loss if it significantly changed from the previous baseline. Significant hematocrit changes will not occur until after 4 hours from the start of hemorrhage (Beneditti, 1996). The client also may exhibit signs of air hunger, anxiety, visual disturbances, and unusual thirst.

The overall goal in postpartum hemorrhage management is to prevent cardiovascular collapse—the bleeding must be controlled quickly. If the cardiac output decreases, renal blood flow will be compromised. The physician will play a major role in evaluating the reason for hemorrhage. A careful exploration of the uterus for retained placental parts and the cervix and vagina for lacerations may show the source of bleeding.

Intravenous access should be available to administer fluids, medications, and replacement blood products, as needed. Pharmacologic agents to control bleeding include oxytocin (Pitocin) and synthetic prostaglandins. Packed methylergonovines (Methergine) most commonly are ordered to expand blood volume; other blood products, such as whole blood, platelets, fresh frozen plasma, and cryoprecipitate, also may be used. A CBC and typing and crossmatching for erythrocytes may be ordered as well as a coagulation profile (prothrombin time, partial thromboplastin time, platelets, fibrinogen, fibrin split products, and a clot retraction test). Blood products normally are given when the hemoglobin is 7 g/dL or less. If all else fails, surgical intervention with laparatomy may be indicated (Beneditti, 1996).

The nurse, along with the provider, should continually try to keep the client informed of her current medical status, especially as interventions are performed in an urgent manner. The nurse should explain what the actions being taken are and why they are being performed. The nurse should assist the client into a supine position, with legs slightly elevated to facilitate blood return to the heart. Other interventions include avoiding administering sedatives, analgesics, or other central nervous system depressants because they depress the vasomotor center. Overheating also should be avoided because it causes vasodilation.

Nursing Alert

Hemabate Precautions

You should not administer carboprost tromethamine (Hemabate) when a client has a history of bronchospasms. Carboprost tromethamine is a prostaglandin that stimulates smooth muscles, such as the lungs, to contract. When given, clients usually develop diarrhea. You may be using medications such as diphenoxylate (Lomotil) and atropine (Atropair) prophylactically to prevent diarrhea.

Late hemorrhage occurs 24 hours or more after delivery and is defined as a sudden increase in bleeding 8 to 14 days postpartum (Bowes, 1996). This is differentiated from normal involution which at this time the lochia transitions to lochia serosa, the client may experience a return to lochia rubra. The bleeding usually lasts for a short period of time and is self-limiting. Subinvolution at the placental site, vulvar hematomas, and infection

Critical Thinking

Beliefs about Blood Transfusions

You must be attuned to the client's cultural or religious values regarding health care. Members of some groups, such as the Jehovah's Witness faith, have deep religious convictions against receiving blood transfusions because doing so directly violates their beliefs. Blood transfusion is forbidden for them by Biblical passages noted in the following citation: "Only flesh with its soul—its blood—you must not eat" (Genesis 9:3-4); "[You must] pour its blood out and cover it with dust" (Leviticus 17:13-14); and "Abstain from . . . fornication and from what is strangled and from blood" (Acts 15:19-21). These beliefs include not accepting homologous or autologous whole blood, packed red blood cells, white blood cells, or platelets. The religious understanding of the Jehovah's Witness does not absolutely prohibit the use of other components such as albumin and immune globulins. Nonblood replacement fluids, such as colloid or crystalloid fluids, are allowed.

Health care professionals face this challenge as a major health issue. There are over half a million (and the numbers are increasing) Jehovah's Witnesses in the United States who do not accept blood transfusions. A liability concern for health care personnel exists; however, Jehovah's Witnesses will take adequate legal steps to relieve liability as to their informed refusal of blood. Many physicians and hospital officials previously viewed refusal of a transfusion as a legal problem and sought court sanctions to proceed as they saw fit medically. Current medical literature indicates changes in attitudes of medical professionals. Nonetheless, the medical community has been trying to adapt other methods of treatment and practice the doctrine of treating the "whole person."

Caring for minors presents the greatest concern, often resulting in legal action against parents under child-neglect statutes. However, many people believe that Jehovah's Witnesses seek good medical care for their children. These parents urge that the legal and medical community give consideration to the family's religious beliefs.

How would you feel if your client is bleeding heavily and urgently needs a blood transfusion to replace her volume deficit?

(endometritis) are some of the reasons for the delayed or late bleeding. Of all cases, 40% are caused by retained placental parts (Bowes, 1996). Ultrasonography assists in identifying retained placental fragments, and suction evacuation is performed to remove the fragments.

Pelvic Hematoma

Perineal pain that does not go away despite treatment with analgesics should be examined more closely. A common cause of severe perineal pain is the presence of a hematoma. This condition is potentially dangerous because blood loss may not be visible. Hematomas may be categorized into three types: vulvar, vaginal, and retroperitoneal. It is not always possible to visualize a hematoma, so when a hematoma is suspected, the doctor or midwife should be notified. Medical management of a hematoma usually includes a combination of surgical drainage, antibiotics, and pain medication.

The most common hematoma is located on the vulva, which forms when ruptured arteries and veins in the superficial fascia seep into the nearby vulvar tissue (Benedetti, 1996). Signs of a vulvar hematoma are local pressure; discoloration, such as ecchymosis (bluish-purplish); and a visible outline of a hematoma (Figure 17-1). Blood loss is subacute and the client may complain of perineal pain. Management involves surgical incision and evacuation of the blood and clots. Once sutured, the space is compressed with a large sterile dressing. An indwelling urinary catheter inserted at the start of the procedure should remain in place for 24 to 36 hours.

Trauma to maternal soft tissues during delivery (e.g., by the use of forceps) may result in formation of a vaginal hematoma. Large amounts of blood usually do not form. The client frequently complains of severe, unrelenting rectal pain. On examination, a large bulging mass may be protruding into the vagina. A large enough vaginal hematoma can make urination difficult. A vaginal hematoma is treated with incision and evacuation. The incision need not be closed; a vaginal pack is used to put pressure on the incision edges and is removed after 12 to 18 hours (Beneditti, 1996).

Least common but most dangerous to the mother are retroperitoneal hematomas. They occur when one of the vessels from the hypogastric artery is lacerated. A large amount of bleeding may ensue until the signs and symptoms of hypotension or shock are noted. Treating this life-threatening hematoma requires surgical exploration and ligation of the lacerated vessels (Beneditti, 1996).

It is important for the nurse to examine the perineal area with the client in a supine as well as side-lying positioning to adequately detect a hematoma, especially when a new mother presents with severe perineal pain. Opened

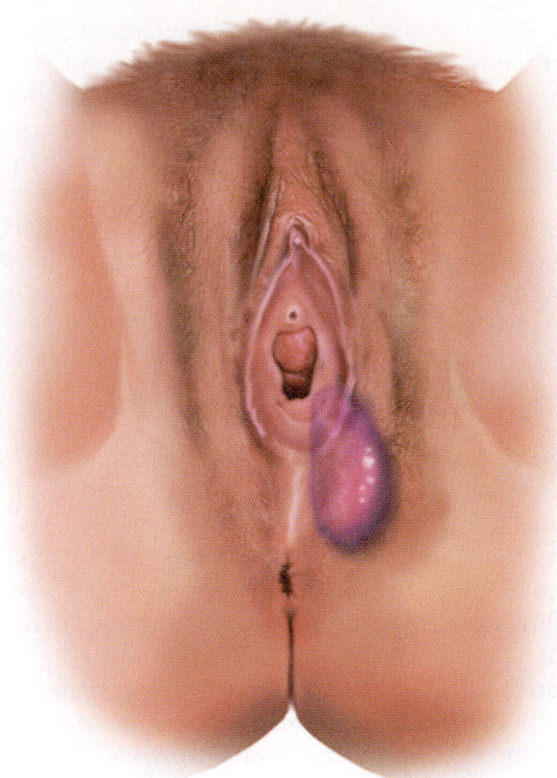

Figure 17-1 Hematoma of the vulva.

hematoma sites should be kept clean, with frequent pad changes. Smaller hematomas usually are allowed to resolve spontaneously, with ice packs used for comfort.

Many health care providers may order a postpartum CBC to evaluate hemoglobin and hematocrit values, especially if blood loss is significant. Otherwise, no other laboratory tests are required until clinical indications dictate.

Postpartum Infections

Postpartum infections, commonly known as **puerperal sepsis**, involve infections of the genital organs that occur during the first 6 weeks after childbirth. Postpartum infections are the leading cause of nosocomial infections and maternal morbidity and mortality (Clark, 1995). Postpartum infection is significant in that it may interfere with mother-infant attachment and breastfeeding, the hospital stay is prolonged, or readmission occurs. Nurses have the opportunity to identify women at risk for infection and recognize the subtle and early signs and symptoms. Because of early discharge, the nurse also must provide preventive care and anticipatory teaching to minimize the risks.

The classic definition of postpartum infection is an oral temperature greater than 38°C (100.4°F) taken twice 6

Nursing Tip   *Postpartum Urine Cultures*

Postpartum women often have midstream urine contaminated with lochia. When obtaining a clean-catch urine specimen to evaluate the client for a urinary tract infection, you should instruct the client in the proper technique. Because catheterization increases the risk of infection, it should be avoided when possible.

To obtain a clean-catch urine specimen, instruct the client to separate the labia with two fingers of one hand. Using the other free hand, she should clean the labia with sterile wipes, moving from front to back. The client should try to wipe three times: once on each side of the urethra along the labia and the third in the middle, cleansing the urethra. The specimen can then be collected.

■ Long labors with frequent vaginal examinations (greater chance of introducing microorganisms)

■ Prolonged delivery after rupture of membranes (>24 hours)

■ Internal fetal monitoring (fetal scalp electrodes, intrauterine pressure catheter)

■ Positive amniotic fluid culture (*Escherichia coli* and *Klebsiella* are commonly obtained from cultures of amniotic fluid)

■ History of UTIs, GBS, STDs

Physical examination of the client with a suspected infection includes assessment of a change in the color, amount, odor, and consistency of the lochia. The episiotomy, if present, should be examined for redness, warmth, edema, tenderness, or disruption in the wound incision. The nurse should assess for fundal tenderness or pain when massaged. Costovertebral tenderness that may suggest pyelonephritis should be ruled out. Vital signs may indicate elevated temperature and tachycardia. Laboratory findings from blood, cultures, urinalysis, and culture and sensitivity tests may indicate the presence of infection. Culture reports will help determine the diagnosis and type of antibiotic therapy needed.

General Approach to Management of Infection

Infection with a single organism is rare. Broad spectrum antibiotics directed at multiple organisms often are administered prophylactically for cesarean sections and prolonged rupture of membranes. The issues of treatment and timing of the treatment, however, vary among health care providers. General nursing practice in preventing infection is targeted at maintaining health with diet, exercise, and diligent hygiene practices, such as good handwashing technique.

The nurse can provide anticipatory teaching to help clients prevent infection. The client should be instructed on how to use a squeeze-bottle with warm water after using the toilet to better cleanse the area and on how to wipe anteriorly to posteriorly. Perineal pads should be changed in the same manner, that is, removed from anterior to posterior, and should be replaced each time she goes to the bathroom. Client education includes the side effects of therapy, prevention of spread of infection, maintenance of adequate fluid intake, adherence to the prescribed treatment regimen, the signs and symptoms of worsening infection, and when to contact her provider.

Caregivers also should be cognizant of preventing the transmission of infection among staff and clients. Standard precautions and careful conscientious handwashing should be practiced. Shared equipment (e.g.,

hours apart on any 2 of the first 10 days postpartum, excluding the first 24 hours after delivery (Bowes, 1996). Postpartum infections may occur within or outside of the pelvis. Pelvic infections include endometritis (the most common), pelvic cellulitis, pelvic abscesses, hematomas, and septic pelvic thrombophlebitis. Extrapelvic infections are those that occur in the urinary tract, at the episiotomy site, in the breasts (mastitis), or in the legs (thrombophlebitis). Refer to Table 17-4 for a description of the most common postpartum infections. Cesarean birth is the single most significant risk for postpartum infections (20 times greater than vaginal birth). Prolonged rupture of membranes is the second most common cause of postpartum infections followed by prolonged labor. Eight vaginal exams during labor puts the client at the same infection risk as having ruptured membranes for 18 hours or greater.

The causes of postpartum infections are related to anatomic and microbiologic factors. Microorganisms may enter the body at the site of the placental implantation. The infection then becomes systemic. With prolonged rupture of membranes, endogenous or exogenous flora may enter and ascend the vagina, causing infection. Dilation of the cervical canal after delivery makes it susceptible to bacterial invasion from normal flora.

The duration of labor (>18 hours), route of delivery, and colonization of amniotic fluid are the strongest predictors of developing a puerperal infection. Other factors that predispose clients to infections are obesity, anemia, malnourishment, cigarette smoking, diabetes, drug abuse, and immunosuppression. Other risk factors for developing infection include the following (Bowes, 1996):

Table 17-4   Common Postpartum Infections

INFECTION	CHARACTERISTICS	CLINICAL FINDINGS	MANAGEMENT AND TEACHING
Endometritis • Infection of endometrium, lining of uterus • Causative organisms: —*Escherichia coli* —*Chlamydia trachomatis* —*Gardnerella vaginalis* —*Mycoplasma hominis*	• Major risk factor: cesarean section (especially after laboring or rupture of membrane [ROM]) • Incidence increases with presence of bacterial vaginosis • Degree of fever can indicate extent of infection	• Uterine distention or tenderness • Abdominal pain • Malaise, lethargy • Nausea and vomiting • Anorexia • Foul-smelling lochia • Fever, chills • Tachycardia • Anemia • Increased leukocytes with shift to the left • Increased erythrocyte sedimentation rate	• Broad-spectrum antibiotics (double or triple) • If single antibiotics: high-dose clindamycin (Cleocin) or cephalosporins (Keflex) for 24–72 h • Supportive treatments • Rest • Hydration • Analgesia
Mastitis • Infection of lactating breast • Causative organism: —*Staphylococcus aureus*	• Preventable infection • Found most often in Caucasian multiparous women • Found in 7%–11% of lactating women • Symptoms usually occur 2–4 weeks postpartum • Presentation might be mild and almost chronic, or severe and acute • Risk factors: —Damaged nipples —Failure to empty breasts adequately —Primiparity —Stress —Breast abnormalities —Skin infections —Increased maternal age	• Sudden onset of flulike symptoms • Chills, fever • Tachycardia • Achiness • Headache • Malaise • Nausea and vomiting • Unilateral local breast pain • Warmth, swelling, redness • Axillary adenopathy • Clogged milk ducts • Endemic mastitis • Red, inflamed V-shaped area • Leukocytosis	• Antibiotics • Dicloxacillin • Complete emptying of breasts • Use of breast pumps • If not breastfeeding, bind breasts • Supportive measures • Moist heat or ice to the local area • Hydration • Analgesics • Assess breastfeeding technique • Client teaching on preventive measures • Proper infant position for correct latch-on and sucking • Breastfeed every 2–3 h • Avoid nipple shields • Try to avoid supplemental feedings and pacifier use • Change wet nursing pads • Avoid tight clothing, underwire bras, infant carriers that may block milk ducts or prevent breasts from emptying adequately • Avoid practices that put pressure on breasts: —Sleeping on stomach —Gripping breasts tightly when nursing —Resting infant on the breast while supine —Pressing breast tissue away from infant's nose during feeding —Stopping milk flow by pressing on areola • Empty breasts completely; avoid milk stasis • Manually express milk if milk duct is blocked • Avoid cracked nipples • Use larger or different cut of bra for comfort

Table 17-4 *(Continued)*

INFECTION	CHARACTERISTICS	CLINICAL FINDINGS	MANAGEMENT AND TEACHING
Thrombophlebitis (so-called milk legs): —Septic pelvic thrombophlebitis (SPT) —Deep vein thrombosis (DVT) —Inflammation of lining of blood vessel owing to blood clot formation, usually in deep veins in legs, thighs, or pelvis	• SPT is the least common infection • SPT frequently occurs with wound infection, especially when no client response to antibiotics • DVT incidence: —1:1,000 in vaginal deliveries —3–4:1,000 in assisted deliveries —25:1,000 in cesarean sections • Risk factors for SPT and DVT: —Venous stasis from remaining in bed for prolonged period —Increased coagulopathy —Blood vessel damage	**SPT** • Pain 2–4h postpartum in groin, upper or lower abdomen, flank area • Moderate fever • Guarding • Tachycardia • Ropelike, tender mass near uterus • Gastrointestinal distress • Decreased bowel sounds **DVT** • Rapid onset • Severe pain and swelling • Redness, warmth, tenderness in calves or legs • Hardness or nodules along a vein • Varicosities • Positive Homan's sign	**SPT** • Laboratory tests: complete blood count, chemistry, coagulation profile, cultures • Chest X-ray film, computerized tomography scan • Readmission • Anticoagulation therapy with heparin • Antibiotics • Supportive care • Rest • Hydration • Analgesia • Evaluation of respiratory status every 2–4 h • Breath sounds • Rales (from pulmonary edema) • Monitoring of coagulation profile • Prothrombin time, partial thromboplastin time
Urinary tract infection (UTI) • Infection of bladder or ureters • Causative organisms: —*E. coli* —*Other gram-negative aerobic bacilli* —*Other enterococci*	• Most common extrapelvic infection • Risk factors: —Bladder hypotonia —Urinary stasis —Intermittent catheterization —Epidural anesthesia • High number of pelvic examinations • Genital tract injury • History of UTI • Bacteriuria • Operative delivery • Anatomic disorders • Impaired bladder function; bacteria ascends from perineal or vaginal site into urethra	• Manifestations of lower UTI: —Dysuria —Frequency —Urgency —Low-grade fever —Bladder overdistention • Suprapubic pain • Urinary retention • Hematuria • Pyuria • Manifestations of upper UTI: —Flank pain —Costovertebral tenderness —Urinalysis —Leukocytes —Nitrites —Bacteria >100,000/mL in a CCUA	• Monitor for client complaints of infrequent or insufficient urination, discomfort, burning, foul-smelling urine • 10 day antibiotic therapy • Ampicillin • Cephalosporin • Analgesia • Hydration • Outpatient treatment (except for pyelonephritis) • Client teaching • Monitor temperature, pulse, bladder function, urine appearance • Self-care measures • Report complications • Preventive measures • Avoid carbonated drinks (increased alkalinity) • Drink acidic fluids (cranberry, plum, apricot, prune juices) • Wipe from "front to back" • Increase fluid intake • Urinate frequently

(continues)

Table 17-4 (*Continued*)

INFECTION	CHARACTERISTICS	CLINICAL FINDINGS	MANAGEMENT AND TEACHING
Wound site infections • Encompasses infections of cesarean section, episiotomy, lacerations, and so on • Causative organisms: —*E. coli* —*Mixed group A streptococcus* —*Clostridium perfringens*	• Usually develops after hospital discharge • Risk factors: —Obesity —Diabetes —Prolonged labor —Prolonged ROM —Frequent vaginal examinations —Chorioamnionitis —Immunodeficiency —Hematoma formation	• White line along the episiotomy • Edema • Skin discoloration • Erythema • Warmth • Tenderness • Seropurulent drainage • Wound edge separation • Fever • Pain • Lochia odor • Lochia color change	• Readmission • Debride wound; excise all necrotic tissue • Open and drain abdominal wound; pack as required • Antibiotics such as cephalosporins, penicillin-resistant drugs, and vancomycin (Vancocin) • Comfort measures such as frequent perineal care, sitz baths, and warm compresses • Client teaching • Frequent pad changes • Good handwashing technique • Wipe "front to back" (avoid cross-contamination) • Modify activities • No isolation precautions from infant • Self-care • Adequate diet and fluids

heat lamps and tubs) should be thoroughly cleaned and disinfected. Staff members with signs of infection (i.e., respiratory infection) should refrain from providing direct client care.

Endometritis

Endometritis is an infection of the uterine lining occurring from pathogens that ascend from the lower genital tract (Bowes, 1996). Endometritis occurs in 2% of vaginal deliveries and 10% to 15% of cesarean deliveries. When endometritis presents after 1 to 2 days after delivery, the causative agent usually is group A streptococcus. Infections that occur after 3 or 4 days usually are caused by anaerobic organisms, such as *Escherichia coli* (Bowes, 1996).

The client with endometritis may complain of symptoms of lower abdominal pain, chills, anorexia, malaise, and a malodorous vaginal discharge. The nurse should assess for fever, abdominal tenderness, and mucopurulent vaginal discharge. Laboratory studies will include a CBC, urine culture, and blood cultures.

Prompt IV antibiotic therapy is used to treat suspected endometritis. Treatment is continued until all symptoms have been resolved for 48 hours, including fever. A combination of clindamycin and gentamicin usually is ordered, which will provide coverage for aerobic and anaerobic organisms (Bowes, 1996). Single antibiotic therapy may be prescribed with either a cepholasporin or extended spectrum penicillin (Bowes, 1996).

Mastitis

An infection of the breast, mastitis, usually involves the ducts and lactiferous glands of the breast. Mastitis usually is endemic in nature, resulting from *Staphylococcus aureas*, which comes from the infant's mouth (Clark, 1995). The most common reason for mastitis is improper latching-on. If the baby does not latch on correctly, some sores and openings develop in the areola, which allow bacteria to enter the breast tissue. It is not harmful to the infant. Other causes of mastitis include missed or shortened feedings, and consistent pressure placed on the breast (Lawrence, 1999). Incomplete emptying of the breast will result in the breasts being overly full and, subsequently, development of plugged milk ducts. The nurse should teach the client steps to prevent mastitis.

Mastitis can occur as early as 7 to 10 days postpartum, though the client most often will present with complaints of swollen tender breasts around 5 or 6 weeks postpartum (Bowes, 1996). The breast (normally unilateral) will feel very warm, with areas that may appear reddened with hardened nodules. The client may report a sudden onset of flulike symptoms, including aching joints, malaise, nausea, vomiting, severe headache, chills, and fever (Overfield & Tully, 1997). Mastitis resulting from an endemic nature may be characterized by a demarcated V-shaped area of redness and inflammation (Clark, 1995).

The nurse should instruct the client with mastitis to continue breastfeeding. If she prefers, the client may

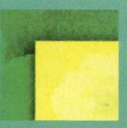

CASE STUDY/CARE PLAN
THE CLIENT WITH POSTPARTUM BLEEDING AND PAIN

Cristina, grava 4, para 4, is a married, 32-year-old Hispanic woman who gave birth to a healthy, term baby boy at 8:48 a.m. by forceps delivery. Her membranes ruptured 6 hours before the start of active labor. She had an episiotomy with a second-degree laceration. The estimated blood loss was 450 mL. Apgar scores were 8 and 9 at 1 and 5 minutes after birth. No resuscitation was required. The infant weighed 9 lb, 10 oz., and was 21 in long. During the intrapartum course, Cristina received only IV analgesia for pain relief. She was catheterized once when she was unable to urinate. She quickly progressed through labor, totaling only 5 hours and 22 minutes for the entire labor. Her perineum was moderately swollen.

During fundal massage the first hour after childbirth, the nurse noted the peripad was saturated with a large amount of lochia rubra. The fundus was boggy, firmed up on massage, but became soft again once massage was discontinued. The location of the fundus was U+2 deviated to the right side. Cristina had not voided for the past 4 hours. The client was awake, alert, and mildly tired after labor. Vital signs were as follows: blood pressure 105/72 mmHg, pulse 94 bpm, respirations 20 bpm, and temperature 99.2°F. An IV of lactated Ringer's solution with 20 U of oxytocin is infusing at 125 mL/h. Bowel sounds are present and active. She complains of moderate cramping. She plans to breastfeed. Her husband is at her bedside holding their new baby.

Assessment

Cristina presents with two major nursing problems related to bleeding and pain. First, she delivered a large infant by forceps delivery, making her at risk for bleeding. The bleeding may be caused by atony secondary to uterine distention and lacerations from the use of forceps. Having a full bladder and delivering rapidly also are risk factors for bleeding. Second, the client is a multipara who previously has experienced very uncomfortable afterpains. Her discomfort is increased with her episiotomy and, most likely, the full bladder.

Nursing Diagnosis

Deficient fluid volume related to postpartum hemorrhage secondary to uterine atony.

Expected Outcomes	● Maintain a firm fundus within normal assessment parameters.
	● Saturate no more than one pad an hour during the recovery period.
	● Maintain normal fluid balance as evidenced by vital signs and hematocrit within normal limits.
Planning	Closely observe normal fluid volume balance within the first 24 to 28 hours following delivery.
NOC	Fluid balance
NIC	Fluid monitoring

Nursing Interventions	Rationales
1. Monitor fundal height, position, and tone per the protocol. Massage as appropriate.	1. Ensures the uterus remains firmly contracted.
2. Monitor amount, color, and type of lochia as per the protocol. Note the amount of blood saturated on the peripad and on the pad under the buttocks and bed sheets. Weigh peripads as necessary.	2. Obtains an accurate estimate of blood loss.
3. Observe for vital sign changes and report acute or critical values to the primary care provider.	3. Ensures prompt identification and treatment of complications.
4. Ensure adequate IV access. Administer IV fluids with oxytocin as ordered.	4. Maintains uterine tone and involution after delivery.

(continues)

Nursing Interventions	Rationales
5. Interventions beyond nursing may be necessary.	5. Administer other medications as needed if bleeding continues. If bleeding continues despite above actions, notify provider for further evaluation.
6. Obtain hemoglobin and hematocrit levels as ordered. Ensure or prepare for administration of blood or blood products. Obtain blood for typing and cross-matching.	6. To prepare for transfusion if needed.

Evaluation   Cristina's bleeding may decrease to a small amount of lochia rubra 12 hours after delivery; however, the nurse must continue to assess for bleeding until discharge. Ongoing evaluation may demonstrate that although the fundus remains firm, the continuation of moderate vaginal bleeding and changing vital signs may indicate bleeding coming from an overt site, such as an overlooked vaginal or cervical laceration.

Nursing Diagnosis

Urinary retention related to trauma to tissues secondary to childbirth and perineal discomfort.

Expected Outcome   Resume normal bladder function as evidenced by minimal urinary output of greater than 150 mL per voiding and absence of urinary distention.

Planning   Work with client to set time-bound goals for voiding.

NOC   Urinary elimination

NIC   Urinary elimination management

Nursing Interventions	Rationales
1. Assess the time and amount of last voiding.	1. Provides baseline data.
2. Palpate symphysis pubis and evaluate location of fundus in relation to the umbilicus the first 8 hours after delivery.	2. Notes bladder distention.
3. Assist client to ambulate to bathroom if able, providing privacy as needed. Palpate bladder after voiding.	3. To ensure adequate emptying.
4. Offer various methods to encourage urination. Use ice packs to decrease perineal discomfort.	4. Instructing in various bladder management techniques increases likelihood of client finding successful method.
5. If unable to void, perform straight catheterization as ordered.	5. To avoid urinary stasis and retention.
6. Encourage minimum fluid intake of 2,000 mL/d.	6. Maintains hydration.

Evaluation   If Cristina continues to experience urinary retention, she may be discharged with an indwelling catheter or be taught self-catheterization. Cristina's input and output are within targeted parameters within 6 hours.

Nursing Diagnosis

Acute pain related to uterine cramping (normal uterine involution), perineal pain, and breast tenderness.

Expected Outcomes
- Experience pain relief or moderate control of pain.
- Verbalize methods of satisfactory pain relief.
- Obtain restful pain-free periods and the ability to return to normal activities of daily living and self-care.

Planning   Plan care procedures to minimize disruptions in client rest; ask client about her preferred methods of pain management (therapy, guided imagery, medications, and so forth).

NOC   Pain level

NIC   Pain management

(continues)

Nursing Interventions	**Rationales**
1. Assess location, intensity, and duration of pain. Determine pain intensity by asking the client to describe her pain on a scale from 1 to 10, with 10 being the strongest intensity of pain.	1. Clarifies client's interpretation of the pain experience.
2. Administer the appropriate prescribed analgesia to the client. A combination of different prescribed medication also may be effective in controlling pain if the client is very uncomfortable (e.g., nursing frequently).	2. Regularly administered medications may control the pain more effectively.
3. Support client's use of nonpharmaceutical pain control, such as patterned breathing, touch therapies, and visualization.	3. These may provide effective pain relief, avoiding rests associated with medications.
4. Provide ice packs to the perineum for the first 24 hours after delivery, then warm therapy with sitz baths afterward.	4. Reduces inflammation and promotes healing.
5. Provide ordered anesthetic sprays or creams as desired.	5. Reduces discomfort.
6. Instruct the client to position herself differently while sitting or lying in bed.	6. Position changes may alter pain levels.
7. Ensure proper positioning and latch-on when breastfeeding. Instruct client to massage colostrum into nipples to soothe them.	7. Proper positioning and breast care will alleviate discomfort.
8. Encourage rest and relaxation strategies.	8. These will help reduce pain and tension and facilitate let-down response.

Evaluation   Cristina continued to experience uterine cramping 6 hours after delivery; it intensified significantly when she breastfed her son. Lying on her side to nurse seemed to dull the intensity of the afterpains.

continue to express milk either though pumping or manual expression to ensure complete emptying of the affected breast. The client will require increased fluids and ample time to rest. The nurse should instruct the client to place warm compresses on the affected area and take NSAIDs to relieve pain and fever. The mother should avoid supplementing with infant formula, nipple shields, and pacifiers (Clark, 1995). Nursing pads should be changed when they become wet. Antibiotic therapy using penicillin, ampicillin, or dicloxacillin (Bowes, 1996) often is prescribed to complete the treatment. When mastitis recurs, the infant's throat may be cultured to determine if the baby is reinfecting the mother. Reassure the mother that although the course of mastitis may be very painful and frustrating for her and her baby, the infection will eventually resolve within a few days of antibiotic treatment.

Client Education

Preventing Mastitis

You should instruct the breastfeeding mother to avoid missing or shortening feeding times. She should be mindful of the times her baby begins to suddenly sleep longer at night, begins an irregular nursing pattern (nursing a lot one day and less the next), she begins to supplement feedings with formula, or she begins to give the baby a pacifier frequently.

The client should be instructed to avoid putting pressure on the breasts. She should try not to sleep on her stomach or hold her baby too tight against her chest while feeding. She should be told that shoulder straps from purses and diaper bags may place pressure on her breast. The client should make sure her bra fits correctly. Underwire bras may cause a problem. Thick breast pads or breast shells also may make her bra too tight.

Instruct the client to pay attention to proper positioning and how her baby is latching on. She can massage the hardened area to try to open plugged milk ducts. Finally, she should be sure to take care of herself by getting enough rest. Mastitis often is the first sign a new mother is doing too much and not taking care of herself. She should try cutting back on activities and start relying on family members and friends to help.

POSTPARTUM PSYCHOLOGIC DISORDERS

The postpartum adjustment involves psychologic and social adaptations as well as physiologic changes. There are several psychiatric problems that may arise in the postpartal period. Although psychiatric diagnoses specific to postpartum are still controversial, mood disorder classifications with a postpartum-onset have been identified in the *Diagnostic and Statistical Manual of Mental Disorders, 4th Edition, (DSM-IV)* (American Psychological Association, 2000). The *DSM-IV* lists three subclasses under mood disorders with a postpartum onset: (1) adjustment reaction with depressed mood; (2) postpartum major mood disorder; and (3) postpartum psychosis. Beck (2001) has researched postpartum psychiatric disorders and has been instrumental in the position statement by AWHONN.

Postpartum Blues

Adjustment reaction with depressed mood, often called postpartum blues, is a common reaction of postpartum women, occurring in 50% to 80% of new mothers (Ugarriza & Robinson, 1997). This is generally transient and resolves without treatment. Blues typically occur in the early postpartum period, often within 3 to 10 days after delivery. The symptoms include feeling overwhelmed, tearful, fatigued, irritable, oversensitive, anxious, and having poor concentration or poor appetite. Episodic tearfulness, often with no discernible reason, is characteristic of blues. Etiology is thought to be a combination of physiologic changes, especially the changes in hormonal levels after birth, and adjustment to motherhood. If the blues last longer than 2 weeks or the woman exhibits other signs of a more serious depression, she should seek medical attention.

Blues appear to be more severe in primiparas. It is helpful to prepare new mothers prior to discharge for the possibility of blues, and to provide information for family members so they can offer assistance with infant care during episodes. If the symptoms do not quickly resolve or if there are signs of a more serious psychiatric disorder, it is important for family members to assist the woman in receiving the help she needs to protect herself and her baby.

Postpartum Depression

Postpartum major mood disorder depression, or postpartum depression (PPD), affects from 10% to 16% of postpartal women (Ugarriza & Robinson, 1997; Beck, 2002). The actual number may be larger because not all women are diagnosed. The onset is slow and generally later than the blues, often around the fourth week postpartum and

may occur anytime within the first year. Symptoms begin with a depressed mood or loss of interest or pleasure, and are followed by weight loss or gain, psychomotor agitation or retardation, fatigue and loss of energy, feelings of worthlessness, impaired concentration, and intrusive thoughts of death or suicide. For a diagnosis to be made, at least four of the symptoms should be present most of the day, every day for at least 2 weeks (American Psychological Association, 2000). Generally, women with postpartum depression have no ideation of hurting their infants, though their infants may suffer from failure to thrive resulting from neglect.

Risk factors include personal or family history of depression or mood disorder, lack of support system or stable relationship with partner or parents, no or poor relationship with partner, history of abuse, low self-esteem, and marked ambivalence regarding the pregnancy. Additional factors associated with postpartum depression are history of infertility, early menarche (before age 11), unrealistic expectations of mothering, and adverse reactions to oral contraceptives. Women with any of these risk factors should be monitored for signs of depression. Because the majority of women who develop postpartum depression have no identified risk factors, all women should be screened for signs and symptoms of depression. Education regarding depression or the "blues" should ideally occur as part of prenatal education. Mothers will often hide symptoms of depression because they feel a sense of guilt. It is important for the nurse to provide reassurance that PPD is a medical condition and that treatment is available. Education should include both the new mother and family members. They should have information on community resources and be

---

Nursing Alert

AWHONN Position Paper on Postpartum Depression

AWHONN (1999) has developed a position statement regarding the "Role of the Nurse in Postpartum Depression." The nurse and other health providers working with pregnant women, new mothers, and newborns should integrate the following protocols related to postpartum depression into standard practices:

- Routine screening protocols for clients exhibiting symptoms of mood disorders.
- Routine educational mechanisms for staff and clients.

encouraged to contact their primary care provider at the earliest signs of depression. Treatment may include psychotherapy, medications, and hospitalization.

Postpartum Psychosis

Postpartum psychosis (PPP) is the most serious psychiatric condition. It occurs in one to two women per 1,000 births (Ugarriza & Robinson, 1997). The symptoms generally appear after the second week postpartum, and include sleep and eating disturbances; agitation and confusion; difficulty remembering or concentrating; extreme mood lability; insomnia; irrationality; poor judgment, and, often, delusions or hallucinations. Risk factors include previous postpartum psychosis, history of bipolar or manic depressive disorders, and family history of severe psychiatric disorders. This condition is life threatening and, if not treated, may result in suicide or infanticide. Treatment may include hospitalization, antipsychotic medications, and psychotherapy. With appropriate treatment, the majority of mothers may recover, although there is a high risk of recurrence in subsequent pregnancies. The onset of postpartum psychosis in a woman represents a true emergency because there is a real possibility of harm to her infant. Her thought process will be disordered and chaotic. She is likely to hallucinate and become delusional. Delusions are often about God and the devil. She may be convinced that the only way to save her baby from "the fires of hell" is to kill her baby. This illness is a very frightening condition and needs immediate treatment.

NURSING IMPLICATIONS AND PREPARATION FOR DISCHARGE

Other psychiatric disorders with a postpartum onset include postpartum panic disorder and postpartum obsessive-compulsive disorder. The symptoms are similar to the basic psychiatric disorders; however, much of the ideation is focused on the mother's relationship with her infant. Most of the symptoms occur after discharge; therefore, this material should be included as part of discharge planning. Most women will see their obstetrician for only one or more follow-up appointments in the first 2 months postpartum, and then for their annual checkup within the year. Should depressive symptoms develop, it is important for the woman and her family to realize that treatment is indicated.

CLIENT EDUCATION

Nurses must monitor closely all postpartum women for signs of hemorrhage and infection and PPP. Preventive measures and early intervention need to be a top priority

in nursing care of the postpartal family. Before being discharged the new mother must learn how to care for herself and her infant (Figure 17-2). Self-care topics include those activities that help her to manage, anticipate, and recognize health problems or danger signs. Infant care encompasses activities such as feeding, dressing, and recognition of health problems.

General instructions, in addition to other client education discussed throughout this chapter, should be given to the client. The nurse should also instruct the client on warning signs of complications after delivery. Suggestions for client education on discharge are included in Box 17-1.

As part of the discharge process, the nurse may use a facility-specific checklist to ensure all care has been provided (e.g., birth certificate completed, laboratory testing obtained, and teaching handouts and pertinent information received). The nurse should ensure the client is instructed on any discharge medications ordered and where to obtain them. Some women may continue to take their prenatal vitamins and iron until the postpartum checkup, especially if their hematocrit is low. If the woman experienced a third- or fourth-degree laceration, she may be

> ### Nursing Tip | Sleep Disturbances and Postpartum Depression
>
> One of the key symptoms associated with postpartum depression is sleep disturbances. Most new mothers are able to fall asleep easily and may be able to catch up on their sleep by napping. When mothers cannot fall asleep easily, they should be screened for other signs of depression. If any signs are present, these women should be referred for further evaluation.

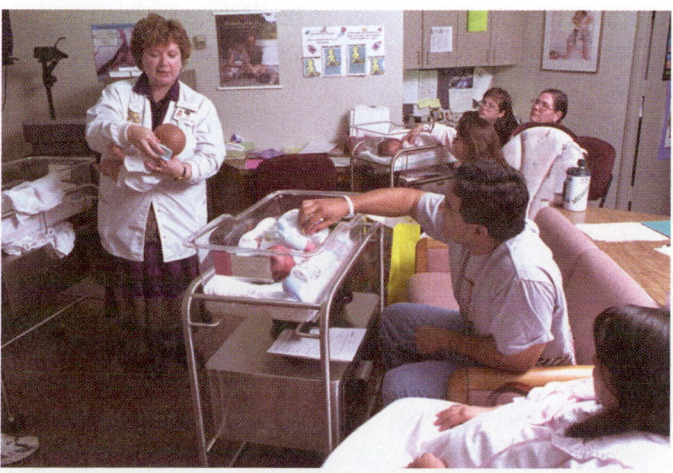

Figure 17-2 Infant care, self-care, and family adaptation are topics typically covered in postpartum education classes.

Client Education

Warning Signs of Illness after Delivery

You should inform the client to call her provider if she experiences any of the warning signs of sickness after she is discharged from the hospital:

- Fever greater than 100.4°F
- Severe pain, redness, or swelling in the episiotomy or cesarean section incision
- Foul-smelling vaginal discharge
- Increased bleeding; soaking of a peripad more than once an hour or a large amount of bright-red lochia after discharge has turned dark red or pink
- Passing of several large clots greater than the size of a half dollar coin
- Backache or severe abdominal pain or cramping (unrelieved by medication), or pain in the episiotomy or perineal area
- Reddened, tender, swollen breasts that may have hardened lumps (may be related to flulike symptoms)
- Pain, redness, and swelling of the legs
- Burning on urination, or frequent urination
- The blues or crying that lasts for several days
- Depression that is severe or does not go away
- Thoughts of harming the baby
- Suicidal thoughts
- Insomnia
- Loss of energy
- Impaired concentration
- Feelings of worthlessness

Box 17-1

Predictors of Postpartum Depression

Beck (2001, 2002) conducted a meta-analysis of studies on postpartum depression and identified the following characteristics as predictors of postpartum depression:

- Prenatal depression
- Childcare stress
- Prenatal anxiety
- Life stress
- Lack of social support
- Marital dissatisfaction
- History of previous depression
- Low compatibility with infant temperment
- Maternity blues
- Low self-esteem
- Marital status (single)
- Socioeconomic status (low)
- Unplanned/unwanted pregnancy

Reflections from a Mother

My baby was 2 weeks old and I had just returned from the store. I was putting away groceries, trying to get the food in the freezer before it melted. The baby was crying and needed to be fed. My 3-year-old just spilled her milk all over the floor, the phone was ringing, then the doorbell rang. I started to cry and thought I had lost it. I just sat down and sobbed. My husband came home and reminded me that this was normal blues and helped fix dinner and take care of the children.

Reflections from a Father

About a week after my wife came home with our second child, I was going to take my mother, who was visiting, out to play bingo at the local church. My wife was sitting on the couch folding laundry and our 2-year-old was playing nearby. The baby cried and she started breastfeeding. All of a sudden she burst into tears, saying everyone was abandoning her and she would never be able to deal with 2 babies. I was stunned. She was very capable, had just made us a great meal, done laundry, taken care of two children and a neighbor's child for the afternoon. I couldn't imagine what had come over her. When I got back about 20 minutes later, she was fine, and then I remembered what they had told me in our prepared childbirth class about postpartum blues .

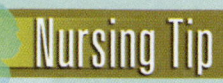

Nursing Tip

Assessment of Light Bleeding Weeks after Delivery

At the 6-week postpartum checkup the provider will perform a Pap smear, which may cause light bleeding.

Some women may experience light bleeding for up to 3 months postpartum, which is considered normal when the following criteria are present:

- The uterus has returned to its normal size.
- No fever is present.
- Clots or tissue are not being passed.
- The client is not feeling exceptionally fatigued.
- No foul odor is associated with the bleeding.

Postpartum bleeding also can be caused by exercise, sexual intercourse, and breastfeeding. Certain oral contraceptives and Depo-Provera (medroxyprogesterone) cause postpartum spotting. The bleeding also can be the start of the first menstrual period.

prescribed a stool softener. The provider may order over-the-counter or prescription pain medication for home use.

Before discharge the new mother should leave the hospital with a follow-up clinic appointment already in hand or with clear instructions on how to obtain one. A postpartum follow-up examination usually is scheduled for 6 weeks after delivery. The examination may be scheduled for as early as 2 or 4 weeks if the client has experienced complications.

LOSSES IN THE POSTPARTUM

Perinatal nursing is an exciting and busy specialty that encompasses the best in working with clients as they begin their families. By definition, the perinatal period is the interval from about 28 weeks' gestation to about 28 days after birth (Anderson, 1998). Perinatal nurses work with clients in low- and high-risk obstretrical units, at infertility clinics, and in the high-tech world of neonatal intensive care. Perinatal nurses work with clients during the physical and emotional adjustments of postpartum life.

An early miscarriage or the unexpected experience of a death during the perinatal period also is part of perinatal nursing. The way in which caregivers support the client and family can make a profound difference in their grief work and their future health. The grieving parents are experiencing the death of their infant along with the end of all their hopes and dreams for that infant.

When an unexpected death occurs, there is disappointment and loss of what could have been. A person's response to the loss results from a combination of factors:

life experience, education, culture, traditions, and beliefs. The feeling of being in crisis and the need for support can depend on the type of loss experienced and on the background and beliefs of the person.

Grief and Neonatal Death

Grief is an intense and personal experience in response to a loss. Grief, as a response of sadness to a death, has common characteristics, although the process is very individual. A person's response to a death or loss depends on culture, traditions, reaction to past losses, circumstances surrounding the death, and the perceived available support networks.

Pathologic grief is a distortion of the normal bereavement process. **Grief work** has three components: accepting the painful emotions involved, actively reviewing the experiences and events, and testing new patterns of interaction and role relationships. The behaviors found in normal grief work are listed in Box 17-2. Lindemann's classic work was translated by Davidson (1984) to describe the response of the survivors-parents experiencing a perinatal death (Table 17-5). The four stages identified by Davidson are shock and numbness, searching and yearning, disorientation, and reorganization. Shock and numbness can occur when a prenatal or postnatal diagnosis of a fatal disease or anomaly is made. Grieving parents report walking around "as if in a daze."

Box 17-2

Symptomatology of Normal Grief

- Acute grief: sensations of somatic distress occurring in waves and lasting 20 to 60 minutes
- Feeling of tightness in the throat
- Choking, with shortness of breath
- Need for sighing (recovering the oxygen level in the body)
- Empty feeling in the abdomen
- Lack of muscular power
- Intense subjective distress described as tension
- Frequent crying
- Slight sense of unreality
- Preoccupation with the image of the deceased
- Preoccupation with guilt ("If only . . .")
- Irritability and anger
- Restlessness
- Lack of energy

Note. From "Symptomatology and Management of Acute Grief," by E. Lindemann, 1944, *American Journal of Psychiatry*, 101, pp. 141–148.

Table 17-5 Normal Characteristics of Stages of Grief

STAGE OF GRIEF	CHARACTERISTICS
Shock and numbness (age: 24 h–3 wk)	• Resistance to stimuli and denial • Difficulty in making judgments • Impeded functioning • Emotional outbursts • Stunned feelings • Extreme sensitivity to stimuli
Searching and yearning (3 wk–4 mo, with occasional recurrences)	• Anger and guilt • Restlessness and impatience • Ambiguity • Testing of reality
Disorientation (intensity lifts by 7 mo)	• Disorganization • Depression and lowered self-esteem • Guilt • Anorexia • Awareness of reality and increasing acceptance of death
Reorganization (age: 18–24 mo)	• Sense of release • Renewed energy and the ability to plan for the future • Better judgment • Stable eating and sleeping patterns • Stabilization of old relationships and formation of new ones

Note. From *Understanding Mourning*, by G. W. Davidson, 1984, Minneapolis, MN: Augsburg.

Reflections from a Client

I felt as if a weight had been lifted. I didn't miss her any less, it just was different. I didn't think of her with sadness every moment of the day. Now when I think of her, it may be about what we might have been doing if she were here. She's always in my heart. I'll always carry her with me.

As the shock and numbness stage comes to an end, around 3 weeks to 3 months, searching and yearning begin. Davidson describes the searching and yearning phase as being characterized by restlessness, anger, guilt, and ambiguity. The need to have questions answered and to gather mementos takes on renewed energy. It is an ideal time for parents to consider joining a group for support, to hear about the experiences of others, and to see how other parents are coping.

According to Davidson, just as the searching comes to an end, a sense of disorientation is felt. Disorientation usually occurs 5 to 6 months after the death and peaks just before the first anniversary. Clients may feel disorganized and depressed and may speak of feelings of guilt. This reaction is common; it is at this point that they are aware of the reality of the death and emptiness this loss has brought and no longer are testing what is true. As the first 18 months pass, there is a sense of release and a pattern of stable eating and sleeping habits. This begins to occur because clients have survived the cycle of firsts and now have life experience without their "wished for" child (Davidson, 1979). At the end of the second year, the client and family begin to understand what has happened and reconcile this into their lives. By no means are they over the death. They have only just begun to understand the impact of and will forever be changed by these events.

Reproductive Loss

Reproductive loss can include the inability to conceive, spontaneous miscarriage and ectopic pregnancy, preterm delivery, birth of an infant with a congenital anomaly (physical or neurological), death of one or more of a multiple gestation, intrauterine fetal demise, neonatal death, relinquishment (voluntary and involuntary), and sudden infant death syndrome (SIDS). Nurses, in various roles, are able to assist the survivors as they work through their grief and incorporate the meaning of the loss into their lives.

Spontaneous abortion is the most commonly occurring reproductive loss and occurs in one out of two pregnancies. Post miscarriage distress is identified by perceived physical and emotional trauma at delivery and emotional distress related to poor follow-up (Lee & Slade, 1996). Persistent miscarriage and infertility are also triggers for the grieving process. Written resources and telephone numbers should be part of the discharge information. Many women would benefit from a referral to a counselor.

Perinatal death triggers many obvious signs of the grieving process. Feelings of guilt and anger are the more common manifestations in families who are grieving. Davidson, in combination with Sr. Jane Marie Lamb, created the basis for the first international perinatal grief support program called SHARE Pregnancy and Infant Loss Support, Inc. This program has been a model for professionals and a critical link for families since the late 1970s.

Delivery of an infant with a congenital anomaly or an infant who is relinquished are considered incomplete losses and may lead to a chronic grief state. Expectations and dreams of the infant are never fulfilled. Opportunities to discuss these unfulfilled dreams are an important part of the grieving process for the family.

RESOLVE is the National Infertility Association with chapters nationwide. They provide advocacy, support,

Reflections from a Client

Why me? All my friends are sexually active. Why was I the one to get pregnant? It's so unfair to me and my baby. I couldn't even look at a couple with a new baby without getting angry. I knew adoption was the right thing to do for my baby, but deep down I still did not want to give him up.

and education for women and men with infertility concerns. Support groups are established in many cities. They have a helpline at 888-623-0744 and their email address is info@RESOLVE.org.

Loss of the Perfect Baby

Once the pregnancy test result is positive, a woman begins to plan. She knows the possible due date and begins to fantasize about her child's future. This trajectory of hopes and dreams that may extend into the child's adult years can be halted abruptly by the birth of an infant who does not meet parents' expectations or by the death of the infant. Parents will grieve the loss of their expectations: a full-term healthy boy or girl with certain features. They also must grieve the loss of the idealized infant before they will be able to adapt and attach to the real child. Parents of premature infants and infants who have anomalies or deformities will ask themselves how a thing such as this could have happened. As the parents attempt to attach, they also have concerns that the child may not survive. The roller coaster of emotions may be overwhelming. Nurses can be most helpful by listening to parents without making judgments. The degree of their grief reaction may not be equal to the level of severity or critical state of the child. It is the personal meaning of the anomaly or the reaction to the shock of not having the child they imagined that will give form to the grief.

It is frightening to see one's infant for the first time attached to equipment and wires. Most staff of neonatal intensive care units (NICUs) have a good working knowledge of what it takes to orient parents to the unit and the importance of getting them involved as early as possible as parents (Figure 17-3). Supporting the new mother to provide breast milk for her infant from the beginning—even though it may be weeks before it can be used—helps foster the parental role. Care of the infant by parents continues to show results in the infant through improved weight gain and response to therapy (Figure 17-4). If the infant were to die in the NICU, the interdisciplinary care team would continue to work with the parents to assist them in making the transition from having the hope of taking their infant home to having the needs involved in the death of a child. The death of an infant will have a lifelong effect on the family. The care provided to them in the hospital and the follow-up care during the first 18 months after the death will shape their future.

Sudden Infant Death

If the child is healthy at birth or is premature and survives the neonatal period, graduating from the NICU, the

Critical Thinking

Fetal Demise

How do you feel about entering the room of a client whose infant is dying? Will your need to "make it better" cause you to use clichés or try to find a reason for parents? Will you choose to limit your contact with the client because of your discomfort? Or, can you sit down and listen to the family's story?

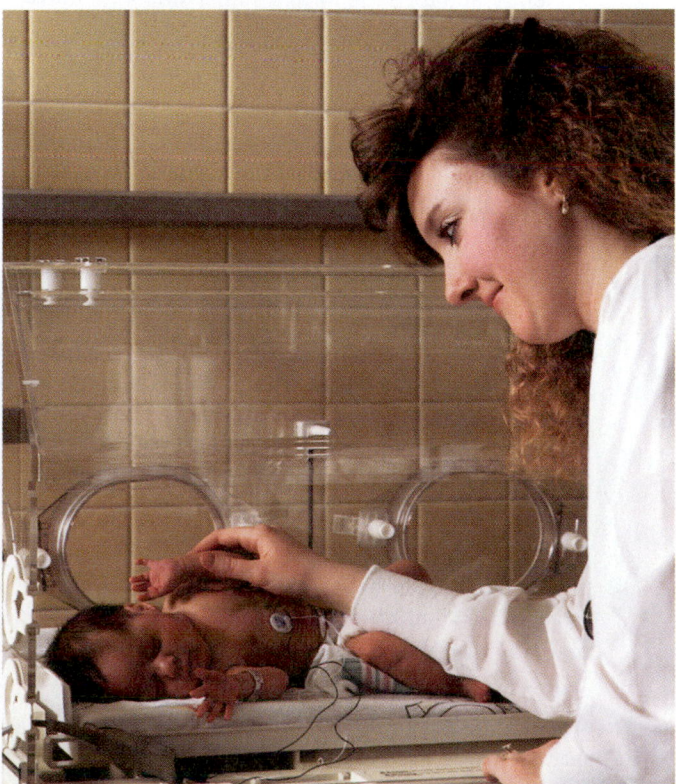

Figure 17-3   Nurses should help parents of high-risk infants to find ways to bond with and comfort their newborns.

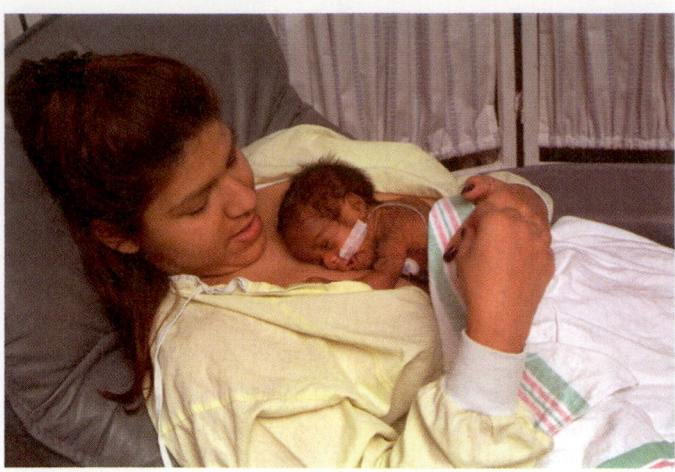

Figure 17-4   Kangaroo care (skin-to-skin contact) promotes bonding and attachment, which is especially important for the premature infant.

family will be given instructions on what to do to decrease the risk of SIDS. **Sudden infant death syndrome**, or **SIDS**, refers to any death of an infant that is unexpected and in which a thorough postmortem examination, medical history, and case study demonstrate adequate care before death (www:sidsalliance.org). Infants are most at risk for SIDS during the first 6 months of life. SIDS usually occurs during sleep, with no evidence of disease.

Relinquishment

Relinquishment refers to a mother's decision to give up her right to parent her child. Doing so may cause silent grieving that needs recognition. By carrying an infant to term, the feelings of attachment and detachment are simultaneous. A woman who goes through the birth process and

---

Nursing Tip   *Key Actions for Working with Mothers Who are Relinquishing Their Babies*

1. Prepare the birth parents for hospitalization and delivery. Explain their rights, discuss their options for contact with the child, and ensure that decisions and information are provided in written form. Include information on the grief process early in all discussions.

2. Validate the importance of the birth parents' roles. Recognize the birth mother's contribution to the child's life through caring for herself during the pregnancy and the work of delivery. Naming the infant is another way to validate the experience and give the birth parents someone for whom to grieve.

3. Encourage the birth parents to see, hold, and spend time in private with the baby. According to Roles (1997), one of the main regrets of parents who give up the right to parent their child is the decision not to see the infant.

4. Reconfirm the commitment to the adoption decision. Doubts that arise must be discussed immediately with the social worker or counselor before consent forms are signed. Parents need to understand the adoption law that rules the waiting period, that they have the opportunity to change their minds, and the irrevocability of the consent once the form is signed.

5. Assist the birth parents in creating memories. Just as it is recommended that mementos be created for parents grieving the death of an infant, the same rationale applies here.

6. Acknowledge the birth mother's role. Give ample opportunity during the postpartum period for the birth mother to discuss the pregnancy, labor, and birth, especially because the opportunity may be limited once she returns home.

7. Treat birth mothers with respect. When mothers are able to care for their infants for a short time after the birth, they may have less guilt in the future. When they choose this option, birth mothers will need the support, reassurance, and teaching provided to all new mothers.

8. Validate the significance of the loss. Be aware of the normal grief response and provide education about it to birth mothers. Offer resources that can be used immediately after discharge.

9. Be creative in ways the birth parents might say good-bye. There are booklets, such as "Service in Giving a Child in Love," and "Given in Love," by Maureen Connelly from the Centering Corporation, that offer suggestions. Beginning to write in a journal or writing a letter to the adoptive parents and one to the child explaining why this choice was made and including the birth parents' medical histories can be helpful for all involved.

10. Encourage open dialogue and support. Refer the parents for family counseling.

11. Act as a neutral advocate. Facilitate information about issues, such as legal rights and rights to information, while birth mothers are in the hospital.

Note. Adapted from "Birth Parents' Grief: Relinquishing a Baby for Adoption" by P. Roles, 1997, In *Loss during Pregnancy or in the Newborn Period: Principles of Care with Clinical Cases and Analysis*, by J. R. Wood and J. L. Esposito (Eds.). Pitman, NJ: Jannetti.

Nursing Alert

Postpartum Risk

When you hear something that sounds like a flat affect or hopelessness during a follow-up phone call following a perinatal loss, you need to document and act on the observation. You can say, "I am concerned, and I would like you to talk with someone. Are you willing?" If the concern is severe, do not hang up. Instead, ask to speak with a family member and suggest bringing the client to the emergency room. Contact social services or a nursing psychiatric liaison to support your efforts.

Box 17-3

Behaviors in Pathologic Grief

- Overactivity without a sense of loss, or activities that bear a resemblance to those of the deceased
- Symptoms belonging to those of the deceased
- Initial episodes or exacerbations of diseases known to be associated with stress or psychosomatic conditions, such as ulcerative colitis, rheumatoid arthritis, and asthma
- Alterations in relationships with friends and relatives owing to feelings of irritability and a marked desire to be left alone, which leads to progressive social isolation
- Furious hostility against a specific person, particularly professionals, such as physicians and nurses
- Affectivity and conduct resembling schizophrenic behavior often as a result of attempting to hide hostility
- Lasting loss of social interaction patterns that also can include lack of decision making and lack of initiative to participate in social activities without the intervention of a friend
- Activities detrimental to personal economic and social existence, including spending large sums of money or engaging in activities, such as excessive drinking, leading to job loss
- Agitated depression, including tension, agitation, insomnia, feelings of worthlessness, bitter self-accusation, and suicidal tendencies

then relinquishes her infant will experience a grief process that is prolonged and that may intensify over time (Davis, 1994; Askren & Bloom, 1999). This incomplete loss may contribute to the chronic aspect of the grief. The nurse must recognize that the mother will experience shock as she goes through the confusing feelings of pride and joy when she gives birth and the feelings of pain and sadness in the process of letting go. Nurses must also be sensitive to mothers who are forced to relinquish their infants due to substance abuse, a history of child abuse, or incarceration, as these women may also experience feelings of loss and despair.

Because many birth mothers do not realize they will experience a grief reaction, an opportunity exists for education and preparation. Clients may experience **anticipatory grieving**, which is an emotional response based on the perception of a potential or expected loss. When clients are hospitalized and faced with reality, it is important to have someone there to listen to them and to provide resources so that follow-up and support are available after discharge.

Caring for the Grieving Family

All members of the health care team should have an understanding of normal grief (Box 17-2), as well as some idea of pathologic grief (Box 17-3). In Kavanaugh's (1997) research, behaviors that are perceived by the parents as supportive include accepting parents' feelings and behaviors, being there, and sharing the experience. Families expect they will receive competent care, accurate information, and special attention (Figure 17-5). The continuum of care in supporting a grieving family begins wherever the crisis is first identified and follows the client through the experience. Having some type of structure available during a time of feeling out of control, can be reassuring for all parties involved.

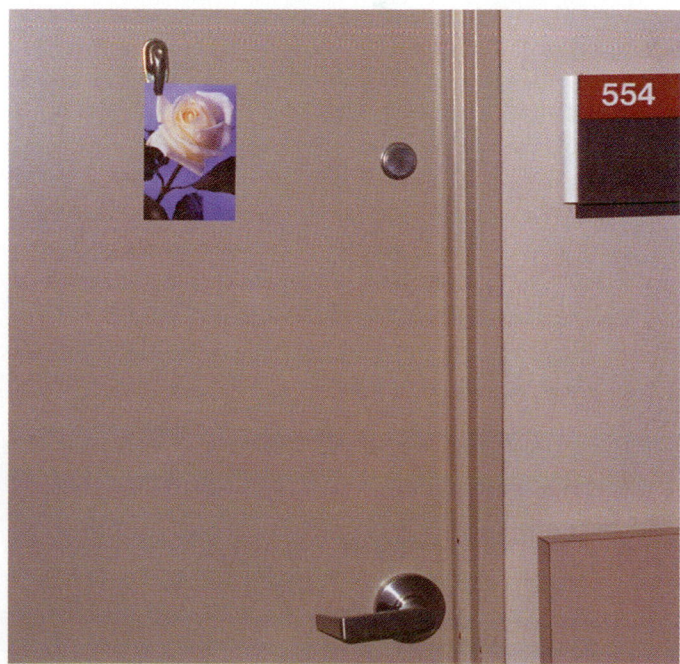

Figure 17-5 Placing a rose or card on the door of a client who has suffered a neonatal loss is a gentle reminder to staff of the need for sensitive care.

Nursing Tip · *Caring for a Bereaved Family*

Many of the behaviors that began in the initial crisis period must continue through the continuum of care. The following are tips for nursing care of a bereaved family:

- Recognize the initial confusion and shock.

- Provide ample time for taking-in the information.

- Repeat information as needed. Encourage parents to repeat or summarize what they have heard. Prepare written information.

- Prepare other health care workers and support their work with parents in a caring way whenever they need care in an area of the facility other than the obstetrics.

- Help parents with the logistics of admission to the facility.

- Acknowledge the difficulty in concentrating and understanding.

- Encourage the presence of a support person.

- Identify important cultural and spiritual practices.

- Provide opportunities for the client to tell her story.

- Recognize the unique aspects of the infant that bind the infant to the family, and treat the infant with respect.

- Identify and address fears as defined by the client.

- Be attentive during labor of a baby dead in utero, even though the baby cannot be saved.

- Provide comfort measures, such as music, massage, whirlpool baths, and family support.

- Support the client to experience the many emotions that may arise during labor.

- Refrain from comments that attempt to fix or minimize the parents' experience.

- Facilitate holding the baby as the parents desire.

- Create mementos consistent with hospital practices.

- Support sharing the experience with other family members.

- Discuss options regarding funeral or memorial services.

COLLABORATIVE CARE

Collaborative Team for Families Experiencing Neonatal Loss

In cases in which either the mother or the newborn is ill, or the parents are relinquishing the neonate or the baby dies, a number of health care providers are involved as a team to support the parents. In addition to the nurse caring for the mother, this team may include some of the following health care professionals:

- Advanced practice nurses
- Obstetricians
- Neonatologists
- Social workers
- Bereavement counselors

Multiple nurses are often involved, including several postpartum nurses and neonatal nurses. It is important that nurses find therapeutic ways to communicate and coordinate their care in supporting the family through this difficult period.

Creating Memories and Finding Meaning

In perinatal loss, couples need ways to create memories. In harmony with their beliefs, a blessing, baptism, or naming ceremony can be created to recognize the infant-individual for whom they are grieving. If the ceremony is to be performed before the baby is born (or surgical procedure is begun), it can be done on the mother's abdomen. Prayers, chants, and readings can be done by the family in the informal setting of the client's room, chapel, or later in their place of worship. Resources to assist in planning a farewell service are available, such as *Bittersweet, Hello . . . Goodbye*, edited by Sr. Jane Marie Lamb (1988). These types of rituals are important to families who want to celebrate a life and keep the memory of these moments in their hearts forever (Figure 17-6).

Staff Education and Support

Few nursing care situations produce more anxiety than being left alone with a grieving client or family. The first few times a nurse cares for such a client, an experienced nurse or the bereavement resource person should be present. The nurse needs to feel supported to sort through

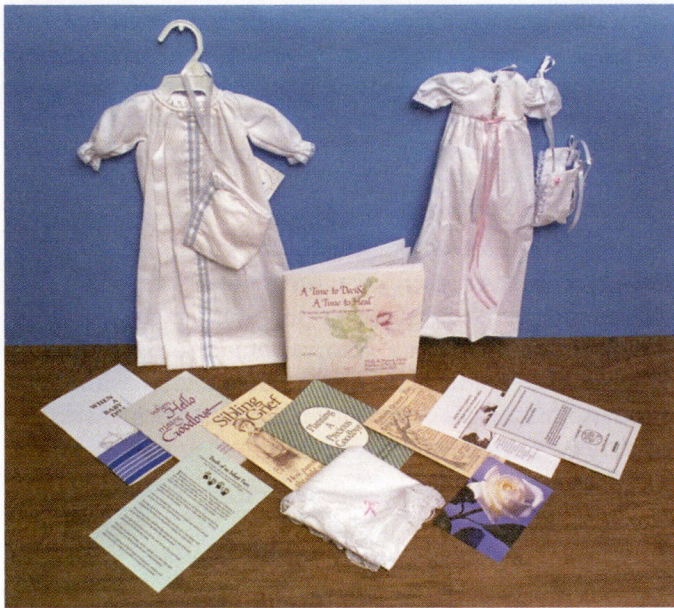

Figure 17-6   A memory kit may help grieving families preserve precious mementos of their baby.

Nursing Tip   *Grief Process*

Well-meaning family members can be guided to assist by recognizing the parents' need to experience the pain and tears to begin healthy grief. Part of the grief process includes telling the story of their pregnancy and infant's birth and subsequent death along with the tears. Grieving also includes the process of creating mementos and putting away baby items when the parents are ready, not when everyone else thinks they should be ready.

Critical Thinking

Grief Process

Many parents experiencing the death of an infant are in shock emotionally. They initially think it would be easier not to see and hold their baby, have a photograph, name their baby, or have a private burial.

- Do you think these activities can assist the parents in their grief process by identifying the infant?
- How would you assist them to recognize the importance of mementos and rituals in their grief process and still support their needs?

the feelings and responses stimulated by working with parents in intense psychologic pain who are in shock and denial. An overview of the bereavement program also should be included in new staff orientation for nurses

Client Education

Neonatal Loss

Because many couples separate or divorce after a perinatal loss, nurses can be instrumental in facilitating coping. It is often helpful to inform families of the following:

- That there are patterns of grieving, such as those described by Davidson.
- That individuals grieve according to their own timetable.
- That the grieving process is not linear and many times a person may have conflicting feelings.
- That the mother and father may be experiencing different feelings at a given time and this sometimes leads to conflict. For example, one person is experiencing anger, whereas the other is experiencing guilt.
- That men and women express their grief and feelings in gender-scripted ways. For example, women may be more comfortable expressing sadness and crying than men; conversely, men may be more comfortable expressing anger than women.
- That an understanding of these aspects of the grief process is the basis for the couple to communicate and support each other through the grieving process.
- That if there are other children in the family, their understanding and expression of grief and loss varies with their age.
- That resources are available to help the couple with grief and to help them work with their children.

Reflections from Families

I will never forget the nurse who came in and spent time with us. I know she had other patients and it probably would have been easy to say she was busy. I feel she spent quality time with us by listening to us, allowing us to piece together what happened, and even crying with us. She validated that what happened was very significant and that our baby was very precious. No matter what the gestation or diagnosis, he still was our baby.

and physicians. This overview could include the philosophy and goals of the program; the process used to support families (such as checklists, books, consultants, and mementos); and most importantly, an organized opportunity to discuss concerns and past experiences. The rights of the family when a baby dies are described in Box 17-4.

Ongoing education and support for staff, even in tertiary care centers in which death may occur more frequently, is pivotal to the well-being of the staff. An example of supportive education is a discussion that focuses on case studies and ethical issues emphasizing difficult situations. Key points in these discussions might include those found in Box 17-5.

Box 17-4

The Rights of Parents and Baby When an Infant Dies

Rights of Parents When a Baby Dies

- To be given the opportunity to see, hold, and touch their baby at any time before or after death within reason.
- To have photographs taken of their baby and made available or held in security until the parents wish to see them.
- To be given as many mementos as possible, that is, the crib card, baby beads, ultrasound pictures and photographs, a lock of hair, feet prints and handprints, and a record of the baby's weight and length.
- To name their child and bond with their child.
- To observe cultural and religious practices.
- To be cared for by an empathetic staff who respects their feelings, thoughts, beliefs, and individual requests.
- To be with each other as much as possible throughout the hospitalization.
- To be informed of the grieving process.

- To be given time alone with their baby, allowing for individual needs.
- To request an autopsy. In case of miscarriage, to request to have or not have an autopsy or pathology examination performed as determined by applicable law.
- To have information presented in terminology understandable to the parents regarding their baby's status and cause of death, including autopsy and pathology reports and medical records.
- To plan a farewell ritual, burial, or cremation in compliance with local and state regulations and according to their personal beliefs, religious beliefs, or cultural traditions.
- To be provided with information about support resources that assist in the healing process, that is, support groups, counseling, reading materials, and perinatal loss newsletters.

Rights of the Baby

- To be recognized as a person who was born and died.
- To be named.
- To be seen, touched, and held by the family.

- To have the ending of life acknowledged.
- To be put to rest with dignity.

Rights of Children When a Sibling Dies

- To be acknowledged as persons who have feelings that need to be expressed.
- To be given the choice to see and hold the baby before and after the death within reason.
- To have the option of being considered in the choices parents make.

- To be informed about the feelings of grief in our terms, giving us the choice of a support group or counselor.
- To be recognized by our society that we will always love and miss our sibling.

Note. From "Rights of Children When a Sibling Dies," by C. Lammert, 1999, *SHARE Pregnancy and Infant Loss Support, Inc., 1*(2).

Box 17-5

Key Discussion Points in an Educational Session after a Stillborn or Newborn Loss

- Never underestimate the supportive power of your peers.
- Offer opportunities to express emotions and gain an understanding of the management of the case.
- Schedule debriefing sessions as close as possible to a major incident.
- Encourage staff to hear all sides of the situation without judgment.
- Work to establish feelings of trust and support.
- Recognize your own response regarding how you can learn and grow from the experience.
- Work to build confidence in the staff in supporting grieving parents.
- Perform an annual review of the program, philosophy, and goals, with input from staff.
- Create a clinical competency that ensures all staff, including the nurse, doctor, social workers and chaplains, have a basic understanding of perinatal grief.

NURSING PROCESS

Implementation of the nursing process is very useful in working with bereaved parents and their family and friends. The nursing process provides a structure to make certain that all steps in caring for a family experiencing loss are addressed. The following example utilizes the nursing process to help nurses begin thinking in this way about perinatal loss.

Assessment

When making an assessment, the nursing history is the first step. The areas that are important can be discovered by asking the following:

- Did the parents have advanced warning that the baby was dead or very ill? Are there medical complications for the mother?
- Was the pregnancy wanted or unwanted? When a pregnancy is unwanted, one or both parents can exhibit a combination of guilt and relief that appears different from the feelings exhibited in a planned pregnancy.
- Were there multiple losses? Parents who have had other pregnancy losses or other significant losses often feel overwhelmed and lack fundamental coping mechanisms.
- How do their religious beliefs or culture support them? Parents who have very strong religious or

cultural beliefs often have a structure of support that can be very helpful.
- Are there close friends or family who share the same culture or beliefs, and are they able to help? Seek information from family and friends regarding beliefs and customs.
- What are the social connections within the network of friends and family? What is the relationship between the infant's mother and father?
- How do the parents, family, and friends express their feelings regarding the loss? Does evidence exist of anger, tears, guilt, sadness, shock, and numbness?

Nursing Diagnosis

Problems need to be identified on an individual basis because each family unit will cope with loss differently. Examples of some general nursing diagnoses include the following:

- Fear related to the initial diagnosis of infant death as evidenced by increased tension and expression of horror or dread.
- Ineffective coping related to inadequate social support, a high degree of threat, as evidenced by a lack of goal-directed behavior, poor concentration, destructive behavior toward self or others, or fatigue.
- Spiritual distress related to perinatal loss as evidenced by energy-consuming anxiety, physical or psychologic stress, loss of a loved one, or poor relationships.
- Health-seeking behaviors related to effective managing of adaptive tasks by the family as evidenced by the family moving in the direction of a health-promoting and enriching lifestyle that supports maturational processes.

Outcome Identification/Planning

Planning for desired outcomes must be constructed with the participation of the mother and her partner. Planning also could involve friends and family:

- Mother and father will be able to work through the bereavement process, each at their own pace, with understanding and support for one another.
- At 1 or 2 years after the loss, the parents will be able to identify positive growth for themselves from the experience.

Nursing Intervention

The nurse needs to take the following actions with the client and her partner:

- Physical care. After delivery, the mother has the same needs as does a mother whose baby was born alive. Do not forget breast engorgement because there is not an infant to empty the breasts. Sleeping medication is not usually helpful because it dulls the feelings and delays coping until after the client has left the hospital, when she cannot receive help as easily.

■ Psychologic and emotional care. Keep parents and families informed and together. Support seeing and holding the infant and create memories, including photographs and mementos. Support decision-making regarding paperwork and disposition of the infant's body. Encourage choices and an increased sense of control. Listen.

■ Educational care. Provide educational pamphlets and booklists. Discuss the bereavement process. Encourage questions. Address issues, such as burial arrangements, funeral, or memorial service; and telling the other children, family, friends, and strangers who know the mother was pregnant. Identify the available resources, such as support groups, reading materials, and Web sites.

■ Follow-up. With much briefer hospital stays today than in the past, follow-up is even more important. It is critical to have a physician follow-up visit scheduled. There may be community follow-up available with a public health nurse. Some facilities have a perinatal loss clinic in which clients receive special attention.

Evaluation

Ongoing evaluation of the bereavement process is important. Encourage couples to seek help and support. Often nurses, or a designated bereavement nurse, will phone the family at key periods for follow-up. Referral to Social Services may also be appropriate.

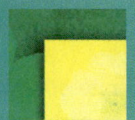

CASE STUDY/CARE PLAN
CLIENT EXPERIENCING INTRAUTERINE FETAL DEMISE

Bonnie is a registered nurse in a labor and delivery ward of a busy county hospital. She has her bachelor's degree and has been working on this particular ward for 2 years. Her morning assignment includes care of a laboring client, Mrs. Kay, a 29-year-old Caucasian American, gravida 1, para 0, with an intrauterine fetal demise (IUFD) at 36 weeks' gestation. Mrs. Kay entered the hospital last night at 3 a.m. with complaints of contractions. She and her husband were not aware there was a problem with the baby because her pregnancy had been without complications. Mrs. Kay was diagnosed with a term IUFD shortly after admission. Owing to the rapid progression of her labor, Mrs. Kay has not had much time to grieve. She is currently dilated at 6 cm. The report from the night shift reveals that Mrs. Kay received intravenous Demerol (meperidine), which had been controlling her pain until the last 30 minutes or so when she started becoming restless. No support services were activated because the admission had been in the middle of the night. Mr. and Mrs. Kay are new to the area; all their family and friends live 500 miles away. Although their immediate families have been notified, there are no plans for them to come at this time.

Assessment

Mrs. Kay lay in the labor bed staring out of the window. Her face is stained with tears. Her husband is sitting quietly with his hand on hers, and there is no verbal communication between the two. Her contractions are coming every 3 minutes, and she breathes hard and cries out with each contraction. Between contractions, Mrs. Kay tells Bonnie that she is in terrible pain and that she is frightened about delivering the baby. Mrs. Kay also states that she and her husband would like to see a member of the clergy.

Nursing Diagnosis

Pain related to contractions associated with active labor as evidenced by crying out and an accelerated respiratory rate.

Expected Outcomes	The client-family will be able to manage the pain experience through partner support, breathing techniques, and medications.
Planning	Pain management and support are interventions aimed at assisting the client now.
NOC	Pain control
NIC	Pain management

(continues)

Nursing Interventions	Rationales
1. Use pain medications that do not alter alertness.	1. Although the client may feel distressed at this particular time, mind-altering medications will only prolong the grieving process. The woman also may grieve the inability to remember her baby.

Evaluation — As is the healing process, evaluation is ongoing. Management of pain in the intrapartum period while soothing fears and anxiety may be monitored by the labor nurse. Effective management of the client may be evidenced by the client stating she has little pain or is pain-free while also monitoring mental alertness.

Nursing Diagnosis

Fear related to delivering a dead infant, as evidenced by the client's apprehension and increased tension

Expected Outcomes — The couple supports each other through the labor process, with help of the nurse, clergy, physician, and other support members.

Planning — The nurse must plan interventions aimed at assisting the client and family with immediate and future needs.

NOC — Fear level

NIC — Coping enhancement

Nursing Interventions	Rationales
1. Use coaching techniques for labor and encourage use. Speak softly and respectfully.	1. The client's response during labor usually is focused on what is happening from moment to moment. By providing support, encouragement, and direction, the nurse may help ease the client's anxiety and fear.

Evaluation — Levels of anxiety and fear may be monitored by verbal and nonverbal cues from the client and family.

Nursing Diagnosis

Spiritual distress related to perinatal loss as evidenced by energy-consuming anxiety, psychologic stress, and loss of a loved one.

Expected Outcomes — Work through the grieving process at their own pace with understanding and support for each other.
Identify positive growth for themselves from the experience.

Planning — Consultations with the clergy and grief counselor may assist the client and family in the near future.

NOC — Grief resolution

NIC — Counseling

Nursing Interventions	Rationales
1. Follow institution guidelines to create mementos: footprints, photographs, and certificates.	1. Mementos are helpful in assisting the family to move through the grieving process. Parents may desire to look at these reminders of their baby for years to come.

Evaluation — The family is meeting with a grief counselor and/or clergy; this is just the first step in a long journey.

WEB ACTIVITIES

• • • Develop a plan of care for a family with a single parent, siblings, and grandparents who are coping with a perinatal loss.

• • • Visit three of the grief Web sites listed in this chapter. Compare the information they offer for families and health care providers.

• • • Which online site provides information on recovering from labor and delivery?

• • • Which resources on the Internet can you find regarding general postpartum care?

• • • Visit AWHONN's Web site and look up postpartum care.

• • • Visit the American Psychological Association's Web site at http://www.apa.org and look up postpartum depression.

Key Concepts

■ Postpartum hemorrhage, often attributable to uterine atony, is most often prevented with astute fundal and lochia monitoring.

■ Postpartum infection can occur in several sites and must be quickly diagnosed and treated.

■ Postpartum depression usually emerges after discharge; therefore, nurses need to give information to the family prior to discharge.

■ Nursing care and support for parents and families when a pregnancy ends or a baby dies constitutes a difficult nursing intervention in an environment that is supposed to be happy, exciting, and focused on new life.

■ When caring for clients at any point during a reproductive loss, it is the individualization of the plan that will give the family the best opportunity to successfully grieve the loss.

■ Reproductive loss can be meaningful, growth-producing and may have positive aspects when the nursing staff can look at this death and loss and create the best possible experience for this family, given the intensely painful situation.

Review Questions and Activities

The first two review questions relate to the previous case study on p. 671. Melanie Jones is the day shift registered nurse caring for Cristina for the first 12 hours after delivery.

1. Cristina was unable to urinate 4 hours after delivery. Which risk factors did she have that would predispose her to having problems?
   a. Delivery of a male infant
   b. Forceps delivery
   c. Blood loss of 450 mL
   d. Rapid labor

   The correct answer is b.

2. Which intrapartum factor put Cristina at risk for increased bleeding?
   a. Ruptured membranes more than 4 hours before the start of active labor
   b. Catheterization
   c. Overdistended uterus
   d. Administration of a narcotic analgesic

   The correct answer is c.

3. Compare and contrast postpartum blues, depression, and psychosis.

4. There are some identifiable phases in the bereavement process that always occur in the same order, one step at a time. True or False?

   The correct response is false.

5. Saying. "I know how you feel," will help the family to know that you care and will ease the expression of their grief. True or False?

   The correct response is false.

6. Mementos and pictures are important for grieving parents. True or False?

   The correct response is true.

7. Parents should be encouraged to join an infant loss support group. True or False?

   The correct response is true.

8. List the four phases of the grief process as described in this chapter.

References

American College of Obstetrics and Gynecology (ACOG). (1990). *Diagnosis and management of postpartum hemorrhage* (Tech. Bulletin No. 143). pp. 1–5. Washington, DC: Author.

American Psychological Association. (2000). *Diagnostic and Statistical Manual of Mental Disorders* (4th ed. text revision). Washington, DC: Author.

Anderson, K. (Ed.). (1998). Mosby's medical, nursing and allied health dicitionery, (5th ed.). Chicago, IL: Mosby.

Askren, H. A., & Bloom, K. C. (1999). Postadaptive reactions of the relinquishing mother: A review. *Journal of Obstetric, Gynecologic, and Neonatal Nursing, 28*(4), 395–400.

Association of Women's Health, Obstetrics, and Neonatal Nurses (AWHONN). (1999). *AWHONN position statement: The role of the nurse in postpartum depression.* Retrieved April 8, 2004, from http://www.awhonn.org/awhonn/?pg=875-4730-4770

Beck, C. T. (2001). Predictions of postpartum depression: An update. *Nursing Research, 501*(5), 275–285.

Beck, C. T. (2002). Revision of the postpartum depression inventory. *Journal of Obstetric, Gynecological, and Neonatal Nursing, 31*(14), 394–402.

Beneditti, T. J. (1996). Obstetric hemorrhage. In S. G. Gabbe, J. R. Niebyl, & J. L. Simpson (Eds.), *Obstetrics: Normal and problem pregnancies* (pp. 692–713). New York: Churchill Livingston.

Bowes, W. A. (1996). Postpartum care. In S. G. Gabbe, J. R. Niebyl, & J. L. Simpson (Eds.), *Obstetrics: Normal and problem pregnancies* (pp. 692–713). New York: Churchill Livingston.

Clark, R. A. (1995). Infections during the postpartum period. *Journal of Obstetric, Gynecologic, and Neonatal Nurses, 24*(6), 542–548.

Davidson, G. W. (1979). *Understanding death of the wished-for child.* Springfield, IL: OGR Service Corp.

Davidson, G. W. (1984). *Understanding mourning.* Minneapolis, MN: Augsburg.

Davis, C. E. (1994). Separation loss in relinquishing birth mothers. *The International Journal of Psychiatric Nursing Research, 1*(2), 63–70.

Jehovah's Witnesses: The surgical/ethical challenge. (1981). *Journal of the American Medical Association, 246*(21), 2471–2472. Retrieved 2000, from http://www.watchtower.org/library/hb/jw_surgical_ethical.htm

Kavanaugh, K. (1997). Parents experiences surrounding the death of a newborn whose birth is at the margin of viability. *Journal of Obstetric, Gynecologic, and Neonatal Nursing, 26,* 43–51.

Lamb, J. M. Ed. (1988). *Bittersweet; Hello . . . goodbye: A resource in planning farewell rituals when a baby dies.* Belleville, IL: National Share Office.

Lammert, C. (1991). Rights of children when a sibling dies. *SHARE Pregnancy and Infant Loss Support, Inc., 1*(2).

Lawrence, R. (1999). *Breastfeeding: A guide for the medical profession* (5th ed.). St. Louis, MO: Mosby.

Lee, C., & Slade, P. (1996). Miscarriage as a traumatic event: A review of the literature and new implications for intervention. *Journal of Psychosomatic Research, 40*(3), 235–244.

Lindemann, E. (1944). Symptomatology and management of acute grief. *American Journal of Psychiatry, 101,* 141–148.

Overfield, M. L., & Tully, M. R. (1997). Newborn nutrition and feeding. In D. L. Lowdermilk, S. E. Perry, & I. M. Bobak. *Maternity and women's health care* (6th ed.). St. Louis, MO: Mosby.

Roles, P. (1997). Birth parents' grief: Relinquishing a baby for adoption. In J. R. Wood & J. L. Esposito (Eds.), *Loss during pregnancy or in the newborn period: Principles of care with clinical cases and analysis.* Pitman, NJ: Jannetti.

Ugarriza, D. N., & Robinson, M. K. (1997). Assessment of postpartum depression: A review of the literature. *The Online Journal of Knowledge Synthesis in Nursing, 4*(6).

Suggested Readings

Alspach, J. G., & Williams, S. M. (1995). *Core curriculum for critical care nursing.* Philadelphia: W. B. Saunders.

American Academy of Pediatrics & American College of Gynecologists. (1997). *Guidelines for perinatal care* (4th ed.). Elk Grove, IL: Authors.

Association of Women's Health, Obstetric, and Neonatal Nurses (AWHONN). (1996). *Compendium of postpartum care.* Washington, DC: Author.

Association of Women's Health, Obstetric, and Neonatal Nurses (AWHONN) Committee on Practice. (1997). *Guidelines for providing care to the family experiencing perinatal loss and fetal death.* Washington, DC: Author.

Borg, S., & Lasker, J. (1981). *When pregnancy fails: Families coping with miscarriage, stillbirth and infant death.* Boston: Beacon Press.

Calhoun, L. K. (1994). Parents' perceptions of nursing support following neonatal loss. *Journal of Perinatal and Neonatal Nursing, 8*(2), 57–66.

Davis, D. L. (1996). *Empty cradle, broken heart: Surviving the death of your baby* (Rev. ed.). Golden, CO: Fulcrum.

Doenges, M. E., & Moorhouse, M. F. (1996). *Nurses pocket guide: Nursing diagnoses with interventions* (5th ed.). Philadelphia: F. A. Davis.

Duff, P. (1996). Maternal and perinatal infection. In S. G. Gabbe, J. R. Niebyl, & J. L. Simpson (Eds.), *Obstetrics: Normal and problem pregnancies* (pp. 692–713). New York: Churchill Livingston.

Grollman, E. (1967). *Explaining death to children* (p. 102). Boston: Beacon Press.

Gunderson, J. M., & Harris, D. E. (Eds.). (1990). *Quietus: A story of stillbirth.* Omaha, NE: Centering Corp.

Harrigan, R., Naber, M. M., & Jensen, K. A. (1993). Perinatal grief: Response to the loss of an infant. *Neonatal Network, 12*(5), 25–31.

Higgins, P. (2000). Postpartum complications. In S. Mattson, & J. E. Smith (Eds.), *Core curriculum for maternal-newborn nursing* (2nd ed.). Philadelphia: W. B. Saunders.

Hutti, M. H. (1998). A quick reference table of interventions to assist families to cope with pregnancy loss or perinatal death. *Birth: Issues in Perinatal Care and Education, 15,* 33–35.

Ilse, S., & Furrh, C. B. (1988). Development of a comprehensive follow-up care plan after perinatal and neonatal loss. *Journal of Perinatal and Neonatal Nursing, 2*(2), 23–33.

Kushner, H. S. (1981). *When bad things happen to good people.* New York: Collier Books.

Leoni, L. C. (1997). The nurse's role: Care of patients after pregnancy loss. In J. R. Woods Jr., & J. L. E. Woods (Eds.), *Loss during pregnancy or in the newborn period* (pp. 361–386). Pitman, NJ: Jannetti.

Mattson, S., & Smith, J. E. (Eds.). (2004). *Core curriculum for maternal-newborn nursing* (3rd ed.). Philadelphia: W. B. Saunders.

Primeau, M. R., & Lamb, J. M. (1995). When a baby dies. *Journal of Obstetrics, Gynecology, and Neonatal Nursing, 24,* 206–208.

Rando, T. A. (1986). *Parental loss of a child.* Champaign, IL: Research Press.

Spratto, G. R., & Woods, A. L. (2005). *PDR nurse's drug handbook.* Clifton Park, NY: Thomson Delmar Learning.

Wheeler, L. (1997). *Nurse-midwifery handbook: A practical guide to prenatal and postpartum care.* Philadelphia: Lippincott Williams & Wilkins.

Woods, Jr., J. J. (1997). Pregnancy loss counseling: The challenge to the obstetrician. In J. R. Woods, Jr., & J. L. Woods (Eds.), *Loss during pregnancy or in the newborn period* (p. 84). Pitman, NJ: Jannetti.

Resources

Engender Health, 440 Ninth Avenue, New York, NY 10001; 212-561-8000; Fax: 212-561-8067; http://www.engenderhealth.com

Kimberly-Clark Corporation, Dept. INT, P.O. Box 2020, Neenah, WI 54957-2020; 888-525-8388; http://www.depend.com

Parents Place, http://www.parentsplace.com

National Organizations: Parents Experiencing Perinatal Death

Association of Death Education and Counseling, Professional organization and certification, 342 N. Main St., West Hartford, CT 06117, http://www.adec.org

Bereaved Parents of the USA, National Headquarters, P.O. Box 95, Park Forest, IL 60466

Bereavement Services—RTS, Gundersen Lutheran Medical Center, 1910 South Ave., LaCrosse, WI 54601, 800-362-9567, x4767

Center for Loss in Multiple Births (CLIMB), P.O. Box 91377, Anchorage, AK 99405

The Centering Corporation (books and videos), 7230 Maple Street, Omaha, NE 68134, 402-553-1200

National Funeral Directors Association (NFDA), Marketplace (books and videos), 13625 Bishops Drive, Brookfield, WI 53005

National Organization for Rare Disorders (NORD), 800-999-6673

Paraclete Press & Paraclete Video Productions (book and videos), P.O. Box 1568, Orleans, MA 02653, 800-451-5006

Resolve, Inc. Infertility, 1310 Broadway, Somerville, MA 02144-1779, 888-623-0744, http://www.resolve.org

SHARE, Pregnancy & Infant Loss Support, Inc., St. Joseph Health Center, 300 First Capital Drive, St. Charles, MO 63301-2893, 800-821-6819, http://www.NationalSHAREoffice.com

Sidelines National Support Network, P.O. Box 1808, Laguna Beach, CA 92652, 888-447-4754, http://www.sidelines.org

SIDS Alliance, 1314 Bedord Ave., Suite 210, Baltimore, MD 21208, 800-221-SIDS

The Compassionate Friends (TCF) National Office, P.O. Box 3696, Oak Brook, IL 60522-3696, 877-869-0010, http://www.compassionatefriends.org

The Self-Help Center, A Division of the Mental Health Association of Illinois, 217-352-0099

Wisconsin Stillbirth Service Program: Life and Death before Birth (for professional use). Wisconsin Stillbirth Service Program: University of Wisconsin Clinical Cenetics Center, Waisman Center, Room 343, 1500 Highland Ave., Madison, WI 53705-2280.

1: Stillbirth, 23 minutes

2: Justification for stillbirth assessment and evaluation, 21 minutes

3: Practical guide to stillbirth evaluation, 21 minutes

4: Summarization data of the 10-year study, 17 minutes

5: Case studies of evaluations

Pediatrics Bereavement Support Groups Centers and Publications

The Bobbi Burrow: A Center for Grieving Children of All Ages, 403 Walnut Street, St. Charles, IL 60174, 603-513-8327

The Compassionate Friends, Inc., P.O. Box 3696, Oak Brook, IL 60522-3696, 877-869-0010, Theresa Goodrich, http://www.compassionatefriends.org

The Dougy Center: The National Center for Grieving Children and Families, 3909 S.E. 52nd Ave., P.O. Box 86852, Portland, OR 97206, 503-775-5683, Fax: 503-777-3097, http://www.dougy.org

Suggested Readings for Children

Brown, L. K., & Brown, M. (1996). *When dinosuars die: A guide to understanding death.* Boston: Little, Brown.

Buscalia, L. (1983). *The fall of Freddy the leaf.*

Coh, J. (1987). *I had a friend named Peter: Talking to children about the death of a friend.* New York: Morrow Junior Books.

Cohn, J. (1994). *Molly's rosebush.* Morton Grove, IL: Whitman & Co. ISBN #08075-5213-5

Collins, P. L. (1990). *Waiting for baby Joe.* ICEA Publication #FC9201.

Dodge, N. C. (1984). *Thump's story: A story of love and grief shared by Thumpy, the Bunny.* Springfield, IL: Prairie Lark Press.

Grollman, E. A. (1970). *Talking about death: A dialogue between parent and child.* Boston: Beacon Press.

Gryte, M. (1988). *No new baby.* ICEA Publication FC#8811.

O'Connor, J. (1997). *Heaven's not a crying place: Teaching your child about funerals, death and the life beyond.* Grand Rapids, MI: Baker Book House.

O'Toole, D. (1988). *Aarvy Aardvark finds hope.* Burnsville, NC: Celo Press.

Palmer, P. (1994). *I wish I could hold your hand: A child's guide to grief and loss.* San Luis, CA: Impact.

Roberts, J., & Johnson, J. (1994). *Thank-you for coming to say goodbye.* Omaha, NE: Centering Corp.

Slater, R. C. (1978). *Tell me, papa.* Omaha, NE: Centering Corp.

Van-Si, L., & Powers, L. (1994). *Helping children heal from loss: A keepsake book of special memories.* Portland, OR: Portland State University/Continuing Education Press.

Grief Websites

Association of Women's Health, Obstetric, and Neonatal Nurses (AWHONN): http://www.awhonn.org

Bereavement and hospice directory: http://www.ubalt.edu

Care plans, library, forum, and tips on patient education: http://www.rncentral.com

The Changing Face of Women's Health: http://www.whealth.org

Cremation Society: locations: http://www.cremation.org

The Dougy Center: The National Center for Grieving Children and Families: http://www.dougy.org

For Women, 800-994-9662: http://www.4women.gov

GriefNet: http://rivendell.org

Growth House: directory, end of life care: http://www.growthhouse.org

Kids' Health: http://www.kidshealth.org

CHAPTER 18

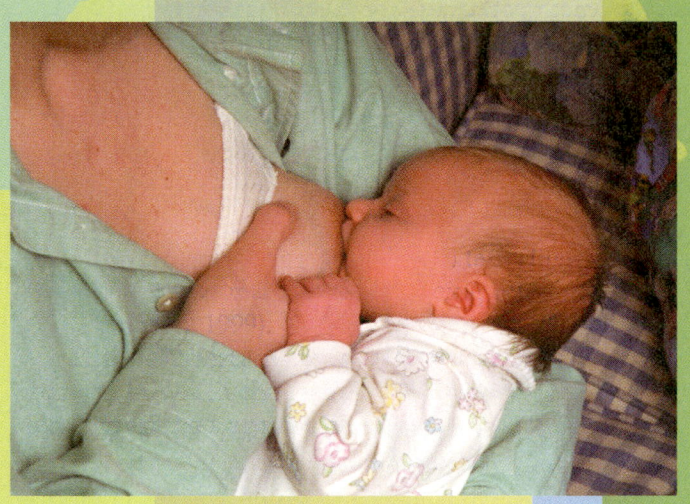

LACTATION AND NEWBORN NUTRITION

Guidelines from the American Academy of Pediatrics recommend breastfeeding and human milk as the standard for optimal infant nutrition in the first year of life. These guidelines are emphasized and current alternatives are presented for infants when breastfeeding and human milk feeding are not possible. Use the following questions to examine your knowledge and attitudes about infant nutrition:

- Do I really believe that "breast is best"?
- Which feeding method would I choose for my own infant?
- Do I feel embarrassed to see a woman breastfeed in public?
- How do I feel when trying to help a woman breastfeed for the first time?
- Do I feel angry when a client doesn't do what I think is best for her or her infant?
- Can I allow a client to tell me how she really feels without judging her?
- Do I respect cultural beliefs about breastfeeding that may not be scientifically sound?

Key Terms

Alveoli	Let-down reflex
Antioxidant	Macronutrients
Areola	Mammogenesis
Bioavailability	Mastitis
Colostrum	Mature milk
Engorgement	Micronutrients
Foremilk	Oxytocin
Galactopoiesis	Prolactin
Hindmilk	Reducing agent
Lactation consultant	Renal solute load
Lactogenesis	Rooting reflex
Latching-on	Transitional milk
La Leche League	Weaning

Competencies

Upon completion of this chapter, the reader should be able to:

1. Discuss the composition and function of basic nutrients in human milk compared with artificial infant formula.
2. Describe the expected growth rates for normal full-term infants based on type of milk (human or artificial formula) received in the early months of life.
3. Identify the health and financial benefits of both breast and formula feeding.
4. Explore the motivations and perceived barriers related to breastfeeding.
5. Describe effective strategies to promote breastfeeding in a culturally sensitive manner.
6. Develop interventions that lead to successful breastfeeding outcomes.
7. Delineate nursing responsibilities for client education and informed consent related to breastfeeding and formula feeding decisions.
8. Assess the nutritional status of the breastfed infant.
9. Describe the physiology of lactation.
10. Discuss selection of formulas.
11. Discuss preparation of formula and bottle feeding.
12. Discuss interventions to support the formula feeding mother.

*T*he newborn infant requires dietary energy for adequate growth and development. Determining the optimal nutrition for the healthy newborn infant has required extensive scientific investigation for decades. Infant nutrition research repeatedly concludes that human milk and breastfeeding are the gold standard to which all other forms of infant feeding alternatives should be compared.

INFANT NUTRITION

Breastfeeding is the infant feeding method recommended by the American Academy of Pediatrics, American Public Health Association, and American Dietetic Association for the first 12 months after birth (American Academy of Pe-

diatrics, 1997). The practice guidelines of the American Academy of Pediatrics are straightforward and supported by solid research. These recommendations include the following:

■ Newborns should be nursed when they show signs of hunger (crying is identified as a late sign of hunger). Newborns should be nursed approximately 8 to 12 times every 24 hours until satiety.

■ No supplements should be given to newborns unless a medical indication exists. Supplements and pacifiers should be avoided if used at all, and only used after breastfeeding is well established.

■ Exclusive breastfeeding is ideal and sufficient to support optimal growth and development for approximately 6 months.

- Gradual introduction of iron-enriched solid foods in the second half of the first year should complement breast milk.

- Breastfeeding should continue for at least 12 months, and thereafter for as long as mutually desired.

Breastfeeding provides the optimal nutrition for infants during the first year of life when there is rapid physical and developmental growth. In addition to providing essential nutrients, breastfeeding provides unique opportunities for positive interactions and bonding between infants and mothers. A woman's decision to breastfeed is determined by many factors. Feeding her new infant can be an exciting, satisfying, and personally empowering experience for many women. The nurse can provide vital support to women who choose to breastfeed and do not have role models in their families who have successfully breastfed.

GROWTH AND DEVELOPMENT

Growth is the standard by which infant nutrition is judged. Birth weight triples and length increases by 50% during the first year. Infant growth is especially rapid during the first few months of life when weekly weight and length gains approximate 200 g and 1 cm, respectively. Brain growth is profound, tripling in size during infancy to reach 90% of adult size at 2 years of age (Dobbing & Sands, 1973; Widdowson, 1991). Scientific evidence is emerging that different diets in early infancy can have long-term consequences (Barker, 1992; Sultan & Barker, 1994).

Human milk has the distinct capability of providing not only energy to fuel growth but unique properties benefiting the infant's immune system and health status. Immune properties, most specifically secretory immunoglobulin A (sIgA), present in human milk, protect the infant from infection (Wold & Hanson, 1994).

Growth charts are used to monitor individual infant growth patterns. Charts currently used throughout the world are based on the U.S. National Center for Health Statistics (NCHS) reference data (U.S. Department of Health, Education and Welfare, 1977), which are normed on formula-fed infants.

It has been demonstrated in several studies that the growth patterns of breastfed infants differ from the NCHS reference data (Binns, Senturia, LeBailly, Donovan, & Kaufer, 1996; Dewey, Heinig, & Nommsen-Rivers, 1995; Dewey, Heinig, Nommsen-Rivers, Beerson, & Lonnerdal, 1992; Hitchcock, Gracey, & Gilmour, 1985). Breastfed infants showed as rapid or more rapid weight gains compared with formula-fed infants during the first 2 to 3 months; however, formula-fed infants weigh more than breastfed infants during the later months of the first year.

Until new growth references are available, health care providers need to take into account differences in growth rates based on feeding mode (Figure 18-1). Misinterpreting the growth patterns of healthy breastfed infants by advising mothers to supplement unnecessarily or to stop breastfeeding altogether has profound public health significance. A general guideline is to note weight gain of 20 to 30 g/d ($\frac{1}{3}$ to $\frac{1}{2}$ lb/wk) for the first 5 months, with a length gain of 0.80 to 1.07 mm/d (0.28 in/wk) and a head circumference increment of 0.3 cm/wk (Guo et al., 1991; Hamill et al., 1979).

Energy

Carbohydrates and fat meet the primary energy requirements for growth, metabolism, and activity. Protein also may provide energy. The most important function of protein in growth, however, is to provide the amino acids

Reflections from a Nurse

For years, I routinely promoted bottle-feeding because it was easy to see how much formula the babies consumed. It also was easy to teach mothers how to prepare the formula. Then I began to learn more about how formula was developed and how the formula companies were researching the composition of breast milk. I became convinced that, whenever possible, the best food for infants is their mother's milk. After more reading, I now feel that the babies whose mothers are not breast-feeding, for whatever reason, also are getting good nutrition as the infant formulas are getting more and more sophisticated.

Nursing Tip *Infant Assessment*

A general approach to infant nutritional assessment follows:

1. Use an accurate electronic scale to measure weight.
2. Use a length board.

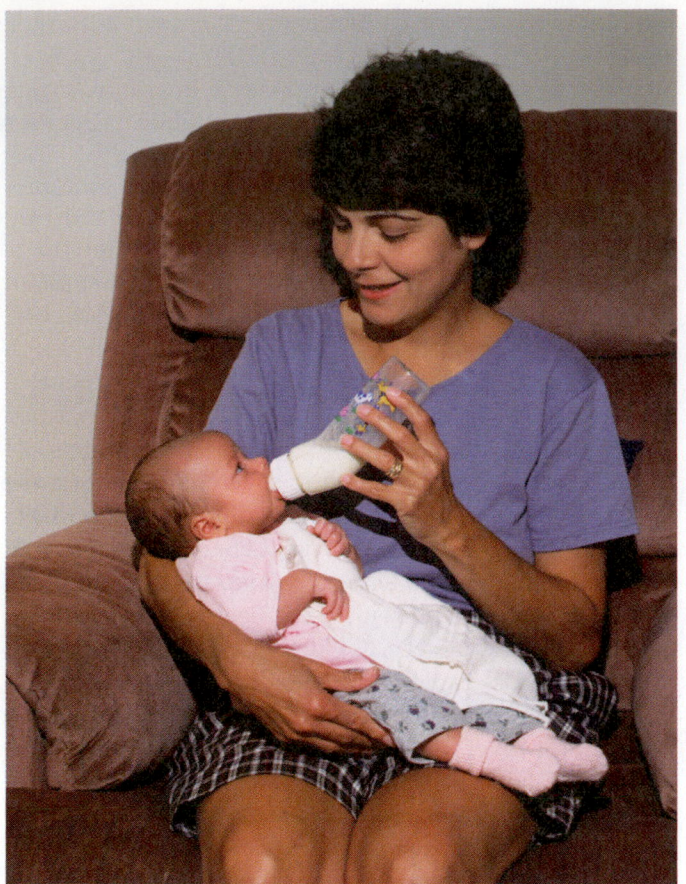

Figure 18-1   Adequate nutritional intake is noted by an infant's overall healthy appearance and steady growth rate.

necessary for synthesis of body proteins and the hormones and enzymes that regulate metabolism (Carlson & Barness, 1996).

The current recommendations for energy requirements for a term infant are 108 kcal and 100 kcal per kilogram of body weight from birth through 6 months and 6 months through 12 months, respectively (Food and Nutrition Board, 1989). The general compositions of human, bovine, and several infant formulas are compared in Table 18-1.

Protein

The amount of total energy intake utilized for growth is higher during the first 2 months of life than at any other time. During this most rapid period of postnatal growth, infants may use 60% of the protein they consume in producing new tissue.

There are significant differences in the digestibility and quality of human milk proteins compared with those of bovine milk-based formulas. The proportion of whey (supernatant) and casein (curd) in human milk is of interest. Human milk is more whey-dominant, with a whey-to-casein ratio of approximately 70:30 compared with 18:82 in bovine milk. In general, the whey fraction of soluble proteins is more easily digested and promotes more rapid gastric emptying (Billeaud, Guillet, & Sandler, 1990).

Fat

The fats in human milk provide approximately 50% of the calories in the milk. The lipid profile consists of 98% triglycerides, 1% phospholipids, and 0.5% cholesterol and cholesterol esters (Jensen & Jensen, 1992). In addition, fats are an integral part of all cell membranes, provide fatty acids necessary for brain development, and are the sole

Table 18-1   Composition of Human Milk and Formulas*

SELECTED NUTRIENTS (100 ML)	HUMAN MILK	FORMULAS**			
		STANDARD COW'S MILK–BASED	SOY	ELEMENTAL	PRETERM
Kcal	68	68	68	68	81
Carbohydrates (g)	7.2	7.0–7.3	7.0	7–9.1	9.0
Protein (g)	1.0	1.5	1.7–2.0	1.6–1.9	2.2–2.4
Fat (g)	3.9	3.6–3.8	3.6–3.7	2.7–3.9	4.1–4.4
Sodium (mEq)	0.78	0.8–0.96	0.9–1.4	0.7–1.4	1.4–1.5
Potassium (mEq)	1.34	1.43–1.87	1.9–2.1	1.7–2.0	2.1–2.7
Calcium (mEq)	28	42–51.9	60–71	43–71	134–146
Iron (mg)	0.03	1.2–1.3	1.2–1.3	1.2–1.3	1.5

*Commercial formulas average content: read individual labels for up-to-date quantity (Ross, Mead Johnson, and Store Brand formulas).

**Formulas with iron.

vehicle for fat-soluble vitamins and hormones in milk (Hamosh, 1988). The total fat content of human milk is approximately 3.5% to 4.5%; however, it is the most variable component of milk, varying in content throughout lactation, and within and between feedings. The fat content of human milk increases markedly during a single feeding from a breast, with the concentration of *hindmilk* (that milk produced toward the end of a nursing interval) typically being twice that of *foremilk* (lower-fat milk secreted from the breast prior to milk ejection). In addition, fat content increases during the day, with early morning milk having the lowest fat content. Total fat content increases gradually from colostrum (2.0%) through transitional milk (2.5% to 3.0%) to mature milk (3.5% to 4.5%) (Bitman et al., 1986).

Carbohydrates

Carbohydrates provide fuel for neonatal metabolism, supplying both immediately usable and stored energy. The neonatal brain is the major consumer of glucose, relying almost exclusively on glucose for its metabolism.

Lactose is the principal carbohydrate in human milk and provides approximately 50% of the energy content. Human milk carbohydrates have been shown to enhance infant immunity and brain development.

Water and Electrolytes

Water represents the largest component in human milk, providing approximately 89 mL of preformed water in each 100 mL of milk consumed. Water is required by the infant to replace evaporative losses of water from skin and lungs and excretory losses from feces and urine. The infant's first priority for water is through evaporative loss. The second priority is for urinary water necessary for the excretion of solutes.

The amount of water excreted in the urine is determined by the renal solute load and renal concentrating

Table 18-2	Electrolyte Composition of Human and Bovine Milks	
COMPONENT (mg/dL)	**HUMAN**	**BOVINE**
Sodium	15	58
Chloride	43	103
Potassium	55	138

ability. The sum of solutes that must be excreted by the kidney is termed the **renal solute load**. The renal solute load is of considerable importance in circumstances such as low fluid intake; abnormally high losses of water, for example, as those occurring with fever; hyperventilation; and diarrhea (Foman, 1993).

The electrolyte compositions of human and bovine milks are given in Table 18-2.

Minerals

Calcium (Ca), phosphorus (P), and magnesium (Mg) homeostasis in the newborn involves hormonal influences that regulate the concentrations of these minerals in the infant.

Calcium homeostasis is closely linked with that of P and Mg. Human milk provides optimal Ca, P, and Mg content for bone mineralization in term newborns. Cow's milk-based formulas generally have higher Ca content than does human milk to compensate for the poorer absorption rates of the formulas. Infants receive an average of 240 mg of Ca from 750 mL of human milk, approximately two thirds of which they retain. The retention of Ca from infant formulas based on cow's milk is less than one half. These differences in retention are reflected in the recommendations for Ca, P, and Mg for breastfed and formula-fed infants outlined in Table 18-3.

Table 18-3	Recommended Dietary Intake of Calcium, Phosphorus, and Magnesium for Breastfed and Formula-Fed Infants				
AGE	1–6 MO		6–12 MO		
MINERAL	BREASTFED (mg)	FORMULA-FED (mg)	BREASTFED (mg)	FORMULA-FED (mg)	
Calcium	300	400	500	600	
Phosphorus	300	300	500	500	
Magnesium	40	60	40	60	

Note. Adapted from *Recommended Dietary Allowances* by the National Academy of Science Food and Nutrition Board, 1989, Washington, DC: Author.

Trace Elements

The macronutrients (protein, fat, carbohydrates, and major minerals) are essential components of body structure and energy sources. Micronutrients provide protection against oxidative damage during cellular metabolism and have major roles in immune function. **Macronutrients** are any of the chemical elements, such as carbon, required in relatively large quantities for growth. **Micronutrients** are any of the chemical elements, such as iron and other minerals, required in minute quantities for growth.

Iron, zinc, copper, manganese, selenium, molybdenum, chromium, and iodine are generally considered to be the essential trace minerals. Table 18-4 outlines the recommended daily intake of trace elements for infants.

Iron is a powerful oxidant and a constituent of hemoglobin, myoglobin, and a number of enzymes and, therefore, an essential nutrient for the infant. With stored iron, the term infant can maintain satisfactory hemoglobin levels from human milk without other iron sources during the first 4 months of life. Unlike bottle-fed infants, breast-fed babies do not require iron supplementation until 6 months of age, because breast milk contains lactoferrin. After 6 months of age, infants should consume iron-fortified foods or iron-fortified formula to ensure adequate iron stores (Haschke et al., 1993). The recommended daily allowance (RDA) from 6 months to 3 years of age is set at 10 mg/d per kilogram of body weight for healthy infants and should not exceed a maximum of 15 mg/d. Iron deficiency anemia has been associated with impaired mental and motor development and should be prevented (Scheard, 1994).

Zinc is an essential component of many enzymes and plays a role in cellular immune function (Prasad, 1991). Because full-term infants who are exclusively breastfed rarely show signs of zinc depletion, requirements must be satisfied by maternal milk levels. The dietary zinc requirement of infants consuming formula is higher than that of breastfed infants because of lower bioavailability of the formula (Lonnerdal, Cederblad, Davidsson, & Sandstrom, 1984).

The remaining trace elements have received less investigation but are no less important in the enzymatic activity of the body. One consistent finding from studies of levels of trace elements in human milk is their variability between individuals and stages of lactation.

Water-Soluble Vitamins

The water-soluble vitamins (B and C vitamins) are, for the most part, present in the serum and, as the name implies, the fluid compartments of the body. The RDAs for water-soluble vitamins for infants are presented in Table 18-5.

Vitamin C (ascorbic acid) functions primarily as an antioxidant and a reducing agent. An **antioxidant** is a substance that slows down the oxidation of hydrocarbons, oils, fats, and so on, thus helping to check deterioration. A **reducing agent** is a substance that reduces another one, or brings about reduction, and is itself oxidized in the process. In addition, vitamin C enhances iron absorption from the GI tract. Human milk is a rich source of vitamin C. It is recommended that infant formulas contain at least 8 mg/100 kcal of vitamin C.

Thiamin, riboflavin, and niacin are three B vitamins essential to the body's metabolism. Thiamin serves primarily as a cofactor for three enzyme complexes involved in carbohydrate metabolism (Moran & Greene, 1987).

Riboflavin serves as an essential component of flavoproteins, which function as hydrogen carriers in a number of critical oxidation-reduction reactions.

Niacin is converted in the liver to the active cofactors that play central roles in body metabolism in a wide range of oxidation-reduction reactions.

Table 18-4	Estimated Trace Element Requirements for Healthy Infants	
TRACE ELEMENT	**1–6 MO**	**6–12 MO**
Iron	6 mg	10 mg
Zinc	5 mg	5 mg
Copper	0.4–0.6 mg	0.6–0.7 mg
Manganese	0.3–0.6 mg	0.6–1.0 mg
Selenium	10 mEq	15 mEq
Molybdenum	15–30 mEq	20–40 mEq
Chromium	10–40 mEq	20–60 mEq
Iodine	40 mEq	50 mEq

Note. Adapted from *Recommended Dietary Allowances* by the Food and Nutrition Board, 1989, National Academy of Science, Washington, DC: Author.

Table 18-5	Recommended Daily Dietary Allowances for Water-Soluble Vitamins for Infants	
VITAMIN	**0–6 MO**	**6–12 MO**
Vitamin C	30 mg	35 mg
Thiamin	0.3 mg	0.4 mg
Riboflavin	0.4 mg	0.5 mg
Niacin	5 mg NE	6 mg NE
Vitamin B_6	0.3 mg	0.6 mg
Folic acid	25 µg	35 µg
Vitamin B_{12}	0.3 µg	0.5 µg

Note. Adapted from *Recommended Dietary Allowances* by the Food and Nutrition Board, 1989, National Academy of Science, Washington, DC: Author.

COLLABORATIVE CARE

Collaborative Team for Infant Feeding

Multiple professionals may be involved with a family regarding infant feeding:

- Nurse: The nurse is in very close contact with mothers and infants in the immediate postpartum period and can be in a pivotal position to help a new mother initiate breastfeeding.

- Obstetrician: The physician may be involved, especially if the mother has any medical problems. It is very important for the nurse to keep the physician informed if the mother is breastfeeding. For example, if the mother is having a treatment or procedure that keeps her away from the infant, breast pumping may need to be arranged. If the mother is receiving any medication, it is important for the physician to know if she is breastfeeding.

- Social worker: Many clients have social workers on their team, especially if the social worker might be involved in helping the family obtain food supplements through government programs such as WIC (Women, Infants, and Children). The nurse can utilize the social worker to assist the family in the area of infant nutrition, whether breast or formula feeding is chosen.

- Lactation consultant: Many hospitals and clinics have lactation consultants who work intensely with mothers in successfully starting and maintaining breastfeeding. These lactation consultants may be laypeople with special background in breastfeeding or nurses who have specialized in this area.

- Pediatrician: Infant feeding is an integral part of the care of the infant. Pediatricians will be very important to the success of breastfeeding or for the selection of any specialized formula that the infant may require. If the infant is preterm or has other health problems, the neonatalogist or pediatrician will be closely involved in monitoring the nutrition of the infant.

- Nutritionist: Some institutions have nutritionists that work with lactating mothers, ensuring that they have adequate nutritional intake. If the newborn has health problems, the nutritionist may also become involved in assisting the family to meet their infant's nutritional needs.

Advanced practice nurses may also be members of the health care team, monitoring the mother or infant separately, or together as a couple.

Vitamins B_6 and B_{12}, and folic acid, aid in metabolism of essential amino acids. Vitamin B_6 serves as a cofactor for a large number of reactions involved in the synthesis, interconversion, and catabolism of amino acids and neurotransmission (McCormick, 1989).

Folates function metabolically as coenzymes that transport single carbon fragments from one compound to another in amino acid metabolism and nucleic acid synthesis. The needs of infants are adequately met by milk from humans and cow's milk.

Vitamin B_{12} functions as an enzyme in amino acid metabolism. The minimum RDA for infants is 0.3 µg/d the first year of life, when growth is rapid.

Fat-Soluble Vitamins

Vitamins A, D, E, and K are the fat-soluble vitamins. Fat-soluble vitamins are found in the fat component of milk and other foods and tend to move into the liver and adipose tissue for storage, rather than the excess being excreted as is the case for water-soluble vitamins. Table 18-6 outlines the RDAs for the fat-soluble vitamins.

Vitamin A is essential for vision, growth, cellular differentiation, reproduction, and the integrity of the immune system (Goodman, 1984; West, Rombout, Van der Zijpp, & Sijtsma, 1991).

Vitamin D is essential for proper formation of bone and mineralization. Vitamin D is unique among nutrients

Table 18-6   Recommended Daily Dietary Allowances for Fat-Soluble Vitamins for Infants

AGE (MO)	VITAMIN A (µg RE)*	VITAMIN D (µg)**	VITAMIN E (mg)	VITAMIN K (µg)
0–6	395	7.5	3	5
6–12	375	10	4	10

*1 retinol equivalent (RE) of vitamin A equals 3, 33 IU.

**10 g of vitamin D equals 400 IU.

Note. Adapted from *Recommended Dietary Allowances* by the Food and Nutrition Board, 1989, National Academy of Science, Washington, DC: Author.

because the body can synthesize it with exposure to sunlight.

Vitamin E is an antioxidant similar in function to vitamin C but is fat-soluble. Its primary function is as a scavenger of free radicals, thereby protecting cellular membranes against oxidative destruction (Kelleher, 1991).

Vitamin K is a group of compounds essential for the formation of prothrombin and other proteins involved in the regulation of blood clotting. Owing to the low concentrations of vitamin K reported in human milk (2 µg/L), it is recommended that exclusively breastfed infants receive a supplement at birth. Additionally, infant formulas should contain 4 mg/100 kcal of vitamin K (AAP, 1985).

BREASTFEEDING

As previously stated, breastfeeding is the optimal choice of infant feeding by all major societies and agencies, including the American Academy of Pediatrics (AAP), American Dietetics Association, and the World Health Organization (WHO). These groups base their recommendations on the strong scientific evidence of decreased infant mortality in developing countries and decreased morbidity in developed countries seen in exclusively breastfed infants compared with those fed human milk substitutes.

Lactation is a complex physiologic process under neuroendocrine control, whereas breastfeeding is the process by which milk is transferred from the maternal breast to the infant. Understanding the difference in these two interrelated processes is important when counseling the mother. Most lactation and breastfeeding problems are preventable and can be overcome with proper knowledge and technical skills. Prenatal visits should include discussion about infant feeding choice to provide an opportunity for parents to make an informed decision and obtain information.

Critical Thinking

Cultural Views on Colostrum

Clients from some cultures, such as Hispanic, Navajo, Filipino, and Vietnamese, will not give their infants colostrum. These women begin breastfeeding only after the transitional milk comes in and, therefore, will reject attempts to begin breastfeeding behavior in the immediate postpartum period.

How can nurses ensure good breastfeeding outcomes and still respect cultural differences, values, and beliefs?

Biology of Lactation

Lactation is the biologic completion of the reproductive cycle. Starting at about 16 weeks' gestation the breast develops and prepares for full lactation. In the first few postpartal hours and days the breast responds to hormones and the stimulation of the infant's sucking to produce and release milk.

Anatomy of the Breast

Nurses caring for new mothers need to have accurate knowledge about the anatomy and physiology of the lactating breast. The breasts are composed of adipose, fibrous, and glandular tissues. Deep within the glandular tissue are the treelike branching **alveoli** (secretory units of the mammary gland in which milk production takes place), or acini, arranged in a series of 15 to 42 lobes. Lobes are separated by adipose and fibrous tissues and are arranged like spokes converging on the central nipple. Each lobe is made up of many lobules. The lobules are made of many grapelike clusters of alveoli (acini) around small ducts. The ducts combine to form larger lactiferous ducts that open on the surface of the nipple (Figure 18-2).

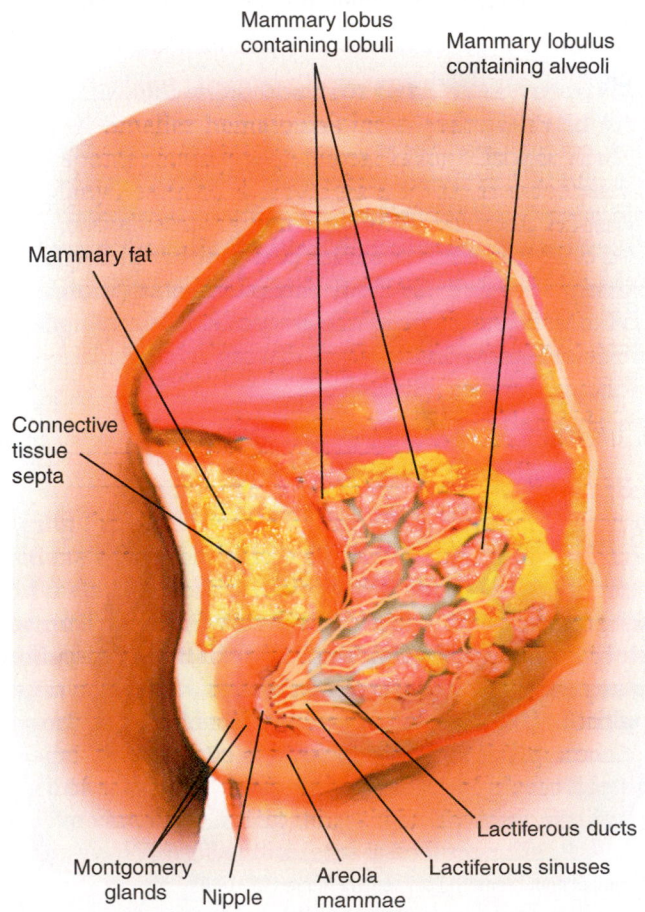

Figure 18-2 Anatomy of the breast.

At the center of each breast is the nipple, a conic elevation composed of erectile tissue that becomes more rigid during lactation, pregnancy, and sexual excitement. Each nipple contains 15 to 25 lactiferous ducts that end as small orifices near the tip of the nipple (Figure 18-3). The tissue surrounding the nipple is heavily pigmented and called the **areola**. Montgomery's tubercles, small papillae, are located in the areola. These tubercles secrete a substance that lubricates the nipples and areola during pregnancy and lactation.

Physiology of Lactation: Hormones and Processes

One of the biologic functions of the breasts is to supply nourishment and protective antibodies to infants during the lactation process. The hormonal control of lactation can be described under three main headings: **mammogenesis**, or mammary growth; **lactogenesis**, or initiation of milk secretion; and **galactopoiesis**, or the maintenance of established milk secretion. The nonpregnant breast does not ordinarily secrete any milklike substance but may enlarge slightly during the menstrual cycle. During pregnancy, changing levels of circulating hormones profoundly change the growth of the ducts, alveoli, and lobes in the breasts.

Mammogenesis

During lactation, the breast tissue is characterized by large numbers of alveoli. After lactation, when milk is no longer removed from the breast by the infant, the alveoli gradually collapse and adipose tissue increases.

Lactogenesis

Complex nervous and endocrine factors are involved in the establishment of milk production in the first 2 to 5 days postpartum (lactogenesis). Childbirth results in a rapid decrease in estrogen and progesterone and an increase in prolactin secretion. **Prolactin** is a hormone produced by the pituitary gland that triggers milk production by stimulating the alveolar cells of the breast. Prolactin levels increase in response to tactile stimulation of the breast and sucking by the infant. The increase in prolactin results in the synthesis of milk within the cells of the acini (Figure 18-4).

Let-down Reflex and Milk Ejection

The infant's sucking also stimulates the release of oxytocin. **Oxytocin** is a hormone produced by the posterior pituitary that stimulates uterine contractions and release of milk from the mammary glands. Oxytocin increases the contractility of the myoepthelial cells that line the walls of the mammary ducts, resulting in the let-down reflex (Figure 18-5). The **let-down reflex** is the ejection of milk from the breast and milk flow toward the nipple triggered by nipple stimulation or emotional response to the infant.

Milk ejection involves both neural and endocrinologic stimulation and response. Interference with the ejection reflex usually is due to psychologic inhibition caused by stress of some kind, such as disapproval of breastfeeding by a family member. Once lactation is well established, prolactin decreases, while oxytocin and suckling continue to be important in maintaining milk supply.

Establishment of Milk Supply

The nurse also needs to instruct the new mother that because breast milk is based on supply and demand, the best way to increase breast milk supply is for the infant to demand more by nursing often. Therefore, supplementation with formula or glucose water decreases the demand, and the supply diminishes. The nurse should advise the new mother to avoid giving supplemental bottles because doing so will interfere with establishing her milk supply and may lead to *nipple preference* (the refusal of the infant to go from bottle to breast and vice versa). Encouraging night feedings and preparing the client for infant growth spurts (that usually occur at 10 to 14 days, 6 weeks, 3 to 4

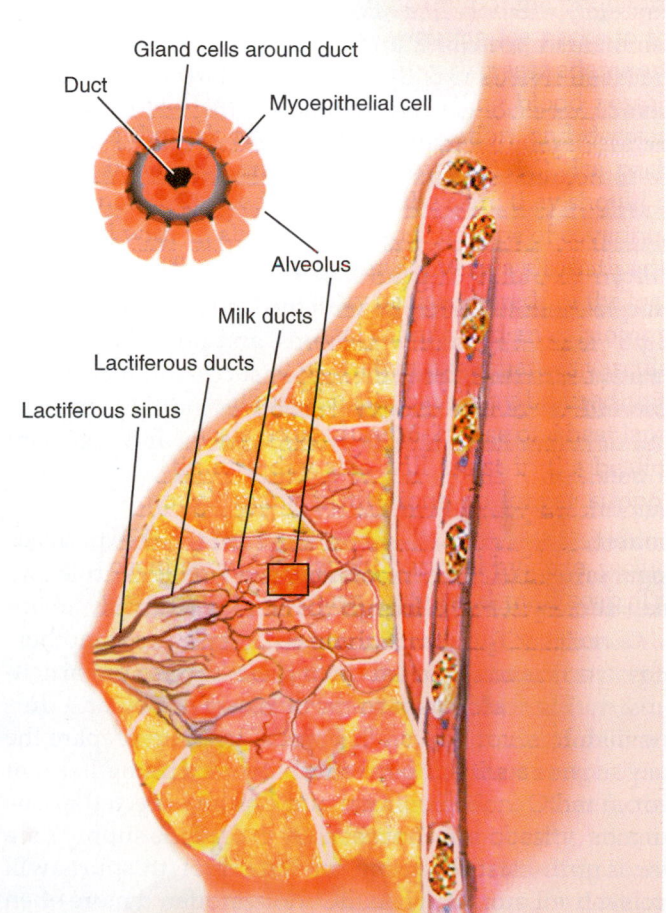

Figure 18-3 Duct system of the breast.

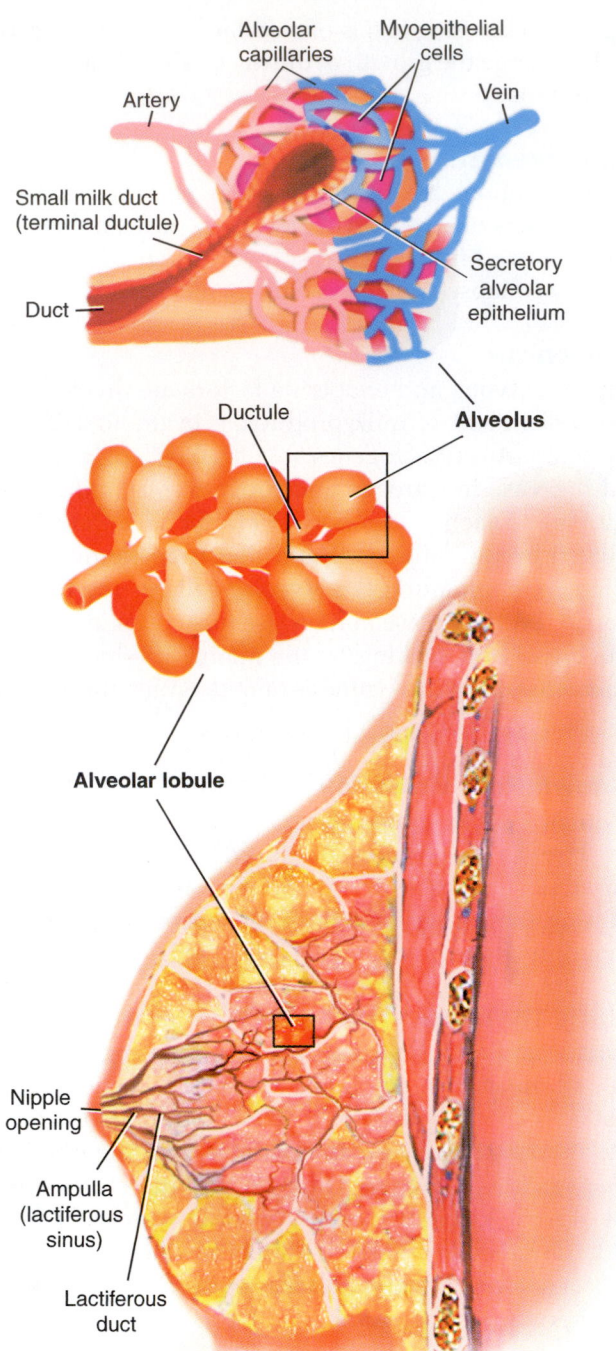

Figure 18-4 Physiology of lactation.

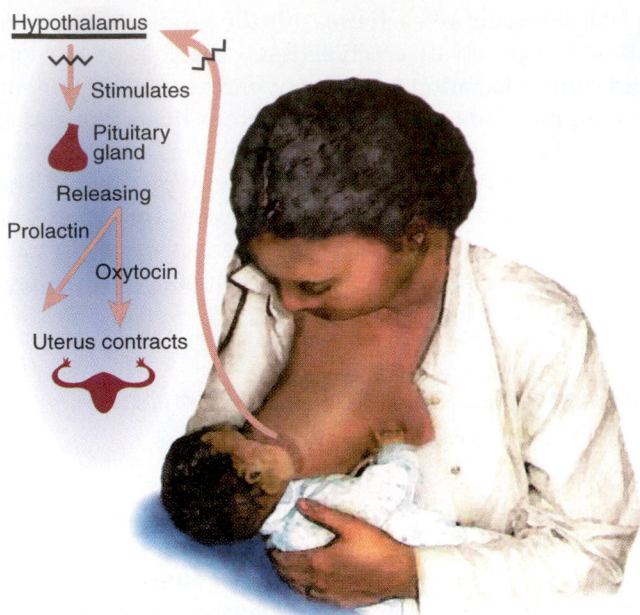

Figure 18-5 Physiology of the let-down reflex.

tentment after breastfeeding. The stools of breastfed infants differ from those of formula-fed infants in color and consistency. Stools from the breastfed infant are golden yellow, sweet smelling, and loose or liquid in consistency. Breastfed infants usually regain their birth weight by 14 days of age, then gain approximately 15 g/d (0.5 oz/d) in the first 6 months of life. Birth weight usually is doubled by approximately 5 months of age (Riordan & Auerbach, 1999).

Interference with Lactation

Many factors can interfere with the lactation process. Maternal anxiety, medical conditions, and poor diet, all can contribute to the success or lack of success in breastfeeding Additional factors might include pendulous breasts, flat or inverted nipples, post-op pain, and deficient knowledge.

Anxiety Mothers who are breastfeeding may experience some problems coping with their new maternal role and may develop fears or anxieties. The nurse can play an important role in diminishing anxiety. For example, mothers may worry about not producing enough milk, particularly during the first few days of breastfeeding and during infant growth spurts. The nurse can help prepare the new mother to handle these fears by reminding her that these emotions are common and can be expected as the infant's demand may occasionally exceed the supply for a few days. Milk production for these growth spurts will correct itself quickly when the breast is offered more often and for longer periods of time.

months, and 6 months) will reduce concern about the lack of an adequate milk supply.

The client also needs to be taught that infants usually feed every 2 to 3 hours during the first 3 to 4 weeks. Frequent demand for feedings may concern the new parents, and they may wonder if the infant is getting enough to eat. Signs of adequate intake include 8 to 10 wet diapers in 24 hours, frequent stooling, steady weight gain, and con-

Medical Problems The breastfeeding mother who has a serious medical condition or who suddenly develops a condition that requires hospitalization or management with surgery presents an unusual situation. It is obvious that the medical condition must be addressed promptly; however, it is also important to treat the mother as a lactating woman. Questions must be answered such as whether or not the condition is life-threatening or contagious and whether the drugs necessary for treatment will pass into the breast milk and adversely affect the infant. The other questions that must be taken into consideration are the prognosis for recovery and how long recovery will take. When the prognosis is poor and drugs prescribed for the mother are contraindicated in the infant, the decision to discontinue breastfeeding may be the only alternative. If breastfeeding must be discontinued abruptly, this can lead to engorgement and cause an influenza-like syndrome in the mother that may confuse the medical picture (Lawrence, 1999).

Nutrition and Fluid Intake Breastfeeding mothers will need approximately 500 additional calories per day compared with mothers feeding their infants formula (Figure 18-6). An average of 2,500 calories per day are needed while lactating. This calorie intake can be met through a properly balanced diet. The increase is met through certain food groups, especially protein sources and dairy products. Lactating women should also increase their intake of fluids, calcium, and folic acid. A proper diet promotes a good supply of milk and maintains maternal health. Prenatal vitamins are usually continued during the lactation period. Fluid requirements can be met by drinking at least six 8 oz glasses of water or caffeine-free drinks every day (Figure 18-7). Increasing fluid intake above normal levels, however, will not increase the milk supply (Reifsnider & Gill, 2000).

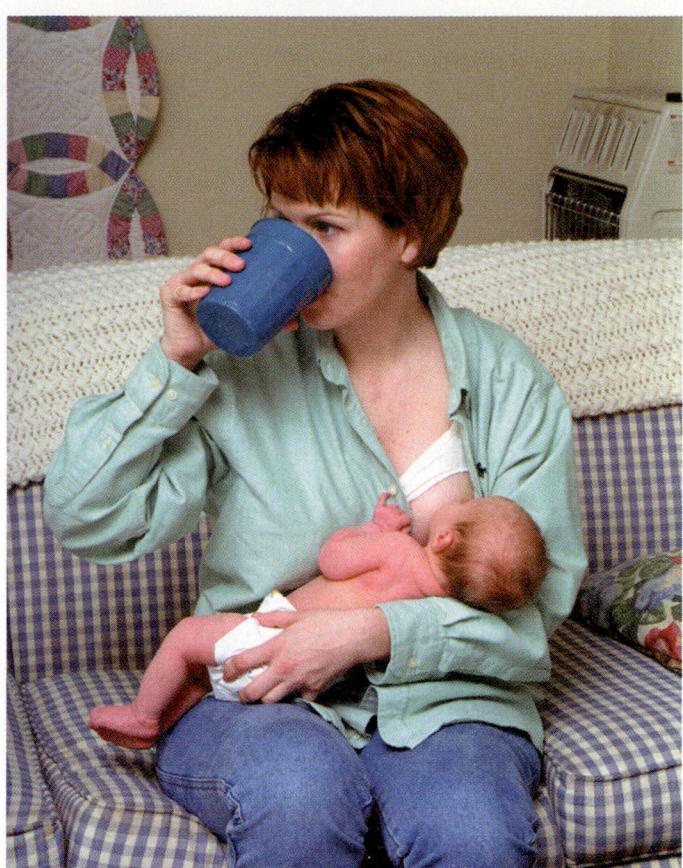

Figure 18-7 Increased fluid intake is especially important for the breastfeeding woman.

Promoting Successful Breastfeeding

Although breastfeeding is a natural process, breastfeeding skills must be learned and practiced. It may help to tell the new mother that she and her infant are both learning new skills. The nurse can promote successful breastfeeding through timely interventions to correct any problems before they undermine the mother's confidence in her ability to feed her baby. The nurse assisting the new

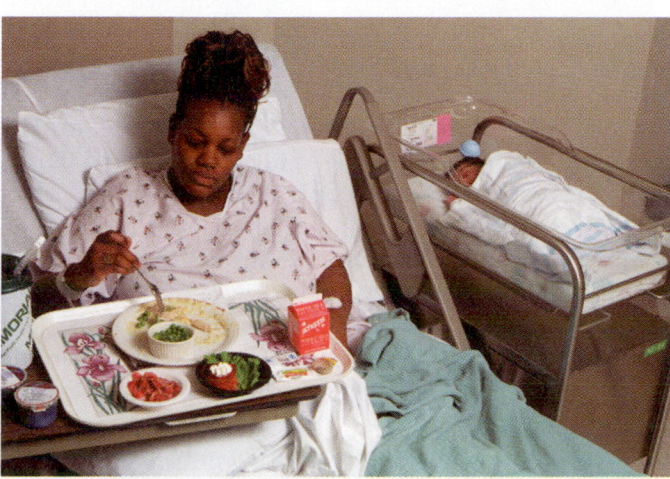

Figure 18-6 Breastfeeding mothers need an additional 500 cal/d.

Reflections from a Father

My wife breastfed all three of our children. I enjoyed watching her develop a close bond with each child as they nursed. I admit that sometimes, as a new dad, I felt left out. So we decided that my role was to burp the baby during and after each feeding. I loved this! Feedings became a family event, each of us with our own important role to play.

mother needs to assess the woman's prior experience with breastfeeding (through self, family, or friends). This individualizes the content of instruction and the type of assistance for each breastfeeding mother.

Maternal

The mother needs to find a comfortable position before beginning so that she can relax. She will enjoy breastfeeding much more and experience the let-down reflex more easily when comfortable. Next, she must position her infant so that she and her infant are comfortable and the breast is supported. She needs to cup her breast in one hand with all four fingers underneath and the thumb on top, making sure that the fingers and thumb are not touching the areola, while supporting the baby's head with the other hand (Figure 18-8).

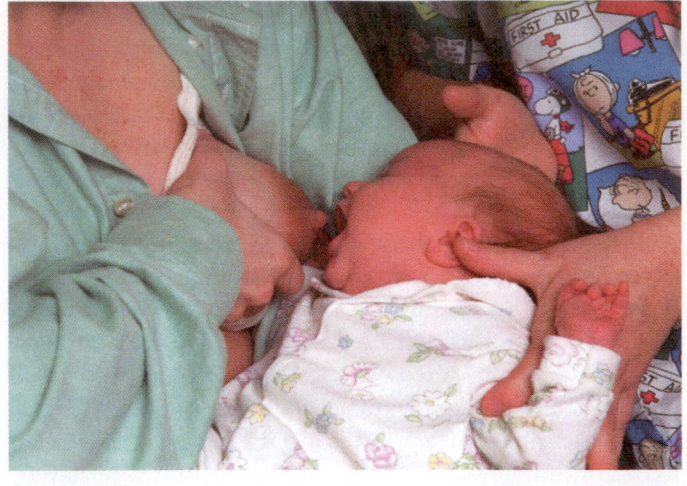

A.

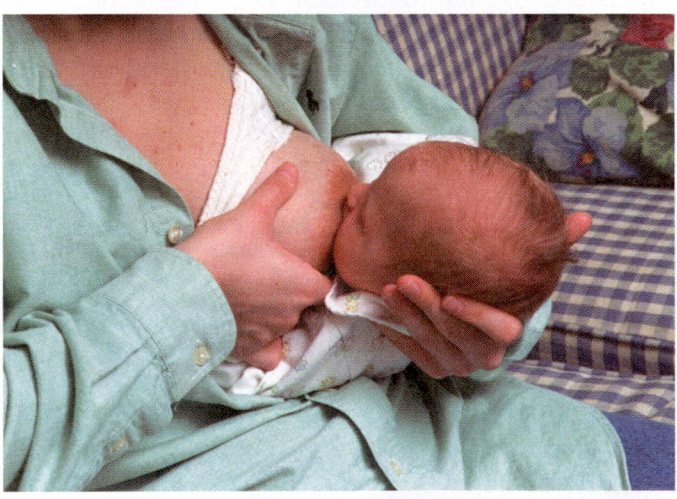

B.

Figure 18-9   Initiating latch-on. A. Touching the baby's lips with the nipple stimulates the rooting reflex. B. Once the baby opens the mouth wide, the mother can pull the baby's head to her breast.

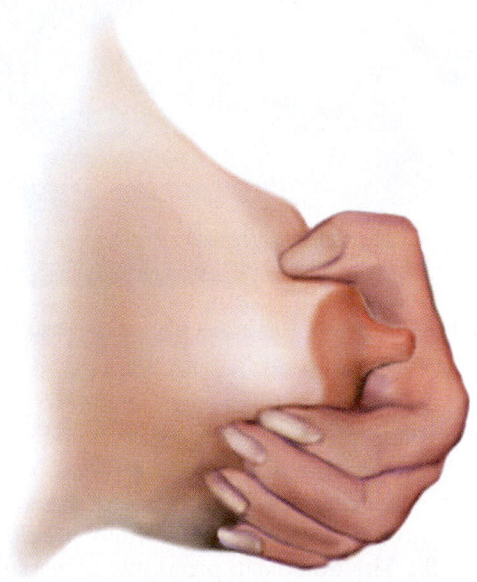

A.

B.

Figure 18-8   C-hold technique. A. Hand placement. B. Position of infant.

When the mother touches the baby's lips with her nipple she will activate the rooting reflex in her baby, and the infant will open the mouth wide (Figure 18-9a). The mother can pull the baby's head to her breast, and the infant will latch on to the nipple (Figure 18-9b). Correct latching-on will occur when the nipple and most of the areola are in the baby's mouth, and the baby's lips are pursed out as opposed to tucked under, forming solid suction. The sucking may cause discomfort for the first few seconds; however, the discomfort will stop when the baby settles into a rhythmic sucking pattern (Methodist Hospital, 1999).

Research suggests that nipple soreness is not related to the length of time the infant is at the breast but to improper positioning or improper removal of the infant from the breast (Mohrbacher & Stock, 1997). Inserting a finger into the corner of the sucking infant's mouth to break the suction will facilitate removing the infant without damage to the nipple (Figure 18-10).

After removing the infant from the breast, the mother needs to be taught how the infant may be burped in any one of three positions (Figure 18-11). Burping will allow any swallowed air to be released from the infant's stomach. The mother should position the infant upright, with the head resting on the mother's shoulder. The mother can then rub or pat the infant's back with her hand, while supporting the infant's buttocks with her other hand. A mother may prefer to burp the infant by placing the infant face down across the mother's lap. While holding the infant's head with one hand, the mother can rub or pat the infant's back with the other. An infant also may be burped by holding the infant upright on the mother's lap, supporting the head from the front with one hand and patting or rubbing the back with the other.

Infant

It is important to determine the gestational age of the neonate, as this can affect his nursing ability. In order to determine if the neonate is ready to be breastfed, the nurse or mother can test the rooting and sucking reflexes (Figure 18-12). Stimulation of the rooting reflex can be accomplished by stroking the infant's cheek toward the lips. The infant should turn toward the side that is being stroked. The mother can insert her finger into the infant's mouth and gently stroke the soft palate to trigger the sucking reflex. Sucking should be strong, and the tongue should curve around the finger. When the infant sucks strongly on the mother's finger, breastfeeding can begin. Sucking patterns differ in bottle-fed versus breastfed infants. In breastfeeding the tongue presses the nipple against the hard palate, forcing milk from the ducts and sinuses (Figure 18-13).

Latching-on

The nurse can help the new mother by teaching her to position her infant's nose at the level of her own nipple and then to brush the nipple across the baby's lower lip. Doing so will cause the infant to open the mouth wide (**rooting reflex**), allowing the mother to bring her nipple in toward the upper part of the infant's mouth. The rooting reflex is the normal response of the newborn to move toward whatever touches the area around the mouth. The rooting reflex facilitates proper **latching-on** (attachment of the infant to the breast for feeding) to the entire areola, not just the end of the nipple. Riordan and Auerbach (1999) state that both breasts should be offered at each feeding to more rapidly stimulate milk production quickly. Each breast should be offered frequently for at least 15 minutes every 2 hours or on demand, whichever occurs first. After breastfeeding is established the client should let the infant complete a feeding on one breast before offering the other.

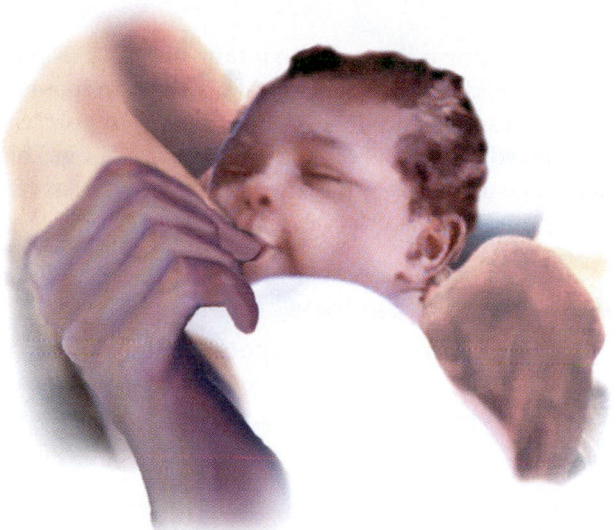

Figure 18-10   Removing the infant from the breast.

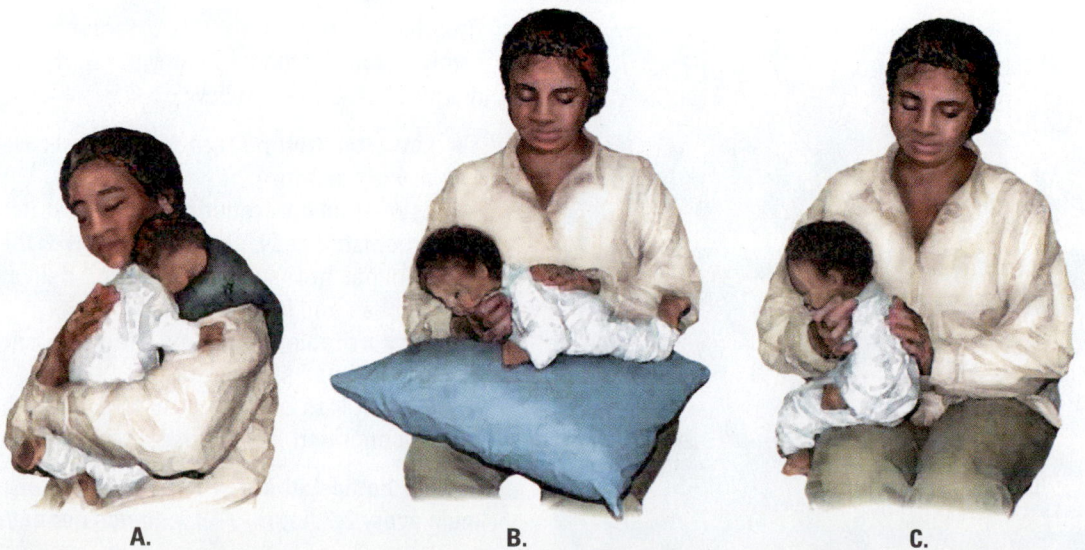

   A.   B.   C.

Figure 18-11   Burping positions. A. Supported on the shoulder. B. Face down across the lap. C. Upright on the lap.

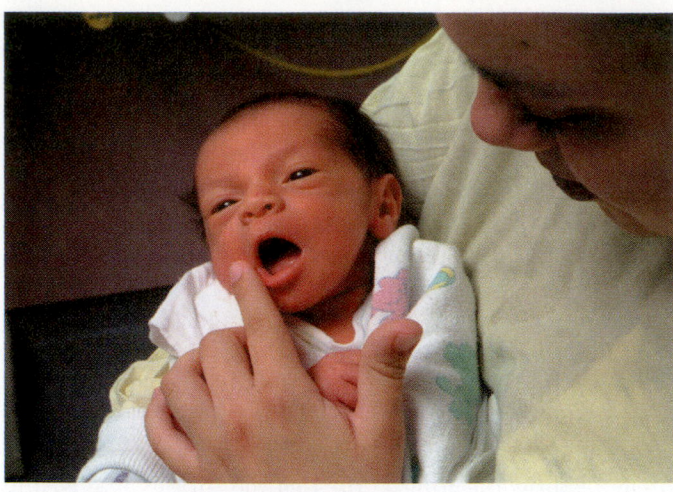

A.

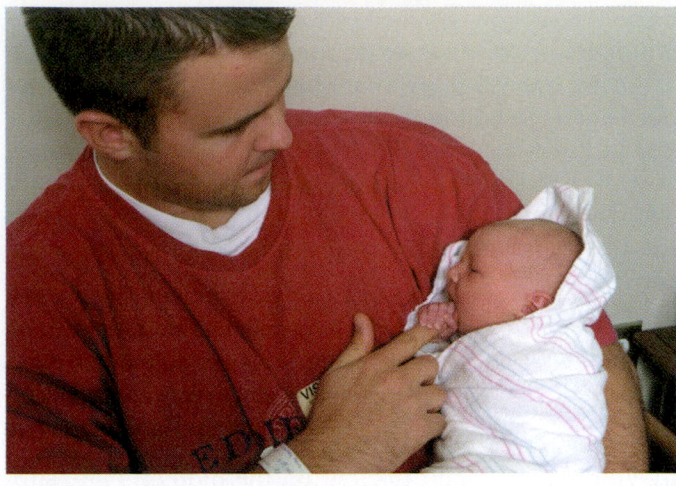

B.

Figure 18-12   Judging readiness to nurse. A. Stroking the cheek next to the baby's mouth elicits the rooting reflex. B. This newborn is attempting to suck on her father's finger.

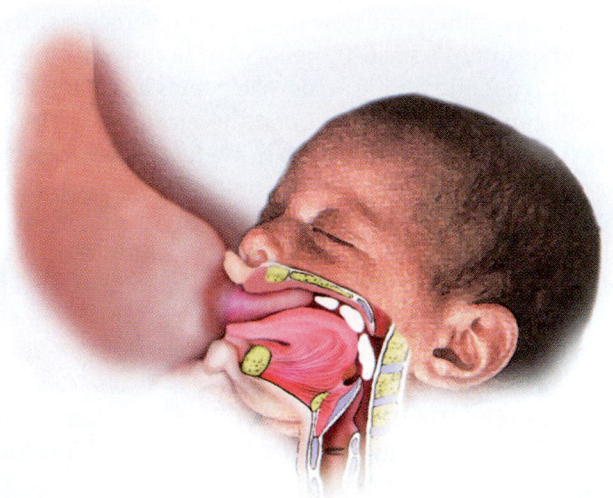

Figure 18-13   Proper positioning for successful latch-on.

As milk volume adjusts to the infant's needs this pattern may change, depending on the infant's requirements during growth spurts. Frequently, mothers will report feeling very relaxed, almost sleepy, during breastfeeding. This relaxed state is a side benefit of the hormone oxytocin, which promotes maternal rest.

Nursing Implications

Whether or not an infant is responsive and eager to suck immediately after delivery can be affected by external factors such as epidural anesthesia, narcotics, tocolytics, and

Client Education

Feeding Readiness Cues

Confirm that parents know to respond to early feeding readiness cues:

- Sucking movements
- Sucking sounds
- Hand-to-mouth movements
- Rapid eye movements
- Soft cooing or sighing sounds
- Fussiness

Nursing Tip   *Infant Assessment for Insufficient Lactation*

Possible signs of insufficient lactation in the exclusively breastfeeding infant-mother dyad in the first month after delivery follow:

- Low urination pattern (at least six wet diapers a day is the norm)
- Low stooling frequency (at least three yellow-greenish, seedy, soft stools a day is the norm)
- Minimal breast changes after delivery (such as fullness and leaking of milk)
- Very irritable or sleepy infant, nursing less than seven times a day
- Weight loss of more than 10% of the birth weight, or continued weight loss after day 10 of life

For the bottle-fed infant intake of 4 oz or more of formula every 2-3 hours, 6-10 feedings per day is the norm.

length of labor. For the healthy full-term newborn, no contraindications exist to feeding immediately after delivery. Most infants are highly responsive and eager to suck during the first 30 minutes after delivery. The nurse can use this time to teach and help initiate successful breastfeeding behaviors.

When working with a new mother, the nurse should always stay at her eye level to decrease the anxiety that any new activity causes the learner. Proper positioning at the breast can decrease the problem of ineffective breastfeeding by teaching the mother different comfortable positions that enhance feeding behaviors. The mother should be made as comfortable as possible either in her bed or chair and given as much privacy as needed. Mothers who have delivered by cesarean section usually need more help to find a comfortable position because of the abdominal incision and the pain related to movement. The woman may need to void before beginning to breastfeed, and she should be instructed to wash her hands each time she nurses her infant.

There are three common breastfeeding positions that can be used by most mothers. These positions are the cradle hold, the football hold, and the side-lying position (Figure 18-14).

Issues Related to Breastfeeding

According to the American Academy of Pediatrics policy statement (1997, pp. 1035–1039), "Extensive research, especially in recent years, documents diverse and compelling advantages to infants, mothers, families, and society from breastfeeding and the use of human milk for infant feeding. These include health, nutritional,

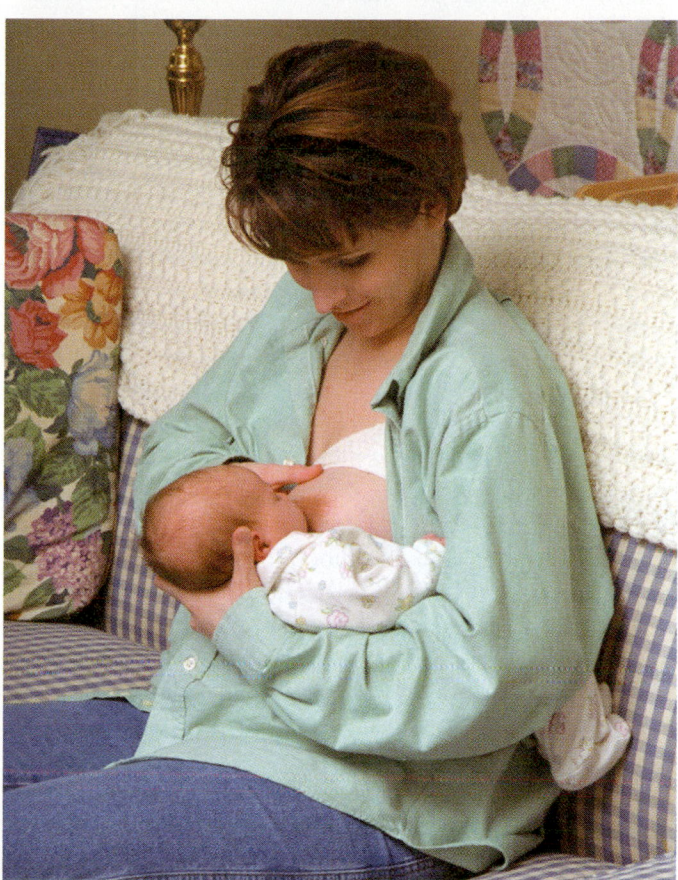

B.

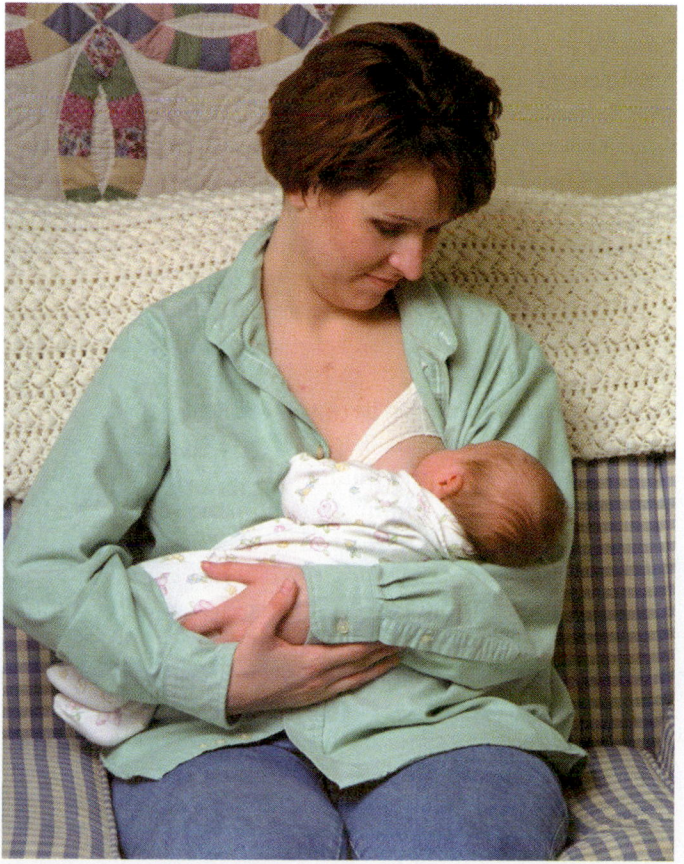

A.

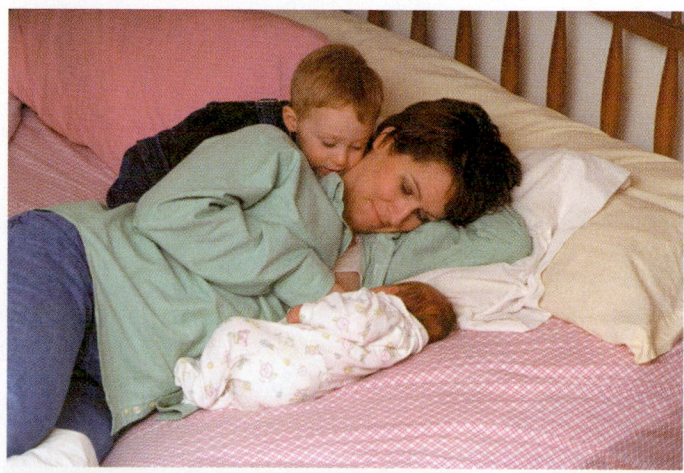

C.

Figure 18-14   Breastfeeding holds. A. Cradle hold. B. Football hold. C. Side-lying hold.

immunologic, developmental, psychological, social, economic, and environmental benefits."

Benefits

The benefits of breastfeeding include but are not limited to the fact that it provides for optimum infant growth, health, and development. Breast milk also has been shown to decrease the incidence and severity of many childhood illnesses, provide a protective effect against several diseases, and enhance cognitive development. A number of research studies indicate there are health benefits to breastfeeding, including a decrease in maternal and infant morbidity and mortality. Research studies also have found a link between breastfeeding and a decrease in the development of breast cancer in women who have breastfed. In addition to these individual benefits, breastfeeding provides significant social and economic benefits to the nation. These include reduced health care costs and reduced employee absenteeism (American Academy of Pediatrics, 1997).

Benefits to the Mother

Maternal benefits include lactational amenorrhea, which promotes a longer period of decreased fertility after the birth of an infant, and less blood loss from menstruation. New research demonstrates that lactating women have an earlier return to prepregnant weight, improved bone remineralization, reduction in hip fractures in the postmenopausal period, and reduced rates of ovarian cancer and premenopausal breast cancer (American Academy of Pediatrics, 1997).

The release of oxytocin during breastfeeding causes the uterus to contract, hastening the involution of the uterus to its prepregnant state (Figure 18-15). This same action also reduces the chances of postpartal hemorrhage by keeping the uterus contracted.

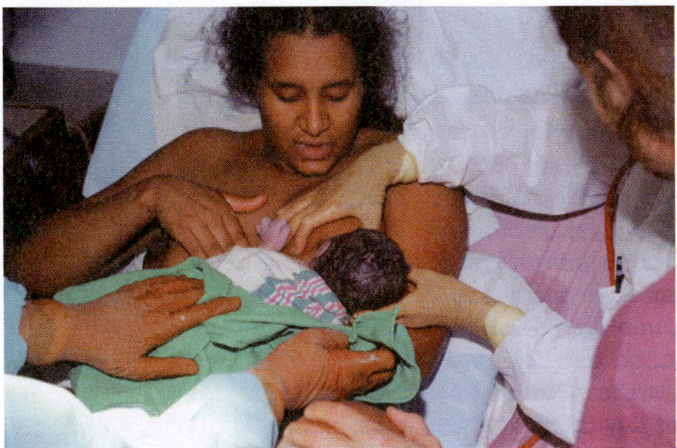

Figure 18-15 Breastfeeding immediately after delivery stimulates involution of the uterus.

Critical Thinking

Comparison of Breast Milk with Formula

- Breast milk is nutritionally superior to formula.
- Breast milk contains immunoglobulins, enzymes, and leukocytes to protect against infection.
- Breast milk is less expensive than formula.
- Breast milk is easily available at a perfect temperature and with no preparation.
- Breast milk may reduce allergies.
- Breastfeeding may enhance mother-infant attachment.
- Breastfeeding promotes the development of jaw and facial muscles.
- Breast milk reduces the risk of bacterial contamination.

How can a nurse help promote breastfeeding among all women of childbearing age?

Breastfeeding promotes weight loss after delivery because of the greater expenditure of energy and calories needed during lactation. Breastfeeding also provides new mothers with many psychosocial advantages. The increased levels of oxytocin in the nursing mother's bloodstream are believed to coincide with more even mood responses and increased feelings of maternal well-being (Lawrence, 1999). Many researchers believe that increased levels of oxytocin promote maternal-infant bonding and protective behaviors. Attachment is the development of an enduring relationship between the infant and the caregiver (Klaus, Kennell, & Klaus, 1995). Breastfeeding increases the quantity and quality of early contact between the mother and her infant, thus enhancing the strength of the relationship. Klaus et al. (1995) have stated that early and continuous mother-infant contact appears to decrease infant abandonment and increase the length and success of breastfeeding.

Exclusive breastfeeding has been found to delay ovulation and thus acts as a natural birth control method. Breastfeeding makes a woman less likely to conceive; however, the degree of protection depends on many variables, such as hormonal levels, nipple stimulation, and frequency of feedings. Ovulation and a return to fertility typically will occur within 4 to 6 weeks in the nonnursing mother. Breastfeeding extends the normal period of anovulation by sending impulses to the hypothalamus that decrease the release of gonadotropins. The woman who desires the use of this method of contraception needs to continue to fully or nearly fully breastfeed her infant, must remain amenorrheic, and must be feeding frequently (including during the night) for the method to work (Lawrence, 1999).

The cost of formula is about twice that of the extra food needed by the lactating mother (Jarosz, 1993.)

The costs of increased morbidity and mortality associated with formula feeding include medical costs, physician visits, medicine, and hospitalizations. The hidden costs associated with these problems are lost wages to parents of sick children and increased premiums for health care insurance.

Benefits to the Infant

Breast milk has been called the perfect food for infants because it contains all necessary nutrients in readily bioavailable forms, while providing many immunologic components at the same time. Human milk is considered a living tissue, such as blood, and is capable of affecting biochemical systems, increasing immunity, and even destroying pathogens (Newman, 1995). The main selling point for manufacturers of infant formula continues to be the comparison of how closely the product conforms to the gold standard of breast milk.

Natural Variation in Composition of Human Milk.

Over 200 constituents have been identified in breast milk, and researchers are just beginning to understand the impact that these changing constituents have on the infant. Moreover, milk composition changes as the infant nurses at each feeding.

Transitional milk is produced at the end of colostrum production and immediately before mature milk comes into the breast. **Foremilk** is the thin, watery breast milk secreted at the beginning of a feeding. Foremilk is low in calories but high in water-soluble vitamins. **Hindmilk** is the thick, high-fat breast milk secreted at the end of a feeding. Hindmilk is ejected approximately 10 to 15 minutes after the initial "let down" and has the highest concentratation of calories. Hindmilk is thicker and richer in appearance than is foremilk owing to its higher fat content essential for the infant's proper growth and development. **Mature milk** is breast milk that contains 10% solids for energy and growth.

The nutritional needs of the infant vary with the unique differences of each stage of the new baby's development. Breast milk supplies all of the nutrients to meet the ever-changing demands of the baby from newborn to toddler stage. The infant's diet must provide adequate calories and must include sufficient protein, carbohydrates, fat, water, vitamins, and minerals to meet the rapid rate of both physical and mental growth and development (Lawrence, 1999).

Epidemiologic research shows that human milk may provide a possible protective effect against sudden infant death syndrome (SIDS), insulin-dependent diabetes mellitus, lymphoma, Crohn's disease, ulcerative colitis, allergic diseases, and other chronic digestive diseases. Breastfeeding also has been related to enhancement of intelligence and visual acuity (American Academy of Pediatrics, 1997).

The immunologic benefits of breastfeeding for infants are well-known and include varying degrees of protection against many types of infections. Breastfeeding has a positive effect on the overall health of the infant because it provides increased protection from meningitis, sepsis, otitis media, and respiratory and gastrointestinal (GI) diseases. These benefits are due to the many components of colostrum and breast milk present in varying amounts, depending on the specific environment of the mother-baby dyad. **Colostrum** is the thin fluid present in the breast from pregnancy into the early pospartal period. Colostrum is rich in antibodies, which provide protection from many diseases; high in protein, which binds bilirubin; and acts as a laxative, speeding the elimination of meconium and helping loosen mucus.

Researchers have shown that colostrum and human milk contain a specific factor called bifidus factor that supports the growth of *Lactobacillus bifidum*, which offers protection against many intestinal disorders. Exclusive breastfeeding also reduces the likelihood of exposure to infection that arises when contaminated food is introduced (Kovar, Serdula, Marks, & Fraser, 1984).

The collection of antibodies transmitted to the infant is highly targeted against pathogens in the child's immediate surroundings. The mother synthesizes specific antibodies when she inhales or ingests an environmental disease-causing agent, thus protecting the infant against

Nursing Alert

Assisting with Breastfeeding

When teaching clients about breastfeeding, you should wear disposable gloves while:

- Assisting new mothers to breastfeed immediately after delivery
- Handling the mother's breasts during expression of milk
- Handling breast pads
- Handling breast milk for storage or milk banking

You must wash your hands before and after gloving!

those specific infectious agents most likely to cause illness (Newman, 1995).

Working with Barriers to Breastfeeding

Barriers or deterrents to breastfeeding may be biologic, psychologic, social, or cultural in nature. The risk-to-benefit ratio of breastfeeding compared with bottle-feeding must be assessed by the woman and her health care provider to arrive at the best decision for both the mother and her infant.

Biologic Barriers

Although most women are physically capable of breast-feeding, a biologic problem may occasionally interfere with lactation. The problem can be due to abnormal breast anatomy such as unilateral or bilateral hypoplasia. Acquired abnormalities of the breasts from trauma, burns, or radiation also may interfere with lactation. Clients with biologic barriers must be carefully evaluated on a case-by-case basis to determine if lactation is possible.

Maternal Barriers. Maternal barriers to breastfeeding can be due to physical problems, medical or disease conditions, hormonal factors, or psychiatric disorders. Insufficient milk supply may be attributed to many factors, including insufficient glandular tissue, diet, illness, fatigue, psychologic factors, drugs, and smoking. When these factors have been ruled out, the cause may involve imbalances in hormone production or secretion. The most common reason for insufficient milk supply, however, is the early use of supplemental feedings, which results in decreased nursing time.

Maternal Breast Surgery. Augmentation mammoplasty has become an acceptable surgical procedure that can have implications for the breastfeeding mother. Breast-feeding can be successful when there is no destruction of breast tissue or interruption of ducts, nerve supply, or blood supply to the breast tissue or nipple.

Reduction mammoplasty is a surgical procedure to reduce the size of very large breasts. This type of surgery is more destructive to breast tissue than is augmentation because of the necessity of replacing the nipples symmetrically, which requires interruption of the milk ducts. There are many new surgical methods now for both breast reduction and breast augmentation that are designed to improve the likelihood of successful breastfeeding.

Breast surgery for nonmalignant tumors usually does not preclude breastfeeding unless the ductal structure has been interrupted. Women with a periareolar incision have a fivefold risk of lactation insufficiency (Lawrence, 1999).

Nipple Inversion. Flat or inverted nipples do not preclude breastfeeding and may respond to breast shells. Breast shells are vented plastic disks with holes in the center and a dome cover that allows the nipples to evert (Figure 18-16). The shell is slipped into the cup of a brassiere. The shells can be worn during the last trimester. However, research has shown no significant difference between groups of women who have used breast shells and groups who have used exercises that pull and stretch the nipple (Hoffman exercises) before delivery. Physicians caution women to avoid nipple stimulation because of the possibility of causing uterine contractions or preterm labor (Lawrence, 1999).

Nipple shields made of silicone are now frequently used to allow the infant to latch on to a nipple that is more difficult to grasp (Figure 18-17). The mother is taught to pump her breasts after each nursing session to build up her milk supply while using the nipple shields. After the nipples are everted and the milk supply is built up the mother is encouraged to gradually wean the infant to the bare nipple (Martin, 2000).

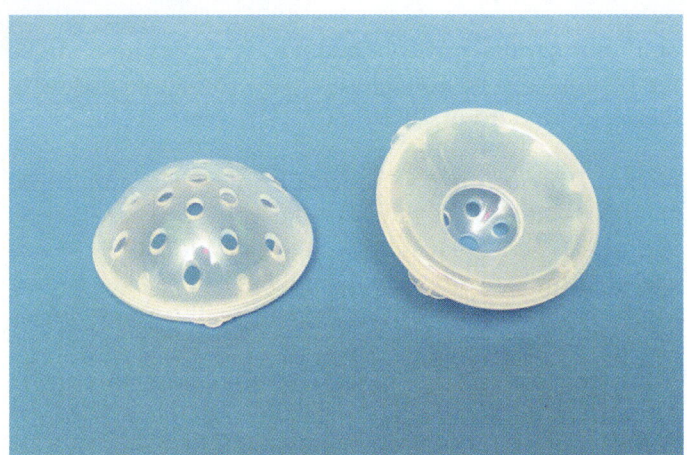

Figure 18-16 Breast shells.

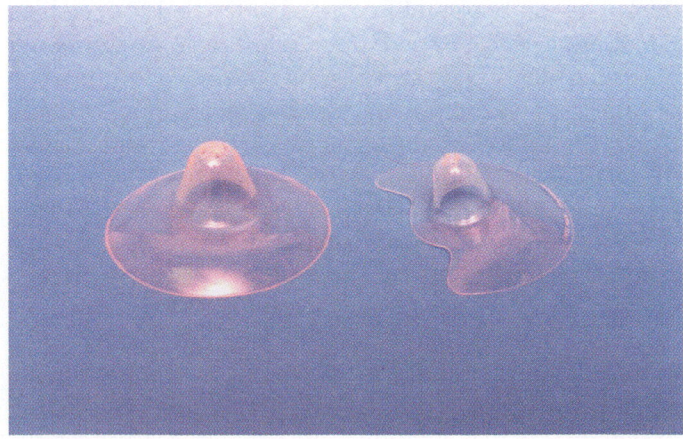

Figure 18-17 Nipple shields.

Contraceptive Use. Use of a contraceptive method in a breastfeeding mother is a particularly important decision, because ovulation may occur before the onset of menses. Nonhormonal methods, such as condoms, cervical caps, and diaphragms, can be effective in preventing pregnancy when used correctly and consistently. Spermicides also may be used in the postpartum period.

Intrauterine devices (IUDs) are a very effective method of contraception available to nursing mothers and can be inserted only after uterine involution is complete.

Hormonal contraceptive methods must be used in the breastfeeding mother with caution because some hormonal methods will interfere with milk production. Oral contraceptives containing only progestin are very effective when used in combination with breastfeeding. They also have a minimal effect on milk production.

In 1981, the American Academy of Pediatrics approved the use of combination oral contraceptives in women electing to breastfeed once lactation is well established. Estrogen has been reported to reduce milk supply in several studies (Lawrence, 1999; Riordan & Auerbach, 1999). Therefore, alternative contraceptive methods should be considered as a first choice in lactating women, particularly during the first 6 weeks postpartum. The WHO has suggested that the combination oral contraceptive should not be the first choice for women who are lactating (World Health Organization, 1988, 1994).

Depot medroxyprogesterone acetate (Depo-Provera) does not significantly suppress milk production when administered to the lactating woman after the milk supply is established (4-6 weeks postpartum), and is an effective contraceptive method for breastfeeding women. Subdermal implants that contain progestin do not affect the breastfed infant and may be inserted at 6 weeks postpartum after lactation is established (Lawrence, 1999). Vaginal dryness from hormonal influences during breastfeeding may cause dyspareunia for some nursing mothers. Vaginal lubricants, such K-Y jelly, can sometimes help alleviate this problem. A sudden change in vaginal lubrication can sometimes indicate ovulation.

Infant Barriers. Most normal full-term infants can breastfeed with only minor adjustments. The infant with a medical or surgical problem presents a need for special interventions that ensure adequate newborn nutrition.

Prematurity. Low-birth-weight and premature infants present unique nutritional problems. Optimal growth for premature infants is considered to be the growth curve they would have normally followed if they had remained inside the uterus. Although human milk provides the ideal nutrients, it would require an inordinate volume to achieve adequate amounts of some nutrients. These needs can be met by artificial formula or supplementation.

Preterm milk has been found to contain special properties that are uniquely suited to meet the needs of the premature infant (Figure 18-18). Preterm milk contains higher levels of fat, protein, and other necessary nutrients than term milk. Many mothers of preterm infants require instructions on how to build up their milk supply with electric breast pumps. The milk may be used to feed very low-birth-weight infants by feeding tube until the infant is strong enough to nurse on his own.

The protective properties of human milk against infection are considered a very important reason to provide human milk to preterm infants. An acute inflammatory disease of the GI mucosa commonly seen in the premature infant is called necrotizing enterocolitis (NEC).

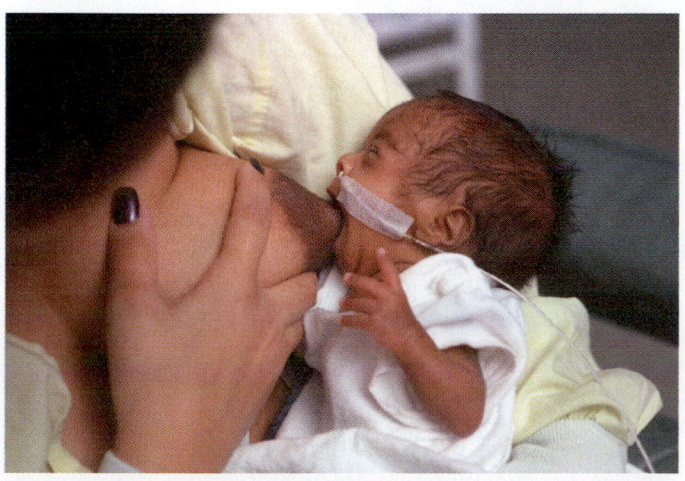

A.

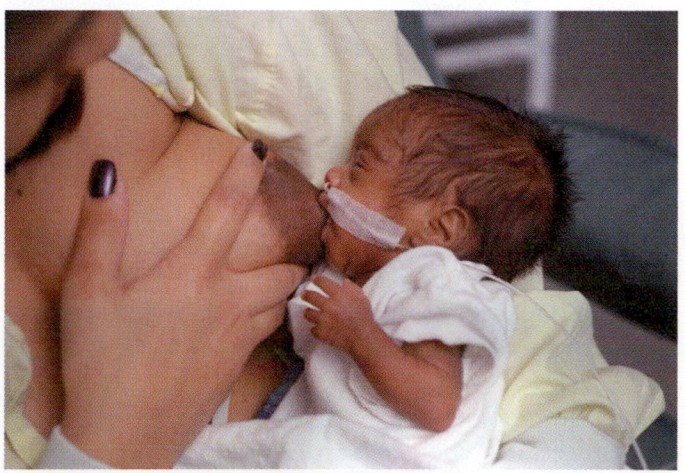

B.

Figure 18-18   This preterm infant, who has been gavage feeding, is trying breastfeeding for the first time. A. The mother elicits the rooting reflex, and the baby responds by opening the mouth wide. B. The baby gets the nipple into the mouth but not much of the areola.

Human milk has been associated with a decreased incidence of this life-threatening condition (Lawrence, 1999).

Recent research has demonstrated that the use of small, thin, silicone nipple shields in preterm infants significantly increases milk transfer (Meier et al., 2000). The nipple shield makes it easier for the preterm infant to stay latched on to the breast and extract milk.

Illness and Disability. Infants with meconium aspiration or transient tachypnea of the newborn (TTN) are focused on establishing adequate oxygenation via a compromised respiratory system. These infants are often initially bottle fed breast milk or formula. Breastfeeding mothers of these infants may require assistance with the latching-on process when allowed to nurse their infants.

Down syndrome or other congenital anomalies may make breastfeeding more difficult. Down syndrome infants have a thicker tongue, which may not curl around the mother's nipple as easily.

Hypoglycemia. Hypoglycemia during the early neonatal period of a term infant is defined as a blood glucose concentration of less than 35 mg/dL, or a plasma concentration of less than 40 mg/dL.

Hypoglycemia during the first 3 hours after delivery usually has a physiologic cause. Early, frequent breastfeeding helps prevent lowered blood glucose levels. Because colostrum contains 18 cal/oz compared with 6 cal/oz for 5% glucose water, newborns are less likely to experience hypoglycemia when feeding is not supplemented with glucose water after delivery. Colostrum also has higher levels of protein than does glucose water and therefore has a stabilizing effect on blood glucose levels (ILCA, 1999).

Jaundice. Physiologic jaundice is a normal occurrence in 50% of term and 80% of preterm newborns and appears 24 hours after delivery. Neonatal jaundice occurs because the newborn has a high rate of bilirubin production, the result of the normal decomposition of fetal erythrocytes as the neonate transitions. Meconium is extremely high in bilirubin. Delayed stooling increases the amount of reabsorbed bilirubin. Colostrum is a natural laxative and promotes the excretion of meconium, thus decreasing bilirubin levels. More frequent breastfeedings also lowers the bilirubin level (Lawrence, 1999). Nursing at least 8 or more times a day increases fluid intake.

Psychologic Barriers

A number of psychologic barriers to breastfeeding exist. Bryant (1992) identified the following perceived barriers keeping women from breastfeeding:

- Lack of confidence in their ability to breastfeed
- Embarrassment

Nursing Alert

Management of Early Physiologic Jaundice While Breastfeeding

You should:

- Monitor all infants for initial stooling.
- Initiate breastfeeding early and frequently.
- Discourage water, dextrose water, and formula supplementation.
- Monitor weight, voidings, and stooling associated with breastfeeding.
- When the bilirubin level approaches 15 mg/dL, stimulate stooling by feeding the infant more often and stimulate breast milk production with pumping. When the bilirubin level exceeds 20 mg/dL, use phototherapy.

No evidence exists that early jaundice is associated with an abnormality of the breast milk; therefore, withdrawing breast milk is indicated only when jaundice persists for more than 6 days, the bilirubin level increases to above 20 mg/dL, or the mother has a history of having had an affected infant (Lawrence, 1999).

- Loss of freedom
- Concerns about dietary and health practices
- Influence of family and friends
- Other concerns, such as pain, fear of disfigurement, sexual feelings about breasts, invalid medical concerns, and a lack of social support

Modesty. Many women view their breasts as sexual objects and associate them with their ability to attract and please men. Because of these feelings many women are apprehensive about breastfeeding in front of other people, particularly men. Women may worry that nursing their infant in public will arouse men, make their husbands or boyfriends jealous, or look disgusting to others. Finding a private place to breastfeed while out in public is a very real concern for many women.

The nurse can help allay these fears by teaching the woman how to breastfeed discreetly by demonstrating how to cover her breasts while she is nursing and assuring her that most women are apprehensive about breastfeeding in front of others but usually adjust quickly once they begin to nurse. Most maternity shops sell blouses and tops that assist the new mother in breastfeeding discreetly. If she is one of the women who does not adjust,

Client Education

Sexuality and the Breastfeeding Woman

Sexual stimulus can trigger the milk ejection reflex in breastfeeding women, particularly during orgasm. This "let-down" of milk during sexual relations may have either a negative or positive effect on the sexual partner. Psychologic conflicts in the partner may be a result of misunderstanding of the let-down reflex. Practical solutions to unwanted spraying of milk during sexual relations include the following:

- Breastfeeding the infant immediately before sexual relations

- Expressing milk before beginning sexual relations

- Explaining the biologic phenomenon to couples, thus avoiding negative reactions

- Teaching couples that oral and manual manipulation and fondling of the breasts during lovemaking need not be restricted (Lawrence, 1999)

she can pump her breast milk and give the baby a bottle when she is in public.

Lack of Confidence. Some women lack confidence in their abilities to produce an adequate supply of nutritious breast milk. Few women understand the mechanics of breast milk production and are easily influenced by stories from other women whose milk "dried up" or couldn't satisfy their child's nutritional needs because it was too weak, blue in color, or too thin. If these stories come from an important social influence, such as a grandmother, they may take on special significance because of the possibility that the problem may have been passed on genetically to the new mother.

When women lack confidence in their own ability to make adequate and nutritious breast milk, they frequently will begin supplementing with formula. Doing so creates a downward spiral in breast milk production that becomes a self-fulfilling prophecy. Because infant formulas have labels that list the ingredients, many women will trust these products more than their own bodies. Not being able to accurately measure the amount of breast milk the infant is taking during nursing also seems less scientific than being able to measure formula taken in ounces, leading women to worry about the amount of milk being produced.

Social Barriers

Social support can be provided by a nurse, a lactation consultant, a family member, friends, peers, or a significant other. The attitude of the baby's father, health care providers, family, and friends all play a significant role in the establishment and continuation of breastfeeding. Organizations such as La Leche League can also be a tremendous help in overcoming barriers to breastfeeding (Figure 18-19). The nurse plays an important role in facilitating the new skills necessary to promote successful breastfeeding because the nurse frequently has the most direct and personal contact with new mothers.

The negative influence of family and friends or lack of social support is associated with a decrease in breastfeeding initiation and duration (Raj & Plichta, 1998). Studies of socioeconomic factors associated with lower breastfeeding rates include women who are unmarried, single, widowed, or divorced.

Nurses need to elicit the client's misconceptions and misperceptions to deal with them effectively. Simply saying, "Tell me what you have been told about breastfeeding" will help the client state her concerns in a nonthreatening environment (Bryant, 1992).

In addition to personal barriers to breastfeeding, subliminal messages linked to specific hospital policies and institutional procedures also can play an important role in feeding decisions.

Hospital Policies

Many studies have looked at the effect of institutional promotion of formula supplementation on breastfeeding outcomes. Most of these studies have reported a decrease in milk supply that seems to be directly related to the amount of supplementation of formula. Mothers who were given formula discharge packs were significantly less likely to be breastfeeding at 1 month and were more likely to have introduced solid foods by 2 months.

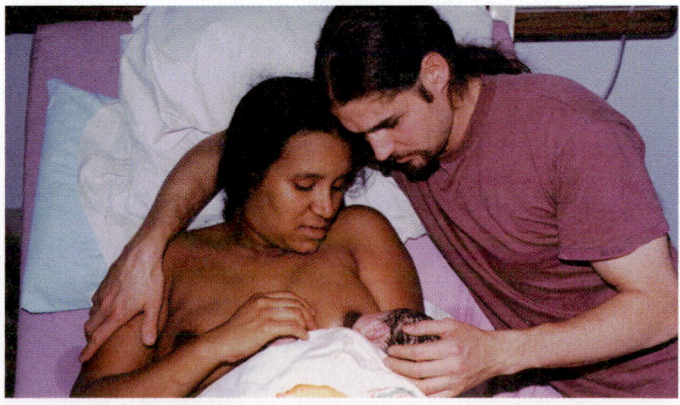

Figure 18-19   Involvement of the baby's father or other support persons in the breastfeeding process is more likely to result in successful breastfeeding.

Critical Thinking

Breastfeeding Myths

Can you answer clients' questions about breastfeeding myths? What information would you offer to counter each myth? Research and continue to dispel myths about breastfeeding.

- Women need to drink large amounts of fluids to produce large amounts of breast milk.

  Advice is simple: Drink fluids when thirsty.

- Women need to restrict the food they eat while breastfeeding.

  Advice is simple: There is no need to eliminate foods from the diet unless consumption of a certain food, such as onions, is followed by symptoms in the breastfed baby, such as excessive crying or gas.

- A mother cannot drink alcohol and continue breastfeeding.

  Advice is simple: There is no need to completely eliminate drinking alcohol while breastfeeding.

- Mothers and babies cannot sleep together.

  Advice is simple: Co-sleeping is safe and facilitates breastfeeding for mother and baby. The infant should be kept supine and soft materials are not allowed in the bed.

- Breastfeeding does not make breasts sag or become disfigured.

  Advice is simple: Wear a good supportive bra.

- A mother's anger will ruin or curdle her milk.

  Advice is simple: Angry feelings may cause mothers to feel tense and the infant may sense this tension; however, the quality of the breast milk will not be affected (Lamaze International, 1998).

Client Education

Working and Breastfeeding

You should teach the client to consider the following information for successfully combining working with breastfeeding:

- Take full advantage of maternity leave to establish a supply of milk.

- Keep in mind that breastfeeding can reduce the amount of sick days taken because breastfed infants usually are sick less often than are formula-fed infants.

- Try to introduce a bottle once you have a milk supply established (in 4 to 6 weeks) to prepare the baby for bottle-feeding during the day by someone else.

- Purchase or rent a high-quality, automatic, electric breast pump.

- Purchase a double-pumping kit with the electric pump so that both breasts can be expressed simultaneously in only 10 to 15 minutes (Figure 18-20).

- Gradually become familiar with the process by simulating the pumping schedule to be used at work for 2 weeks before returning to work.

- Breastfeed once in the morning; pump every 2 to 3 hours at work; and then breastfeed as soon as possible on returning home, during the evening, and at bedtime.

- Try to find a private area if a pumping room is not available at your place of employment.

- Store the breast milk pumped at work in a refrigerator or cooler. Milk can be kept refrigerated for 72 hours; it also can be labeled, dated, and frozen for 6 months when kept in the deep-freeze section of the freezer.

You can teach the mother to keep the following in mind:

- Pumping the breasts at work can be easy, fast, and painless.

- Many working mothers combine breastfeeding and bottle-feeding with few problems.

- Your child-care provider can feed the baby breast milk from a bottle while you are at work.

- Breastfeeding creates a special bond between you and the baby that no one else can have.

- Plan and commit yourself to breastfeeding because it is a worthwhile endeavor for your baby.

Other hospital policies that can negatively affect breastfeeding include taking the newborn to a transitional nursery immediately after delivery, no rooming-in policy, routine supplementation of breastfeeding infants in the nursery, inconsistent or contradictory advice from hospital staff, and infants being allowed to nurse only on a strict hospital schedule. The woman who wants to breastfeed her infant may need to find out about the breastfeeding policies of the hospital before she chooses where to deliver.

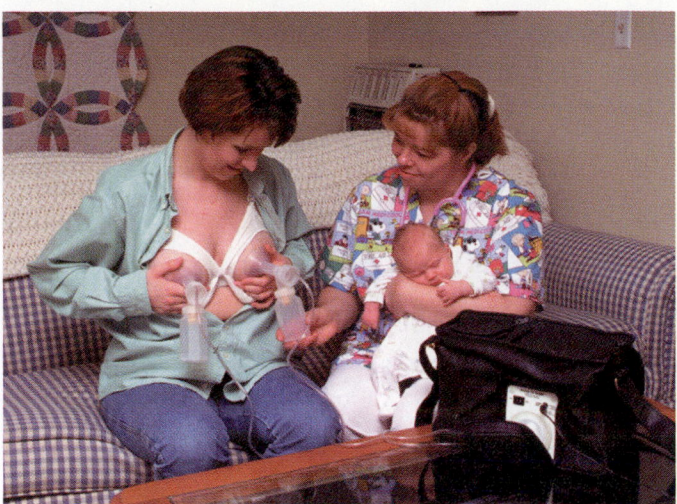

Figure 18-20 Expressing milk from both breasts simultaneously is a time-saver for the busy mother.

Return to Work

The largest number of women choosing to breastfeed today are women who intend to return to work (Bar-Yam, 1998). Some women may feel that returning to work is a barrier to breastfeeding because of the added commitment and effort needed to combine work and breastfeeding the baby. Although breastfeeding will require some extra commitment and effort, many women find that the rewards far outweigh the difficulties. See Client Education Box on working and breastfeeding.

The client can breastfeed when she is home and pump her milk while at work. She can leave breast milk for the infant to be given by a babysitter while she is away. The client's work wardrobe should include clothing that will allow her easy and private access to her breasts so that pumping while at work will be as easy as possible. Breasts may also leak during the first few weeks after returning to work. To help minimize leakage, instruct the client to press against the nipples when she feels the tingling feeling associated with the let-down reflex. The

---

Reflections of a New Mother of Twins

During an interview with a new mother of twins, she was asked how in the world she could possibly breast-feed twins. The mother replied with absolute sincerity: "I breast-feed because it is the easiest way to feed two babies. How would I ever keep up with bottles and formula for both of them? This way I can nurse both of them at once. It just makes good sense!"

---

client also may want to place breast pads in her bra so that the milk will not stain her clothing. Wearing patterned clothing or bringing along a sweater to wear over other clothes also will prevent embarrassment if leaking occurs.

Tandem Nursing and Breastfeeding Multiples

Many women may wonder if pregnancy, multiple births, or being unable to establish lactation immediately after delivery are barriers to successful breastfeeding. Pregnancy can and does occur while lactating. It is possible to nurse one child throughout a subsequent pregnancy and then to breastfeed both infants once delivery has occurred. This is known as tandem nursing.

It is also possible for a mother to nurse twins and triplets (Figure 18-21). The breast is capable of responding to nutritional demands placed on it by more than one infant. If the mother can nurse both twins simultaneously, the time needed to feed twins can be minimized. The mother will need adequate nutrition, rest, help, and support from relatives and friends to breastfeed twins during the first busy year of life. Many mothers of twins report that breastfeeding is much easier than trying to keep up with bottles for more than one infant.

Contraindications to Breastfeeding

When discussing the contraindications to breastfeeding, it is necessary to examine the specific conditions that put the mother or infant at risk. The risk-to-benefit ratios must be weighed by the clinician and mother to arrive at the best decision for both mother and child. Life-threatening or severely debilitating illnesses in the mother may necessitate avoiding lactation. Inborn errors of metabolism, once diagnosed, may also necessitate cessation of lactation.

Maternal Contraindications

A new mother with a diagnosis of breast cancer should not nurse her infant so that the mother can begin definitive treatment for the disease. Breastfeeding is incompatible with chemotherapeutic agents.

Hepatitis B virus is transmitted from mother to infant via breastfeeding. All infants born to mothers who have active disease or are carriers now receive hepatitis B immune globulin (HBIG) immediately after birth plus a dose of human hepatitis B vaccine, followed by a second dose at a week of age or later. These infants may be breastfed (Lawrence, 1999). Hepatitis C virus in the mother is a contraindication for breastfeeding.

Cytomegalovirus (CMV) is not a contraindication because the milk also contains appropriate antibodies that protect the infant.

The Centers for Disease Control and Prevention (CDC) and the U.S. Public Health Service recommend that women in the United States who test positive for the HIV

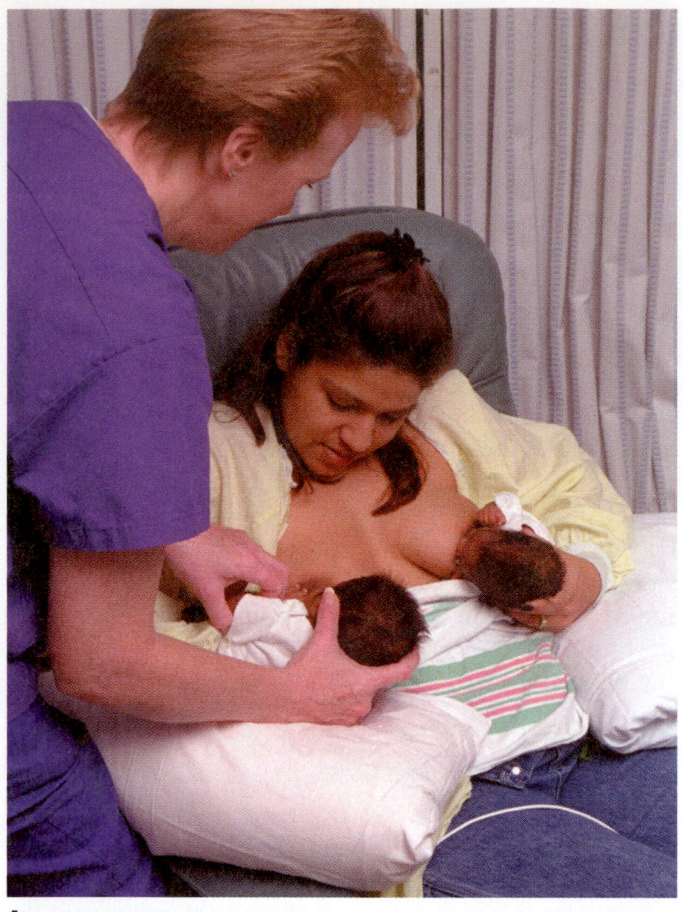

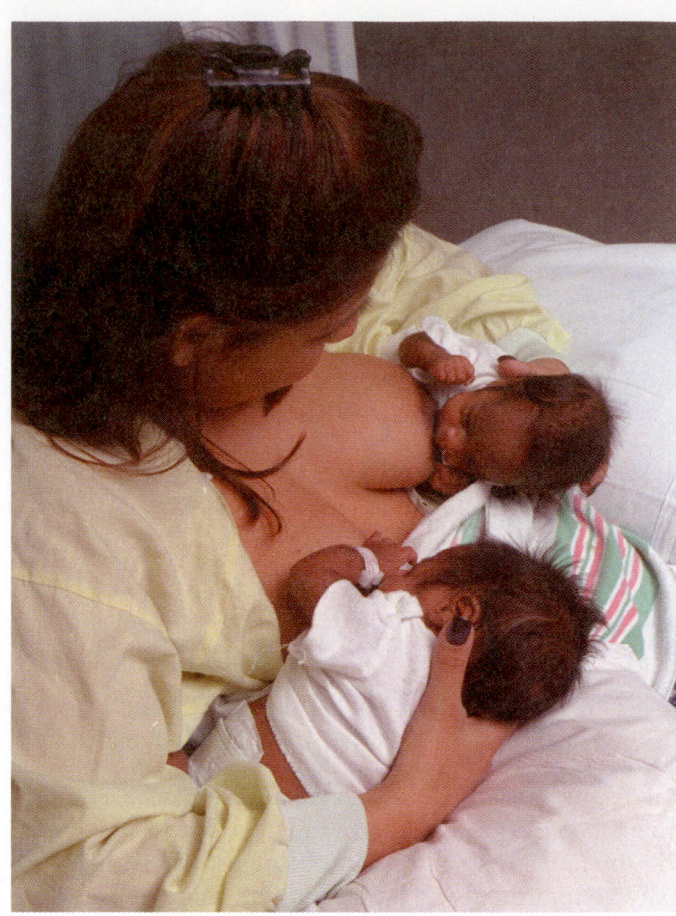

A.

B.

Figure 18-21 Breastfeeding multiples. A. The nurse is helping this mother of triplets with her efforts at breastfeeding two babies at once. B. This mother and her babies will learn how to breastfeed together.

antibody should not breastfeed to avoid postnatal transmission (Bangkok Collaborative, 1999).

Breastfeeding is not recommended for women who test positive for HTLV-I and for any mother who is abusing drugs because of the possibility of the infant receiving substantial amounts of the drug through breast milk (Lawrence, 1999).

Pharmacologic Considerations

Riordan and Auerbach (1999) emphasize the three "knows" about drugs and human milk:

1. Most drugs pass into breast milk.
2. Most medications appear only in small amounts in breast milk.
3. Few drugs are contraindicated for breastfeeding mothers.

Many variables affect the passage of drugs into breast milk: amount of drug taken, frequency and route of administration, timing of the dose in relationship to feeding the infant, and characteristics of the drug involved.

The mother who is breastfeeding should always inform her primary care provider that she is lactating to avoid harming the infant. Information on potential effects of drugs given during lactation can be obtained from the American Academy of Pediatrics Committee on Drugs, 1994.

Herbs and herbal teas currently are very popular remedies for a variety of problems. Many herbs have been reported to enhance milk production (Lawrence, 1999). Mothers should be aware of the effects of herbal compounds that are ingested and the possible reaction in the breastfeeding infant. The nurse needs to inquire about all foods and beverages when taking a history.

According to the National Institute on Drug Abuse (1998), persons with the highest rate of illicit drug use are those between the ages of 18 and 25 years. It is important that the nurse have accurate information to inform these women about the possible adverse effects of specific drugs on breastfeeding and newborns (Riordan & Auerbach, 1999).

Cocaine use in the United States has dramatically increased because it has become less expensive, and the

Nursing Tip   *Assessment Checklist for the Breastfeeding Mother*

You should document the following in the breastfeeding client:

1. Maternal vital signs
2. Maternal and infant intake and output
3. Maternal position and comfort level during breast-feeding
4. Condition of nipples and breasts
5. Maternal sensations during breastfeeding (tingling)
6. Maternal understanding of breast care and nutrition
7. Maternal understanding of assessment of adequate infant intake
8. Maternal understanding of proper infant positioning
9. Maternal understanding of pumping methods
10. Maternal and paternal attitudes toward breastfeeding
11. Maternal age and education
12. Maternal parity and personal experience with breast-feeding

You should teach the mother the signs that the infant needs to be seen by a health care provider:

1. The infant is putting out scant or no urine.
2. The infant has infrequent stools, less than four a day by end of first week.
3. The infant is very fretful and never appears satisfied after feedings.
4. The infant is lethargic, that is, hard to awaken.
5. The infant does not make swallowing sounds during feedings.
6. The infant is not gaining weight.

Initially the neonate's intestines contain meconium, which is a dark, thick, greenish-black tarry stool. Normally, the infant will pass the first meconium stool within the first 24 hours. Early and frequent breastfeeding stimulates the passage of stool much earlier and helps decrease bilirubin reabsorption from the meconium in the infant's intestinal tract. The type of infant feeding determines the characteristics of subsequent stools. Formula-fed infants pass pasty, pale-yellow stools with a strong odor. Formula-fed infants may have problems with constipation owing to a more solid stool formation than breastfed infants. Breastfed infants pass stools that are golden yellow, sweet smelling, and more liquid in consistency. Breastfed infants have more frequent bowel movements than do formula-fed infants because breast milk is more easily digested than formula.

You should assess the following factors in the infant:

- Excessive drooling, coughing, gagging, or respiratory distress
- Time spent at the breast
- Sucking reflex
- Signs of lactose intolerance, for example, cramping, distention, and diarrhea
- Response after a feeding session

---

more popular form known as crack cocaine has emerged. Cocaine harms the fetus and the nursing infant. Therefore, the recommendation is very clear: cocaine should never be used by a mother who is breastfeeding.

The effects of alcohol on the infant of a mother who is breastfeeding seem to be directly related to the amount of alcohol ingested by the mother. When the mother who is breastfeeding drinks a small amount of alcohol, the alcohol may not affect the infant or may cause a little sedation. One study in mothers who were breastfeeding and who drank alcohol found the motor development of their infants to be slower; however, no effect on the infants' mental development was noted (Little, 1989).

While all efforts should be taken to encourage pregnant women and new mothers to quit smoking to avoid harm to both themselves and their infants, for women who do not quit smoking, some of the harm to the infant from smoking may be offset by breastfeeding. A new study suggests that children of smoking mothers who were breastfed scored better in tests of mental development than those whose mothers smoked and did not breastfeed (Batsra, Nealeman, & Hadders-Algra, 2003). Some of the hormones in breast milk may help infants overcome the negative effects of maternal smoking. Therefore, these mothers should be encouraged to breastfeed.

Common Problems Encountered with Breastfeeding

Many of the so-called breastfeeding "problems" are merely normal phenomena that proper instruction and support can alleviate. Nurses can offer anticipatory guidance to new mothers prenatally and postpartally as well as informing them of referral services available after discharge, as needed.

Client Education

Milk Supply

You must teach clients to cope with fears about adequate milk supply:

- Remember that the more milk the baby removes from the breasts, the more will be produced.

- Expect to breastfeed every 2 to 3 hours until the milk supply is established.

- Do not skip feedings or supplement feedings. Night feedings are necessary to establish adequate milk supply for the first few weeks after delivery.

- Breastfeed for at least 15 to 20 minutes so that the baby will receive the rich hindmilk.

- Try to rest and relax as often as possible, and accept offers from friends and family for help.

- Offer both breasts to the infant at every feeding.

- Eat an adequate healthy diet, and drink plenty of liquids.

- Remember that infant growth spurts are to be expected and are only temporary.

Reflections from a Client

When talking to a new mother who had been breastfeeding for 3 months, she shared this story of how difficult it was to learn to trust her body to make good-quality and an adequate quantity of breast milk.

"During the first 4 weeks I would breastfeed my baby every 1 to 2 hours all day long. By nighttime my breasts felt completely empty. I was afraid to put my baby to sleep for the night when she might be hungry or starving to death, so each night I would breastfeed first and then offer a bottle of formula. She would sometimes take one ounce and then go off to sleep. When I took her back for her well-baby check-up at 6 weeks, her weight was off the top of the chart. I decided to confess to the pediatrician that I had been supplementing. When I told him how much formula she was taking each day, he laughed and said, 'If you think your baby is gaining this much weight from one ounce of formula a day, you must be kidding me.' Then he said, 'Your breast milk is what is making this child gain weight so well.' From that day on, I never supplemented again because I finally trusted and believed in my own body. It was just a matter of gaining confidence in myself."

The nurse's role in working with the woman who is breastfeeding includes developing a plan of care that includes teaching of proper feeding techniques and interventions to correct any related problems.

Cracked or Sore Nipples

Although some nipple soreness is normal during the first few days or weeks of breastfeeding, sore nipples usually are due to improper infant latching-on. Probably the most important intervention for this concern is observing the placement of the infant on the breast and helping the mother to ensure the infant is on the areola and not just the nipple. Letting the nipples air dry after feeding, applying a few drops of breast milk to the nipples after feeding, and avoiding soaps and other drying agents usually will relieve soreness.

Nipple soreness may be decreased by encouraging the mother to rotate positions when feeding the infant. Changing position alters the focus of greatest stress and promotes more complete breast emptying. Nipple soreness also can develop because of faulty infant sucking habits. Nipples can develop bruises, scabs, or blisters during improper sucking episodes when the nipple is rubbing against the roof of the infant's mouth. Nipples can be chewed because of improper positioning when the baby is latched on the nipple and not the areola, resulting in cracked and tender areas near the base. Mothers need to be taught how to get the baby's mouth wide open and on the areola and how to remove the infant without causing more damage to the nipple. Nipple soreness also can result in cracked nipples. Cracked nipples need to be assessed for fissures, and the breastfeeding position must be observed. The mother may want to begin the feeding session with the nipple that is less sore or may need to temporarily use a nipple shield made of silicone to allow time for the nipple to heal.

The mother needs to be made aware that nipple soreness is most uncomfortable during the first few minutes of breastfeeding. Because the let-down reflex takes a few minutes to occur, she needs to try to keep nursing long enough for the milk to begin flowing. When the infant is overeager because of extreme hunger, nipple pain can be compounded. Feeding more often and applying ice to the nipples before beginning may help.

The best way to care for the nipples is simply to apply some breast milk to them at the end of the feeding and allow them to air dry. The use of creams or ointments is discouraged. Washing the nipples with plain water (no soap) prevents drying and helps healing. If the mother's nipples are irritated by clothing, breast shields or pads may be worn under the bra.

When a mother has persistent sore nipples, candidiasis is a possibility. It is caused by a fungus, *Candida albicans*, also called *Monilia* or thrush when it occurs orally. This condition should be suspected when the mother has been breastfeeding without discomfort and then suddenly complains of very sore nipples, itching, burning, or pain deep in the breast. When the mother has signs of deep pink inflammation on her nipples, the infant's mouth also needs assessment for signs of white patches. Treatment of all infected areas in both mother and baby is necessary to eliminate the infection and prevent reinfection (Heinig & Francis, 1999). Antifungal medication is given by mouth to the infant, and the mother must apply antifungal cream to her nipples before each breastfeeding (Riordan & Auerbach, 1999).

Breast Engorgement

Swelling and fullness occur from 3 to 7 days after delivery in all women who are lactating. This condition is known as breast **engorgement**. Engorgement usually involves the vascular and lymph systems as the breasts prepare for milk production after delivery (Figure 18-22). The breasts are described as full, warm, and uncomfortable. This type of engorgement will subside on its own within 3 to 5 days and is a natural response.

A more uncommon type of engorgement involves overdistention of breast milk in the alveola. This overdistention may be due to restricted sucking time, large volumes of milk, or incorrect infant attachment. Some mothers experience plugging of one or more milk ducts, especially during or after engorgement. This problem is manifested by a lumpy, reddened area of tenderness in the breast and is sometimes referred to as "caked breasts." Treatment consists of the use of moist heat, breast massage, and frequent breastfeeding to ensure complete emptying of the breast (Lawrence, 1999).

Client Education

Prevention and Treatment of Engorgement

You should teach the client how to prevent engorgement:

- Breastfeed the infant frequently, 8 to 12 times in 24 hours to prevent discomfort and mastitis.
- Avoid supplements of water or formula for the first 3 to 4 weeks.
- Express milk when feedings are missed.
- Gradually wean the baby.
- Wear a good-fitting supportive bra.

You should teach the client how to treat engorgement:

- Apply hot, moist towels to the breasts for 2 to 5 minutes, or take a hot shower before nursing.
- Hand express some milk to soften the areola after using moist heat, making it easier for the baby to attach to the breast.
- Use gentle breast massage before and during breastfeeding.
- Avoid bottles, pacifiers, and nipple shields during this period, which can cause nipple confusion for the infant.
- Apply cold compresses to the breasts after feeding to relieve discomfort.
- Use relaxation techniques before and during feeding.
- When the baby will take only one breast at a feeding, use a breast pump or hand express milk from the other breast during engorgement periods.
- Use a breast pump or hand express milk to soften the areola when the baby cannot latch on to the nipples because the breasts are too full.

Mastitis

Mastitis is an infection of the breast generally caused by *Staphylococcus aureus* and seen primarily in women who are breastfeeding. The most common source of the bacteria is the infant's mouth. This infection usually occurs after discharge from the hospital; therefore, the client

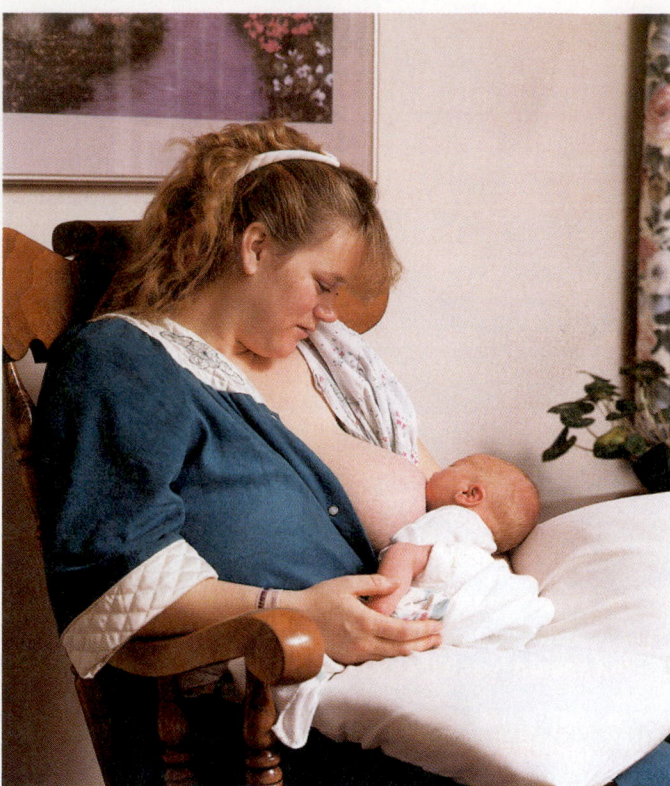

Figure 18-22 Breastfeeding is the best relief for breast engorgement.

needs to be taught symptoms and preventive measures before discharge. The symptoms of mastitis are erythema, swelling, and pain, usually occurring in the upper outer quadrant of the breast. Enlarged and painful axillary lymph nodes also may be present. The woman with infectious mastitis may also present with influenza-like symptoms, such as fever, and a headache, along with a reddened and painful area in the breast.

Nursing Alert

Mastitis

Evaluating outcomes of nursing care for the client with mastitis include the following:

- Client has knowledge of proper breastfeeding techniques.
- Client is aware of signs and symptoms of mastitis.
- Client reports the condition early.
- Treatment is successful.
- Client is able to maintain milk supply and continue breastfeeding.
- Client understands preventive measures to avoid recurrence.

Many factors contribute to the development of mastitis and most can be prevented: poor drainage of milk; cracked or damaged nipples; a tight bra or improper breast support; poor hygiene; engorgement; or a change in the infant's feeding habits, such as sleeping through the night or being ill. By instructing the woman in proper breastfeeding techniques, encouraging mothers who are breastfeeding to wear a good supportive bra, and checking to make sure that all areas of the breast are empty after each feeding, nurses are able to emphasize the prevention of mastitis and milk stasis.

New mothers should contact their physician, nurse practitioner, or Certified Nurse Midwife immediately if they experience signs of mastitis. A diagnosis of mastitis usually is based on symptoms and physical examination. Treatment consists of feeding the baby frequently or pumping the breasts, bed rest, increased fluid intake, a supportive bra, local application of heat, medications for pain, and with a 10-day course of antibiotics (Lawrence, 1999). Most antibiotics are safe for the breastfeeding mother. If the antibiotic can be given to an infant, it is then safe to give the breastfeeding mother. However, because most antibiotics transfer into breast milk, the antibiotic may cause loose stools or candidiasis in both the mother and infant (Riordan & Auerbach, 1999).

Mastitis occasionally may develop into an abcess that needs to be incised and cultured. If breastfeeding is not possible, the mother should be encouraged to pump her breasts to maintain her milk supply until breastfeeding can be resumed and also to prevent engorgement.

Alternative Therapy for Breastfeeding Problems

Applying tea bags moistened in warm water is receiving new acceptance. The tannic acid in the tea helps toughen the nipples, and the warmth promotes healing. Tea bags can also be applied cold if the woman prefers. The tea bag should be discarded after 24 hours because of a tendency to cultivate mold.

Lawrence (1999) reports that application of cabbage leaves is a favorite treatment for breast engorgement that has been handed down for generations. Two reports in the literature are cited. Treatment consists of application of refrigerated cabbage leaves to the breast, leaving the nipple exposed. The leaves are left on for 20 minutes or until wilted. Whether it is the coolness of the leaves or some innate property of the leaves that helps the engorgement is yet to be proved.

Many herbs and foods have been used to encourage and promote the flow of milk and to treat some of the problems of breastfeeding. Simple teas such as raspberry leaf and alfalfa are used to stimulate a plentiful supply of breast milk and a relaxed mother and infant. All leafy greens such as parsley, watercress, and green beans are considered helpful in maintaining lactation. However, many other common herbs are considered dangerous and should be avoided while breastfeeding: aloe vera, basil, black cohosh, bladderwrack, comfrey, ginseng, licorice, and golden seal (Kopec, 1999).

The use of relaxation techniques, such as deep breathing, imagery, and body massage, also can be used to promote relaxation and thus the "let-down" reflex. Accupressure massage techniques also can be used to help create relaxation and decrease stress and anxiety. Many women find that they need a quiet, private place to breastfeed their infant to allow the flow of milk to occur. A warm, relaxing bath or shower also will stimulate the flow of milk. After the first few weeks, the let-down reflex occurs more easily and just the thought, sight, or sound of the infant frequently will trigger milk flow.

Pumping, Storing, and Supplementation

When a mother wishes to breastfeed and is unable to nurse her baby because the infant is premature or she must return to work, she can express the milk either manually or with a breast pump. During the postpartum period, if a baby is unable to nurse at the breast, the mother needs frequent breast stimulation to help establish her milk supply. She should use an electric breast pump with a double setup (pumps both breasts at once) at least 8 times in a 24-hour period (Riordan & Auerbach, 1999). The milk obtained can be refrigerated and given by gavage or fed from a tiny plastic cup made especially for premies, until the infant is able to nurse on its own.

There are many kinds of breast pumps on the market (Figure 18-23). The new mother should be taught to first wash her hands and gather all equipment, which should also be clean. The let-down reflex can be triggered before beginning to pump by rolling the nipple between the thumb and forefinger for a minute or two, or by focusing on a photograph of the infant. Pumping, using an electric pump on each breast for at least 10 minutes every 3 to 4 hours around the clock, will stimulate milk production. Milk can then be transferred to sterile containers and frozen until needed. Breast pumps can be hand pumps, which are inexpensive but also inefficient. Battery-operated pumps are more efficient than hand pumps but also are more expensive. Electric pumps are the most efficient but are the most expensive. Most agencies now offer clients the option of renting an electric breast pump that is easy to use and very efficient in collecting and stimulating milk production. Most hospitals offer new mothers a list of suppliers of these types of pumps.

Milk also can be expressed manually by squeezing toward the nipple using the thumb and fingers around and above the areola and rotating 360 degrees around the breast (Figure 18-24). Massaging the breasts and nipples to stimulate the let-down reflex will help make the milk flow more readily.

Client Education

Breast Milk Storage

For the client to successfully store breast milk, the nurse must teach the following about storage and preparation of the breast milk:

1. Refrigerated breast milk must be stored at 40°F or below and used within 72 hours.

2. Frozen breast milk must be stored at 0°F or below and used within 6 months.

3. To thaw frozen breast milk, run warm water over the container and shake it to return the milk to suspension.

4. Frozen breast milk that is thawed must be refrigerated at 40° or below and used within 24 hours.

Breast milk should be stored in clean plastic containers because leukocytes in the milk adhere to glass containers and thus their protective effect may be lost. To safely use frozen breast milk, it must be thawed by running warm water over the container and then shaking it well to return the milk to suspension. It should not be warmed in a microwave oven because doing so causes uneven heating that may burn the infant; it also destroys the proteins in the milk.

Many businesses are now starting to provide comfortable, private places that allow new mothers to nurse their infants or to pump breast milk to be given to their infant at a later time. These pumping rooms, with breast pumps and refrigerators for breast milk storage, are being offered to employees by companies that realize the health benefits and resulting cost savings that can result from encouraging their female employees to breastfeed their infants. Because many new mothers must return to work before they are ready to wean their infants, it is imperative that these mothers be allowed the time and opportunity to remove the breast milk to prevent the breast engorgement. The newest electric pumps are extremely effective in removing the milk, and most mothers can finish pumping in 20 to 30 minutes. This type of support from employers can enable new mothers to continue their commitment to breastfeeding while maintaining their commitment to their jobs.

Weaning

The decision to stop breastfeeding and either place the infant on a bottle or a cup (weaning) may be considered a potential problem by the mother. Women who are

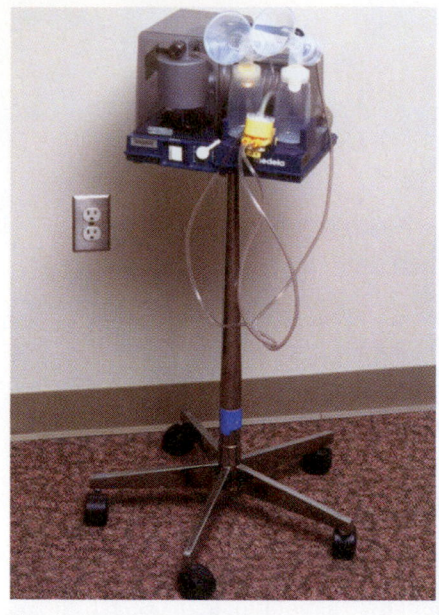
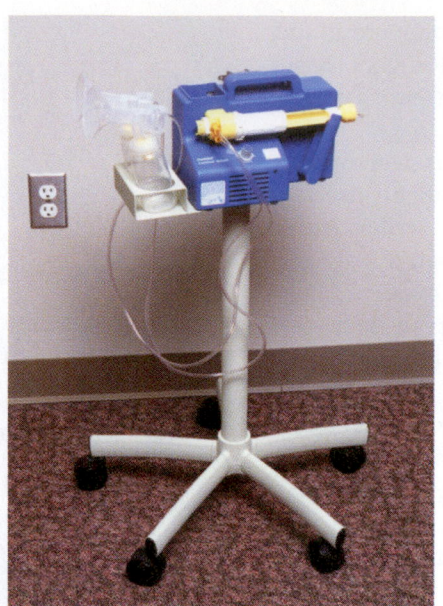

A.

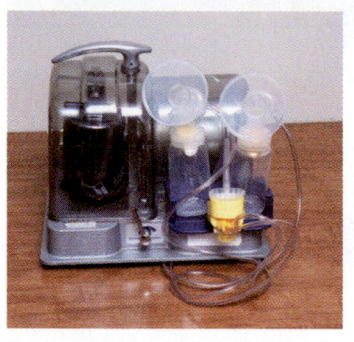
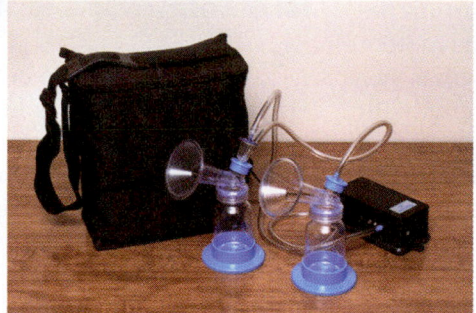
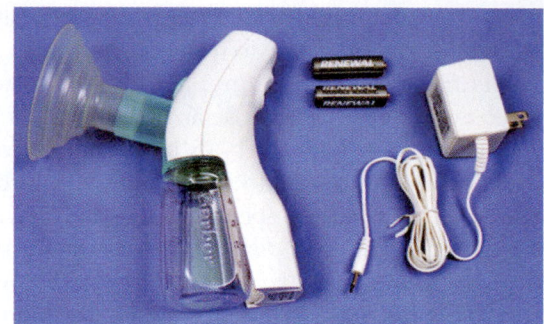

B.

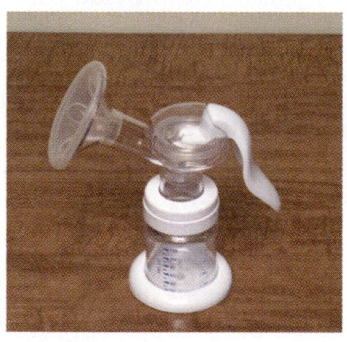
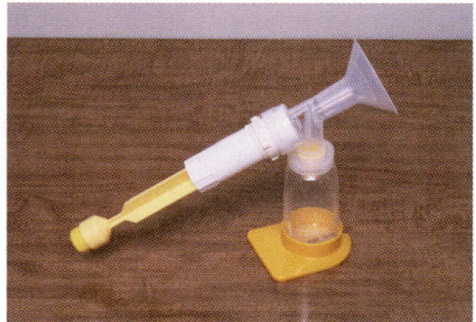
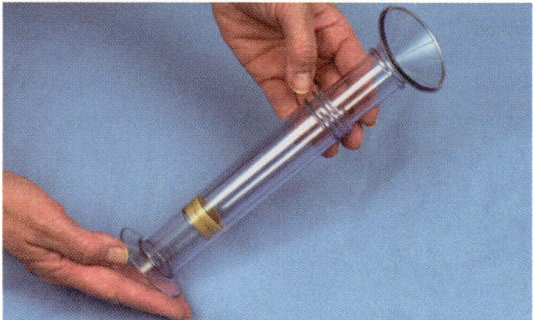

C.

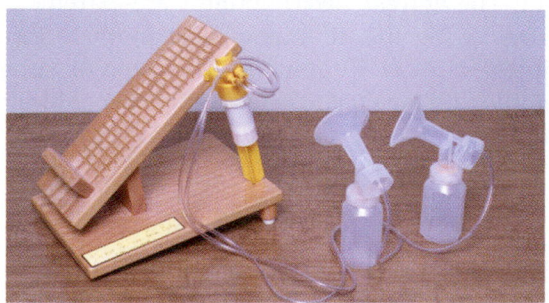

D.

Figure 18-23 Breast pumps. A. Hospital pumps. B. Electric and battery-operated pumps. C. Manual pumps. D. Foot-operated pump

comfortable with breastfeeding and understand the weaning process will know when the time comes to wean because of sensitivity to the child's cues. The latest recommendation from the American Academy of Pediatrics is to breastfeed for one year (American Academy of Pediatrics, 1997). The slow method of weaning by gradually substituting one cup or one bottle for one breastfeeding session over days or weeks helps prevent breast engorgement and allows the infant to slowly adapt to the new feeding method (Lawrence, 1999).

The timing and type of weaning can affect the infant's health and may even be associated with a feeling of being rejected in either the infant or the mother. It is important to help the mother understand that weaning can be initiated by either the mother or the infant, or both.

Resources for Breastfeeding Mothers

An important breastfeeding promotion strategy that has developed to help provide support for women's breastfeeding efforts is the lactation consultant. **Lactation consultants** are specially trained health care providers whose primary focus is assisting new mothers in establishing breastfeeding. These consultants provide a variety of services, including individual consultations, collaboration with other health care providers to develop a plan of care for new mothers, teaching classes, and instruction on the use of products such as breast pumps. These consultants also serve as informational sources, researchers, and data

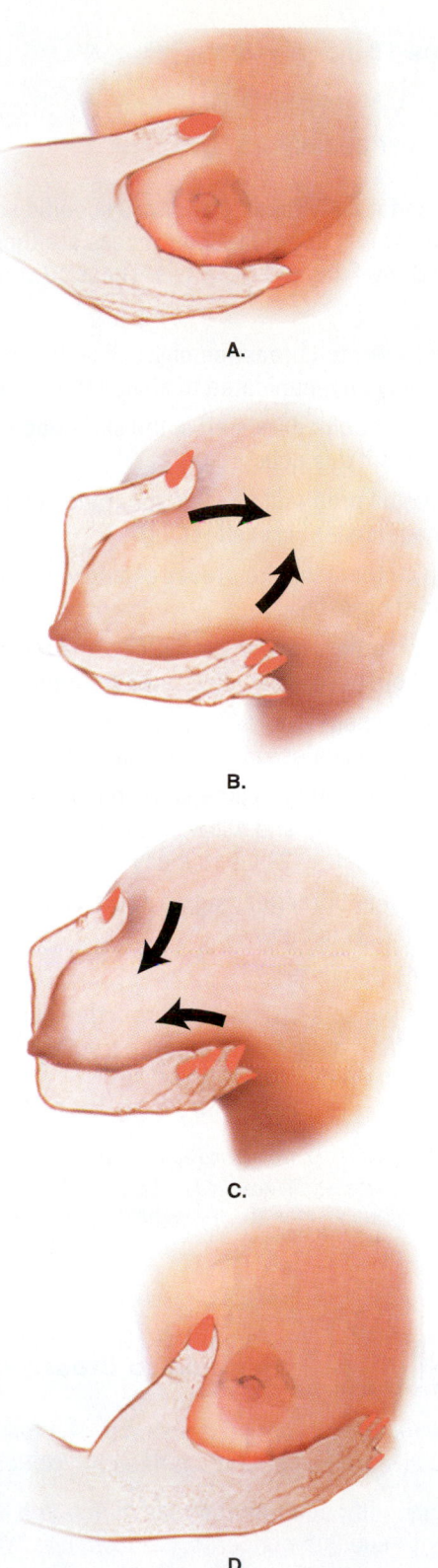

Figure 18-24   Manual expression of breast milk. A. Grasp your breast in a C-hold. B. Squeeze your thumb and fingers together while pushing fingers toward the chest wall. C. Maintain hand position, and push your fingers toward the nipple. D. Shift thumb and fingers an inch away from their first location and repeat the process, working your way around the entire breast.

> **Nursing Tip**   *La Leche League*
>
> **La Leche League** is a self-help group for breastfeeding mothers with members around the world. La Leche sponsors workshops and has an extensive publication list. The organization consists of small neighborhood groups in all major cities and rural areas. La Leche group leaders also are available for additional information and support. The groups usually have a lending library and newsletter, and participation is free.

> **Nursing Tip**   *ILCA*
>
> The International Lactation Consultant Association (ILCA) promotes breastfeeding awareness among health care providers and the public. The ILCA also helps define the scope of practice of lactation consultants. The ILCA publishes the *Journal of Human Lactation*.

collectors and may help in developing special breastfeeding programs.

Nursing Implications

Although most women in the United States know that breast milk is best for infants, the breastfeeding rates still remain low. Traditional education programs that promote breastfeeding have not adequately influenced the adoption of breastfeeding in a large segment of the population.

Overcoming Barriers

Prenatal education should begin as early as possible so that breastfeeding information can be presented to each client as often as possible to clear up misinformation and resolve doubts.

Education

Most women decide on an infant feeding method either before getting pregnant or during the first trimester. Therefore breastfeeding education programs need to be designed to provide information either preconceptually or during the early prenatal period. Breastfeeding education can be accomplished by formal classes, informal discussions, printed materials, video tapes, and even by way of the Internet (Riordan, 2000). Educational programs should emphasize the benefits of breastfeeding. A complete promotion program has two essential components. First, counseling on how to overcome barriers to breastfeeding must be provided. Second, educational sessions must be held covering the mechanics of breastfeeding, how to deal with common breastfeeding problems, and how to assess adequate nutrition in the infant.

Another attempt to increase breastfeeding initiation in hospitals is shown in Box 18-1.

Cultural Negotiations

The nurse and other health care providers need to provide culturally appropriate care and guidance when helping new mothers breastfeed. The nurse needs to consider breastfeeding beliefs about health, support or resource persons, parenting responsibilities, and infant care. Because breastfeeding is a sensitive and personal matter for all women, it is important to assess attitudes toward modesty and cultural norms for each woman. Breastfeeding in a public place or in the presence of other people is an extremely sensitive issue for most women. Teaching women that breastfeeding can be accomplished in a modest manner and acknowledging variations in comfort are essential to successful feeding experiences. The right to breastfeed in public is protected by law in most states.

In many cultures, colostrum is viewed as "old" milk that is not healthy for infants. In other cultures, this first

---

Box 18-1

The WHO/UNICEF "Ten Steps to Successful Breastfeeding"

Hospitals that are willing to adopt 10 specific steps and complete an accreditation process are then named "Baby-Friendly" hospitals. These 10 steps follow:

1. Have a written breastfeeding policy that is routinely communicated to all health care staff.
2. Train all health care staff in the skills necessary to implement this policy.
3. Inform all pregnant women about the benefits and management of breastfeeding.
4. Help mothers initiate breastfeeding within a half hour of birth.
5. Show mothers how to breastfeed and maintain lactation, even when separated from their infants.
6. Give newborn infants no food or drink other than breast milk, unless medically indicated.
7. Practice rooming-in (keeping the infant in the mother's room), and allow mothers and infants to remain together 24 hours a day.
8. Encourage breastfeeding on demand (whenever the infant is hungry).
9. Give no pacifiers.
10. Foster the establishment of breastfeeding support and refer mothers on discharge from the hospital or clinic.

Note. From *Protecting, Promoting and Supporting Breastfeeding: The Special Role of Maternity Services. A Joint Statement by WHO/UNICEF, 1989,* by WHO/UNICEF, 1994, Geneva: World Health Organization.

Nursing Tip   *Decision to Breastfeed*

When working with pregnant women who may be interested in learning about breastfeeding, you can:

- Begin with open-ended questions to elicit the client's specific concerns. For example, "What do you know about breastfeeding?"
- Acknowledge her concerns and reassure her that her feelings are normal. For example, "Many women worry about that same thing."
- Educate each woman using carefully targeted messages that address specific concerns.

Nursing Tip

Supporting Breastfeeding

You should encourage breastfeeding by:

- Enthusiastically promoting and supporting breastfeeding.
- Simplifying breastfeeding. There is no need to eat or drink differently because only an additional 500 cal/d are needed along with a normal amount of fluid, six 8 oz glasses a day.
- Helping women understand the ability of their infant to communicate readiness to feed, latch on, and breastfeed well.
- Talking about parenting styles that promote and facilitate breastfeeding, such as holding and cosleeping.
- Communicating the rewards and benefits of breastfeeding after returning to work.
- Discussing ways women can influence their workplace to become breastfeeding-friendly.
- Working to change hospital practices that sabotage initiation of breastfeeding, for example, providing formula discharge packs, separation from the baby, and lack of adequate help to initiate breastfeeding.
- Encouraging the media to present breastfeeding as positive and normal.
- Keeping informed regarding new breastfeeding knowledge.

Note. From "A Special Report on Breastfeeding," by Lamaze International, ASPO/Lamaze, 1(7), p. 3.

Critical Thinking

Informed Consent for Infant Feeding Decisions

In order for women to make an informed decision about infant feeding methods, mothers must be given facts about the nutritional and immunologic needs of the infant that can best be met by human milk and potential benefits to the mother. The nurse is required to give the parents complete information, document that she has done so, and record the mother's choice in her medical record.

How can you make sure that your client makes informed decisions regarding health care for herself and her family?

milk is viewed as "poison" or "pus" that must not be given to babies. Nurses need to assess beliefs about colostrum in each client and attempt to educate the client while being careful not to insult her cultural beliefs. Well-meaning efforts to acculturate women to the nurse's beliefs may actually disrupt breastfeeding efforts. It is important to demonstrate understanding and value of the client's beliefs while helping her establish successful breastfeeding behaviors (Riordan & Auerbach, 1999).

Prenatal Decision Making

The most effective time to prepare for breastfeeding is early in the prenatal period or even preconceptually. An examination of the breasts is part of good prenatal care. If any anatomic abnormalities are observed, they can be discussed at that time.

The First Feeding

Early feedings after birth are important for several reasons. The infant's suckling stimulates uterine contractions, helps control postpartal bleeding, and hastens involution of the uterus. The infant will be most interested in breastfeeding within the first 20 to 30 minutes after birth, and the colostrum will begin to provide immunologic benefits immediately. The infant's digestive system will be stimulated by 19 different GI hormones, and passage of meconium will be enhanced by the ingestion of colostrum. The milk supply will be stimulated, and attachment between mother and baby will be increased (Ivnas-Mobert, 1989).

Early Postpartum Period

This is a good time to teach new parents about the cues that infants may use to communicate their needs. Breastfeeding is designed to be led by the baby. Babies are born capable of communicating readiness to eat in many ways. Crying is actually a late sign of hunger. Early signs of hunger include rapid eye movements, hand to mouth movements, mouth and tongue movements, body movements, and small sounds. Responding to these feeding cues, rather than waiting for crying, results in a baby and mother who are relaxed and a baby who is not too frantic to latch on and feed properly (Lamaze International, 1998). For a sleepy baby it may be necessary to show the new mother some easy ways of increasing the infant's alertness. Activities such as rubbing gently, taking the infant out of the blanket, and moving and talking to the infant usually will stimulate infants to come to a more awake state. For an overly hungry or upset infant, rocking or talking quietly may provide an opportunity for the infant to calm down so that breastfeeding can begin.

Discharge Planning

Early discharge from the hospital markedly reduces the time to teach beginning breastfeeding skills and assess

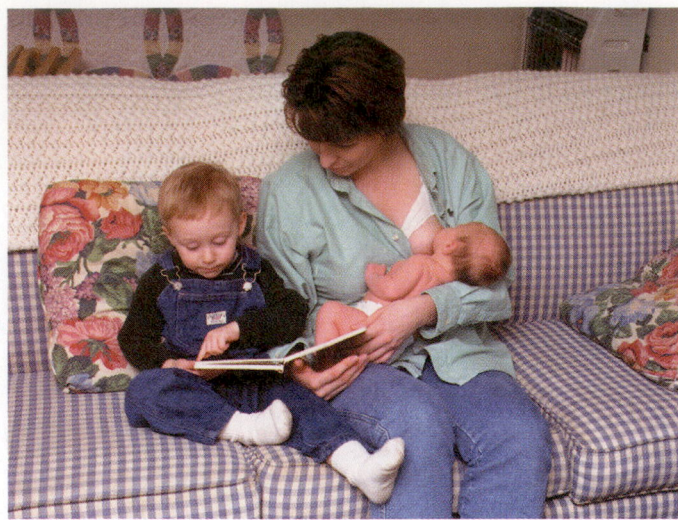

Figure 18-25 Nurses can help new mothers learn to balance the many demands on their time.

Critical Thinking

Bottle Propping

Feeding the infant by propping the bottle as the infant lies in the crib is not recommended. What are some of the reasons that this is not a good idea?

- The infant may regurgitate and aspirate the formula.
- Infants who nurse from propped bottles may develop bottle mouth syndrome.

Which other negative effects can you think of that are related to this manner of feeding?

how well the baby is nursing. Many hospitals are now beginning to provide support and follow-up by using telephone calls and home visits. In endeavoring to prevent premature weaning and help new mothers deal with common problems (Figure 18-25), hospitals are now providing written instructions on breastfeeding and telephone numbers of community referrals and resources (Riordan & Auerbach, 1999).

COMMERCIAL INFANT FORMULA

No commercially processed infant formula has been developed that reproduces the immunologic properties, nutrient **bioavailability** (rate at which a nutrient enters the blood stream and is circulated to specific organs or tissues), digestibility, and nutritional effects of human milk. The composition of infant formula, however, has im-

proved tremendously in the past 50 years as a result of a greater understanding of infant nutrient requirements, absorption, and metabolic activities. Continual research is under way to qualitatively enhance infant formulas (Lo & Kleinman, 1996).

When used as the sole source of infant nutrition, infant formula must meet all the energy and nutrient requirements for the healthy term infant. The AAP Committee on Nutrition has developed infant formula standards. The Food and Drug Administration regulations for infant formula are based on these standards. Additionally, the Infant Formula Act mandates adherence to standards and quality control and requires that quantitative label declaration be made for 38 nutrients. The amount of each nutrient is added in formulas at higher concentrations than human milk to compensate for the lower bioavailability of nutrients from infant formula.

Commercially available infant formulas fall into several categories: 1) Standard cow's milk-based formulas; 2) soy-based and lactose-free formulas; 3) elemental,

Client Education

Preparation of Infant Formula

- **The equipment should be gathered:**
  - Bottles may be made of plastic or glass, or have plastic liners.
  - Nipples should allow a steady flow of formula but should not be so large as to cause the infant to swallow too fast.
  - Formula may be in ready-to-feed, concentrate, or powder form.
- **The label should be checked to make sure the formula is in ready-to-feed or concentrate form.**
- **When powder or concentrate forms are used, they must be mixed according to the directions on the bottle.**
- **Either the ready-to-feed formula is poured directly into the bottles, or the concentrated or powdered formula is mixed with water in a clean container and then poured into the bottles.**
- **Once prepared, the formula may be stored in the refrigerator for up to 24 hours; if not used in 24 hours, it should be discarded.**
- **Formula may be left at room temperature for up to an hour and then should be discarded.**

Client Education

Bottle-Feeding the Neonate

- The bottle should be prepared (see Client Education Box: Preparation of Infant Formula) and allowed to come to room temperature, either by sitting out for half an hour or running warm water over the bottle.

- The neonate should be held in a comfortable position with the head elevated.

- The bottle should be held so the formula fills the nipple and no air is in the neck of the bottle (Figure 18-26).

- The infant should be burped at least twice during the feeding:

  — The infant may be upright on the shoulder.

  — The infant may be placed in a sitting position, with one hand supporting the chin and the other gently rubbing the back. This is the preferred position as it allows one to watch for regurgitation.

  — After a few minutes, resume feeding.

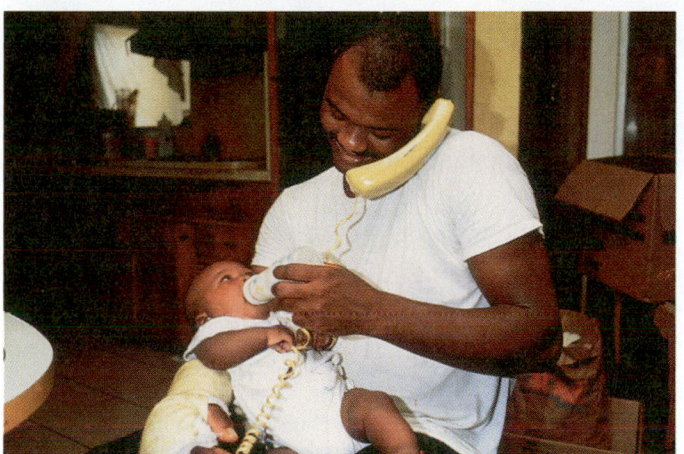

A.

hydrolyzed protein, and free amino acid formulas; 4) premature infant formulas; and 5) specialty infant formulas, including those for metabolic disorders (Table 18-7). These formulas come in powder, concentrate, or ready-to-feed forms. Health care providers should make sure that parents understand how to mix these formulas correctly to avoid hyperosmolar or overly dilute preparations, which can be dangerous (Wilcox, Florello, & Glick, 1993). When using a ready-to-feed formula after the infant is 6 months of age or living in an area with nonfluorinated water, a fluoride supplement may be required (AAP, 1985).

Standard cow's milk-based formula is the formula of choice for routine feeding when human milk or breastfeeding is not available (Klish, 1990) (Figure 18-27). These

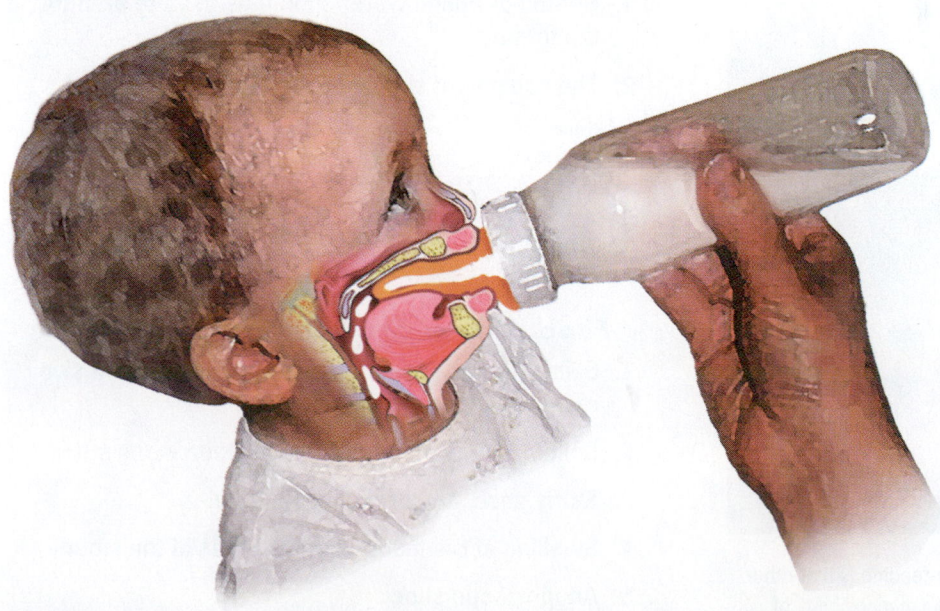

Figure 18-26   Proper bottle position for feeding. A. The baby should be held in a comfortable position with the head elevated. B. The bottle should be angled so that the nipple is completely covered with milk, preventing the baby from sucking air.

B.

Table 18-7 Commercial Infant Formula Selection	
FORMULA	**CRITERIA**
Standard, cow's milk–based	Human milk not available
Soy, lactose-free	Galactose deficiency
	Vegan
Elemental, protein hydrolysate	Cow's milk allergy
	Intestinal malabsorption
Premature	Premature, low-birth-weight infants
Specialty	Metabolic disorders

formulations modify whole cow's milk to reduce protein and renal solute load. Iron-fortified standard formulas generally are well tolerated (Nelson, Ziegler, Copeland, Edwards, & Foman, 1988) and should be used to provide adequate iron. With a caloric density of 67 to 70 kcal/dL (20 kcal/oz) these formulas should be offered as needed. The usual intake of 150 to 200 mL/d per kilogram of body

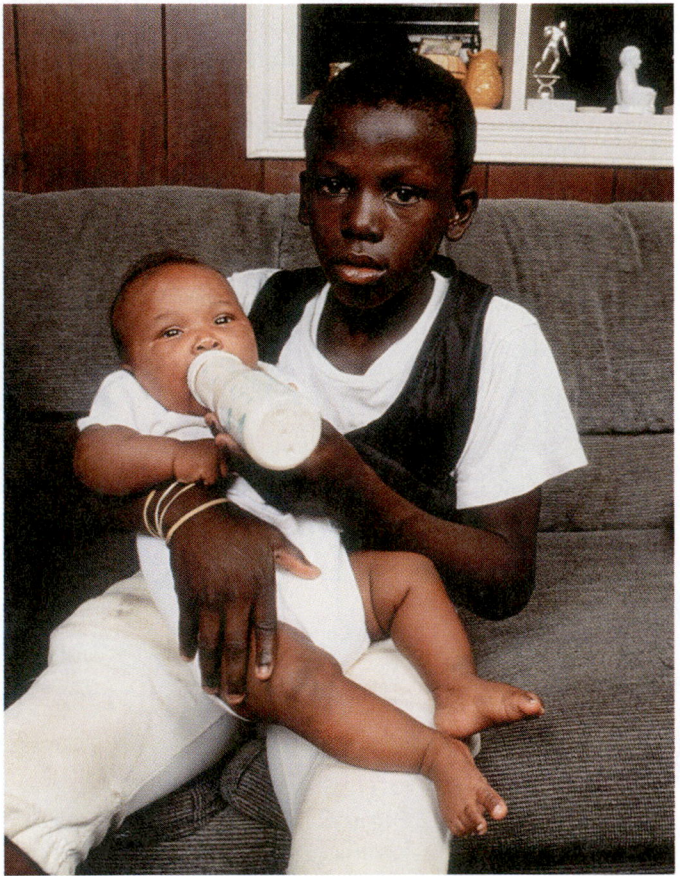

Figure 18-27 One of the benefits of bottle-feeding is that other family members, including siblings, can share in the responsibility of feeding the baby.

Nursing Alert

Clean Bottles

It is important to make sure that the bottles are clean and contain no dried milk before sterilization, because this can contaminate the formula. Bottles can be washed in the dishwasher.

Nursing Tip Cost of Formula

Powdered or concentrated formula is less expensive than the ready-to-feed form.

weight provides 100 to 130 kcal/d per kilogram of body weight, resulting in a goal target weight gain of 20 to 30 g/d. Client education is important to help new mothers prepare and feed their infants safely. Family members can also participate (Figure 18-27).

Nursing Alert

Water for Formula

If the water supply is not purified or there is any question about cleanliness, then:

1. Bottled or boiled water should be used to prepare the formula.

2. The equipment should be sterilized.

Nursing Alert

Food Allergy Symptoms

1. Skin symptoms, such as swelling, hives, and skin rashes

2. Colicky behavior, diarrhea, and blood in the stool

3. Stuffy nose, and breathing difficulties

4. Swelling of the mucous membranes of the mouth

5. Anaphylactic shock

Client Education

Methods for Infant Formula and Equipment Sterilization

Bottles must be sterilized if there is any question about the cleanliness of the water. There are two methods of bottle sterilization

Terminal Method

- The equipment is washed with soap and water.

- The formula is prepared according to directions.

- Bottles are filled; nipples are inverted, with caps loosely applied.

- Bottles are placed in a large pan, with 2 to 3 inches of water or in a bottle sterilizer.

- The pan is covered, and the water is boiled for 25 minutes.

- The bottles are allowed to cool, the lids screwed on, and the bottles stored in the refrigerator.

Aseptic Method

- The equipment is washed in soap and water and placed in a large pan or sterilizer.

- The equipment is boiled for 5 minutes.

- The water for mixing the formula is boiled separately for 5 minutes.

- The equipment is removed with tongs, and the formula is mixed in the sterilized pitcher.

- The prepared formula is poured into the bottles, lids applied, and stored in the refrigerator.

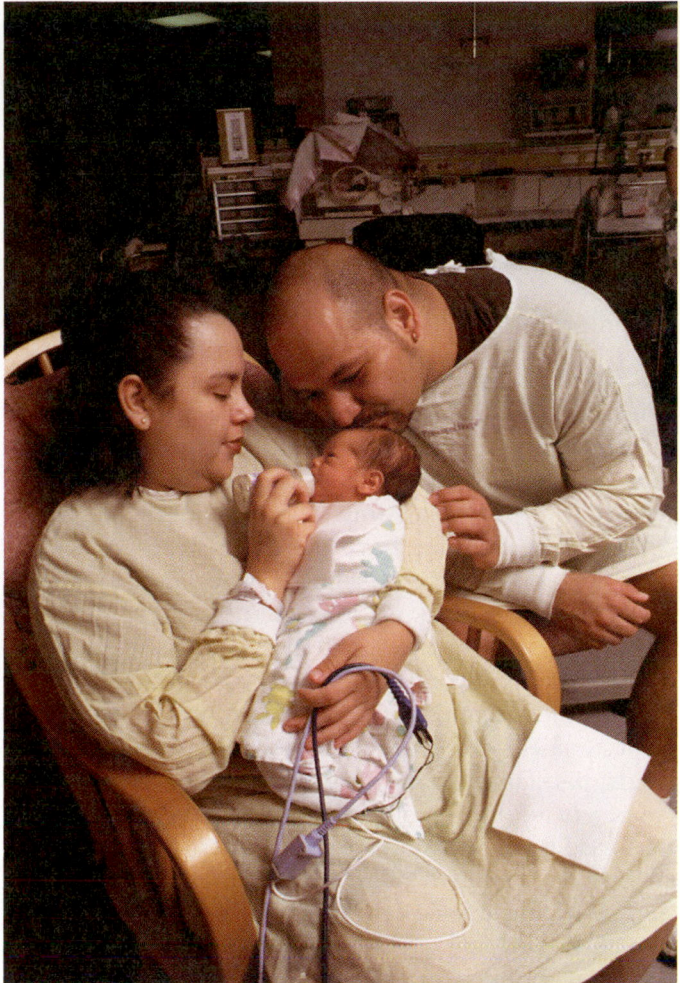

Figure 18-28   Special formulas are available for premature and high-risk infants.

Specialized Formulas

Specialty formulas are made for infants with severe nutrient sensitivities (e.g., 3232A), or specific inborn errors of metabolism (e.g., phenol-free for infants with phenylketonuria). These products should only be used in consultation with a metabolic dietician.

Premature formulas (Enfamil Premature Formula, Mead-Johnson; Similac Special Care, Ross) are designed specifically for the immature infant at high risk (Figure 18-28). Low-birth-weight infants are born without the benefit of the last trimester's supply of fat, minerals, and trace elements; therefore, requirements for intake are specialized to meet their needs (Neu, Valentine, & Meetze, 1990).

Introduction of Solid Foods

The introduction of semisolid foods should not take place too early for several reasons. Developmentally, the infant has an extrusion tongue reflex until 4 to 6 months of age, making solid feeding inappropriate. This protective reflex results in the infant pushing out with the tongue any semisolid or solid bolus of food. The practice of solid additions to the bottle, or so-called infant feeders, should also be avoided. In addition, solid foods add to the renal solute load and may contribute to higher plasma concentrations of sodium and urea (Wharton & Scott, 1996). As a result the infant will either reduce milk intake, which will compromise normal growth and development, or consume more calories than are needed, increasing the risk of

Nursing Alert

Choking Prevention

Avoid small items that can easily lodge in infant's airway, such as grapes, nuts, popcorn, watermelon, and seeds. Hotdogs also should be avoided.

childhood obesity. Some parents have started solids early believing that this practice will help the infant sleep through the night. However, feeding infants solids at bedtime is not related to nighttime sleeping patterns. Several well-controlled studies found that infants who receive solids before bedtime have the same sleep patterns as those who do not receive solids (Keane, Charney, Straus, & Roberts, 1988; Macknin, Medendorp, & Maier, 1989).

Conversely, the introduction of solids should not be delayed much beyond 6 months of age (AAP, 1980). For the breastfed infant, mother's milk alone may be insufficient to meet the recommended energy and nutrient needs, particularly in terms of vitamin D, iron, zinc, and copper. In addition, some infants who have not started to take food from a spoon by 6 months of age subsequently show considerable delay in adapting to the chewing and tongue-rolling action of the weaning from the milking action of the suckling.

Most mothers initially use manufactured weaning foods because of their convenience and their physical and nutritional properties. Because of the infant's need for iron at 6 months, iron-fortified rice cereal should be introduced first in quantities of 1 to 2 tablespoons/d mixed

Nursing Tip *Vitamin Supplements*

Generally, routine vitamin supplements are not necessary for the fully breastfed or formula-fed infant drinking 32 oz/d. Breastfed infants receiving a limited amount of sunshine may require 44 IU/d of vitamin D. After 4 to 6 months, both breastfed and formula-fed infants need iron; however, this need can be met by an iron-enriched diet or iron-fortified formula. Fluoride supplementation at 0.25 mg/d should be started once the teeth erupt (Foman and Ekshard, 1993) if the infants do not receive an adequate source of fluorinated water (AAP, 1986). Parents and caregivers should call their local water service to check how much fluoride is in the water.

Critical Thinking

Infant Nutrition

You are asked to attend medical rounds in the neonatal unit. Infant nutrition is discussed. Several of the nurses, doctors, and residents have questions about the comparison of human milk and prepared formulas. How will you prepare for a continued discussion of this topic the next week?

- When comparing the constituents of human milk and formula, what are the benefits of human milk?
- What are some of the specialty formula preparations, and how do they differ from standard infant formula?
- What are some of the reasons that prepared formula would be used or recommended?

with breast milk or formula (Poskitt, 1983; AAP, 1980). One food at a time should be introduced, waiting at least 3 days between each new food to watch for allergic reactions (e.g., hives, wheezing, gas, and blood in the stool). Oatmeal and barley cereal can then be introduced into the diet, again with portion sizes of 1 to 2 tablespoon per day. Orange, yellow, and green vegetables should be used next to provide increased vitamins A and C. Fruits can then be initiated, avoiding citris fruits (e.g., oranges and orange juice) until after 9 months of age. At 8 months of age, egg yolks and meats can be added to the diet. Avoid egg whites and fish until after 1 year of age because these foods can be highly allergenic. See Table 18-8 for a suggested schedule for introducing solid foods.

Careful attention to food preparation is essential when using commercially prepared foods to avoid exposure to botulism or lead from cans. Honey should be avoided because botulism spores tend to contaminate this product and can make the infant very ill. Other foods to avoid include nuts, grapes, popcorn, hard chopped carrots, celery, white bread (which can be very sticky), hard candy, and seeds. Cow's milk, whole milk, is recommended to begin after 1 year of age (AAP, 1992). Infants that begin too early are found to be iron deficient. Cow's milk also is an inadequate source of folate, copper, linoleic acid, and vitamin C.

Infants on vegan diets should be assessed by a nutritionist because energy, protein, vitamin D, vitamin B_{12}, calcium, and zinc can be limited in their meals (Nutrition Standing Committee of the British Pediatric Association,

Table 18-8	Recommended Timetable for Introducing Solid Foods
AGE (MO)	GOAL INTAKE
6	1–2 tbsp/d of iron-fortified rice cereal, increase to 4–5 tbsp/d, rice, oatmeal, or barley
7	Add 1–2 tbsp/d of yellow, green, or orange vegetables
8	Add 1–2 tbsp/d of strained meats or egg yolk
12	Add whole cow's milk Egg whites Seafood Orange juice

Nursing Alert

Is the Infant Getting Enough Milk?

You should assess the infant's nutritional status:

- The infant should be breastfed from 8 to 12 times in 24 hours.
- The infant should swallow every two to three sucks when attached properly, and the mother should see and hear the swallowing.
- The infant should gain weight.
- The infant should have at least six wet diapers in a 24-hour period by day 5 to 7.
- The infant should have frequent stooling, that is, four stools a day.
- Infants older than 3 weeks may have fewer stools but should continue to have six or more heavy, wet diapers a day.

1988). Menus and supplements should be provided to the caregivers to help them plan adequate nutrition. A sample menu for a 7-month-old infant is presented in Box 18-2.

Nursing Implications

The nurse needs to assess the particular nutritional needs of the infant. Prematurity, metabolic disorders, or sensitivities may require a specialized formula. The nurse also needs to assess the parent's choice of feeding. It is important to discuss this decision because the mother may have made the decision without adequate knowledge. Once

these data have been gathered, the nurse may formulate nursing diagnoses regarding the infant's intake and the mother's knowledge and ability to feed the infant. One of the most important interventions is to teach the mother to safely feed the infant, whether breastfeeding or formula feeding. The nurse must monitor the infant feeding to ensure the infant is receiving adequate nutrition. The nurse can determine if the mother is able to prepare and properly feed her infant.

Box 18-2

Sample Menu for a 7-Month-Old Infant

A.M.	6 oz of milk (*nursing time)
10 A.M.	2 oz of apple juice
Noon	1–2 tbsp of rice cereal
	1–2 tbsp of apple juice mixed in cereal
	6 oz of milk (*breast milk)
3 P.M.	1–2 tbsp of banana
Dinner	1–2 tbsp of rice cereal
	1–2 tbsp of strained squash or pumpkin
Evening	6 oz of milk (*breast milk)

*May be nursing or expressed breast milk or formula

NURSING PROCESS

The nurse can use the nursing process to provide a framework to help guide the assessment, nursing diagnosis, planning, implementation, and evaluation of the nursing pair.

Infant feeding is an interdependent, constantly evolving, and reciprocal relationship between mother and infant. Nurturing mothers and babies during the initiation of breastfeeding or formula feeding can help new mothers learn the skills necessary for successful and satisfactory infant feeding.

Assessment of the Nursing Pair

An assessment of the health of mother and infant as well as family preferences and perceptions is necessary.

Nursing Diagnoses

Nursing diagnoses provide the basis for the selection and implementation of nursing interventions to help the client achieve satisfactory outcomes. The following are potential nursing diagnoses for the client who is breastfeeding. The following nursing diagnoses related to infant feeding are diagnostic labels approved by the North American Nursing Diagnosis Association (NANDA):

- Effective breastfeeding: the state in which a mother-infant dyad/family exhibits adequate proficiency and satisfaction with the breastfeeding process
- Ineffective breastfeeding: the state in which a mother or child experiences difficulty with the breastfeeding process
- Nutrition, imbalanced: less than body requirements (potential)
- Interrupted breastfeeding: a break in the continuity of the breastfeeding process as a result of the inability or inadvisability to put the baby to breast for feeding
- Deficient knowledge related to formula preparation and feeding

Outcome Identification

A client outcome is a statement of the progression toward goal achievement. Collaborative planning with the new mother helps promote goal attainment. The mother would expect to progress toward the outcome of providing her infant with optimal nutrition.

Planning

After assessing the client and formulating the nursing diagnoses, the nurse must develop and implement a plan of care. Interventions are planned strategies, based on scientific rationale, devised by the nurse to assist the client in meeting the client's desired outcomes. Planning for breastfeeding clients would include discussion of proper feeding methods and infant positioning, and client demonstration of breastfeeding to assess the client's abilities. Planning for formula feeding includes preparation and feeding the infant.

Nursing Intervention

Implementation is the execution of the interventions that were devised during the planning stage. The nurse should use respect, empathy, and understanding when working with clients to encourage collaboration in this planning process. Interventions can include providing information for decision making or implementing feeding methods as well as specific help and techniques of breast or formula feeding and referrals to ongoing support resources.

Evaluation

Evaluation is the last phase of the nursing process. During the evaluation, the client's progress in reaching outcomes is determined. The nurse, in collaboration with the client, evaluates the effectiveness of the plan of care. The nurse evaluates both subjective and objective data on an ongoing basis. When the client's outcome goals have been met, then the plan of care has been effective. When the client's outcome goals have not been met, then the nurse and client must revise the nursing plan to include different interventions.

Evaluation of the feeding plan of care would include statements such as the following:

- The client was able to demonstrate proper breastfeeding techniques.
- The client was able to demonstrate proper bottle-feeding techniques.
- The client was able to demonstrate proper formula preparation.
- The client was able to demonstrate proper pumping techniques.
- The client was able to list the signs that her infant was obtaining adequate milk.
- The client showed no signs of breast problems.
- The client was able to state support systems available to her after discharge.

WEB ACTIVITIES

••• Which resources can you locate on the Internet for new mothers experiencing difficulties initiating breastfeeding?

••• Where can a new mother locate a lactation consultant?

••• Where can a new mother locate an electric breast pump?

••• Where can a pregnant woman find a hospital that is "breast friendly"?

••• Where can a mother find information on formula feeding her infant?

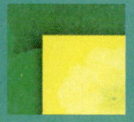

CASE STUDY/CARE PLAN
THE CLIENT WITH INTERRUPTED BREASTFEEDING

Judy Martin, aged 31, delivered her first child, a boy weighing 7 lb, 4 oz, 15 hours ago. Ms. Martin had a traumatic delivery and ran an elevated temperature of 102°F during the birth. Her infant was taken to the neonatal intensive care unit (NICU) for a sepsis workup to rule out infection. During Ms. Martin's first attempt at breastfeeding in the NICU, the infant had a difficult time latching on and both became agitated and anxious. Ms. Martin's nipples are slightly inverted, and her infant is having trouble latching on. Ms. Martin calls the nurse and is crying and very upset. She says that every time she attempts to nurse her infant, "He acts like I am killing him." She says either she has to have help today or she is going to quit breastfeeding.

Assessment

Subjective Data

- Client denies prenatal problems.
- Client states that because she had an elevated temperature (102°F) during a prolonged (more than 20 hours) labor and vaginal delivery, her infant was taken to NICU to rule out sepsis.
- Client states that the nurses have told her that her infant cannot be brought to her room for 48 hours.
- Client states that she had a very traumatic delivery, has a fourth-degree episiotomy, and is in pain.
- Client states she is a registered nurse and "really wants to breastfeed as soon as possible because she knows it is best for the baby."

Objective Data

- Client is a para 1, gravida 1, delivered at 39 weeks' gestation.
- Client vital signs: temperature, 98.8°F; pulse, 90; respirations, 20; blood pressure 110/80 mmHg.
- Client has an intravenous infusion of 1,000 mL lactated Ringer's with ampicillin, 500 mg, dripping at 100 mL/h.
- Client appears to be in pain when moving or sitting and needs help with ambulation.
- Breasts are soft; nipples have no cracks and are slightly inverted.
- Client is 15 hours postdelivery.
- Infant is male, appropriate for gestational age.
- Infant's Apgar scores were 8 and 9.
- Gestational age assessment was 39 weeks.
- Infant weight is 7 lb, 4 oz, and length is 21 inches.
- Infant temperature is 98.2°F rectally.

Nursing Diagnosis

Interrupted breastfeeding related to possible illness in infant.

Expected Outcome   Client wants to breastfeed her infant successfully as soon as possible and plans on breastfeeding for 6 months.

Planning   Before leaving the hospital, the client will do the following:

1. Initiate breastfeeding behaviors as soon as the infant's condition allows.
2. Demonstrate proper breastfeeding techniques.
3. List three positions for breastfeeding.
4. Demonstrate appropriate techniques for attaching the infant to the breast.
5. Maintain close contact with her infant.
6. Explain criteria to assess infant's hydration and weight gain status.

(continues)

7. List proper pumping and storage techniques.

8. Discuss support resources she can use after hospital discharge.

NOC   Breastfeeding maintenance

NIC   Emotional support

Nursing Interventions	Rationales
1. Assist client to the NICU in a wheelchair to hold and breastfeed her infant as soon as permitted.	1. Client's physical condition requires assistance for ambulation.
2. Teach the client breastfeeding techniques, including positions and proper latching-on.	2. Many new mothers need help with the skills and techniques that must be learned for successful breastfeeding.
3. Provide the client with privacy and help in the NICU, as needed.	3. Privacy helps to allay some embarrassment and anxiety associated with breastfeeding for the first time.
4. Teach the client with information on infant nutritional assessment in short sessions using appropriate terms and language.	4. Teaching clients in short sessions helps prevent information overload and allows the client to process and remember the material presented.
5. Instruct the client on the use of breast pumps and milk storage.	5. The client may need to establish a milk supply with a pump and store her milk until the infant is discharged from the NICU.
6. Provide lists of breastfeeding resources and support available after discharge.	6. Written material allows the client to review information after discharge. Support for breastfeeding has been found to be an essential element in successful lactation.

Evaluation

- Client was taken to the NICU 15 hours after delivery to hold her infant and initiate breastfeeding.
- Client demonstrated proper breastfeeding techniques behind a movable screen, which provided privacy from the rest of the nursery.
- Client became anxious because her infant was unable to latch on because of inverted nipples.
- Client was able to explain information provided to her, including proper pumping and storage of breast milk.
- Client stored the written materials in her suitcase for use after discharge.

Nursing Diagnosis

Ineffective breastfeeding related to poor latching-on.

Expected Outcome   Client will effectively breastfeed her infant.

Planning

1. Nurse will call a lactation consultant today to obtain a visit to assess the breastfeeding pair.

2. Client will pump breast milk and use a specially designed nipple to feed the infant until the infant is able to latch on (a nipple specially designed to mimic the breast in both form and function).

3. Client will use a breast shield made of silicone to help the infant latch on and to stimulate the nipples to evert.

4. Client will use an electric breast pump to help maintain an adequate milk supply and to help pull out the nipples.

5. Client will have someone in her family take care of her and her infant when she is discharged to home to encourage rest and relaxation.

NOC   Breastfeeding establishment: Infant

NIC   Breastfeeding assistance

(continues)

Nursing Interventions

1. Use a silicone breast shield to facilitate infant latching-on.

2. Apply ice compresses to the nipples just before feeding to stimulate them.
3. Lubricate the nipples with a few drops of expressed milk before feeding.
4. Let the nipples dry thoroughly after feeding.
5. Apply warm tea bags to the nipples if soreness occurs.

6. Avoid applying soaps to the nipples.

7. Encourage frequent feeding.

8. Use prophylactic breast massage after each feeding.

9. Express milk by using an electric breast pump, if necessary.

10. Take a warm shower.

Rationales

1. A silicone breast shield can protect sore nipples from further damage and make the nipples easier for the infant to grasp.
2. Ice numbs the nipples and makes them firmer and easier for the infant to grasp.
3. Expressed breast milk put on the nipples helps prevent dryness.
4. Air drying helps promote healing and comfort.
5. Tannic acid in warm tea bags toughens the nipples, and the warmth promotes healing.
6. Soaps directly applied to the nipples can cause drying and cracking.
7. Frequent feedings help stimulate milk production, prevent stasis of breast milk, and reduce the risk of mastitis.
8. Breast massage helps prevent breast engorgement and stasis and promotes the let-down reflex and milk flow.
9. Expression of milk using an electric pump relieves overdistention and promotes milk drainage while maintaining the milk supply.
10. Warm water promotes the let-down reflex and milk flow and enhances relaxation in the mother.

Evaluation

Ms. Martin met with the lactation consultant that day and felt very encouraged and more positive about continuing breastfeeding. Ms. Martin's infant nursed well with the breast shields in place and latched on well. Ms. Martin was aware that using breast shields can decrease milk supply and was instructed to gradually wean her infant off the shields. She was also instructed that she should continue to pump after nursing to maintain milk supply. Ms. Martin continued to successfully breastfeed her infant and gradually weaned her infant to her own nipples.

Key Concepts

- Breastfeeding provides unparalleled health benefits for infants and cost savings for mothers, families, the health care system, and taxpayers.

- Understanding the motivations and perceived barriers felt by many women can help health care professionals develop effective infant feeding.

- Interventions that lead to successful breastfeeding and formula feeding need to be individualized to fit the needs of each client.

- Promotion of successful breastfeeding requires that the nurse be sensitive to the needs of the mother so that a trusting relationship will permit the sharing of knowledge about techniques to facilitate lactation.

- Informed consent can only be obtained by providing women with both the advantages and disadvantages of breast- and formula feeding.

- Although breastfeeding is a natural process, the necessary skills must be taught and learned by both mother and baby.

- There are significant differences related to growth and development when comparing breastfed and formula-fed infants.

- Infant formulas are designed to meet the energy and nutrient requirements based on human milk as the gold standard or attend to particular needs such as prematurity and allergies.

Review Questions and Activities

1. Compared with prepared formulas, which benefit does mature breast milk have?
   a. A thicker consistency
   b. More calories per ounce
   c. Greater immunologic value
   d. More nitrogenous wastes

   The correct answer is c.

2. The milk protein whey is much easier to digest than is casein. In comparing human milk with bovine milk (the base for many formula preparations), the

whey-to-casein ratio is different. Which ratio of whey to casein is best representative of human milk?
a. 70:30
b. 50:50
c. 18:82
d. 40:60

The correct answer is a.

3. Within what time frame after birth is colostrum replaced by transitional milk?
a. 8 hours
b. 12 to 24 hours
c. 2 to 4 days
d. 1 week

The correct answer is c.

4. At what time in the perinatal period should the nurse first provide information about breastfeeding?
a. First trimester
b. Second trimester
c. Third trimester
d. First attempt at breastfeeding

The correct answer is a.

5. Which of the following actions would help reduce or prevent engorgement in the breastfeeding mother?
a. Reducing fluid intake for 24 hours
b. Breastfeeding her infant every 1 to 2 hours
c. Avoiding use of a breast pump
d. Skipping feedings to let her breasts rest

The correct answer is b.

6. A new breastfeeding mother asks, "Is it true that breast milk will prevent my baby from catching colds and other infections?" Which reply can the nurse give that will reflect the results of current research?
a. Breastfed infants will have increased resistance to illness but may still get sick.
b. Mothers of breastfed infants do not have to worry about exposure to contagious diseases until breastfeeding stops.
c. Breast milk offers no greater protection to breast-fed infants than does formula.
d. Breast milk will give infants protection from all illnesses to which the mother is immune.

The correct answer is a.

7. A breastfeeding mother tells the nurse, "Something must be wrong. Every time I breastfeed my baby I feel like I am having labor pains again." What is the nurse's best response?
a. "Your breasts are secreting a hormone that causes your abdominal muscles to contract."
b. "Prolactin hormone is causing more blood to go to your uterus, resulting in pain."

c. "The same hormone that is released in response to your baby's sucking and that causes the milk to flow also causes your uterus to contract."
d. "You may have a small blood clot in your uterus, and you are trying to expel it."

The correct answer is c.

8. What is the normal interval between feedings when breastfeeding a newborn?
a. Every 4 hours
b. Every hour
c. Every 2 to 3 hours
d. Every 3 hours

The correct answer is c.

9. Which of the following observations will allow a new mother to feel confident that her breastfed infant is receiving enough milk?
a. Six wet diapers in 24 hours, and four stools a day
b. Three to four wet diapers in 24 hours and two stools a day
c. One to two wet diapers in 24 hours, and six to eight stools a day
d. No problem sleeping after nursing

The correct answer is a.

10. A new mother is planning to bottle feed her infant. Which is the safest and easiest type of formula?
a. One that is prepared from powdered milk
b. A ready-to-feed formula
c. A concentrated formula without dilution
d. Fresh milk with added sugar

The correct answer is b.

11. If preparing formula in advance, formula needs to be refrigerated. How long can the formula be refrigerated before it should be discarded?
a. 4 hours
b. 12 hours
c. 24 hours
d. 48 hours

The correct answer is c.

12. Infants who are bottle feeding are prone to swallowing air. Which of the following is a technique that minimizes this?
a. Holding the infant upside down for a minute after feeding
b. Holding the bottle at an angle where the nipple is full
c. Lay the infant on the left side and pound on the back to force a burp
d. Feed in segments of no longer than 2 minutes to avoid swallowing air

The correct answer is b.

13. Adequate carbohydrate intake is required by the infant for the following activities except:
    a. Energy for metabolism
    b. Energy for colonic bacteria
    c. Brain development
    d. Protein catabolism

    The correct answer is d.

14. What are the fluid and electrolyte consequences of feeding an infant concentrated formula?

References

American Academy of Pediatrics Committee on Nutrition. (1980). Vitamin and mineral supplemental needs in normal children in the United States. *Pediatrics, 66,* 1015.

American Academy of Pediatrics Committee on Nutrition. (1981). Nutrition and Lactation. *Pediatrics, 68*(3), 435–443.

American Academy of Pediatrics. (1985). *Pediatric nutrition handbook* (2nd ed.). Elk Grove Village, IL: Author.

American Academy of Pediatrics Committee on Nutrition. (1986). Fluoride supplementation. *Pediatrics, 77*(5), 758.

American Academy of Pediatrics Committee on Nutrition. (1992). The use of whole cow's milk in infancy. *Pediatrics, 89,* 1105.

American Academy of Pediatrics Committee on Drugs. (1994). The transfer of drugs and other chemicals into human milk (RE 9403). *Pediatrics, 93*(1), 137–150.

American Academy of Pediatrics Work Group on Breastfeeding. (1997). Breastfeeding and the use of human milk. *Pediatrics, 100,* 1035–1039.

Bangkok Collaborative Perinatal HIV Transmission Study Group. (1999, December). *Counseling pregnant women and new mothers about HIV: Counseling practices at Siriraj and Rajavithi Hospitals and Queen Sirikit National Institute for Child Health, Bangkok, 1999:* Section 8: Formula Feeding Counseling for Children Born to HIV-Seropositive Mothers. (Nonthaburi, Thailand: HIV/AIDS Collaboration.) Retrieved April 15, 2004, from U.S. Centers for Disease Control and Prevention Web site: http://www.cdc.gov/hiv/pubs/HAC-PCG/section8.htm.

Barker, D. J. (1992). *Fetal and infant origins of adult disease.* London: British Medical Journal Publishing Groups.

Bar-Yam, N. B. (1998). Workplace Lactation support, Part I: A return-to-work breastfeeding assessment tool. *Journal of Human Lactation, 14*(3): 249–254.

Batstra, L., Neeleman, J., & Hadders-Algra, M. (2003). Can breast feeding modify the adverse effects of smoking during pregnancy on the child's cognitive development? *Journal of Epidemiology and Community Health, 57,* 403–404.

Billeaud, C., Guillet, J., & Sandler, B. (1990). Gastric empeying in infants with or without gastro-esophageal reflux according to the type of milk. *European Journal of Clinical Nutrition, 44,* 577–583.

Binns, H. J., Senturia, Y. D., LeBailly, S., Donovan, M., & Kaufer, C. K. (1996). Growth of Chicago area infants, 1985 through 1987. *Archives of Pediatric Adolescent Medicine, 150,* 842–849.

Bitman, J., Freed, L. M., Neville, M. C., Wood, D. L., Hamosh, P., & Hamosh, M. (1986). Lipid composition of prepartum human mammary secretion and postpartum milk. *Journal of Pediatric Gastroenterology & Nutrition, 5*(4), 608–615.

Bryant, C. (1992). A strategy for promoting breastfeeding among economically disadvantaged women and adolescents. *NAACOG'S Clinical Issues in Perinatal & Women's Health Nursing, 3,* 723–730.

Carlson, S. E., & Barness, L. A. (1996). Macronutrient requirements for growth. In W. A. Walker & J. B. Watkins (Eds.), *Nutrition in Pediatrics* (2nd ed., pp. 81–90). Boston: Blackwell Science.

Centers for Disease Control and Prevention. (1998). Guidelines for treatment of sexually transmitted diseases. *Morbidity and Mortality Weekly Report, 47,* 1–117.

Dewey, K. G., Heinig, M. J., & Nommsen-Rivers, L. A., Peerson, J. M., & Lonnerdal, B. (1992). Growth of breast-fed and formula-fed infants from 0 to 18 months: The DARLING study. *Pediatrics, 89,* 1035–1041.

Dewey, K. G., Heinig, M. J., & Nommsen-Rivers, L. A. (1995). Differences in morbidity between breast-fed and formula-fed infants. *Journal of Pediatrics, 126,* 696–702.

Dobbing, J., & Sands, J. (1973). The quantitative growth and development of the human brain. *Archives of Diseases of Children, 48,* 757–767.

Foman, S. J. (1993). *Nutrition of normal infants.* St. Louis, MO: Mosby-Year Book.

Foman, S. J., & Ekshard, J. (1993). Fluoride. In S. J. Foman (Ed.) (pp. 299–310). *Nutrition of normal infants.* St. Louis, MO: Mosby-Year Book.

Food and Nutrition Board. (1989). *Recommended Dietary Allowances.* National Research Council. Commission on Life Sciences. Washington, DC: National Academy Press.

Goodman, D. S. (1984). Vitamin A and retinoids in health and disease. *New England Journal of Medicine, 310,* 1023–1031.

Guo, S., Roche, A. F., Foman, S. J., Nelsen, S. E., Chumlea, W. C., Rogers, R. R., et al. (1991). Reference data on gains in weight and length during the first two years of life. *Journal of Pediatrics, 119,* 355–362.

Hamill, P. B., Drizd, T. A., Johnson, C. L., Reed, R. B., Roche, A. F., & Moore, W. M. (1979). Physical growth: National Center for Health Statistics percentiles. *American Journal of Clinical Nutrition, 32,* 607–629.

Hamosh, M. (1988). Fat needs for term and preterm infants. In R. C. Tsang & B. L. Nichols (Eds.), *Nutrition during infancy* (pp. 133–159). Philadelphia: Hanley & Belfus.

Haschke, F., Vanura, H., Male, C., Owen, G., Pietschnig, B., Schuster, I., et al. (1993). Iron nutrition and growth of breast and formula-fed infants during the first 9 months of life. *Journal of Pediatric Gastroenterology and Nutrition, 16*(2), 151–156.

Heinig, M. J., & Francis, J. (1999). Mammary candidosis in lactating women. *Journal of Human Lactation, 15*(4), 281–288.

Heinig, M. J. (2000). Bed sharing and infant mortality: Guilt by association? *Journal of Human Lactation, 16*(3), 189–191.

Hitchcock, N. E., Gracey, M., & Gilmour, A. I. (1985). The growth of breastfed and artificially fed infants from birth to twelve months. *Acta Paediatrica Scandinavica, 74*(2), 240–245.

International Lactation Consultants Association. (1999). Evidence-based guidelines for breastfeeding management during the first fourteen days. Raleigh, NC: Author.

Ivnas-Mobert, K. (1989). The effects of breastfeeding on gastrointestinal absorption. *Scientific American, 7,* 78–83.

Jarosz, L. (1993). Breast-feeding versus formula: Cost comparison. *Hawaii Medical Journal, 52*(1), 14–18.

Jensen, R. G., & Jensen, G. L. (1992). Specialty lipids for infant nutrition. I. Milks and formulas. *Journal of Pediatric Gastroenterology and Nutrition, 1*, 232–245.

Keane, V., Charney, J., Straus, J., & Roberts, K. (1988). Do solids help baby sleep through the night? *American Journal of Diseases of Children, 142*, 404–405.

Kelleher, J. (1991). Vitamin E and the immune response. *Proceedings of Nutrition Society, 50*, 245–249.

Klaus, M., Kennell, J., & Klaus, P. (1995). *Bonding: Building the foundation of a secure attachment and independence.* Reading, MA: Perseus Books.

Klish, W. J. (1990). Special infant formulas. *Pediatrics in Review, 12*(2), 55–62.

Kopec, K. (1999). Herbal medications and breastfeeding. *Journal of Human Lactation, 15*(2), 157–161.

Kovar, M., Serdula, M., Marks, J., & Fraser, D. (1984). Review of the epidemiologic evidence for an association between infant feeding and infant health. *Pediatrics* (Task Force on Infant Feeding Practices), 615–638.

Lamaze International. (1998). A special report on breastfeeding. *ASPO/Lamaze, 1*(7), 3.

Lawrence, R. (1999). *Breastfeeding: A guide for the medical profession* (5th ed.). St. Louis, MO: Mosby.

Little, R. E. (1989). Maternal alcohol use during breast-feeding and infant mental and mother development at one year. *New England Journal of Medicine, 321*, 425–430.

Lo, C. W., & Kleinman, R. E. (1996). Infant formula, past and future: Opportunities for improvement. *American Journal of Clinical Nutrition, 63*, 6465–6505.

Lonnerdal, B., Cederblad, A., Davidsson, L., & Sandstrom, B. (1984). The effect of individual components of soy formula and cows' milk formula on zinc bioavailability. *American Journal of Clinical Nutrition, 40*, 1064–1070.

Macknin, M. L., Medendorp, S. V., & Maier, M. C. (1989). Infant sleep and bedtime cereal. *American Journal of Diseases of Children, 143*, 1066–1068.

Martin, C. (2000). *The nursing mother's problem solver.* New York: Fireside.

McCormick, D. B. (1989). Vitamin B$_6$. In M. E. Shils & V. Young (Eds.), *Modern nutrition in health and disease* (7th ed., pp. 376–382). Philadelphia: Lea and Febiger.

Meier, P., Brown, L., Hurst, N., Spatz, D., Engstrom, J, Borucki, L., et al. (2000). Nipple shields for preterm infants: Effect on milk transfer and duration of breastfeeding. *Journal of Human Lactation, 16*(2), 106–114.

Methodist Hospital. (1999). *Guidelines for breastfeeding your baby.* Houston, TX: Methodist Press.

Mohrbacher, N., & Stock, J. (1997). *The breastfeeding answer book.* Schaumburg, IL: La Leche League International.

Moran, J. R., & Greene, H. L. (1987). Nutritional biochemistry of water-soluble vitamins. In R. J. Grand, J. L. Sutphen, & W. H. Dietz, Jr. (Eds.), *Pediatric nutrition: Theory and practice* (pp. 51–67). Boston: Butterworths.

National Academy of Science Food and Nutrition Board. (1989). *Recommended dietary allowances.* Washington, DC: Author.

National Institute on Drug Abuse. (1998). *Drug abuse statistics: 1998 population estimates*, Washington, DC: Alcohol, Drug Abuse, and Mental Health, U.S. Public Health Service.

Nelson, S. E., Ziegler, E. E., Copeland, A. M., Edwards, B. B., & Foman, S. J. (1988). Lack of adverse reactions to iron-fortified formula. *Pediatrics, 81*(3), 360–364.

Neu, J., Valentine, C. J., & Meetze, W. (1990). Scientific-based strategies for nutrition of the high risk low birth weight infant. *European Journal of Pediatrics, 150*, 2–13.

Newman, J. (1995). How breast milk protects newborns. *Scientific American*, 76–79.

Nutrition Standing Committee of the British Pediatric Association. (1988). Vegetarian weaning. *Archives of Diseases of Children, 63*, 1286–1292.

Poskitt, E. M. (1983). Infant feeding. A review. *Human Nutrition Applied Nutrition, 37*(4), 271–286.

Prasad, A. S. (1991). Discovery of human zinc deficiency and studies in an experimental human model. *American Journal of Clinical Nutrition, 53*, 403–412.

Raj, V., & Plichta, S. (1998). The role of social support in breast-feeding promotion: A literature review. *Journal of Human Lactation, 14*(1), 41–45.

Reifsnider, E., & Gill, S. (2000). Nutrition for the Childbearing Years. *Journal of Obstetric, Gynecologic, and Neonatal Nursing, 29*(1), 43–55.

Riordan, J. (2000). Teaching breastfeeding on the Web. *Journal of Human Lactation, 16*(3), 231–234.

Riordan, J., & Auerbach, K. (1999). *Breastfeeding and human lactation.* Sudbury, MA: Jones & Barlett.

Scheard, N. F. (1994). Iron deficiency and infant development. *Nutrition Reviews, 52*(4), 137–146.

Sultan,, H. Y., & Barker, D. J. P. (1994). Programming the baby. In Barker, D. J. P. (Ed.), *Mothers, babies and disease in later life* (pp. 14–36). London: British Medical Journal Publishing Group.

U.S. Department of Health, Education and Welfare. (1977). *NCHS growth curves for children, birth–18 years.* (PHS 78-1650). Washington, DC: U.S. Government Printing Office.

West, C. E., Rombout, J. H. W. M., Van der Zijpp, A. J., & Sijtsma, S. R. (1991). Vitamin A and immune function. *Proceedings of the Nutrition Society, 50*(2), 251–262.

Wharton, B. A. & Scott, P. H. (1996). Distinctive aspects of metabolism and nutrition in infancy. *Clinical Biochemistry, 29*(5), 419–428.

World Health Organization. (1988). Special task force on oral contraceptives: Effects of hormonal contraceptives on breast milk composition and infant growth. *Study of Family Planning, 19*, 361–369.

World Health Organization. (1994). Progestin only contraceptives during lactation: Infant growth. *Contraception, 50*, 55–58.

WHO/UNICEF. (1994). *Protecting, promoting, and supporting breastfeeding: The special role of maternity hospitals. A Joint Statement by WHO/UNICEF, 1989.* Geneva: World Health Organization.

Widdowson, E. M. (1991). Growth and body composition in childhood. In E. Brunser, R. F. Carrazza, M. Gracey, B. L. Nichols, & J. Senterre (Eds.), *Clinical nutrition of the young child.* New York: Raven Press.

Wilcox, P. T., Florello, A. B., & Glick, P. L. (1993). Hypovolemic shock and intestinal ischemia: A preventable complication of incomplete formula labeling. *Journal of Pediatrics, 122*(1), 103–104.

Wold, A. E., & Hanson, L. A. (1994). Defense factors in human milk. *Current Opinions in Gastroenterology, 10*, 652–658.

Worthington-Roberts, B., & Williams, S. (1993). *Nutrition in pregnancy and lactation* (5th ed.). St. Louis, MO: C.V. Mosby.

Suggested Readings

Auerbach, G., & Riordan, J. (2000). *Clinical lactation: A visual guide.* Sudbury, MA: Jones & Barlett.

Biancuzzo, M. (1998). *Breastfeeding the newborn: Clinical strategies for nurses.* St. Louis, MO: Mosby.

Healthy People 2010. (1999). *Healthy people 2010 objectives.* Retrieved July 2000, from http://web.health.gov./healthypeople/2010/object.htm

Pryor, G. (1999). *Nursing mother, working mother: The essential guide for breastfeeding and staying close to your baby when you return to work.* New York: Harvard Common Press.

Stuart-Macadam, P., & Dettwyler, K. (Eds). (1995). *Breastfeeding biocultural perspectives.* New York: Aldine De Gruyer.

UNICEF. (1994, April). *Barriers and solutions to the global 10 steps to successful breastfeeding: A summary of in depth interviews with hospitals participating in the WHO/UNICEF baby friendly hospital initiative interim program in the United States.* U.S. Committee for UNICEF.

Weinberg, G. (2000). The dilemma of postnatal mother-to-child transmission of HIV: To breastfeed or not? *Birth, 27*(3), 199–205.

World Health Organization Working Group on Infant Growth. (1995). An evaluation of infant growth. *Bulletin WHO, 73,* 165–174.

Wright, A. L., Holberg, C. J., Taussig, L. M., & Martinez, F. D. (1995). Relationship of infant feeding to recurrent wheezing at age 6 year. *Archives of Pediatric Adolescent Medicine, 149,* 758–763.

Resources

The Academy of Breastfeeding Medicine, ABM Executive Office, 191 Clarksville Road, Princeton Junction, NJ 08850, 877-836-9947, http://www.bfmed.org

American Academy of Pediatrics, 141 Northwest Point Boulevard, Elk Grove Village, IL 60007-1098, 847-228-5005, http://www.aap.org, http://www.pediatrics.org

American Dietetic Association, 120 S. Riverside Plaza, Suite 2000, Chicago, IL 60606, 800-877-1600, http://www.eatright.org

Association of Women's Health, Obstetrics and Neonatal Nurses (AWHONN), 2000 L Street NW, Suite 740, Washington, DC 20036, 800-673-8499, http://www.awhonn.org

Baby Friendly Hospital Initiative, Baby Friendly USA, 327 Quaker Meeting House Road, East Sandwich, MA 02537, 508-888-8092

The Cochrane Pregnancy and Childbirth database is an ongoing meta-analysis of evidence documenting effective health care practices for childbearing women and their neonates, http://www.hcn.net.au/

Doulas of North America, P.O. Box 626, Jasper, IN 47547, 888-788-DONA, http://www.dona.com

Healthy People 2010 Document, http://www.healthypeople.gov

Human Milk Banking Association of North America, 1500 Sunday Drive, Suite 102, Raleigh, NC 27607, 919-861-4530

International Lactation Consultant Association, 1500 Sunday Drive, Suite 102, Raleigh, NC 27605, 919-861-5577, http://www.ilca.org

La Leche League International, 1400 N. Meacham Road, Schaumburg, IL 60173, 847-519-7730, http://www.lalecheleague.org

National Guideline Clearinghouse, 5200 Butler Pike, Plymouth Meeting, PA 19462, http://www.guideline.gov

Special Supplemental Nutrition Program for Women, Infants, and Children (WIC), Food and Consumer Service, 3101 Park Center Drive, Room 819, Alexandria, VA 22302, 703-305-2286, http://www.usda.gov

U.S. Representative Carolyn Maloney, Breastfeeding legislation in the 106th Congress, http://www.house.gov.

World Breastfeeding Week, World Alliance for Breastfeeding Action (WABA), P.O. Box 1200, 10850 Penang, Malaysia

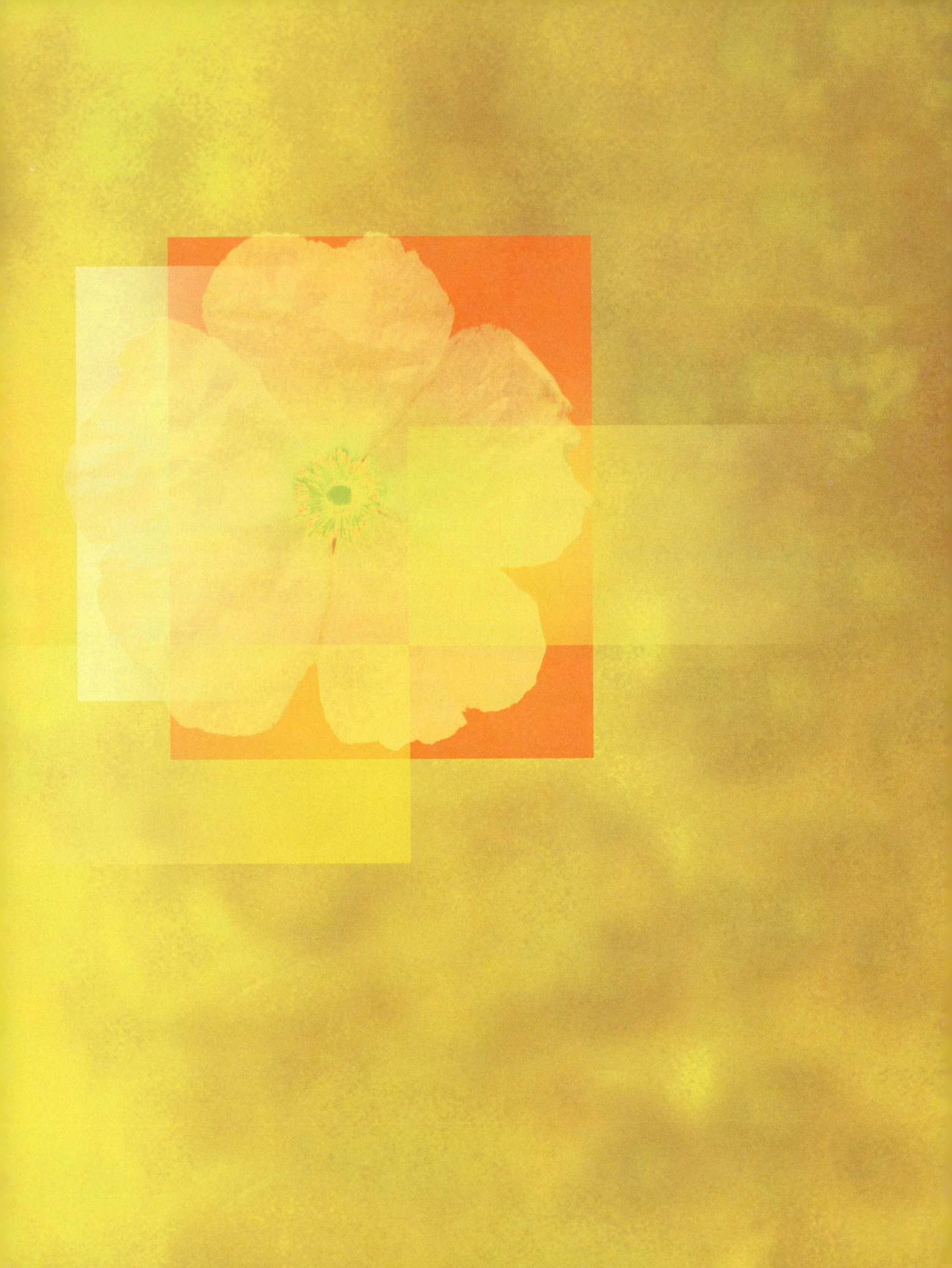

UNIT 7

Newborn Development and Nursing Care

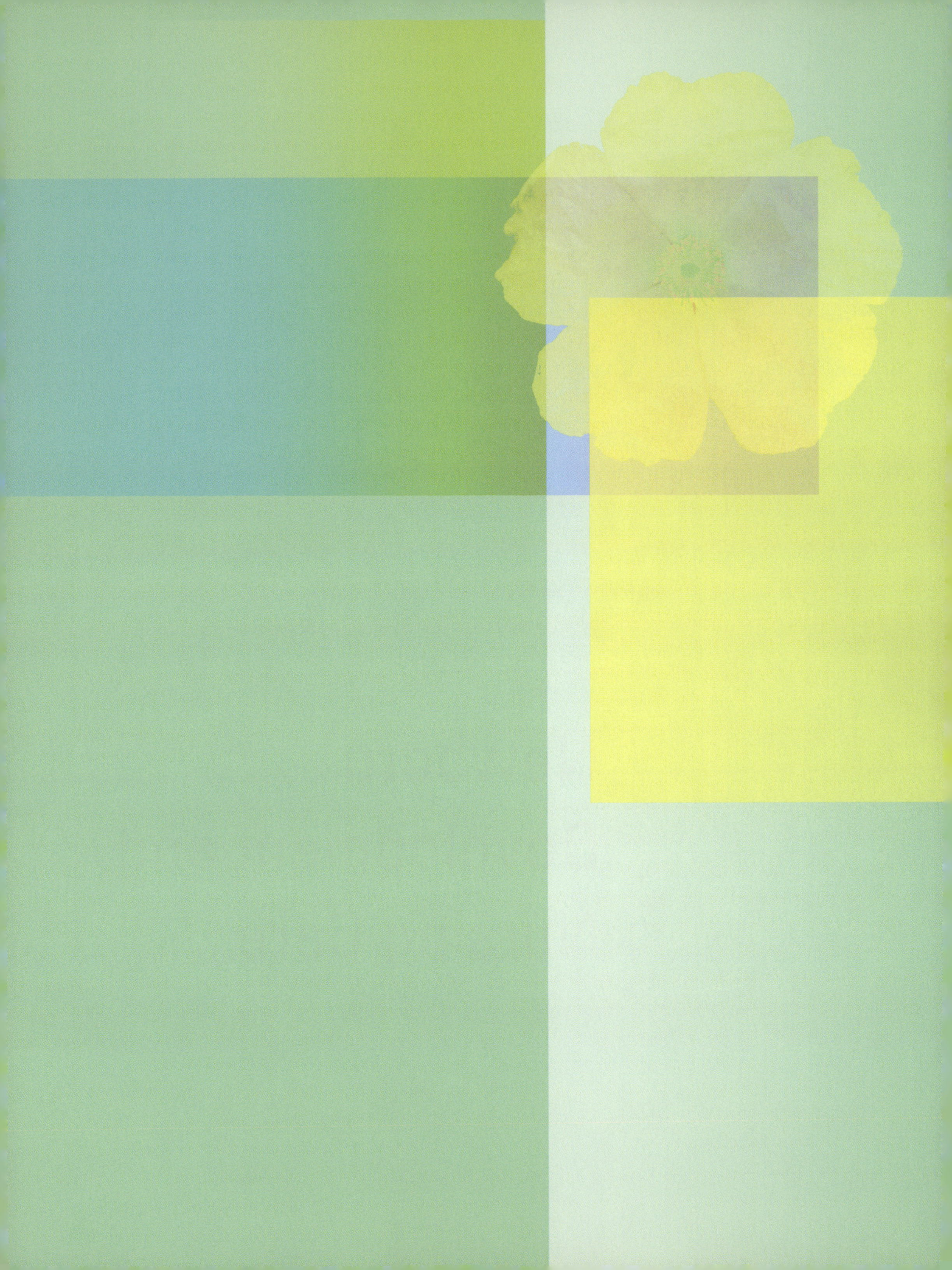

CHAPTER 19

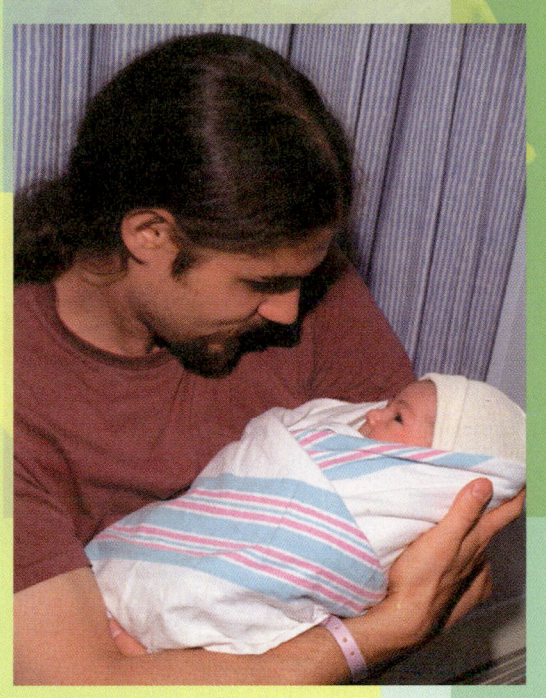

TRANSITION TO EXTRAUTERINE LIFE

The journey to birth is nothing more than an incredible miracle of life. This journey requires a number of successful transitions if the newborn is to survive. In utero, the fetus is entirely dependent on the placenta to sustain physiologic functions and to provide nutrition necessary for optimal growth and development. Following birth, a number of major physiologic changes must occur if the infant is to make a successful transition to extrauterine life, including pulmonary, cardiovascular, and gastrointestinal changes.

The first few hours after birth of a baby are also a time of transition for the parents. Perinatal nurses play an important role in helping parents to make a successful transition to parenthood by facilitating positive parent-infant interactions and providing education on routine baby care. Anticipatory guidance and crisis intervention are also important aspects of the perinatal nurses' role in caring for parents who experience delivery complications or the birth of a sick newborn.

Key Terms

Asphyxia
Behavioral state
Congenital heart defects
Diaphragmatic hernia
Ductus arteriosus
Ductus venosus
Extrauterine life
Fetal circulation
Foramen ovale
Habituation
Hypoglycemia
Hypothermia
Hypovolemia
Meconium staining

Neutral thermal environment
Postnatal circulation
Preterm
Primary apnea
Pulmonary vascular resistance
Resuscitation
Secondary apnea
Sepsis
Thermoregulation
Transient tachypnea of the newborn

Competencies

Upon completion of this chapter, the reader should be able to:

1. Describe the primary features of the fetal pulmonary and cardiac systems.
2. Identify the physiologic changes that occur at birth as the newborn makes the transition to extrauterine life.
3. Describe the neurobehavioral changes that occur during the first 12 hours after birth as the newborn makes the transition to extrauterine life.
4. Discuss the parenting and family issues that occur during the period of newborn transition to extrauterine life.
5. Understand the major complications that can occur during the transition process.
6. Discuss the effects of prematurity on the transition to extrauterine life.
7. Understand the role and responsibilities of the nurse during the transition process.
8. Discuss appropriate role of the nurse in resuscitation of the asphyxiated infant.

Transitions by nature are challenging, but this is never more true than it is for transition from intrauterine to extrauterine life. In fact, the essence of life depends on this successful transition. Successful transition requires the initiation of spontaneous breathing; significant cardiopulmonary changes, including the shift from fetal to postnatal circulation; and a variety of other important adaptations, including, but not limited to, thermoregulatory and metabolic adjustments. Failure of the infant to make a successful transition may result in varying degrees of morbidity or mortality.

Two major factors have contributed to today's awareness of the importance of the process of the infant's transition to extrauterine life in the first critical hours after birth. First, the technology and assessment techniques available to monitor the well-being of the fetus and the neonate have increased in sophistication, availability, and routine use. Strategies, such as fetal monitoring, sonography, and development of training and certification in the assessment of fetal heart rate monitoring and resuscitation, have all heightened the awareness of the complexity of the physiologic changes the neonate undergoes in the hours before, during, and after birth. Second, the changes in health care policy that have led to shorter and shorter hospital stays for

mothers and babies have created an increased need for careful assessment of the infant's transition process during the hours before discharge from the hospital (Behram, Moschler, Sayegh, Garguillo, & Mann, 1998).

This chapter explores the physiologic changes that occur during the newborn's adaptation to extrauterine life. It discusses common newborn complications that interfere with the newborn's ability to adapt successfully. First, this chapter explores physiologic and neurobehavioral transitions of the newborn at and immediately following birth. Common neonatal conditions and diseases that may interfere with the newborn's smooth transition to extrauterine life and require resuscitation and stabilization in the delivery room are discussed. The effect of prematurity on pulmonary and cardiac transition also is discussed. Finally, resuscitation of newborns in the delivery room is discussed.

PHYSIOLOGIC TRANSITIONS OF MAJOR SYSTEMS

Physiologic transition from intrauterine to extrauterine life involves a number of major changes that are necessary for newborn survival. These include pulmonary, cardiac, thermoregulation, metabolic, and gastrointestinal changes.

Pulmonary System Transition

During uterine development, the placenta is the organ of respiration, with the lungs receiving little of the cardiac output (Guyton & Hall, 2001). The blood bypasses the lungs through shunt pathways, such as the ductus venosus, the ductus arteriosus, and the foramen ovale. This occurs primarily because of pressure gradient differences between pulmonary and systemic vascular systems. In the fetus, the lungs are a high-resistance, low-flow organ (Guyton & Hall, 2001).

Pulmonary vascular resistance (PVR) is the resistance in the pulmonary vascular bed against which the right ventricle must eject blood. High levels of fetal PVR are caused by a number of interrelated factors that promote constriction of the pulmonary capillaries.

This constriction of pulmonary vessels keeps blood from flowing through the fetal lungs and causes oxygenation to occur in the placenta. The exchange of oxygen (O_2) and carbon dioxide (CO_2) within the placenta occurs by simple diffusion at the intervillous space (Sansoucie & Cavaliere, 1997).

In addition to simple diffusion processes, differences in O_2 content (i.e., dissolved and hemoglobin-bound O_2) and higher concentrations of fetal Hgb also serve to facilitate oxygenation in the fetus. Oxygen-carrying capacity is enhanced by the increased presence of fetal Hgb. Fetal Hgb has a higher affinity for oxygen than does maternal adult Hgb (Guyton & Hall, 2001; Sansoucie & Cavaliere, 1997).

Pulmonary adaptation at birth is accomplished via a complex series of events that switches the function of respiration from the placenta to the lungs. Various metabolic and environmental factors are responsible for the onset of breathing in the neonate. Mild hypercapnia, hypoxia, and acidosis act as powerful stimuli for the onset of breathing in the newly born infant and result from the intermittent cessation of uteroplacental perfusion during contractions, which occurs during normal labor (Guyton & Hall, 2001; Nelson, 1994). Other external stimuli that also enhance rhythmic breathing at delivery include the environmental factors of cold, light, noise, and touch (Nelson, 1994).

During pulmonary transition, fluid within the lung must also be cleared. During labor, fetal lung fluid is beginning to be reabsorbed. During vaginal delivery, the chest wall is compressed and approximately one-third of the fetal lung fluid is expelled via the trachea. Following delivery of the chest, the chest wall recoils, causing inspiration of air and expansion of the lungs (Nelson, 1994). The transpulmonary pressure generated by the first breath drives the remaining fetal lung fluid into the inter-

stitium, where it is absorbed through the lymphatic and pulmonary circulation (Donn & Faix, 1996; Guyton & Hall, 2001; Nelson, 1994).

With initial lung expansion, the pulmonary arterioles dilate in response to the increase in oxygen levels, and the PVR level falls, and pulmonary blood flow increases (Guyton & Hall, 2001). Lung compliance continues to improve in the hours after delivery.

Cardiac System Transition

Cardiac transition from intrauterine to extrauterine life involves closure of fetal circulatory pathways and other cardiovascular adaptations that promote increased blood flow to the lungs for oxygenation and switch the fetal circulation to a postnatal (adult) circulatory pathway.

Fetal Circulatory Pathways

Fetal circulation is anatomically and physiologically different than that of the newborn. This difference allows the oxygenation of the fetus to occur in the placenta rather than in the lungs. Among the important differences are the existence of three anatomic shunts that, in utero, allow the most highly oxygenated blood to be delivered from the placenta to the brain and heart, while being diverted from the lungs (Donn & Faix, 1996; Guyton & Hall, 2001; Nelson, 1994; Sansoucie & Cavaliere, 1997). The three fetal circulatory shunts include the ductus venosus, the foramen ovale, and the ductus arteriosus. The ductus venosus, which connects the umbilical vein to the inferior vena cava, allows blood to bypass the liver. The foramen ovale allows blood entering the right atrium of the heart to go directly through the left atrium, left ventricle, and out the ascending aorta to immediately supply the brain, heart, and upper extremities. The ductus arteriosus shunts blood from the pulmonary artery to the descending aorta, bypassing the lung, to perfuse the lower body and return to the placenta for oxygenation. Figure 19-1 illustrates fetal circulation.

Cardiovascular Adaptation

The first breath has significant effects on cardiovascular function. With the onset of breathing, there is a decrease in PVR and an increase in pulmonary blood flow (Nelson, 1994; Sansoucie & Cavaliere, 1997). As a result of the pulmonary changes, the pressure in the right side of the heart falls and pulmonary venous return increases to the left atrium (Nelson, 1994).

With cord clamping and the loss of placenta circulation, pressures within the aorta and left heart increase significantly. The reversal of pressures leads to diminished right-to-left shunting across the foramen ovale, causing

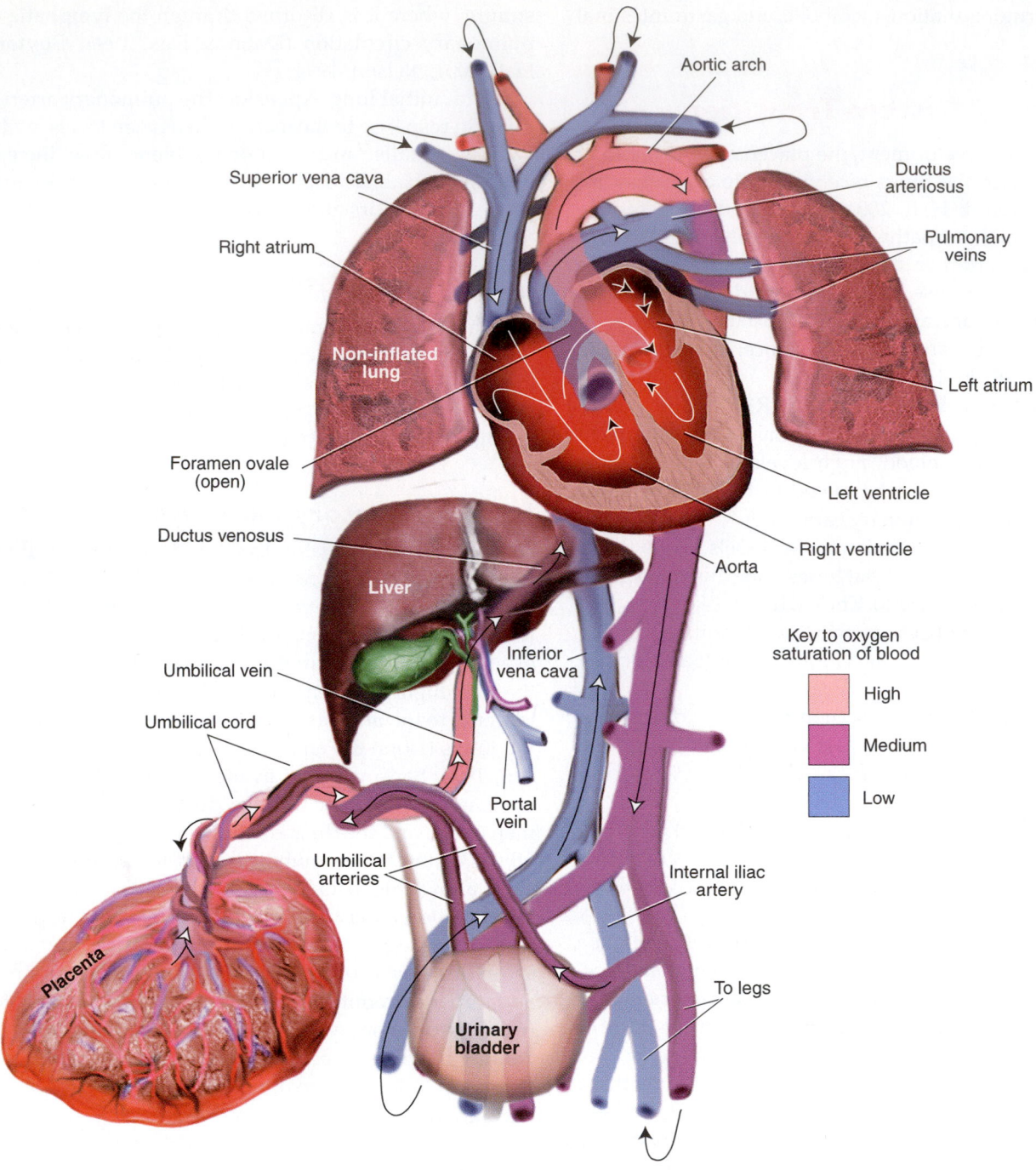

Figure 19-1 Fetal circulation.

the flap to shut between the two atria within minutes or hours after birth (Donn & Faix, 1996; Guyton & Hall, 2001; Sansoucie & Cavaliere, 1997). Until the foramen ovale is anatomically sealed, anything that produces a significant increase in right atrial pressure can reopen the foramen ovale and allow a right-to-left shunt.

The ductus arteriosus also undergoes rapid change after birth. In contrast to the pulmonary arterioles, the muscular ductus arteriosus becomes smaller. Pressure changes within the cardiac chambers also lead to diminished flow

across the ductus arteriosus. Blood flow through the ductus arteriosus reverses and blood flows from left to right (from the descending aorta to pulmonary artery) (Guyton & Hall, 2001). Functional closure of the ductus is usually achieved within 96 hours in healthy, term newborns, and anatomic closure is generally completed within 4 months through endothelial and fibrous tissue proliferation (Guyton & Hall, 2001; Sansoucie & Cavaliere, 1997). As with the foramen ovale, during the functional closure stage, the ductus may be reopened under certain cardiopulmonary dysfunctions that result in a return to fetal circulation.

The third anatomic shunt, the ductus venosus, also undergoes change during the transition to extrauterine life. When the placenta is removed after birth, the ductus venosus constricts, as blood stops flowing through the umbilical vein (Guyton & Hall, 2001). Functional closure occurs within 2 to 3 days. Anatomic closure is achieved by fibrosis and is generally completed within 7 days, with

the structure becoming the ligamentum venosum. Figure 19-2 shows the changes that shift fetal circulation to a postnatal (adult) circulatory pathway.

Postnatal Circulation

Once the placenta is removed, the neonate must change from a fetal circulatory pathway to a **postnatal** (or adult) **circulation** to survive in the extrauterine world. Systemic

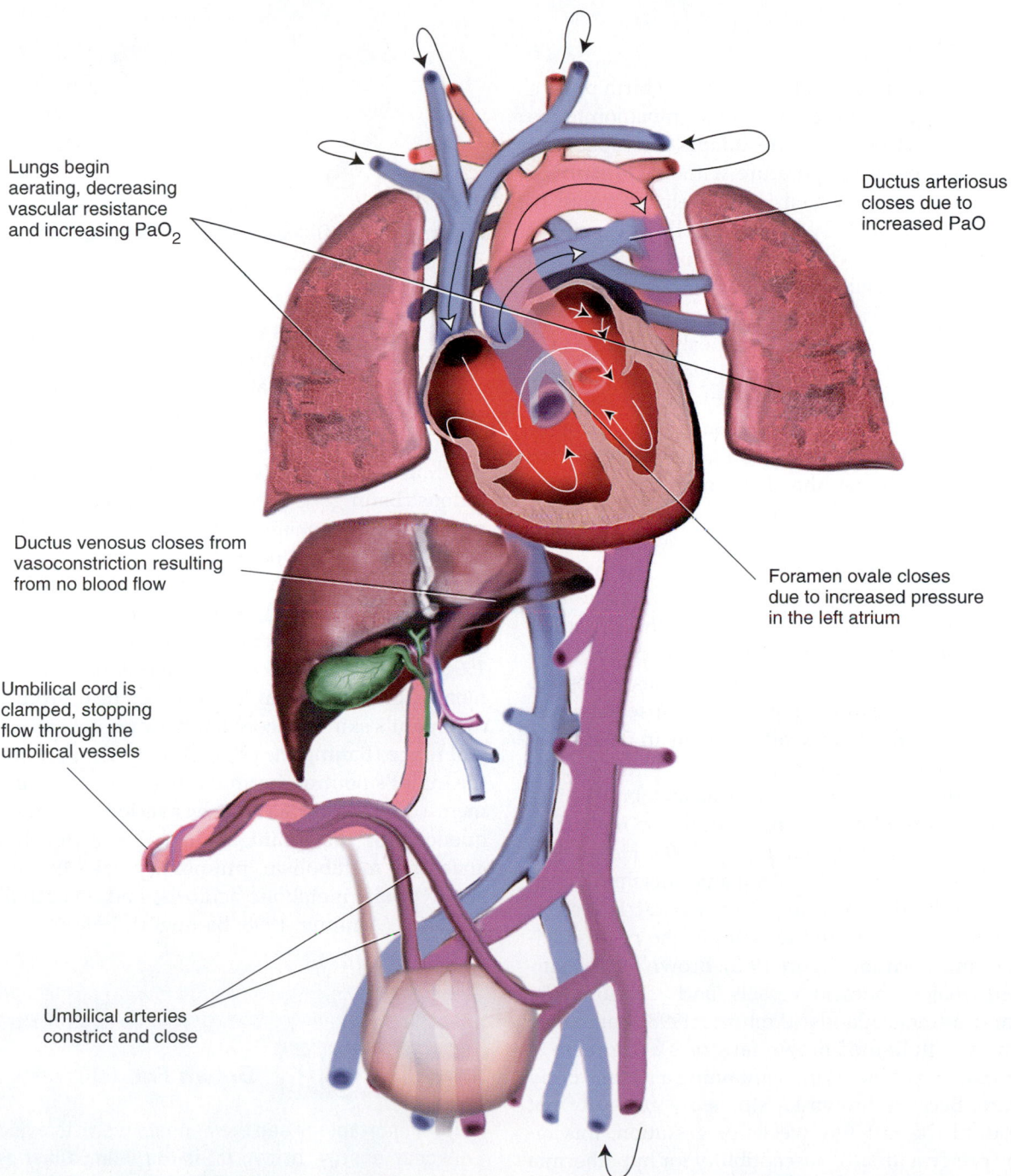

Lungs begin aerating, decreasing vascular resistance and increasing PaO_2

Ductus arteriosus closes due to increased PaO

Ductus venosus closes from vasoconstriction resulting from no blood flow

Foramen ovale closes due to increased pressure in the left atrium

Umbilical cord is clamped, stopping flow through the umbilical vessels

Umbilical arteries constrict and close

Figure 19-2   The modifications that change fetal circulation to postnatal (adult) circulation.

venous blood enters the right atrium from the superior vena cava and the inferior vena cava. Poorly oxygenated blood enters the right ventricle and passes through the pulmonary artery into the pulmonary circulation for oxygenation. The oxygenated blood returns to the left atrium through the pulmonary veins. This blood passes through the left ventricle and into the aorta to supply the systemic circulation. Following the oxygenation and perfusion of tissue beds, the blood returns to the right heart and the circulatory pathway is repeated.

Thermoregulation

Effective thermal management at the time of birth plays a significant role in promoting an optimal transition to extrauterine life. Most healthy term infants are capable of reaching a stable body temperature without difficulty if proper methods are employed in the delivery room to prevent heat loss postnatally. Newborns, however, are at a distinct disadvantage when it comes to their ability to maintain normal **thermoregulation** as compared with the older infant or child. First, the neonate has a much greater potential for losing body heat, primarily because of a large body surface area in relation to weight, as well as poor thermal insulation resulting from limited neonatal fat stores (Amlung, 1998; Guyton & Hall, 2001). Another disadvantage is that the neonate has a limited capacity for heat production. Although the older child may use shivering to generate heat in the presence of thermal stress, the neonate has almost no ability to produce heat in this manner (Amlung, 1998; Baumgart, 1996). The healthy, full-term neonate may use, to a limited extent, voluntary muscle activity to assume flexed postures, thereby minimizing heat loss through a reduction of exposed body surface area. The preterm infant, however, has almost no ability to generate heat through increased muscular activity, because motor immaturity often results in flaccid, extended postures (Amlung, 1998).

In the healthy newborn, brown-fat metabolism is a primary mechanism of heat energy production in the first days of life (Amlung, 1998; Baumgart, 1996; Hey, 1994). Although brown fat is stored in small amounts throughout the infant's body, the majority of brown fat is located around the blood vessels and muscles in the neck, clavicles, axillae, and sternum (Figure 19-3). Brown fat also surrounds the major thoracic vessels and envelops the kidneys and adrenal glands (Amlung; 1998; Baumgart; 1996). Infants with limited brown-fat stores at birth are at particular risk for problems in maintaining a normal body temperature. Because brown-fat stores are generally not complete until the last few weeks of gestation, this increases the preterm infant's susceptibility for hypothermia (Amlung, 1998; Baumgart, 1996). In addition, brown-fat stores may have been consumed in utero for energy needs

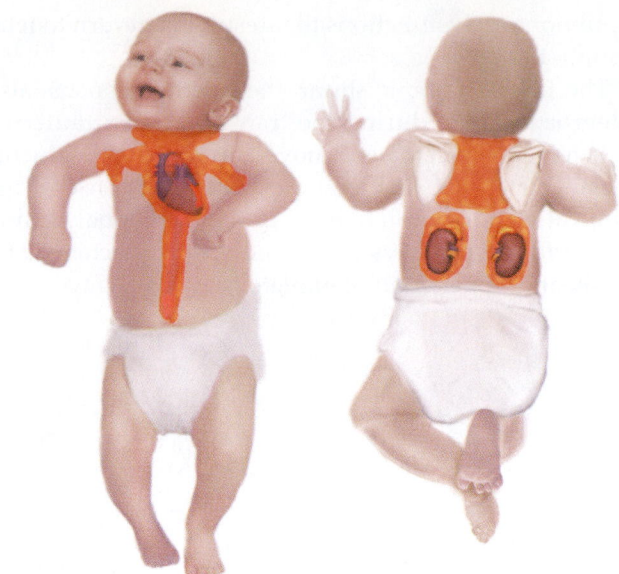

Figure 19-3   Distribution of brown fat in the newborn.

before birth in infants who are small for gestational age or who experience intrauterine growth restriction, thus also placing them at thermal risk (Amlung, 1998).

It has been estimated that heat loss in the delivery room may be as high as 0.4°F to 1.8°F per minute, depending on the infant's maturity and environmental conditions (Baumgart, 1996). This far exceeds maximal heat production in neonates and rapidly gives rise to the deleterious effects of hypothermia and cold stress. **Hypothermia** is defined as a rectal or axillary temperature below 97°F. In a cold environment, there is first a rise in oxygen consumption and endogenous heat production (Baumgart, 1996). If appropriate thermal interventions are not implemented promptly, heat loss exceeds heat production and the infant's skin and core temperature fall below the normal range (Baumgart, 1996). A body temperature outside the infant's neutral thermal range may result in development of hypothermia that has serious metabolic consequences for the infant, including the development of anaerobic metabolism, pulmonary vasoconstriction, tissue hypoxia, metabolic acidosis, and, eventually, hypoglycemia (Amlung, 1998; Baumgart, 1996).

Nursing Tip   *Brown Fat*

It is important to keep the neonate warm to avoid using excess energy. Brown fat is the infant's last defense mechanism against hypothermia.

Throughout delivery and the neonatal period, every newborn's thermoregulation needs must be carefully managed. The goal is to keep the infant in a **neutral thermal environment**, while maintaining a normal body temperature (Amlung, 1998; Baumgart, 1996). In a neutral thermal environment, the infant's axillary temperature is usually maintained in the range of 97°F to 99.5°F.

Nursing Process: Preventing Hypothermia and Maintaining a Neutral Thermal Environment

Full-term and preterm neonates are at risk for altered thermoregulation during the immediate postnatal period. This nursing process focuses on maintaining a neutral thermal environment for these infants.

Assessment

1. Assess factors related to the infant's risk of temperature fluctuation, including prematurity, sepsis, asphyxia, caregiving procedures, and high or low environmental temperatures. Assessment offers an opportunity to prevent cold stress.
2. Assess for potential or actual hypothermia by monitoring the infant's axillary temperature every 30 to 60 minutes after delivery until stable and then every 4 hours per nursery routine.
3. Monitor environmental room temperatures within the delivery room and nursery areas and readjust to avoid convective heat loss.

Nursing Diagnoses

Risk for imbalanced body temperature related to prematurity, abnormal disorders at birth, and exposure to cool environments.

Outcome Identification

Infant maintains an axillary temperature between 97°F and 99.5°F.

Planning

1. Identify the infant at risk for potential or actual temperature instability.
2. Prevent conditions that precipitate cold stress.
3. Provide a neutral thermal environment.
4. Teach parents how to maintain the infant's temperature.

Nursing Interventions

1. Minimize evaporative heat loss at delivery by immediately drying the infant and removing wet blankets.
2. Use a hat and warm blankets to swaddle infant during parent bonding.
3. Avoid placing the infant directly in contact with cold surfaces, such as a radiant warmer table or infant scale. This prevents heat loss by conduction.
4. Avoid placing the infant in drafts. This prevents heat loss by convection.
5. If body temperature is unstable, place the infant under a radiant warmer or in an incubator.
6. Use heat source when bathing the infant. Wash only small sections of the body at a time, being careful to immediately dry the area before proceeding to the next area.
7. When placing the infant in an open bassinet in the nursery, dress the infant warmly and cover with two or more blankets, as needed, to maintain normal axillary temperature.
8. Teach parents how to take their infant's axillary temperature and have them demonstrate the procedure. Talk with parents about causes of temperature fluctuation in newborns and how to prevent heat loss by appropriate clothing, avoiding drafts, and bathing techniques.

Evaluation

1. Assess and record the infant's axillary temperature every 30 to 60 minutes after delivery until stable and then every 4 hours per nursery routine.
2. Assess infant caregiving techniques in the delivery room and nursery and modify as necessary to prevent cold stress.
3. Assess the infant's immediate environment for adequacy of thermal support, such as clothing and number of blankets.
4. Encourage parents' questions and requests for clarifications, and give demonstrations to ensure their knowledge of the infant's thermoregulation needs.

Healthy term infants are typically quite capable of thermal self-regulation when clothed and provided with a few ancillary support measures, such as swaddling. Swaddling minimizes heat loss by increasing insulation at the skin surface (Baumgart, 1996). Stocking caps may also assist the term infant in maintaining a normal body temperature, because they decrease heat loss from the large surface area of the head (Amlung, 1998; Baumgart, 1996).

Metabolic Transition

In utero, the fetus is supplied with the necessary nutrients for growth and metabolic processes by the placenta and begins to prepare for postnatal energy demands. Primarily in the third trimester, the fetus begins the process of storing glycogen in the liver for conversion back to glucose during the immediate postnatal period (Brooks,

1997; Ogata, 1994). Although the fetal insulin response to maternal glucose load remains somewhat immature throughout gestation, fetal insulin also plays a role in stimulating fetal growth and body-fat deposition that is later used to maintain postnatal glucose homeostasis (Brooks, 1997; Ogata, 1994).

At birth, the continuous supply of glucose that diffused across the placenta is abruptly terminated. Although immediate newborn glucose levels are roughly equal to those of the mother, levels fall rapidly and reach their lowest point (approximately 40 mg/dL) within 1 to 3 hours in the healthy term newborn. Glucose levels begin to stabilize by 4 to 6 hours and typically are maintained in the range of 45 to 80 mg/dL. The transition to free fatty acids as the alternate fuel source is normally accomplished without incident in healthy term infants. However, the normal achievement of postnatal glucose homeostasis can be disrupted in high-risk infants who have low glycogen or fat stores, an increased glucose need, or immature hormonal regulation of glucose. These complications are discussed later in this chapter.

Gastrointestinal System Transition

The gastrointestinal tract undergoes major changes immediately after birth as a function of the beginning of respiration and the introduction of the first nutrients into the infant's gastrointestinal system. At birth, the infant's abdomen is relatively flat and bowel sounds are absent. With the start of respiration, the intestinal tract begins to fill up with air, the abdomen becomes more rounded and soft, and bowel sounds become audible with the stethoscope. This usually occurs within the first 15 minutes of life. Peristalsis may not be continuously audible over the next few hours but should be clearly initiated during the first period of reactivity. Some infants may pass meconium during this time.

NEUROBEHAVIORAL TRANSITION IN THE FIRST 12 HOURS

The transition to extrauterine life begins with the birth of the infant and extends through the first 12 to 24 hours of life. It is a process in which the infant moves from a homeostatic metabolic state in the uterine environment to a homeostatic state in the extrauterine environment. It is a defined progression of events that is probably triggered by stimuli from the external environment.

First Period of Reactivity

During the first few minutes after birth, the infant undergoes an intense period of activity and alertness that probably represents a sympathetic nervous system response to the intense stimulation of the labor and delivery process. The infant often responds with bursts of rapid, jerky movements of the extremities, alternating with periods of relative immobility. The infant may show high muscular tone during this period and demonstrate behaviors, such as finger splaying, arching, and hyperextension. The period is characterized by myoclonic movements of the eyeball, spontaneous startles and Moro reflexes, sucking activity, chewing, smacking and rooting, and fine tremors of the extremities. All of these behaviors indicate the infant's stress in coping with the sudden increase in environmental stimuli. During this period, the infant enters a state of alertness, peering intently at the surrounding people and environment. This may allow the infant to achieve and maintain eye contact with the parents or caregivers for brief periods of time.

This period of reactivity is also characterized by tachycardia and tachypnea. The infant's heart rate peaks in the first 2 to 3 minutes after delivery and typically falls over the first 30 minutes to 120 to 140 bpm. The respiratory rate remains rapid over the first hour, typically peaking at 1 hour and decreasing during the quiet period that follows the first period of reactivity. Some transient nasal flaring, chest retractions, and grunting are not unusual but should be decreasing by the end of the first period of reactivity. Fine rales and rhonchi are often heard in the first period of reactivity, usually clearing spontaneously within the first 15 minutes after vaginal birth.

Implications for Parent, Family, and Newborn Interaction

The first period of reactivity provides a unique opportunity to promote early family and newborn interaction. Two elements of the infant's behavior during this period are particularly conducive to this process. First, the infant is alert and responding to the immediate environment. This is a time in the infant's normal transition process when it is possible for the mother and father to hold and interact with the baby. If both mother and baby are stable, the family should be allowed a quiet time and place to be with their baby. The infant may be placed in the parents' arms in an "en face" (face-to-face) position to promote eye contact between parent and infant (Figure 19-4). This time of physical closeness and quiet interaction has been found to be intensely emotionally gratifying for many parents. The mother may also enjoy having skin-to-skin contact with the infant. The infant, clad only in a diaper, may be placed on the mother's chest and then covered with a blanket to maintain body temperature. This physical contact may also enhance the infant's physiologic organization (Ludington-Hoe, Hadeed, & Anderson, 1991).

Additional infant characteristics that may contribute to family and newborn interaction in this period of reac-

period. Muscle tone, which was high in the first period of reactivity, should begin to moderate. Movements should become smoother, less jerky, and less frequent. The infant's heart and respiratory rates decline, and heart rate variability decreases. Respiratory symptoms, such as grunting, chest retractions, brief apneic periods, rales, and rhonchi, may still occur but should be diminishing during this period.

Implications for Parent, Family, and Newborn Interaction

Depending on hospital policy, mothers and infants may remain together during this period, or the infant may be taken to an observation nursery, where some of the initial assessment data are collected. This may be an opportunity for the parents to have some quiet time together and for the mother to rest. If the mother indicates a readiness to learn about her baby during this period, some teaching about the process of the baby's adjustment to extrauterine

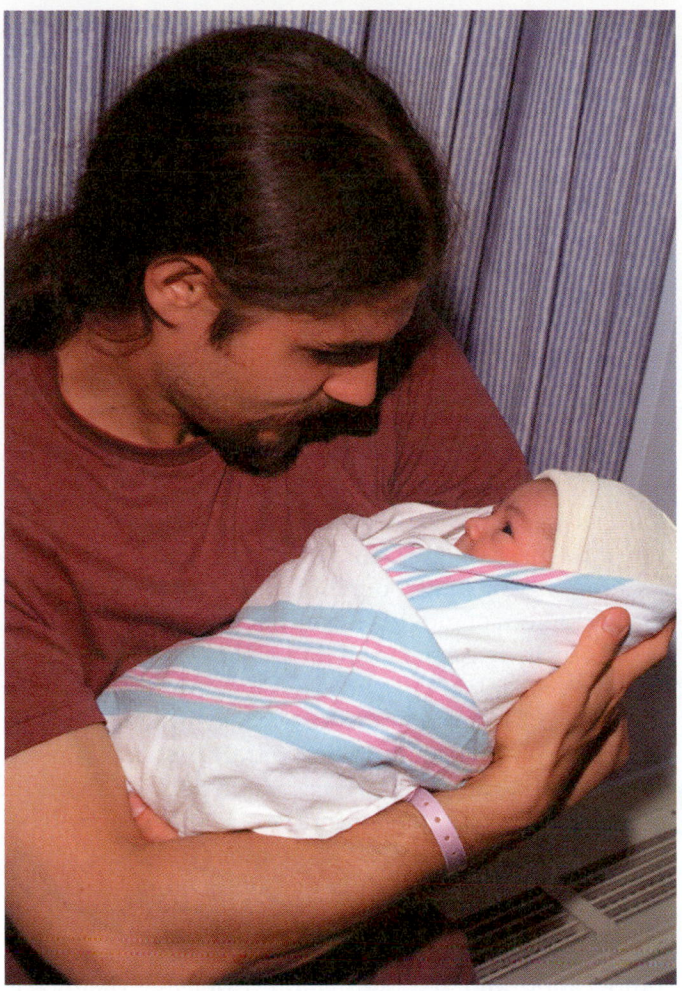

Figure 19-4   Father interacting with his alert newborn infant in the "en face" position.

tivity are sucking, rooting, and chewing behaviors. If the infant is to be breastfed, this is an opportune time to start suckling, using the infant's normal behaviors to promote a successful experience (Figure 19-5). Again, the determination of whether or not to start breastfeeding at this time must be made through the assessment of the physiologic stability of both the mother and the infant and the mother's emotional readiness and preferences.

Period of Decreased Activity

This period follows the first period of reactivity and probably represents a parasympathetic nervous system response as the environmental activity decreases and the infant's ability to cope with stimuli increases. During this period the infant's alertness gradually decreases and sleep may occur. Motor activity may reach a peak and then decline over this period. The infant continues to demonstrate some tics, twitches, and involuntary startles, although these should gradually diminish throughout this

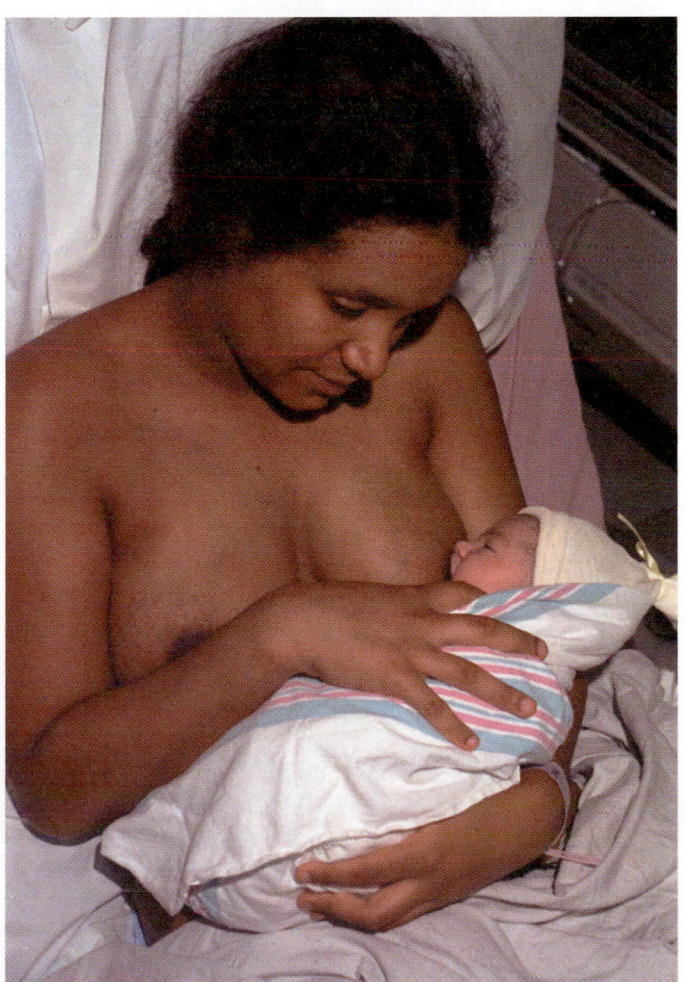

Figure 19-5   Full-term infant ready for breastfeeding at 30 minutes of age.

life, the initial assessment process, and the meaning of some of the infant's behaviors may be appropriate.

Second Period of Reactivity

The second period of reactivity begins as the baby awakens and shows an increased responsiveness to environmental stimuli. At this time the infant may show both heart and respiratory accelerations, particularly in response to environmental stimuli, such as loud noises, bright lights, voices, and touch. There may also be an increase in respiratory symptoms, such as transient grunting, retractions, rales, and rhonchi, although the frequency and severity should be less than that of the first period of reactivity and should gradually diminish throughout this second period. This period is also characterized by an increase in peristalsis and, frequently, the first passage of meconium, although this may have occurred earlier. At the same time, infants may show an increase in hiccoughs, gagging, and spitting up as they become more interactive with the environment and challenged by it. Motor activity increases during this stage but should not reach the level achieved in the first period of reactivity. Motor activity should also be smoother and more organized than in the first period. Muscle tone may increase in comparison to the period of decreased activity but should continue to moderate throughout this period.

Implications for Parent, Family, and Newborn Interaction

The pace and rhythm of parent, family, and newborn interaction during this transition period depends on the readiness and availability of all the involved parties for interaction. The onset of the second period of reactivity represents a time when the newborn is alert, active, and available. The mother's readiness or availability depends on her fatigue levels, her recovery from the delivery process, the amount and type of medication she has received, and her emotional status. It is common for the mother to desire to have her baby close and to want to participate in feeding and caring for the baby. It is equally normal for the mother to express a need for rest and recovery and to have minimal contact with the baby during this time. If the mother is ready for interaction with her baby, they should be provided with a quiet, comfortable environment in which to be together. The mother and father may have questions about behaviors they see in the baby at this time. If necessary, the parents should be helped to position the baby in a face-to-face position to promote interaction. Helping them to feed the baby or change a diaper are ways of strengthening their sense of competence in caring for their infant. Parents may also be encouraged to examine the baby and to ask any questions they may have.

Assessment Strategies and Newborn Competencies

The most widely used assessment strategies in this neonatal period are the Apgar score and the assessment of gestational age. Both of these assessment tools are discussed in detail elsewhere in this text and represent commonly used and valid one-time "snapshots" of the infant's status (Jepson, Talashek, & Tichy, 1991). However, adequate assessment of an infant's progress through the process of adjustment to extrauterine life requires that the nurse engage in serial observations of the infant. The determination that the infant is progressing normally through this transition period is based not on the observations of symptoms at one time point but on the observation of an infant's pattern of moving toward more organized behaviors and an increase in the infant's ability to regulate his or her own physiologic responses. As an example, it is not uncommon for an infant to display symptoms such as grunting with respirations, chest retractions, or brief periods of apnea throughout the transition period. However, these symptoms should become less frequent and less severe over time. If these same symptoms appear to increase in frequency or severity over time, to continue beyond a normal transition period, or to be unresponsive to routine interventions, they may indicate a more serious medical complication and require a more extensive diagnostic workup and treatment.

Two infant neurobehavioral competencies, infant state and habituation, provide additional information regarding an infant's adjustment to extrauterine life. Infant state, or **behavioral state**, refers to the quality and level of alertness the infant demonstrates. Infant state is viewed as a range of alertness levels from sound quiet sleep through levels of drowsiness to levels of wakeful attentiveness and, finally, to hyperalert, agitated, or crying states. Infant state stability provides a valuable window into the maturing nervous system and a useful assessment measure for evaluating neurobehavioral stabilization over the first 24 hours. Behavioral state is evaluated in terms of the range of states the infant is able to achieve and their duration and stability. In the first stage of reactivity, most infants are able to achieve an alert, wakeful state and are able to focus on a face or object for brief periods of time. These periods of alertness, however, may be interrupted by agitated movements, respiratory disturbances, and other signs of disorganization. The infant is likely to be distracted and reactive to environmental stimuli and to move rapidly from alert to drowsy to fussy states. During the period of decreased activity, the infant is likely to sleep but may continue to demonstrate involuntary movements and respiratory disturbances during the sleep state, rather than achieving a quiet, well-organized sleep state. Throughout the first 24 hours, the infant's ability to achieve and maintain an organized, quiet alert state and an organized quiet sleep state, as well as all of the intermediate states, should gradually increase. The nurse's observation of the change in the duration, stability, and range of the infant's state control is a valuable indicator of the infant's neurobehavioral intactness.

The concept of **habituation** refers to the ability of the infant to become adjusted or adapted to a specific environmental stimulus. When an infant is first confronted with an unexpected environmental stimulus, the infant responds with startles, twitches, tics, or respiratory instability. In a mature, well-organized baby, the reaction to the stimulus gradually decreases and the startles, twitches, and other behaviors subside. This is called habituation. In the period immediately after birth, many infants are not able to habituate to an environmental stimulus. The startle reactions continue until the stimulus stops. Over the first 24 hours, the infant should increase the ability to habituate to environmental stimuli. This process, again, provides a useful indicator of the infant's neurobehavioral intactness.

COMPLICATIONS OF TRANSITION

Most healthy term newborns make the transition to extrauterine life without difficulty. However, this complex process does not always occur uneventfully. Complications occur that may be transient and require only minimal intervention or may represent a significant threat to the infant's well-being.

Common Complications

Conditions that may interfere with the newborn's smooth transition to extrauterine life include asphyxia, meconium staining, transient tachypnea of the newborn, hypoglycemia, and hypovolemia (shock).

Asphyxia

One of the most serious of the complications of the transition process is asphyxia. **Asphyxia** is a metabolic process that arises from failure of the respiratory organ in the fetus or neonate. Failure of the organ of respiration leads to impairment of oxygen and carbon dioxide exchange. This results in hypoxemia, hypercarbia, and, subsequently, acute respiratory acidosis. If such circumstances persist for a prolonged period, tissue hypoxia occurs, with superimposed metabolic acidosis. Without appropriate caregiver interventions to reverse and restore optimal gas exchange within the placenta or lung, permanent brain or

other major organ injury or death may result (Fisher & Paton, 1986; Kattwinkel, 2000).

A classic series of events occurs when an infant becomes asphyxiated in utero or postnatally. The progressively severe clinical phases of asphyxia include primary apnea, gasping, and secondary, or terminal, apnea.

During the initial period of deprivation of oxygen, the infant exhibits rapid breathing. If hypoxic conditions persist, the heart rate begins to fall, and the infant's respiratory efforts cease. This is referred to as **primary apnea**. During this period, blood pressure is normal or slightly elevated and pulses are palpable. Although the infant's tone gradually diminishes, the infant is still responsive to tactile stimulation and oxygen. If resuscitation is provided at this point, the infant responds quickly with gasping respirations, rapidly followed by the establishment of normal oxygenation (Fisher & Paton, 1986; Kattwinkel, 2000).

If the asphyxia progresses, the infant begins to demonstrate deep gasping respirations. If the asphyxia continues, the infant's heart rate progressively falls, the infant's blood pressure begins to drop, and the infant becomes almost flaccid. The infant's respiratory efforts become progressively weaker until respirations cease, and the infant enters into the period of **secondary apnea**. During this period, metabolic derangements are severe, with marked hypoxemia, hypercarbia, and acidemia. Heart rate is extremely low, pulses are absent, and, without prompt intervention, death occurs. Tactile stimulation is ineffective for resuscitation of an infant in secondary apnea, thus requiring quick initiation of positive pressure ventilation with 100% oxygen. The infant usually becomes pink before the reestablishment of spontaneous respirations, because oxygenation is restored sooner than the brain can recover from the severely hypoxic event (Fisher & Paton, 1986; Kattwinkel, 2000).

Because primary and secondary apnea are often difficult to distinguish from one another, the health care provider should always assume the latter and initiate respirations using assisted ventilation. This approach facilitates rapid response to resuscitation efforts, ensures more rapid establishment of spontaneous respirations, and minimizes the potential for adverse neurologic outcomes (Fisher & Paton, 1986; Kattwinkel, 2000).

While the Apgar score has been widely used in the delivery room to evaluate the overall health status of the newly born infant, the Apgar score neither establishes nor rules out the presence of asphyxia. Apgar scoring frequently correlates poorly with the underlying acid-base status of the infant at birth. The need for resuscitation can be more accurately assessed by the evaluation of the infant's heart rate, respiratory activity, and color than by the Apgar score. Resuscitation, therefore, should not be delayed for the assessment of the 1-minute score but should be initiated immediately. Resuscitation of the newborn consists of emergency life-support measures, including airway management, positive pressure ventilation, chest compressions, medications, and thermal support.

Meconium Staining

Meconium staining of amniotic fluid occurs in 10% to 15% of all deliveries (Whitsett, Pryhuber, Rice, Warner, & Wert, 1994). Meconium staining occurs when the fetus passes meconium close to or during the labor or birth process, usually in response to some distress, such as an episode of asphyxia. It is most common in infants born postterm and occurs less commonly with decreasing gestational age. Meconium staining rarely occurs in infants born before 34 weeks' gestation.

The concern in the case of meconium-stained amniotic fluid is the possibility that the infant may aspirate the meconium. Aspiration of meconium can be a cause of serious pulmonary disease in neonates, either by causing an obstruction of the airways or by producing a chemical pneumonitis. These conditions may be severe and life threatening, even in the healthy full-term infant. Complications resulting from meconium aspiration are increased if: (1) passage of meconium occurs before the second stage of labor, thus increasing the possibility that aspiration will occur; or (2) the meconium-stained amniotic fluid is thick, increasing the severity of airway obstruction if aspiration occurs. Symptoms of clinical disease may be immediate and severe, requiring resuscitation in the delivery room, or may occur gradually over the first few hours after birth with the infant demonstrating respiratory distress and hypoxemia.

When meconium-stained amniotic fluid is noted, special measures should be taken to prepare for the delivery. An extra person may be necessary to help with the suctioning procedure, including assembling endotracheal tubes and suctioning equipment and monitoring the infant's physiologic status. Some institutions have a neonatal resuscitation team (usually a NICU nurse and respiratory therapist). If possible, the mouth, nose, and posterior pharynx should be suctioned immediately after the head is delivered and while the chest is still compressed in the birth canal. After birth, the need for tracheal suctioning of the infant's airway is determined by whether or not the infant is vigorous at birth (defined by strong respiratory effort, good muscle tone, and a heart rate of more than 100 bpm) (Kattwinkel, 2000). If tracheal suctioning is required, the infant should not be stimulated to cry or inhale until the infant is intubated and suctioning has been performed.

Parents are often unprepared for complications at delivery. In the accompanying box, a father shares the experiences of one family whose baby had thick meconium

Critical Thinking

Newborn Resuscitation

Parents are often restricted from being present while their infant is being resuscitated in the newborn stabilization area adjacent to the delivery room. Ask yourself if this practice is done for the benefit of the newborn infant or for the comfort level of the health care team? Also ask yourself: If this was your baby, how would you feel if you were excluded from the newborn stabilization area while the health care team attempted to resuscitate or stabilize your infant? Would you be more frightened by the procedures being performed or by not knowing how your infant was responding to the intervention measures?

staining and respiratory depression at birth. Nurses must partner with parents to ensure that hospital policies and practices facilitate the parents' right to be with their baby and to participate in their infant's care, as the clinical situation allows.

Transient Tachypnea of the Newborn

Transient tachypnea of the newborn (TTN) is a condition in which the infant presents with grunting, retractions, and an elevated respiratory rate at birth or shortly after. The condition is self-limiting, usually resolving within 5 days. Because the condition is self-limiting, infants with TTN usually require only supportive care, mainly oxygen therapy and intravenous fluid supplementation. Rarely is short-term ventilation necessary. In addition, if maternal risk factors for sepsis or other causes for respiratory distress cannot be ruled out, infants are usually treated prophylactically with broad-spectrum antibiotics.

Although the symptoms of TTN are similar to behaviors in the normal process of transition to extrauterine life, the clinical progression is quite different. Shortly after delivery, infants with TTN demonstrate tachypnea, grunting, nasal flaring, rib retraction, and varying degrees of cyanosis. Many healthy infants also demonstrate some respiratory grunting and chest retractions initially, but these symptoms are usually resolved and the respiratory rate should be stabilizing by the end of the second period of reactivity. During the end of the second period of reactivity, grunting, retraction, and increased respiratory rate should occur primarily in response to environmental stimuli, not when the infant is at rest. The increased respiratory efforts normally noted in the first and second pe-

Reflections from a Father

We were so excited that the time had finally come for my wife to deliver our firstborn son. Everyone was there, even my parents who lived 2 hours away by car. When my wife went into labor, the doctor said everything was fine. What we had not prepared for was meconium staining which the health care team members noted when my wife's bag of water broke. When he was delivered, the neonatal team 'whisked' our baby away to a separate room. The neonatal doctor said that I could come be with my baby as soon as they were certain that everything was okay. I didn't understand why I couldn't go with them. What were they doing to my baby that I shouldn't see? I think my wife and I were more frightened by not knowing what was going on and how our son was doing, than we would have been if I would have been allowed to go with them and observe and be with my son.

riods of reactivity are related to the clearance of fetal fluid from the infant's lungs after birth and are not usually accompanied by cyanosis. In TTN, these symptoms may persist for several days and occur even when the baby is at rest. Nursing observations of the infant, then, should focus on whether these respiratory symptoms appear to be resolving through the first and second periods of reactivity or persisting at the same level or increasing in severity and whether the distress results in the need for oxygen therapy.

Hypoglycemia

Hypoglycemia is a relatively common complication in the early newborn period and one for which the nurse should be continually alert. Plasma glucose levels of less than 40 mg/dL should be considered hypoglycemic, although this level is somewhat arbitrary and has not been correlated with the glucose use rate of the infant or with severity of symptoms. Symptoms of hypoglycemia include jitteriness, tremors, apnea, cyanosis, limpness or lethargy, and, in severe cases, convulsions.

Several groups of neonates are at particular risk for hypoglycemia. Infants who are born small for gestational age (SGA) have inadequate hepatic glycogen stores at birth. During intrauterine life, the nutrients available to these infants were necessarily channeled toward growth rather than being set aside for glycogen storage. At birth, then, little glycogen reserve is available to meet the infant's metabolic needs. Hypoglycemia is usually short-lived in these infants as nutrient intake is increased. Infants born prematurely are, similar to SGA infants, born with inadequate glycogen stores and are also vulnerable to hypoglycemic episodes. These infants have missed all or part of the third trimester of intrauterine development, during which much of the hepatic glycogen is stored. The younger the gestational age at birth, the less glycogen is present and the greater the risk for hypoglycemia. Furthermore, infants who are born both SGA and premature are at extremely high risk for hypoglycemia.

A third group of infants who have low glycogen stores at birth are those who have experienced perinatal stress. Stressful events, such as hypoxia, acidosis, and fluctuations in fetal blood pressure and flow, can increase catecholamine secretion in utero and subsequently increase mobilization of hepatic glycogen stores. At birth, these infants may have significantly depleted glycogen stores and are at increased risk for hypoglycemia.

Infants who experience a hyperinsulin state during intrauterine development, most commonly infants of diabetic mothers (IDM), carry over this hyperinsulin response to the extrauterine state. IDMs develop hyperinsulinism in utero in response to the mother's hyperglycemic state. In the neonatal period, the infants often have elevated plasma insulin concentrations and are hyperresponsive to increases in glucose levels. Infants with other conditions, including disorders of the pancreas and certain syndromes, may also have experienced a hyperinsulin state in utero and subsequently are at an increased risk for hypoglycemia postnatally.

Another group of infants at risk for hypoglycemia are those experiencing sepsis. Although the underlying mechanisms of this are not well understood, hypoglycemia or hyperglycemia are often the first indicators of sepsis in a neonate. An evaluation for sepsis should always be considered for infants with unexplained hypoglycemia.

The clinical management of infants susceptible to hypoglycemia begins with prevention and early identification. Although many neonates are asymptomatic, the symptoms most often described consist of respiratory distress, lethargy, apnea, or marked jitteriness (Brooks, 1997). Once the newborn is stabilized in the delivery room, feedings can be initiated as soon as possible after birth in healthy term infants. Such infants may be offered early breastfeeding or oral feedings with formula or glucose. Whenever hypoglycemic symptoms are observed or risk factors are present, glucose screening should be performed using a glucose oxidase strip or an approved blood glucose reflectance meter. LGA infants are often screened due to possible risk of hypoglycemia from undiagnosed maternal diabetes. If the screening test value is below 40 mg/dL, results should be confirmed with a laboratory venous blood glucose determination (Brooks, 1997; Ogata, 1994). Because asymptomatic or symptomatic hypoglycemia can result in serious neurologic sequelae to the neonate if untreated, it is recommended that therapy be started before obtaining the blood glucose test results. Asymptomatic infants may be offered a feeding and a glucose determination repeated 30 minutes after the feeding. Management of symptomatic infants is usually best accomplished by treatment with an intravenous bolus of glucose, followed by a continuous glucose infusion (Brooks, 1997; Levitt-Katz & Stanley, 1996). Blood glucose levels should be checked 20 minutes after intravenous therapy is begun and should be monitored until stable.

Hypovolemia

Hypovolemia (shock), or low blood volume, is a relatively uncommon but critical complication for the newborn. Acute hypovolemia may occur as a result of blood loss from the fetal side of the placenta secondary to placenta previa or abruptio placentae. These two maternal emergencies are discussed elsewhere in this text, but can lead to a severely compromised infant at delivery. The delivery room management of these infants is a critical part of their survival. Resuscitation equipment and personnel trained in neonatal resuscitation must be present in the delivery room as soon as one of these maternal emergencies is identified. Other possible causes of fetal or neonatal hemorrhage include umbilical cord rupture (secondary to precipitous delivery) or superficially implanted umbilical vessels. Hypovolemia may also be seen with intrauterine asphyxia without evidence of frank hemorrhage. While the healthy newborn can compensate for some blood loss, asphyxia disrupts the infant's ability to do so. In spite of this, most infants experiencing asphyxia do not progress to hypovolemia. However, almost all infants who develop hypovolemia have a history of intrauterine asphyxia.

Babies with hypovolemia appear pale and have weak pulses. They may have a persistently high or low heart rate. Their extremities may feel cold and they may have delayed filling of the capillaries after blanching under normal pressure (provided that core temperature is normal). Infants with hypovolemia may have persistent metabolic acidosis and their circulatory status often does not improve in response to effective ventilation, chest compressions, and epinephrine during resuscitation. The treatment for hypovolemia is blood volume expansion through repeated small infusions of normal saline,

Ringer's lactate, or O-negative blood that has been cross-matched with mother's blood (if time permits before delivery).

Major Pathologies That Affect Transition

Three major diseases that may interfere with the newborn's smooth transition to extrauterine life include congenital heart defects, sepsis, and diaphragmatic hernia. Congenital heart defects, diaphragmatic hernia, and other structural defects are often found prenatally during routine obstetrical ultrasound. When prenatal diagnosis is possible, this allows the family to prepare for transport of the newborn immediately after birth or to make plans to deliver in an institution with a level III nursery.

Congenital Heart Defects

Congenital heart defects, or structural malformations of the heart in the developing fetus, may limit or prevent the neonate from making a successful transition to extrauterine life. Difficulties in transition may not become apparent until the organ of respiration changes from the placenta to the lungs and fetal circulatory shunts close, particularly the ductus arteriosus (Sansoucie & Cavaliere, 1997). In neonates with congenital heart malformations, the ductus arteriosus often maintains blood flow between the pulmonary and systemic circulations after birth, allowing the cardiac defect to go unrecognized. With spontaneous closure of the ductus arteriosus during transition to extrauterine life, the status of a previously asymptomatic neonate may suddenly deteriorate as blood flow between the pulmonary and systemic circulations is abruptly terminated (Sansoucie & Cavaliere, 1997).

Characteristics of cardiac blood flow in utero have an important influence on the structure of the developing heart (Sansoucie & Cavaliere, 1997). Aberrant flow patterns in utero significantly affect the size and shape of the heart postnatally (Serwer, 1992). For example, if blood flow from the right to left atrium is decreased in fetal circulation, diminished growth of the left atrium and ventricle may result and the infant may demonstrate signs of hypoplastic left heart in the early newborn period, such as poor perfusion and a mottled appearance of the skin.

Development of the pulmonary vascular bed may also be affected by structural malformations of the heart. A fetus with pulmonary atresia in utero may have an underdeveloped pulmonary vascular bed that leads to devastating and often fatal problems in the immediate postnatal period. Many of these defects can be diagnosed prenatally by ultrasound (usually after 24 weeks' gestation).

Sepsis

Successful transition to extrauterine life may also be affected by the presence of viral or bacterial endotoxins that are acquired in utero, at birth, or during the early newborn period. Sepsis is defined as a clinical syndrome of systemic illness accompanied by bacteremia. Infants at risk for complications related to sepsis include the preterm infant and the infant born to a mother who experiences a prolonged period between rupture of membranes and delivery, fever, chorioamnionitis, or other characteristics suggesting infection (Lott & Kenner, 1998).

Circulating bacterial endotoxins, particularly group B streptococcal endotoxin, can exert effects on both systemic and pulmonary circulations, making the neonate vulnerable to the effects of septic shock and possibly even compromising the infant's survival, if aggressive medical interventions are not rapidly instituted. The infant who has sepsis at birth may exhibit apnea, poor respiratory effort, cyanosis, persistent hypoglycemia, or frank signs of respiratory distress (Freij & McCracken, 1994). These infants may require initiation of oxygen and respiratory support, and all require the prompt initiation of antibiotics.

Diaphragmatic Hernia

Conditions requiring surgery may compromise the infant's ability to make a successful transition to extrauterine life. One of the most critical conditions requiring intense surgical intervention after delivery is the infant born with a diaphragmatic hernia. Diaphragmatic hernia is a condition in which the contents of the abdominal cavity are herniated into the thoracic cavity through a defect in the diaphragm. The herniation of the intestines into the chest cavity results in hypoplasia of the developing lung. The timing of the entry and the amount of abdominal contents that are herniated into the chest both determine the degree of pulmonary hypoplasia and degree of respiratory embarrassment experienced by the infant at birth. Diaphragmatic hernia is now diagnosed antenatally by ultrasound as early as 16 weeks. Most infants present with respiratory distress at birth or shortly after birth. Symptoms include cyanosis, increased work of breathing, and decreased breath sounds on the affected side. Heart tones may also be shifted from their normal point of maximal impulse. The abdomen is scaphoid as a result of the absence of intestines, and bowel sounds may be heard within the thoracic cavity. If the defect goes unrecognized, the infant is at serious risk for persistence of fetal circulation and pulmonary hypertension. The establishment of adequate oxygenation and systemic circulation are key components to infant survival, and most infants require some measure of respiratory support, including oxygen, intubation, and positive pressure ventilation (Guzzetta, et al., 1994). If the infant with suspected diaphragmatic hernia requires prolonged positive pressure ventilation, ventilation should be delivered with an endotracheal tube rather than a bag and mask to prevent further respiratory embarrassment, which may result from distention of the gastrointestinal tract (Kattwinkel, 2000).

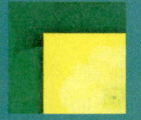

CASE STUDY/CARE PLAN

BIRTH OF INFANT WITH CONGENITAL DIAPHRAGMATIC HERNIA

A 3,940-gram male infant was born to a 24-year-old woman at 40 weeks' gestation by spontaneous vaginal delivery. Apgar scores were 8 at 1 minute and 8 at 5 minutes. The infant did well initially; however, shortly after birth he developed cyanosis and respiratory distress and, 15 minutes later, required intubation and ventilatory support. On physical assessment, the abdomen was unusually flat (scaphoid). Breath sounds were diminished on the left, and heart sounds were shifted to the right side of the thorax. A chest X-ray film was done and revealed air-filled loops of intestine within the left side of the chest, confirming the presence of a left-side congenital diaphragmatic hernia. The priority nursing diagnosis is discussed below, though several other diagnoses would also apply.

Assessment

Term infant with respiratory distress, as evidenced by presence of cyanosis, ineffective breathing pattern requiring ventilatory support, and diminished breath sounds.

Nursing Diagnosis

Impaired gas exchange related to presence of congenital diaphragmatic hernia.

(continues)

Expected Outcomes	Infant will maintain adequate gas exchange (until surgery can be performed) as evidenced by lack of cyanosis, maintenance of arterial PO_2 of more than 60 mmHg and PCO_2 of less than 45 mmHg, clear breath sounds on unaffected side of chest, respiratory rate within normal limits (40 to 60 breaths per minute).
Planning	• Frequent assessments to determine adequacy of gas exchange. • Provision of interventions (based on assessments and medical orders) to optimize effectiveness of breathing pattern and gas exchange.
NOC	Respiratory status: Gas exchange
NIC	Airway management

Nursing Interventions	Rationales
1. Assess and record respiratory rate, breath sounds, and signs and symptoms of respiratory distress every 1 to 2 hours.	1. Monitors respiratory status.
2. Take samples and record results of arterial blood gas tests when indicated.	2. Determines adequacy of gas exchange.
3. Check and record oxygen and ventilator settings every 1 to 2 hours.	3. Provides baseline and measure of changing oxygen needs.
4. Assess patency of endotracheal tube by listening to breath sounds every 1 to 2 hours. Suction endotracheal tube, using sterile technique, as clinically indicated. Record characteristics of secretions and tolerance of procedure.	4. Ensures patency of ET tube.
5. Position infant on left side with head of bed elevated.	5. Optimizes gas exchange of unaffected lung and helps to encourage downward displacement of the abdominal contents.
6. Prevent infant from crying whenever possible by using comfort measures and sedation if ordered.	6. Crying allows the infant to swallow air, which will result in gastric and intestinal distention and increased respiratory distress.
7. Ensure nasogastric tube is placed correctly and connected to suction.	7. Decompresses the stomach and minimizes respiratory distress.
8. Administer antibiotics as ordered.	8. Minimizes potential for infection related to planned surgery and invasive procedures.
9. Check and record results of chest X-ray film, if available.	9. Identifies existence of congenital diaphragmatic hernia.

Evaluation	Describe breath sounds and any signs or symptoms of impaired gas exchange and any successful measures used to decrease crying. Record nasogastric suction pressures and characteristics of drainage. Record medications administered as ordered, including antibiotic and sedative agents.

TRANSITION OF THE PREMATURE INFANT

A **preterm** neonate is defined as an infant born at less than 37 weeks' gestation. Successful transition to extrauterine life is much more complicated in infants born prematurely. In this section, the effects of developmental immaturity of the pulmonary and cardiac systems on adaptation of the preterm neonate to extrauterine life are discussed. The general approach to education of prospective parents of preterm neonates in the delivery room is also discussed.

Complications of Pulmonary System Transition

Developmental characteristics of premature newborns predispose them to respiratory complications in the transition to extrauterine life. One such characteristic is the developmental stage of the alveolar structures in the lungs. At the beginning of the third trimester of fetal development, the respiratory system of the fetus has reached the end of the canalicular period. This period, at about 24 to 26 weeks of gestation, is the first point at which respiration is possible, because some but not all of the infant's alveolar ducts have developed into thin-walled, vascularized terminal sacs. This developmental period determines the lower limits of viability for the premature infant. By the 28th week of gestation, most preterm infants have sufficient terminal air sac development to permit survival. However, the process of terminal sac development continues through the next period of lung development, called the terminal sac or saccular period (24 to 36 weeks' gestational age). Throughout this period, the surface available for the exchange of oxygen and carbon dioxide is increasing correspondingly with the infant's capacity to sustain independent respiratory function. In the period from 36 weeks' gestation through early childhood, the pulmonary system is considered to be within the alveolar period of development, during which the walls of the terminal air sacs become extremely thin and take on the form of the mature pulmonary alveoli (Moore & Persaud, 1993).

Another major factor influencing the respiratory transition of the premature infant is the presence or absence of surfactant in the lungs. Surfactant is a substance secreted by the epithelial cells in the terminal air sacs, beginning at about the 28th week of gestation. This substance provides a surface tension–reducing action in the alveoli, which allows the alveoli to expand more easily on inspiration and prevents their collapse on expiration. The lack of adequate surfactant in the infant's alveoli is a primary reason for the development of respiratory distress in the premature infant and the need for mechanical ventilation. Synthetic forms of surfactant have now been developed. They are administered shortly after birth and have greatly reduced the need for mechanical ventilation (Lott, 1998).

An infant born early in the third trimester of gestation experiences compromised respiration not because of any existing disease but because of the normal immaturity of the developing respiratory system. It is the combination of inadequate terminal sac development, incomplete vascular development, and inadequate surfactant secretion that leads to the development of the life-threatening condition of respiratory distress syndrome (RDS), formerly called hyaline membrane disease. RDS is a primary cause of mortality and morbidity in the premature infant. The lower the gestational age of the infant at birth, the higher the incidence of RDS and, generally, the greater the severity of the condition. Infants with RDS present, at birth or within a few hours of birth, with signs of respiratory distress, including grunting, chest retractions, cyanosis, rales, nasal flaring, use of the accessory muscles of breathing, and an increasing oxygen requirement.

Complications of Cardiac System Transition

One of the common complications of cardiac transition to extrauterine life in the premature infant is the occurrence of a persistent patent ductus arteriosus (PDA). In the fetus, the ductus arteriosus forms a bridge between the pulmonary artery and the dorsal aorta, inserting at the aortic isthmus. At birth, the ductus is a muscular contractile structure. The closure of the ductus at birth depends on multiple factors, including the increase in oxygen tension, the level of circulating prostaglandins, and the available ductal muscle mass. Each of these factors is compromised by premature birth. Prostaglandin E_2 (PGE_2) appears to be responsible for maintaining the patency of the ductus arteriosus during fetal life. Before term birth, there is a reduction in the levels of circulating PGE_2 that allows the constriction of the ductus. Infants born prematurely have high levels of circulating PGE_2, which tend to maintain the patency of the ductus after delivery (Lott, 1998).

Clinical manifestations of PDA depend in part on the size of the ductus (mild PDA may be asymptomatic) and the PVR level. Clinical presentation may include the classic continuous murmur (most commonly heard in the small premature infant) or a crescendo systolic murmur. Infants with severe PDA may demonstrate bounding peripheral pulses and widened pulse pressures and a hyperactive precordium. If the PDA persists, the infant may show signs of increasing congestive heart failure.

Indomethacin (Indocin I.V.), administered intravenously, is used in the treatment of PDA in premature infants. If given early, indomethacin has been found effective in closing nearly 85% of PDAs (Flanagan & Fyler, 1994). Indomethacin acts to inhibit the production of PGE_2 and thereby promotes the closure of the ductus. Indomethacin is toxic to the kidneys and is contraindicated in infants with renal compromise, bleeding disorders, hyperbilirubinemia, and necrotizing enterocolitis. Surgical ligation of the PDA is indicated when treatment with indomethacin has not been successful or when such treatment is contraindicated.

Anticipatory Guidance for Prospective Parents

Parents are often unprepared for emergency situations that occur during the birth of their infant. Because of the unanticipated nature of preterm births, parent counseling before delivery is often performed under less than ideal circumstances. However, every effort should be made to communicate effectively with the prospective parents. Medical terms, abbreviations, and percentages should be avoided as much as possible. Discuss with parents what to expect at delivery, possible complications, and the range of possible outcomes. The infant's chances for survival should also be discussed, and the uncertainties regarding the infant's outcome should be acknowledged. Most importantly, repetition may be necessary for parents to understand all this information, and an opportunity to review the information and ask questions should be provided. If neonatal intensive care unit (NICU) admission is anticipated, an opportunity to tour the NICU should be offered, if time permits (Gomella, Cunningham, Eyal, & Zenk, 1999). Grief counseling should also be made available to parents of infants with congenital anomalies.

RESUSCITATION AND STABILIZATION IN THE DELIVERY ROOM

After delivery of a healthy term infant, routine care should be provided, including warmth, clearing of the infant's airway, and drying to prevent heat loss. In addition, because of the concern about the transmission of communicable diseases through blood or body fluid contact, strict universal precautions should be followed for all infants.

Resuscitation of an infant should be provided if meconium is present, the infant is not breathing or crying, the infant lacks good muscle tone, the infant is cyanotic, or the infant is delivered prematurely. Initial steps in the resuscitation include thermal management, positioning, suctioning, and tactile stimulation. First, the infant should be placed under a preheated radiant warmer to prevent heat loss. The infant should be positioned on his or her back or side with the neck slightly extended to ensure an open airway. If meconium was present in the amniotic fluid and the baby is not vigorous at birth (defined by strong respiratory effort, good muscle tone, and a heart rate of more than 100 bpm), tracheal suctioning should be performed (Kattwinkel, 2000). The infant's mouth, and then the nose, should be gently suctioned, using either a bulb syringe or mechanical suction (Figure 19-6). The infant should then be dried and the wet linens removed.

Once the infant has been dried, suctioned, and positioned, resuscitative personnel should simultaneously evaluate the infant's respiratory effort, heart rate, and color (Kattwinkel, 2000). If central cyanosis is present but the infant is breathing spontaneously with a heart rate of more than 100 bpm, free-flow oxygen should be administered at 5 to 10 L/min, using either an oxygen mask or oxygen tubing held with a cupped hand over the infant's face (Kattwinkel, 2000) (Figure 19-7). If the infant remains cyanotic despite 100% free-flow oxygen, positive pressure ventilation should be initiated.

If the infant is not breathing or has inadequate respirations, tactile stimulation can be briefly provided by gently slapping the soles of the infant's feet or rubbing the infant's back. If the infant does not respond, mask-bag ventilation should be provided at a rate of 40 to 60 breaths per minute and continued until spontaneous respirations are established. Bag-mask ventilation should be given with enough pressure to provide an easy rise and fall of

Client Education

Anticipatory Guidance for Expectant Parents of Premature Infants

Anticipatory guidance for prospective parents of preterm neonates should be geared toward brief explanations about the infant's probable condition, expected outcome, length of hospital stay, equipment, and policies and procedures of the NICU (Gomella, et al., 1999). Some points that may be discussed with parents of preterm infants include:

1. Most extremely preterm neonates have respiratory distress and require oxygen and ventilatory support to breathe effectively. Other problems commonly experienced by preterm neonates include metabolic problems, infection, necrotizing enterocolotis, patent ductus arteriosus, intraventricular hemorrhage, apnea, and bradycardia.

2. Chronic complications of prematurity include chronic lung disease, periventricular leukomalacia, intraparenchymal cysts, hydrocephalus, malnutrition, retinopathy of prematurity, and hearing impairment.

3. Although the risk of disability is higher in preterm infants than in the general population, the majority of preterm children do not develop a major disability. Learning disability, attention deficit disorder, minor neuromotor dysfunction, and behavior problems are more frequent in school-aged children who were preterm than in full-term controls.

4. The expected length of hospital stay for most preterm neonates is estimated to be 2 weeks before or after the baby's estimated due date.

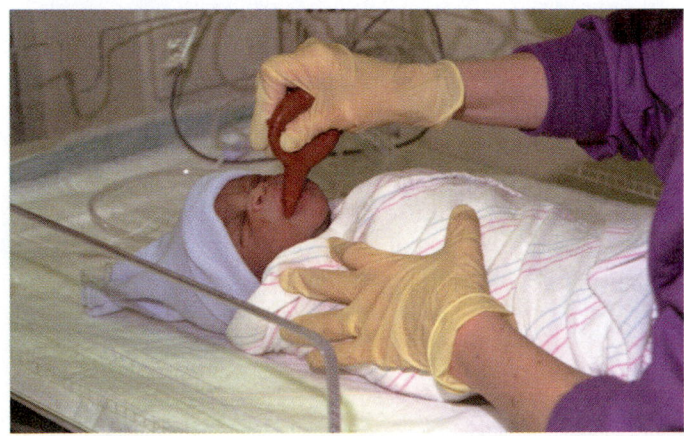

Figure 19-6   Bulb suction of post-term infant in delivery room.

Nursing Alert

Universal Precautions

When performing neonatal resuscitation in the delivery room, the infectious status of the mother and baby is often unknown and the risk of exposure to potentially harmful body fluids is relatively high. The Centers for Disease Control and Prevention recommends that all bodily fluids be treated as potentially infectious, including blood, urine, stool, saliva, vomitus, and, in the case at delivery, amniotic fluid. Masks and protective eyewear or face shields should be worn during procedures that are likely to generate droplets of blood or other bodily fluids, which are especially common during the birth process. Gloves and protective gowns should be worn during resuscitation and when handling the newborn immediately after delivery. Mechanical devices should be used when suctioning the baby's nose, mouth, and pharynx and when suctioning the infant for meconium. Bag-mask devices should be used instead of mouth-to-mouth resuscitation when positive pressure ventilation is required. Although relatively uncommon, endotracheal suctioning or umbilical catheter placement has at times produced potentially infectious splashes of sputum or blood, respectively, thus requiring caregivers to exercise extreme caution and proper precautions when performing these procedures on a newborn.

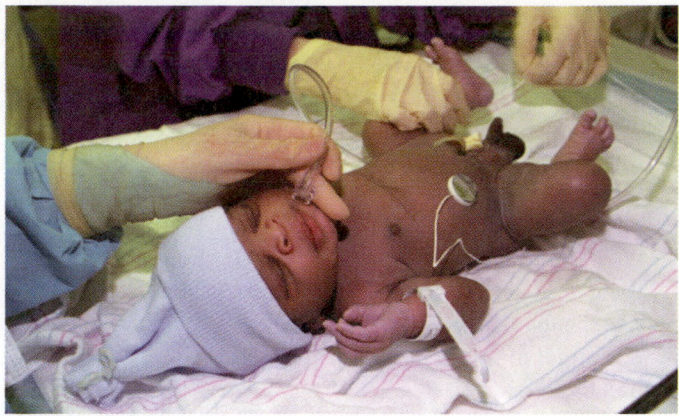

Figure 19-7   Newborn receiving free-flow oxygen in delivery room as therapy for central cyanosis.

Positive pressure ventilation should also be performed any time that the heart rate is less than 100 bpm. If the heart rate is less than 60 bpm, despite 30 seconds of effective positive pressure ventilation with 100% oxygen, chest compressions should be initiated. The lower third of the infant's sternum, immediately above the xyphoid process, should be compressed to a depth of one-third the anterior-posterior diameter of the infant's chest and at a rate of 90/sec in conjunction with a ventilation rate of 30 breaths per minute (Kattwinkel, 2000).

Positive response of the infant to resuscitative efforts is indicated by increasing heart rate, spontaneous respirations, and improving color. If the infant's condition continues to deteriorate or fails to improve despite assisted ventilation, the resuscitative team should check the adequacy of ventilation. If the chest movement is adequate and 100% oxygen is being administered, the infant may require endotracheal intubation to further stabilize his or her condition.

Although medications are rarely needed in newborn resuscitation, if the heart rate remains less than 60 bpm, despite 30 seconds of ventilation and another 30 seconds of coordinated chest compressions and ventilation, drugs may be indicated to improve the infant's circulatory status (Table 19-1). Although the umbilical vein is the preferred route of administration in the delivery room,

the chest and produce breath sounds. If bag-mask ventilation is performed for longer than a few minutes, an orogastric tube should be inserted and left in place, thereby preventing distention of the stomach and intestines and decreasing the risk of aspiration of gastric contents. If the infant is suspected of having a diaphragmatic hernia, prolonged positive pressure ventilation should be performed using a bag and endotracheal tube (Kattwinkel, 2000).

Table 19-1	Medications for Neonatal Resuscitation		
MEDICATION	DOSE	ROUTE	RATE
Epinephrine (1:10,000)	0.1–0.3 mL/kg	Endotracheal tube Umbilical vein or other intravenous route	Rapid push
If hypovolemia, normal saline or Ringer's lactate or O-negative blood	10 mL/kg	Umbilical vein or other intravenous route	Over 5–10 minutes
If severe metabolic acidosis, sodium bicarbonate, 0.5 mEq/mL (4.2% solution)	2 mEq/kg	Umbilical vein or other intravenous route	Slowly; no faster than 1 mEq/kg/min

Nursing Tip — *Positive Pressure Ventilation*

Since establishing effective ventilation is the key to nearly all successful newborn resuscitations, the caregiver must be prepared to troubleshoot if the infant is not responding to positive pressure ventilation (Kattwinkel, 2000). Assessment must be done to ensure that chest movement is adequate. Common reasons why the chest may not be rising with each squeeze of the bag include:

- Inadequate face mask seal
- Airway blocked because of improper head position or secretions
- Not enough pressure being used to ventilate the infant

If this happens when you are attempting to provide positive pressure ventilation, try using the following techniques:

- Reapply the mask to the infant's face.
- Reposition the infant's head.
- Suction secretions from the infant's nose, mouth, or oropharynx.
- Increase ventilation pressure until there is an easy rise and fall of the chest.

epinephrine may also be administered by an endotracheal tube if an umbilical venous catheter or other intravenous catheter is not already in place.

If the infant continues to deteriorate despite effective resuscitative efforts, other possible causes that should be explored include depressed respiratory drive, airway malformations, congenital heart disease, and lung problems, such as pneumothorax or diaphragmatic hernia.

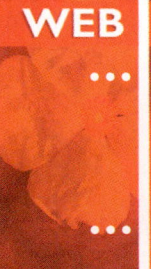

WEB ACTIVITIES

••• What information can you locate on the Internet about transition to extrauterine life that both parents and nurses can use?

••• What parent support groups can you locate on the Internet for families of full-term or preterm infants who require neonatal intensive care?

Key Concepts

- Fetal circulation differs from that in the newborn in three major respects: minimal blood flow through the lungs, presence of placental circulation, and presence of anatomic shunts.

- Three anatomic shunts divert oxygenated blood to organs performing life-sustaining functions. The ductus venosus connects the umbilical vein to the inferior vena cava and allows blood to bypass the liver; the foramen ovale allows blood entering the right atrium of the heart to go directly to the left atrium, left ventricle, and out the ascending aorta to immediately supply the brain; and the ductus arteriosus shunts blood from the pulmonary artery to the descending aorta, thus bypassing the lungs.

- Effective thermal management at the time of birth plays a significant role in promoting an optimal transition by the neonate to extrauterine life.

- Physiologic and behavioral transition to extrauterine life in the immediate newborn period occurs in three phases: initial period of reactivity, period of relative inactivity, and second period of reactivity.

- Conditions that may interfere with the newborn's smooth transition to extrauterine life include asphyxia, meconium staining, transient tachypnea of the newborn, hypoglycemia, and hypovolemia (shock).

- Asphyxia is a metabolic process that arises from failure of the respiratory organ in the fetus or neonate. This impaired gas exchange results in a complex combination of hypoxemia, hypercapnia, acidosis, and ischemia.

- The Apgar score neither establishes nor rules out the presence of asphyxia. Resuscitation should be immediately initiated when indicated and not delayed for assessment of 1-minute Apgar score.

- Major pathologies that may interfere with the newborn's smooth transition to extrauterine life include congenital heart defects, sepsis, and diaphragmatic hernia.

- Developmental immaturity of the pulmonary and cardiac systems may interfere with the preterm neonate's adaptation to extrauterine life.

- Nurses must partner with parents to ensure that hospital policies and practices facilitate the parent's right to be with their baby during the crisis period and to participate in their infant's care, as guided by parent preference and the clinical situation.

Review Questions and Activities

1. An infant in primary apnea would exhibit which of the following signs?
   a. Gasping before becoming pink
   b. Heart rate around 50 bpm
   c. Pulses poor or absent
   d. No response to tactile stimuli

   The correct answer is a.

2. Which of the following statements is true concerning asphyxia?
   a. The Apgar score is a good indicator of the presence or absence of asphyxia
   b. Poor perfusion accompanied by asphyxia is caused by volume depletion
   c. The acidosis associated with asphyxia is primarily metabolic in origin
   d. Ischemia has a more profound effect on tissue oxygenation than hypoxemia

   The correct answer is d.

3. In the delivery room, an infant presenting with no spontaneous respiratory effort and an Apgar score of 2 probably has:
   a. Primary apnea
   b. Secondary apnea
   c. Narcotic depression
   d. Retained fetal lung fluid

   The correct answer is b.

4. A term infant develops severe respiratory distress within minutes after birth. On physical examination, the chest is hyperexpanded and the point of maximal impulse (PMI) is shifted to the right. Which of the following is the most likely cause for this infant's respiratory distress?
   a. Diaphragmatic hernia
   b. Congenital pneumonia
   c. Right-sided pneumothorax
   d. Meconium aspiration

   The correct answer is a.

5. Which of the following statements is *true* concerning thermoregulation in the newborn?
   a. The infant's core body temperature is an accurate assessment of neutral thermal environment
   b. Hypoxia blunts the infant's metabolic response to cold stress
   c. An infant in an incubator is in a neutral thermal environment when the randomly set air temperature maintains the infant's axillary temperature at 97.5°F to 99.5°F

   d. The zone of thermal neutrality is wider in the infant with a very low birth weight

   The correct answer is b.

6. The method of heat loss in which heat is lost to cool surfaces in direct contact with the infant is called:
   a. Radiation
   b. Convection
   c. Conduction
   d. Evaporation

   The correct answer is c.

7. The neonate with an axillary temperature of 96.5°F is at increased risk of developing all of the following *except*:
   a. Metabolic acidosis
   b. Hypoglycemia
   c. Hypotension
   d. Hypoxemia

   The correct answer is c.

References

Amlung, S. R. (1998). Neonatal thermoregulation. In C. Kenner, J. W. Lott, & A. A. Flandemeyer (Eds.), *Comprehensive neonatal nursing: A physiologic perspective* (2nd ed., pp. 207–219). Philadelphia: W. B. Saunders.

Baumgart, S. (1996). Thermal regulation in the fetus and newborn. In A. R. Spitzer (Ed.), *Intensive care of the fetus and neonate*, (pp. 401–416). St. Louis, MO: Mosby.

Behram, S., Moschler, E. F., Sayegh, S. K., Garguillo, F. P., & Mann, W. J. (1998). Implementation of early discharges after uncomplicated vaginal deliveries: Maternal and infant complications. *Southern Medical Journal, 91*(6), 541–545.

Brooks, C. (1997). Neonatal hypoglycemia. *Neonatal Network, 16*(2), 15–21.

Donn, S. M., & Faix, R. G. (1996). Delivery room resuscitation. In A. R. Spitzer (Ed.), *Intensive care of the fetus and neonate*, (pp. 326–336). St. Louis, MO: Mosby.

Fisher, D. E., & Paton, J. B. (1986). Resuscitation of the newborn infant. In M. H. Klaus & A. A. Fanaroff (Eds.), *Care of the high-risk neonate* (3rd ed., pp. 31–50). Philadelphia: W. B. Saunders.

Flanagan, M. F., & Fyler, D. C. (1994). Cardiac disease. In G. B. Avery, M. A. Fletcher, & M. G. MacDonald (Eds.), *Neonatology: Pathophysiology and management of the newborn* (4th ed., pp. 516–559). Philadelphia: J. B. Lippincott.

Freij, B., & McCracken, G. (1994). Acute infections. In G. B. Avery, M. A. Fletcher, & M. G. MacDonald (Eds.), *Neonatology: Pathophysiology and management of the newborn* (4th ed., pp. 1082–1116). Philadelphia: J. B. Lippincott.

Gomella, T. L., Cunningham, M. D., Eyal, F. G., & Zenk, K. E. (Eds.) (1999). *Neonatology: Management, procedures, on-call problems, diseases, and drugs* (4th ed., pp. 209–212). Stamford, CT: Appleton & Lange.

Guyton, A., & Hall, J. (2001). *Textbook of medical physiology* (10th ed.). Philadelphia: W. B. Saunders.

Guzzetta, P. C., Anderson, K. D., Eichelberger, M. R., Newman, K. D., Rouse, T. M., Schnitzer, J. J., et al. (1994). General surgery. In G. B. Avery, M. A. Fletcher, & M. G. MacDonald (Eds.), *Neonatology: Pathophysiology and management of the newborn* (4th ed., pp. 914–951). Philadelphia: J. B. Lippincott.

Hey, E. (1994). Thermoregulation. In G. B. Avery, M. A. Fletcher, & M. G. MacDonald (Eds.), *Neonatology: Pathophysiology and management of the newborn* (4th ed., pp. 357–365). Philadelphia: J. B. Lippincott.

Jepson, H. A., Talashek, M. L., & Tichy, A. M. (1991). The Apgar score: Evolution, limitations, and scoring guidelines. *Birth 18*(2), 83–91.

Kattwinkel, J. (Ed.) (2000). *Textbook of neonatal resuscitation* (4th ed.). Elk Grove Village, IL: American Academy of Pediatrics & American Heart Association.

Levitt-Katz, L. E., & Stanley, C. (1996). Disorders of glucose and other sugars. In A. R. Spitzer (Ed.), *Intensive care of the fetus and neonate* (pp. 982–992). St. Louis, MO: Mosby.

Lott, J. W. (1998). Assessment and management of cardiovascular dysfunction. In C. Kenner, J. W. Lott, & A. A. Flandemeyer (Eds.), *Comprehensive neonatal nursing: A physiologic perspective* (2nd ed., pp. 306–335). Philadelphia: W. B. Saunders.

Lott, J. W., & Kenner, C. (1998). Assessment and management of immunologic dysfunction. In C. Kenner, J. W. Lott, & A. A. Flandemeyer (Eds.), *Comprehensive neonatal nursing: A physiologic perspective* (2nd ed., pp. 496–519). Philadelphia: W. B. Saunders.

Ludington-Hoe, S. M., Hadeed, A. J., & Anderson, G. C. (1991). Physiological responses to skin-to-skin contact in hospitalized premature infants. *Journal of Perinatology, 11*(1), 19–24.

Moore, K. L., & Persaud, T. V. N. (1993). *The developing human: Clinically oriented embryology* (5th ed., pp. 226–236). Philadelphia: W. B. Saunders.

Nelson, N. (1994). Physiology of transition. In G. B. Avery, M. A. Fletcher, & M. G. MacDonald (Eds.), *Neonatology: Pathophysiology and management of the newborn* (4th ed., pp. 223–247). Philadelphia: J. B. Lippincott.

Ogata, E. (1994). Carbohydrate homeostasis. In G. B. Avery, M. A. Fletcher, & M. G. MacDonald (Eds.), *Neonatology: Pathophysiology and management of the newborn* (4th ed., pp. 568–584). Philadelphia: J. B. Lippincott.

Sansoucie, D. A., & Cavaliere, T. A. (1997). Transition from fetal to extrauterine circulation. *Neonatal Network, 16*(2), 5–12.

Serwer, G. A. (1992). Postnatal circulatory adjustments. In R. A. Polin & W. W. Fox (Eds.), *Fetal and neonatal physiology* (pp. 710–721). Philadelphia: W. B. Saunders.

Whitsett, J. A., Pryhuber, G. S., Rice, W. R., Warner, B. B., & Wert, S. E. (1994). Acute respiratory disorders. In G. B. Avery, M. A. Fletcher, & M. G. MacDonald (Eds.), *Neonatology: Pathophysiology and management of the newborn* (4th ed., pp. 429–452). Philadelphia: J. B. Lippincott.

Suggested Readings

McCollum, L. (1998). Resuscitation and stabilization of the neonate. In C. Kenner, J. W. Lott, & A. A. Flandemeyer (Eds.), *Comprehensive neonatal nursing: A physiologic perspective* (2nd ed., pp. 190–206). Philadelphia: W. B. Saunders.

Varda, K., & Behnke, R. (2000). The effect of timing of initial bath on newborn's temperature. *Journal of Obstetric, Gynecological, and Neonatal Nurses, 29*, 27–32.

Zabloudil, C. (1999). Adaptation to extrauterine life. In J. Deacon & P. O'Neill (Eds.), *Core curriculum for neonatal intensive care nursing* (2nd ed., pp. 40–62). Philadelphia: W. B. Saunders.

Resources

National Association of Neonatal Nurses, 4700 W. Lake Avenue, Glenview, IL 60026-1485, 800-451-3795 or 847-375-3660, http://www.nann.org

CHAPTER 20

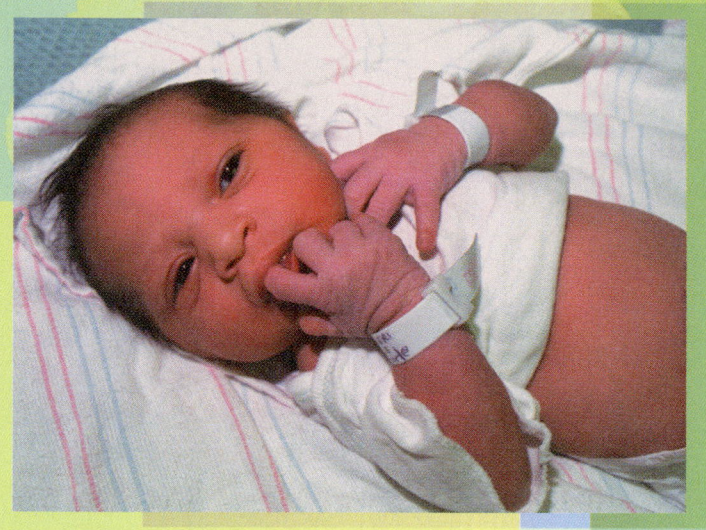

NURSING CARE OF THE NORMAL NEWBORN

Nursing care of mothers and their newborn infants is often thought to be the most joyous and rewarding experience for the nurse because a brand new person is welcomed into the world. Although nursing care of the newborn after transition is focused on the health of the infant, the nurse has the opportunity to be involved with the parents of the infant and to interact with other family members to plan for the infant's future well-being within the family unit. Use the following questions to examine your personal feelings regarding nursing care of newborn infants:

- How would I feel if I were the nurse caring for an infant who would not stop crying?
- How would I feel as a new mother if no one were to tell me whether my baby was doing well and what I needed to do to care for him?
- How would I feel as a nurse if I were caring for an infant who was not feeding well?
- How would I feel if I were the nurse caring for a mother and her newborn and I overheard a family member say something to the mother that might affect the infant's health and safety at home?
- How do I feel about caring for a newborn infant?

Key Terms

Acrocyanosis

Anal wink reflex

Anterior fontanel

Caput succedaneum

Cephalhematoma

Chorioamnionitis

Coarctation of the aorta

Cyanosis

Developmental dysplasia
of the hip (DDH)

Erythema toxicum

Imperforate anus

Lanugo

Macrocephaly

Meconium

Microcephaly

Milia

Mongolian spots

Mottling

Patent ductus arteriosus
(PDA)

Polydactyly

Posterior fontanel

Post-term infant

Preterm infant

Pustular melanosis

Syndactyly

Tachycardia

Tachypnea

Term infant

Competencies

Upon completion of this chapter, the reader should be able to:

1. Perform a full physical examination and gestational age assessment on a newborn infant to provide an accurate account of the infant's status to his or her mother and father.

2. Describe the unique characteristics and behaviors of a newborn infant to his or her parents and other family members.

3. Demonstrate to all family members proper holding and positioning of infants for safety and to prevent injury.

4. Discuss factors with the parents and family that may place the infant at risk for illness, and suggest parental interventions for illness prevention.

5. Explain feeding and elimination schedules to parents to lessen any concerns.

6. Anticipate parental anxieties related to caring for their new infant during the neonatal period and develop a teaching plan for parents to address these anxieties.

7. Incorporate family values and ethnic and religious perspectives into teaching plans for infant care and health maintenance visits.

Preparing for a healthy infant preoccupies a mother-to-be during the time that she is pregnant until the time of delivery, when the physiologic forces of contractions and the process of labor disrupt her fantasies and redirect her attentions. Her first glimpse of her infant reassures her that the journey from the womb to the world was accomplished safely (Rubin, 1984). As the mother holds her newborn for the first time, she may celebrate this new life with the infant's father and other family members. The nurse in charge of the infant's care can safeguard this moment in family life by not intruding or interrupting the family's opportunity to be with their newest member.

After the parents and family members have the opportunity to touch, hold, and interact with their infant, the nurse can address any concerns related to the infant's condition or behavior. The interaction of the nurse with all family members at this time forms the basis for the nursing assessment of the family's ethnic or cultural perspectives regarding the infant. This assessment is incorporated into the nurse's teaching plans for the parents and the family regarding caring for the infant at home.

Before the introduction of the infant to the parents and the family, the nurse uses assessment skills to determine the physical health of the infant and his or her physiologic stability after transition. This chapter describes the complete examination of the infant and the gestational age determination with size parameters that describe the physical condition of the infant. Findings that may place the infant at risk for injury or infection or that warrant further investigation alert the nurse to develop strategies for intervention. In addition, guidelines are presented for continued nursing assessments of the infant while the infant remains under the nurse's care. Finally, factors to consider in determining parental and family perspectives are described to provide a comprehensive assessment of the parental and family environment. This chapter provides knowledge of the skills in newborn assessment so that the nurse can intervene when necessary and implement infant care strategies that address parental concerns and family considerations. Specific assessments are done during transition, full assessment, shift assessments, and periodic assessments.

ASSESSMENT AFTER TRANSITION

Nursing assessment of the newborn infant during and after transition continues to be a critical factor in determining the infant's adjustment to the extrauterine environment. Transition of the newborn immediately after delivery in the nursery or in another special care environment is conducted according to the institutional protocol. Time frames for this transitional period are adjusted for the individual infant's condition and accurate assessment of the infant's physiologic stability. Transition of newborn infants usually encompasses the first 4 to 6 hours of life (Seidel, Rosenstein, & Pathak, 2001). Nursing concerns after the transitional period are directed toward balancing the need for observation and assessment of the newborn infant with the needs of the mother and family to have their infant with them.

Temperature

During the transitional period, the nurse determines that the infant is physiologically stable by skilled examination and assessment of the infant's thermoregulatory effort, cardiac system, and respiratory system. Infants received from the delivery room are usually swaddled in warmed blankets with stocking caps to prevent chilling (Figure 20-1). To maintain body temperature, the infants are placed immediately in a temperature-controlled isolette on a radiant warmer, or skin-to-skin with the mother. Body temperature is assessed by recording axillary tem-

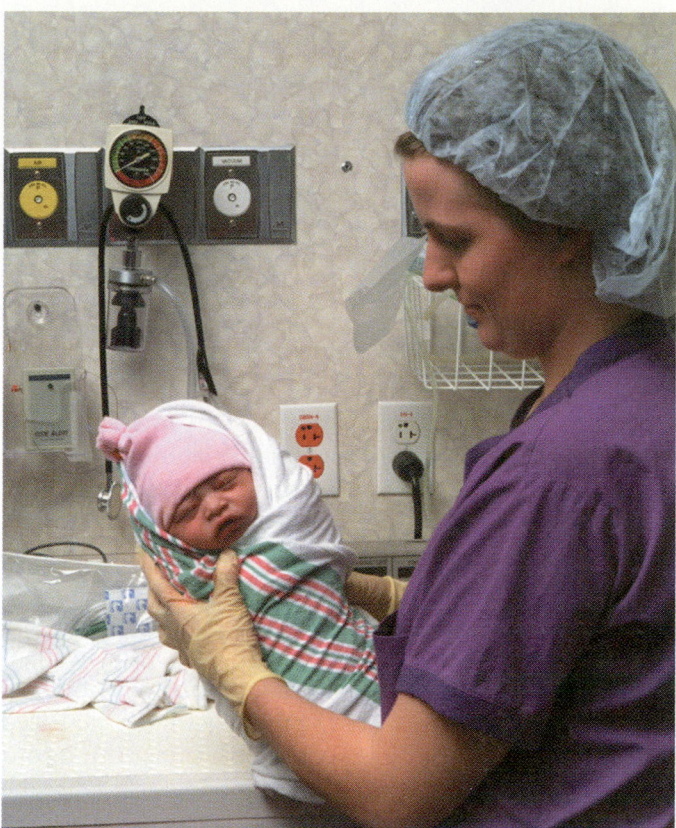

Figure 20-1   Knit caps and swaddling in a blanket help newborns maintain body heat.

perature or attaching the infant to a thermoprobe and recording monitor. Rectal temperatures are no longer routinely done on infants because the insertion of the rectal thermometer into the anus of an infant risks damage to the rectal lining, may break the thermometer, and may stimulate the vagal response, lowering the heart rate. Anal patency is no longer confirmed by insertion of a thermometer. It is assessed by examination of the anus and visual confirmation of stool being excreted through the anal opening (Seidel et al., 2001). Axillary infant temperature should be maintained between 97°F and 99.5°F.

The infant's ability to maintain body heat is related to controlling the factors that produce heat loss in the newborn infant. The organ system that occupies the largest surface area on an infant is the skin, placing the infant at risk for heat loss by evaporation to the environment. Placing the infant in a warm environment minimizes this risk. In spite of the rise in newborn birth weight, leading to larger infants, the subcutaneous fat layer is thin, offering no insulation against heat loss and no adequate energy source to raise body temperature. Warm environments coupled with decreased infant stimulation and energy expenditures assist the infant in maintaining body temperature. Infants who are chilled are not able to produce body heat through shivering but can produce body heat

Reflections from a Nursery Nurse

I had gone to the mother's room to pick up her infant for the end of shift report. The mother was adamant that her infant was not going anywhere. She informed me that this was her baby, and if I touched her baby, she would call hospital security and accuse me of kidnapping. I was speechless. I didn't know what to do, so I left her infant in her room and made my report to the next shift. I went home and thought about what the mother had said, her rights as the mother of this infant, and hospital policies interfering with parental rights to their infants. I decided that my role as a nurse was to facilitate the opportunities for infants, mothers, and families to be together and that I needed to adjust my thinking and approach to accomplish this.

through an alternative mechanism. This alternative mechanism involves stimulating the metabolism of brown fat as discussed in Chapter 19. The location of brown fat in the axillae may cause a transient rise in axillary temperature that the nurse may misinterpret as a rise in infant core body temperature. Assessments of infant temperature after transition provide the nurse ample opportunities for a determination of the infant's ability to control his or her temperature within the environment.

Cardiovascular System

Assessment of the cardiovascular system after the transitional period is directed to the infant's ability to convert fetal circulation to postnatal circulation. Fetal circulation during pregnancy was dependent on shunting blood flow through the foramen ovale, the ductus arteriosus, and the ductus venosus. As the infant breathes on his or her own, the inspired oxygen enters the pulmonary vasculature. Pulmonary vascular resistance decreases, leading to an increase in pulmonary blood flow and to the chambers on the left side of the heart. This, coupled with the increased systemic blood circulation from the placenta during cord clamping, leads to reversal of fetal blood flow because the heart now undergoes postnatal ventricular contraction (Hockenberry et al., 2003). Reversing blood flow through the fetal shunts ultimately results in their closure, and backflow through the shunts results in heart murmurs that are often called "flow murmurs." The nurse monitors these events by carefully auscultating heart sounds, determining heart rate, checking peripheral pulses, and observing skin color changes indicative of improving cardiac perfusion to the extremities.

During the course of transition, the nurse would expect the infant's heart rate to decrease from highs of 150 to 160 bpm to a regular pattern and rate between 130 and 140 bpm. The infant heart adjusts to the increased blood flow through the ventricles and becomes more efficient at pumping blood through them. Peripheral perfusion is evaluated by the presence of peripheral pulses, capillary refill, and skin color. The nurse identifies the characteristics of peripheral pulses related to strength, rhythm, and bounding qualities; compares pulses bilaterally; and times capillary refill (rapid refill is 3 seconds or less). Skin color should remain flushed or healthy and may appear "rosy" as capillary circulation improves.

Respiratory System

Nursing assessment of the infant's respiratory system after transition begins with observing the infant's respiratory effort, listening to the sounds made while the infant is breathing, and auscultating all lung fields. Air entering the infant's lungs after delivery competes with fluid remaining in the alveolar spaces. The majority of this fluid in the lungs and alveoli is removed by pulmonary capillaries, the lymphatic system, and the labor and delivery process. Surfactant reduces the surface tension of the fluid and allows air to enter the alveoli for gas exchange (Hockenberry et al., 2003). Fluid remaining in the lungs may cause a condition called transient tachypnea of the newborn (TTN) characterized by a rapid respiratory rate (above 60 breaths per minute; normal respiratory rates in the newborn are 40 to 60 breaths per minute) with no other symptoms of respiratory distress, for example, intercostal or sternal retractions, nasal flaring, or expiratory grunting. Expiratory grunting is an audible sound made by the infant while undergoing expiration. Normal breathing occurs quietly. Normally, with no treatment other than careful observation, there is resolution and clearing of the fluid within 24 hours.

Observation of the infant in the supine position assists the nurse in the evaluation of the infant's respiratory effort. Symmetrical chest movements, use of accessory muscles, a labored or unlabored appearance, and intercostal or sternal retractions are noted. Infants breathe primarily through their nose, and visual inspection can confirm this. Those infants who have evidence of bubbles around the mouth or who appear to be blowing bubbles through their nares can be relieved by using a bulb syringe to clear the oropharynx or the nasal passages (Figure 20-2). Lung fields should be auscultated anteriorly and posteriorly while gently rolling the infant onto each side. Breath sounds are noisy, and the sound radiates and echoes throughout the entire chest because of the thinness of the chest wall. Until respiratory and hemodynamic stability is achieved, at approximately 12 to 24 hours of life, it is difficult to determine the presence of rales or rhonchi in lung fields because of the echoing and radiation of the auscultated sounds.

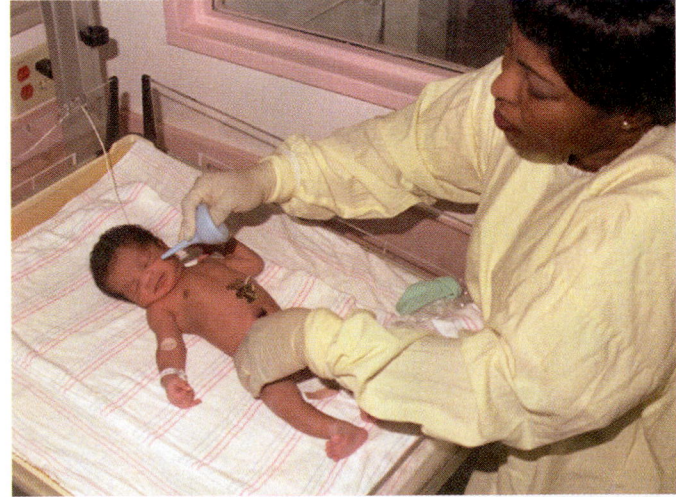

Figure 20-2   Infants who blow bubbles through their mouth or nose should be suctioned with a bulb syringe.

Nursing Alert

Tachypnea

Tachypnea is usually defined as a respiratory rate of 70 or more breaths per minute. Respiratory rates between 60 and 70 breaths per minute are called borderline tachypnea and the infant should be observed carefully. Any newborn infant with respiratory rates that are borderline or tachypneic beyond 24 hours of life should be evaluated immediately for infection.

Nasal patency can be confirmed by gently blocking off one naris at a time with the infant's mouth closed and observing for a rise in the chest, which indicates the infant's ability to inhale air into the lungs through an intact nasal passageway. Infants who have difficulty with this maneuver may have choanal atresia, a malformation of the bucconasal membrane, leading to obstruction of the nasal passageway. Choanal atresia is confirmed by being unable to insert a small catheter (a No. 8 French feeding tube is preferred in newborns) into an infant's nares. Bilateral choanal atresia produces cyanosis when the infant's mouth is closed and disappears when the mouth is open or the infant is crying. Unilateral choanal atresia may not be identified until rhinorrhea (nasal discharge) occurs in early childhood, obstructing the naris that is patent (Seidel et al., 2001). Choanal atresia is a developmental anomaly occurring during gestation, and it may be accompanied by other defects. Positive findings of choanal atresia should be reported immediately, and the infant should be examined for other anomalies.

General Nursing Care

Once the nursing assessment of body temperature and the cardiac and respiratory systems is made and established as stable over time, the nurse notes whether the infant has received ophthalmic and vitamin K prophylaxis and a first bath.

Nursing Tip *Clearing Air Passages*

Auscultation of the infant's nose and mouth may reveal noisy breath sounds indicative of obstruction of air flow through the nares or oropharynx. Suctioning with the bulb syringe may remove fluid and debris that clutters these passageways. The nurse should subsequently hear decreased noise on auscultation.

Nursing Alert

Eye Discharge

Any eye irritation or discharge persisting for more than 24 hours should be reported immediately to rule out chemical conjunctivitis from eye prophylaxis.

Ophthalmic Prophylaxis

Ophthalmic prophylaxis is given according to institutional protocol in ointment or drop form to prevent gonococcal and chlamydial infection in neonates (Figure 20-3). Choices for ointments or drops include 0.5% erythromycin (ERYC), 1% silver nitrate solution, and 1% tetracycline (Tetracyn), which are effective against infection. Silver nitrate solution stains the periorbital area black when the infant blinks and can be removed with a moist wipe. All three medications may cause a chemical conjunctivitis of the eyes within the first 24 hours of life. The nurse observes a matting of the eyelashes and, possibly, a yellowish discharge that can be removed with a moist wipe. The discharge and irritation to the eyes ceases after 24 hours.

Vitamin K Prophylaxis

Prophylactic injection of vitamin K (0.5 to 1.0 mg phytonadione) is given by intramuscular injection into the infant's thigh during the first hour of life to stimulate production of vitamin K by the bacteria in the infant's intestine (Figure 20-4). At delivery, the intestine of the infant is considered to be sterile, or without normal bacteria. Once the **meconium** stool has passed, the intestinal lining and mucosal

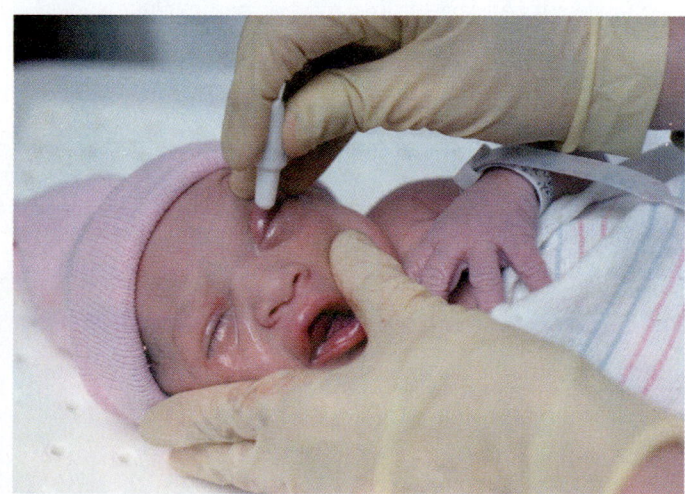

Figure 20-3 Ophthalmic prophylaxis prevents gonococcal and chlamydial infection in the newborn.

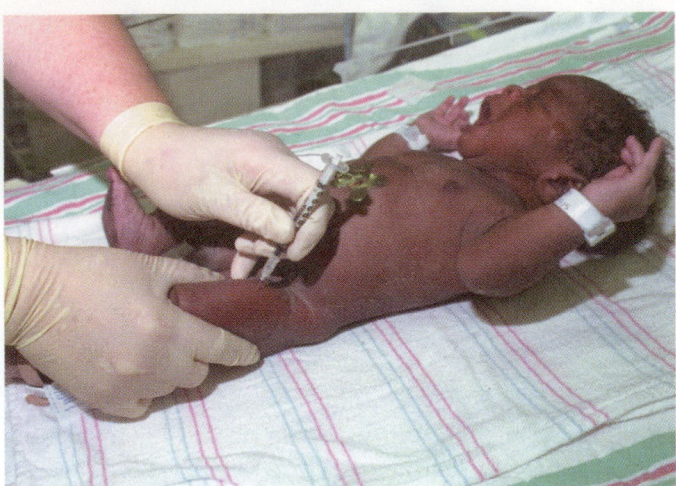

Figure 20-4   Administration of vitamin K.

Reflections from a Nurse

I was the nurse caring for a mother and her newborn son in the rooming-in area of our postpartum unit. I remembered this mother because she was so upset that she delivered here instead of at home. All she wanted to do was go home. She didn't want anything done for the baby. I think she was worried about it costing more money. I brought her the consent form to sign for the vitamin K injection and the eye ointment and she refused. She said her baby didn't need it. I went back to the nurse practitioner in charge, who subsequently conferred with the physician. The nurse practitioner and I went back to see the mother and explain to her that she had the right not to sign the consent form but that she needed to be fully informed before she made that decision. The nurse practitioner told the mother that there was a 10% risk of intraventricular hemorrhage in her baby's head during the first year of life without prophylaxis vitamin K and also explained the importance of the eye ointment to protect her baby's corneas. Mom said she would think about it. Later that day, before she left with her infant, she asked for both the eye ointment and vitamin K for her baby. I thought to myself, "I'm so glad she thought about what her baby needed, instead of her own frustration at being here."

cells rapidly adjust to metabolize food and excrete food by-products. Bacterial formation stimulates production of vitamin K, a cofactor in the normal clotting process. Rarely, infants may develop a vitamin K deficiency within 2 to 3 days following birth if the vitamin K prophylaxis is not given. Severe consequences may occur in infants not given vitamin K, because central nervous system hemorrhages commonly occur (Taeusch & Ballard, 1998).

First Bath

The first bath is given in warm water with a mild soap to remove amniotic fluid, blood, vaginal secretions, and other residues on the skin, using standard precautions (Figure 20-5). The nurse should anticipate any chilling effect from the circulating air or the bath and take precautions to ensure that the infant is kept warm and dried quickly.

After being bathed and swaddled in blankets, the infant is ready to be examined in more detail. Nurses perform several different assessments on newborns after delivery. The first assessment is accomplished during the transition, the first 4 to 6 hours of the infant's life. The infant is monitored for temperature and cardiac and respiratory stability during transition. During or after transition, the nurse performs a full physical examination, including a general assessment and physical examination. Gestational age assessment is usually performed on a preterm infant. For term infants, refer to institutional policy if gestational age assessment is routinely performed. Once this examination has been completed, the infant is monitored for any changes through periodic nursing assessments done at each nursing shift, brief examinations two or three times during the shift, and interactional assessments with the mother, father, and other family members. The purpose of all these assessments is to ensure the

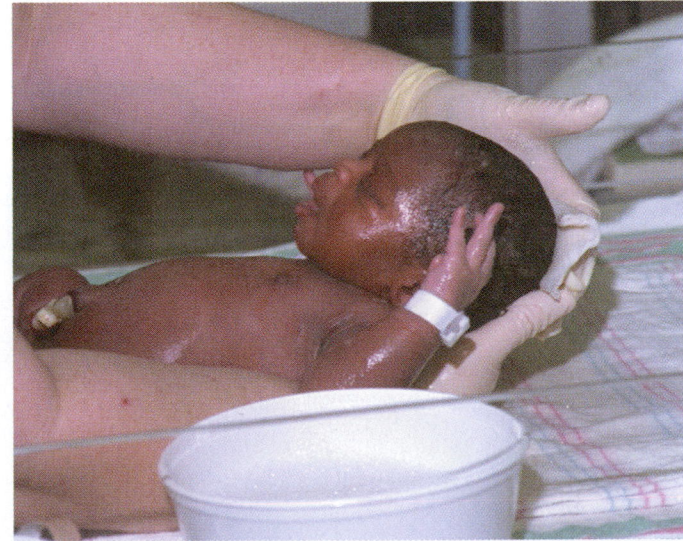

Figure 20-5   A newborn's first bath.

Nursing Tip   *Umbilical Cord Vessels*

The infant should have an umbilical cord with three vessels, two arteries, and one vein. Two-vessel cords (one artery, one vein) must be reported immediately: they are associated with renal and cardiac anomalies. Ultrasound examinations and echocardiograms are recommended in these cases to confirm any abnormality that might be present. The most common renal abnormality characterized by a two-vessel cord is renal agenesis, which affects the infant's urinary output because a kidney, usually the left, fails to develop normally in utero.

infant's physical and biologic stability and assist the nurse in planning for the family's adaptation to and care for the infant (Table 20-1).

GENERAL ASSESSMENT

Visual inspection of the infant in the crib forms the basis for a general nursing assessment. From inspection, the nurse can determine the infant's body position, skin color, respiratory effort, relative size and length, and state of mind (asleep, awake, quiet-alert, or alert) and evaluate security measures in place to guarantee the identity of the infant and protect him or her from abduction. Infants in the nursery have nurses who are charged with the care of infants who are not at mother's bedside. Infants rooming in with mother are cared for by the mother with the assistance of the nursing staff when needed.

Position

A newborn's position leaves clues as to its innate position of comfort. Many infants adopt their in utero position after delivery to enhance their feelings of security after separating from mother during the birth process. The normal body position of the newborn is flexion of both upper and lower extremities. The flexion of the upper extremities allows infants to touch their face with their hands, suck their fingers, and explore their new environment. Assessment of position of the neonate also gives some indication of tone: hypertonic (tense), normal tone or hypotonic (flaccid).

Lower extremities may be extended, fixed in one position from delivery position, or flexed. Usually, positioning in newborn infants is symmetrical. Asymmetrical positioning may suggest an initial nursing assessment of injury related to birth trauma and may warrant further investigation. Failure to move an extremity or diminished extremity movement, unilaterally or bilaterally, would be a cause for concern.

Nursing Tip   *Positioning of Infants*

The American Academy of Pediatrics (2000) recommends that all infants be placed to sleep in a nonprone position to prevent sudden infant death syndrome (SIDS). Placing infants in the supine position offers the best protection against SIDS.

Skin Color

Skin color becomes a vital part of the general nursing assessment because the newly born infant may show signs of jaundice or cardiovascular instability in the first several days of life. Jaundice in the newborn is characterized by a gradual yellowing of the skin that develops from head to toe. Visual jaundice in a newborn infant less than 24 hours old is considered to be "pathologic jaundice" or "hemolytic jaundice" and most likely results from serious blood incompatibility between the mother and the infant. "Physiologic jaundice" or "non-hemolytic" jaundice is the gradual yellowing of the skin in newborn infants that occurs after 24 hours of life, which may have a non-hemolytic cause. The three most common of these causes are (1) the failure to adequately process bilirubin through inadequate intake or elimination, (2) traumatic birth injuries, and (3) minor blood incompatibilities. The neonatal jaundice that occurs with breastfeeding is usually not seen in the early postpartum period; this type of jaundice becomes visible in newborns who are approximately 1 week old and may persist during the entire course of breastfeeding.

Additionally, congenital heart defects may be initially detected by skin pallor that does not improve with time. Skin color in all infants should be pink or flushed, indicating successful cardiac perfusion to the extremities. Acrocyanosis is common in newborns, localized to the hands and feet (Figure 20-6). Central cyanosis in the newborn has been described as a blue tint of the lips, gums, tongue, fingertips, and toes, with pallor noted underneath the eyes and on the cheeks. This is an indication that the

Nursing Alert

Jaundice

Visible jaundice in a newborn infant under 24 hours of age must be reported immediately. A rate of rise in bilirubin levels of more than 0.5 mg/dL per hour should be investigated.

Table 20-1 Critical Pathway for Timing of Newborn Assessment

ASSESSMENT	AGE (HR)					
	0–4	4–8	8–12	12–24	24–36	36–48
Laboratory	Blood type Coombs' test[1] (cord blood) Glucose blood level[2]	—	—	—	—	—
Assessment						
Gestational age	—	—	X	—	—	—
Physical	—	—	X	X	X	X
Vital signs[3]	HR >130	HR 100–130	X	X	X	X
	RR <60	X	X	RR 40–60	X	X
	T >97°F	X	X	X	X	X
Skin color	Pink, flushed	Pink, flushed	X	X	X	X
Interventions	Radiant warmer Blankets	Feeding	Position	X	X	X
Nutrition	None or breastfeeding	Formula or breast	Formula or breast	X	X	X
Medication	Vitamin K Eye prophylaxis	Cord dye if used, or alcohol	—	—	Hepatitis B vaccine	X
Activity	Sleep	Awake	Active-alert	X	X	X
Safety	Airway identification	Position	X	X	X	X
Teaching	—	Bulb syringe First bath	Feeding	Cord care Breastfeeding	Skin care Illness	Diaper rash Follow-up
Discharge planning	—	—	—	Feeding	X	Car seat
	—	—	—	Car seat	X	Follow-up[5]
	—	—	—	Neonatal screening[4]	X	
	—	—	—	Follow-up	X	

[1]Not all hospitals do Coombs' test. Nurse needs to handle cord blood according to hospital policy.
[2]Glucose blood level test is not routine in all hospitals, but may be on infants small for gestational age, large for gestational age, or infants of diabetic mothers.
[3]RR, respiratory rate; HR, heart rate; T, temperature
[4]Second neonatal screening done at 2-wk follow-up visit.
[5]Many are discharged between 24–36h. Nurse needs to ensure all teaching is done before discharge.

newborn has a circulatory problem and needs immediate attention and investigation into the suspected cause of the cyanosis. Stimulating the infant to cry, changing the infant's position to increase movement, or gently patting the soles of the feet should result in a rapid pinking of the skin to a red color as the infant increases respiratory and heart rate. The length of time the infant takes to return to the previous skin color forms the basis for the visual nursing assessment of the infant's cardiovascular system.

While the development of jaundice and pallor are the most critical problems found during the nursing assessment of skin, neither jaundice nor pallor of the skin can be determined accurately without knowing the infant's normal skin color. Infants of color, particularly Black and Hispanic infants, may have skin colors that have yellow tones that may make it difficult for the nurse to determine normal skin color. Strategies to improve the accuracy of as-

sessment of infant skin include using more than one light source, examining all skin surface areas of the infant, and palpating over bony prominences. Light sources in areas where infants are examined vary in intensity from overhead room lights and hallway lights to lights in radiant warmers and fluorescent lights. Nurses who examine infants using more than one light source can identify skin color more accurately. Examination of the entire skin surface of the infant, paying particular attention to the palms, soles of the feet, lips, and behind the ears, adds to the accuracy of the determination of normal skin color for the infant. Brief palpation of the infant's bony prominences, including the nose, sternum, sacrum, wrist, and ankle, by applying gentle pressure for 1 second yields the normal white color of blanching (first stage), followed by the "true skin color" (second stage), and ending with the skin color that reflects the ethnic heritage of the infant (third

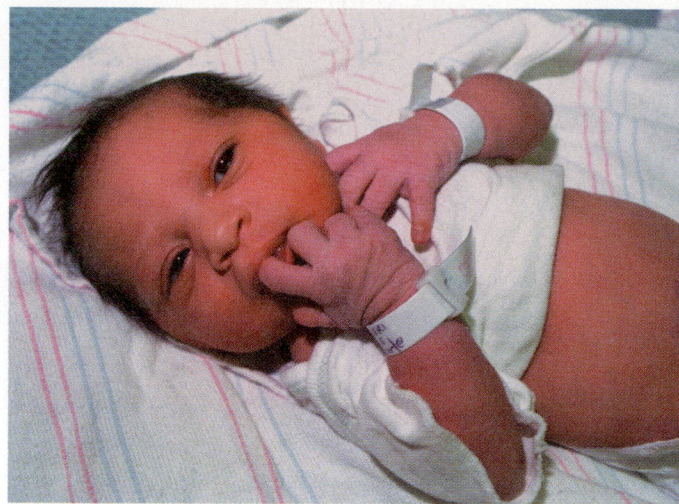

Figure 20-6   This newborn's hands show acrocyanosis.

stage). Second-stage skin color (determined by using this method) that is not pink-white or true skin-color and remains yellow or pale white indicates jaundice or pallor.

Body Size

Infant size is visually approximated for head-to-toe length and abdominal girth. The nurse's opinion as to whether the infant is small, medium, or large is later correlated with the graphed size classification. These physical parameters form the foundation for all future assessments of growth and development. The nurse also visually confirms that the head of the infant appears to be the largest body part.

Reactivity

The infant's reactions confirm the neuromuscular development of the infant. Is the infant asleep, awake, awake and quiet, or alert? Is the infant beginning to respond to the nurse by looking and moving extremities? Or is the infant actively alert, starting to fuss and cry? These are all discrete behavioral levels of awareness, or states (Brazelton, 1973), and require the infant to progress or regress from one to the other. The official behavioral state terms are deep sleep, light sleep, drowsy, quiet alert, considerable motor activity, and crying (Brazelton, 1973) (Figure 20-7). This assessment implies that the term infant has developed a mature neuro-organizational system that eases the transition from one behavioral state to another (D'Apolito, 1991). Term infants exposed to cocaine in utero have lost the ability to change behavior levels in an orderly manner. Their behavior is erratic and disorganized, with excessive responses to stimuli and lengthy or absent transition periods between behaviors (Napiorkowski, et al., 1996).

Reflections from a Nurse

It was two days before St. Patrick's Day and I had just finished the physical examination on a newborn girl with bright red hair and creamy white skin. I showed her off to everyone in the nursery, because you just don't see a lot of newborns with red hair. We (the nurses) joked that she came just in time for St. Patrick's Day. When I took her to her mother, I had to go in the room twice because I didn't see any Caucasian mothers in the room. I pulled her mother's chart and checked the ID bracelets just to make sure. I presented her to her mother, who was a very dark-skinned Black woman. She told me that all her babies had been born with red hair and this one looked like all of her other babies! I admitted my awkwardness and it gave me the opportunity to talk with this mother on a completely different level about her baby and her other children. I was so glad I had this experience. It totally changed my thinking about skin color in babies.

Observing the infant's response to the presence and voice of the nurse confirms the infant's responsiveness and behavioral organization levels. Infants who are irritable or who appear to be overreacting to voices, touch, or movement need comforting to assist them in calming their behavior. Swaddling in blankets, cuddling, rocking, and holding infants are interventions that the nurse can implement in the nursery. A complete physical examination should not be done on infants who are already irritated, because the examination leads to further disruption and disorganization of the infant's behavior.

Identification

All infants born in birthing centers, health care institutions, or hospitals are monitored to prevent misidentification, switching, or abduction. It is estimated that 12 to 18 infants are abducted by non–family members or strangers from health care facilities each year (Schuman, 1999). All nurses must become familiar with the infant security system used in their area of practice. Identification bracelets, "name-alert" cards for mothers with the identical last name, video cameras, door alarms, name badges to identify institutional personnel, and other sensing devices are often used to allay parental fears about the whereabouts and safety of their infant (Figure 20-8). Postpartum nursing units and nurseries

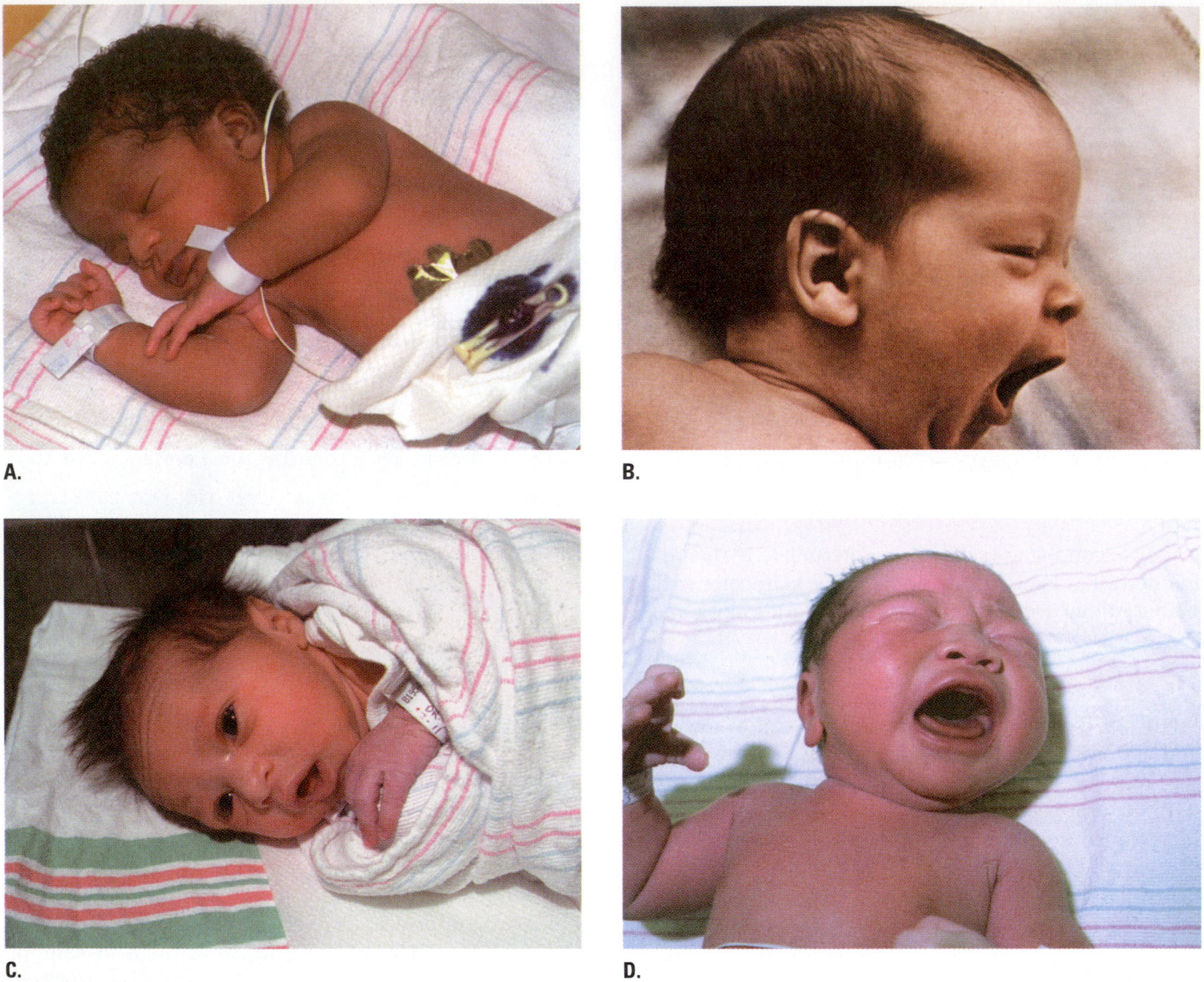

A.

B.

C.

D.

Figure 20-7   Behavioral states of the newborn. A. Light sleep; B. Drowsy *(Courtesy of Mead Johnson Nutritionals)*; C. Quiet alert; D. Crying.

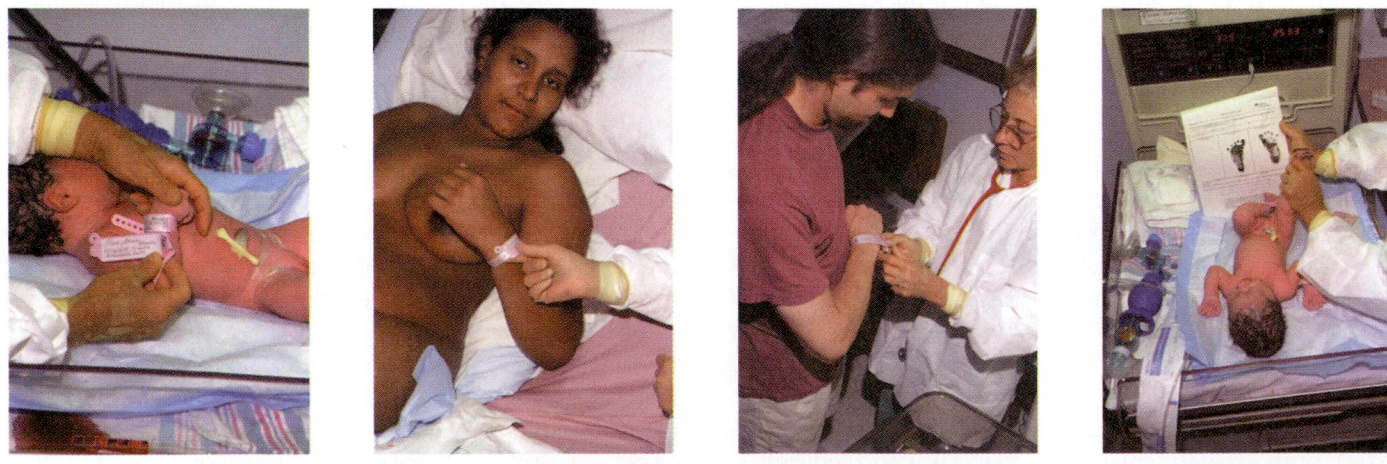

Figure 20-8   Matching identification bands are placed on infant, mother, and father; infant is footprinted.

traditionally receive many daily visitors because friends and family members want to welcome and see the new arrival. Increased traffic patterns between these two nursing units lead to crowding and increased opportunities for security violations. Nurses must also be alert to the location of the infant at all times and continually share this knowledge with the mother. Refer to Box 20-1.

PHYSICAL EXAMINATION

After the general nursing assessment is complete, the nurse begins the physical examination of the infant if the infant appears calm or resting. The manipulation and examination of the infant should not stress or irritate the infant.

Box 20-1

Preventing Infant Abductions

1. The identity of mothers of newborn infants is verified by their identification bracelet or other institutional device for identification.

2. Infants are identified by wearing two identification bracelets or one bracelet and another device (sensor or tag) (Figure 20-9). These security devices are placed on the infant in the delivery room. The nurse must verify that all identification devices, in addition to name cards, paperwork, charts, or anything else placed in proximity to an infant, belongs to that infant.

3. All identification devices of a mother and her infant are checked by the nursing staff before an infant is matched to his or her mother for visits or rooming-in. These devices are continuously rechecked by the nursing staff at the end and at the beginning of each nursing shift.

4. Transportation of infants from one unit to another or to another department for examination should be done only by authorized nursing staff, who should remain with the infant until the examination is complete and return the infant to his or her original location.

5. The infant should not be left by nursing staff with anyone but the birth mother, unless an official agency involved with parents and family has stipulated to the contrary. This includes persons claiming to be the mother's sister or spouse, father of the infant, grandmother, family relative, or adoptive mother.

6. When the birth mother is ill and is unable to take care of her infant, the father assumes responsibility for the infant and receives an identification bracelet to be matched with the infant's. In many hospitals, the father routinely

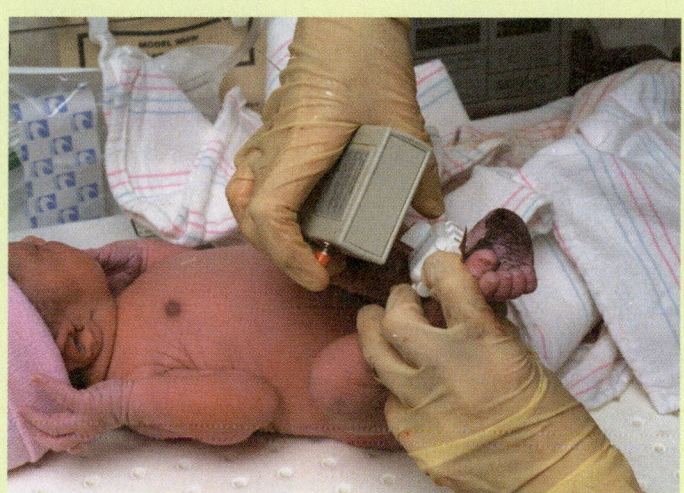

Figure 20-9   Application of a heel sensor.

receives an ID bracelet as well.

7. Family members or relatives may see the infant only while he or she is in the nursery. The mother's written permission is required for them to be able to hold or feed her infant in the nursery under nursing staff supervision.

8. The mother of the infant is instructed by the nursing staff never to give her permission to let someone she does not know take or hold her infant.

9. All nursing staff are identified through their identification badges, not by the clothes they wear. Nursing staff must continually reinforce their identity with mothers of newborns and be available to accompany them at all times for their security and safety.

10. All nursing staff should be aware of the institutional code for infant abduction and the procedures to follow should this event occur.

Weight, Measurement, and Vital Signs

The infant's weight in grams and length in centimeters was determined in the delivery room and during the transitional period. Average weight for a term newborn infant is 3,400 g (range, 2,500 to 4,300 g) and average length is 49.6 cm (range, 45 to 54 cm) (Fox, 1997). The frontal-occipital circumference (FOC) is measured in centimeters with a measuring tape to determine head size. The measuring tape is gently placed around the infant's head at the largest part of the occipital area and gathered over the forehead, resting on top of the eyebrows. The largest of three attempts is recorded by the nurse. Normal head circumference for a term infant at birth ranges from 33 to 38 cm (Johnson & Oski, 1997). Infants with FOC greater than the 90th percentile have **macrocephaly** and those with FOC less than the 10th percentile are considered to have **microcephaly**. The weight, length, and head circumference measurements are plotted against the gestational age of the infant to determine the size category of the infant (Figure 20-10). Size categories are small for gestational age (SGA) (< 10th percentile), appropriate for gestational age (AGA) (10th to 90th percentile), and large for gestational age (LGA) (> 90th percentile).

Vital signs are taken by the nurse and charted. Heart rate and respiratory rate are determined by auscultation. Temperature is recorded with an axillary thermometer or tympanic membrane thermometer. Blood pressure is checked on both the thigh and the arm of the infant. Systolic blood pressures range from 50 to 90 mmHg and diastolic blood pressures range from 20 to 60 mmHg (Fox, 1997). The systolic blood pressure of both the thigh and arm should be equal. A decrease of 10 mmHg or more in the thigh in comparison to the arm may indicate **coarctation of the aorta**. This may also be indicated with a systolic blood pressure of more than 90 mmHg (Fox, 1997).

Nursing Tip

Calculating Pounds from Grams and Inches from Centimeters

Infant weight is usually a whole number indicating how many grams the infant weighs. Divide this number by 1000: 1000 g = 1 kg = 2.2 lb. Multiplication of the number of kilograms by 2.2 yields the number of pounds of infant weight. Less than 1 pound can be converted to ounces by remembering that 16 ounces = 1 pound. One can multiply the grams by 0.0022 to convert to pounds. To convert grams to ounces, divide the grams by 28.35. For example, a 7 pound 8 oz baby would be 3,402 grams. The length of the infant in centimeters is divided by 2.5 to convert centimeters to inches: 1 in. = 2.5 cm.

Gestational Age Assessment

Since 1967, when the American Academy of Pediatrics recommended that all newborns be classified by birth weight and gestational age, the modification of the Dubowitz scoring system by Ballard, et al. (1991) remains the most popular method for determining gestational age. This examination provides a score of neuromuscular and physical maturity that can be mathematically projected onto a corresponding age scale to reveal the gestational age in weeks. Approximation of gestational age at delivery can be obtained by date of the mother's last menstrual cycle. This information is not as accurate as physical examination for gestational age. Gestational age assessments are often done by nurses on normal newborns and reported in the infant's chart.

The Ballard Gestational Age by Maturity Rating (Ballard et al., 1991) consists of two scoring systems: neuromuscular maturity and physical maturity of six to seven characteristics each. Scores from each system are added together and mathematically projected on the maturity rating scale to determine the gestational age by examination (Figure 20-11). The systems scored reflect the decreasing flexibility of muscles and joints in prematurity and the return to original positioning after movement indicative of a mature term infant. This examination is usually performed by the nurse within the first 12 hours of life and is more accurate when done on term infants between 10 and 36 hours of life (Gagliardi, 1993). It is not necessary to perform this examination in any order of categories to be assessed.

Maturity may occur at different rates among these categories. A score of 4 in one category does not mean that all subsequent categories must be scored as a 4. The examiner may strongly feel that a half-score is needed in one particular category because the infant exhibits a characteristic that falls between two scoring options. This is a valid choice, and half-scores are seen quite often in these assessments. These assessments are illustrated in the accompanying photo story.

Posture: Posture is the natural position that the infant assumes on its back. Both arm and leg positions are assessed in this category, and this is matched to the best picture of upper and lower extremities for scoring.

Square window: Wearing gloves, the examiner uses his or her thumb to gently press the infant's wrist and palm toward the infant's forearm. Either the angle that the wrist and the third and fourth fingers make against the forearm or the angle that the wrist and thumb make against the forearm is used for scoring purposes.

Arm recoil: This category is scored by the lateral or inferior extension of both arms after flexing them at chest

Newborn Assessment

O nce the infant enters the nursery, the nurse conducts a complete head-to-toe physical assessment to determine the infant's health status.

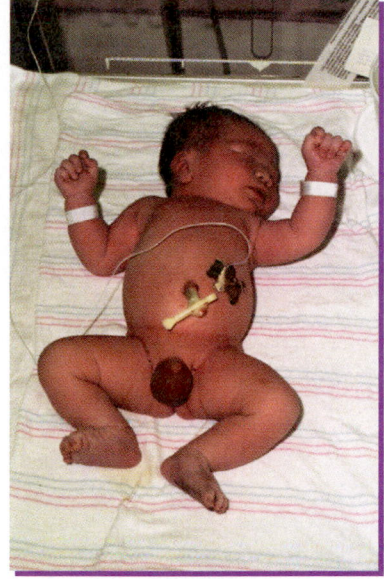

A general inspection is done first to identify abnormalities. A normal newborn assumes a flexed position.

Skin is inspected for color and texture. A full-term infant may display signs of skin dryness and cracking. Acrocyanosis may be present in the hands and feet but should diminish.

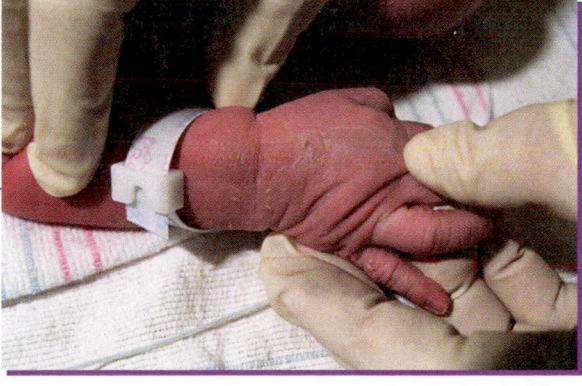

The newborn's heart is auscultated for rate and rhythm.

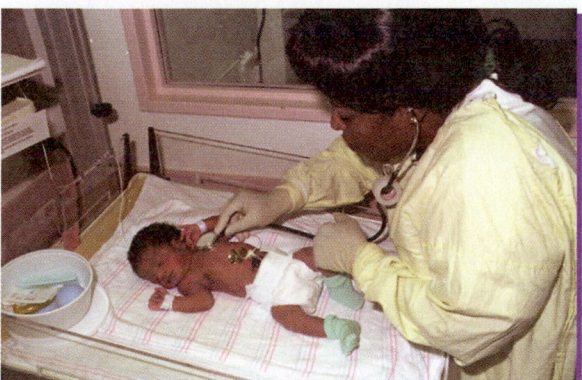

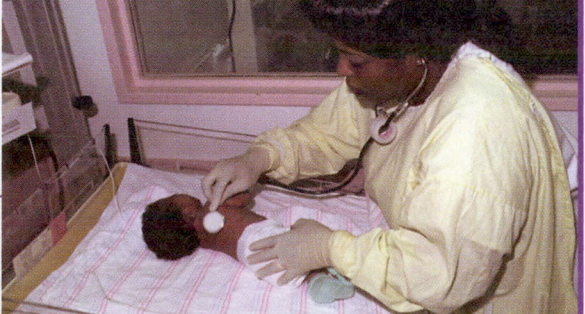

The lungs are auscultated to ensure expansion of both lungs and equal breath sounds.

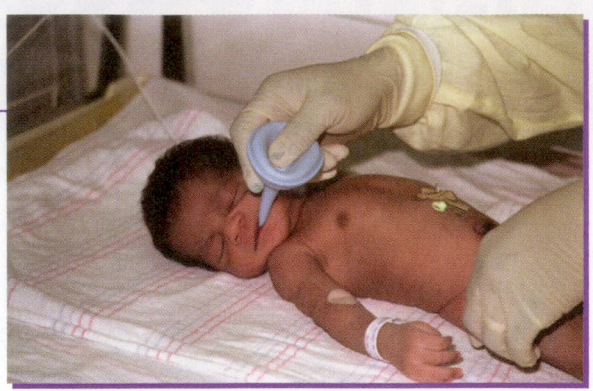

Sometimes suctioning is required to remove residual fluid from the infant's mouth.

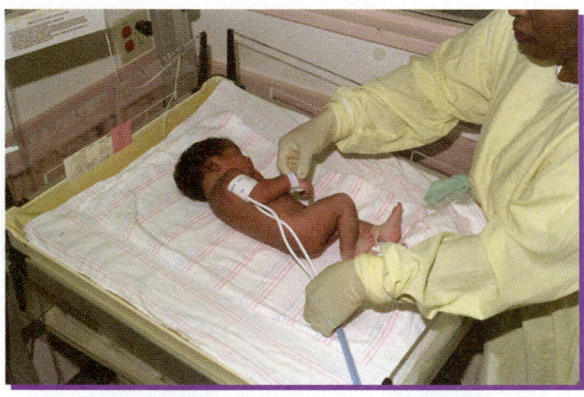

The newborn's first blood pressure measurement is taken.

The axillary body temperature is taken.

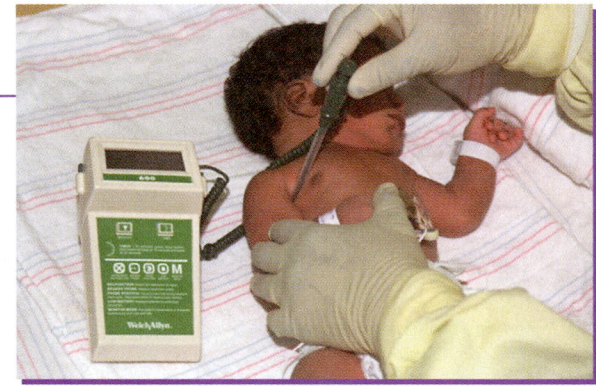

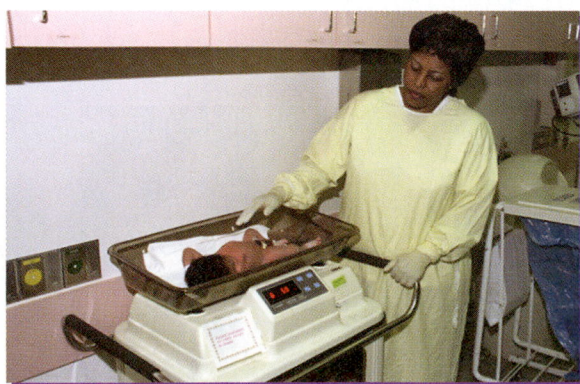

The newborn is weighed.

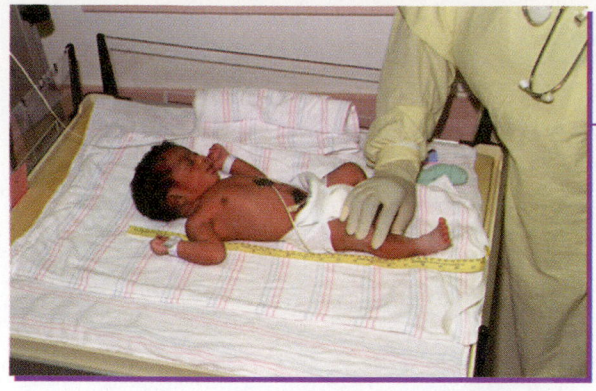

The infant's head-to-toe length is measured.

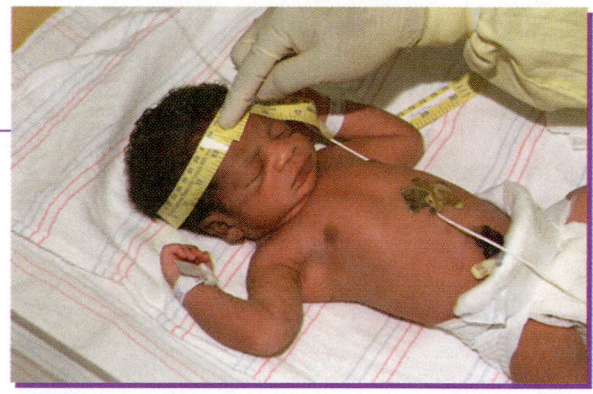

The infant's head circumference is measured (frontol occiptal circumference [FOC]).

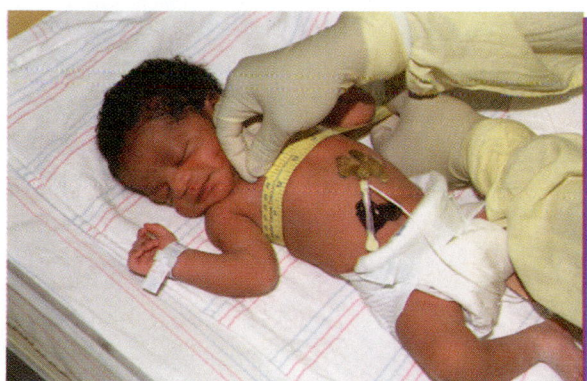

The infant's chest circumference is measured.

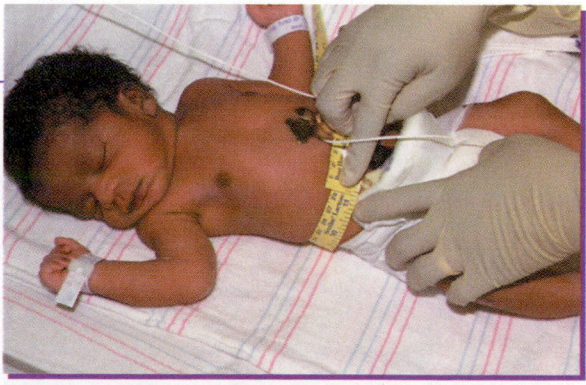

The infant's abdominal circumference is measured.

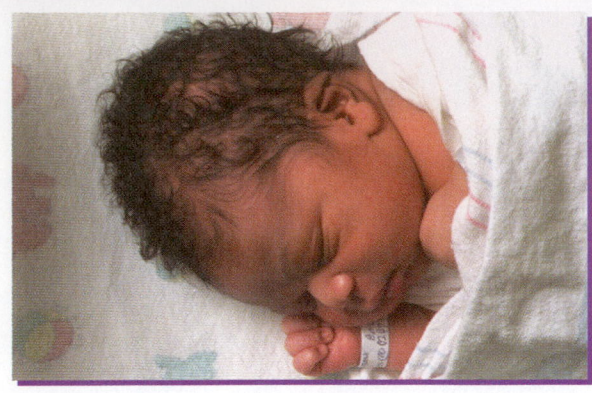

The infant's head is inspected for molding, and suture lines are palpated.

The face is inspected for symmetry, birth marks, milia, and nevi ("stork bites") over the forehead and eyelids.

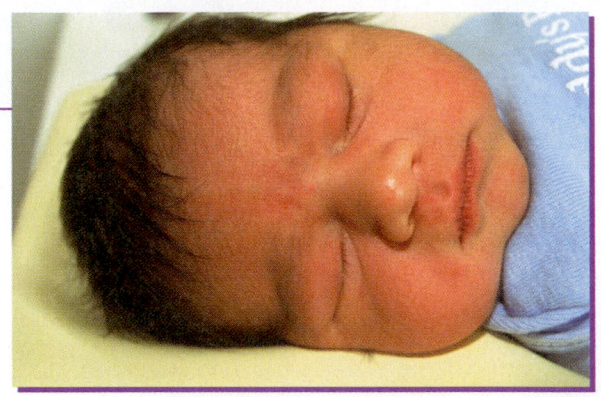

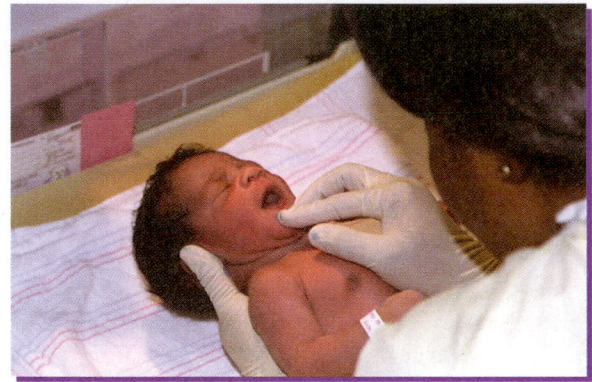

The mouth is inspected for natal teeth and abnormalities of the hard and soft palate; the tongue should be at midline.

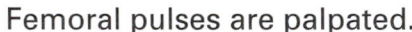

Femoral pulses are palpated.

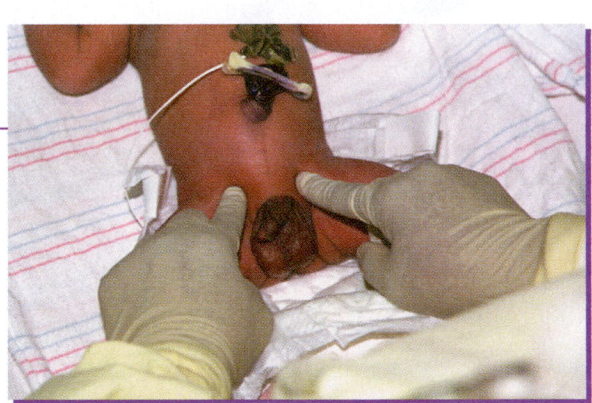

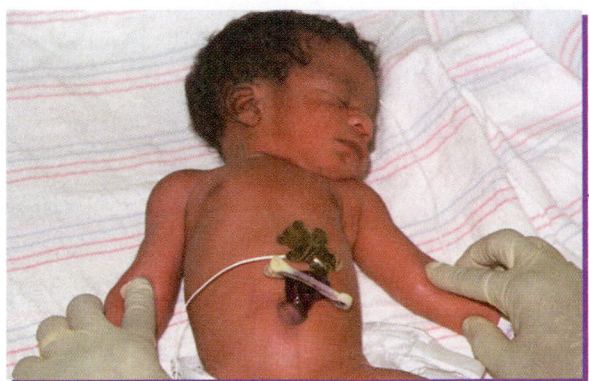

Brachial pulses are palpated.

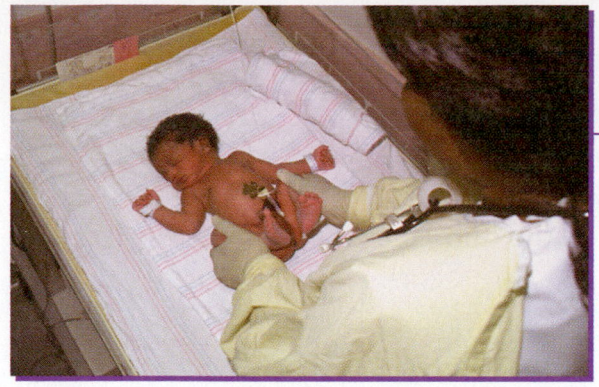

Ortolani's maneuver is done to check for hip dislocation.

Inspection of the genitalia. The nurse is palpating the scrotum to check for descent of the testes.

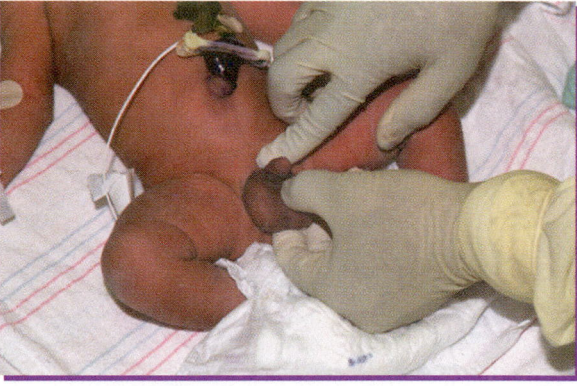

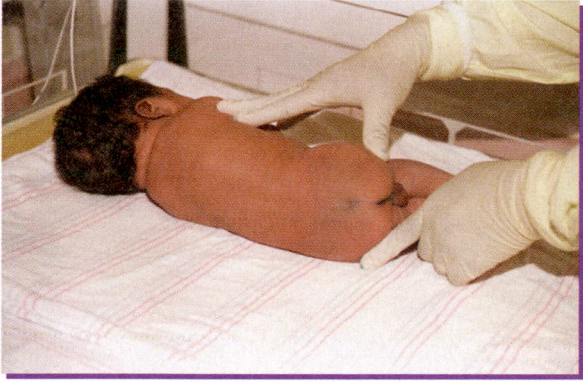

The spine and skin on the back are inspected for alignment, breaks in skin, moles, birth marks, or markers along the spinal column. This infant has a Mongolian spot near the base of the spine; this is a normal finding.

During the examination, the nurse will check certain reflexes. The presence of these reflexes suggests maturity of the neonatal neurological system.

This is the rooting reflex. The infant turns his head and opens his mouth when the perioral area is stimulated.

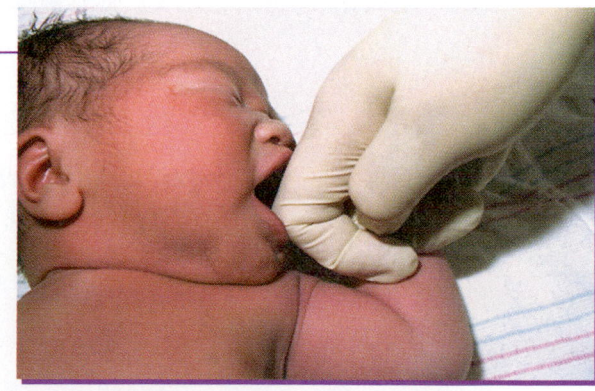

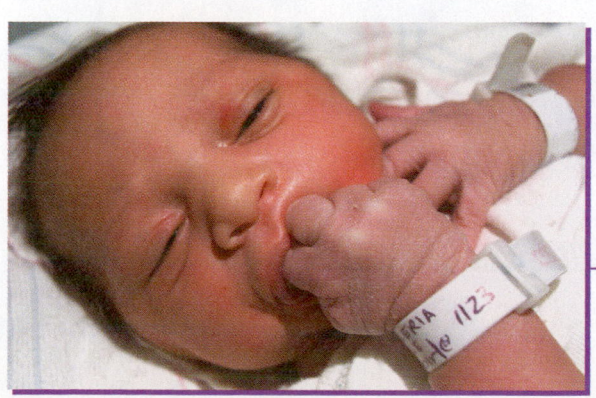

Sucking reflex is sometimes demonstrated spontaneously during the examination.

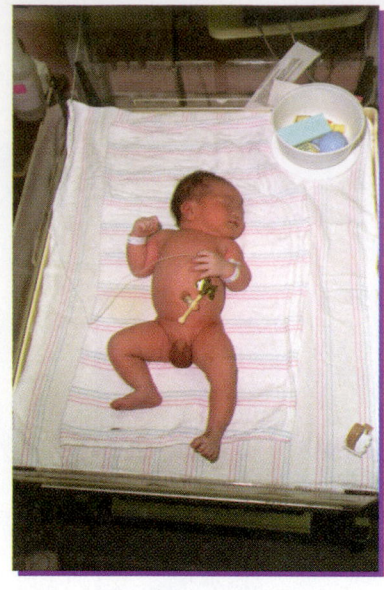

The tonic neck or fencing reflex—note the leg extension and the partial extension of the arm on the side the head is turned to, and the flexion of the arm and leg on the opposite side.

The grasp reflex is assessed.

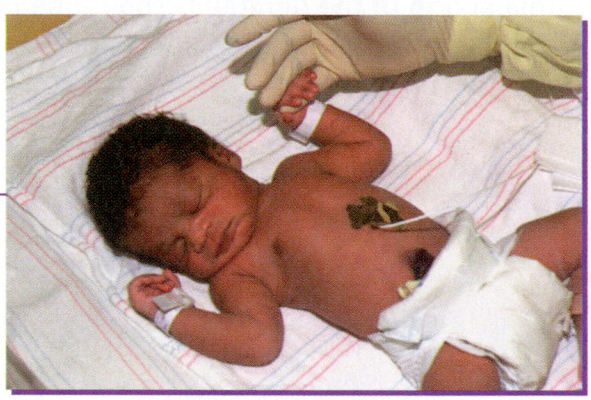

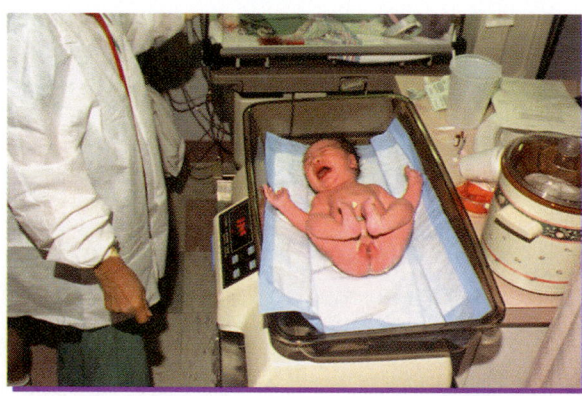

The Moro reflex is assessed.

The head lag or traction reflex is assessed.

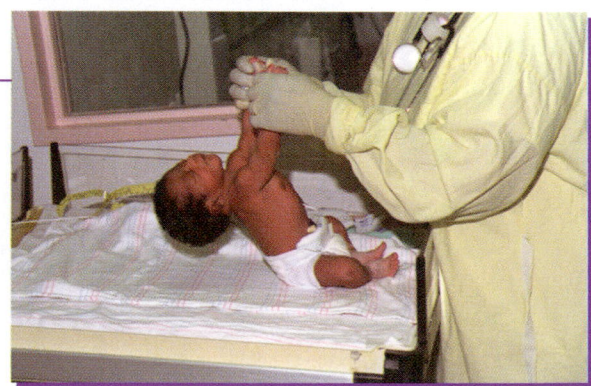

Assessment of Physical Maturity Using the Ballard Scale

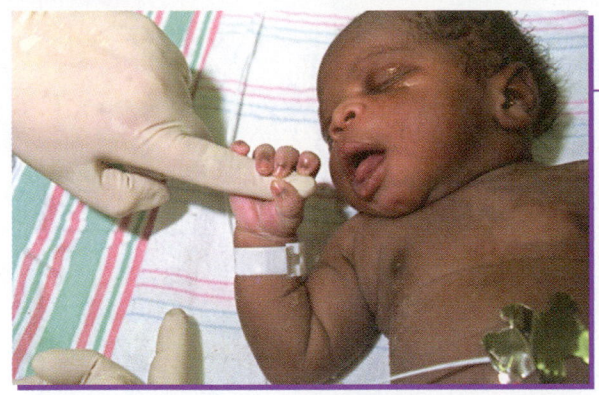

Skin is assessed using the parameters of the Ballard Scale. This post-term newborn shows skin cracking and peeling.

The amount of lanugo is estimated using the six parameters of the Ballard Scale.

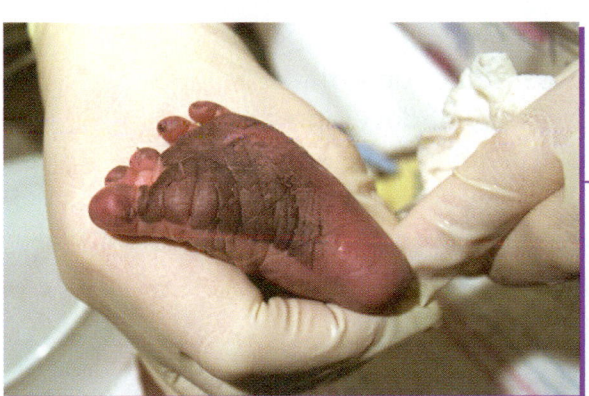

The plantar surface of the foot is assessed for creases.

Maturity of nipple buds is estimated.

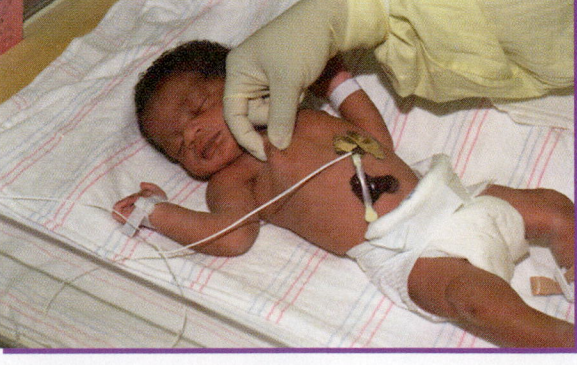

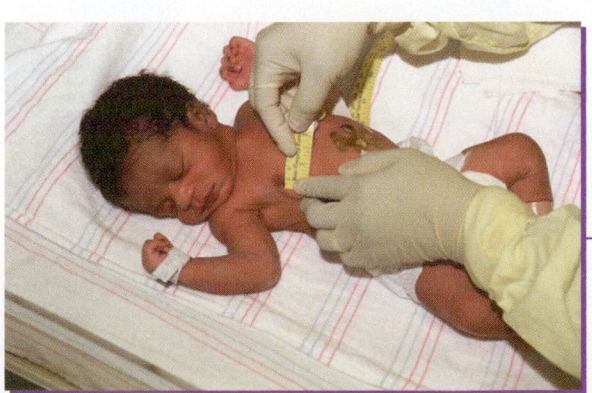

Nipples are measured.

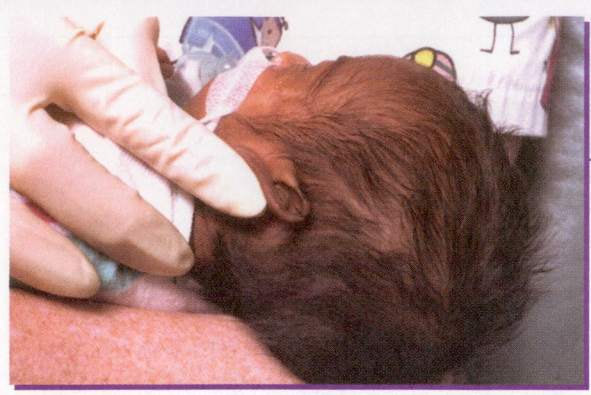

The amount of cartilage in the ear is assessed.

The male genitalia are assessed to determine if the testes have descended and if rugae are present.

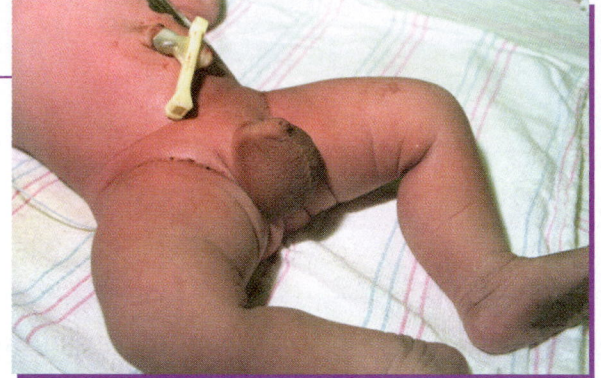

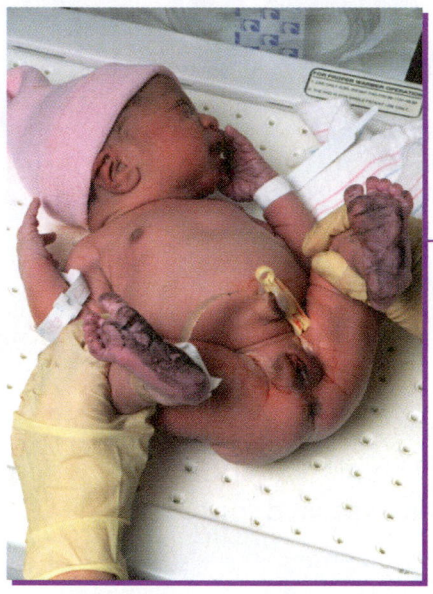

The female genitalia are assessed to determine maturity of development of the labia and clitoris.

*A*ssessment of Neuromuscular Maturity

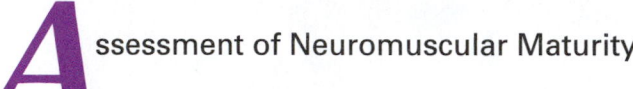

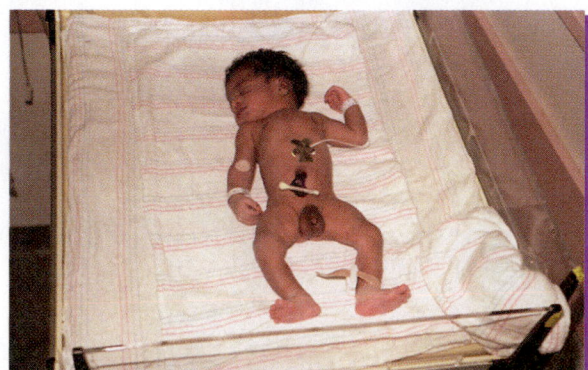

Degree of flexion is determined.

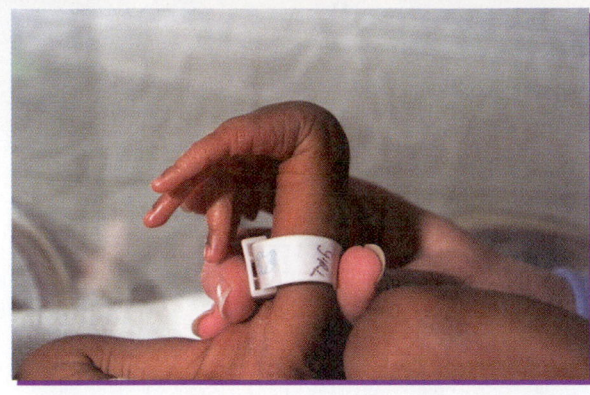

Square window determination.

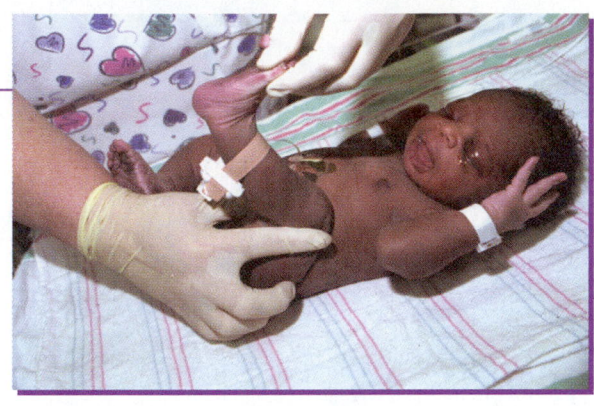

Popliteal angle.

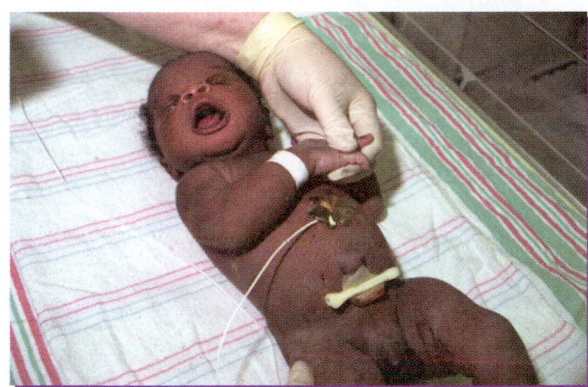

Scarf sign in term infant.

Scarf sign in preterm infant.

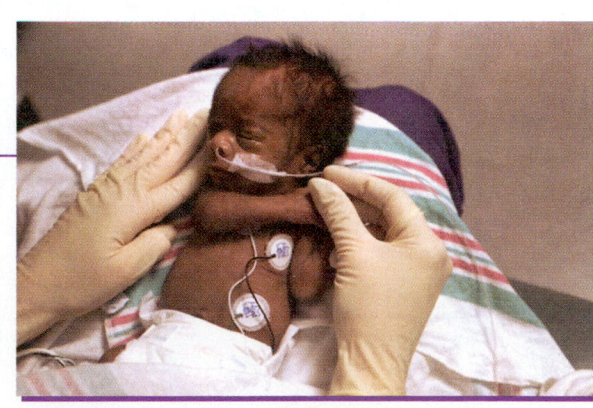

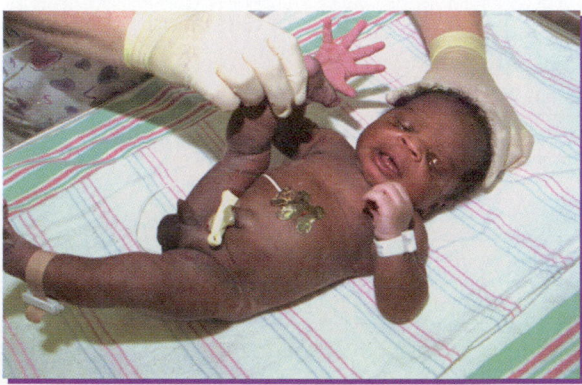

Heel to ear.

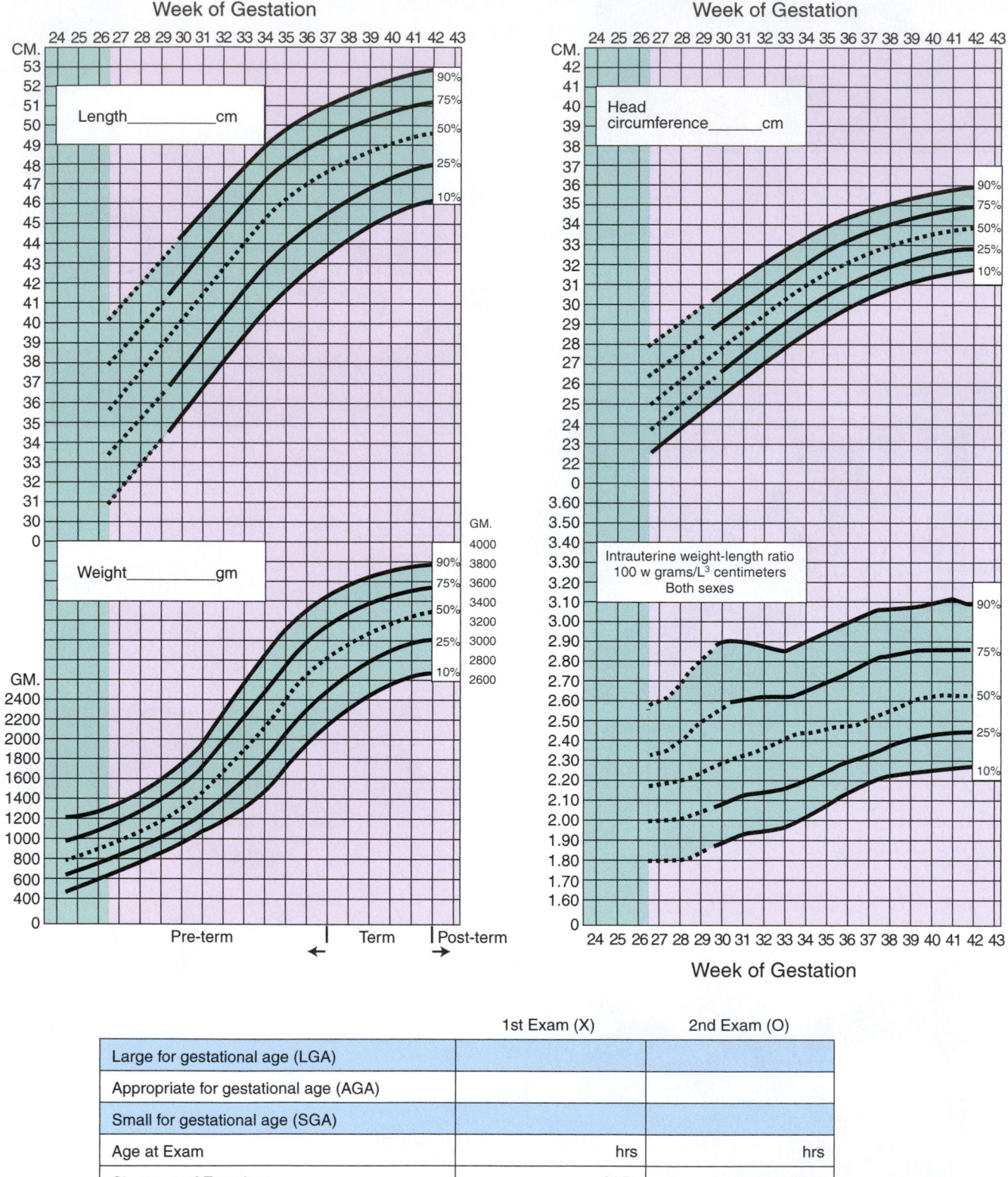

Figure 20-10 Gestational age assessment *(Courtesy of Mead Johnson Nutritionals)*.

NEWBORN MATURITY RATING & CLASSIFICATION

ESTIMATION OF GESTATIONAL AGE BY MATURITY RATING
SYMBOLS: X - 1ST EXAM   O - 2ND EXAM

Gestation by Dates _____ wks

Birth Date _____ Hour _____ am/pm

APGAR _____ 1 min _____ 5 min

NEUROMUSCULAR MATURITY

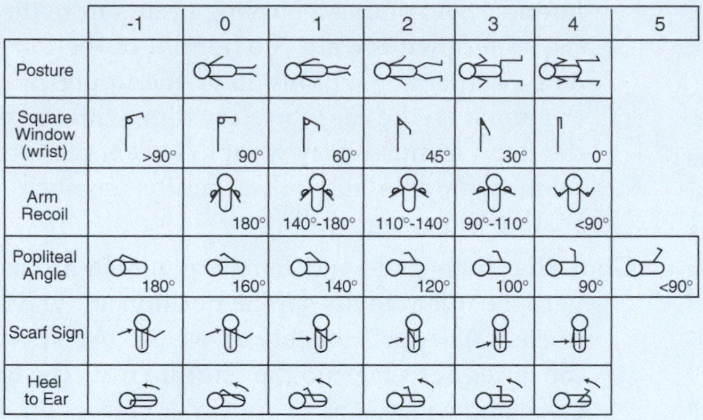

	-1	0	1	2	3	4	5
Posture							
Square Window (wrist)	>90°	90°	60°	45°	30°	0°	
Arm Recoil		180°	140°-180°	110°-140°	90°-110°	<90°	
Popliteal Angle	180°	160°	140°	120°	100°	90°	<90°
Scarf Sign							
Heel to Ear							

MATURITY RATING

score	weeks
-10	20
-5	22
0	24
5	26
10	28
15	30
20	32
25	34
30	36
35	38
40	40
45	42
50	44

PHYSICAL MATURITY

Skin	sticky friable transparent	gelatinous red, translucent	smooth pink, visible veins	superficial peeling and or rash few veins	cracking pale areas rare veins	parchment deep cracking no vessels	feathery cracked wrinkled
Lanugo	none	sparse	abundant	thinning	bald areas	mostly bald	
Planiar Surface	heel-toe 40-50min: -1 <40 min: -2	>50mm no crease	faint red marks	anterior transverse crease only	creases ant. 2/3	creases over entire sole	
Breast	imperceptible	barely perceptible	flat areola no bud	stippled areola 1-2mm bud	raised areola 3-4mm bud	full areola 5-10mm bud	
Eye/Ear	lids fused loosely: -1 tightly: -2	lids open pinna flat stays folded	sl. curved pinna; soft slow recoil	well curved pinna; soft but ready recoil	formed and firm instant recoil	thick cartilage ear stiff	
Genitals Male	scrotum flat, smooth	scrotum empty faint rugae	testes in upper canal rare rugae	testes descending few rugae	testes down good rugae	testes pendulous deep rugae	
Genitals Female	clitoris prominent labia flat	prominent clitoris small labia minora	prominent clitoris enlarging minora	majora & minora equally prominent	majora large minora small	majora cover clitoris and minors	

SCORING SECTION

	1st Exam=X	2nd Exam=O
Estimating Gest Age by Maturity Rating	_____ Weeks	_____ Weeks
Time of Exam	Date ____ Hour ____ am/pm	Date ____ Hour ____ am/pm
Age at Exam	_____ Hours	_____ Hours
Signature of Examiner	_____ M.D.	_____ M.D.

Figure 20-11   New Ballard score *(Courtesy of Mead Johnson Nutritionals).*

level. After release from extension, the amount of return to original position is observed by the nurse and scored. This assessment is often used to confirm brachial plexus injuries or fractured clavicles in the newborn when movements of the arms are observed to be unequal.

Popliteal angle: This is the assessment of the angle created when the knee is extended. The infant is assessed in the supine position with the pelvis flat and the thigh of one leg resting on the abdomen while the knee is extended by exerting upward pressure on the heel of the leg with the examiner's finger until resistance is met.

Scarf sign: This is placement of the infant's hand to the opposite shoulder. It is scored by observing where the elbow of the arm that was moved falls. The dotted line in the scoring category picture represents the sternal border or midline. In the supine position, the infant's hand is grasped between the thumb and first finger of the nurse's hand and, in one sweeping movement, the nurse attempts to place the hand on the opposite shoulder. Using a finger, the nurse marks on the infant's chest where the elbow of the infant falls and scores this category accordingly.

Heel-to-ear: This category assesses hip flexibility in infants. With the infant in the supine position, with the pelvis on a flat surface, one leg is gently extended and moved toward the infant's head on the corresponding side. When resistance is met, the visual distance between the ear on the infant's head and the great toe of the foot, along with the leg position, is scored. Infants who experienced breech positioning or who are suspected of having **developmental dysplasia of the hip (DDH)** may show a great amount of flexibility in this category.

Skin: Scoring in this category is based on palpation and visual inspection. Skin texture, transparency, relative thickness, and flaking and peeling of the epidermis are noted. Transparency, defined as skin through which veins can be seen, is evident in premature (preterm) infants and disappears with increasing maturity. Flaking of skin and peeling with wrinkles occurs in post-term infants.

Lanugo: **Lanugo** is the fine hair seen mostly on the backs and arms of premature infants. It eventually thins out in the lumbar region and disappears, leaving small traces on the shoulders. Stroking the infant's back while in the prone position will assist the nurse in identifying the lanugo that still exists apart from the infant's natural body hair. Mexican-American infants normally have thin, dark body hair that may cover their entire back and shoulders. This needs to be distinguished from real lanugo, which is lighter in color and softer and curls at the ends.

Plantar surface: Creases on the soles of both feet are scored according to the extent to which the creases cover the soles. The best way to visualize the extent of plantar creases is to gently curl the infant's toes toward the heel, and determine the score.

Breast: The amount of breast tissue is approximated by gently measuring the tissue present on the infant using a measuring tape in millimeters or by grasping the tissue between the examiner's thumb and forefinger. In addition, the bud and areola are inspected for size and stippling. Lastly, the area of breast tissue is palpated to determine its elevation from the chest wall.

Eye and ear: Eyelids should be open and should open easily in the mature infant. Ears are inspected for incurving of the pinna and palpated for a determination of the thickness of cartilage. The upper lobe recoil is performed bilaterally to validate the return to the posterior upright position when moved anteriorly and inferiorly. As pinnal incurving occurs from the top of the lobe down toward the bottom of the lobe, some mature infants may only have the upper portion of the pinna on the ear lobe curved in, with the remainder flat. The nurse may want to look at the ears of the infant's parents and other family members before scoring this category.

Genitalia: Both male and female genitalia are assessed with the infant in the supine position and the legs abducted. At approximately 35 weeks' gestational age, the testes descend into the scrotum from the inguinal canal and rugae start to appear as creases on the surface of the scrotum. Deep creases gradually develop as crevices on the scrotum as the infant becomes more mature. Visualization of a pendulous scrotum occurs in the supine position with the lower extremities abducted. In this same position, female infants can be assessed for the covering of the clitoris and the size of the labia majora. The distance between the edges of the labia majora and how much of the female genitalia is covered can also be visualized and scored.

Once the scoring is complete on the Ballard Newborn Maturity Rating, the scores from both the neuromuscular and physical maturity categories are totaled. This score is compared mathematically to the gestational age (in weeks) through a simple proportionate formula that equates the score range with the gestational age in weeks and calculates the exact position of the score within that range. Nurses should note that maturity scoring does not

Nursing Tip

How to Calculate Gestational Age

Your newborn's gestational age examination score of 34 falls between the scores 30 and 35 and occupies 4/5 of the score range from 30 to 35. Correspondingly, the exact age in weeks must also occupy 4/5 of the age score range of 2 between 36 and 38. Solving this simple ratio equation, you note that 4/5 of 2 equals $1\frac{3}{5}$, which, multiplied by 7 (days in a week) and added to 36, reveals a gestational age of $37\frac{4}{7}$ weeks for a maturity score of 34.

directly translate to gestational age in weeks. Often examiners make this mistake and estimate an infant's age at birth to be much younger than it is. An infant determined to be less than 37 weeks' gestational age is called **preterm**, or premature. An infant whose score falls between 37 weeks' and 42 weeks' gestational age is called **term**, and the infant that is scored beyond 42 weeks' gestation is called **post-term**.

Systems Assessment

The nursing assessment of the newborn infant's physical characteristics begins after completion of the general assessment and the gestational age assessment. The examination is initiated by placing the infant in the supine position and usually proceeds from the assessment of the skin first, followed by a head-to-toe examination. The examination may be performed on a radiant warmer to preserve infant temperature stability, in the infant's crib in the nursery.

Integumentary System

The skin and all the other elements of the integumentary system, that is, hair and nails, are examined for color, texture, distribution, disruptions, eruptions, and distinguishing characteristics or birth marks. When performing the skin assessment, the nurse should make sure that the room is well lit and be willing to use extra light sources for accuracy. The color of a newborn's skin should be flushed and appropriate to ethnic heritage, indicating good peripheral cardiac perfusion. After blanching over bony prominences, the underlying skin color should be pink-white before it returns to its natural pigmentation. Skin color can also be assessed by a visual inspection of the infant's mouth, tongue, and gums. These areas should always display a healthy pink-red color, darkening to bright red when the infant is crying.

Common Findings

Wearing gloves, the nurse inspects and lightly palpates the scalp and body hair for texture and distribution. Mexican-American, Asian, and Black infants are often born with a full head of scalp hair and have some body hair on their back, shoulders, and buttocks. Hair is described as fine, thick, curly, or straight and the color and location are noted (Figure 20-12). Mexican-American and Asian newborns have dark, straight hair at birth. The hair on Black newborns is usually tightly curled and softer in texture. Eyelashes and brows, if present, are also inspected. Nail beds are examined on both fingers and toes for shape, length, and color. Many infants are born with long fingernails that may cause facial scratches as the infant feels and explores using fingers. Scratching by a newborn infant is controlled by placing mittens on the hands because newborn nails are very soft and flexible and difficult to trim with accuracy.

Infant skin should feel soft and smooth in term infants, and leathery with cracking and peeling in post-term infants. Breaks in the skin are noted to be either disruptions or eruptions. Disruptions include any break in skin integrity, including lacerations, electrode marks, and peeling layers. Forceps deliveries or vacuum extractions may break the skin on the scalp or face, leaving marks or bruises. Scalp electrode monitors leave small puncture sites in the infant's scalp that may not have a scab covering them at the time of the nursing assessment. Skin peeling is common in those infants classified as post-term. Frequently, infants are born with a condition called **pustular melanosis**. These small pustules are formed before delivery. The pustule disintegrates, leaving behind a small

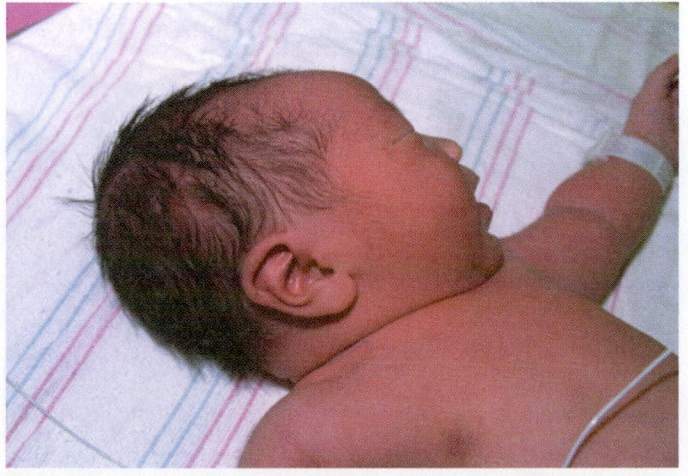

A.

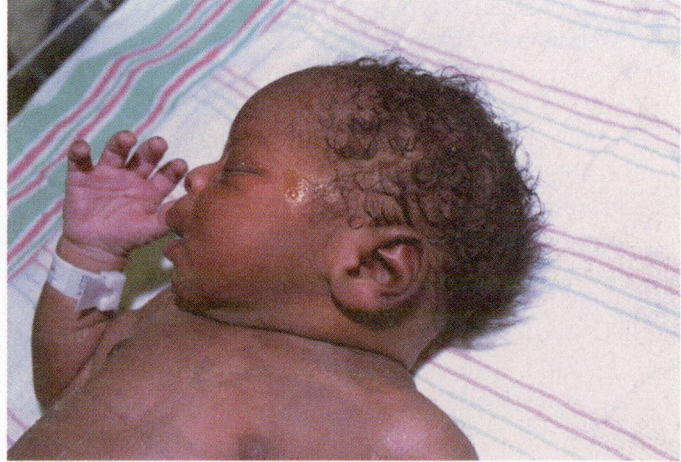

B.

Figure 20-12   Newborn hair varies in texture, from straight (A) to curly (B).

Nursing Tip — Nail Length in Newborns

Nurses who are experienced in examining newborns report: "the longer the nails, the more mature the baby." They are basing this observation on the time of development of fingernails and toe nails, which occurs late in the third trimester of pregnancy.

A greenish color around the nail bed of a finger or toe may indicate meconium staining from in utero exposure to meconium before or during delivery. Two other places where the nurse would see meconium staining on a newborn infant are the umbilical cord and the ear canals.

residue (scale) in the shape of the pustule, which later develops into a small flat spot called a macule, 1 to 2 mm in diameter. These small macules are numerous, look brown similar to freckles, are located on the chest and extremities, and appear to be a rash (but are not). Pustular melanosis is more commonly seen on Black infants than on Caucasian infants.

Some of the skin eruptions that occur in the early neonatal period are classified as normal variations. Small, singular, white papules that appear to be tiny pimples may be seen on a newborn's face, particularly on the chin. This skin condition is called **milia** and is one form of a sebaceous cyst. One or two white, pinhead-sized inclusion cysts may be seen on the penis or the scrotum of male infants or on the areola of female infants. Separate from milia and inclusion cysts, the infant may have acne, a skin eruption that usually occurs with puberty but, in infancy, is related to excessive amounts of maternal hormones. Neonatal acne eventually disappear from the infant's cheeks and chest. The most common normal skin eruption seen in newborns is **erythema toxicum**, a rash that generally occurs on the face and chest first and spreads to the rest of the body. The cause of this rash is unknown, and it may persist on the infant for a month after delivery. It begins with small, irregular, flat patches of redness on the cheeks and progresses to singular, small, yellow pimples on an erythematous base, as it moves to the chest, abdomen, and extremities. This skin condition appears particularly disturbing and frustrating to parents because there is no treatment to speed up its departure. It appears, remains, and disappears on its own schedule.

Another skin eruption is a blister formation on the fingers, wrist, or upper lip of the infant from sucking before and after delivery. These are not cause for alarm, and parents need to be reassured that these blisters or calluses will go away.

Distinguishing characteristics of the newborn's skin are either normal variations in skin color, birth marks, or evidence of birth trauma from the delivery. Normal variations in skin color include the dark blue, gray, or purple diffuse color seen on the buttocks of infants called **Mongolian spots**, which also appear on their shoulders, forearms, wrists, and ankles (Figure 20-13). These spots will fade and may disappear as the infant grows older. Some newborn skin shows a "cobblestone" appearance of pink-white areas outlined with a darker pink border (Figure 20-14). This **mottling** (called cutis marmorata) of the skin is common in newborns and results from the infant's vasomotor response to a lowered environmental temperature outside the womb. As the newborn adjusts to extrauterine life, this mottling disappears. Additionally, maternal hormones during labor and delivery may cause a normal darkening of the skin in the genital areas of both male and female infants.

Birth marks on a newborn infant are different from other marks that are the result of trauma to the infant from the delivery process. Birth marks are usually small,

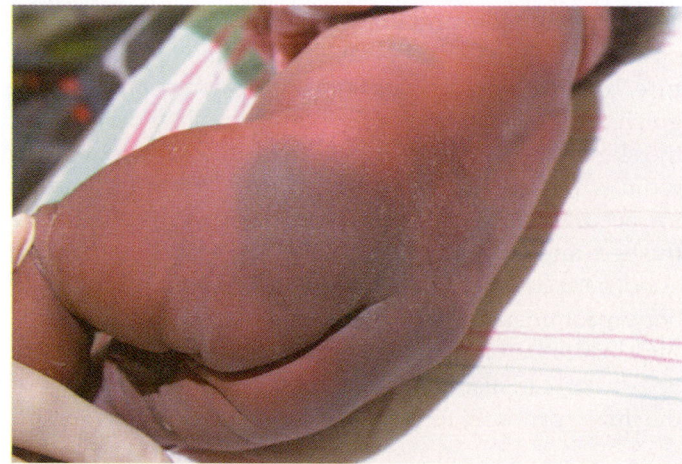

Figure 20-13 Mongolian spots.

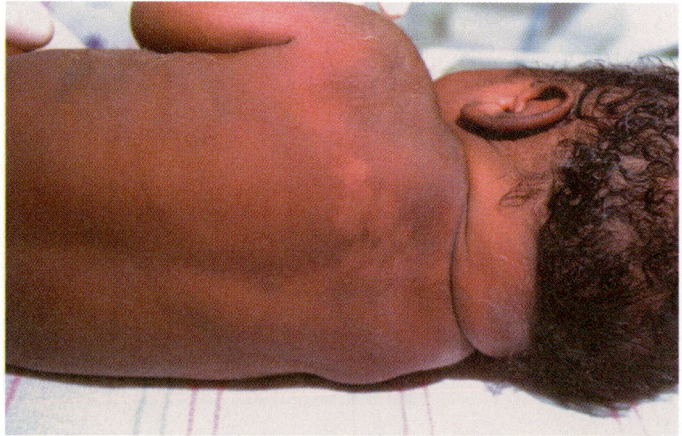

Figure 20-14 Mottling.

flat areas of color that may be white, tan, brown, red, or blue. Borders may be irregular. The nurse documents the location and color of the birth mark (Figure 20-15). Any area of colored skin that contains hair or is located at the midline of the infant anteriorly or posteriorly should be investigated for underlying tissue involvement. A white or pale patch of skin usually represents an area of hypopigmentation and, by itself, is not an indicator for concern. However, numerous areas of hypopigmentation, including patches that have a leaf pattern, must be reported immediately. These patches may be found on the chest, back, extremities, and in the axilla. A neurologic condition, tuberous sclerosis, may be suspected in infants who have a hypopigmented skin patch that resembles a patterned leaf. Tan spots on the skin are often called cafe-au-lait marks and are very difficult to see on a Black infant. Many infants are born with these, and it is only a significant finding when the nurse counts six or more that are larger than 0.5 cm in diameter. Infants with these large cafe-au-lait spots at birth may be at risk for developing type I neurofibromatosis and need observation during infancy for any tumors that develop underneath the skin.

Brown skin marks or brown nevi (singular, *nevus*) are birth marks in which the color may vary from brown to intense black. Nevi have been thought to be an early form of a precancerous lesion (Seidel et al., 2001), and parents are taught by nurses to observe and report any change in color, shape, size, or elevation of these marks during the lifetime of their child.

A red birth mark, or nevus flammeus, is often seen at the nape of the neck ("stork bite") and on the face between the eyebrows or on the eyelids, nose, or upper lip. Appearing pale red in color, the nevus flammeus often has an irregular border or "splash mark" appearance. Red birth marks often turn bright red when the infant is crying, and gradually fade as the infant gets older. Other red birth marks observed in infancy are capillary heman-giomas, which may appear as red, raised lesions anywhere on the infant's body. They also contain areas of purple, blue, or white skin within the lesion. The nurse can address the parents' concern about this lesion by explaining that it will grow larger, undergo a process of involution, and then gradually disappear during the first 7 years of life. These lesions are not surgically removed unless they interfere with a vital system or are located on the face.

A blue nevus is a small, discrete blue or blue-black birth mark. It is usually found on the buttocks and hands and feet. This nevus is often mistaken for a Mongolian spot when located on the buttocks. It is differentiated from a Mongolian spot by its distinct borders and brighter color, which is different from the darker diffuse purple-blue-gray coloring over a general area characteristic of Mongolian spots. They are usually no larger than one centimeter in diameter.

Common Problems

Marks on an infant that are the result of birth trauma are usually characterized by the initial red imprint of the traumatizing instrument (e.g., forceps) and their color follows the normal progression of the skin color changes like it would with a bruise. Common areas to inspect for birth injuries are the scalp, face, shoulders, arms, legs, and feet. Marks from birth trauma are commonly seen in large infants when it is difficult to deliver the head or rotate the shoulders. Infants whose delivery position is breech or whose presenting parts are either the legs or feet can often show extensive bruising or edema from attempts to deliver the infant. In some cases, birth trauma may not be evident by a difference in skin color or edema at the injury site. These infants become extremely irritable when their position is changed or during simple extremity movements. Observation of infant behavior when the nurse examines the skin of the infant in the prone and supine position may lead the nurse to further investigate additional areas. The following may need further investigation:

- *Petechiae*. The presence of petechiae on the infant's skin that cannot be attributed to birth injury or trauma must be investigated further. Petechiae may represent an underlying infection, a hemorrhagic process, or congenital condition (congenital rubella). Petechiae should be reported immediately because many of the causes may be life-threatening to the infant if left untreated.

- *Port wine stains*. Purple or dark red marks that are extensive and differ from nevus flammeus are called port wine stains. Port wine stains are usually found on the head over the eyelid along the trigeminal nerve tract. These birth marks usually do not cross the midline and may be seen on the trunk or

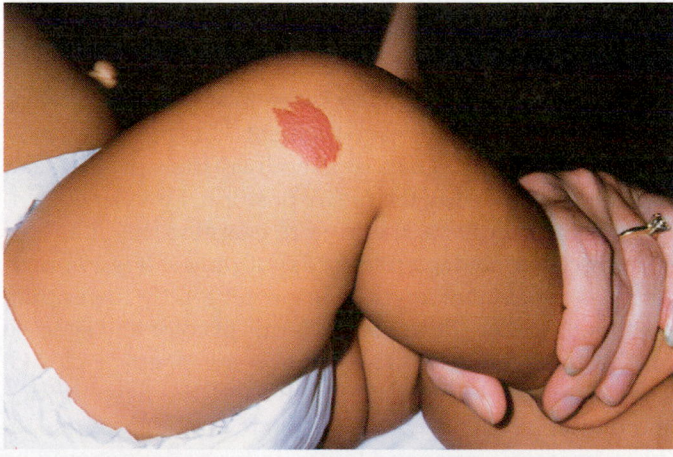

Figure 20-15   Nevus vasculosus (strawberry mark).

extremities. Neurologic assessments should be performed on all infants with port wine stains. Parents can be reassured that pulse-dye laser surgery can achieve cosmetic correction of the lesion at a later age (Seidel et al., 2001).

■ *Extensive lesions.* Colored skin lesions that contain two distinct areas of color, are extensive, cover a large amount of body surface, or contain hairs or a tuft of hair should be evaluated by a dermatologist. These skin lesions may indicate a defect in the underlying structures, and often ultrasound is indicated to evaluate the tissue underneath the skin. Skin nevi that contain hairs or a tuft of hair are called hairy nevi and, when present on the posterior surface midline in conjunction with the spinal column, may indicate a vertebral defect. The nurse should inspect and palpate the spinal column and sacrum for dimpling or depressions in the skin that may also be an indication of a vertebral defect. Spinal ultrasound examination of the spinal vertebrae is necessary to confirm any defects that would indicate the presence of spina bifida or spina bifida occulta.

■ *Blisters.* Small crops of blisters or a single blister found on full examination may require further evaluation. Blisters that are not located on the thumb or hand (sucking blisters) or on the extremities in conjunction with other lesions indicative of pustular melanosis are a cause for concern. Groups or crops of blisters on a presenting part of the infant's body are often caused by exposure to herpes as the infant passed through the birth canal. The most common location for these blisters is on the infant's scalp, near the hairline, or around the scalp electrode monitor site. Because this condition can be lifethreatening to the infant, this finding must be reported immediately.

■ *Plethora.* Newborn skin color that remains red or dark pink may be an indication of plethora. Plethora may be caused by polycythemia vera or hyperthermia. Polycythemia vera is a condition in which an increased number of red blood cells in the infant's bloodstream occurs as a result of backflow of maternal blood into the infant when the cord was cut. This diagnosis can be confirmed by a capillary hematocrit value of 65 or greater and a venous hematocrit of 60 or more (Seidel et al., 2001). Treatment of polycythemia vera includes admission to the intensive care unit for monitoring and a partial exchange transfusion.

■ *Hair distribution.* Hair patterns may present a problem in infancy. Hair distribution is described in the nursing assessment, and the nurse notes the texture, color, and distribution. Visually, the nurse determines any disruptions to the distribution of hair or any areas that contain hair that is not uniformly distributed over the scalp with distinct hairlines. Hair that extends over the forehead, blurring the forehead and shortening the distance between the hairline and the eyebrows, raises a concern because of its association with congenital syndromes. Particular attention should be directed toward those areas of hair that are lighter in color, sections of hair colored very differently in comparison to the rest of the scalp hair, and hair patterns that appear to have a circular design (whorls). White hair patches in the midst of darker colored scalp hair and circular hair patterns may indicate a defect in underlying structures or be initial findings in congenital syndromes. These findings should be documented by the nurse and reported immediately for further evaluation.

Nursing Implications

An accurate assessment of the infant's skin allows the nurse the opportunity to prepare for conditions that might adversely affect the infant and to show common skin variations on the infant to the parents and any other family members that are present. New parents are especially concerned about "marks" or "spots" on their babies, and the nurse can address these concerns as well as remove any fears that the parents or family members may have voiced.

Head, Ears, Eyes, Nose, and Throat

The head, ears, eyes, nose, and throat (HEENT) of the infant are examined next, after the skin has been assessed. Visual inspection guides the nursing assessment of this system. The nurse inspects the face for symmetry and placement of eyes, nose, lips, mouth, and ears. The shape of the eyes, nose, and mouth are also examined, and any movements of the lips and eyelids are observed. Damage to cranial nerve VII (facial nerve) from trauma during the delivery process can result in one side of the mouth or tongue drooping, unequal cheek muscle movement, or lack of appropriate eyelid movement. Ear shape, size, and position on the head can be examined from profile head positioning as well as the *en face* position. Low-set ears bilaterally may indicate the need to examine the infant for other physical characteristics of syndromes. It is common for infants to be born with one ear set a little lower than the other. Eyes are described in terms of color and spacing on the forehead, and whether lids are open or closed. Nares should be open bilaterally, and the nasal bridge should not have a lateral deviation resulting from the delivery process. Upper and lower lip formations should be approximately the same size with the same color as the

Nursing Tip   **Newborn Examination**

The nurse should wash her hands and don clean gloves before touching the newborn during the examination.

tongue and buccal mucosa inside the mouth. A chin should be visible and more prominent when the infant's head is placed in the profile position. A small jaw (micrognathia) viewed from the profile position may cause concern about proper tooth development, sucking, swallowing, and later tongue movement inside the mouth for speech.

Common Findings

Palpation begins with the head to determine the spaces between suture lines, the width of the fontanels, and the location and extent of edema from the delivery process. The sutures are felt as bony ridges, with spacing between them to indicate the distance between the borders (Figure 20-16). The **anterior fontanel** is a diamond-shaped open space formed by the anterior-posterior sagittal and frontal sutures and the lateral coronal suture. The area of the fontanel can be determined by feeling its borders and using the nurse's finger for measurements; 2.5 cm, or 1 inch, is the distance from the tip of the finger to the first finger joint. Some infants may have fairly large anterior fontanels (from 5 to 7 cm), and, conversely, others may have small anterior fontanels (from 1 to 2 cm). The **posterior fontanel** is a small, triangular-shaped space formed by the sagittal suture and the posterior lateral suture and called the lambdoidal suture. This fontanel is usually 1 cm at its widest point and, on palpation, may be closed, with only a slight indentation at the initial examination. This is not an unusual finding. The anterior fontanel must be open to provide for the expansion of the bones of the skull for brain growth during the first year of life. Spaces between suture lines are reflective of the molding process necessary to deliver the head of the infant and may extend to all suture lines, including the frontal suture in the middle of the forehead. Fontanels should be palpated by the nurse for an assessment of intracranial pressure. Fullness without bulging, either palpated or visible, is a sign of normal intracranial pressure. Bulging fontanels in infants with large head circumferences are characteristic of increased intracranial pressures, most likely associated with hydrocephalus.

Soft-tissue edema or swelling from delivery may be palpated during the examination of the head (Figure 2017). Edema that is fairly diffuse and crosses suture lines is called **caput succedaneum** and usually disappears dur-

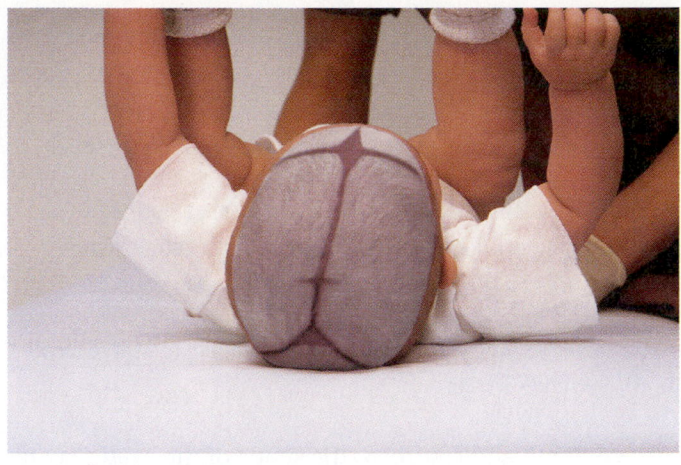

Figure 20-16   Sutures and fontanels.

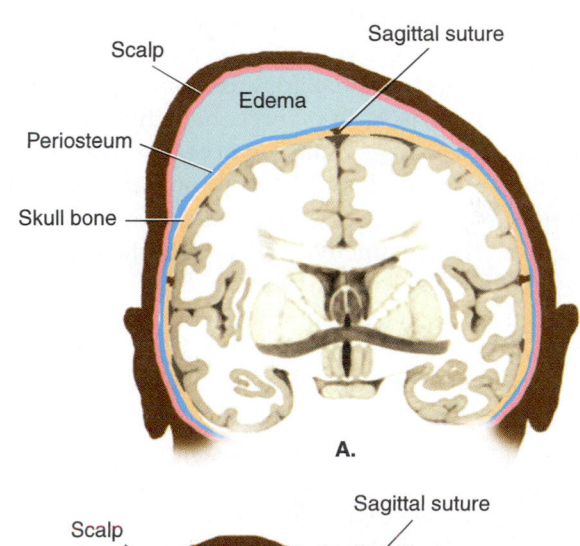

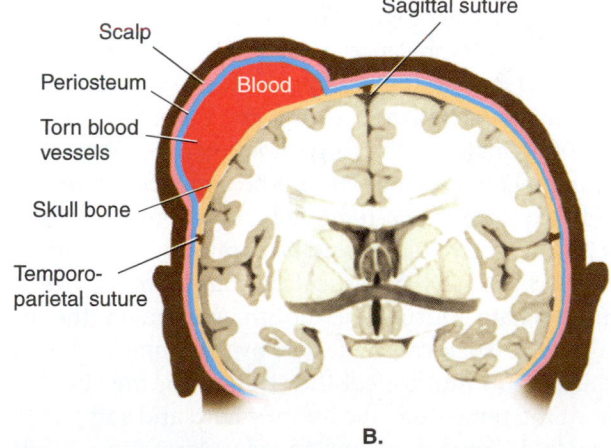

Figure 20-17   A. Caput succedaneum; B. Cephalhematoma.

ing the first several days of life. Edema that appears to be localized, giving the infant's head the appearance of growing a horn on one side, is called a **cephalhematoma**. This represents a subperiosteal hemorrhage that does not cross suture lines (Table 20-2). The skin in the area may or may not have a reddened color. As this material is slowly

Table 20-2	Comparison of Caput Succedaneum and Cephalohematoma	
CAPUT SUCCEDANEUM	**CEPHALOHEMATOMA**
Soft tissue edema	Subperiosteal hemorrhage
Can cross suture lines	Does not cross suture lines
Disappears in a few days	May last for several weeks
Self-resolving with little symptoms	May have jaundice as it resolves

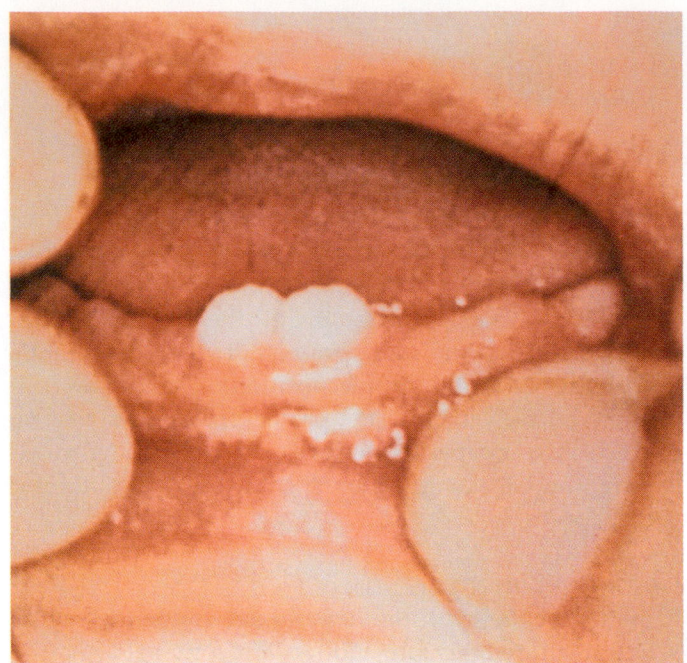

Figure 20-18 Neonatal teeth or precocious teeth *(Courtesy of Mead Johnson).*

broken down and resorbed, the shape of the head may remain "lumpy" for 3 to 4 months after birth and the infant may show signs of jaundice from the metabolism of broken red blood cells from the hemorrhage.

The face, including eyes, nose, and ears, is palpated to confirm shape and size. Eyelids are opened manually to check color of the iris, sclera, and conjunctiva. Tiny pinpoint scleral hemorrhages may be noted in the inner or outer canthus of the eyes and are common after delivery. Small amounts of a yellowish discharge that appear to originate from the conjunctiva and stick to the eyelashes, along with swollen eyelids, indicate that the infant has received eye prophylaxis. Bilateral red reflexes are assessed with an ophthalmoscope and recorded.

Gross vision in the infant may be evaluated by holding the examiner's face approximately 8 to 10 inches from the infant's face and determining the infant's ability to direct his or her gaze to the nurse's face and readjust the gaze when the nurse moves. The nasal bridge is palpated for symmetry and presence of any fracture that might have occurred during the delivery process. The mouth is opened and inspected and gums are palpated for the presence of neonatal teeth lying underneath the gum surface. Visible neonatal teeth should be assessed for looseness and may have to be removed to prevent aspiration (Figure 20-18). The uvula should be at midline. A bivalved or two-lobed uvula is an indication that there may be a cleft in the palate. During the mouth assessment, the infant's ability to suck can be tested by inserting a gloved finger into the mouth to feel the strength of the sucking motion. At the same time, the infant's hard and soft palate can be assessed for size, shape, and cleft formations. Cleft formations may be palpated as an actual opening or a notched ridge. High-arched palates may be an indication of difficulties in swallowing and may affect later speech development. The gag reflex should also be elicited and the back of the mouth, throat, tongue, and uvula visualized. The throat is palpated externally to check for the presence of an enlarged thyroid gland and to ensure the trachea is at midline. Neck rotation is assessed through inspection of head movement and with gentle passive ro-

tation by the examiner. Limitations to neck rotation may be a torticollis, which manifests as the head held to one side with the chin pointing to the other side, or a congenital defect in the cervical vertebrae. Since any limitation in neck movement has serious consequences for the infant, this must be reported immediately.

The ears are palpated to determine the thickness of the ear lobe and pinna, and irregular or unsymmetrical shapes are noted. Two common preauricular ear malformations are ear pits and ear tags. Ear pits are tiny pinholes located near the upper curved border of the pinna. These may represent a small sinus tract between the skin and underlying structures. The nurse should examine ear pits carefully to determine if there is a layer of skin covering the opening or the pit is open at its bottom. Ear pits that are draining fluid or appear to be at risk for infection require surgical repair. Preauricular skin tags are tags of

Nursing Tip *Absence of Red Reflex*

Absence of a red reflex on physical examination of a newborn infant on one or both eyes constitutes an ophthalmic emergency because of the interference with the transmission of light to the retina. Appropriate nursing and medical personnel are notified immediately: early suppression of optic nerve function from obstructed light pathways may cause blindness.

skin shaped like bulbs that project from the surface of the skin. Removal by a plastic surgeon for cosmetic purposes is recommended because these areas often contain microcapillaries that bleed when severed. Ear canals are inspected for patency and universal hearing screening is done before discharge.

Common Problems

HEENT findings that necessitate further investigation are asymmetrical, unusual, or may be indicative of defects in underlying structures or congenital syndromes. The examination findings that are the most problematic for the infant are those that are immediately visible to the nurse examiner. Down syndrome is often identified in the early newborn period during the HEENT exam by the positive physical findings of a flattened (not round) occiput; a broad nasal bridge; upward slanted eyes with epicanthal folds; low-set ears; a prominent, enlarged tongue; a high, arched palate; and a small chin. In addition, the infant may exhibit Brushfield's spots, which are whitish spots on the iris of the eye. Cleft lip and cleft palate appear as open separations of the lip, mouth, nose, and hard or soft palate and are associated with a bivalved uvula. These clefts involve facial disfigurement, and the parents and family members are sensitive to other persons observing their infant. Malformations of the ears that involve missing lobes or lack of an ear canal also increase parental sensitivity unless they are covered by the infant's hair.

A careful nursing assessment of the eyes reveals several conditions that have the potential to adversely affect the infant's condition. In the visual inspection of the eye, any deviation from the normal white color of the sclera should be noted. Sclera that appear to have a bluish color may be indicative of a congenital condition called osteogenesis imperfecta, which affects the integrity of the structure of the bones. Infants with this condition may already have fractures from the trauma of delivery and must be handled carefully. Yellowing of the sclera appears last in the progression of jaundice in the newborn infant. The yellow color should alert the nurse to increased bilirubin levels in the newborn and the possible need for immediate intervention, including intravenous fluids and phototherapy. Examination of the iris of the eye may show a disruption, called a coloboma, that looks like a keyhole in the distinct circle of the iris and pupil that will affect vision in that eye. A yellow or white shadowy covering of the iris and pupil that occludes the red reflex may be a congenital cataract, which requires immediate referral. A red reflex that appears to be white in color, called *leukocoria* or "white eye," instead of the normal red or red-orange color may be caused by a neuroblastoma, which requires immediate medical attention. Congenital glaucoma manifests as eyes that appear to be protruding slightly from the periorbital area and feel hard and firm on palpation.

This is an ophthalmic emergency because eye drops are required to decrease intraocular pressure to preserve vision.

A detailed examination of the eyes, nose, and upper lip may also reveal facial features characteristic of alcohol-related birth defects (ARBD). Short palpebral fissures, a small upturned nose, a flattened nasal bridge, and a thin upper lip with a wide, smooth philtrum are the most prominent features of ARBD (Jones, 1997). These infants demonstrate poor growth, microcephaly, small chins, and mental retardation (Taeusch & Ballard, 1998). Previously, these characteristics were referred to as fetal alcohol syndrome (FAS) or fetal alcohol effects (FAE), indicating the range of physical and mental effects that maternal alcohol consumption has on the developing fetus. The incidence of ARBD is 1 to 2 infants per 1,000 live births and it may occur with the consumption of as little as 3 ounces of alcohol per day (Taeusch & Ballard, 1998). The incidence is much higher (1 in 50 live births) in Native American populations (Abel & Sokol, 1987). After delivery, these infants may exhibit jitteriness, irritability, and poor feeding that are related to their alcohol exposure. Nursing care of these infants is directed toward comforting mechanisms and decreasing environmental stimuli that would surprise or startle an infant prone to irritability.

Nursing Implications

The examination of the head, face, eyes, ears, nose, and throat is one of the most important examinations for nursing. The infant's head and face are the only body parts that are visible to the outside world when the infant is wrapped in or covered with blankets. The parents, family visitors, and strangers form their impression of the infant by viewing the head and face. Unfortunately, many congenital defects and syndromes affect parts of the head and face. Normal variations (for example, large or protruding ears, hair color, and birth marks) that often are the result of familial inheritance are also compared to other infants. Accurate assessments of the head and face will guide the nurse to address parental concerns.

Respiratory System

The infant's respiratory efforts are first assessed visually by the nurse noting the symmetry of chest movements. At this time, the chest is also inspected for placement and size of breast tissue. Maternal hormones crossing the placenta during labor and delivery may cause an enlargement of breast tissue even in male infants. Breast tissue and nipples should be aligned with the mid-clavicular line, which is an imaginary line that is one-half the distance from midline (the sternum) to the lateral border of the chest wall formed by the rib cage. Breast tissue that is placed between the mid-clavicular line and the lateral

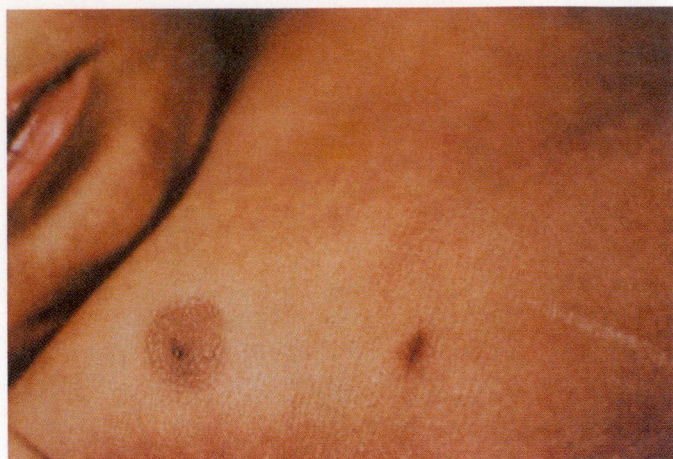

Figure 20-19   Accessory nipple *(Courtesy of Mead Johnson).*

chest wall is called "wide-spaced nipples." Wide-spaced nipples have been associated with several congenital syndromes, particularly Down syndrome. Additionally, the infant may have smaller extra nipples either above or below the primary nipples. The extra nipples, called accessory nipples, do not enlarge with puberty and may be removed at a later age for cosmetic reasons (Figure 20-19).

Common Findings

Relative ease of breathing can be determined by examining the infant lying in a supine position and observing the pattern of breathing, counting the respirations, and determining whether or not accessory muscles are needed for quiet breathing. The nurse may notice very slight sternal retractions during normal respirations in the infant. On palpation, the xiphoid process may be prominent or appear to protrude underneath the skin. Parents need reassurance that as the infant grows, this small piece of the sternum will not get bigger or pierce the skin. Infants are known to have irregular breathing rates with apneic spells that may last up to 15 seconds. Parents need to be warned by the nurse that infants do have apneic spells with normal breathing. Otherwise, they may become frightened that their infant is not breathing. Taking several respiratory rates during the physical examination may be required to get an accurate picture of the infant's respiratory effort. Count rate for a full minute to get a clear picture because of normal periodic breathing. Respiratory rates under 60 breaths per minute in a term newborn infant are considered normal. Rates between 60 and 70 breaths per minute that are not caused by crying episodes and that persist need further examination.

Common Problems

Infants who appear to have marked sternal or intercostal retractions with breathing and look like they are expend-

ing energy ("working hard to breathe") need a prompt respiratory assessment. Palpation of the anterior lung fields may reveal a birth injury, a fractured clavicle or rib, which may be causing an increased respiratory rate resulting from pain at the injury site. Rib injuries may also be visualized as asymmetrical respiratory movements of the chest wall. The shape of the chest may be inspected for deformities that might interfere with normal lung expansion. Funnel chest (pectus excavatum) and pigeon chest (pectus carinatum) result from an abnormal development of the ribs and sternum. Auscultation of all lung fields anteriorly and posteriorly can confirm the respiratory rate (instead of counting abdominal movements) as well as detect adventitious breath sounds from congestion. Upper airway congestion from mucus and residual amniotic fluid can be differentiated from lower airway congestion by auscultation of the infant's nose. Noisy breath sounds heard from the nose are usually indicators that the congestion exists in the nasal passages, throat, and upper bronchus rather than in the middle or lower lobes of the lungs. The nurse can use a bulb syringe to clear nasal and throat passages of fluid and mucus to ease breathing efforts by the infant. Retractions decrease as breathing becomes easier.

Retractions that do not disappear may be an indicator of respiratory distress in the infant. Respiratory distress is a symptom of many conditions in the newborn infant that should be investigated immediately. The infant may have a congenital respiratory condition, which is usually a narrowing of an airway; a congenital heart condition that interferes with the capacity of the lungs to supply oxygen to the blood for circulation; or an infection acquired from the mother. All of these conditions are life-threatening to the infant, and they require nursing and medical interventions.

Nursing Implications

Respiratory rates in newborns between 60 and 70 breaths per minute require continual observation by the nurse. The infant breathes faster when moving, irritated, or crying. The respiratory rate should be taken when the infant is calm or quiet. As with transient tachypnea of the newborn, a rapid respiratory rate in a quiet infant may be a temporary adjustment to extrauterine life. However, the nurse must be alert to the development of additional symptoms, that is, nasal flaring, grunting, or intercostal retractions, that would indicate the development of a more serious condition (Figure 20-20). The nurse should monitor skin color and capillary refill of both upper and lower extremities to complete the nursing assessment of the efficiency of the respiratory system. The nurse must determine whether additional symptoms indicate a condition of respiratory distress in the infant or whether the absence of additional symptoms indicates that the infant is approaching respiratory stability.

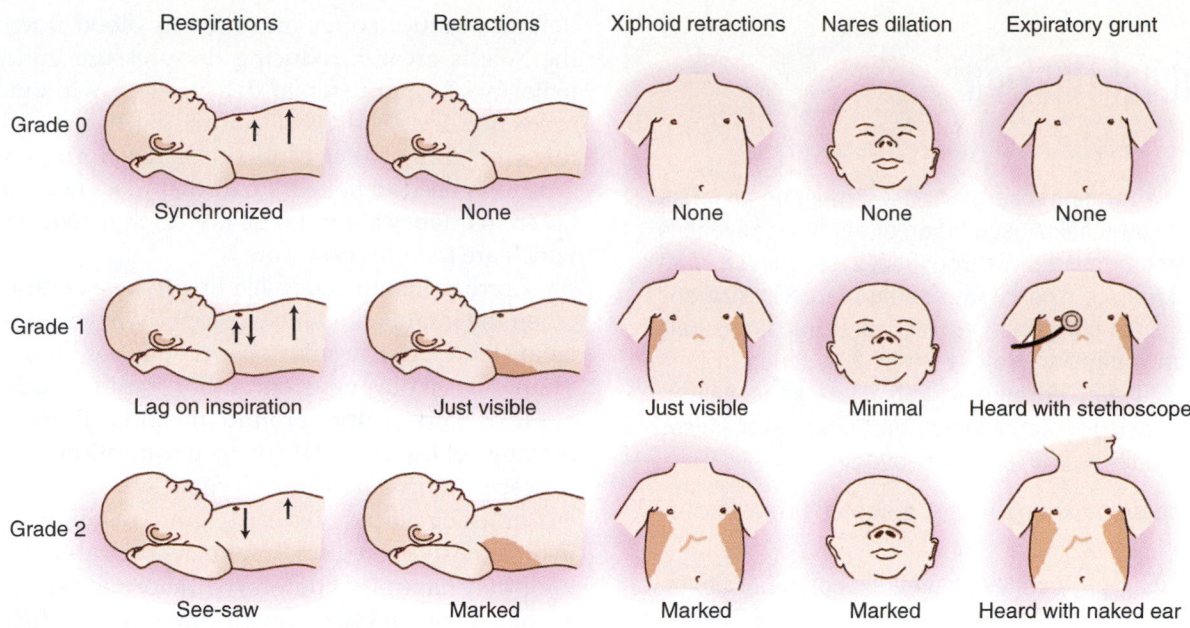

	Respirations	Retractions	Xiphoid retractions	Nares dilation	Expiratory grunt
Grade 0	Synchronized	None	None	None	None
Grade 1	Lag on inspiration	Just visible	Just visible	Minimal	Heard with stethoscope
Grade 2	See-saw	Marked	Marked	Marked	Heard with naked ear

Figure 20-20 Silverman-Anderson index of respiratory distress. *Reprinted with permission from* Pediatrics, 17, 1–10, Copyright 1956.

Cardiovascular System

The cardiovascular system is best assessed by the nurse visually and by auscultation. Visual assessment includes skin color of the trunk of the infant and the skin color of the extremities. Color should be ethnically appropriate and darken when the infant cries or moves its extremities. Visual inspection of the lips, mouth, gums, and buccal mucosa is the best indicator of cardiac perfusion. The chest is palpated for any thrills, heaves, and the point of maximum impulse (PMI). In newborns, the PMI by auscultation occurs at the apex of the heart near the third or fourth left intercostal space. Heart rate is counted for a full minute and heart rates above 160 bpm are called **tachycardia**. The heart rate normally should fall in the range of between 120 and 150 bpm. Capillary refill in fingers and toes is examined by pinching the end of the finger or toe and counting the seconds until the skin returns to its normal color. Normal refill times are less than 3 seconds. Refill times of more than 3 seconds may indicate a shunting of the circulation away from the periphery toward the trunk of the infant. All peripheral pulses are palpated for bilateral symmetry, strength, and rate. Pulses that continue to be strong and bounding as distance from the heart increases may be an indication of a cardiovascular problem. Special attention is given to femoral pulses. These are checked one at a time and compared to the brachial pulses. Any decrease in the strength of the pulse between the brachial pulses and the femoral pulses may be an indication for a cardiac condition called coarctation of the aorta. Coarctation of the aorta is a narrowing of a portion of the aortic arch. The aorta is the main transport vessel for oxygenated blood to the upper and lower portions of the body. A narrowing of the aortic arch causes diminished blood flow patterns and may be suspected in infants with diminished or decreased femoral pulses.

Common Findings

All areas of the heart, that is, the aortic, pulmonic, tricuspid, mitral, base, and apex, are examined by auscultation. Infant heart rates vary: they slow down with rest and speed up with activity or crying. Term infants usually maintain a heart rate of between 110 and 160 bpm; rates lower than 100 bpm indicate bradycardia and rates higher than 160 bpm are considered to be tachycardia (Seidel et al., 2001). Either persistent bradycardia or tachycardia must be reported to the nursing staff responsible for the infant. Initially, infant heart rates are difficult to hear. The chest wall in infancy is thin and heart sound transmission has a tendency to be noisy and obscured by the infants' respirations. Patience and continued listening by the nurse are often necessary to determine the heart rate as well as any extra sounds or murmurs. Murmurs are often heard in newborns less than 24 hours old near the sternal border at the level of the left second or third intercostal space. An increasing amount of sound (crescendo) occurring through systole is the usual sound pattern heard. The sound from an infant with **patent ductus arteriosus (PDA)** will gradually disappear when the ductus closes, within 2 to 3 days. Murmurs that persist beyond the second day of life and whose sound has changed to a more definitive whoosh pattern are not characteristic of an open ductus and require a cardiac evaluation.

Critical Thinking

The Newborn after Transition

You are performing a cardiac assessment on an infant who is 8 hours old. Auscultation of the heart reveals a soft heart murmur heard throughout systole and a heart rate of 170 bpm. The infant appears large in size and has no visible congenital anomalies. Skin color is pale pink with a capillary refill time of 3 seconds in both upper and lower extremities. Pulses are equal bilaterally, rhythm is regular, and you note that pedal pulses are especially strong, close to bounding.

- What do bounding pulses mean in a newborn infant?
- Are your physical exam findings normal or abnormal at this time?
- Which is the best nursing action to take next?
  1. Continue observation of this infant and repeat your assessment in 30 minutes.
  2. Ask a nursing colleague to verify your physical examination findings before the shift is over.
  3. Report your findings to the medical staff immediately.
  4. Repeat your assessment to confirm your findings.

The best response is 3. Bounding pedal pulses, a heart rate increased above normal, and a soft systolic murmur indicate increased cardiac contractility in the presence of blood backflow through fetal shunts. This "increased workload" for the heart may lead to cardiac failure if not evaluated immediately. While confirmation of findings may be an appropriate action, examination findings can always be confirmed by the medical staff on duty. The nurse must learn to trust her own assessment skills and judgment in patient care situations that require immediate decisions. Signs of cardiac failure in newborns infants may be very subtle at first, and the nurse must be alert to any cardiac findings that are questionable.

Common Problems

The most common heart murmur in infancy is the ventricular septal defect (VSD) in which there is a small hole in the wall of the ventricle between the right and left chambers of the heart. The sound of the murmur is created by the heart pumping blood and the blood leaking through this hole. Small defects produce louder murmurs because of the buildup in pressure in the chambers from the blood leaking through with each contraction. Large defects produce softer murmurs as blood flow through the hole is greater, reducing the pressure buildup. The majority of ventral septal defects close without surgical correction as a result of the normal cardiac growth during the first year of life. Mothers of newborns with heart murmurs need to be reassured that most heart murmurs noted in infancy are not fatal nor do they require surgery, which are their biggest fears.

Cardiac insufficiency, leading to heart failure, occurs when the infant is unable to properly oxygenate and circulate blood. Nurses may suspect this condition in irritable infants with persistent pallor, rapid breathing, and **cyanosis** (blue color) around the lips. Pulse oximetry readings of less than 94% oxygen saturation are cause for concern. An infant whose oxygen saturation falls below 90% must be placed on a cardiac and respiratory monitor in an intensive care unit. Infants who exhibit these symptoms may have heart defects with normal heart functions as long as the ductus remains open. As the ductus starts to close on day 2 or 3 of life, their cardiac condition becomes unstable and compromised. In these infants, a murmur develops on day 2 of life, which is the first indication of a cardiac problem. Infants who develop cardiac instability within the first 2 days of life are those infants who have a genetic karyotype of trisomy 13, 18, or 21 or tetralogy of Fallot. Tetralogy of Fallot consists of four specific cardiac anomalies: transposition of the aorta and pulmonary artery, right ventricular hypertrophy, pulmonary stenosis, and ventricular septal defect (Taeusch and Ballard, 1998). Newborns with tetralogy of Fallot are stable after birth, have no murmurs on auscultation, and maintain cardiac perfusion as long as their ductus arteriosus remains open. Medical and nursing staff refer to these infants as "pink tets." When the ductus begins to close after 24 hours of life, severe cardiac instability occurs, with the development of central cyanosis. These infants are placed on a cardiac monitor in an intensive care unit, receive intravenous fluids with medication to preserve cardiac output, and undergo a full cardiac and surgical evaluation.

Nursing Implications

The accurate assessment of the heart and cardiovascular system in a newborn is necessary for the determination of present and future cardiac stability of the infant. Nurses who examine newborns develop the knowledge and expertise to detect cardiac conditions often before the medical staff is aware of them. Nurses are also the key personnel that parents and family members contact who have concerns about the health of their infant. Cardiac problems in infancy cause severe anxiety in both parents. The major role of nurses beyond the cardiac assessment of newborns is to develop skills in communication to convey to parents and other family members the nature of the

Critical Thinking

Newborn Heart Defect: What Do You Say?

You are reading an infant's chart and discover that the health care provider suspects a cardiac defect, has ordered an ECG, and has called a pediatric cardiologist to examine the infant. When you bring the infant to the mother, she tells you that she feels great, is ready to go home, and has called the father of the baby to come pick them up.

- What would you say to this mother?
- What might you say to the physician?

Reflections from a Nurse

It was late in my shift and I was rushing to deliver a newborn to the mother before shift change. The mother had indicated in the chart that she wanted to breastfeed her infant, and I was determined to get her baby to her to make that happen before the next shift came on duty. As I brought the baby to her bedside, the mother greeted me and told me she was so glad I was there, and she had been waiting for me to come. I was so surprised. She told me that I had taken care of her first baby who had something wrong with his heart. She said that she will always remember me sitting down with her and explaining to her about the heart, and how it worked. "I've kept the drawing you gave me all these years," she said. "I've had all my babies at this hospital because I wanted you to take care of them," she continued. I left her room with a big smile on my face. I never realized how much talking to mothers about their babies really meant to them.

problem, the steps being taken, and the health and welfare of their infant.

Abdomen

The abdomen of a newborn infant in the supine position appears round, full, and bilaterally symmetrical. The umbilical cord should be clamped securely with no oozing of blood or it will need to be reclamped. The cord should be examined for the presence of three vessels, two arteries, and one vein. The arteries are smaller than the vein. Umbilical cords with fewer than three vessels should be reported to the charge nurse and medical staff. Large cords that have thickened areas of gelatinous material are referred to as having Wharton's jelly. Infants' abdomens may look distended from the presence of stool that has not yet been eliminated. After inspection of the relative size and shape of the abdomen, and watching abdominal breathing patterns, auscultation for bowel sounds in all four quadrants is begun. Several areas in each quadrant are assessed, because bowel obstruction in the newborn may present initially as a lack of bowel sounds in a small area of the bowel. Auscultation for the gastric bubble and the heart sounds of the abdominal aorta completes this part of the examination.

Common Findings

Light and deep palpation of the abdomen allows the nurse the opportunity to assess the integrity of the abdominal contents of the infant. Light palpation begins with the end of the sternum and the xiphoid process, proceeding midline to the seat of the umbilicus on the abdomen. As palpation proceeds along the midline, a diastasis rectus, or a thinning of the abdominal wall along the midline may be palpated. A diastasis rectus can also be visualized as a "furrow" formation, or elongated lump, at midline when

the infant is crying. Last, the circumference of the umbilicus can be palpated for hernias. The umbilical cord should be firmly seated in the abdominal wall, but there may be a separation between the cord and the abdominal wall, called a hernia. Hernias are measured by fingertips to determine if they are large or small. Umbilical hernias are common in newborn infants, and small ones often close on their own when infants grow larger. Palpation is continued along the midline below the umbilicus to the symphysis pubis. Some umbilical hernias extend inferiorly and the size of the hernia may be misjudged.

Light palpation of the abdomen continues from midline to the costal margins (rib cage) to determine the presence of masses or enlarged organs. The small size of the newborn abdomen facilitates this examination as a result of the lack of space for enlarged organs or extra material (tumors or masses). Deep palpation is used to outline specific organs and their borders. The liver border, felt just below the right costal margin should be smooth and firm and not extend more than 2 cm below this margin. The spleen, tucked underneath the left costal margin, is only palpable at the tip of the organ, 1 cm below the costal margin. Positive palpation findings on a newborn's spleen are a cause for concern because organ enlargement must be present for the spleen to be palpated beyond its tip. Kidneys may be palpated at a right angle to the umbilicus at midline, located 1 to 2 cm above the umbilicus. However, they may be missed because of their small size. The bladder wall should be smooth and can be palpated at midline, inferior to the umbilicus.

Common Problems

Assessment findings that indicate a serious abdominal condition in the newborn are abdominal distention, absent bowel sounds, discharge from the umbilical cord or site, and palpation of an abdominal mass. Abdominal distention may appear to involve the entire abdominal surface or small areas of bulging. The nurse may notice enlarged abdominal veins in a distended abdomen. Light and deep palpation may reveal stool in the colon, which is not cause for alarm. Areas of abdominal bulging that shift when the infant is moved in the supine position may indicate the presence of fluid in the abdomen. Light pressure on the abdomen below the costal margin may generate a fluid wave to the opposite costal margin. This requires immediate attention by the medical staff to determine the source of the fluid in the abdomen.

Auscultatory sounds that are diminished or absent in the abdomen are indicators of potential circulatory problems. Auscultation of the abdominal aorta at midline above the umbilicus gives the listener an impression of circulation to the abdominal organs and lower extremities. Diminished sounds may indicate decreased circulatory efforts, as in coarctation of the aorta. Decreased blood flow would affect the kidney's ability to filter blood and form urine, and the bowel's ability to digest nutrients and undergo peristalsis. Absent bowel sounds in an area of the abdomen would indicate a portion of the bowel that is not functioning and requires immediate attention. Necrotizing enterocolitis is a severe abdominal condition of newborns, resulting from inadequate circulation to the bowel, the destruction of the intestinal mucosa, and complete loss of bowel function. Loss of bowel function leads to intestinal obstruction and secretion of toxins from tissue that has been destroyed. This condition is life-threatening and requires immediate surgical intervention.

Inspection of the umbilicus and umbilical cord for discharge or leakage is done to detect signs of infection. Umbilical cords that have not been stained with the bacteriostatic dye are pale yellow. Green staining of umbilical cords occurs when the infant has passed meconium before delivery. The base of the umbilical cord should be clean and dry with no discharge or leakage of blood. The presence of a discharge must be reported immediately because it is an indicator of infection. Stool and urine from the diaper area should not leak out of the diaper and be in contact with the cord or the base of the cord. When this occurs, careful cleansing is required. An extra cord clamp can be applied if there is a blood leak. The abdominal wall surrounding the seat of the cord is inspected for redness. A circular area of redness around the base of the cord on the abdomen is a symptom of omphalitis, an infection of the base of the cord that requires antibiotic therapy.

Palpation of an abdominal mass or an enlarged abdominal organ in the newborn is facilitated by the infant's usually small abdominal girth. Masses or enlarged organs require immediate attention and investigation. The mass can be confirmed by an ultrasound examination, and medical management can be instituted at this time. In the newborn period, abdominal masses are usually a form of neuroblastoma, and the cause can be confirmed by biopsy. The most common enlarged abdominal organs are the liver, spleen, and kidneys. These findings can also be confirmed by ultrasound examination. The organs may be enlarged from an associated obstructive process or congenital malformation.

Nursing Implications

In addition to the cardiac and respiratory assessment, the assessment of the abdomen is vitally important in the newborn as the site of digestion and the beginning processes of elimination. The nurse develops auscultation and palpation skills to ensure the integrity of the abdominal organs and to detect any causes for concern. The nurse can anticipate the parental expectation that a round, full "tummy" on their baby indicates a healthy baby, and teach the parents the signs and symptoms of abnormal conditions of the abdomen.

Genitalia and Anus

Both male and female genitalia are visualized and assessed with the infant in the supine position with its hips abducted. The scrotum of male infants in this position can be determined to be pendulous with descended testes. Flattened or depressed areas of the scrotal sac may indicate that a testis that has not descended. Testes are pal-

---

Nursing Alert

Distended Abdomen

The essential tool for nursing assessment of the distended abdomen in a newborn is palpation. Abdomens that are distended can be palpated easily; they feel soft and pliable. A distended abdomen that the nurse is unable to palpate because of the rigidity of the abdominal wall is a medical emergency. This condition is often referred to as "acute abdomen," and the infant is often inconsolable.

pated in the scrotal sac by placing the nurse's second finger at the posterior midline of the scrotum and the thumb on the anterior midline. The index finger and thumb can easily palpate the left side of the scrotum for the presence of a testis, and the third finger and the thumb can likewise palpate for a testis on the right scrotum. Palpation in this manner ensures that one testis is not mistaken for two by being passed from side to side. This technique also allows for gently stroking of the inguinal canal with the respective finger and thumb if a testis is not felt in the scrotal sac. The nurse can bathe the inguinal canal with warm soapy water when a testis cannot be located. Warm water has a tendency to make a testis "pop up" in the canal and become more visible. One or both undescended testes that cannot be located in the inguinal canal in an infant older than 35 weeks' gestational age is an indication for a urologic evaluation of the infant.

Female genitalia are inspected with the hips of the infant abducted while lying in a supine position. The labia majora are visualized first and the extent to which they cover the remaining tissues of the female genitalia indicates the maturity of the infant. In most female infants at term, the borders of the labia majora meet and the clitoris is covered completely. In some term infants, the development of the genitalia may lag behind other systems and the nurse may see the labia minora and the clitoris uncovered.

Inspection of the anus and palpation of the anal opening occurs at the same time as the genitalia are assessed. Hopefully, the infant will have a stool during the nurse's examination, so that the nurse can validate that the anus is patent and that the stool does, indeed, come out of one and only one anal opening. Stool appearing in a female infant from the vaginal opening results from a rectovaginal fistula, an opening between the rectum and the vagina. The anus is palpated by spreading the tissue around the anal opening and feeling the musculature around the opening. At this time, any rectal tears from the passage of stool in the anal ring may be noted and the **anal wink reflex** elicited. While the infant is in the prone position, the buttocks are stroked from side to side with the index finger of the nurse. The buttocks draw together and "wink" at the point of the anal opening, validating the anatomic position. This reflex is used to evaluate anal openings in females that are closer than 1 cm from the vaginal opening. Anal openings too close to vaginal openings do not develop the appropriate muscle strength needed to assist in evacuating the rectum as the infant grows older. The "wink" reflex indicates where the normal anal opening should be positioned for future surgical correction.

Common Findings

In male infants, the nurse may discover that palpation of the scrotum for testes is impossible because the scrotal sac is swollen and distended, preventing accurate palpation. Fluid accumulation in the scrotal sac causes this and can be verified by transillumination of the scrotum. However, the nurse must first verify that the enlarged scrotum does not contain trapped bowel. Careful auscultation of the scrotum for bowel sounds will confirm this condition. If bowel sounds are present, it must be reported and confirmed immediately because this a medical emergency for the infant. If bowel sounds are not present, the nurse can then proceed with transillumination of the scrotum. A penlight or an ophthalmoscope is used as the light source pressed against the scrotum to transilluminate it in a darkened room. Fluid appears as a yellow-orange reflection and, occasionally, a small, dark, round testis can be seen. The nurse must note that a scrotal or testicular mass does not transilluminate and report it immediately. Fluid in the scrotal sac is gradually reabsorbed over the infant's first several weeks of life, and the mother can be reassured that the scrotum will eventually have a more normal size and appearance.

Palpation continues in male infants to include the shaft of the penis in order to estimate penile length. Normal male infants are born at term with a penis that measures about 2 cm. The foreskin (prepuce) is lightly retracted to inspect the urethral opening and the location of the opening on the glans. The nurse may notice a cheesy coating, called *smegma*, of the glans underneath the foreskin.

Many female infants have a white, thick cheesy substance, called vernix caseosa, between the labia; this is not a cause for concern. A small, triangular-shaped piece of tissue may be visualized between the labia. This is a *hymenal tag* and decreases in size as the infant grows larger. Gentle palpation of the labia majora and labia minora allows for visualization of the hymenal area. It is not unusual at this time to see a white mucoid discharge in the vaginal area as well as a small amount of blood. Maternal hormones crossing the placenta create this discharge and bleeding that mimics a period in female infants. This is normal, and parents need to know how to clean the genitalia of their infants and not to be frightened when they see small amounts of blood. It usually takes about a week for a female infant to eliminate the influence of maternal hormones. Females may also have a smegma discharge between the labia.

Common Problems

The nursing assessment of the male genitalia is focused on the determination of whether they are normal. Swelling or edema from the delivery process may impede this assessment. Bruising of the scrotum can occur with breech presentations, and palpation must be done carefully. Infants of color, particularly Black infants, have dark-skinned scrotums. Examination of the scrotal sac should reveal two testes. Undescended testes may be located in the inguinal canal and become problematic when they do not descend into the scrotal sac. Inguinal hernias are difficult to palpate in infancy. They are usually discovered when a loop of the infant's bowel becomes trapped in the scrotal sac. The scrotum enlarges, does not transilluminate, and exhibits characteristic bowel sounds when auscultated. This condition must be reported immediately, because surgical repair is necessary to save the bowel. A darkened area of the scrotum surrounding one testis with edema may be testicular torsion, in which the spermatic cord and tunica vaginalis twist before attachment of the tunica vaginalis to the scrotum (Juretschke, 2000). This condition in infancy is extremely rare, carries a high risk of testicular loss, and requires immediate surgical intervention (Juretschke, 2000).

Inspection and palpation of the penis determines penile length and completes the assessment of normal male genitalia. A penis less than 2 cm long indicates *micropenis* and may be associated with a pituitary tumor or insufficiency. Structures that resemble a penis in a female or ridges that mimic labia on a male require immediate investigation as ambiguous genitalia. In cases in which definite genitalia of either sex cannot be determined, genetic studies are performed in addition to testing for adrenal insufficiencies. Labeling of the infant as a "boy" or a "girl" prematurely leads the parents to treat the infant according to the label already given, which may be contrary to the genetic evidence.

The two most prominent concerns in the assessment of the female genitalia are an enlarged clitoral hood and imperforate hymen. Hormones crossing the placenta may cause the clitoris to be slightly enlarged. A large clitoris that appears hood-shaped and elongated, resembling a penis, may be the result of excess androgen stimulation. This is one symptom of congenital adrenal hyperplasia. Tests for precursors of adrenal corticosteroids and electrolytes for normal kidney function need to be initiated immediately. Edema from the birthing process may interfere with the examination of the labia majora and labia minora. Careful separation of the labia should reveal the urethral opening and an intact vaginal introitus. An imperforate hymen is a muscle wall that obstructs the vagi-

nal opening. This condition will need surgical correction for future release of menses during normal menstrual cycles.

Inspection of the anal opening in both male and female newborns may reveal skin tags on the anal ring or an anal ring without an opening. The skin tags or other hemorrhoid-like tissues may cause discomfort or bleeding in the diaper when the infant is stooling. The lack of either an anal ring or an opening in the anal ring is a condition called **imperforate anus**. This condition in the newborn is a surgical emergency because the newborn is unable to evacuate stool from the rectum. In 50% of newborns who have imperforate anus, this condition occurs as an isolated event and is not associated with other congenital malformations or syndromes (Taeusch & Ballard, 1998). A common congenital syndrome associated with anal malformations is VATER association. Three or more of the major abnormalities must be present to make the diagnosis, and prognosis for normal development is enhanced after surgical correction (Taeusch & Ballard, 1998). Characteristics of VATER association in the newborn include:

V = vertebral abnormalities

A = anal abnormalities (imperforate anus)

T = tracheal abnormalities

E = esophageal abnormalities (tracheoesophageal fistulas)

R = renal and radial abnormalities

Nursing care of newborns with VATER association is directed toward proper newborn positioning for arm and spinal defects as well as promotion of breathing effort through a partially compromised trachea. Additional nursing efforts to ensure nutritional intake and elimination are emphasized.

Nursing Implications

Nursing assessment of the genitalia of newborns forms the basis for parental interaction with the infant. The determination of sex is done briefly by inspection only in the delivery room and communicated to the parents. A detailed inspection and further examination is the responsibility of the nurse in charge of the newborn's care. Parents want to see that their infant is normal and looks normal. Any observed difference increases their anxiety. The nurse must have the sensitivity to address these issues with the parents and be prepared to correct misinformation that would affect the parents' ability to interact with their infant in a positive manner.

Circumcision of Male Infants

Circumcision of male infants is usually performed in the nursery and is the personal choice of parents based on their cultural, ethnic, and religious perspectives. Circum-

---

Nursing Tip   *Blood in the Diaper*

Blood in the diaper of a newborn can be a concern for the nurse and frightening for the parents. The location of the blood can indicate the source of the bleeding. Blood that appears near the top of the diaper is most likely oozing from the umbilical cord. Blood that appears in the middle of the diaper in female infants is most likely bleeding that mimics a period from maternal hormones. Blood in the middle of a diaper on a male infant may be the result of a urine stream through a bruised penis from delivery or indicate a more serious problem to be investigated.

Critical Thinking

Ambiguous Genitalia

You are the nurse taking care of twins in the nursery. The twins are the fifth and sixth children of a young couple who desperately wanted to have a boy, since all their previous children were girls. The twins were born weighing 2,200 g and 2,250 g and appear to be normal boys. They have been in the nursery for the last 3 weeks, steadily gaining weight before discharge. As you read through the chart, you notice that one of the nurses palpated a high-arched palate on one twin and described a low-set ear. The medical team ordered chromosomal studies, which were reported last week. There was no evidence of trisomy; however, both of the twins had female karyotypes. Abdominal ultrasound tests revealed the presence of ovaries and a uterus in both infants. Nursing staff conversations with the parents revealed their intentions to raise the infants as boys. What is the best approach for you to take when you talk with the parents today?

- Do you think that the parents are ignoring the test results?
- Do you think the parents will ever accept the test results?
- Which of the following do you think is the best response?

   1. "Do you have any questions for me about the care of your babies?"

   2. "I would like to talk with you about the test results and what they mean for your babies."

   3. "I have made an appointment for you to see the genetics counselor this afternoon about your babies."

   4. "I have asked the genetics counselor to meet with us and help me talk to you about your babies."

The best response is 4. The first response ignores the issue. The second response is repeating the same information the parents have heard before. They are not ready to listen to or hear what the test results mean. The third response takes control away from the parents and places them in a situation that they did not request. The fourth response offers the parents an opportunity to express their feelings and identifies any misunderstandings that they might have.

cisions for religious purposes may be performed at another site, and elective circumcisions during the first 2 weeks of life may be performed in a private office or clinic. This is a decision the parents make and parents need good information to make an informed choice. Risks for the infant include infection, hemorrhage, skin dehiscence, adhesions, urethral fistula, and pain (Hockenberry et al., 2003). Some health care providers may provide anesthetics during the procedure. Benefits to the infant are decreased incidence of urinary tract infections in the first 3 months of life (Schoen, Colby, & Ray, 2000) and possible prevention of penile cancer (Hockenberry et al., 2003). In the circumcision procedure, part of the foreskin is removed by clamping and cutting with a scalpel (Gomco or Mogen clamp) or using a plastic ring with a string tied around it to trim off the excess foreskin (Plastibell). Small sutures or pressure from the plastic ring are used to prevent bleeding and promote wound closure.

Nursing care of the circumcised infant is directed toward providing pain relief before the procedure; comfort before, during, and after the procedure; and skilled observation for bleeding or voiding difficulties. Some infants may not express pain by crying yet still experience pain. It is the responsibility of the nurse to examine the equipment before the procedure for cleanliness and matching parts. Substitute parts that are not made by the same manufacturer may slip and cause the infant additional discomfort. For at least 2 hours before the procedure, the infant is given nothing by mouth to prevent vomiting or aspiration. Pain relief measures to be considered are: a local dorsal penile nerve block; application of EMLA cream (lidocaine) (topical mixture of anesthetics), approximately 1 to 2 g, for 60 minutes before the procedure under an occlusive dressing; and a ring block. EMLA cream is used as a topical anesthetic without nerve blocks and also used with nerve blocks to anesthetize the site of injection. Proper pain relief requires that the cream be applied for at least 1 hour prior to the procedure and the application site varies with the nerve block used. The cream is applied to the foreskin and base of the penis for the dorsal penile nerve block and the foreskin and shaft of the penis for the ring block. The cream should be replaced if the infant urinates during the topical anesthetic period. The penis and scrotum are gently cleaned with a mild soap and warm water and dried. The cream is reapplied to the area required for anesthesia.

The infant is gently restrained during the circumcision procedure on a special board or apparatus with Velcro straps that limit extremity movement near the operative field (see the following circumcision story). The nurse may consider shielding the infants' eyes from the lights, playing soothing music in the background, or

A Circumcision Story

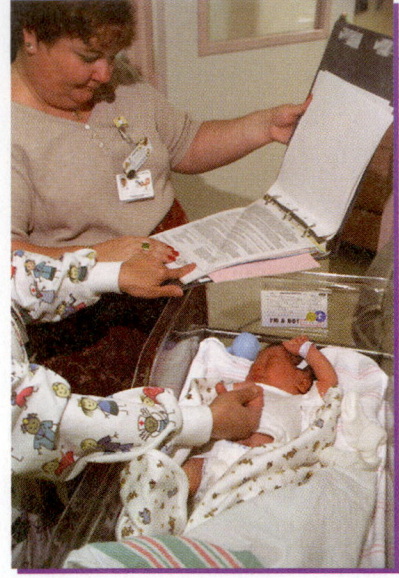

*T*he nurse checks the infant's identification band against the signed consent form.

A circumcision restraint board safely immobilizes the infant during the procedure.

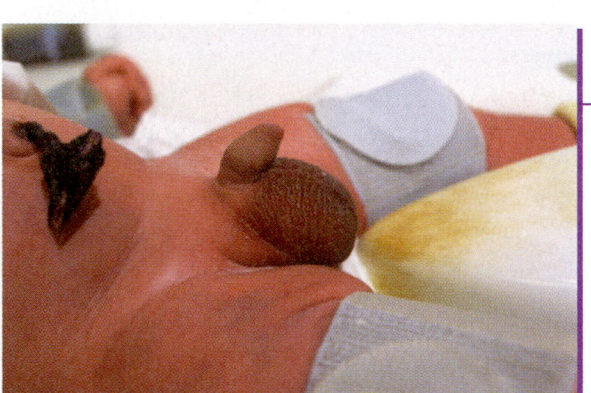

The uncircumcised penis and genital area are exposed.

The physician dons sterile gloves.

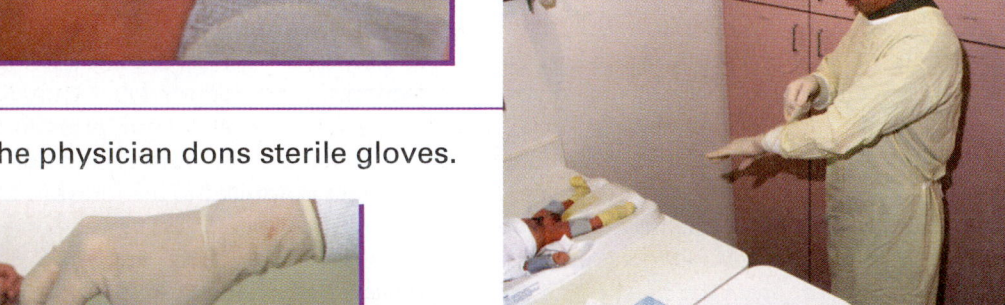

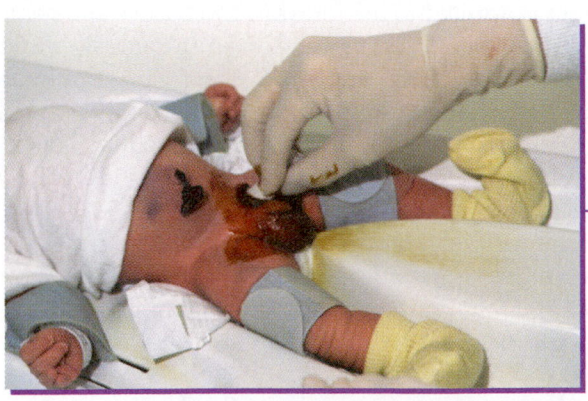

Antiseptic solution is applied to reduce the risk of infection.

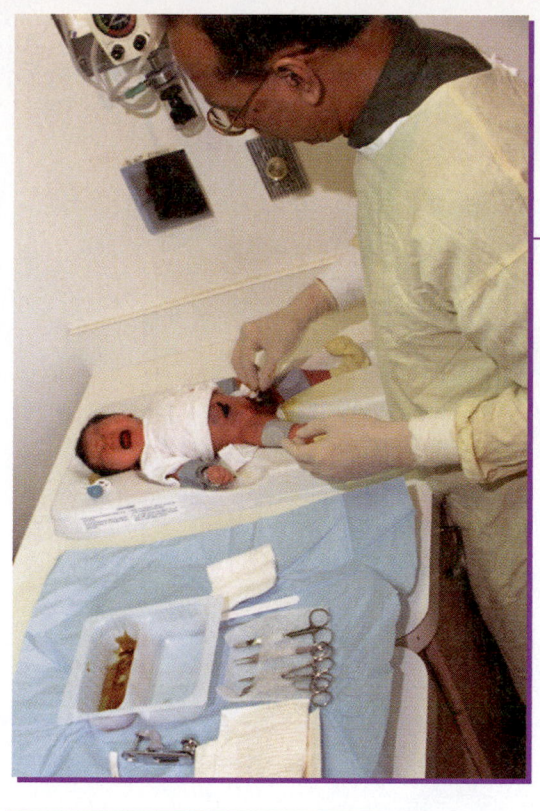

This baby is expressing his opinion of the procedure.

Infants are often offered a pacifier or other soothing measure to help calm them during the procedure.

A sterile drape is applied to provide a sterile field.

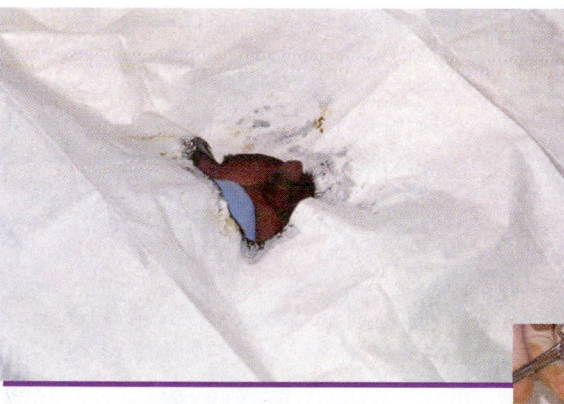

Kelley clamps are used to extend the prepuce.

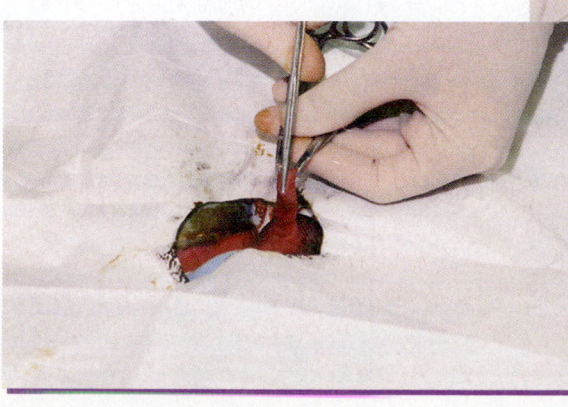

A small incision is made in the prepuce.

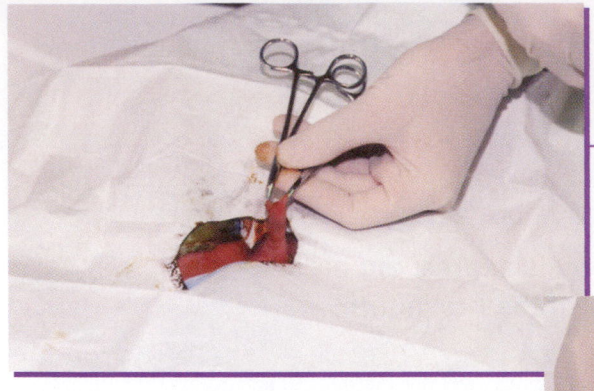

The incision will help accommodate use of the circumcision cone.

The clamps are left in place as the prepuce is retracted over the glans.

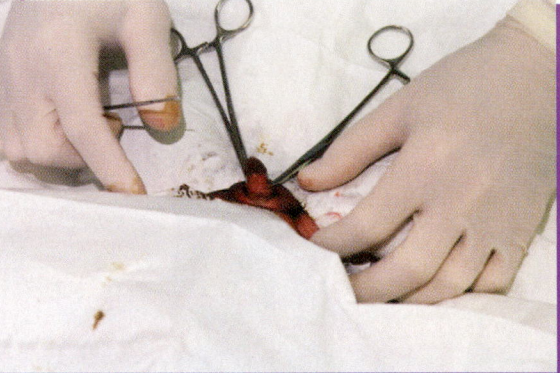

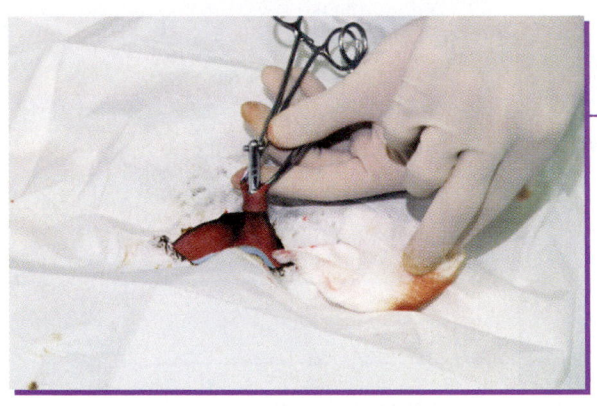

A circumcision cone is placed over the exposed glans penis and the prepuce is drawn up around it.

The clamp is applied and tightened for 3–5 minutes to reduce bleeding and circulation in the prepuce.

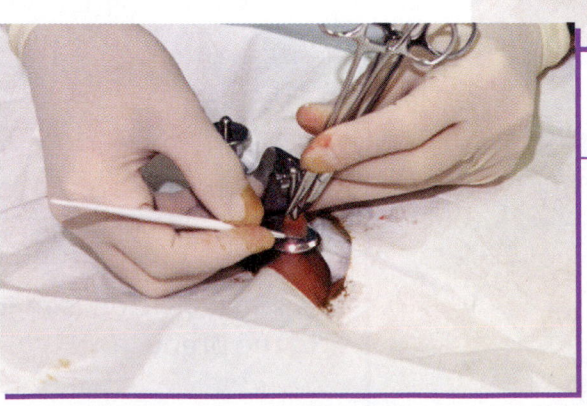

The prepuce is cut away at its base.

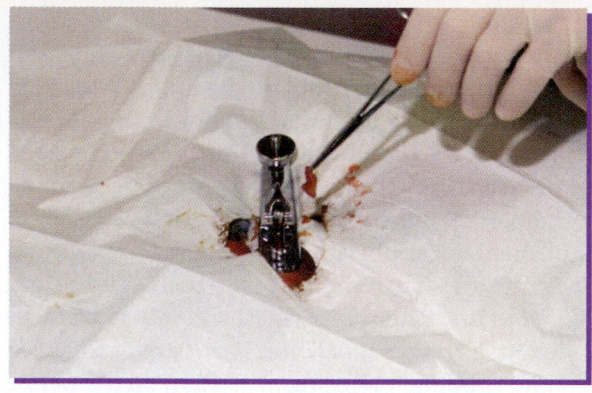

The prepuce is completely removed.

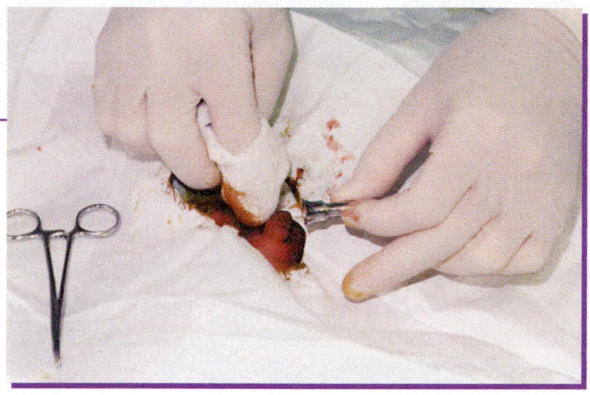

After removal of the cone, the newly exposed glans penis is gently swabbed with sterile gauze.

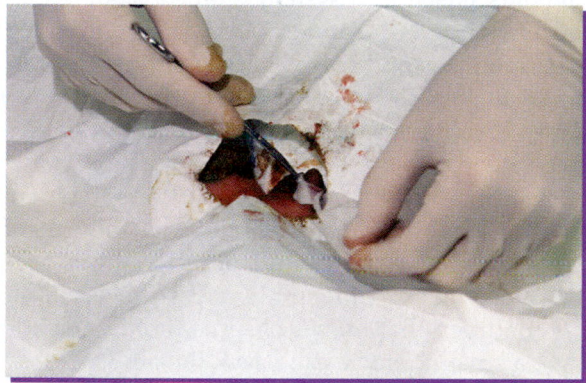

Sterile dressing is carefully applied to protect the circumcision area.

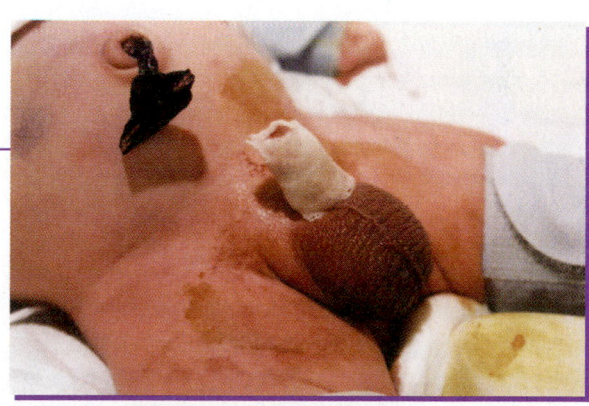

The newly circumcised penis will be completely healed within about a week.

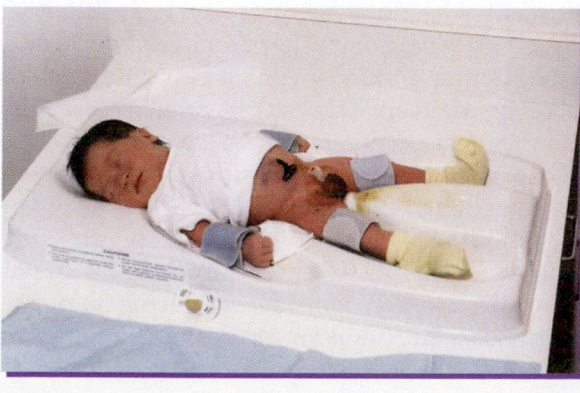

The infant rests following the procedure.

stroking the infant's head, shoulders, or upper extremities during the procedure. Pacifiers soaked in a sugar-water solution (dissolve 1 tablespoon sugar in 4 tablespoons of sterile water) have been shown to be effective in distracting infants from the procedure (Hockenberry et al., 2003).

Client Education

Circumcision Care

The nurse instructs the parents to carefully apply and remove the diaper over the circumcision site to prevent rubbing. During the first 24 hours, it is recommended that the site be checked by the parents or the nurse every 30 minutes for the first 2 hours and then every 2 hours afterward (Williamson, 1997). The site is checked for excess bleeding or swelling, and the diaper can be felt for dampness to indicate the infant has urinated. The infant must demonstrate an ability to void after the procedure, because edema at the operative site may block off the urethra or the urethral meatus. Dressings, if present, are changed at least three times in the first 24 hours. The old dressing is removed; the area gently wiped clean with a warm, damp gauze and dried; and a fresh dressing with jelly or ointment applied. In some institutions, infant acetaminophen (Tylenol) drops can be given every 4 to 6 hours for the first day after the procedure. They are discontinued when the parents feel that their infant is no longer displaying signs of discomfort, pain, or irritability. On the second day, a yellowish exudate appears, which is part of the healing process. The nurse instructs the parents not to remove this or disrupt it when cleansing during the dressing change. Dressing changes are continued for 3 days after the procedure. If the parents do not notice any swelling, discharge, bleeding, or reddening of the penis, they may discontinue dressing changes but need to watch the area very closely for the next week. The parents may want to change the infants' diapers more frequently to avoid the healing penis being exposed to stool in the diaper. The nurse emphasizes that discharge, swelling, or redness indicates signs of infection. Parents who report less than six diaper changes a day need to be concerned that their infant is having difficulty voiding after circumcision. Signs of infection, failure to void adequately, or excessive bleeding from the operative site must be reported immediately to their health care provider.

Once the procedure is complete, the infant is released from the restraints and comforted by the nurse, if the parents are not present. The infant is brought to the parents as soon as possible after the procedure. The choice of dressings or treatments of the circumcision site depends on the method of circumcision. Petroleum jelly (Vaseline) or A & D ointment is applied with 4×4 gauze as a dressing to cover the site when a clamp has been used to cut the foreskin. No dressings are needed when the Plastibell is used. The nurse applies the diaper loosely over this area to prevent any rubbing, pressure, or friction on the penis. When the infant is brought to the parents, the nurse explains the procedure, allows the parents to inspect the circumcision site, addresses their concerns, and instructs both parents on circumcision care. If the infant is uncircumcised, the penis should be kept clean and parents advised to *not* retract the foreskin.

Musculoskeletal System

The musculoskeletal system is on constant display when the infant is moving and exploring its environment. From extending legs and kicking to extending arms and sucking on fingers, the infant is discovering that he or she can move. Visual inspection of the infant reveals any movements that are compromised by injury or birth trauma. Stretching of the extremities often leads the infant to extend the toes and fingers: this confirms movement for the examiner. The nurse carefully observes the extremities for differences in size or length. Achondroplasia is a congenital condition that nurses observe first in newborns who have a small thoracic cage, lack the ability for elbow extension, and appear to have shortening of the humerus and femur (Jones, 1997). These infants are often referred to as dwarfs and have respiratory and neurologic problems in addition to their skeletal anomalies.

Watching the infant move in the supine position and then changing the infant to the prone position gives the nurse a good indication of muscle strength and tone. Failure to move the lower extremities may suggest a lesion or damage to the spinal cord. Asymmetrical movement may indicate nerve damage or a fracture from birth trauma. A newborn infant who does not move or feels "floppy" when turned over may have hypotonia, or decreased muscle tone, from a period of anoxia either in utero or during labor and delivery. Hypertonia, or increased muscle tone, in the presence of small, brief tremors, twitches, or myoclonic jerks, is a characteristic of neonatal abstinence syndrome (Hockenberry et al., 2003). The newborn expresses withdrawal symptoms of drug exposure through these movements. The nurse, through careful inspection and observation, can identify elements of the musculoskeletal examination for further evaluation.

Common Findings

After inspection, palpation of the musculoskeletal system begins with the shoulders and moves inferiorly to the feet. Muscles and bones are palpated for symmetry and amount of tissue present. Joint rotations are checked by gentle passive range of motion. Neck rotation is the first and most important motion to be examined. Infants must exhibit full neck rotation passively. Neck rotation may be hindered by torticollis, in which the head is held to one side with the chin pointing to the other side, or by congenitally missing portions of a cervical vertebra. As infants grow and develop, they turn their head to discover the location of sound and begin "tracking" the sound with their eyes. Proper neck rotation assists in the refinement of hearing and in the development of sight. Head lag is assessed by gently pulling the infant up and watching the head gently fall back as it clears the surface of the crib. In this position, the nurse can also inspect the neck to make sure that there is no thyroid bulge. This maneuver also assists the nurse in evaluating upper body muscle tone and strength in the arms and shoulders.

The second most important joint to assess in newborns is the hip joint. Developmental dysplasia of the hip (DDH) can easily be missed in a newborn and, if not treated, can go on to interfere with the infant's future ability to retain balance and walk. Hips are evaluated by inspection of skin folds on the thighs in the supine and the prone positions. Asymmetrical skin folds may indicate a hip problem. Leg length and knee height are also inspected for unevenness. Palpation of the hips begins with the nurse gently moving the lower extremities in a kicking motion in order to ease the infant's distress during the hip evaluation. The nurse places her hands on the infant's thigh with the tips of her fingers encircling the head of the femur and her thumb and index finger securing the knee joint. From this position, the Barlow maneuver exerts a downward pressure on the head of the femur in an attempt to dislodge the head of the femur from the acetabulum. The Ortolani maneuver is either a circular rotation of the femoral head or an inward-outward motion that attempts to "relocate" the head of the femur displaced by the Barlow maneuver in the acetabulum. Normal hip joints are moved easily and the nurse may feel crepitus or a slight grinding (a hip click) as the head of the femur is manipulated in the socket. Hip dysplasia is very common in infants who had in breech position in utero or breech deliveries. It is confirmed by the inability to move the leg easily in the hip joint and by feeling the head of the femur come out of the hip socket (a hip "clunk"). Many infants who had breech presentations have hyperextended knee joints that give the appearance of hip dysplasia but, on examination, the head of the femur remains firmly in the socket of the acetabulum. These leg positions gradually return to normal flexed positions. The nurse may examine the infant's hips and feel looseness in the hip joint even when the femoral head remains secure in the joint. Maternal hormones during pregnancy and delivery not only cause joint laxity in mothers but also can affect the joints of their infants.

The remaining joints are assessed by passive range of motion and by observing the infant moving or being moved. The last joint to be assessed is the ankle joint. Position of the infant during pregnancy may lead to bowed legs, ankle deformities, or unusual positions of the feet. Pronation (inward turning) of the feet in newborns is common and gently stroking the infant's insole will illustrate for the nurse the ease at which the infant's foot assumes a normal position. A severely pronated foot that the nurse is unable to place in normal alignment is inspected for the posterior alignment of the heel and the knee. Medial displacement of the heel from the posterior knee alignment may indicate the presence of a *club foot*, which can be confirmed on X-ray films. A club foot is usually placed in a cast during the early days of infancy, and parents are instructed by the nurse in the care of the cast. Parents who express concern about their infant's feet "turning in" can be shown a simple exercise (stroking the outside of the infant's foot) that encourages the foot into a straight position.

Common Problems

Before any musculoskeletal assessment of the newborn infant, the nurse must inspect and palpate for broken bones. The infant should not be moved or positioned until this is done. The most common bone fracture is the clavicle, which occurs during delivery when the shoulders of the infant do not rotate easily. Palpation of both clavicles can confirm a separation between the ends of the bone at the fracture site or crepitus. Symptoms of fractures are swelling or edema at the fracture site, a bruise at the site, or infant irritability when moved. Experienced nurses who care for infants recognize the difference between an infant's fussiness at being disturbed and cries of pain. Other common fracture sites include the humerus, the ribs, and the skull. Definitive diagnosis is always made from X-ray films. Fractured clavicles heal by themselves over time, and the mother is taught to position the infant on the side opposite the injury. Special care is taken by the nurse to teach parents how to hold and support their infant's head and shoulders until the fracture heals. Humeral fractures are usually casted; rib fractures may be wrapped; and skull fractures are usually monitored in an intensive care unit.

Developmental dysplasia of the hip (DDH) results from a flattening of the acetabulum during pregnancy from its normal round, cup-like shape. This usually results from the infant in utero remaining in a breech position with legs extended upward during the period when bone growth occurs. The outer portion of the acetabulum becomes flat instead of curling around the head of the femur. The ability to secure the leg in the hip socket is lost. DDH can be diagnosed on physical examination by positive findings on the Barlow and Ortolani maneuvers, unequal leg length, unequal knee height, and abnormal gluteal fold counts anteriorly or posteriorly. Diagnosis is confirmed by X-ray of the hip. Treatment for DDH involves placing the legs of the infant in abduction in a special harness, called a Pavlik harness. This harness remains on the infant for approximately 3 to 6 months, until new bone growth forms around the head of the femur and creates the normal cup-shaped hip socket.

Some infants may have extra digits and toes (**polydactyly**) or digits and toes that appear to be linked together by webbing of the skin (**syndactyly**). Extra digits on the hand are attached to the fourth finger by a thin cord of skin. They appear to have the same size as the fourth finger and may even have a fingernail. These digits need to be palpated by the nurse for the presence of bone. Bone indicates that surgical removal is necessary. The lack of bone is an indication that the extra digit may be tied off with silk suture. Tying off blocks off the capillary, preventing circulation to the digit, and the digit undergoes necrosis and eventually falls off. Keep the extra digit covered with a Bandaid to prevent the infant from sucking on and aspirating the extra digit. Extra digits and toes tend to run in families, and parents will often describe relatives, other infants, or previous personal experiences with them. Webbing of toes does not interfere with balance or walking, and many parents do not choose to have the toes surgically freed from each other. Webbing of fingers is usually corrected for cosmetic and functional reasons.

Hands are inspected for palmar creases. These creases were noted earlier in the gestational age examination of the feet, but not of the hands. Three to four curved palmar creases are usually noted in normal newborns. A single, straight crease appearing in the middle of the palm is called a simian crease. These creases, unilaterally or bilaterally, by themselves are not an indicator of a special condition. However, with the presence of other symptoms, they may be associated with congenital syndromes, particularly Down syndrome.

Nursing Implications

The nursing assessment of the musculoskeletal system identifies the movement abilities of the newborn infant as well as movement limitations resulting from malformations or birth trauma. Through this assessment, the nurse determines the appropriate positioning for the newborn, exercises to enhance future abilities (if needed), and further follow-up or diagnostic evaluations. The nurse can raise parental awareness of their infant's movements, teach parents and family members proper holding and resting positions, and reinforce specific care needs of the newborn after discharge.

Neurologic System

The neurologic assessment concludes the physical assessment of the newborn infant. This assessment consists primarily of reflexes and other movements from which the nurse estimates the level of neurologic function. Reflexes can be divided into minor and major reflexes. Minor reflexes include: finger grasp, toe grasp, rooting, sucking, head righting, stepping, and tonic neck. Major reflexes indicate normal neurologic function; they are the gag reflex and the Babinski, Moro, and Galant reflexes.

Common Findings

Finger or palmar grasp is tested by watching infants curl their fingers around an object (usually the smallest finger of the nurse) placed across the palm. Plantar grasp by the toes is assessed in exactly the same manner, placing the object on the sole of the foot. Rooting and sucking are noted by stroking the infant's cheek and observing the infant turn toward the finger, open his or her mouth, and suck on an object placed in the mouth. Head righting is evaluated by lifting the infant in the prone position and gently stroking the back along the spinal cord. The normal infant attempts to hold the head up and arch the back at the same time. The stepping reflex is demonstrated by holding the infant upright with legs flexed and brushing the soles of the feet on a flat surface. The infant picks up his or her feet and puts them down again in a stepwise fashion, imitating walking. The tonic neck reflex is often called the "fencing" reflex. The infant, in the supine position, extends the arm and leg on the side to which the head and jaw are turned and flexes the arm and leg on the opposite side.

The major reflexes need to be evaluated carefully by the nurse. A successful gag reflex is necessary for an infant to be able to expel material from the back of the throat to avoid choking. Eliciting the Babinski reflex involves the upward stroking of the plantar surface of the foot from the heel to the toe, applying a slight pressure. Proper response to this stimulation is the incurving of the toes as in the plantar grasp with uncurling and fanning out (stretching out) of all the toes. The Moro reflex can be tested at the same time the head lag is assessed. As the infant head is elevated off the surface, a release is mimicked and the bilateral arm extension and leg flexion movements that are indicative of the correct Moro response can be assessed. It is inappropriate to check this reflex in infants by making a loud clap sound to "startle" them. The responses of the infant may not be consistent with the Moro movements

Nursing Tip   *The Galant Reflex*

This reflex occurs when the infant is held securely in the prone position with the infant's arms and legs dangling off the surface of the crib. The infant's legs are gently extended from a flexed position before the reflex motion is attempted. Leg extension is necessary to see the proper incurvation of the trunk and buttocks.

because the infant reacts to the movement of air across his or her body generated by bringing hands together in order to clap or to the sound of the clap itself.

The Galant reflex, or trunk incurvation reflex, is observed when the infant is held in a prone position and the lateral aspect of the leg is slowly stroked from below the knee superiorly to the buttocks. The infant reacts by moving the buttocks toward the side that is stroked in a curving movement. When this reflex is elicited correctly, the reaction is quite dramatic. The nurse can use this reflex to demonstrate to parents the capabilities of their infant.

Common Problems

The most common neurologic injury seen in newborns is at the brachial plexus from difficulties experienced rotating and delivering the infant's shoulders. This injury can be differentiated from shoulder dystocia, which is noted in newborns as temporary decreased movement and muscle tone in a shoulder and upper arm that improves rapidly after delivery. A form of brachial plexus injury, Erb's palsy, is easily detected from the position of the arm in the supine position. The infant's arms are normally flexed and moving. An infant with Erb's palsy has one or both arms extended in the supine position with hand extension. The arm does not spontaneously move into a flexed position. Palpation of the extremity reveals decreased muscle tone, decreased grasp reflex, and negative arm recoil on the affected side. This arm position has been called the "waiter's position" because it imitates a waiter with the arm at the side and the hand held out for a tip. The majority of brachial plexus injuries resolve within the first 2 weeks of life. The nurse assesses grasp and muscle tone frequently in these infants to monitor the resolution. Positioning of the infant requires placing the arm gently in flexed position at rest and supporting the arm while holding. Parents can assist in the resolution of this injury by performing simple arm strengthening exercises that passively flex and extend their infant's arm at each diaper change.

Infants who have severe neurologic injuries from the birthing process or during embryonic development are assessed in neonatal intensive care units. Newborn infants who have difficulty breathing, moving extremities, or lack appropriate muscle tone are monitored closely on this unit. Brain damage or paralysis of extremities may result from periods of *anoxia* (oxygen deprivation) during development or during labor. Oxygen deprivation is one of the causes of cerebral palsy and may result in difficulties with swallowing, breathing, or movement in newborns. Manifestations of cerebral palsy in newborns occur in proportion to the amount of oxygen deprivation. The nurse may notice, at one extreme, an infant with a slight decrease in movement with diminished reflexes, and at the other extreme, no movement and no reflexes, with numerous differences between these extremes.

During the embryonic process, the brain and spinal cord are formed by the closure of the neural tube within the first 30 days of pregnancy. The failure of this tube to close at the posterior end results in a lesion that may contain a fluid or a section of the spinal cord. This condition is called spina bifida and is diagnosed during pregnancy. At birth, spina bifida presents as a skin-covered sac between the fifth lumbar and first sacral vertebrae posteriorly. The sac may contain an extension of the dura mater and fluid called a meningocele and usually does not result in any decrease in motor movement below the waist. A sac that contains dura mater, fluid, and part of the spinal cord is much more serious. This sac is called a myelomeningocele and does result in loss of bladder and lower bowel control and motor function below the waist.

Treatment of spina bifida varies according to the nature of the lesion. Usually, surgical closure of the lesion is required to prevent infection. A variation of spina bifida is called spina bifida occulta, which is a defect in the spinal vertebrae with no protrusion of the dura mater, fluid, or spinal cord that would interfere with motor function.

Incomplete closure of the anterior end of the embryonic neural tube causes a condition called anencephaly, which results in sections of the brain, forehead, skull, and occiput missing. Newborns with this condition are placed on respiratory and cardiac monitors to assess viability and shielded from visitors and curious onlookers.

Nursing Implications

Assessment of the neurologic system in newborns, particularly reflexes, is an important indicator of the newborn's development during pregnancy and the labor and delivery process. The developing fetus and the process of birth are vulnerable periods for the newborn, placing the newborn at risk for neurologic conditions that may be devastating to parents who are expecting a normal child. The nurse can be alerted to subtle changes in infant reactivity or the obvious signs of a neurologic deficit. Changes that warrant further investigation must be carefully communicated to the parents and preparations for care after discharge discussed with the parents and family members.

Body Size Classification

At the end of the physical assessment, the nurse measures the length of the infant from head to heel, with the infant's leg gently extended. This measurement, along with the head circumference and weight obtained in the delivery room, form the basis for the size classification for the infant. These measurements are plotted using the gestational age by examination, as determined earlier (Figure 20-10). Ideally, all three measurements, when plotted, fall on the same portion of the scale. Commonly, two out of the three measurements are similar. The infant's size is determined by noting in which area two out of the three measurements fall, with the weight percentile range given preference. Infants whose scores fall on the graph under the 10th percentile are classified as small for gestational age (SGA). Infants whose scores fall between the 10th and 90th percentile are classified as appropriate for gestational age (AGA), and infants whose scores fall above the 90th percentile are classified as large for gestational age (LGA). Depending on where the graphed points fall, an infant may be additionally described as "borderline" LGA or AGA to illustrate extremes of the classification ranges.

After size classification is determined, the nurse must determine the accuracy of the graphing in comparison to the physical presentation of the infant recently examined. Because these measurements begin all future determinations of infant growth and development from growth curves, the nurse must develop an intuitive feeling that they are accurate.

ADDITIONAL ASSESSMENTS

After the initial physical examination, measurement, and size classification have been completed, the responsibility of the nurse changes to promoting opportunities for the parents and infant to interact and be with each other.

Periodic Shift Assessment

Periodic shift assessments are done at regular times, usually every 4 hours, to ensure infant physiologic stability and to alert the nurse to any changes in the newborn's condition. Parents can provide information, which along with nursing expertise and judgment of the newborn's condition, are all part of ongoing assessment. The medical staff should be informed immediately of any changes in the condition of the newborn.

Periodic assessments include vital signs; body weight; feeding and elimination details; hydration status; respiratory and cardiac function; and hip movements for DDH. Vital signs during the first 24 hours of life include a heart rate that averages between 100 and 130 bpm, a respiratory rate below 60 breaths per minute, and a body temperature above 97°F. Blood pressure is usually not included in the periodic assessment, unless specifically ordered. Weight after the first 24 hours of life should show a loss, as the newborn is expending energy to breathe, maintain cardiac circulation, eat, and eliminate urine and stool. Diapers are checked for urine and the presence and color of stools. Stools should reflect a gradual change in color and consis-

Critical Thinking

Newborn Size

Ask yourself the following questions:

1. What does the graph reveal as the largest part of the infant?

2. What does the physical examination reveal as the largest part of the infant? Is this the same result as the graph?

3. Are the length and head measurements falling at approximately the same percentile range on the graph?

4. Which two out of the three measurements graphed are the closest together in terms of the percentile range and why?

The head of the newborn infant should be the largest part by graph and visual examination. Length and head measurements should fall within the same range on the graph. Embryonic development proceeds from head to toe in utero. Head and length measurements that are close together on the graph suggest that the development of this newborn infant has proceeded normally during this pregnancy.

Any measurement that the nurse suspects is inaccurate should be measured again and plotted on the graph with a notation that the measurement was retaken for the official infant record. Once the physical assessment and size classification are complete, the nurse can report to the parents on the condition and characteristics of their infant. The nurse can bring the completed size graph to the parents to show them exactly where their infant's measurements fall on the graph.

tency, from the dark-colored, thick meconium stools to brown-yellow, pasty transitional stools, and finally to yellow, loosely formed stools (Figure 20-21). Hydration status can be assessed through noting skin turgor and changing diapers. Newborns should have 6 to 10 diaper changes a day for urine, but the stool content in these diapers may vary. The newborn respiratory and cardiac systems are assessed by the nurse at every periodic assessment. The nurse is particularly alert for signs and symptoms of respiratory distress, including intercostal retractions, noisy breathing, sternal retractions, nasal flaring, central cyanosis, tachypnea, and irritability. During the cardiac assessment, the nurse should listen carefully for any arrhythmias and heart murmurs. Murmurs that persist beyond the first 24 hours of life need further evaluation. Positive findings should be reported immediately if the nurse notes new findings at this time. The nurse records in her notes the results of her periodic assessment and tells the parents that the newborn infant is stable and normal.

Quick Examination

Quick examinations are performed when the nurse relieves another nurse and assumes the care of a newborn, either for a short period or for the remainder of the shift. Skin color is assessed for cyanosis, jaundice, or both. The nurse assesses physiologic stability by examining the lungs and heart of the infant and taking its temperature. The nurse compares these findings with the documentation in the newborn's chart and the nursing report received on the status of this newborn. The nurse also should notice the reactivity of the newborn and record the state of the infant as asleep, awake, quiet, active, or irritable. Quick examinations are also performed on newborns when a nurse notices an odd behavior or something in passing that the nurse feels is unusual and should be assessed. This is a skill developed by nurses with experience in caring for newborns. These nurses have the ability to form an opinion about a newborn's condition from a quick look at a newborn at a mother's bedside or in the nursery.

Interactional Assessment

The interactional assessment of the newborn involves an assessment of the infant's reactivity to the environment and parental interaction with the infant. The newborn's reaction to the extrauterine environment fluctuates widely over the first 10 days of life, as the physiologic systems adjust to regular patterns of breathing, circulation, feeding, elimination, and sleeping (Pressler & Hepworth, 1997). There are six behavioral states (Figure 20-7): 1, deep sleep; 2, light sleep; 3, drowsy; 4, quiet alert; 5, considerable motor activity; and 6, crying (Brazelton, 1973). The nurse is aware of these newborn behavioral states and does the handling and examinations of the newborn during state 3 or state 4. Newborns who are at state 5 or state 6 are too irritable to be easily examined, because the examination intensifies and prolongs the motor activity and crying. The nurse can intervene by cuddling the infant, talking to the infant in a soothing voice, and waiting until the infant calms down. During the interactional assessment, the nurse notes the state of the infant, any changes, and the length of time the infant takes to go from one state to another. This timeframe assists the nurse in forming an assessment of the infant's neurologic organization in the early days of life. Substance abuse during pregnancy interferes with

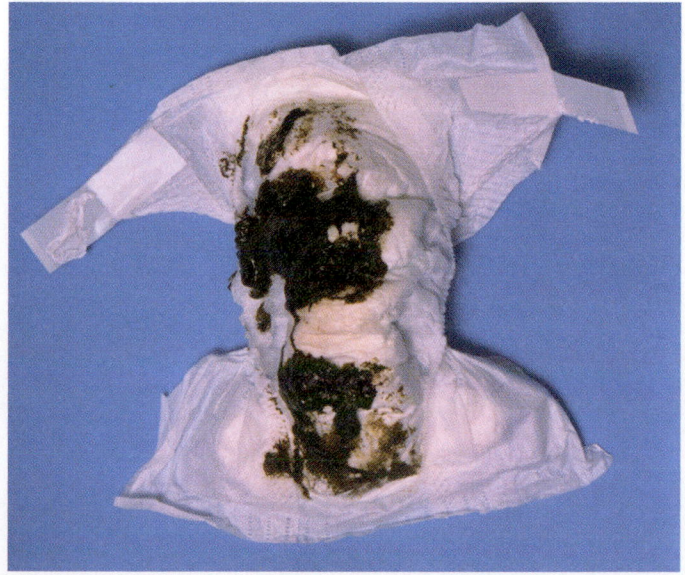

A.

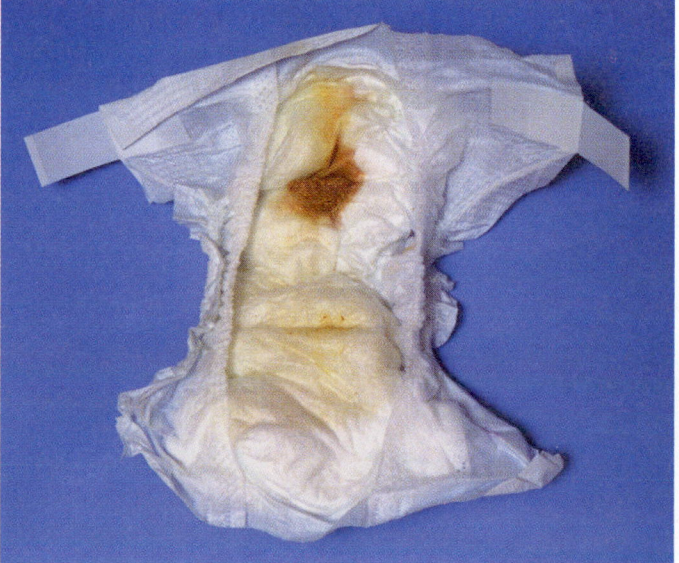

B.

Figure 20-21   A. Meconium stool; B. Breast-milk stool.

and prolongs the newborn's ability to move from one state to another. These newborns are often described as "irritable" or difficult" by parents who spend a great amount of time and effort attempting to calm them.

The nurse observes the interaction between the parents, family members, and the newborn. The nurse initiates attachment of the newborn to the parents and the family and the attachment of the parents and the family to the newborn with the first bedside visit. The newborn is placed in the arms of the parents, and the nurse describes the infant's unique qualities and features. Common parental reactions to newborn infants include touching their infant, exploring and examining all of the body parts, massaging the infant's abdomen, stroking the face, and cuddling (Hockenberry et al., 2003). This process assists the parents in identifying "their baby" and begins the attachment of the mother to the newborn. At this time, the nurse can instruct and demonstrate holding positions for the infant (Figure 20-22).

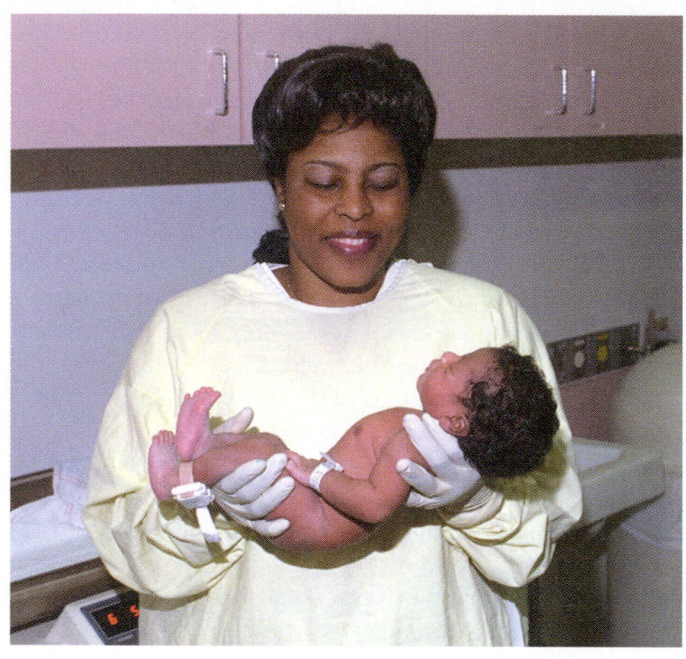

A.

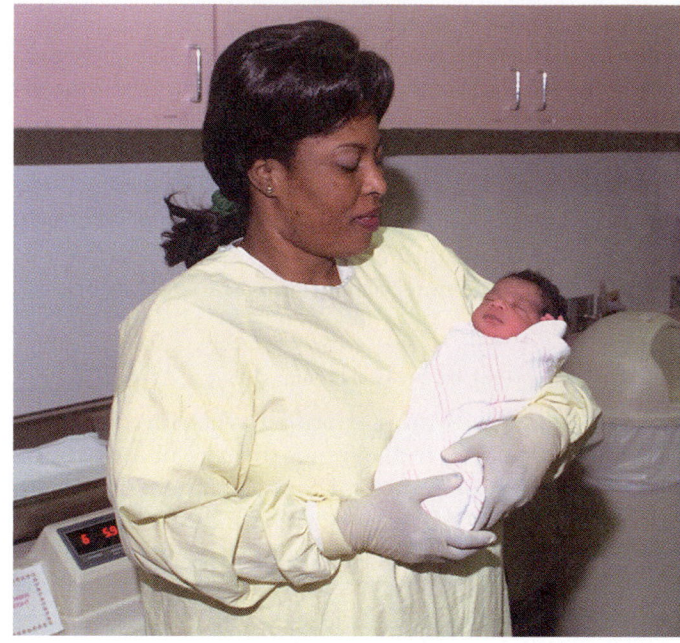

B.

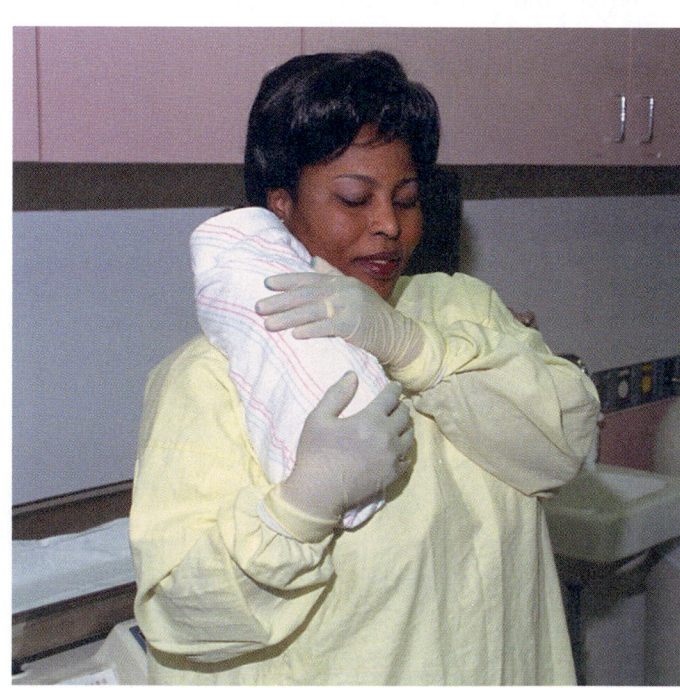

C.

D.

Figure 20-22   Proper holding of a newborn. A. Head and knee supported; B. Cradle hold; C. Football hold; D. Shoulder hold

The involvement of the father and siblings is actively promoted by the nurse as part of the interactional assessment. Paternal engrossment has been defined in the research literature as the father's ability to be preoccupied and interested in the newborn infant (Hockenberry et al., 2003). Fathers want to be able to touch, explore, and hold their infant. The nursing role in promoting the early stages of paternal attachment is to allow private time between both parents and their newborn. The nurse may accomplish this objective by bringing and leaving the newborn at the mother's bedside, closing the door to the mother's room, and taking siblings on a tour of the hospital or down to the cafeteria or gift shop. Children react differently to newborns, depending on their age. School-aged and younger children focus on the newborn's face and touching the infant instead of holding the infant. The nurse can teach siblings proper holding of the infant and infant transfer with the parent's permission.

The interactional assessment of the newborn and the family is accomplished by the nurse at least once a shift. The nurse notes the state of the newborn, the family members present, who is holding the newborn, and the reactions to the newborn by the holder or other family members. The nurse can use this time to address any concerns the parents or family have regarding their infant. The nurse should assess how well the family has understood the instructions on infant holding and positioning and, if necessary, reinforce and support efforts to follow the nursing instructions. Parental or familial interactions that the nurse observes with the infant that are not positive or are neglectful should be reported and confirmed by other nursing staff. This is a good opportunity to teach assessment for pain.

FACTORS THAT PLACE THE INFANT AT RISK

Besides the physical assessment of the infant, the nurse also evaluates other influences and conditions that have an impact on the health and well-being of the infant. These influences and conditions are evaluated for every infant, even those infants who are rooming in with their mothers. It is during this evaluation that the nurse develops a plan of care for the infant and parents.

Physical

Physical factors that are assessed in the newborn period relate to birth injuries, congenital conditions, and temperature control. Bruising, edema, lacerations, and bone fractures are conditions that are detected on the initial physical assessment. The nurse plans care for the infant based on minimizing further injury to the site by proper

---

Client Education

Holding and Transfer Positions

Newborns after delivery are able to see best at a distance of 8 to 10 cm from an object. The holding position for newborns that maintains this distance and that has parent and infant facing each other is called the *en face* position. The advantage of this position is that the newborn can gaze on the holder and attend to something that can be seen. Placement of arms and hands for holding a newborn depends on which side the newborn is to be held. For the left side, the left arm encircles the head and shoulders of the newborn with the left hand holding the left thigh of the infant. The right arm encircles the legs and the right hand supports the newborn's back. The nurse emphasizes that the head of the infant must be supported at all times, because of the inability of the infant's neck muscles to support the head at this time. The nurse can demonstrate head support to the parents by wrapping a hand around the infant's neck and placing the thumb and third or fourth finger underneath the newborn's jaw on both sides of the head. For feeding, the newborn can be held in the parent's lap at a 45° angle to promote swallowing and decrease air going into the newborn's stomach. For transferring the infant from one person to another, the nurse can actively illustrate the transfer. The nurse holds and supports the infant and walks to the parent for transfer. The infant is placed in the parent's outstretched arms and not released until the parent informs the nurse that he or she has control of the infant. Release before that time may cause the infant to be dropped, because the parent does not have a secure enough hold on the infant. The nurse emphasizes that one of the most important aspects of holding positions is the opportunity for parents to interact with and talk to their infant.

---

positioning or protecting the injury site with antibiotic ointment or a gauze bandage. Teaching projects for the parents are designed to alleviate concern and anxieties, continue appropriate care regimens, and emphasize follow-up visits. Congenital physical conditions, such as malformations of the extremities or a cleft lip and palate combination, require special nursing sensitivity to the requirements of the infant. The infant requires special care and protection from curious onlookers who are not family members.

The last physical influence on an infant's health is the infant's ability to maintain body temperature. Infant body temperature should range between 97°F and 99.5°F axillary temperature. Body temperatures of less than this value may indicate that an infant is too cold and needs to be rewrapped. An infant with a body temperature outside this range should be evaluated for possible sepsis. Temperatures are taken about 30 to 45 minutes after nursing interventions. Repetitive low or high temperatures in a newborn infant may indicate an infectious process. Parents can be taught how to read a thermometer and to take their baby's temperature properly. The nurse can give the parents guidance for assessing temperature at home and appropriate actions to take in the event that temperature is outside the normal range.

Psychologic

During the period of recovery from labor and delivery, the mother may be unable to care for the newborn infant and need assistance from the nurse, the father, or other family members. The mother may require intravenous fluids or medication that interfere with her ability to hold, cuddle, or breastfeed her newborn. Pain, uterine cramping, and discomfort from an incision site may contribute to positioning difficulties for the mother. Mothers admitted to intensive care units for observation and monitoring of symptoms experienced during labor and delivery are not able to care for their newborns. Visits to these units for the family members and the newborn are limited by the policies of the unit.

Psychologic conditions that place an infant at risk are those conditions that inhibit interactions between the infant and the parents or primary caretaker, such as separation, rejection, or sensory or neural disorders. Mothers and fathers who are eager to see, hold, stroke, and explore their newborn are learning to accept this new tiny person into their life. Other parents may be disinterested, disappointed in the physical appearance or gender of the infant, or unable to adjust to having an infant with a physical problem. A normal, healthy infant is the dream of all parents. Anything that disrupts this image of the baby, whether it is the physical condition of the infant, medical or nursing statements concerning the infant, or the infant's behavior, may cause the parents to change their responses to the infant (Stern & Hildebrandt, 1986). This places the infant at risk for inappropriate caregiver interaction and possible neglect.

Family

The family constellation and organization are important in planning for care of the newborn. The nurse is able to gather information from parents and other family members concerning their plans after discharge, household arrangements, services needed, and follow-up care. Families with little financial support can be referred to community agencies and services for assistance. This assistance may include formula or food for breastfeeding mothers (Women, Infants, & Children [WIC] programs), diapers, housing or shelter, transportation, and health care for the mother and infant. Young mothers, especially teenagers, may be eligible for teen clinics that provide resources and follow-up services for them.

The nurse can assess the reactions of the siblings to the newborn and initiate interventions to help the parents introduce the infant to siblings. The nurse plans for the care of the infant and designs teaching projects to facilitate the understanding and participation of all family members within the unique family situation that is presented.

Environment

In addition to observing the parental and family dynamics, the nurse plans for newborn care by eliciting information about the home environment. Environmental conditions that place the newborn at risk are smoking in the home, inadequate heating or cooling, lack of kitchen facilities, water from a well, and pets. Infant exposure to second-hand smoke is believed to cause respiratory infections in infancy. Smokers are encouraged not to smoke around the infant and, preferably, to smoke outside rather than in the home, and wash hands and change clothes before holding the infant. Temperature regulation is important for the newborn. Newborns can become chilled or overheated if placed near ceiling fans, window air conditioners, or space heaters or when left in cars. The best position for the newborn is at the opposite end of a room from the fan, air conditioner, or heater. Space heaters are not recommended, owing to the danger of fire. However, many older, unheated homes use them for heat, and parents must be made aware of the danger and the necessity of flame-retardant clothing for infants. Infants should not be left unattended in cars because cars may overheat in the summer. Parents should be asked whether or not they have kitchen facilities, that is, a refrigerator, stove, and running water. Formula and breast milk should be refrigerated and reheated on a stove or under running hot water. Water from a well should be tested every year to make sure that it is safe for consumption. Pets, especially long-haired dogs and cats, carry dander and hairs that might cause future allergies and sensitivities in newborns.

Illness and Infection

Infants of mothers whose delivery took longer than 18 hours after the rupture of membranes are at risk for a septic infection. Infants of mothers who had infections before delivery or who had a body temperature during labor above 100.4°F are at risk for infection (Mitchell, Steffenson, Hogan, & Brooks, 1997a).

The most common maternal illness at delivery is chorioamnionitis, which is an infection of the amniotic fluid surrounding the infant in utero before delivery. It is detected by the appearance of foul-smelling amniotic fluid at delivery, uterine tenderness, maternal fever and tachycardia, and infant tachycardia (Mitchell et al., 1997a). Newborn infants of mothers with these symptoms should be evaluated thoroughly for developing signs and symptoms of infection, which, in newborn infants, include lethargy, decreased appetite, jaundice or pallor, fever or chilling, increased respiratory or heart rate, or a general appearance of not "looking well" (Mitchell, Steffenson, Hogan, & Brooks, 1997b). Newborn infants with suspected infection are examined, tested, and often started on antibiotics. Infants with confirmed infections are placed on a prescribed intravenous antibiotic regimen for 7 to 10 days.

One of the causes of chorioamnionitis is group B streptococcal (GBS) infection, which is the leading cause of bacterial meningitis and sepsis in newborns. GBS and *Escherichia coli* infections account for 70% of all cases; *Listeria monocytogenes* is the causative agent in 5% of cases (Taeusch & Ballard, 1998). Early onset of meningitis in the newborn infant is usually caused by exposure to infection in utero or during passage through the birth canal. Women usually are tested for GBS colonization during their prenatal care, usually after 35 weeks of pregnancy. Many women exhibit no symptoms of infection but can transmit the infection to their fetus during labor and delivery if membranes have ruptured (Mitchell et al., 1997a). Mothers known to be colonized with GBS before delivery are treated with intravenous penicillin G every 4 hours during labor (Mitchell et al., 1997a). Newborn infants of these mothers are monitored closely for the first 48 hours after delivery for early presentation of the infection. Treatments for suspected early-onset infection include immediate in-

travenous antibiotic therapy, obtaining cerebrospinal fluid and blood samples for culture, complete blood cell counts with differential, and a chest X-ray film. Rapid nursing assessment and medical intervention are needed to prevent some of the devastating sequelae from this neonatal infection.

NURSING IMPLICATIONS

Nursing care of the newborn infant after delivery is based on an accurate assessment of the infant's physical condition and any other factors affecting the infant's health and well-being. The infant's physical condition is determined from the physical examination and additional frequent assessments of behavior, feeding, and elimination patterns. Familial and maternal conditions necessitating special procedures or treatment regimens are incorporated into the nursing plan of care.

Promotion of Physiologic Stability

The primary nursing goal in the care of the newborn infant is the maintenance and promotion of physiologic stability. Body temperature control, positioning, creation of a non-stressful environment, and establishing regular routines for newborn infants are the major concerns of nurses during the first several days of life. Creating a non-stressful environment is important for the development of infant behavior and reactivity patterns. Elimination of noise from beepers, monitors, telephones, televisions, and radios help to soothe a distressed infant. Carpeting reduces noise from traffic and dimming the lights reduces glare and assists infants in opening their eyes more easily. Infants who are fussy and irritable require a response from a caregiver that may consist of touching, talking to the infant, or holding or rocking them. The earliest beginnings of Erikson's trust versus mistrust developmental stage are seen shortly after birth, when the infant senses that someone responds to his or her needs. To assist nurses in providing this response, nurseries often encourage foster grandmothers and other volunteers to feed and hold newborn infants when their mothers are unable to do so.

Newborn Care

The care of the healthy newborn focuses on the feeding and elimination pattern of the infant and the parents' adjustment process to the care demands of a new infant. Nurses are able to prepare new parents for their future life at home with a new baby by using anticipatory guidance and by teaching skills in baby care. Nurses are often the first health care provider to answer parents' concerns

> ## Nursing Tip
> ### Culturally Appropriate Care
>
> Optimal care practices for infants should be attuned to the family's cultural and ethnic environment without sacrificing the infant's health and well-being. Achieving this delicate combination results in the provision of culturally sensitive care (Andrews, 1992) and creates a maternal and familial impression that the nurse understands and appreciates the relationship of this newborn infant to the family and their environment.

about their infant. During the period after delivery, the nurse must not only assess the health and well-being of the infant but also determine how well the parents are coping with the new and frequent demands for their attention and time.

Sleep and Activity

Newborn infants spend the majority of their time sleeping and brief periods awake and actively exploring their environment. It is not unusual for newborns to sleep 16 hours a day. Proper sleeping conditions for infants are placement in the supine position on a flat surface without a pillow and covered with a blanket in a crib or bassinet separate from the parents' bed. Sleeping infants should be protected from air currents generated from ceiling fans and air conditioners that may lower their body temperature. Infant sleep-wake periods do not always coincide with a parent's need for rest. Often, parents are awakened several times during the night by an infant needing feeding or attention. The first several months of an infant's life are spent trying to establish a sleep-wake schedule that allows both parents and infant to rest. The most common complaint of parents during the neonatal period is lack of adequate sleep. Encourage parents to rest while their infant is sleeping, instead of catching up on housework, chores, or the demands of other children or the partner (Ruchala & Halstead, 1994). Nurses can play a role in acknowledging parental frustrations during this time by being receptive to inquiries and providing guidance toward positive interactions between infant and family during this time. Infants who are awake and alert can respond to voices and noises and need sound and touch stimulation to begin to explore their environment. The more an infant is able to interact with family members and explore the surrounding environment, the easier it becomes for the infant to achieve developmental milestones and develop a unique personality.

Cord and Skin Care

Umbilical cord and skin care are additional concerns of new parents. The umbilical cord may or may not be stained with a bacteriostatic dye, but it is left clamped when the parents take the infant home. The clamp prevents blood from oozing from the cut cord and remains in place until the cord has dried and shriveled. Nurses can teach parents to look for cord discharge, redness, or oozing, which may be signs of infection. At each diaper change, the cord is swabbed with alcohol on a cotton ball at its base, where it attaches to the umbilicus, and the diaper is folded around the base, leaving the cord exposed to air. Somewhere between 7 and 14 days after delivery,

the cord will fall off, leaving behind a moist stump inside the umbilicus, usually yellow in color. This stump requires application of alcohol or warm water and drying to continue the drying process of the stump for another 3 to 5 days after the cord has fallen off. Some providers do not feel alcohol is effective and don't recommend it.

Many new parents may have cultural practices regarding the umbilical cord. Some families may attach belly bands, coins, cotton balls, or other objects to the umbilical cord to prevent umbilical hernias. Families should be encouraged to keep the area clean, dry, and open to the air as much as possible in keeping with their cultural beliefs.

The nurse can demonstrate proper cleansing of the diaper area with a warm, moist cloth, followed by drying with another cloth, and then replacing the diaper. Infant skin may feel dry to parents; the nurse can recommend a lotion that is hypoallergenic to be applied in a thin coat two or three times a day. Vaseline petroleum jelly and baby oil are not recommended as skin lubricants because they retain moisture and prevent air from contacting the skin. Parents are taught by the nurse to sponge-bathe their infant until the time when the cord falls off. Warm water and a mild soap are used to sponge-bathe the infant from the neck down. The infant's face is cleansed with warm water because the skin on the face has less natural oil and is subject to drying if soap is used. The parents are taught to bathe their infant in sections, drying each section before they proceed to another. This preserves the infant's body heat. Baby shampoo is used for washing the infant's hair. After shampooing and drying, the infant's head is covered. Hooded bath towels are available at stores that specialize in infant clothing and are ideal for keeping the infant's head warm after the bath. Lotion may be applied after the bath. After the cord falls off, the infant can be held securely in a shallow basin for bathing. Bath time can be a special time for parents to interact and play with their infant.

Diaper dermatitis results from mechanical irritation of the skin, the pH of urine, and decreased air circulation inside the diaper. Improper cleaning of the genital area and infrequent changes are all predisposing factors for the development of a diaper rash (Singleton, 1997). Once a reddening of the skin in the irritated area occurs, the best treatment includes washing the area with warm water; drying thoroughly between diaper changes; eliminating cornstarch or other baby powders; leaving the diaper open and the area exposed to air several times a day; and using A & D Ointment or petroleum jelly, which is washed off at each diaper change (Singleton, 1997). Diaper rash that does not improve with these remedies within 2 to 3 days should be evaluated by a health care provider.

WEB | ACTIVITIES

••• Visit the American Academy of Pediatrics Web site for guidelines on newborn care.

••• Search the Internet for the Web site of a hospital in your geographic area. What resources do they include for expectant parents and new parents?

Criteria for Discharge

Newborn infants are often discharged within 24 to 48 hours of delivery, depending on the policies of the institution and preferences of the pediatrician. Federal law requires insurance coverage for newborns for 48 hours after a normal vaginal delivery and 72 hours after a caesarean section delivery. The responsibility of the nurse caring for a newborn is to determine if the infant and the family meet the criteria for discharge. First, the infant must be physiologically stable. The infant should be a term infant; appropriate or large for gestational age; maintain an axillary temperature above 97°F, a heart rate between 100 and 150 bpm, and a respiratory rate of less than 60 per minute; successfully pass urine and stool; feed consistently; and have normal findings on physical examination and periodic assessments (Burns, Brady, Dunn, & Starr, 2000). Second, the parents and family members should be knowledgeable in the care and feeding of the infant, signs and symptoms of illness, community resources for assistance, and locations with appointments for follow-up care. The nurse ensures that the prenatal screening has been done and recommends smoke detectors in the home, a safe sleeping position, and an infant car seat for the trip home (Burns et al., 2000). Infants, parents, and families who meet these criteria can be safely discharged at 48 hours after delivery or less (Banks & Thorne, 1997). Infants who do not meet the criteria should have parents referred to the medical staff for advice and guidance.

Key Concepts

- The newborn's large surface area of skin and thin layer of subcutaneous fat predispose the infant to heat loss. Subsequently, nursing efforts are focused on assessing infant body temperature and maintaining normal temperatures by using blankets or radiant warmers.

- Newborn cardiovascular and respiratory stability in the extrauterine environment is achieved after transition, usually around 12 hours of life.

- The hemodynamic changes in the newborn cardiac system after delivery may lead to "flow murmurs" heard on auscultation, which normally disappear after 24 hours.

- Nurses perform four assessments on newborns when they are physiologically stable. These assessments are the full physical examination, periodic or shift assessment, the quick examination, and the interactional assessment.

- The full physical assessment of the newborn includes a general assessment, measurement of vital signs, body weight and measurements, and a full physical examination.

- The periodic shift assessment is done at regularly scheduled intervals. The nurse evaluates vital signs and weight, feeding and elimination, hydration status, cardiac and respiratory function, and checks for hip DDH.

- The quick examination is performed by the nurse who takes over the care of a newborn from another nurse. This examination is done when a nurse notices a particular behavior or cry from a newborn that needs further investigation. Body temperature, cardiac and respiratory status, and activity and irritability of the infant are assessed.

- The interactional assessment involves an estimate of the newborn's reactivity to being handled and to the environment as well as evaluation of familial interactions.

- The assessment of the newborn's body temperature, skin, and cardiac and respiratory status are the best indicators of newborn physiologic stability.

- The assessment of the musculoskeletal and neurologic systems provides the nurse with indications of disruptions in embryonic development or problems related to trauma experienced during labor and delivery.

- The accurate examination of the newborn genitalia provides parents with an indication of their newborn's gender and the opportunity for the nurse to reinforce what is "normal" with parents.

- Factors that may dispose the newborn to injury or infection are evidence of birth trauma, maternal infection during pregnancy or delivery, and unsafe handling of the infant by family members.

- Family or psychologic factors that place the infant at risk are maternal inability to provide care, paternal noninvolvement, language barriers, and sibling rivalry.

■ Environmental barriers that affect the well-being of newborns include a lack of kitchen and water resources, smokers in the home, pets, and inadequate or dangerous heating or cooling systems.

■ Nursing care of newborns after delivery focuses on the promotion of physiologic stability, providing opportunities for optimal nutrition, protection from injury and infection, and enhancing appropriate interactions between the parents and the infant.

Review Questions and Activities

1. All of the following are assessed by the nurse after transition except:
   a. Temperature
   b. Body weight
   c. Heart rate
   d. Respiratory rate

   The correct answer is b.

2. The best response to a parent's question regarding the skin or hair color of their infant is:
   a. "The color of the skin or hair reflects what the infant inherited from the parents."
   b. "Skin or hair color always darkens during infancy."
   c. "The color of skin or hair in a newborn is not an accurate picture of inherited characteristics."
   d. "Newborn skin and hair color may change so that is difficult for you to picture the changes before they occur."

   The correct answer is d.

3. Which is the true statement regarding heart murmurs in the newborn period?
   a. Heart murmurs that sound the loudest on auscultation indicate large heart defects.
   b. Heart murmurs that are soft and barely audible on auscultation indicate small heart defects.
   c. Heart murmurs that appear on day 2 or 3 of life need further evaluation.
   d. Heart murmurs that are noted on the initial physical examination always disappear by day 2 or 3 of life.

   The correct answer is c.

4. All of the following are signs of respiratory distress in the newborn except:
   a. Hyperglycemia
   b. Nasal flaring
   c. Grunting
   d. Intercostal retractions

The correct answer is a.

5. Which of the following findings on the physical examination of a newborn is the clearest abnormal finding?
   a. Heart murmur
   b. Tachypnea
   c. Pronated feet
   d. Hypotonia

   The correct answer is d.

6. Which of the following findings on the physical examination of the newborn may be normal findings?
   a. Heart murmur
   b. Erb's palsy
   c. Leukocoria
   d. Bivalved uvula

   The correct answer is a.

7. All of the following are assessed during the musculoskeletal examination except:
   a. Muscle tone
   b. Torticollis
   c. Stepping
   d. Range of motion

   The correct answer is c.

8. All of the following may be causes of infant irritability except:
   a. Substance abuse
   b. Hunger
   c. Injury
   d. Heart defects

   The correct answer is d.

9. Which of the following positively influence the care of a newborn by family members?
   a. Feeding the newborn in the supine position in the crib
   b. Leaving the newborn in the nursery to be cared for by nursing staff
   c. Allowing the parents numerous opportunities to be with and care for their infant
   d. Removing all objects and jewelry placed on the infant by family members

   The correct answer is c.

10. The nurse assesses the interaction between the parents and their newborn by observing all of the following except:
    a. Feeding position
    b. Display of affection between the couple
    c. Holding position
    d. Touching and stroking

    The correct answer is b.

References

Abel, E. L., & Sokol, R. J. (1987). Incidence of fetal alcohol syndrome and economic impact of FAS: related anomalies. *Drug and Alcohol Dependence, 19*(1), 51–70.

American Academy of Pediatrics. (2000). Changing concepts of sudden infant death syndrome: Implications for infant sleeping environment and sleep position (RE 9946) *Pediatrics, 105*(3), 650–656.

Andrews, M. M. (1992). Cultural perspectives on nursing in the 21st century. *Journal of Professional Nursing, 8*, 7–15.

Ballard, J. L., Khoury, J. C., Wedig, K., Wang, L., Eilers-Waisman, B. L., & Lipp, R. (1991). New Ballard score, expanded to include extremely premature infants. *Journal of Pediatrics, 119*, 417–423.

Banks, J. M., & Thorne, M. (1997, June). *Early follow-up clinic: An NP clinic for the best start.* Paper presented at the meeting of the American Academy of Nurse Practitioners, New Orleans, LA.

Brazelton, T. B. (1973). *Neonatal behavioral assessment scale.* Philadelphia: Lippincott.

Burns, C. E., Brady, M. A., Dunn, A. M., & Starr, N. B. (2000). *Pediatric primary care* (2nd ed.). Philadelphia: W. B. Saunders.

D'Apolito, K. (1991). What is an organized infant? *Neonatal Network, 10*(1), 23–29.

Fox, J. A. (1997). *Primary health care of children.* St. Louis, MO: Mosby.

Gagliardi, L. (1993). Biased assessment of gestational age at birth when obstetric gestation is known. *Archives of Disease in Childhood, 68*, 32–34.

Hockenberry, M., Wilson, D., Winklestein, M. L., & Kline, N. (2003). *Wong's nursing care of infants and children* (7th ed.). St. Louis, MO: Mosby.

Johnson, K. B., & Oski, F. A. (1997). *Oski's essential pediatrics.* Philadelphia: Lippincott-Raven.

Jones, K. L. (1997). *Smith's recognizable patterns of human malformation* (5th ed.). Philadelphia: W. B. Saunders.

Juretschke, L. J. (2000). Unilateral testicular torsion. *Journal of Obstetric, Gynecologic, and Neonatal Nursing, 29*, 451–456.

Mitchell, A., Steffenson, N., Hogan, H., & Brooks, S. (1997a). Group B streptococcus and pregnancy: Update and recommendations. *Maternal Child Nursing, 22*, 242–248.

Mitchell, A., Steffenson, N., Hogan, H., & Brooks, S. (1997b). Neonatal group B streptococcal disease. *Maternal Child Nursing, 22*, 249–253.

Napiorkowski, B., Lester, B. M., Frier, C., Brunner, S., Dietz, L., Nadra, A., et al. (1996). Effects of in utero substance exposure on infant neurobehavior. *Pediatrics, 98*, 71–75.

Pressler, J. L., & Hepworth, J. T. (1997). Newborn neurological screening using NBAS reflexes. *Neonatal Network, 16*(6), 33–46.

Rubin, R. (1984). *Maternal identity and the maternal experience.* New York: Springer.

Ruchala, P. L., & Halstead, L. (1994). The postpartum experience of low-risk women: A time of adjustment and change. *Maternal-Child Nursing Journal, 22*(3), 83–89.

Schoen, E. J., Colby, C. J., & Ray, G. T. (2000). Newborn circumcision decreases incidence and costs of urinary tract infections during the first year of life. *Pediatrics, 105*, 789–793.

Schuman, A. J. (1999). Infant abductions: Preventing the unthinkable. *Contemporary Pediatrics, 16*(10), 93–110.

Seidel, H. M., Rosenstein, B. J., & Pathak, A. (2001). *Primary care of the newborn* (3rd ed.). St. Louis, MO: Mosby.

Silverman, W. A., & Anderson, D. H. (1956). Evaluation of respiratory status: Silverman and Anderson Index. *Pediatrics, 17*, 1–10.

Singleton, J. K. (1997). Pediatric dermatoses: Three common skin disruptions in infancy. *Nurse Practitioner, 22*(6), 32–50.

Stern, M., & Hildebrandt, K. A. (1986). Prematurely stereotyping: Effects on mother–infant interaction. *Child Development, 57*, 308–315.

Taeusch, H. W., & Ballard, R. A. (1998). *Avery's diseases of the newborn* (7th ed.). Philadelphia: W. B. Saunders.

Williamson, M. L. (1997). Circumcision anesthesia: A study of nursing implications for dorsal penile nerve block. *Pediatric Nursing, 23*, 59–63.

Suggested Readings

Aronson, D. D., Goldberg, M. J., Kling, Jr., T. F., & Roy, D. R. (1994). Developmental dysplasia of the hip. *Pediatrics, 94*, 201–207.

Association of Women's Health, Obstetric, and Neonatal Nurses. (1998). *Standards and guidelines for professional nursing practice in the care of women and newborns* (5th ed.). Washington, DC: Author.

Cottrell, B. H., & Grubbs, L. M. (1994). Women's satisfaction with couplet care nursing compared to traditional postpartum care with rooming-in. *Research in Nursing & Health, 17*, 401–409.

deBecker, C. (1999). *Protecting the gift.* New York: Dial Press.

Dodd, V. (1996). Gestational age assessment. *Neonatal Network, 15*(1), 27–36.

Mercer, R. T. (1995). *Becoming a mother: Research on maternal identity from Rubin to the present.* New York: Springer.

O'Kane, M. (1995). Evaluating cord care. *Nursing Times, 91*(29), 57–58.

Pasquale, J. A., Brittain, L., Lenfestey, C. C., & Jarrett-Pulliam, C. (1996). Breastfeeding, dehydration, and shorter maternity stays. *Neonatal Network, 15*(7), 37–43.

Resources

American Academy of Pediatrics, National Headquarters, 141 Northwest Point Boulevard, Elk Grove Village, IL 60007-1098, 847-434-4000, http://www.aap.org

American Nurses Association, 600 Maryland Avenue, SW, Suite 100, Washington, DC 20024, 800-274-4262, http://www.ana.org

Association of Women's Health, Obstetric, and Neonatal Nurses, 2000 L. Street, NW, Suite 740, Washington, DC 20036, 800-673-8499, http://www.awhonn.org

Information for parents, including a chat room, http://www.babycenter.com

National Association of Neonatal Nurses, 4700 W. Lake Avenue, Glenview, IL 60025-1485, 800-451-3795, http://www.nann.org

Procter and Gamble, http://www.pampers.com

Society of Pediatric Nurses, 7794 Grow Drive, Pensacola, FL 32514, 800-723-2902, http://www.pednurse.org

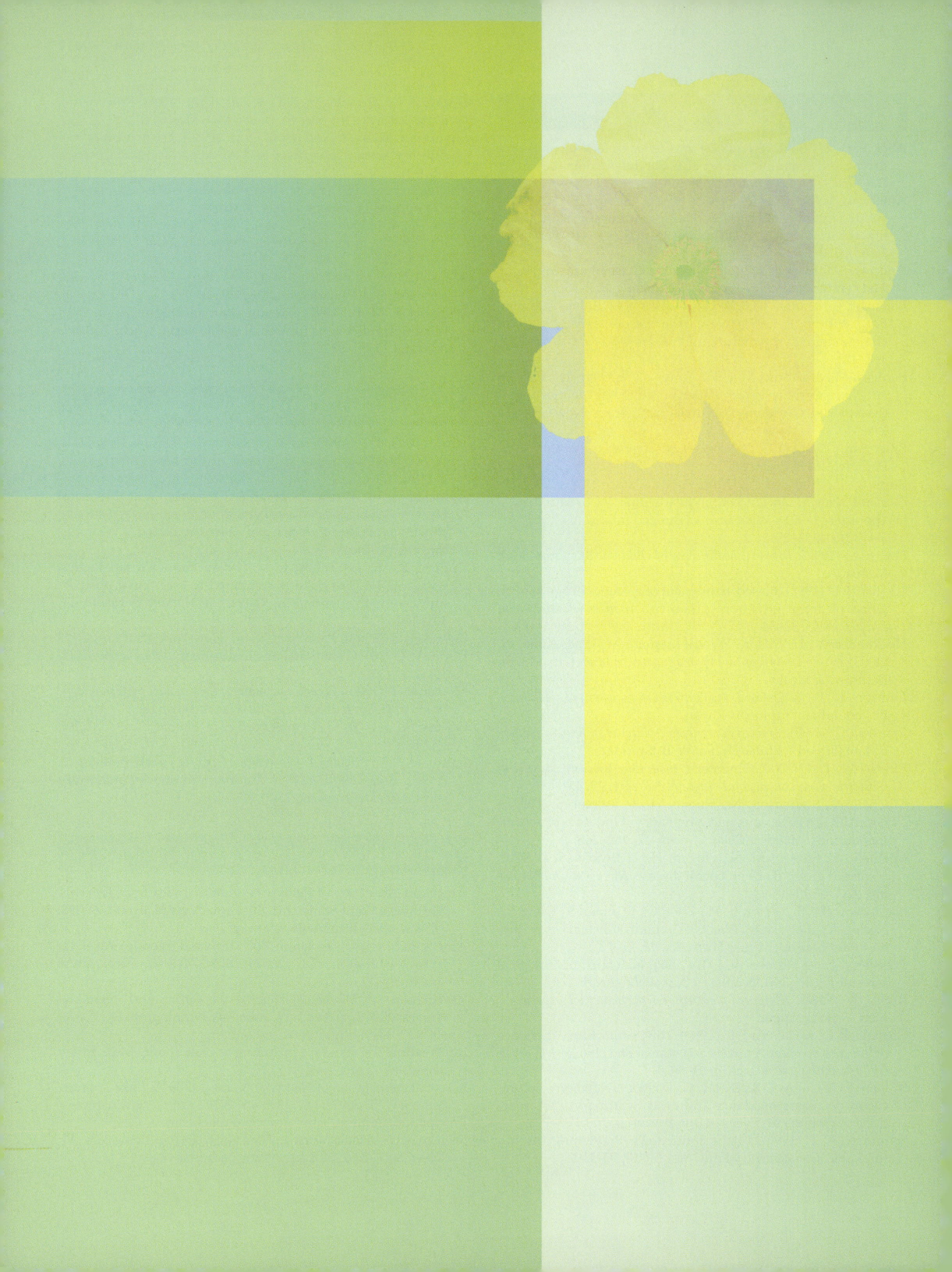

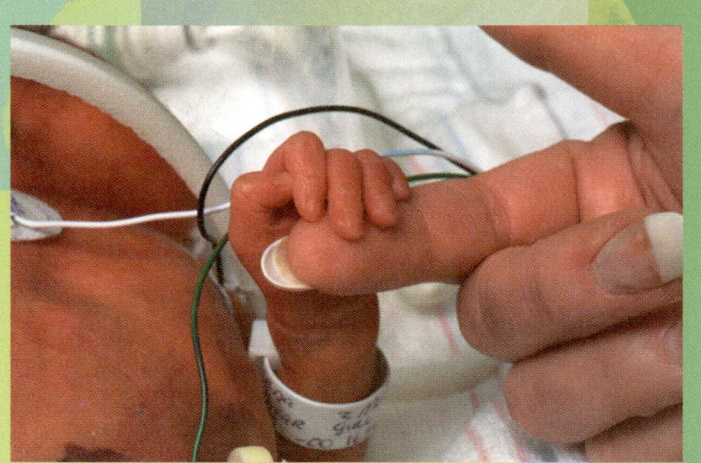

CHAPTER 21

CARE OF NEWBORNS AT RISK RELATED TO BIRTH WEIGHT AND PREMATURE DELIVERY

Nursing care of infants who are at risk for health problems related to low or high birth weight or to prematurity present unique nursing challenges. Although advances in care have improved survival, these infants are medically fragile. To work with these fragile infants, the nurse must be an advocate for neonates who cannot speak for themselves. Understanding the needs of high-risk neonates and their families is the first ingredient to providing effective and sensitive nursing care. Use the following questions to examine your personal feelings about issues that may affect your response to the infant and family.

- How do I feel about caring for an infant with potential long-term morbidity related to complications of prematurity, and who is critically ill?
- How can I make the development of parent-infant bonding easier when an infant is severely ill?
- How do I feel about caring for an infant who has extremely low birth weight?
- How small is too small?
- How can I know if a baby is in distress if he or she cannot cry?
- How important do I think it is for parents to be fully involved in the care of their hospitalized infant?
- The NICU is a very high-technology environment. How does that make me feel?
- What are my ethical questions about aggressive technologic support of the critically ill infant?

Key Terms

Apnea
Asymmetric intrauterine growth restriction
Auditory brain evoked response
Bilirubin
Bronchopulmonary dysplasia (BPD)
Containment
Developmental care
Dysmotility
Extremely low birth weight (ELBW)
Facilitated tucking
Gastroesophageal reflux (GER)
Gavage feeding
Glycosuria
Hyaline membrane disease (HMD)
Hyperglycemia
Hyperkalemia
Hypernatremia
Hypoglycemia
Hyponatremia
Insensible water loss (IWL)
Intrauterine growth restriction (IUGR)
Intraventricular hemorrhage (IVH)
Jaundice
Large for gestational age (LGA)
Low birth weight (LBW)
Macro-environment

Micro-environment
Necrotizing enterocolitis (NEC)
Neutropenia
Oliguria
Opsonization
Osteopenia
Patent ductus arteriosus (PDA)
Perinatal asphyxia profound
Persistent pulmonary hypertension in the newborn (PPHN)
Plethora
Pneumatosis intestinalis
Postconceptional age
Posthemorrhagic hydrocephalus
Prematurity
Preterm birth
Respiratory distress syndrome (RDS)
Retinopathy of prematurity (ROP)
Short bowel syndrome
Small for gestational age (SGA)
Symmetric intrauterine growth restriction
Total parenteral nutrition (TPN)
Ventricular peritoneal shunt (VPS)
Very low birth weight (VLBW)

Competencies

Upon completion of this chapter, the reader should be able to:

1. Compare the clinical characteristics of the infant who is small for gestational age with those of the premature infant.
2. List the problems that frequently affect the preterm infant.
3. Develop a plan of care for the infant who is small or large for gestational age.
4. Illustrate the techniques and strategies that can be used to facilitate parent-infant bonding.
5. Understand the ethical issues that may arise when providing care for the premature infant.
6. Review the long-term medical needs of infants who are small for gestational age or premature.
7. Discuss the rationale for thorough discharge planning to meet the needs of these infants.
8. Identify the elements of developmental care.
9. Discuss the role of the family in the developmental care of the high-risk infant.

This chapter highlights infants who are at risk as a result of low birth weight (LBW), birth weight higher than expected for a given gestational age, and prematurity. Infants who are born at birth weights below or above normal for their **postconceptional age** (age from conception described in weeks) are referred to as having intrauterine growth restriction (IUGR), being small for gestational age (SGA), or being large for gestational age (LGA). These condi-

tions place the infant at risk for health problems, particularly when the infant also is premature. Although alterations in birth weight and prematurity may affect the same infant, the concepts are discussed separately for clarity.

The environment of the intensive care nursery and caregiving practices both affect the process of support for the healthy development of at-risk infants. This chapter also includes discussions of individual developmental care strategies and the role of the family in the care of infants at risk.

THE SMALL FOR GESTATIONAL AGE INFANT

Infants termed small for gestational age (SGA) are those whose birth weight is lower than expected for the infant's gestational age. These infants are at high risk for multiple problems, including growth delays, feeding problems, thermoregulatory problems, respiratory problems, developmental delays, vision disturbances, metabolic problems (glucose, calcium, and bilirubin), and hearing impairment. The potential also exists for disruption of parent-infant bonding (Bernstein, Heimler, & Sasidharan, 1998). Nurses caring for mothers and their newborns should understand the unique challenges these infants and their families face.

Low birth weight often is linked to prematurity (postconceptual age of less than 37 weeks). Infants who are premature have a number of risk factors related to gestational age (Figure 21-1). They also may have risks associated with birth weight that have long-term effects on the infant's health and the family unit. A group of infants at risk for problems separate from and often in conjunction with prematurity are those who are SGA. The infant who is SGA has not met the expected growth parameters for the gestational age at birth. The term implies that some intrinsic or extrinsic factor has affected the ability of the fetus to meet usual growth parameters.

It is important to recognize that the infant who is SGA is at risk for stillbirth, perinatal morbidity, and adverse effects in adulthood (Gardosi, 1997). These infants often require early delivery secondary to a hostile uterine environment. The fetus is compromised by deprivation of ad-

equate nutrients and oxygen and is at risk for intrauterine death (Schaap et al., 1997).

The term low birth weight (LBW) can be defined as a birth weight less than 2,500 g. Each year, 20 million term infants are born with birth weights under 2,500 g (de Onis, Blossner, & Villar, 1998). The infant who is SGA has not achieved his genetic growth potential (Goldenberg & Cliver, 1997). Other terms used interchangeably with SGA are dysmaturity, fetal growth restriction (FGR), and intrauterine growth restriction (IUGR).

Intrauterine Growth Restriction

The term intrauterine growth restriction (IUGR) generally is reserved for infants who are at less than the 10th percentile at birth on standardized graphs in weight, length, and head circumference. Each year 30 million newborns are born who have growth restriction (de Onis, et al., 1998). IUGR is classified as symmetric and asymmetric.

Symmetric Intrauterine Growth Restriction

The term symmetric IUGR is used when the measurements of the head, weight, and length are less than the 10th percentile. Symmetric IUGR implies that the cause of the growth restriction occurred early in pregnancy and was genetic or intrinsic in nature. Symmetric IUGR is more likely to result from an intrinsic cause, that is, something that affects the fetus from within and starts early in gestation. A poor prognosis is associated with major chromosomal disorders and congenital infection.

Asymmetric Intrauterine Growth Restriction

The term asymmetric IUGR is used when the measurements of the head circumference and length are in a higher percentile than is the measurement for weight. This growth pattern occurs later in pregnancy than does symmetric IUGR and may be caused by placental insufficiency, maternal malnutrition, or other extrinsic factors. Extrinsic factors are those that affect the fetus from the outside, such as maternal hypertension and low caloric intake. Outcomes are better in infants who have asymmetric IUGR compared with those who have symmetric IUGR. Asymmetric IUGR is more likely to be caused by extrinsic factors than is symmetric IUGR.

Factors Associated with Fetal Growth Restriction

A number of factors may affect fetal growth, including fetal, maternal, and placental factors. Some of these factors

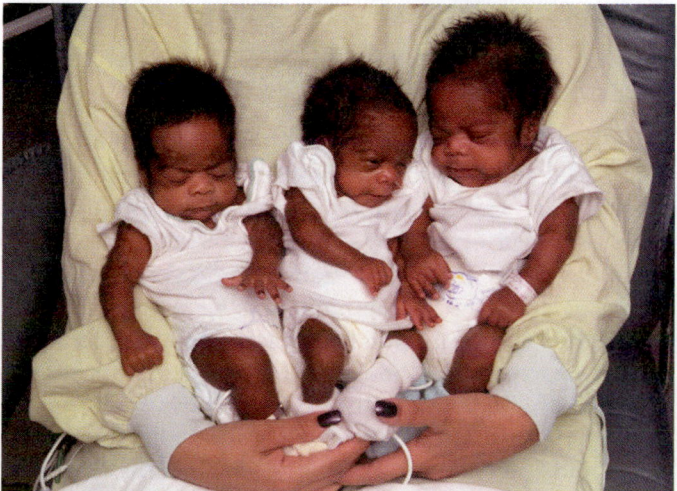

Figure 21-1 These male triplets were delivered before 37 weeks' gestation; now, at 6 weeks of age, they are each showing different rates of growth and weight gain.

are listed in the Nursing Alert. Fetal growth restriction (FGR) may affect perinatal mortality and the infant's short- and long-term morbidity.

Fetal Factors

Fetal factors are those that affect the genetic growth potential of the fetus. This potential may be affected by normal variations, such as race and gender. Multiple gestation also is associated with FGR (Goldenberg & Cliver, 1997; Sherear & Devon, 1997).

Infants with chromosomal anomalies such as trisomy 13 (Patau syndrome), trisomy 18 (Edward syndrome), or trisomy 21 (Down syndrome) may be SGA. Congenital malformations such as anencephaly, gastrointestinal (GI) atresia, renal agenesis, and some cardiovascular defects may be associated with FGR. Congenital infection may be a cause of infants being SGA. Inborn errors of metabolism, such as transient neonatal diabetes, galactosemia, and phenylketonuria, are also associated with small fetal size.

Maternal Factors

Maternal factors include maternal hypoxemia, due to sickle cell disease, respiratory disease, cardiovascular disease, or living in a high-altitude environment. Other maternal factors include short stature, young maternal age, low socioeconomic status, primiparity, grand multiparity, and low pregnancy weight. Maternal exposure to teratogenic agents, such as alcohol, cigarette smoke, and anticonvulsant medications also may be implicated in the cause of FGR.

Placental Factors

Placental insufficiency is the leading cause of infants who are SGA because of the delivery of inadequate nutrients for appropriate fetal growth. Other physical attributes of the placenta and placental circulation also may affect fetal growth. Multiple infarcts, aberrant cord insertions, and small placental size may affect fetal growth.

Complications Associated with the SGA Infant

Infants who are SGA are at risk for a wide range of problems. Knowing that an infant is SGA can assist the nurse to anticipate, prevent, or provide early intervention for problems. To determine whether an infant is at risk for the complications of the SGA infant the gestational age must be determined. See discussion of gestational age assessment in Chapter 20.

Assessment

Information from ultrasonography can be useful in establishing the predelivery diagnosis of IUGR. The fetal bi-

Nursing Alert

Potential Complications Associated with Fetal Growth Restriction

- Hypoxia
- Persistent pulmonary hypertension
- Meconium aspiration syndrome
- Hypothermia
- Hypoglycemia
- Hypocalcemia
- Polycythemia
- Hyperviscosity
- Hyperbilirubinemia

parietal diameter, abdominal circumference, and femur length provide the obstetrician with information to determine appropriate fetal growth. Ultrasonography regarding placental morphology and amniotic fluid assessment and Doppler evaluation of blood flow through the umbilical vessels may contribute to determining the cause of the FGR and assessing the well-being of the fetus before delivery. Fetal lung maturity studies may identify potential respiratory problems.

At birth the infant must be weighed and measured carefully. These measurements are then used to plot the infants' growth against standardized charts. When the gestational age is in question, the New Ballard Score, which has been expanded to include extremely premature infants, may be used to help determine gestational age (see Chapter 20).

Care

Once the infant has been determined to be SGA, steps may be taken to anticipate problems and provide early intervention. Complications may include prematurity, birth asphyxia or birth depression, thermal instability, metabolic imbalances, and hematologic concerns. Birth depression encompasses infants who have low heart rate (HR) at birth. These infants may require intervention from caregivers to establish adequate HR and respirations.

At birth the infant is at risk for hypoxia from perinatal asphyxia profound, persistent pulmonary hypertension, and meconium aspiration syndrome. **Perinatal asphyxia profound** is metabolic acidosis at birth associated with Apgar scores of 3 or less that persist after 5 minutes, multisystem organ dysfunction, and neurologic manifestations. **Persistent pulmonary hypertension in the newborn**

(PPHN) is a condition in which abnormally elevated vascular pressures result in continuation of flow through fetal blood pathways such as the ductus arteriosus and foramen ovale. These infants should be delivered in a location where immediate access to resuscitation equipment and personnel who are expert in the resuscitation of high-risk newborns are available.

After birth, the infant should be stabilized and complications such as hypothermia, hypoglycemia, hypocalcemia, polycythemia, and hyperviscosity should be anticipated, screened for, and corrected early. The infant who is SGA should be observed for respiratory distress and care rendered as needed. Prevention of heat loss is essential. Blood glucose levels should be checked and hypoglycemia corrected promptly. A central hematocrit measurement also is important.

A physical examination should be performed to screen for congenital anomalies. Screening for congenital infection also may be indicated. Families need to be kept informed of the infant's condition and necessary referrals.

Outcome and Follow-up

The mortality risk is significantly higher for the infant who is SGA compared with the infant who is appropriate for gestational age. The infant who is SGA shows more gross motor and minor neurologic dysfunctions over time. Cognitive function also is lower for the infant who is SGA than for the infant who is appropriate for gestational age (Kok, den Ouden, Verloove-Vanhorick, & Brand, 1998). The infant's outcome is determined by the cause of the growth restriction.

THE LARGE FOR GESTATIONAL AGE INFANT

In addition to infants who have low birth weights, those born at birth weights greater than expected for that gestational age may be at significant risk for complications. These complications may occur in utero, during delivery, or postnatally. Infants who are **large for gestational age (LGA)** have birth weights greater than the 90th percentile.

Associated Factors

Infants who are LGA are associated with diabetic mothers, parents who are large, congenital syndromes such as Beckwith-Wiedemann syndrome, or fetal complications such as hydrops fetalis. Mothers who have diabetes or Beckwith-Wiedemann syndrome produce hyperinsulinemic states in utero, thereby causing increased glucose levels in the fetal environment and resulting in increased weight gain by the fetus.

Complications

Infants who are LGA are at risk for macrosomia and resultant cephalopelvic disproportion. Cephalopelvic disproportion may result in difficult vaginal delivery secondary to the inability of the infant to pass through the birth canal, resulting in birth asphyxia or birth trauma. Birth trauma may include brachial plexus injury, a fractured clavicle, facial palsy, or subdural hemorrhage. Postnatally, infants who are LGA are at risk for hypoglycemia, polycythemia, hyperbilirubinemia, respiratory distress, and cardiac and congenital anomalies.

Assessment and Care

Nursing care of the infant who is LGA includes assessment for birth injury or respiratory difficulty, monitoring of glucose levels and other laboratory values, and management of any of these potential medical problems. Parents should be told of the potential complications and informed of changes in the infant's condition. Allowing parents to participate in the care of their infant assists in the bonding process.

THE PREMATURE INFANT

Preterm birth or **prematurity** is defined as delivery before 37 weeks' gestation. Neonatal care has changed dramatically over the past two decades. In the 1980s, viability in infants was defined as those born at 28 weeks' gestation or later. In the 1990s, infants born at 24 to 25 weeks' gestation were surviving with less morbidity. These changes are due to technical advances in ventilatory management, better understanding of the needs of the preterm infant, and improvement in neurodevelopmental care.

Factors Associated with Preterm Delivery

Care of the preterm infant continues to be a challenge in the health care arena. Prematurity continues to be the leading cause of perinatal mortality in the United States. Many risk factors are associated with preterm labor and delivery. Some of these risk factors can be attributed to previous maternal history of a preterm birth, a spontaneous abortion, an incompetent cervix, or other uterine anomalies. Factors that occur during the pregnancy that put a woman at risk for preterm labor and delivery include multiple gestation (Figure 21-2), infection, premature rupture of membranes, adolescent pregnancy, polyhydramnios, and oligohydramnios (American Heart Association [AHA] and the American Academy of Pediatrics [AAP], 2000).

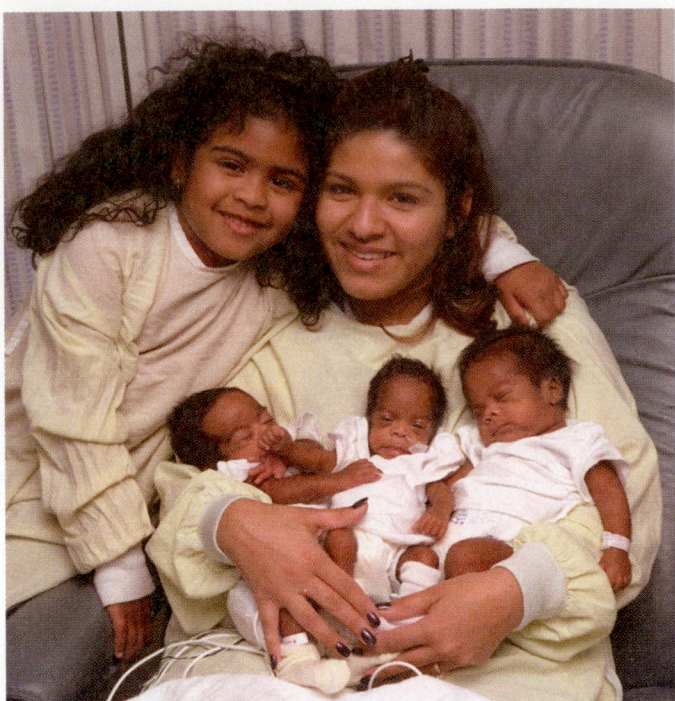

Figure 21-2   Multiple gestation is one risk factor for preterm delivery.

The lack of prenatal care also plays a role in preterm labor and delivery. Maternal habits, such as cigarette smoking, substance abuse, and poor diet are areas associated with poor pregnancy outcomes that could be improved with prenatal education.

Assessment of the Preterm Infant

Assessment of the preterm infant is an important role of the bedside nurse. A systematic approach to the physical assessment of high-risk infants allows the neonatal nurse to determine the infant's condition and approximate gestational age quickly and efficiently. Continued evaluation reveals subtle changes that allow the caregiver to anticipate and manage problems early. It is important to determine the gestational age of the infant because doing so will provide valuable information in interpreting the physical examination and planning age-appropriate care. A careful head-to-toe assessment is important to determine the infant's condition. Ongoing observation allows the nurse to quickly recognize problems before they compromise the infant's well-being.

Gestational Age Assessment

Knowing the infant's gestational age assists the caregiver in anticipating problems that may occur after delivery and must be considered in evaluating posture and muscle tone. The results of the infant's examination may be compared with charts developed by Dubowitz and Ballard, who use a scoring sheet to evaluate neurologic characteristics, such as posture, and physical characteristics, such as skin thickness, to estimate the infant's gestational age (Ballard et al., 1991).

Neurologic Assessment

Neurologic assessment of the newborn includes evaluation of tone, activity, and reflexes. Tone develops by way of a caudalcephalic route. Knowing how reflexes mature with progressing gestational age can aid the nurse in developing a plan of care. For example, an infant's sucking reflex is evident at about 32 weeks' postconception; however, a coordinated suck-swallow-breathe pattern may not develop until about 34 weeks' postconception. Encouraging nonnutritive sucking at 32 weeks' postconception and introducing oral feedings at about 34 weeks' postconception would be included in the care plan of an infant born at less than 32 weeks' gestation.

Physical Characteristics

The skin of a premature infant can be a clue to gestational age. Thin gelatinous skin is associated with infants who are less than 26 weeks' gestation. The skin becomes thicker and less translucent with increased gestational age. The presence or absence of lanugo, plantar creases, breast tissue, and ear cartilage provides other clues to the infant's gestational age (Figure 21-3). Eyes are fused before 24 weeks' gestation. Eyelashes and eyebrows appear at 20 to 23 weeks' gestation. Hair is fine and wooly and sticks together at 28 to 34 weeks' gestation. Before 28 weeks' gestation, the preterm female infant may have a prominent clitoris with small separated labia. Preterm male infants often will have undescended testes and are prone to developing hydroceles and inguinal hernias.

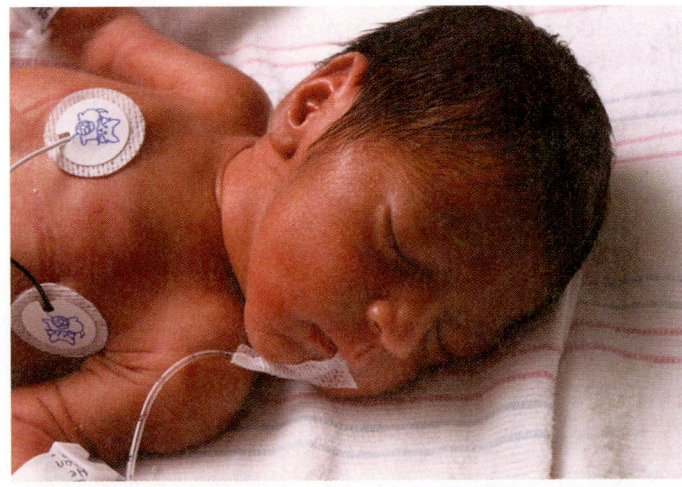

Figure 21-3   This preterm infant still has excess hair on the face, back, and arms.

Reflections from a Nurse

As I wheeled the neonatal transport incubator into the recovery room I mentally prepared myself. I knew it would be a difficult first meeting for this baby and her mother. The mother had been in the hospital for 3 weeks now because of premature labor. It had seemed that the contractions were controlled, at least until tonight. The delivery was very fast; Dad didn't even have time to get to the hospital before the baby was born.

The baby was born at just 26 weeks' gestation, but smaller than expected. So many problems can affect a baby this size. We had to take her to the stabilization area right away; there was no time to show her to her mother. She needed to be warmed, to get oxygen, to be placed on a ventilator, to have IV access—these things are critical in the first minutes of a premature infant's life.

As I looked down at the baby I sighed. Even to me she looked tiny and helpless. A tube in her mouth was secured with tape, almost obscuring her face. Wires attached to electrodes were attached to her chest; a temperature probe was taped to her abdomen. An umbilical artery line for monitoring blood pressure and drawing blood for laboratory tests and an umbilical venous line for administering intravenous fluids and medications were inserted into her umbilical cord and secured with tape. She was curled into the fetal position in a nest of blankets. The constant whoosh of the ventilator and beep of the cardiac monitor accompanied us.

I rolled the incubator to the mother's bedside and positioned it next to the mother's bed. Tears rolled down her face.

"She's so tiny," she said.

"What's her name?" I asked.

"Sara," she answered.

"Would you like to touch Sara?" I offered.

"I'm afraid I will hurt her," she cried.

After assuring the mother that she would not hurt the infant and that in fact, Sara needed her touch, the mother agreed to touch her. I helped the mother to place her hand though the incubator porthole and touch Sara's hand. Sara's tiny fingers curled around her mother's finger. I saw a tiny smile shine through the tears, the first step of a long journey.

Physical Assessment

The physical examination provides an opportunity for early recognition of problems. The nurse must be skilled in assessing the newborn for nonverbal cues. An experienced nurse can process multiple observations while examining individual systems. The nurse should develop a consistent approach to examination of the neonate that covers all major systems. The sequence of the examination should be from least invasive to most invasive; for instance, observation would precede palpation.

A basic physical examination of a preterm infant should include the infant's color and skin condition. The baby's posture, activity, and state of arousal indicate his neurologic status. The respiratory rate and effort, heart rate, and presence or absence of murmurs, pulses, and perfusion are important information in assessing the infant's respiratory and cardiovascular status. The presence or absence of abdominal distension and bowel sounds are indicative of feeding tolerance. Prompt attention should be given to abnormalities observed during assessment.

Examination techniques used with the premature infant include inspection, auscultation, palpation, and transillumination. Observation requires patience and is an important skill to cultivate. Auscultation includes listening to sounds produced by the body that can be heard with the naked ear or a stethoscope. Palpation is examining by touch. Transillumination requires use of an instrument with an intense but cool light source. The light is placed against the infant's skin. Illuminated skin indicates the presence of air or fluid.

When examining an infant, timing is important. The infant should be warm and positioned comfortably and changes in condition evaluated against baseline values. The examination should be clustered with other caregiving activities to provide adequate rest intervals between care and before feedings.

Continuity of care is important in recognizing subtle changes in the infant's physical examination. Parents who visit frequently may be the first to note that something is different about their baby, and their observations should be viewed as important contributions to the evaluation database.

Because all systems are immature, premature infants are at risk for a number of complications. Frequent observations are required to assess an infant for a specific condition common to premature infants. Complications commonly associated with premature infants are discussed in the systems review that follows.

Review of Systems

Potential alterations associated with prematurity are discussed by body system.

Cardiovascular System

The premature infant is at risk for a number of problems associated with the cardiovascular system. Two common problems encountered in the preterm infant are patent ductus arteriosus (PDA) and systemic hypotension.

Patent Ductus Arteriosus. A **patent ductus arteriosus (PDA)** results from the failure of the ductus arteriosus to close or from its reopening after closure. This is often the result of the increased pulmonary tension of the premature infant's lungs. When the ductus arteriosus remains open after birth, a left-to-right shunt through the ductus may occur. This may lead to pulmonary edema and is associated with necrotizing enterocolitis (NEC), bronchopulmonary dysplasia, and intraventricular hemorrhage (IVC) (Davis et al., 1995).

A PDA is common in premature infants. The more premature an infant is, the more likely it is the infant will have a PDA. If left untreated the infant may require extended oxygen and ventilator therapy and may have difficulty gaining weight.

The nurse caring for a premature infant should be aware of the risk of a PDA and monitor the infant for symptoms. These symptoms include a murmur best heard in the second or third intercostal space at the left sternal border, a hyperactive pericardium, bounding peripheral pulses, and a widened pulse pressure.

A PDA is diagnosed by echocardiography. Treatment may be surgical ligation, or closure may be attempted using a prostaglandin inhibitor. The prostaglandin inhibitor commonly used is indomethacin (Indocin I.V.) (Davis et al., 1995).

Hypotension. Hypotension is a complication often seen in premature infants. It usually is associated with vasodilation after rapid rewarming or a response to an illness, such as sepsis or surgery due to fluid shifts from intravascular to extravascular spaces. Morphine used for sedation can also produce hypotension in the preterm infant. Hypotension is associated with hypovolemia after abruptio placentae, cord accidents, and internal bleeding. Cord accidents can occur due to rupture of cord, cord strippers, cutting without clamping, or knot in the end. Symptoms of hypotension include tachycardia, pallor, decreased capillary refill, decreased peripheral pulses, and decreased urine output. Treatment may be with volume expansion using 5% normal saline, albumin, or blood products. Vasopressors may be used to maintain the blood pressure at levels that will maintain renal perfusion and circulation.

Central Nervous System (CNS)

The premature infant is at risk for a number of problems associated with the neurologic system. Common CNS problems associated with prematurity are intraventricular hemorrhage, posthemorrhagic hydrocephalus, and hearing impairment.

Nursing Alert

Clinical Factors Associated with Intraventricular Hemorrhage

- < 34 weeks' postconceptual age
- Low Apgar score at 5 min
- Pneumothorax
- Low birth weight
- Infusion of hyperosmolar solutions
- Asphyxia
- Rapid volume expansion
- Acidosis
- Hypertension
- Hypotension
- Patent ductus arteriosus
- Hypercarbia
- Rapid sodium bicarbonate infusion
- Seizures
- Abnormalities of coagulation

Intraventricular Hemorrhage. An **intraventricular hemorrhage (IVH)** is an intracranial hemorrhage frequently associated with prematurity. The more premature the infant, the more likely it is the infant will have an IVH. The bleeding usually occurs within the first 3 days of life.

The most frequent site of origin is the subependymal germinal matrix (Bernstein et al., 1998). This area of the brain is rich in capillary blood vessels. As the infant grows, the number of blood vessels decreases until about 36 weeks' gestation. The premature infant is unable to regulate blood flow in this area. Thus, changes in blood flow related to asphyxia, trauma, hypercarbia, or rapid fluid infusion may place a strain on the delicate vessels, causing them to rupture and bleed. Clinical factors associated with IVH are listed in the Nursing Alert.

Hypertension has also been implicated as a factor in IVH. Sudden increases in blood pressure can be associated with caregiving. Actions such as suctioning, performing abdominal examinations, lumbar puncture, and starting an intravenous (IV) infusion can increase blood pressure and lead to IVH. Rapid increases in blood pressure also may occur after correction of hypotension. The increased blood pressure may stress the vessel walls in the germinal matrix and lead to IVH.

Prevention of preterm delivery and use of antenatal steroids may reduce the incidence of IVH. Prompt resuscitation in the delivery room is an important factor in the prevention of IVH. Premature infants should be delivered in a location that has equipment and personnel available for expert resuscitation. The nurse caring for an infant who is at risk for IVH should take care to avoid activities that are likely to provoke rapid or excessive changes in the infant's blood pressure. Dim lighting, low noise levels, minimal handling, and care in the administration of fluids and medications are important. The head of the bed should be slightly elevated; the legs of the infant should not be raised higher than the head. Care should be taken especially during diaper changing.

Infants who are at risk for IVH should be monitored for symptoms. These symptoms include a sudden deterioration in condition, oxygen desaturation, hypotension, bulging anterior fontanel, and hyperglycemia. These and other symptoms are listed in the Nursing Alert.

Diagnosis of IVH generally is made with portable ultrasonography using the anterior fontanel as a viewing window. The degree and extent of the IVH are classified from Grades I to IV. The grade describes the location and size of the bleed (Box 21-1). No increase in morbidity or mortality is associated with a Grade I or II IVH. Grade III may be associated with severe developmental delay. Infants with Grade IV are at high risk for death or severe developmental delay.

Intraventricular hemorrhage occurs in 15% to 40% of infants born at less than 32 weeks' gestation and who

Nursing Alert

Signs of Intraventricular Hemorrhage

- Sudden decrease in oxygen saturation
- Sudden deterioration in condition
- Hypotonia
- Hyperglycemia
- Bradycardia
- Hypovolemia
- Metabolic acidosis
- Tense, bulging anterior fontanel
- Significant decrease in hematocrit level
- Seizures
- Apnea

weigh less than 1,500 g at birth. Approximately 35% of infants with IVH develop posthemorrhagic hydrocephalus. In 65% of these infants the progression of ventricular enlargement will arrest spontaneously (Hansen & Snyder, 1998). The long-term outlook for these infants depends more on injury to the parenchyma than on the IVH and hydrocephalus.

Posthemorrhagic Hydrocephalus. After IVH, **posthemorrhagic hydrocephalus** may develop as a result of obstruction at or impaired absorption of the arachnoid villi (Hansen & Snyder, 1998). The obstruction results in overaccumulation of cerebrospinal fluid (CSF).

The daily care of a premature infant who has had an IVH should include keeping the head of the bed slightly elevated and assessing the fontanels and sutures (Roland & Hill, 1997). Head circumference measurements should

Box 21-1

Classification of IVH

Grade I: Subependymal germinal matrix hemorrhage

Grade II: Intraventricular extension without ventricular dilation

Grade III: Intraventricular extension with ventricular dilation

Grade IV: Intraventricular and intraparenchymal hemorrhage

be done weekly. Ventricular enlargement is monitored by serial ultrasonography.

Posthemorrhagic hydrocephalus may be associated with increased intracranial pressure. Signs of increased intracranial pressure include bulging fontanels and separated cranial sutures. Vomiting may be seen and may be forceful. An increase in the frequency and severity of apnea and bradycardia may be noted. Eyes may deviate downward.

Management of posthemorrhagic hydrocephalus depends on the rapidity of progression. A diuretic, such as acetazolamide (Diamox), may reduce CSF production and is usually used in conjunction with furosemide (Lasix). Infants treated with either diuretics or routine removal of CSF should be monitored closely for electrolyte imbalance and metabolic acidosis. Surgical placement of a temporary draining device may be needed until the infant is ready for a **ventricular peritoneal shunt (VPS)** (a tunneled internal drain that empties into the peritoneal cavity).

Before an infant with a VPS is discharged, parents should be taught to watch the infant for signs of increased intracranial pressure that could indicate shunt failure. Parents of infants with arrested posthemorrhagic hydrocephalus should also be taught the signs of increased intracranial pressure, because late progression of hydrocephalus can occur (Hansen & Snyder, 1998).

Hearing Loss. Because premature infants are at risk for otic nerve damage, resulting in hearing loss, it is important to assess the infant's ability to hear. Infants who are born prematurely are physiologically immature and at risk for a number of complications of prematurity, many of which are associated with the risk of hearing impairment. Some of the therapies used in the care of preterm infants are also associated with the risk of hearing loss. Risk factors for hearing impairment are listed in the Nursing Alert.

The nurse should be alert to the infant's responses to sounds. If the infant does not respond to auditory stimuli, a hearing screening test should be performed. Automated oto-acoustic devices are used to screen infants for hearing impairment. An **Auditory Brain Evoked Response** (ABER) test can be performed as well. It is a hearing test designed to screen newborns that records electrical potentials arising from the auditory nervous system. If the infant does not pass the test, follow-up with an audiologist is warranted.

To facilitate cognitive, social, and language development, an infant with hearing deficits may be fitted with hearing devices. The family should be taught communication skills, which will enhance the interactive process (Kenner, Amlung, & Flandermeyer, 1998).

Hematologic System

Nurses caring for preterm infants must have an understanding of the normal and abnormal conditions associ-

Nursing Alert

Risk Factors Associated with Hearing Impairment

- Asphyxia
- Congenital infection
- Hyperbilirubinemia
- Ototoxic drug administration
- Prolonged mechanical ventilation
- Persistent pulmonary hypertension
- Hydrocephalus
- Acidosis
- Sepsis
- High noise levels
- Bacterial meningitis
- Craniofacial anomalies

ated with the hematologic system. Acute and physiologic anemia and polycythemia often are found in the premature infant.

Anemia. Anemia can be defined as hemoglobin less than 13 g/dL in the first 28 days of life. Anemia may be present at birth or develop postnatally. It can be associated with blood loss, hemolysis, or decreased erythrocyte production.

Acute Anemia. Acute anemia is common and also may be associated with hypovolemia. Acute anemia may be caused by intrapartum events or frequent blood sampling for laboratory tests. Conditions related to blood loss in the fetus are fetomaternal transfusion or obstetrical bleeding from abruptio placentae, placenta previa, and abnormal insertion of the umbilical cord. After birth, blood loss may occur from a torn umbilical cord or internal hemorrhage. Internal hemorrhage may include IVH or rupture of the liver or spleen during a traumatic delivery. Anemia also may result from hemolysis from chronic infection, isoimmune hemolytic disease, or inherited defects in the red cell membranes.

Acute anemia should be treated immediately. Symptoms include pallor, tachycardia, hypotension, and shock. The cause should be identified and treated. Laboratory evaluation may be helpful in identifying the cause when the maternal history does not include intrapartum bleeding.

Laboratory evaluation includes measuring hemoglobin and hematocrit levels and obtaining a reticulocyte count. The reticulocyte count indicates if the anemia is chronic, such as in erythroblastosis fetalis. In a chronic anemia the fetus rapidly replaces erythrocytes, which results in an increased reticulocyte count.

Erythrocyte morphology may give a clue to the cause of the anemia. For instance, an increased number of spherocytes may indicate an ABO incompatibility, or an increased number of erythroblasts may suggest hemolytic disease.

Direct and indirect Coombs tests on the infant are important to evaluate for maternal antigens to the infant's blood. These antigens may be seen in Rh disease, ABO incompatibilities, and minor blood group incompatibilities. The mother's blood may be tested to see whether fetal cells are present as seen in fetomaternal transfusions.

Physiologic Anemia.   A physiologic anemia may develop from physiologic changes associated with the change from the production of fetal hemoglobin in utero to that of adult hemoglobin after birth. Physiologic anemia often is seen in the stable premature infant. The hematocrit reaches a natural low point as the infant's body transitions from the production of fetal hemoglobin to that of adult hemoglobin.

The hematocrit reaches a low point at about 6 to 8 weeks in a premature infant. The infant may be pale but usually maintains a heart rate within normal range. Physiologic anemia does not require treatment unless the infant is dependent on oxygen, having frequent blood drawn for monitoring, or symptomatic of anemia. If decreased activity, poor feeding, tachycardia, dyspnea, tachypnea, or poor weight gain are present, the anemia is considered to be symptomatic (Chen, Wu, & Chanlai, 1995). Treatment generally consists of transfusion of packed erythrocytes. Human erythropoietin also may be used for treatment of anemia (Chen et al., 1995; Kenner et al., 1998).

Polycythemia.   Infants with polycythemia will have a peripheral hematocrit value of more than 75% or a central hematocrit value of more than 65%. Infants at risk are those with trisomy 13 (Patau syndrome), trisomy 18 (Edward syndrome), trisomy 21 (Down syndrome), twin-to-twin transfusion syndrome, born to a diabetic mother, and those who receive placental transfusion at birth. Symptoms of polycythemia include lethargy, hypotonia, irritability, tremors, poor feeding, and **plethora** (deep rosy-red skin color). Cyanosis with crying, tachypnea, congestive heart failure, hepatomegaly, cardiomegaly, and jaundice are indicative of polycythemia. Polycythemia may be associated with hypocalcemia, hypoglycemia, and jaundice. When the hematocrit value is less than 70%

and no symptoms are observed, the infant should be monitored. Complications of polycythemia are associated with infarcts in major organs. When the infant is symptomatic the hematocrit may be reduced by a partial exchange transfusion.

Hepatic System

The liver of the preterm infant also is immature. The most common hepatic problem associated with prematurity is hyperbilirubinemia.

Hyperbilirubinemia.   Hyperbilirubinemia implies excessive serum **bilirubin** (product of erythrocyte destruction that may be a result of a natural or a hemolytic process) and, therefore, is associated with a pathologic cause or outcome (Schwoebel & Sakraida, 1997). The physiology and etiology of bilirubin are discussed in Chapter 22.

Premature infants are prone to potentially high levels of bilirubin and may have **jaundice** (yellow tint to the skin related to increased bilirubin levels). Bilirubin levels increase earlier, reach peaks later (5 to 7 days) and remain elevated longer in the preterm infant. The preterm infant is at increased risk of hyperbilirubinemia due to decreased reabsorption of bilirubin from the GI tract because of poor GI motility, inability to feed, feeding intolerance, and delayed stooling.

Phototherapy is the treatment of choice for the management of hyperbilirubinemia in the preterm infant using the same equipment discussed in Chapter 22. Early intervention is recommended, especially for infants who have multiple bruises from delivery or cephalohematomas because serum bilirubin will increase as the blood is broken down.

Issues of importance to the nurse caring for a preterm infant under phototherapy include maintenance of normal body temperature, ensuring eye patches are in place, strict monitoring of intake and output, managing IV fluid, monitoring bilirubin levels, assessing for signs of neurodevelopmental consequences, and educating the parents. Premature infants requiring phototherapy need increased maintenance fluids secondary to an increase in insensible water losses (IWLs).

The premature infant is at increased risk for neurologic injury. Hypoxia and hypoglycemia increase the potential for bilirubin-related kernicterus. There is not a consensus on what bilirubin levels are dangerous to the preterm infant, but cautious management is necessary.

Gastrointestinal System

In utero, the GI tract processes large volumes of amniotic fluid, which aids in maturation. By 20 weeks' gestation the anatomic development of the GI tract is complete, but functional capabilities develop later in gestation. Although some GI function is present at birth, regardless of gestational age, premature infants may have limitations in overall GI function. Common problems related to the immature GI tract include dysmotility, necrotizing enterocolitis, and gastroesophageal reflux.

Dysmotility. The onset of peristalsis is at 28 to 30 weeks' gestation. Once feedings are initiated the infant must be monitored closely for **dysmotility**, or a slow rate of GI peristalsis.

Digestion and absorption of nutrients vary according to gestational age. Protein is remarkably well handled by the preterm infant, whereas carbohydrate absorption is limited. Early low-volume feedings have been shown to increase gut hormones thought to be important in intestinal maturation.

Motility of the GI tract changes during gestation and after birth. The gastroesophageal sphincter pressure increases from 28 weeks' gestation through the first week of life, and peristalsis of the small intestine improves during the third trimester (Merenstein & Gardner, 2002). Gastric emptying is decreased in preterm infants. The more premature the infant, the greater the delay in passage of stool. Enteral feedings promote gastric emptying and the release of hormones that may improve peristalsis (Merenstein & Gardner, 2002).

Necrotizing Enterocolitis. **Necrotizing enterocolitis (NEC)** is a devastating disease process most commonly seen in premature infants but occasionally seen in compromised term infants. NEC is characterized by necrosis of the mucosal and submucosal layers of the GI tract. The risk of mucosal injury in the neonate is associated with perinatal hypoxia; asphyxia; hypovolemia and rapid reperfusion; viscous blood with decreased flow to the GI tract, such as in polycythemia; and hypotension, with resultant decrease in blood flow.

Although prevention of NEC is of primary importance to the practitioner, the lack of a clear cause limits attempts to avoid the disease altogether. Prevention is aimed at preventing factors associated with NEC. Certain factors predispose infants to NEC; these factors are listed in the Nursing Alert. Changes in blood flow patterns to the GI tract are the most common cause of mucosal injury. Once mucosal injury has occurred the bowel lining becomes edematous. Hemorrhage and ulceration occur followed by formation of a false membrane. Introduction of enteral feedings and overgrowth of normal GI flora (bacteria) cause an invasion in this already damaged bowel wall. Gas production occurs, which further weakens the mucosa, and gas becomes trapped in the interspace of the bowel wall. This trapped air is called **pneumatosis intestinalis** and is a hallmark of the disease process.

The infant may have subtle signs and symptoms or may deteriorate rapidly. Early symptoms include abdominal distention, gastric residuals, vomiting, and bloody stools. Lethargy, temperature instability, apnea, and bradycardia also may be present. When these conditions occur, delay in feedings is necessary and the infant should be monitored closely.

As the disease process worsens, fluid shifts from damaged intestinal mucosa into the abdominal cavity. Hypovolemia results, with a decrease in blood pressure and urine output. Late signs include erythema, edema, and abdominal tenderness. Thrombocytopenia occurs as platelets are consumed to help repair damaged bowel mucosa. The infant should be monitored for prolonged bleeding.

Management of this disease process should begin at the earliest signs of difficulty. Management includes stopping feedings and starting IV fluids, gastric decompression with an orogastric tube, antibiotic therapy, strict measurement of intake and output, and replacement intravascular volume with blood or plasma. Resuscitation may be necessary. The infant should be monitored frequently for changes in clinical status. Radiographic views of the abdomen are reviewed every 6 to 8 hours to assess for pneumatosis intestinalis. Laboratory evaluation includes complete blood count (CBC) with differential and platelet count, blood culture, serum electrolytes, blood urea nitrogen (BUN), creatinine, and glucose. A lumbar puncture for culture is done only if the infant's condition permits.

If the infant's condition does not worsen in the first 3 days, feedings are initiated slowly. If symptoms worsen, the infant should not be fed to rest the bowel, and total parenteral nutrition (TPN) with intralipids for nutrition and to promote healing are initiated. IV antibiotics continue for 7 to 14 days when indicated.

Nursing Alert

Risk Factors for Necrotizing Enterocolitis

- Prematurity
- Asphyxia
- Hyperosmolar feedings
- Polycythemia, hyperviscosity
- Rapid increase in the volume of feedings
- Enteric pathogenic microorganisms

The infant is monitored closely for signs of perforation, leading to air in the peritoneal cavity. Surgical intervention is indicated when perforation occurs. Necrotic bowel is resected, and primary anastomosis or stoma is established. All efforts are made to preserve the length of the bowel. When perforation occurs, the mortality rate is 20% to 40%.

Complications of NEC include lactose intolerance, malabsorption, fungal infection, metabolic bone disease, cholestasis, and liver dysfunction. Late complications of NEC include strictures, fistulas, abscesses, chronic electrolyte imbalances, and failure to thrive. **Short bowel syndrome** also may occur in NEC as a result of extensive resection of the GI tract. This results in loss of absorptive surface that, in turn, causes diarrhea, dehydration, and poor growth.

Gastroesophageal Reflux. **Gastroesophageal reflux (GER)** is defined as the return of gastric contents into the esophagus. The premature infant is at great risk for GER secondary to immature muscle tone, poor sphincter control, delay in gastric emptying, and increased intraabdominal pressure. Common signs of GER are vomiting, small wet burps, poor weight gain, apnea and bradycardia, esophagitis, and recurrent aspiration. Collaborative management is essential in GER. Nursing management includes positioning the infant with the head elevated (Figure 21-4), frequent small-volume feedings, frequent burping, monitoring for apnea, and thickening formula. Medical management includes the use of agents to increase gastric emptying time and improve GI motility.

Immune System

One of the many factors that put the preterm infant at high risk for infection is an immature immune system. Two mechanisms responsible for the infant's underdeveloped immune system are qualitative and quantitative neutrophil deficiency and impaired opsonization (Lott, 1994).

Neutropenia (decreased number of neutrophils) is commonly seen in infection. Preterm infants' neutrophils also are less effective than normal during times of stress.

Opsonization (the action of opsonins facilitating phagocytosis) is also impaired. Maternal antibodies are the only source available to aid the preterm infant's immune system and they do not cross the placenta in large quantities before 32 weeks' gestation.

Infection. The most common risk factor for infection in the preterm infant is exposure to infections in utero. These infections are sometimes linked to the onset of preterm labor and delivery. Maternal risk factors for infection in the infant include substance abuse, maternal

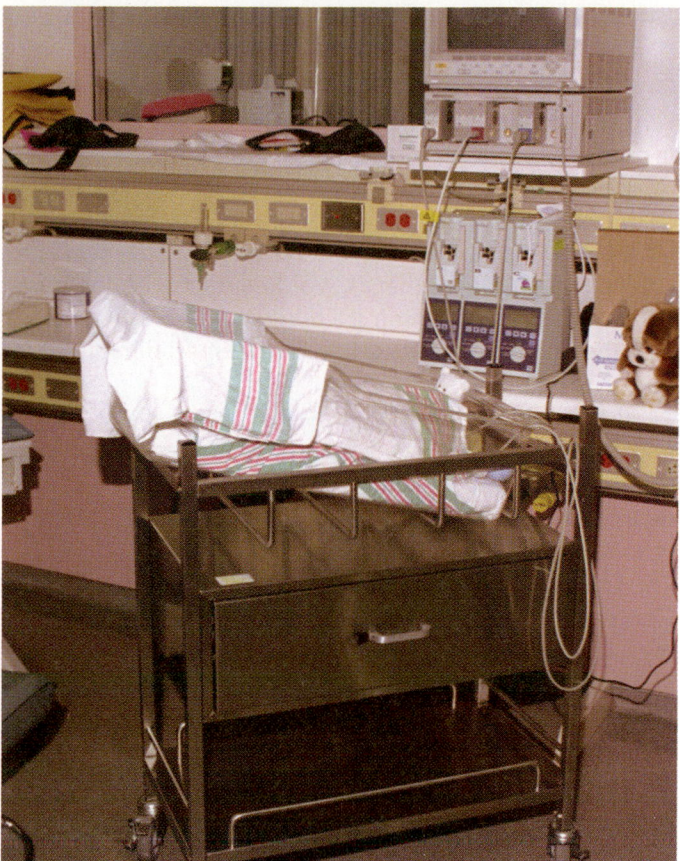

Figure 21-4   Elevating the head is one way of managing care for the infant with gastroesophageal reflux.

illness, colonization with infection, active bacterial or viral infection, premature rupture of membranes, and fever during labor and delivery. Neonatal risk factors include prematurity, male gender, multiple gestation, and congenital anomalies.

Infection should be suspected in all infants born prematurely without a clear cause for the early delivery. Evaluation for infection may include a CBC with differential, blood culture, evaluation of tracheal aspirate (if intubated), Gram stain culture, and a lumbar puncture for culture. Broad-spectrum antibiotic therapy is initiated until the organism is identified. Length of treatment may vary from institution to institution.

The premature infant also is at risk for late-onset infection occurring after the first 5 to 7 days of life. These late-onset infections are commonly nosocomial infections. Underlying illness, poor skin barrier, and immature immune status make the premature infant more susceptible to late-onset infection.

Prevention of late-onset infection is an important aspect of neonatal care. Nurses caring for premature infants must be diligent in good hand-washing techniques and in instructing parents and other health care personnel to wash their hands thoroughly. Equipment should be cleaned before and after use to prevent spread of infection. Each infant should have his or her supplies to prevent cross-contamination. Overcrowding in a nursery also increases the risk for infection. Once an infant is admitted to the nursery, the infant's bed space should not be changed without careful deliberation. The nurse caring for a premature infant also should try to ensure that caregivers and family members avoid contact with the infant when they are ill. Screening siblings for illness when they visit the nursery with their parents is especially important (Figure 21-5).

The evaluation for late-onset infection is the same as for an early infection; plus suprapubic needle aspiration of urine for culture also may be indicated. Increased incidences of meningitis and urinary tract infection are seen in infants who have late-onset infections.

The infant may have varying signs and symptoms. Generalized symptoms are common, such as poor feeding, irritability, lethargy, and temperature instability. Signs of infection often include the following: respiratory symptoms, such as grunting, nasal flaring, retractions, increased respirations, and apnea; cardiovascular symp-

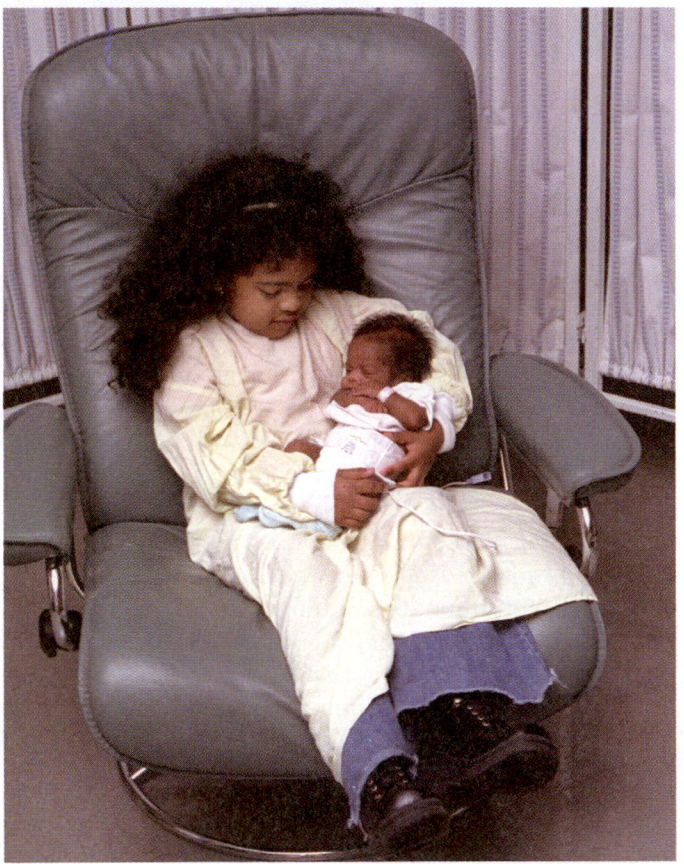

Figure 21-5 The triplet's big sister is allowed to hold only the infant who is showing the best growth rate and adaptation to extrauterine life.

Nursing Tip *Soap for Bathing*

The natural acid mantle of the skin helps keep bacterial growth at a minimum. Nonalkaline soaps should be used for bathing the preterm infant to protect the acid mantle.

toms, such as bradycardia or tachycardia, decreased blood pressure, cyanosis, and mottling; and GI disturbances, such as diarrhea, abdominal distention, emesis, and increased residuals.

As in all pregnancies, mothers delivering premature infants must be screened for sexually transmitted diseases. If the mother has not been tested or if the prenatal chart is not available, the mother must be screened once hospitalized. Follow-up by nursery personnel is essential. Sexually transmitted diseases are treated the same way in preterm infants as they are in term infants.

The preterm infant also is at increased risk for fungal infections for several reasons. Prolonged treatment of the mother with antibiotics may increase yeast colonization in the mother's vaginal canal, thereby increasing the infant's exposure at delivery. These infants have multiple intravascular catheters in place for long periods of time, multiple courses of antibiotic therapy, and an immature immune response. Treatment with antifungal agents is common. These agents have effects on the renal and

Critical Thinking

Protecting Infants from Illness

Calling in sick is discouraged in hospitals. It is especially difficult in a neonatal intensive care unit because the unit may be left short-handed or substitute staff will be provided that cannot provide the level of care a staff nurse is trained to deliver. Even an expert neonatal nurse cannot complete the variety of tasks expected of full-time personnel. Thus, calling in sick places an extra burden on co-workers.

You have read that infants who have low birth weights are susceptible to infection. In balancing personal pressure with the infants and co-workers' needs, what should you do if you wake up one morning with a fever? What should you do if you have had two previous absences and the third means a verbal counseling? What should you do if you know the unit is short-staffed?

hematologic systems. Careful monitoring of potassium, BUN, creatinine, hematocrit, and platelet count is essential for early intervention should side effects occur.

Integumentary System

Skin care is an important aspect of care (Gordon & Montgomery, 1996). Skin functions as a barrier to infection and controls temperature and insensible water loss (Dollison & Beckstrand, 1995). At less than 34 weeks' gestation a preterm infant's skin is immature. Once the infant is born the skin matures over the first couple of weeks and begins to resemble that of a term infant. Because a premature infant's skin is fragile, it is subject to injury. Epidermal stripping, absorption of chemicals applied to the skin, and IV fluid infiltrates are common.

Epidermal Stripping.
The skin of a preterm infant is more permeable because of its thin stratum corneum. The epidermis remains thin until 32 weeks' gestation. Collagen, which provides support to dermal structures and allows the skin to stretch, is unstable. Decreased cohesion between the dermis and epidermis exists. Epidermal stripping occurs easily because the adhesive of bonding agents may be greater than the bond between the epidermis and dermis. When the dermis is stripped, increased chemical absorption and increased fluid loss occur along with the potential for bacterial exposure. The use of pectin-based barriers helps prevent epidermal stripping. Placing the barrier under tape decreases the amount of epidermal stripping (Dollison & Beckstrand, 1995). Pectin-based barriers come in thin sheets that can be cut to the desired size and shape. The sheets stick to skin when warmed. Tape will pull on the barrier rather than the infant's skin.

Absorption of Chemical Agents.
The thin skin of a premature infant allows chemicals to be readily absorbed through the skin. Nursing care includes avoidance or limitation of the use of adhesives and adhesive removers. Table 21-1 lists some chemicals that can be absorbed through the skin. Absorbable chemical agents should be removed from the skin with water.

Table 21-1 Effects of Absorbable Chemical Agents	
ABSORBABLE CHEMICAL	**POTENTIAL EFFECT**
Adhesive remover	Increased blood alcohol levels
Betadine (povidone-iodine)	Transient hypothyroidism
Hexachlorophene	Central nervous system damage
Isopropyl alcohol	Sloughing

Intravenous Fluid Infiltrates.
Intravenous infiltrates are of particular concern in preterm infants because many solutions and medications can cause sloughing of the skin. Infection and scarring also can occur. Many premature infants require IV therapy because of medical conditions that prevent full enteric nutrition or the need for pharmacologic therapy. Properly cleaning the site and protecting the IV to prevent infiltration necessitating multiple IV starts are important considerations. It is important for the nurse to remember that each needle puncture is a break in the integrity of the infant's skin and a potential source of infection.

The IV site should be checked at least every hour. When an IV infiltrate is detected, the IV should be discontinued immediately and the area of infiltrate elevated, if possible.

When the skin breaks down over a joint, scarring and development of a contracture may limit joint mobility in the future. A consultation with plastic surgery often is required for evaluation of the area and for recommendations on steps to take to minimize long-term sequelae.

Ophthalmologic System

As with other body systems, the eyes of a premature infant are still developing. The premature infant, therefore, is at risk for the development of vision problems.

Historically, premature infants developed retrolental fibroplasia (RLF), which resulted in blindness, as a result of exposure to high levels of oxygen. Changes in treatment modalities and development of sensitive monitoring equipment have essentially eliminated this illness; however, it is important for nurses caring for premature infants to be aware of the potential harm of indiscriminate use of oxygen.

With improved methods of treatment and equipment, smaller premature infants are surviving. These infants are at risk for retinopathy of prematurity and other eye problems.

Retinopathy of Prematurity.
One of the most prevalent problems seen in premature infants is **retinopathy of prematurity (ROP)**. Before 32 weeks' gestation, vascularization of the retina is incomplete (Shapiro & Askin, 1999). The younger the infant, the less vascularization has occurred. Once an infant is born, the vessels in the eye continue to grow and extend to the periphery of the retina. As these vessels grow there is risk for abnormal development of the eye vessels. This increase of blood vessels in the eye is known as ROP, which can lead to limited vision or even blindness if not detected and treated early. In severe ROP, treatment includes cryotherapy or laser photocoagulation to limit the development of the abnormal blood vessels. When these treatments fail, the infant may require eye surgery to preserve some sight.

Infants who have birth weights less than 1,500 g or who are born at less than 28 weeks' gestation should be screened by a pediatric ophthalmologist for ROP at 4 to 6 weeks of life and then regularly until vascularization is complete. ROP occurs in 25% to 35% of surviving premature infants. Blindness occurs in 3% to 5% (Bossi & Koerner, 1995; Bernstein et al., 1998).

Other Eye Problems. Infants who have developed ROP at any stage are at risk for late retinal detachment and should be followed closely. Premature infants also are at risk for myopia, amblyopia, glaucoma, and strabismus (Bernstein et al., 1998). Parents should be encouraged to keep postdischarge eye appointments so that vision problems can be identified early to preserve sight. The long-term implications on the quality of life of the infant and family are clear.

Renal System

The kidneys are responsible for elimination of toxins and regulation of fluid, electrolytes, and arterial blood pressure (Seaman, 1995). In utero the placenta acts as the organ of excretion, removing excess fluid and waste products from the fetus. Infants born at less than 36 weeks' gestation have underdeveloped structures and decreased renal function. Renal function increases during the first week of life. Increased renal function results in diuresis at about 5 days of life.

Careful monitoring of the renal status of premature infants is important so that problems are identified early and thus early intervention can be provided. Renal problems most common to premature infants include oliguria and glycosuria.

Oliguria. Urine flow depends on fluid intake. Normal urine output is 1 to 2 mL/h per kilogram of body weight (mL/kg/h). **Oliguria** can be defined as less than 1 mL/kg/h. Oliguria may be a symptom of inadequate fluid intake or acute renal failure. Acute renal failure in premature infants may be associated with perinatal asphyxia and multisystem organ failure. Urine output may be affected by hypoxemia, hypovolemia, acidosis, and mediations that impair renal blood flow. Sepsis sometimes is associated with renal failure.

An accurate urine output measurement is extremely important in monitoring renal well-being in infants; however, accurate measurements may be difficult to obtain. Nurses who care for premature infants have developed creative methods of checking output. One method involves weighing a dry and a wet diaper on a balance scale (Figure 21-6). The difference between the two weights is roughly the urine output.

In severe cases of oliguria a bladder catheter may be required for accurate measurement. In addition to urine

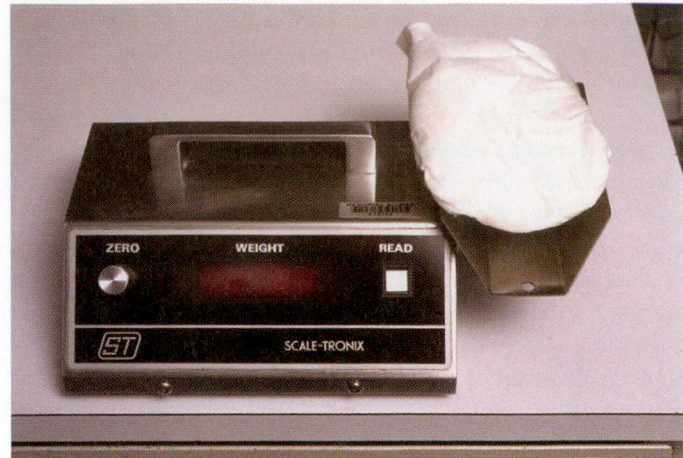

A.

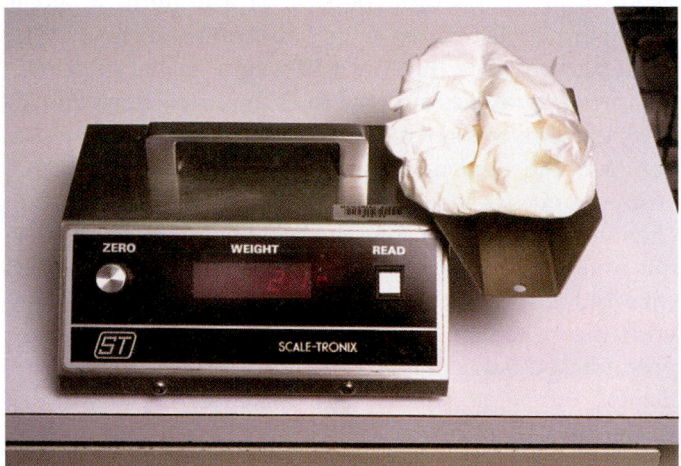

B.

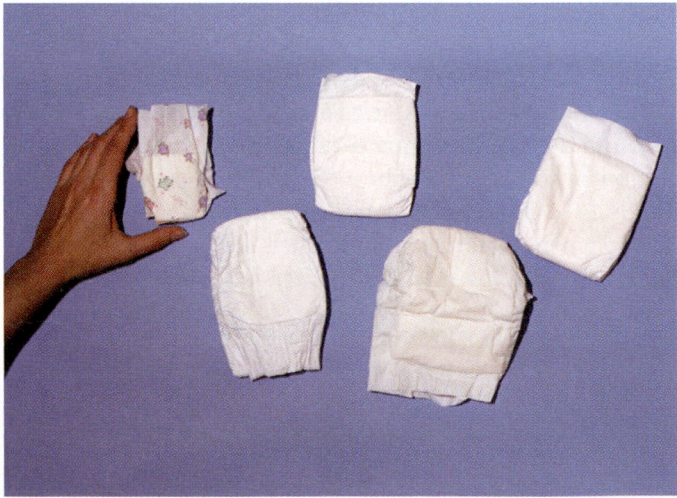

C.

Figure 21-6 Urine output can be measured by first weighing a clean diaper (A) and then a wet diaper (B); the difference is the infant's urine output. (C) The diaper of a premature infant is so small that this method of measuring urine output may prove a challenge.

output, renal function is evaluated by monitoring serum creatinine and hydration by monitoring BUN.

Glycosuria. Term infants may have a trace of glucose in the urine. **Glycosuria** is seen more frequently in premature infants in whom minor elevations in serum glucose allow spillage into the urine. Glucose in the urine sometimes is seen in premature infants who have an infection, IVH, and in those receiving steroids.

An increased frequency of yeast dermatitis has been observed in infants with glycosuria. Keeping the skin area that comes into contact with wet diapers clean and dry is important in preventing cutaneous yeast infections. The nurse caring for the prematue infant should consider each diaper change an opportunity to observe the area for rash and skin breakdown. Yeast infections in the diaper area generally appear as redness in the creases with a papular rash, frequently with satellite lesions, that is, lesions extending beyond the reddened area. The treatment for yeast dermatitis is antifungal cream.

Respiratory System

Before birth the infant's lungs are filled with fluid. The placenta acts as the organ of respiration for the fetus, providing for gas exchange. Fetal lung fluid begins to be absorbed before birth, and the alveolar fluid secretion decreases near term. During labor this process accelerates. When the cord is clamped and with the first breaths, the alveoli are able to fill with air. Thus, lung volume is established. The lung fluid then moves to the interstitial space and is removed by the lymphatic and pulmonary blood vessels. Delivery of a preterm infant interrupts this process and may result in a respiratory disease state.

The most common problem in premature infants is respiratory distress. Premature infants may have respiratory distress syndrome (RDS), bronchopulmonary dysplasia (BPD), apnea of prematurity, or pneumonia. Respiratory problems may occur alone, in combination, or sequentially.

Respiratory Distress Syndrome. Historically called **hyaline membrane disease (HMD), respiratory distress syndrome (RDS)** is the most common cause of respiratory disease in the preterm neonate. The disease manifests as surfactant deficiency characterized by collapsed alveoli and low lung volume. The disease process worsens with decreasing gestational age.

The premature lung is deficient in surfactant. Surfactant is essential in maintaining surface tension and preventing alveolar collapse. As surfactant is used up the premature lung becomes progressively atelectatic and underperfused, resulting in intrapulmonary shunting and hypoxia. Efforts to reduce the incidence and severity of RDS include the use of antenatal steroids and surfactant

replacement therapy. Administering steroids to the mother prenatally seems to accelerate lung growth and maturity. The use of surfactant replacement helps to diminish the severity of RDS once the infant is delivered (Moise & Hansen, 1998; Casey, 1999).

Common forms of treatment include continuous positive airway pressure, positive end expiratory pressure to prevent lung volume loss during expiration, mechanical ventilation, high-frequency oscillatory ventilation, and surfactant replacement therapy (Kenner et al., 1998).

Bronchopulmonary Dysplasia. One of the most common complications of respiratory disease in the preterm infant is **bronchopulmonary dysplasia (BPD)**. Infants who are born prematurely and require mechanical ventilation and oxygen therapy (Figure 21-7) for a prolonged period of time are at risk for damage to the alveoli and lung tissue. The primary cause of BPD is immature pulmonary development with surfactant deficiency. Treatment of this pulmonary disease requires the use of mechanical ventilation, resulting in barotrauma to the small and large airways, interstitial damage, inflammation, fibrosis, and cystic changes.

Prevention of BPD is directed toward prevention of RDS by using prenatal steroids, managing preterm labor, postnatal endotracheal administration of surfactant, and using ventilation strategies designed to reduce the effects of barotrauma. Other management strategies include closure of patent ductus arteriosus, fluid management, early diuretic therapy, and good nutrition. More recent strategies, including vitamin A supplementation, antioxidant therapy, and high-frequency oscillation, have reduced the severity of BPD.

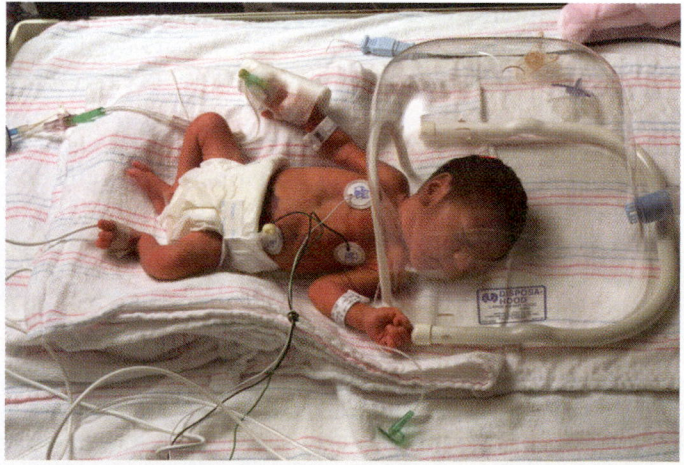

Figure 21-7 Premature infant receiving oxygen therapy through an oxygen hood.

Treatment strategies include a combination of modalities and require a multidisciplinary team approach. Fluid restriction in combination with diuretic therapy while providing adequate nutrition are tremendous challenges for all caregivers. Use of bronchodilators, steroids, and vasodilators is essential in controlling disease progression and managing symptoms.

Nursing care is aimed at providing a stable environment to ensure optimal outcomes. Prevention of hypoxic episodes and close monitoring of the infant's tolerance to procedures and handling are essential. Clustering of care, use of containment during procedures, and sedation often are used to conserve energy expenditure. Energy conservation is extremely important to ensure adequate weight gain and optimal use of calories. Consistent caregivers are important in order to be attuned to subtle changes in the infant's condition that can become serious if early intervention is not provided.

It is essential to have family involvement in the care of these infants. Families must learn to provide the infant's care because many of these infants will go home with monitoring equipment and therapy that may be stressful for the family. A successful transition to home care is dependent on supporting the family structure while the infant is in the hospital. The management and care of these fragile infants with chronic conditions present an ongoing challenge to neonatal caregivers.

Apnea of Prematurity. **Apnea** is defined as the cessation of respirations for more than 20 seconds. Color changes and bradycardia may accompany apnea. Periodic breathing frequently is seen in the premature infant and is described as three or more pauses in respirations, with less than 20 seconds of respirations between pauses.

Apnea may be classified as central or obstructive. Central apnea results secondary to the immature myelination of the neurons in the CNS. The chest wall in the premature infant is highly compliant, resulting in inadequate tidal volume. Obstructive apnea occurs when chest wall movement is evident but no airflow occurs in the nares.

Nursing management is directed toward control of the physical environment through temperature regulation and positioning. When positioning the preterm infant, it is extremely important to avoid neck flexion and, thus, airway obstruction. A good way to position an infant is prone, with neck and shoulder support to decrease flexion.

Exact documentation of the frequency of episodes, duration, severity, resolution, and intervention required is extremely important to determine a pattern, a cause, and adequacy of therapy. Many episodes of apnea may resolve on their own; however, others will require intervention. Intervention may include gentle tactile stimulation, such as stroking the foot. More vigorous stimulation may be needed and can be provided by rubbing the infant's back or soles of the feet. Use care not to rub vigorously enough to bruise the infant. Other interventions include oxygen therapy or positive pressure ventilation with bag and mask.

Medical management of apnea of prematurity includes treatment of the underlying disease process, supportive oxygen therapy, and continuous positive airway pressure. Pharmacologic support is used to stimulate the chemoreceptors in the respiratory center of the CNS, relax bronchial smooth muscle, increase respiratory drive, and increase respiratory muscle activity. The most commonly used methylxanthines are aminophylline, theophylline (Theo-Dur), and caffeine.

Pneumonia. The incidence of pneumonia in the preterm infant is greater than 10% (Lott, 1994) due to immature immune response, extended hospitalizations, and prolonged ventilatory support. The mortality rate for perinatally acquired pneumonia is approximately 20%; for postnatal infections the rate increases to almost 50% (Lott, 1994). The causes of neonatal pneumonia can be divided into three categories: transplacental infections, perinatal infections, and postnatal infections.

Medical treatment requires broad-spectrum antibiotics until the organism is identified. At that time antibiotic therapy is adjusted to suitable drugs for that organism.

SPECIAL CONSIDERATIONS IN CARING FOR THE INFANT AT HIGH RISK

Nurses in the neonatal intensive care unit (NICU) are in a position to provide physical care to infants and psychosocial care to families. This care involves facilitating parent-infant bonding, providing parent education, and serving as advocates for their clients—infants who cannot speak for themselves. Controlling the physical environment, meeting infants' physical and medical needs, and maintaining client records used in medical decision-making are important aspects of the nursing role (Figure 21-8).

Of particular importance in the NICU is alleviating parental anxiety and providing insights into the family's values and cultural preferences for the health care team. The nurse serves as the infant's protector when the parents are not at the bedside and as an interpreter for medical terminology. The following section addresses considerations that affect ill infants whether they are premature, have IUGR, or have other medical conditions.

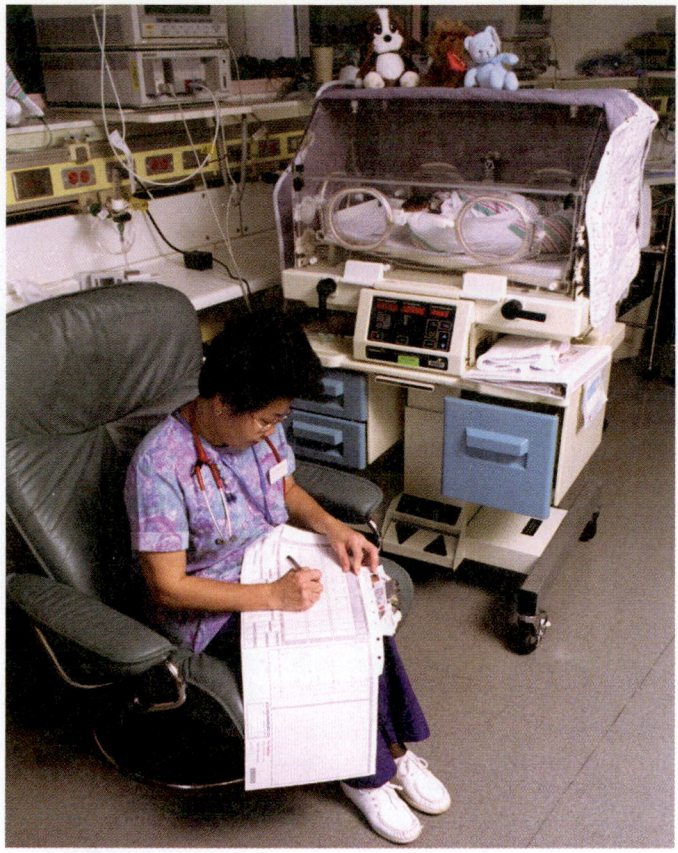

Figure 21-8   Documenting all care given to the high-risk infant is an important nursing responsibility.

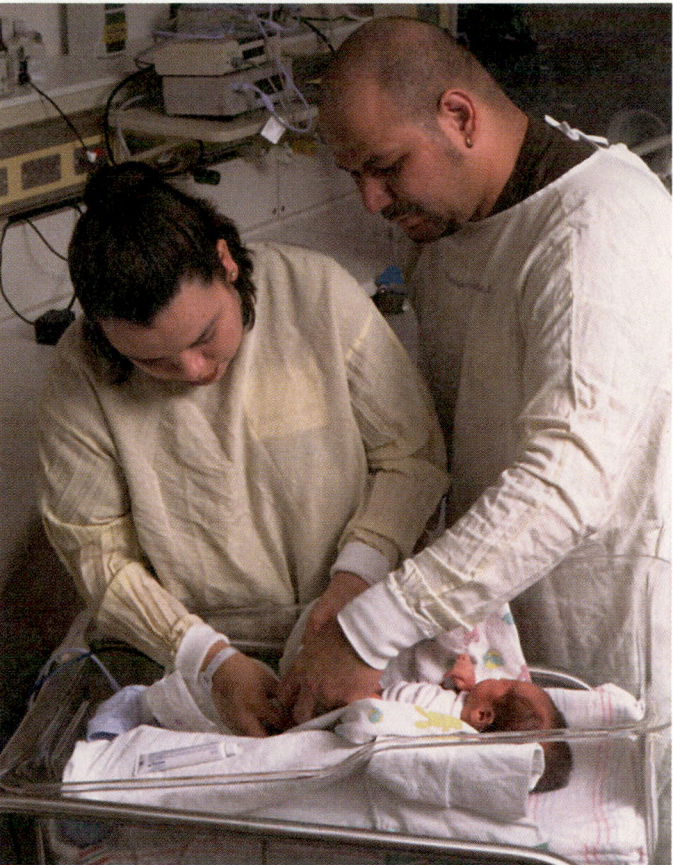

Figure 21-9   Parents of all newborns, especially premature or high-risk newborns, should be encouraged to bond with and care for their new baby.

Families and the High-Risk Infant

Parents play a vital role in shaping the future outcomes of their infants. When an infant is born prematurely and requires intensive care, parents often are not encouraged and facilitated to become active partners in the care of their infant. Parents experience grief over the loss of a full-term healthy newborn and are frequently uncertain about establishing an attachment to the preterm infant because they fear the infant will not survive or they fear the long-term prognosis. Parents with infants in the NICU often need the assistance of the health care team to participate more actively in decisions and in assuming care of their infant. Health care providers must provide opportunities for parents to interact with and care for their infant in developmentally supportive ways. Parental aspects of caregiving for the prematurely born infant can include temperature taking, oral care, diaper changes, and hand swaddling during periods of environmental or procedural stress (Figure 21-9). As the parents gain confidence in caring for their infant and the infant's behavior reflects stability, parental caregiving can evolve to include more complicated tasks, as their infant's care requires.

A key component to parental caregiving in the NICU is helping parents to understand the behavior patterns of premature infants. Parents usually need assistance in interpreting their premature infant's behavior and becoming sensitive and responsive to subtle behavioral and physiologic cues. Parents should be educated to assess their infant for both time-out behaviors and behaviors that support readiness for interaction. Assisting parents to learn appropriate interaction techniques with their preterm infant facilitates ongoing positive social interaction with their infant, allows the parents to contribute to their infant's recovery in a meaningful way, and may set the stage for parental confidence and competence in meeting their infant's needs on discharge to home. As parents become increasingly involved in their infant's care, they can more actively participate in devising their infant's daily plan of care.

Ethical Considerations

The goals of neonatal care are to preserve life, decrease morbidity, and relieve pain and suffering. Technologic

Critical Thinking

Role of Families

When preterm, small, or sick infants are admitted to the NICU, their survival depends on a combination of complex technology and highly skilled caregivers.

- How do you think parents feel when they come into this environment?

- Do you remember the first time you walked into any intensive care unit—adult, pediatric, or neonatal?

- Did you understand the purpose of all the equipment surrounding the client?

- Did you feel comfortable approaching the client the first time?

- How important do you think it is that parents are able to be with their hospitalized newborn?

- Does it matter to the baby?

- Does it matter to the parents?

- Has one of your family members ever been critically ill and hospitalized?

- Was it important to you to be with your family member?

- Was it important for your family member to know you were there?

- What can we do as nurses to make parents feel more welcome in the NICU?

Client Education

Interpreting the Infant's Cues

One of the challenges for parents in caring for their preterm infant is to begin to understand the behavioral cues the baby provides (Figure 21-10). Infants born at full term provide many signals to adults around them that communicate when they are hungry, tired, or ready to interact. These babies cry robustly when hungry or uncomfortable and sleep quietly once they fall asleep. They make eye contact and maintain it, which parents may interpret variously as interest or liking. Parents often respond to such eye contact with deep wonderment and pleasure. In contrast, the preterm infant may produce behavioral cues that are much more ambiguous and difficult for parents to interpret. In the initial period, preterm infants may not be able to be either alertly awake or soundly asleep. Preterm infants often cannot produce the robust cry of the full-term infant to communicate distress. The effort to maintain eye contact with another person also may be overwhelmingly stressful to infants, causing them to avert their eyes (Figure 21-11). At times, parents may interpret this action as rejection or a lack of interest in them (the parents). They may feel that their presence is unimportant to the baby. From the parents' earliest visits to the baby, the nurse should use the opportunity to teach them about the baby's responses. Teach them the signs of stress in their baby and the ways the baby shows comfort and relaxation. For example, show them how the baby's vital signs become more stable, the extremities relax, and movements are smoother. Show them how to change their approach when the baby shows signs of stress, that is, parents' lowering their voices, touching the baby, or talking to the baby (but not doing both at the same time). By using opportunities to help parents get to know their infants throughout the hospitalization, an important part of the discharge planning process will be underway.

advances have been a benefit to many and have improved the mortality and morbidity of premature infants. These advances also have resulted in ethical dilemmas for all parties involved. How small is too small? Whose decision is it to resuscitate an infant born at 23 weeks' gestation? Should infants with lethal anomalies be resuscitated? These are just a few of the questions that face neonatal caregivers.

Nurses are the primary caregivers in the NICU. They need to maintain expertise and objectivity, while providing the family with a supportive and caring environment. These competing obligations make caring for the client more difficult. The role of the nurse should first be as client advocate, to ensure that the care the client is receiving is what is best for that client and the family.

In general, all infants at 24 weeks' gestation and above are considered viable. State and federal laws exist that mandate viability. In all instances, the parents should be given the information that is needed to make informed decisions about therapy and procedures. Most tertiary care centers have ethics committees that can be called on to assist in decision-making processes. The parents or anyone involved in the infant's care can request a committee meeting in which client information is presented, discussion of options occurs, and a collective decision can be made. The caregivers, social services, and support persons of their choice help parents through this process. Of utmost importance is to ensure that the decision is one the parents are comfortable with.

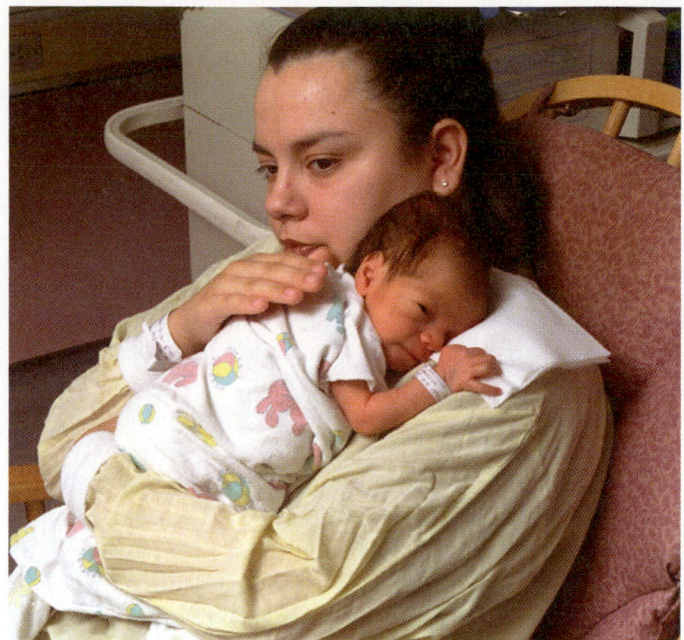

Figure 21-10 Parents will learn the cues to their infant's needs at each visit to the NICU.

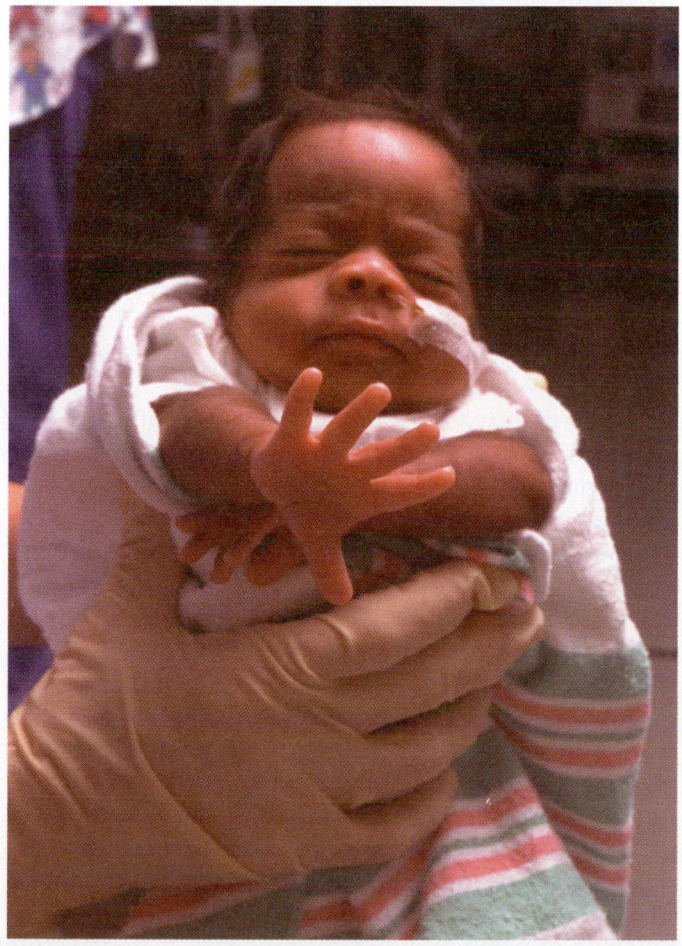

Figure 21-11 Finger splaying is a sign of distress.

Fluid and Nutrition Management

Fluid and nutrition are essential to life. In the newborn who is ill, fluid and nutrition take on added importance. The infant's large surface area, limited storage, and increased metabolic requirements to maintain thermal homeostasis and rapid growth and development greatly increase nutritional needs.

Fluid Management

The management of fluids in the preterm infant may become very complicated. Because of their small size, large surface area, and immature skin barrier, premature infants may have large evaporative losses (insensible water losses). The preterm infant's total body water is 85% to 90%, whereas the term infant's is 80%. The extracellular fluid of the preterm infant is 50% to 55% compared with 45% in the term infant. The major routes of water losses are evaporative from the skin and lungs and excretory from the urinary tract. Mechanisms that increase **insensible water loss (IWL)** include use of radiant warmers and phototherapy.

Fluid losses are inversely proportional to weight and gestational age. The smaller the infant, the greater the fluid losses (Table 21-2). Measures to aid in decreasing IWLs include humidified air and use of plastic blankets or shields.

The overall goal of fluid management is threefold: to maintain normal body fluid composition and volume, to prevent overhydration and dehydration, and to replace ongoing water losses. Fluid needs in the first few days of life usually are higher in infants who have LBW than in larger premature infants or term infants.

Strict monitoring of fluid intake and output is essential. Monitoring the infant's urine output by weighing diapers is necessary to assess fluid status. Evaluating laboratory values also is helpful. The following laboratory tests can assist in maintaining the delicate balance of fluids: serum electrolytes, BUN, and creatinine. Elevated sodium and BUN levels generally indicate a need for fluid. Elevated creatinine indicates renal dysfunction often due to prematurity.

Table 21-2	Fluid Losses in Incubator		
WEIGHT (G)	**INSENSIBLE WATER LOSS (mL/kg)**	**URINE (mL/kg)**	**TOTAL (mL/kg)**
<1,000	65	45	110
1,001–1,250	55	45	100
1,251–1,500	38	45	83
>1,500	17	45	62

All fluids are recorded and considered, including fluids used to mix medications and those used to flush IV lines and catheters. When blood, blood products, and other volume-expanding fluids are used, the measurements also must be included in the infant's daily intake. Electronic pumps designed to administer fluid to a tenth of a milliliter are used to avoid overhydrating an infant. Failing to include medications and blood products in the intake, miscalculating fluid needs, entering an erroneous IV rate, or failing to adjust to decreased urine output in a timely manner can lead to fluid overload. Complications of fluid overload in the premature infant include pulmonary edema, PDA, congestive heart failure, IVH, and BPD.

Weight loss is necessary and expected in the first few days of life (Figure 21-12). Generally, term infants may lose from 10% to 15% of their birth weight, but preterm infants may lose from 15% to 20% of their birth weight. This weight loss is caused by natural diuresis. It is essential to provide adequate nutrition during this time to prevent excess weight loss in an already compromised infant.

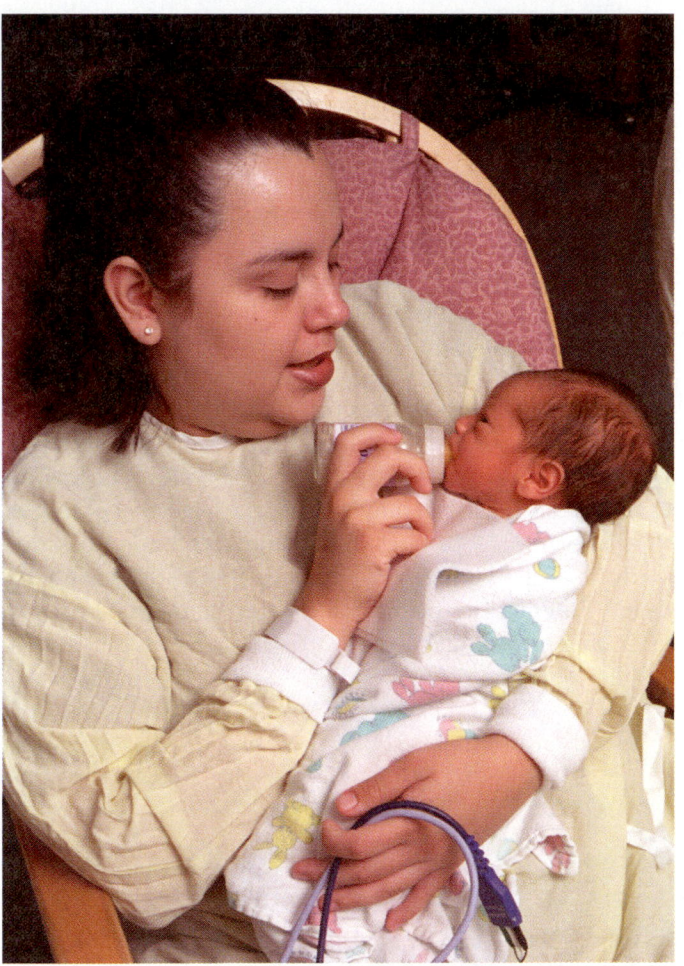

Figure 21-12   At 2 weeks of age, this preterm infant is starting to gain weight.

Fluid management may be divided into short-term and long-term management. Those infants requiring IV fluids for the first few days of life generally are managed on a glucose solution, with the addition of electrolytes and calcium supplements. Very premature and acutely ill infants may require IV fluids for a prolonged period of time. These infants will need a **total parenteral nutrition (TPN)** solution that meets the requirements of carbohydrates, protein, electrolytes, vitamins, and minerals generally received through feedings. These needs generally are met through TPN with intralipids for essential fatty acid requirements.

Various routes are available for parenteral fluid administration in the preterm infant. For short-term access, peripheral lines may be adequate. The nurse generally inserts a small-gauge Teflon catheter into a scalp or peripheral vein. Long-term access is necessary for **very low birth weight (VLBW)** infants, that is, infants weighing 1,500 g or less at birth; **extremely low birth weight (ELBW)** infants, that is, infants weighing 1,000 g or less at birth; and infants who are acutely ill. Long-term access may be achieved with umbilical venous catheters, percutaneous central venous catheters, or central venous catheters. Use of indwelling catheters increases the infant's risk for infection, bleeding, clot formation, and microemboli. Careful monitoring and aseptic technique are necessary.

Electrolyte Management

Electrolyte supplementation usually is not required in the first 24 hours of life and should not be given until urine output is established. The fluid losses from skin, lungs, and urine contain small amounts of electrolytes. By the second day of life maintenance electrolytes are required. At this time, 2 to 4 mEq/kg/d of sodium, potassium, and chloride may be added.

The infant who has VLBW lacks the ability to conserve sodium and potassium. Therefore, sodium requirements may be as high as 9 mEq/kg/d, and potassium requirements 8 to 10 mEq/kg/d.

Hyponatremia (serum sodium less than 125 mg/dL) occurs secondary to sodium wasting with diuretic therapy, GI and renal tubular losses, fluid overload, syndrome of inappropriate antidiuretic hormone, sepsis, and congenital adrenal hyperplasia. **Hypernatremia** (serum sodium greater than 155 mg/dL) is most likely from dehydration or excessive sodium intake (Zenk, Sills, & Koeppel, 2000).

Hyperkalemia (serum potassium greater than 7 mg/dL) occurs as a result of low urine output and immature renal function, specifically distal tubular dysfunction. This condition is life-threatening. Preterm infants may present with electrocardiographic changes. Treatment includes discontinuation of potassium administration, increase in serum glucose levels, and insulin administration.

Glucose Homeostasis

Glucose is the main nutrient necessary for energy, brain metabolism, and CNS integrity. During fetal life, glucose crosses the placenta and is the main source of energy for the growing fetus. After birth, neonates must maintain glucose homeostasis on their own.

Hypoglycemia

Due to immaturity, the preterm infant's metabolism may not be capable of producing and regulating glucose. The preterm infant is at high risk for hypoglycemia secondary to rapid depletion of already low glucose stores and this inability to produce and regulate glucose. **Hypoglycemia** is defined as serum glucose less than 40 mg/dL. Signs and symptoms of hypoglycemia include jitteriness, irritability, cyanosis, seizures, and apnea.

In term infants who are asymptomatic and non-stressed, early feedings can be attempted. This option is less likely for a premature infant because of the inability to suck and lack of nutrients for food absorption. At times, it may be appropriate to provide the early feeding by gavage, retesting 30 minutes after feeding. Infants who are symptomatic and most premature infants will require IV glucose followed by maintenance fluids. Glucose levels are monitored until stable. Treatment of the underlying pathology is essential.

Hyperglycemia

Hyperglycemia is defined as a blood glucose greater than 125 mg/dL in the term infant and greater than 150 mg/dL in the preterm infant. Hyperglycemia is commonly seen in the premature infant. These infants are not able to tolerate a glucose infusion at the same rate as would a more mature infant. This intolerance is due to a decrease in insulin release in response to glucose.

Sepsis, specifically gram-negative sepsis, also increases the risk for hyperglycemia. Certain drugs may cause an increase in glucose levels, including high levels of methylxanthines, which are used in the treatment of apnea of prematurity. Hyperglycemia may be a stress response as

seen in neonates postoperatively. Steroid therapy also produces a hyperglycemic state in preterm infants.

In the infant who has LBW glucose infusions are initiated and increased gradually. Initial fluids are started at 2 to 4 mg/kg/min and gradually increased to 8 to 12 mg/kg/min, depending on the infant's tolerance and needs. The basal metabolic rate in preterm infants is higher than that in term infants and may require higher concentrations of glucose to meet these needs. If the preterm infant is unable to tolerate high glucose concentrations, insulin may be added to the fluids or given as a separate IV drip until levels are under control. In the first few days of life frequent monitoring of glucose levels is extremely important.

Feeding

Nutritional needs for premature infants often are complex. Accelerated needs for calories and minerals cannot always be met through the use of human milk or standard formulas. Approximately 50 to 60 kcal/kg/d are necessary for infants to maintain weight. The term infant may require 100 to 110 kcal/kg/d and the preterm infant from 110 to 140 kcal/kg/d for weight gain.

Formula Feeding

Formulas are available specifically designed for the preterm infant to provide high calorie intake per ounce and extra protein, vitamins, and minerals needed for growth and development (Figure 21-13). Human milk remains the feeding of choice for premature infants. Because of the infant's size and limitations related to the medical conditions, enteral intake may be restricted. Standard formula and human milk at the volumes tolerated by the infant may provide inadequate calories to sustain rapid growth and high metabolic needs. At limited volumes these feedings do not provide adequate minerals for bone mineralization, and **osteopenia** (bone mass below normal levels) may occur.

There are commercial formulas designed for premature infants and commercially prepared fortifiers available to add to expressed human milk that increase the calorie and mineral content of the milk. As the infant grows and is able to tolerate larger volumes of feedings, the formula may be changed to formula designed for term infants or to nonfortified human milk.

Breast Milk Feeding

Mothers who decide to provide breast milk for their infants need encouragement and support. Mothers must be educated on the techniques for expression and correct handling of breast milk. Many hospitals have nurses who specialize in lactation support available to assist these mothers. These lactation consultants are available to

Nursing Alert

Risk Factors for Hypoglycemia

- Decreased nutrient availability
- Endocrine disorders
- Increased utilization
- Sepsis
- Central nervous system abnormalities

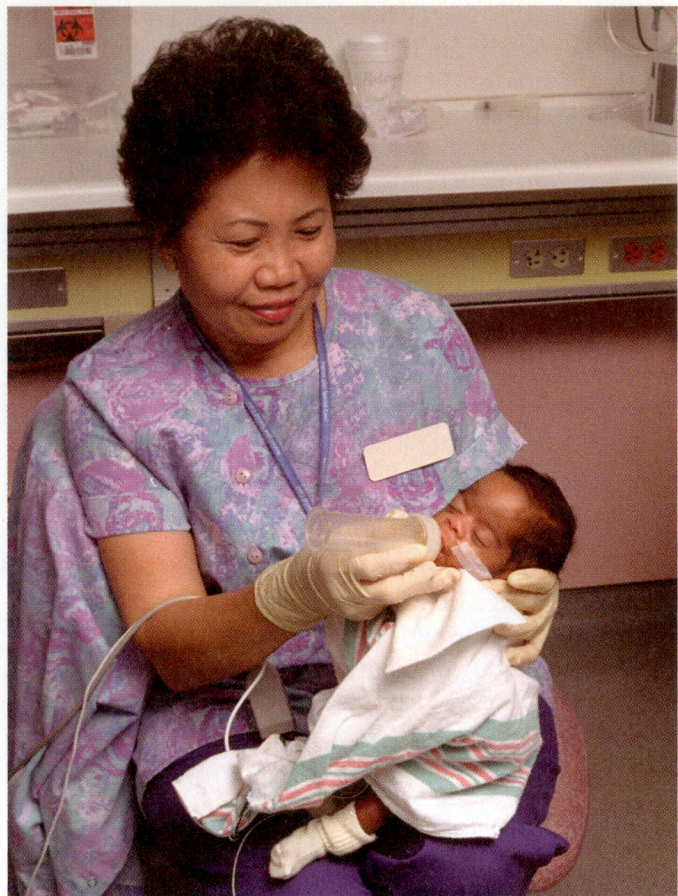

Figure 21-13 This preterm infant receives a specially designed formula to meet his nutritional needs; note placement of a nasogastric tube.

provide support to the mothers during the transition from gavage feedings to breastfeeding.

Initiating Feedings

Determining when to initiate feedings is dependent on several factors: the infant's clinical status, assessment of GI motility, and nutritional needs. Once the infant's condition is stable and stooling has begun, enteral feedings usually may be introduced.

The feeding regimen may vary but generally depends on gestational age and weight. Preterm infants less than 31 week's gestation are unable to coordinate sucking and swallowing with respirations. Therefore, orogastric tube feedings are necessary (Figure 21-14). They may be given as a continuous hourly drip or by intermittent **gavage feedings**, usually every 2 to 3 hours, depending on the infant's tolerance (Box 21-2).

Very premature infants may be started on sterile water, human milk, or half-strength premature formula for the first feedings. These feedings are minute and are used to stimulate GI motility. Larger infants and premature infants who are more mature may be started on

Nursing Tip *Parent Education*

When teaching parents how to check orogastric feeding tube placement, teach them to place the end of the tube in a glass of water after checking placement. The water will bubble with each breath if the tube is in the trachea rather than the stomach. Being able to double-check placement may give parents more confidence in their ability to perform this skill.

human milk or full-strength formula. Once the feedings have been initiated and tolerated, the caloric density and volume of feedings are gradually increased to full-strength 24 cal/oz formula, or fortifiers are added to human milk to increase caloric density to 24 cal/oz. Volume is gradually increased by 15 to 25 mL/kg/d until full feedings are established. A full enteral feeding for a premature infant is 150 to 160 mL/kg/d of premature formula or fortified human milk. Once the infant transitions to 20 cal/oz or nonfortified human milk, the infant must receive at least 180 mL/kg/d.

It is essential for the nurse to watch for the infant's tolerance to feedings and changes in tolerance resulting from an increase in calories or volume. Signs and symptoms of feeding intolerance include increasing gastric residuals, bile in gastric aspirate, blood in gastric contents or stools, abdominal distention, change in bowel pattern or diarrhea, visibly dilated loops of bowel emesis, temperature instability, apnea and bradycardia, and hypoxia.

Infants between 32 and 35 weeks' gestation are generally assessed for readiness to feed by mouth. These include infants born at a younger gestational age and who are now 32 to 35 weeks by postconceptual age and infants who have just been born at this gestational age. If the infant does not demonstrate the ability to coordinate oral

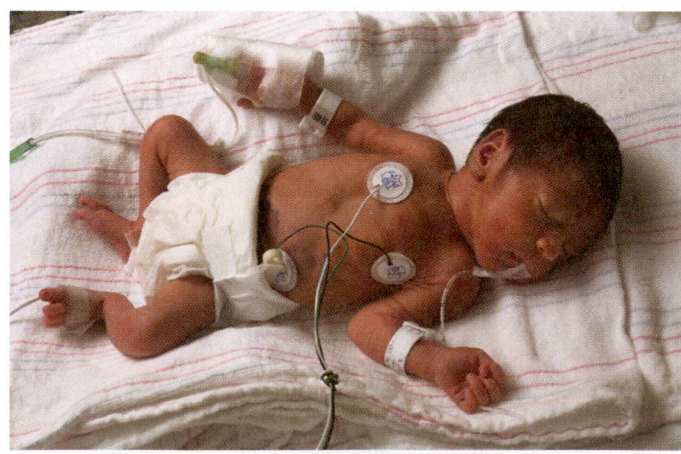

Figure 21-14 Premature infant with orogastric feeding tube.

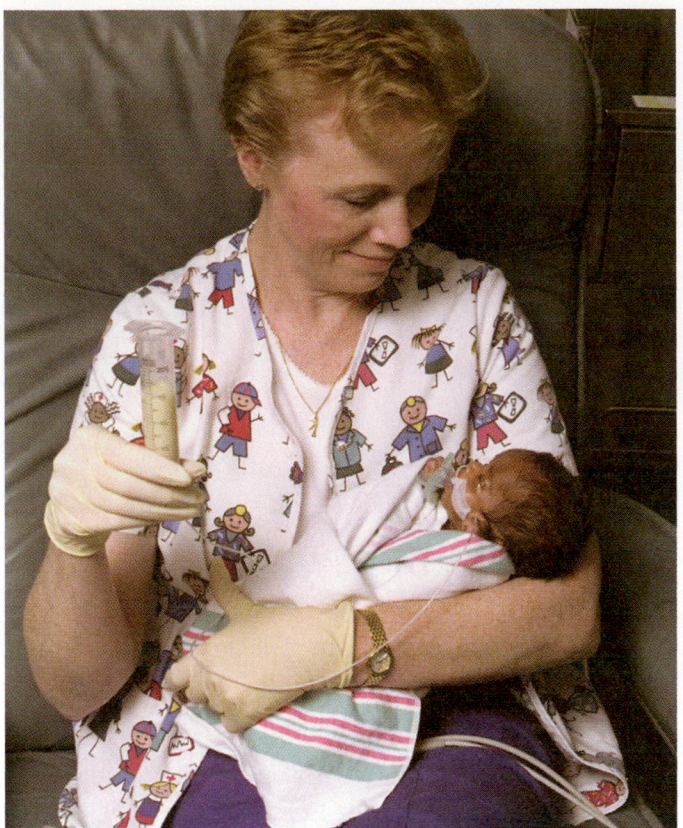

Figure 21-15   This premature infant sucks on a pacifier during his gavage feeding.

feedings (an adequate suck-swallow reflex and breathing) or does not have the stamina to feed orally, gavage feedings are indicated. As discussed previously, volume is increased as tolerated by the infant.

During gavage feedings the infant will require oral stimulation to improve coordination and facial muscle tone. Offering a pacifier during gavage feeds may aid in the development of oral feeding skills (Figure 21-15). Nonnutritive sucking also may be achieved by suckling at the breast once the mother has manually expressed milk.

Occasionally, alternative formulas may be necessary. Because infants who have experienced bowel injury may not tolerate standard or premature formulas, use of elemental or basic formulas may be required. While an important adjunct for feeding high-risk infants, these formulas are not as high in calories and protein as are the premature formulas. When alternative formulas are used, supplementation with carbohydrates and protein is necessary to ensure optimal nutrition.

Pain Assessment and Management

Preterm infants who require specialized neonatal care often are subjected to painful diagnostic and therapeutic procedures. Whereas pain may contribute to immediate

Critical Thinking

Pain in Neonates

In the past, it was thought that newborns were unable to experience pain sensations in the same way as do older children and adults.

- Have you ever watched a newborn when blood was being drawn through a heel stick? How did the baby respond?

- Have you ever had blood drawn or an injection? How did you respond?

- How was your response like or different from the response of the newborn infant?

- Ask yourself what you think is true about a newborn's response to pain.

Critical Thinking

Pain Management

Until just over a decade ago, myths regarding pain in neonates were pervasive in the NICU. Among the two most common myths were that the central nervous system of the preterm neonate was too immature to perceive pain that resulted from common neonatal therapies coupled with the myth that explained the dangers of administering narcotics to neonates. Despite current evidence that neonates have the anatomic and functional capacity to perceive and respond to noxious stimuli, inadequate pain management practices continue to persist within the NICU. Think about it. Would you want to have a chest tube inserted without local and systemic analgesic? Does it make sense when medical care providers say they do not use local anesthesia to perform circumcisions on male infants because the infant cries more when immobilized on the circumcision board than when the prepuce is cut away from the glans penis?

The golden rule of pain management states that what is considered painful for older children and adults must be considered painful in neonates. Think about procedures that are commonly performed on neonates. Which strategies can you use to more effectively advocate for optimal pain management practices within the NICU?

Box 21-2

Oral Gastric Tube Placement

A. Purpose: Provision of enteric feedings when oral feedings are not possible.

B. Action Rationale

1. Immature suck-swallow reflex
2. Abnormal gag reflex secondary to neurologic disease
3. Inability to take full enteric feeding orally
4. Abnormal respiratory pattern
5. For gastric decompression

Contraindications

Recent repair of esophageal fistula or perforation

C. Equipment

1. Cardiac monitor
2. Suction equipment and catheter
3. 5 or 8 F feeding tube
4. 3 or 5 mL syringe
5. Stethoscope
6. Gloves
7. 1/2 in tape, Elastoplast, skin barrier

D. Procedure

1. Wash hands.
2. Put on gloves.
3. Position infant on back.
4. Monitor heart rate, oxygen saturations, and respiratory rate.
5. Gently suction nares and oropharynx.
6. Measure length for insertion by placing catheter tip from tip of the nose to the earlobe to a point just past the xyphoid process and estimating distance (Figure 21-16). Mark length on tube with tape.
7. Moisten end of tube with sterile water.

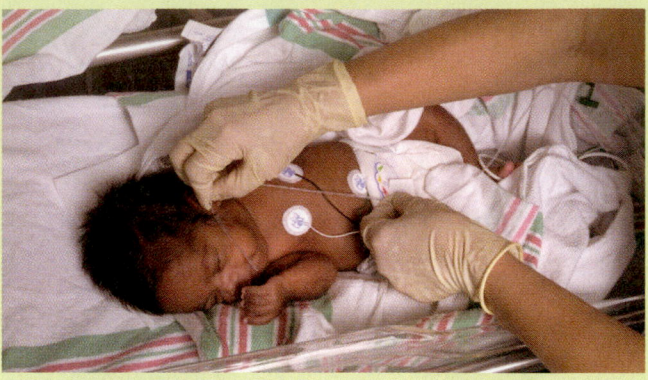

Figure 21-16   Measurement for a nasogastric feeding tube.

8. Place finger on anterior portion of tongue. Stabilize head.
9. Insert tube along finger into oropharynx.
10. Gently advance tube to predetermined length.
11. Use pacifier to stimulate suck-swallow if able.
    a. Do not advance if resistance is met.
    b. Stop procedure if signs of respiratory distress occur.
12. Determine correct placement
    a. Inject 1 mL of air into catheter while auscultating over stomach.
    b. Aspirate contents; note amount and type.
13. Secure catheter to infant's face using pectin-based skin barrier under tape.

E. Follow-up: Observe for the following signs:

1. Apnea or bradycardia
2. Hypoxia
3. Perforation of posterior oropharynx, esophagus, stomach, or duodenum
4. Aspiration or esophagitis
5. Interference with suck reflex

physiologic instability and behavioral state changes, chronic, repeated pain experiences in the NICU also may result in adverse long-term developmental outcomes such as alterations in perceptions of pain in later childhood (Franck & Gregory, 1993; Porter, 1993; Corff, Seideman, Venkataraman, Lutes, & Yates, 1995; Grunau, Whitfield, & Petrie, 1994).

Accurate pain assessment is the first step to optimal pain management. Because pain is a multidimensional phenomenon, pain assessment should incorporate physiologic and behavioral measures. Many physiologic measures of pain have been studied in preterm neonates. The most evidence-based measures include increased heart rate and decreased oxygen saturation (Bozzette, 1993;

> ### Nursing Tip   *Behavioral Signs of Pain in Neonates*
>
> - Cry: change in frequency or pitch
> - Facial changes: brow bulging, vertical furrows, eye squeezing, nasolabial furrow, and open lips
> - Gross motor: attempt to withdraw from painful stimuli (near term infants),
> - Limpness or flaccidity (preterm infants)

Craig, Whitfield, Grunau, Linton, & Hadjistavropoulos, 1993; McIntosh, van Veen, & Brameyer, 1994; Stevens & Johnston, 1994; Stevens, Johnston, & Horton, 1993). Whereas physiologic measures provide greater objectivity in the assessment of pain responses, behavioral measures have been demonstrated to offer more specificity in terms of the pain experience, particularly facial actions. Brow bulge, eye squeeze, nasolabial furrow, and open mouth are the four most common facial patterns demonstrated by both preterm and full-term neonates (Bozzette, 1993; Stevens, Johnston, & Horton, 1993; 1994).

Studies of full-term and preterm infants provide evidence that pain responses vary within the context in which pain is experienced. Therefore, the nurse also must consider contextual factors when assessing for pain in the neonate. Gestational age and behavioral state are the two most powerful contextual modifiers of the pain response in neonates (Craig et al., 1993; Johnston, Stevens, Craig, & Grunau, 1993; Stevens & Johnston, 1994; Stevens et al., 1993; 1994). For example, whereas term infants may respond to painful stimuli with crying and localized deliberate withdrawal responses, 26% to 90% of preterm neonates between 26 and 36 weeks' postconceptional age will not cry in response to noxious stimuli (Johnston, Stevens, Yang & Horton, 1995; Stevens et al., 1994). Infants in awake or alert states also demonstrate a more robust reaction to painful stimuli than do infants in sleep states. Therefore, gestational age and behavioral state may contribute to a less vigorous response pattern, requiring the caregiver to be an astute observer. In order to provide optimal pain management within the NICU, it must be assumed that what is painful to older children and adults is similarly painful to the preterm neonate who has limited behavioral capabilities to respond because of immaturity. It is particularly important to teach parents of hospitalized infants how to assess the pain cues of their child. Parents who are accustomed to seeing pain responses of full-term infants and older children may well not recognize the pain responses of a premature or sick baby.

Instruments for Pain Assessment in Infants

Several multidimensional instruments to assess pain in neonates have been published. The Pain Assessment Tool (PAT) is a multidimensional instrument designed for assessing postoperative pain in preterm and full-term neonates (Hodgkinson, Bear, Thorn, & Van Blaricum, 1994). The PAT includes four behavioral indicators of pain (posture and tone, sleep pattern, facial expression, and cry); four physiologic measures (respiration, heart rate, oxygen saturation, and blood pressure); color; and the nurses' perception of the neonate's pain. Bildner and Krechel (1996) developed the CRIES scale for assessing postoperative pain in preterm and full-term neonates. The acronym CRIES indicates five categories that are scored on a three-point scale (0, 1, 2) and includes *c*rying, *r*equires oxygen to maintain saturation greater than 95%, *i*ncreased vital signs, *e*xpression, and *s*leepless. The third instrument, the Premature Infant Pain Profile (PIPP), developed by Stevens, Johnston, Petryshen, and Taddio (1996), includes two physiologic indicators of pain (heart rate and oxygen saturation), three behavioral variables (brow bulge, eye squeeze, and nasolabial furrow), and two contextual factors (gestational age and behavioral state). The PIPP is scored on a point scale from 0 to 3. Because the PIPP currently is the only multidimensional instrument that incorporates contextual factors that modify the pain response, it may serve to be a very useful instrument in assessing pain in preterm neonates in the NICU.

Management Strategies

In the NICU, critically ill neonates are subjected to frequent painful procedures required for clinical monitoring and intervention. Considering the long-term negative impact of frequent and prolonged pain in preterm infants, strategies to prevent pain must be of paramount concern to health care providers in the NICU. The primary strategy to prevent pain in the high-risk neonate involves the change from protocol-based care to individualized strategic planning, which first evaluates the medical necessity of invasive procedures. This approach would promote caregiving techniques such as the minimal use of tape, use of noninvasive monitoring devices when possible, and tracheal suctioning on an as-needed basis only instead of as a routine procedure. Furthermore, for those procedures deemed medically necessary, careful coordination of painful procedures, such as grouping blood drawings, should be performed to minimize the number of heel sticks and venipunctures per day (Figure 21-17).

Another goal of pain management in infants is to minimize the intensity, duration, and physiologic cost of painful experiences. The intensity and duration of pain

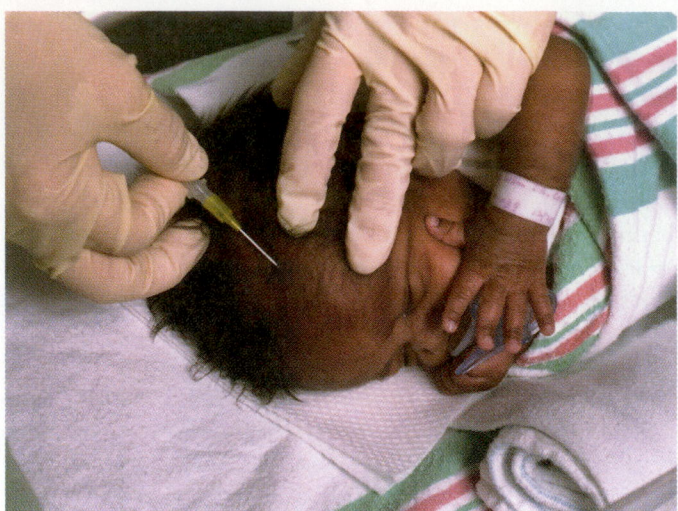

Figure 21-17 Offering a pacifier during a painful procedure, such as venipuncture, can help calm and reassure the infant.

often can be minimized through the use of quick, efficient, and skilled execution of invasive procedures. This goal can be facilitated in units that routinely monitor the competence of their laboratory and nursing staff personnel or units that use only expert staff to attempt invasive procedures, such as intravenous placement, on the most unstable infants or those with a history of difficult intravenous access. Other interventions, such as swaddling, facilitating hand-to-mouth contact, nonnutritive sucking, and touch therapies, also may assist the infant in coping with noxious stimuli. Parents also can play an active role in relieving the stress of their infants in the NICU and should be encouraged to participate in the provision of nonpharmacologic comfort measures whenever possible.

Although nonpharmacologic measures may be used appropriately to manage pain in many circumstances in the NICU, pharmacologic agents should be used when severe or prolonged pain is assessed or anticipated. Optimal treatment of pain in infants in the NICU often has been hindered by persistent fears of health care providers regarding safety, addiction, and respiratory depression associated with the administration of opioids. Although infants younger than 1 month of age and preterm infants generally metabolize pharmacologic agents more slowly and have prolonged elimination times of the drug from their systems, it is believed that analgesic and anesthetic agents can be administered with relative safety in the NICU.

Opioid analgesics are considered the most effective agents to treat moderate to severe pain in neonates. A variety of analgesics is available. The most commonly used analgesics for neonates include morphine and fentanyl (Sublimaze). Although the use of acetaminophen (Tylenol) in neonates is limited by the constraints of the route of administration, acetaminophen may remain an option for treating mild pain in some infants. A summary of the routes of administration, recommended dosages for neonates, and side effects is provided in Table 21-3.

Although sedative and other adjuvant drugs often are used in combination with analgesics, no research is available regarding the efficacy or safety of combining these drugs in the neonatal population. It also must be remembered that sedatives have no analgesic effect and may depress the behavioral expression of pain. Therefore, sedation should be used only if sedation—not pain relief—is required.

Recommendations for Practice

The difficulty with pain measurement in preterm infants arises not from lack of empirical and clinical evidence to support that preterm infants do experience pain, but in the bedside practitioner's ability to accurately assess pain and to determine the potential impact of the experience on any given individual infant. Assessment of pain in the preverbal infant is entirely dependent on the caregiver's ability to properly evaluate pain and is a prerequisite for providing optimal pain management. Unfortunately, because of immaturity, clinical conditions, or therapeutic programs, not all infants respond to pain with clear, robust behaviors. Thus, no single physiologic or behavioral measure should be used in isolation as an exclusive criterion to assess the presence and impact of pain in preterm infants. By combining physiologic and behavioral measures while considering contextual factors, health care

Nursing Tip *Opioid Use in Infants*

Opioids remain the cornerstone of pharmacologic management of moderate to severe pain in neonates. Health care professionals must examine their own personal beliefs about pain management in neonates and acknowledge the prevailing myths that may persist within the NICU in which they practice. Multidisciplinary focus groups may serve as a vehicle to open dialogue and discussions about current practices and to formulate strategies to improve pain management practices within the NICU. Nurses also must continue to systematically study the effectiveness of frequently used nonpharmacologic measures (cuddling, swaddling, touch, hands-off periods, and nonnutritive sucking) to comfort infants undergoing minor painful procedures. As advocates for their small, preverbal clients, nurses must continue to play a major role in conducting research in the area of pain management for preterm infants.

Table 21-3	Drugs, Routes, Recommended Dosages, and Side Effects of Pharmacologic Pain Agents in Neonates			
DRUG	**ROUTES***	**DOSAGE**	**FREQUENCY**	**SIDE EFFECTS**
Morphine	Intermittent IV	0.05–0.2 mg/kg over at least 5 min	As required (usually every 4 h)	• Respiratory depression • Hypotension • Ileus and delayed gastric emptying • Urine retention • Seizures
	Continuous IV infusion IM, SQ	Loading dose 100 μg/kg over 1 h; then 0.01–0.03 mg/kg/h 0.05–0.2 mg/kg	Continuous	
Fentanyl	Intermittent IV	1–4 μg/kg slow IV push	As required (usually every 4 h)	• Respiratory depression • Muscle rigidity • Seizures • Hypotension • Bradycardia
	Continuous IV infusion	1–5.0 μg/kg/h	Continuous IV	• Tolerance with prolonged use • Withdrawal symptoms after 5 days of continuous infusion
Acetaminophen	PO	10–15 mg/kg	Every 6–8 h	• Limited data in neonates • Liver toxicity • Rash
	PR	20–25 mg/kg	Every 6–8 h	• Fever • Thrombocytopenia • Leukopenia • Neutropenia

*IV—intravenous; IM—intramuscular; SQ—subcutaneous; PO—by mouth; PR—per rectum

Note. From *NeoFax: A Manual of Drugs Used in Neonatal Care* (10th ed.) by T. Young and O. Mangum, 1997, Raleigh, NC: Acorn. Copyright 1997 Thomas E. Young and O. Barry Mangum.

providers can better assess pain in preterm infants. Better assessment can best be achieved through the use of a valid and reliable multidimensional pain instrument.

Drug Metabolism and Excretion

The liver and the kidneys are the major organs responsible for removal of drugs from the body. Whereas the metabolism and excretion of therapeutic drugs is well studied in healthy adults, the use of drugs in neonates is not well understood. Drug therapy must be carefully monitored for its tolerance and effect. In discussing drug metabolism absorption, distribution, clearance, and elimination must be considered.

Many factors affect drug absorption in the neonate. The route by which the drug is given plays an important part. For example, for oral administration, the surface area of the intestinal tract is relatively small and the gastric emptying time is prolonged. The bile salt pool size is decreased, and bacterial colonization is not conducive to absorption. IM injection is not feasible long term because of small muscle mass, poor peripheral perfusion, and de-

creased muscle activity. IV drug therapy is best tolerated by the neonate but in most cases requires prolonged IV placement with increased risk for infection.

Factors affecting drug distribution include increased body and extracellular water, decreased amount of plasma protein available for binding, decreased serum pH, and altered cardiac output.

In the preterm infant the liver and all other systems are immature. Hepatic function is decreased in neonates. There are varied hepatic pathways that mature at different points in gestation. Drug metabolism and elimination in the liver, therefore, depend on gestational age.

Renal elimination is directly correlated with the GFR. Extreme caution must be used in administering and monitoring drugs in premature infants. Drug therapy is tailored to the infant and may change daily.

Drug metabolism and elimination must be carefully monitored. Monitoring for therapeutic levels is essential to ensure that treatment is adequate and toxic levels are not reached. Standardized dosing regimens are common in neonates and calculated daily based on the infant's weight.

Complementary Therapy

Neonatal nurses must be prepared to provide holistic family-centered care to the infants in their charge. Nurses can nurture clients and families by their caring and insight. There are nonpharmacologic therapies to enhance the experience of the infant and the family. Some are described in this section. The emphasis is on the premature infant and the infant's family because these infants are often hospitalized for long periods of time.

Developmental Care

Developmental care is a philosophic approach to the care of the premature infant. Premature infants may be hospitalized for a prolonged period of time and are subjected to many tests, procedures, and therapies during hospitalization. Developmental care is an approach designed to support the infant's efforts toward self-regulation.

The term developmental care is used broadly to describe any infant care protocol designed to promote optimal physical, cognitive, and emotional development in the first weeks or months of life. Whereas the protocols described as developmental care differ from one setting to another, they generally address issues of environmental light, sound, and temperature levels; infant position, containment, and handling strategies; nonnutritive sucking; and managing twins.

Elements of Developmental Care

The elements considered part of developmental care can and do vary somewhat among clinical sites. In general, however, these elements can be divided into those related to the total nursery environment, such as light and sound (macro-environment), and those related to the individual infant's environment or care experiences, such as positioning and handling (micro-environment).

Nursing Tip *Individualized Developmental Care*

Individualized Developmental Care refers to the modification of the nursery environment and caregiving practices to support the infant's optimal development. This approach to care includes the reduction of excessive environmental stimuli by lowering light and sound levels in the NICU; organizing caregiving activities to provide periods of rest and recovery for the infant; positioning the infant in a flexed, contained position; modifying caregiving practices based on an assessment of what the individual infant finds least distressing; and supporting the infant's efforts to provide self-comfort and maintain physiologic stability and organization.

Macro-environment Components

The macro-environment of the high-risk infant is considered to be all of those elements that define the caregiving milieu, that is, the conditions that define the surrounding space in which caregiving occurs. This macro-environment has been found to have a major impact on the development of prematurely born and high-risk infants. The macro-environment is one aspect of the infant's neonatal experience in which nursing has a major responsibility. The macro-environmental components to be discussed include the levels and patterns of NICU light and sound and temperature control.

Light. One element common to many developmental care protocols is the control of light levels in the infant's environment. Some protocols prescribe consistently dim lights throughout the 24-hour day, whereas others recommend regularly scheduled times when the lights are dimmed.

Peak light exposure for the infant is associated with supplementary light sources such as phototherapy lamps, treatment lamps, and, most dramatically, extensive direct window exposure supplementing artificial lighting. Within hospitals, illumination levels were found to be highest in the areas of highest infant acuity and perhaps greatest infant vulnerability to negative effects of excessive illumination.

The level of illumination for any particular infant in a nursery also may vary according to placement of the incubator in relation to windows, overhead lighting, and other nursery equipment. The total light exposure of an infant also depends on factors such as the use of eye shields, frequency with which the fluorescent tubes are changed in both the phototherapy unit and rooms of the unit, and use of additional lighting for instrumentation and other procedures. The position of the infant's head also can influence light exposure. When the infant is in a side-lying position, the lower eye receives less light exposure than does the upper eye. The potential exists for

---

Critical Thinking

Light Patterns

When you are thinking about the effects of lighting levels and patterns in the NICU, ask yourself how light affects you. Which kind of lighting is restful or quieting? When you are ill or tired, which kind of lighting do you prefer? What do you know about the effects of continuous lighting on adults? How do you think light levels affect sound levels?

infants lying in a supine position to be staring directly into the overhead lights. Therefore, illumination levels described for a NICU may or may not be representative of the conditions experienced by an individual infant, and comparisons between nurseries are difficult to make.

Recommendations for Practice

In the past, continuous lighting levels of 60 to 100 ft-c (approximately the light level in an office or classroom) were thought to be necessary to allow adequate evaluation of the infant's skin color and perfusion from any area of the NICU. Although, at this time there is no established standard for light levels in the NICU, within the concept of developmental care lower light levels (±20 ft-c) are recommended. Current standards for NICU lighting recommend that light levels be adjustable over a range of 1 to 60 ft-c (Consensus Committee to Establish Recommended Standards for Nursery ICU Design, 1999). At this time no recommendation can be made for the implementation of light-dark cycles in the nursery. Specific strategies for reducing the effects of lighting on the infant in the NICU include the following:

- Avoid the use of overhead lights unless necessary. Use individual lighting at the infant's bedside for caregiving.

- Incubator covers can be used during times when the infant is at rest. Small, thin receiving-type blankets may not provide optimal light shielding for the infant. Opaque covers that cover the top and the sides of the incubator are preferable.

- Outside windows often are the source of the highest light levels in the NICU. When outside windows are present, opaque shades of some type should be available to allow modifications of light levels, and incubators should be placed away from direct sunlight.

- When overhead phototherapy lights are used, ensure that the infants in adjacent incubators are screened from any increase in light levels.

- Shield the infant's eyes when using treatment lights for procedures or caregiving. Place a screen between the treatment light and adjacent incubators to protect those infants from random light exposure.

- When the infant is placed in a supine or side-lying position with the face upward, ensure that the infant is not directly under an overhead light. Preterm infants may not have the ability to turn their heads away from the light or to adequately shield their eyes by closing them.

- Education of the family about the infant's development and caregiving needs should include explanations of the concerns about light levels and the precautions taken to protect the baby from excessive light. The nurse may help the family reflect on their own practices in relation to light levels in an infant's environment. Do they darken the room in which an infant is sleeping? Do they protect a baby's eyes from bright sunlight?

Sound. Over the past 3 decades researchers have repeatedly documented consistent sound levels of 50 to 90 dB in the NICU, with excursions to as high as 120 dB (Robertson & Philbin, 1996). For the purpose of comparison, 50 dB is about the sound level of light traffic and 90 dB is about that generated by light machinery (Figure 21-18). According to the Occupational Safety and Health Administration standards, 80 dB is the highest sound level that

---

Critical Thinking

Effects of Sound

Sound levels or sharp unexpected noises can negatively affect the sick or immature infant.

- How do you respond when you hear an unexpected sharp noise such as a car backfiring nearby or a door slamming? Do you startle?

- What happens to your heart rate and breathing?

- How do you feel when you have been in a very noisy environment for several hours?

- Do you think a premature or sick baby will respond differently or in the same way as you do?

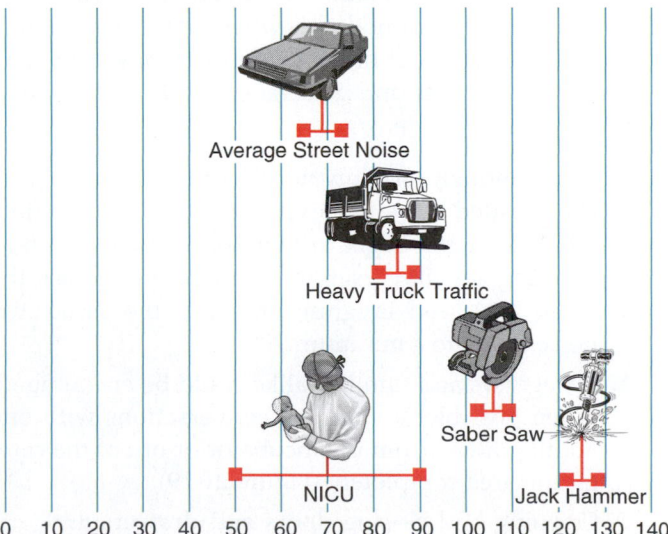

Figure 21-18 NICU sound levels (in dB) relative to other common environments.

Nursing Alert

Ototoxic Drugs in the NICU

Sound levels in the NICU have not been proved to have a negative effect on the development of hearing in the hospitalized preterm infant. Particular concern, however, is focused on the interaction of excessive ambient sound levels with ototoxic drugs the infant may receive while hospitalized. These drugs include but are not limited to the aminoglycosides, such as gentamicin, kanamycin (Kantrex), streptomycin, and tobramycin (Nebcin), when used for more than 5 days. An additional ototoxic effect may occur when loop diuretics (diuretics acting on the loop of Henle), such as furosemide (Lasix), ethacrynic acid (Edecrin), bumetanide (Bumex) and others, are given with aminoglycosides. Nurses should be alert to the possible risks posed to infants by these drugs alone or in interaction with the NICU environment.

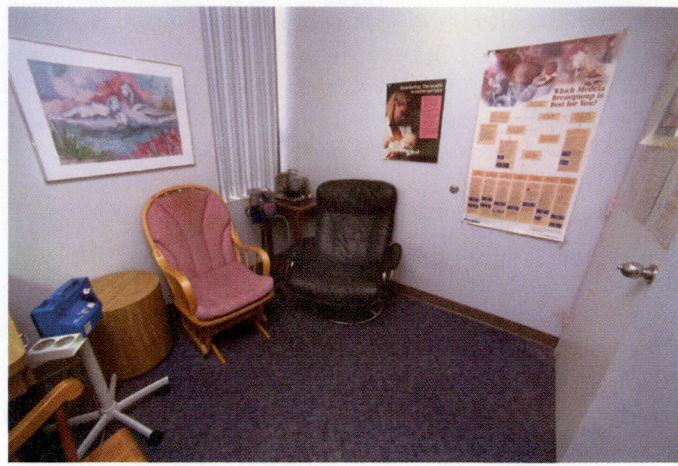

Figure 21-19   Many NICUs have a separate room in which families can spend quiet time with their newborn.

does not produce measurable damage, regardless of the duration of the sound, and 90 dB is the limit imposed in industrial standards as the highest safe level for an 8-hour period for adults. The NICU noise level also has been found to demonstrate little diurnal variation and fluctuations in sound.

Recommendations for Practice

A review of the research related to the effect of nursery sound on the developing low-birth-weight infant does provide support for realistic concern and justification for the modification of sound levels where possible, although it does not provide definitive evidence of any long-term effects of excessive sound. Several suggestions for sound reduction can be made:

- Some, though certainly not all, of the noxious noise is generated by staff activities that can be modified. NICU staff can begin to monitor activities, such as carrying on conversations with people across the room and loud laughing, to keep the associated noise levels to a minimum.

- Caregivers and families alike could be encouraged, when possible, to conduct conversations with one another away from the incubator or out of the caregiving area completely (Figure 21-19).

- Opening and closing doors and drawers and manipulating equipment can be done in ways that keep noise to a minimum. One source of noise could be minimized simply by depressing the latch on the in-

cubator ports before closing them or applying some felt stripping around the incubator doors.

- Where possible, metal equipment such as wastebaskets could be replaced with plastic to reduce the associated noise level.

- Radios, intercoms, and other extraneous sound could be eliminated from the NICU.

- Equipment used in the nursery could be modified where possible to reduce the sound reaching the baby. Computer printers could be equipped with soundproofed covers. Telephones could be placed away from the caregiving area or equipped with flashers rather than ringers. Monitor alarms could be replaced with quieter audible alarms or flashing alarms.

- The use of carpeting and acoustical ceilings where possible can significantly reduce noise levels.

- When considering new or replacement equipment or other items for the nursery, the noise level generated by those items or equipment should be a primary consideration. Sound levels inside the incubator certainly are determined in large part by the noise of the machinery itself, and such noise levels should become part of the selection criteria.

- Specific guidelines for acceptable noise levels should be established for the NICU. These could be used as a standard when selecting nursery equipment and would serve to encourage manufacturers to design and develop quieter equipment for use in the NICU. Such guidelines also could be used to evaluate caregiving procedures.

Temperature.   Maintenance of a normal body temperature is an extremely important aspect of nursing care of the preterm neonate. A healthy term infant is able to initiate temperature regulation by heat production within a few hours after birth. Term and preterm infants who are ill do not have this ability. The newborn can produce heat through four mechanisms: metabolic processes, voluntary muscle activity, peripheral vasoconstriction, and nonshivering thermogenesis (Kenner et al., 1998). The preterm infant is limited in the ability to produce heat as a result of decreased glycogen stores in the liver, decreased brown fat availability, small muscle mass, and increased body surface area.

The infant can lose heat by four modes of heat transfer: evaporation, conduction, convection, and radiation. It is important for nurses caring for premature infants to understand these concepts to prevent cold stress in infants (Box 21-3).

Evaporation is the loss of heat as water is lost from the skin to the environment. It is important to dry an infant rapidly after birth to prevent evaporative heat loss and cold stress. *Conduction* is the transfer of heat from one object to another when in direct contact. For example, placement on a cold scale to weigh the infant will result in heat from the infant's body being transferred to the scale. Placing a warm blanket on the scale first, and returning the dial to zero, before weighing the infant helps prevent conductive heat loss. Electronically warmed scales are available to help maintain the infant's temperature.

Convection is the loss of heat from an object to the environment. The use of servo-controlled incubators and neutral thermal temperature charts determines the best incubator temperature to prevent heat loss and minimize oxygen and calorie consumption so important in the care of the premature infant. When caring for an infant, use of portholes instead of opening the incubator door prevents rapid heat loss from the incubator. Open only the portholes of the incubator on one side at a time to prevent cross-ventilation and heat loss from the incubator. When nursed in a bassinet or on a warmer, the infant should be protected from drafts.

Radiation is the loss of heat between objects that are not in direct contact. A cold window near the infant's incubator would allow the wall of the incubator to cool. The infant would then lose heat to the cool incubator wall. The use of double-walled incubators and incubator covers helps prevent heat loss by radiation.

Once these conditions are controlled in the environment of a preterm infant, maintenance of body temperature is easier. Signs and symptoms of hypothermia and hyperthermia are outlined in Box 21-4. The consequences of hypothermia include hypoglycemia, pulmonary vasoconstriction, altered surfactant production, metabolic acidosis, hypoxia, and weight loss or poor weight gain (Blackburn, 2003).

Box 21-3

Preventing Cold Stress in the Premature Infant

Evaporation
- Dry at delivery.
- Dry after bathing.
- Keep linens dry.
- Use plastic-wrap blankets.
- Use heat shields.
- Use humidified air.

Conduction
- Prewarm the bedding.
- Use a warmed scale.
- Cover X-ray plates.
- Warm the diapers.
- Warm the water and cleansers.

Convection
- Warm the environment.
- Avoid drafts.
- Cover up the infant.
- Use head caps.

Radiation
- Avoid windows.
- Use incubator covers.
- Use a double-walled incubator.

Box 21-4

Signs of Thermal Stress

Hypothermia
- Mottling, pallor
- Acrocyanosis
- Cyanosis
- Bradycardia
- Tachypnea
- Apnea
- Lethargy
- Hypotonia
- Poor feeding or feeding intolerance

Hyperthermia
- Flushing
- Hypotension
- Diaphoresis
- Tachycardia
- Tachypnea
- Apnea
- Irritability

Nursing Tip **Maintaining an Appropriate Thermal Environment**

Maintenance of a neutral thermal environment is extremely important in the management of all aspects of caring for a premature infant.

When rewarming an infant who has been stressed by cold, it is important to increase the temperature gradually. Rapid rewarming may result in hypotension from peripheral vasodilation and apnea.

Consequences of hyperthermia include an increased metabolic rate, leading to increased oxygen consumption and dehydration from increased insensible water loss. Peripheral vasodilation may result in hypotension (Kenner et al., 1998). Seizures and apnea also may occur (Merenstein & Gardner, 2002).

All types of warming devices used in the care of preterm infants have benefits and risks. Shown in Figure 21-20 are a radiant warmer and one type of incubator. Heat shields, plastic-wrap blankets, hats, warming pads, and skin protectors are useful tools in temperature regulation. Skin-to-skin holding also is of benefit in heat conservation for infants and is discussed later in this chapter.

Recommendations for Practice

Understanding the sources of heat loss has enabled nurses to modify the infant's environment to minimize such losses. Some suggested interventions follow:

- Place incubators or radiant warmers away from external wall and windows and away from drafts.
- Use thermal shades on windows.
- Prewarm incubators and radiant warmers before placing the infant in them.
- Ensure use of double-walled incubators.
- Place warmed blankets on surfaces, such as scales, that will be in contact with the infant.
- Warm blankets before wrapping the infant.
- Avoid opening the incubator unnecessarily.
- Use the plastic sleeves on the portholes when caring for the baby. It also is important to teach families to use the sleeves on the portholes.
- Use side guards to protect the baby from air currents when using a radiant warmer.
- Keep infants in incubators swaddled (Figure 21-21).
- Keep the baby's head covered. Many nurseries use soft knit hats for this purpose.
- Replace wet blankets immediately with dry, warmed ones.

- Warm and humidify oxygen before administration.
- Prewarm solutions for the infant that are either applied externally or used internally such as intravenous medications.

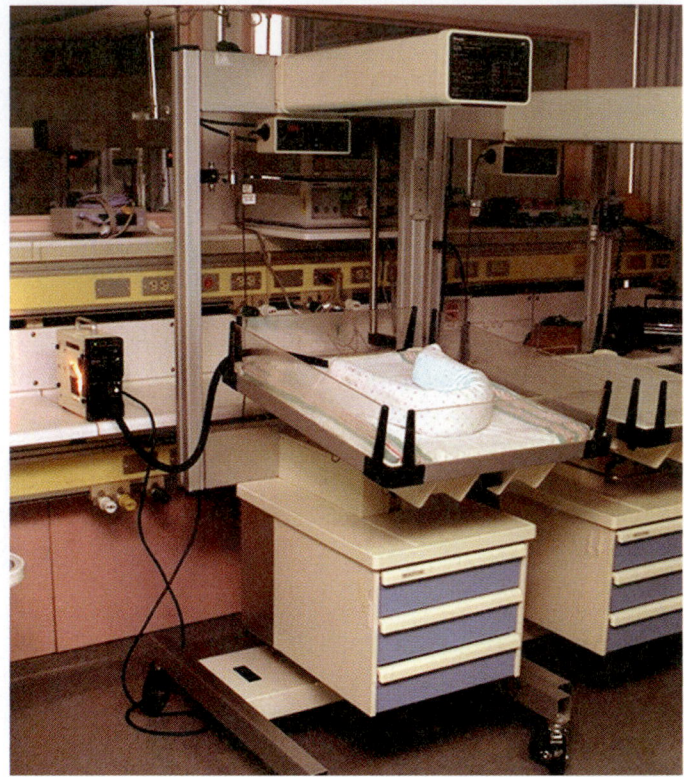

A.

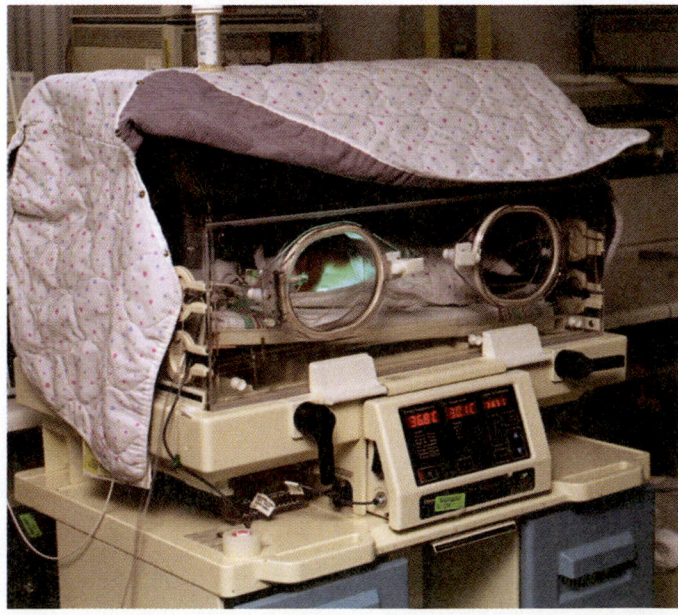

B.

Figure 21-20 A. Radiant warmer. B. Covered incubator with portholes.

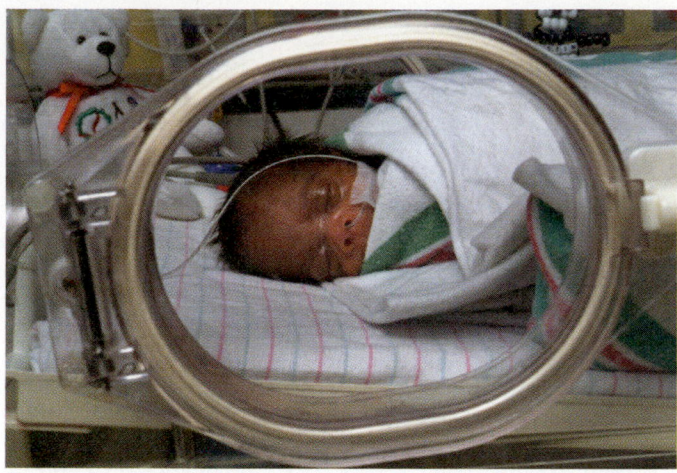

Figure 21-21   Infants in incubators should be swaddled comfortably to prevent heat loss.

Micro-environment Components

The second set of elements included in developmental care protocols are those specifically related to the environment or care experiences of the individual infant. As a group these components can be considered the **microenvironment** or individual sensory environment of the infant. The components of the micro-environment discussed include positioning and containment strategies, handling and touching, and nonnutritive sucking.

Positioning and Containment Strategies. Current thought related to neonatal positioning in the NICU has evolved primarily from the study of the intrauterine posture of the fetus. The intrauterine environment is such that the fetus is aided in maintaining a position of flexion as well as midline posture. This flexed, midline position is important for normal motor development but also serves to facilitate hand-to-face and mouth behaviors, which provide opportunities for sucking and self-calming behaviors. Increasing evidence suggests that supportive positioning and handling of preterm neonates in the NICU may promote more normal motor development and minimize the chances of developing abnormal movement patterns (Jorgensen, 1993; Perez-Woods, Malloy, & Tse, 1992).

   Containment is the use of the hands to support the infant in a midline position during painful or noxious procedures. Also referred to as facilitated touch or gentle human touch, containment consists of a caregiver placing one hand on the infant's head and the other on either the infant's bottom or legs in a tucked position, and providing firm but gentle pressure (Figure 21-22). Containment has been shown to increase the infant's tolerance of procedures; provide faster return to baseline levels of vital signs on completion; cause less hypoxia, tachypnea, and tachycardia; and result in less energy expenditure.

Nursing Alert

Recommendations for Infant Positioning Related to Sudden Infant Death Syndrome

Until 1992, the standard of practice for positioning was to place the infant in a prone position, particularly after feeding. The rationale was that the prone position decreased the infant's risks for aspiration of vomitus. In preterm infants, the prone position also was found to produce longer sleep periods, improved respiratory effort, and decreased heart rate compared with the supine position (Masterson, Zucker, & Schulze, 1987). In the early 1990s, studies of Sudden Infant Death Syndrome (SIDS) began to link the prone position when sleeping with a significantly increased risk for SIDS. As these data emerged, the American Academy of Pediatrics (2000) issued a recommendation that the prone sleeping position no longer be used for healthy infants under 6 months of age. Whereas these recommendations are not specific to the hospitalized preterm infant, they have raised concerns about the use of the prone position for this population. These concerns have resulted in an increased use of the side-lying position in developmental care protocols, although few data are available describing the effects of the side-lying position on heart rate, respiratory rate, sleep duration, or infant state compared with the prone or supine sleeping positions. Discharge planning for all infants including the preterm or high-risk infant should include teaching the parents about the risks for SIDS and the precautions to take.

Recommendations for Practice

The primary goal of supportive positioning for the preterm infant is to encourage a balance between flexion and extension (Figure 21-23). Careful attention also should be paid to maintaining body symmetry while enhancing midline orientation of extremities. The goals of

Nursing Tip   *Prone Position*

Although the prone position often is preferred to enhance physiologic stability in preterm infants, you need to accustom infants to side- or supine-lying positions before discharge because these positions will be recommended to parents to reduce the risk for SIDS.

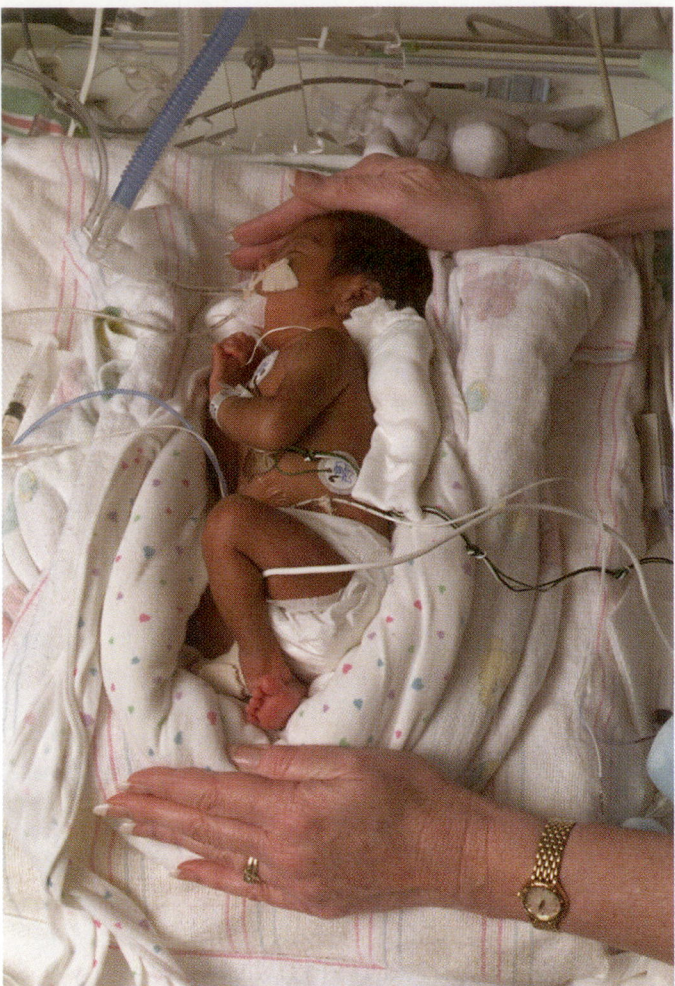

Figure 21-22   This premature infant is sleeping in the side-lying position; the nurse is containing the infant with her hands to offer a sense of warmth and security.

Critical Thinking

Positioning and Containment

Preterm infants are growing and developing in the hospital nursery environment during a period of time when they normally still would be growing and developing in their mother's uterus. It is this uterine environment that is most appropriate for the fetus and in which the fetus will grow and develop optimally. Think about how different the NICU environment is from the uterine environment. In the third trimester, the developing fetus would maintain a curled up flexed position, held there by the uterine walls. In contrast, in the NICU infants often are put in a supine, open position, which has been thought to make caregiving easier.

In the third trimester, the developing fetus also would feel the surrounding uterine walls as barriers or boundaries. As the fetus moves or kicks, the fetus impacts the uterine wall and feels the resistance and containment of that barrier. In contrast, in the NICU infants often are positioned in the center of the incubator or warmer bed, away from any barrier that could provide a sense of containment comparable with the uterine environment.

- How can the developmental care strategies for positioning and containment provide sensory input similar to that which infants would have received if they had remained in the uterus until gestational term?

- Which behavioral changes would you expect to see in preterm infants as you implement the positioning and containment strategies that are part of developmental care?

developmentally supportive positioning can be accomplished in a variety of prone, lateral, and supine positions. Some developmentally supportive positioning interventions include the following:

- Provide boundaries that maintain the infant's position in flexion while allowing the infant adequate room for extension (Figure 21-24).

- Whenever possible, encourage side-lying positions for the acutely ill or recovering preterm infant.

- Provide midline orientation to facilitate hand-to-mouth activities and prevent shoulder retraction.

- To avoid head molding, use gel products or water pillows and reposition frequently.

- Use the smallest diaper available to prevent hip abduction.

- When positioning the infant in the prone position, prevent external hip rotation by placing a roll under the hips, thus supporting the pelvis and allowing the knees to be flexed and tucked in. An additional blanket roll that encircles the lower extremities and extends up to the upper thorax will provide opportunities for the infant to brace against as well as facilitate hand-to-mouth behaviors. To avoid hyperextension of the neck, the head should be kept in a neutral position or with the chin tucked slightly toward the chest.

- The side-lying position may be used to make midline orientation easier and allow opportunities for the infant to engage in sucking and self-calming behaviors. The infant can be properly positioned in the lateral position by placing a wedge or blanket roll

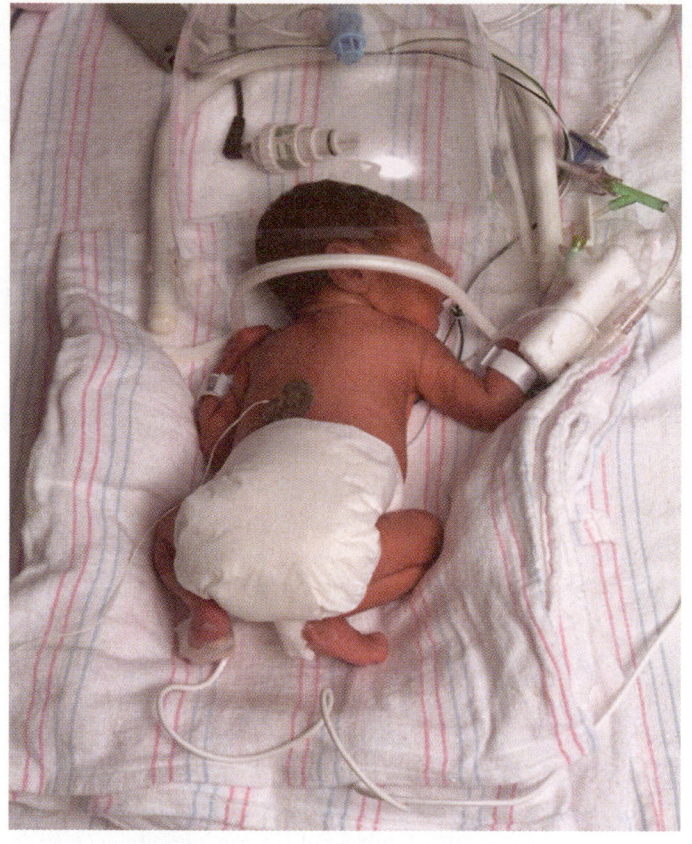

A.

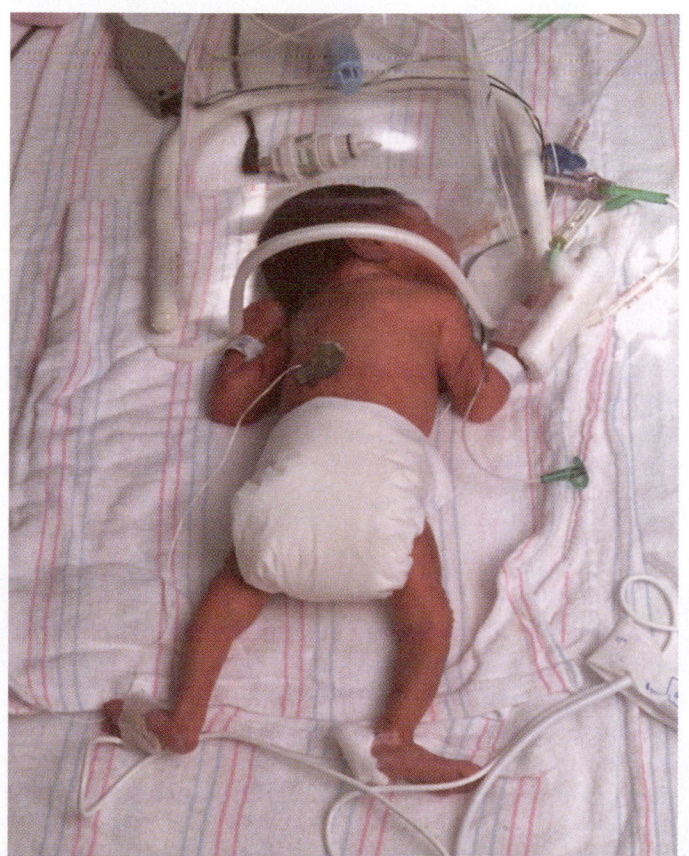

B.

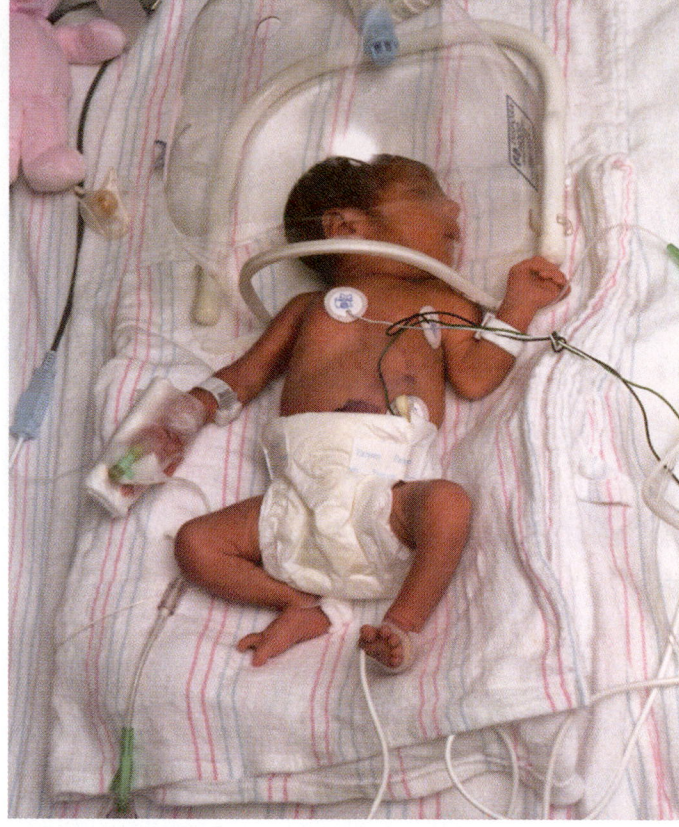

C.

Figure 21-23   Developmental positioning of the preterm infant
A. Prone, flexed (frog-legged position) B. Prone, extended position
C. Supine position.

Client Education

Infant Positioning

When parents are present, talk with them as you position the baby. This is an opportunity to teach them how to position their infant and to practice positioning the baby with you there to support them. Talk with them about where the baby will sleep at home and how they will be able to position the baby with the supplies available to them in the home environment. A variety of positioning aids have become available on the commercial market to assist in developmentally supportive positioning, although many of these represent a significant expense. Point out to parents that although you may use some specialized equipment in the hospital, they will be able to position their baby appropriately using blanket rolls or small receiving blankets. Also discuss some of the concerns about using pillows and loose blankets in the crib with the infant (AAP, 2000).

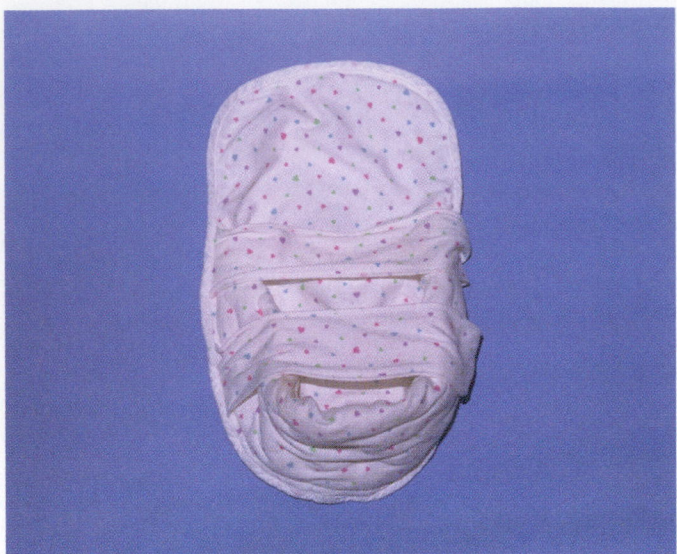

Figure 21-24 Swaddling-type bedding provides soft boundaries for the newborn.

behind the infant's back, with a folded sheet placed across the pelvis and tucked into the bedding. Doing so will facilitate flexion of extremities and maintain the trunk perpendicular to the bed surface. Neutral lower extremity positioning also may be made easier by placing a soft roll between the infant's legs. Furthermore, a soft, thin blanket roll or small stuffed toy can be positioned at the anterior midline to encourage slight forward rounding of the spine and to prevent trunk arching. Finally, the head should be kept in midline or with the chin tucked slightly toward the chest.

■ Supine positioning may be required for the provision of necessary medical care in the acutely ill preterm infant. In the supine position, the head, body, and feet can be supported midline, using soft blanket rolls positioned close to the infant. Lateral rolls should make rounding of the shoulders easier by gently lifting and supporting the arms off the bed. A small roll under the knees will make hip and knee flexion easier, thereby preventing hip abduction. Finally, a blanket roll placed at the bottom of the feet will provide containment and improve muscle tone by providing a surface against which to flex.

Handling and Touching. Adequate rest is a primary prerequisite for optimal recovery of human beings experiencing acute and chronic conditions. Preterm infants in the NICU, however, often are subjected to frequent caregiving episodes. Indeed, the NICU is an environment in which the caregiving episodes are not only frequent but also intense, often painful or stressful, and involve multiple caregivers.

Critical Thinking

Patterns of Caregiving

To provide optimal developmental support, any approach to caregiving must be embraced by all caregivers who come into contact with the infant. The care of the high-risk neonate involves the coordinated efforts of a full multidisciplinary team, including nurses, pharmacists, physicians, medicine, respiratory therapists, and X-ray technicians. Each member of the team has an important role in the care of the infant; however, all members may not be aware of the total demands on the infant's limited energy reserves. Neonatal nurses are in a key position to act as advocates for high-risk neonates to protect them from unnecessary handling or to structure the necessary care to provide for optimal rest and recovery.

● If you felt that the caregiving activities for an infant in your care were not allowing the infant to have periods of rest and recovery, how would you begin to modify those patterns?

■ How would you work with caregivers from other disciplines in organizing the care activities of an infant?

Although most of the caregiving activities are a necessary part of medical care, some disruptions of the infant that occur daily in the NICU could be deemed unnecessary and poorly timed. Adverse physiologic changes noted with handling include hypoxemia, tachycardia, bradycardia, tachypnea, apnea, and increased intracranial pressures. Frequent caregiver handling also has been associated with behavioral distress and may interfere with normal sleep patterns that are important for neurologic organization and growth (Appleton, 1997). Conversely, developmentally supportive handling allows for longer periods of sleep; results in earlier transition to oral feedings; and reduces hospital stays, with improved long-term outcomes (Lotas & Walden, 1996).

Organization of Care

Two strategies are necessary in reducing the infant's stress with handling during caregiving. First, all routine caregiving actions should be evaluated and unnecessary ones eliminated. Another strategy used by nurses to modify this continuous activity level is to cluster or group the infant's care in a way that protects some blocks of time for the baby to rest. This effort is based on two critical components: timing of caregiving and individualization of caregiving approaches to provide optimal rest and recovery for the infant. Neonatal nurses must coordinate the infant's care to decrease the frequency of disruptive contacts while providing periods of uninterrupted rest. To accomplish this, many NICUs have implemented hands-off times during which all nonemergency procedures are postponed to ensure infants an opportunity for undisturbed sleep. Caregiving activities are grouped together and typically timed to coincide with scheduled events such as feedings (Figure 21-25). Optimally, caregiving would also coincide with the infant's awake or more alert periods. Such clustering of care activities, although providing the infant with increased opportunities for undisturbed sleep, may not be tolerated by the acutely ill neonate. Since physiologically unstable infants may become easily stressed with handling, infant cues such as grimacing, changes in muscle tone, heart rate, respiratory rate, and color should be used to evaluate the individual infant's tolerance for caregiving activities at a particular time. An infant's tolerance to handling may be observed through behavioral cues suggesting stress and disorganization (Table 21-4). Developmentally supportive caregiving individualizes care so that infant stress behaviors are minimized and self-regulatory behaviors facilitated.

Touch Therapies

Although the negative effects of excessive handling on preterm infants are well documented, several researchers have argued that certain kinds of supplemental touch therapies may be beneficial to preterm neonates. Some researchers have reported that supplemental tactile stimulation, such as infant massage, results in improved performance on developmental tests, increased growth and weight gain, early discharge, reduced behavioral distress, and improved parental bonding and attachment (Field et al., 1986; Field, Scafid, & Schanberg, 1987; Whitley & Cowan, 1991; Nelson, Heitman, & Jennings, 1986;

Harrison and Woods, 1991; Paterson, 1990; Russell, 1993). These studies were performed with medically stable preterm infants, however, and may not be appropriate for younger, sicker preterm neonates.

Other forms of touch have been found to be therapeutic in supporting or facilitating the infant in maintaining or regaining physiologic organization or stability when stressed, for example, the use of touching to provide gentle containment of the infant's extremities during a stressful procedure and allowing the infant to hold the caregiver's finger. It is important to recognize that touching is a powerful stimulus that can be both stressful and disorganizing, or soothing and organizing. Sensitive evaluation of the infant's individual response to a specific stimulus at a particular time is the most important skill for the nurse to develop in approaching the care of the preterm infant.

Kangaroo Care

Kangaroo care originated in Bogota, Columbia, as a necessity for providing preterm infants with warmth and closeness with the mother. Kangaroo care consists of a parent holding an infant, unclothed except for a diaper, upright on the mother's or father's chest. The parents are instructed to wear a shirt that opens in the front. This technique also is called skin-to-skin holding (Figure 21-26).

The benefits for the parents include feelings of well-being, feeling a part of their infant's care, enhanced parent-infant attachment, and self-confidence and self-esteem. The benefits for the infant include better weight gain, temperature regulation, decreased apnea, improved oxygenation, earlier discharge, increase in breastfeeding and increased supply, and earlier time to oral feeding. Kangaroo care, once viewed as an alternative therapy, is now common in most NICUs (Victor & Person, 1994).

Recommendations for Practice

Guidelines for appropriate handling of preterm infants are based on the characteristics of handling, the timing of caregiving activities, and individualizing care based on

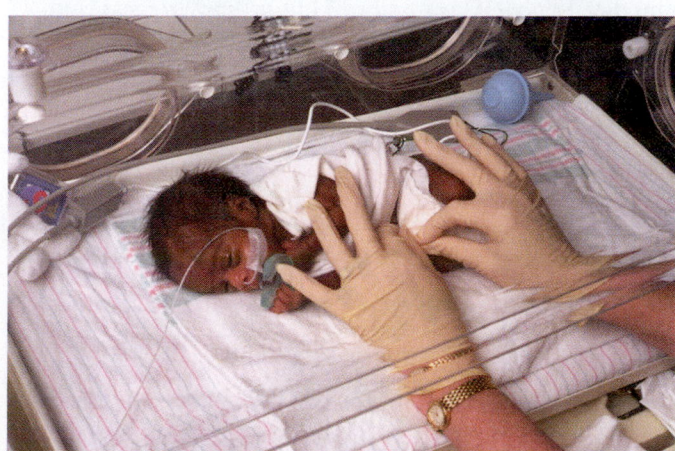

Figure 21-25   While this infant is awake, the nurse offers him a pacifier and schedules routine activities such as diaper changes.

Nursing Tip   *Touch Therapies*

Therapeutic touch and healing touch are very different from infant massage because they may use very gentle tactile stimulation or even may provide no physical contact. These touch therapies may be useful in the high-risk neonate because they are less likely to cause overstimulation.

Table 21-4 **Stress Signals and Self-Regulatory Behaviors for Autonomic, Motor, and State Subsystems of Functions**

SUBSYSTEM	BEHAVIOR	STRESS	SELF-REGULATORY
Autonomic	Respiratory	Irregular, slow, fast, pauses	Regular
	Color	Pale (gray), webbed, red, dusky, blue	Pink
	Instability-related patterns	Tremors, startles, twitches, yawning, sneezing	Absence of tremors, startles, twitches, yawning, sneezing
	Visceral and respiratory	Spitting up, gagging, hiccoughing, bowel movement grunting, sounds, sighing, gasping	Stable viscera as evidenced by absence of visceral and respiratory stress behaviors
Motor	General extremity and trunk	Flaccidity: arms, legs, postural hyperextension, arching, stretch-down, diffuse squirming	Flexed, tucked arms and legs; well-regulated tone; trunk tucking; leg and foot bracing
	Face	Gape face, tongue extensions, grimacing; mouthing; frowning	Hand on face, suck searching, sucking
	Specific extremity movement	Finger splaying, airplaning, saluting, sitting on air, fisting	Hand clasping, foot clasping, hand-to-mouth, grasping, holding on
State	Sleep-awake states	Diffuse sleep-awake states, eye floating, fussing; discharge; smiling	Clear, robust sleep states

Note. Adapted from "Toward a Synactive Theory of Development: Promise for the Assessment and Support of Infant Individuality," by H. Als, 1982, *Infant Mental Health Journal, 3*(4), pp. 237–238. Copyright 1982 Michigan Association for Infant Mental Health.

Reflections from a Mother

I couldn't think the first time they took me into the NICU to see my son. There were so many machines, so many people, so many other babies. All the babies were very quiet and still. When I saw my son I was terrified. He didn't look like I thought he would, like any other baby I had ever seen, or like me or like my husband. I didn't see how he could ever live or be normal. He was so small. I just felt helpless and wanted to cry.

The nurses said the next time I came in I could hold him, but I didn't know if I wanted to. I knew I should feel something different—like other mothers do. I should be overwhelmed with love for him, but he didn't seem to be a part of me. I wanted to feel like a mother, but I couldn't. All I could do was cry. The nurses said that when I came back the second time I could do "kangaroo care" with him. They explained what I needed to do and said that I would hold my baby on my chest between my breasts.

When I came back, the nurses had me stand by my baby's incubator while they picked him up, nestled him into my chest, and helped me sit down in a large comfortable chair. As he nestled in, they covered both of us with a soft warm blanket. He squirmed a little. I could feel him move against me—almost like when he was in the womb. Then he fell asleep. He looked very comfortable, and I wasn't afraid anymore. The nurse showed me how his heart rate, temperature, and everything else was stable—just like it should be. I just kept looking and looking at him. It was like I couldn't get enough of him. I think he has my husband's chin and my long fingers.

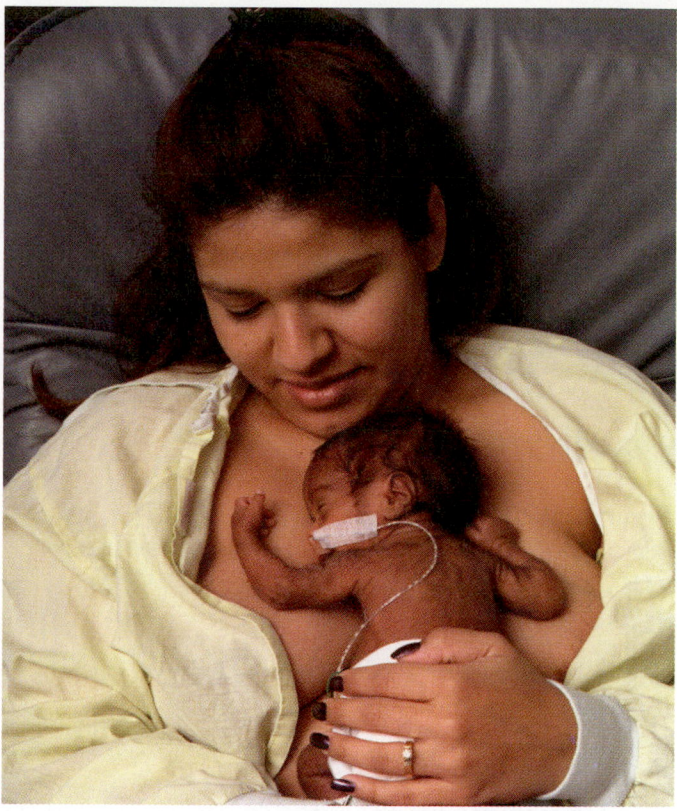

Figure 21-26   Kangaroo care, or skin-to-skin holding, has many benefits for the parent and infant.

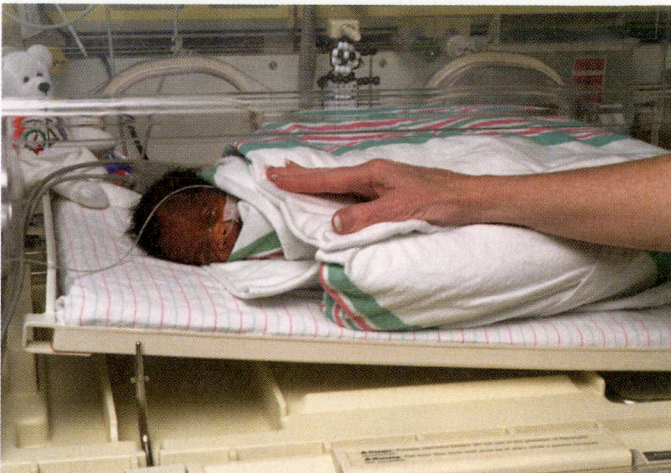

Figure 21-27   The nurse gently places a hand on the infant to signal the start of caregiving.

the infant's physiologic and behavioral responses to caregiving. Recommendations for handling of preterm neonates during caregiving follow:

Characteristics of Handling

- Use slow, gentle movements when handling the preterm infant.
- Use alerting techniques, that is, speaking softly to the infant or gently placing your hand on the infant, to prevent startling and signal the start of caregiving (Figure 21-27).
- Perform caregiving activities in an unhurried manner and allow time outs when the infant shows marked signs of stress.
- Provide extra caregiving hands or boundary support during difficult and uncomfortable procedures.
- Provide **facilitated tucking** with caregiving hands or boundary support until the infant settles after care, remaining at the bedside for at least 2 to 5 minutes after completion of any procedure.
- Bathe the infant while providing support with swaddling.

- Perform caregiving with the infant in a prone or side-lying position to minimizing the need for repositioning, thereby reducing handling and stress.
- Weigh the infant while swaddled or in a containment device to maintain the infant's level of physiologic organization. The blanket or other containment device can be weighed separately so that its weight can be deducted from the infant's weight.

Timing of Care

- Time caregiving activities around the sleep-wake cycles of the infant.
- Protect periods of sleep, providing 2 to 3 hours of uninterrupted sleep.
- Use electronic monitoring devices for continuous display and routine assessment of physiologic parameters. Perform hands-on assessment of vital signs once per shift to correlate monitor readings, thereby minimizing infant handling.
- Cluster caregiving activities as much as possible without evoking a stress response in the infant.
- Gather all necessary supplies before disturbing the infant.
- Use signs at the bedside to remind all caregivers of scheduled touch times, thereby promoting periods of undisturbed sleep.

Evaluate Infant Responses

- Assess all caregiving activities for necessity, and avoid the use of routine procedures.
- Recognize stress behaviors, and use these in organizing the infant's care according to individual tolerance levels.

- Document and communicate an individualized plan of care based on infant behavioral cues of stress and self-regulation.

Recommendations for Kangaroo Care

- Kangaroo care is an important intervention for preterm and high-risk infants. Before initiating kangaroo care with a mother and infant, it is important that the nurse be thoroughly knowledgeable about the process and that the process be explained fully to the parent.

- An in-service program by a clinician experienced in the use of kangaroo care would be an important step in preparing to implement this procedure in a nursery.

- Before implementing kangaroo care, ensure that you have a comfortable chair and, if possible, arrange for some privacy for the parent. A screen around the isolette can be used to provide some sense of private space.

- Arrange the timing of the kangaroo care in relation to other caregiving activities so that it is not necessary for anyone to interrupt the mother while she holds her baby.

- If the mother is planning to breast-feed, the period of kangaroo care can be an opportunity to initiate feeding. Evaluate for this before the beginning of kangaroo care.

- Kangaroo care also has been found to be beneficial for fathers in terms of facilitating their developing relationship with the baby. Offer the opportunity for kangaroo care to fathers when possible.

Nonnutritive Sucking. Nonnutritive sucking has been associated with numerous positive outcomes for preterm neonates (Figure 21-28). Positive benefits documented from nonnutritive sucking include improved oxygenation levels during gavage feedings and at rest, enhanced weight gain, earlier transition from gavage to oral feedings, increased levels of alertness before feedings, and shorter hospital stays (McCain, 1992). The benefits of nonnutritive sucking have been well documented; however, caregivers have noted that the smallest infants in the nursery who could benefit from nonnutritive sucking have difficulty owing to the size of most available pacifiers. Pacifiers designed for the term infant, and even those appropriately sized for the older premature infant (those born at 30 weeks' gestational age or older), may be too large for the younger preterm infant. Pacifiers, such as the Wee Thumbie, designed for very small preterm infants allow the nurse to provide important sucking opportunities for these babies. This pacifier was designed from developmental theories to simulate thumb sucking

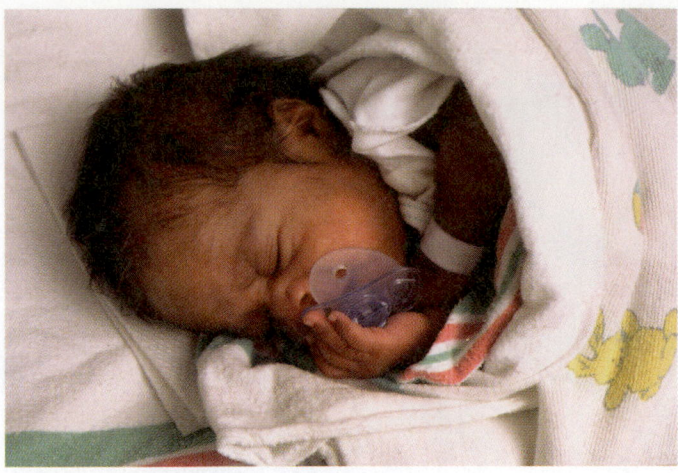

Figure 21-28   Nonnutritive sucking on a Wee-Thumbie pacifier helps this infant who has low birth weight remain calm and conserve energy.

in utero. It has been tested on low-birth-weight infants (Engebretson & Wardell, 1997).

Recommendations for Practice

- Experiment with the available pacifiers to find the one best suited for an individual baby. Infants may demonstrate more effective sucking behavior with a particular size and style of pacifier.

- When infants are given bolus gavage feeding, nonnutritive sucking opportunities should be provided before initiation of the feeding and continued for a few minutes after the feeding is completed.

- When infants are continuously fed, nonnutritive sucking opportunities should be offered on a regular schedule such as 20 minutes every 3 to 4 hours.

- Nonnutritive sucking opportunities should be offered to even very immature infants who are not able to demonstrate a sustained organized suck. These early sucking behaviors may be important in stimulating the neurobehavioral development of the infant.

- Offer a pacifier to the infant who is fussy, restless, or irritable. Nonnutritive sucking is one of the mechanisms infants use to calm and comfort themselves.

- Do not provide an empty nipple or one stuffed with cotton to the infant. Use only an approved pacifier that meets federal safety standards.

Co-Bedding of Twins

Placing newborn twins together may provide support for the infants during transition to extrauterine life. Twins may be born with unique expectation of what constitutes

Critical Thinking

Nonnutritive Sucking

Infants in utero are able to bring their hands to their mouths by the middle of the second trimester. Often, sonograms taken during the second trimester show the fetus apparently sucking its thumb. Preterm infants, however, rarely show any spontaneous thumb sucking. Unlike in the watery uterine environment in which they can move freely and their flexed position helps bring their hands to their mouths, preterm infants in the NICU rarely are able to get their hands to their mouths. Think about it. If sucking often is seen on sonography in the second trimester, it must be a common behavior. If sucking is a common behavior in the developing fetus, is it just a chance occurrence or is it, in some way, important to fetal development? If it is important to fetal development, then is it important for the development of the preterm infant in the NICU? In studying this question, researchers have found that when preterm infants were given regular opportunities for nonnutritive sucking, they demonstrated more rapid weight gain and shorter hospital stays as well as changes in infant behavioral state and activity (McCain, 1992).

a normal habitat, and their transition to extrauterine life may be facilitated by maintaining contact with each other. This contact is thought to be supportive in nature (coregulating) (Nyquist & Lutes, 1998). Co-bedding is based on the premise that extrauterine adaptation of twin neonates is enhanced by continued physical contact with the other twin rather than the sudden deprivation of such stimuli (Nyquist & Lutes, 1998).

An improvement in temperature regulation and behavioral states has been observed in co-bedding. Cobedding may facilitate the development of similar circadian rhythm patterns and sleep-wake cycles. The effects of co-bedding and the value of supporting synchronized behavior in twins require additional evaluation (Nyquist & Lutes, 1998).

NEONATAL TRANSPORT

Because care of small and premature infants requires specialized equipment and highly trained personnel, many infants require transport to regional centers where the needs of the infants can be met. Moving these infants requires a well-integrated system of assessment and perinatal transport.

Perinatal centers are designated according to their ability to handle complicated maternal and neonatal conditions. A level I center generally is a community hospital that is designed to care for the normal pregnant woman and delivery of a well newborn. A level II center is designed to handle more complex pregnancies and deliveries, and the nursery is prepared to care for infants with mild and intermediate conditions. A level III center is one that cares for the most complex obstetric and neonatal complications and conditions. A level III center also has the latest diagnostic techniques and the subspecialists necessary to care for infants with uncommon illnesses.

Maternal Transport versus Neonatal Transport

When a pregnancy is determined to be at high risk, plans can be made early to deliver the infant in a tertiary center. Mothers who go into premature labor may have no problems before the onset of labor. Transport of the pregnant mother to a center equipped to care for both her and the infant is the preferred method of transport.

When an infant is transported inside the womb there is no risk of exposure to cold stress or hypoglycemia, which are serious potential risks of neonatal transport. Transferring the pregnant woman who is in preterm labor allows the possibility of stopping labor on arrival at the tertiary care center.

Because high-risk deliveries may follow uneventful pregnancies, all hospitals must be set up to resuscitate and stabilize newborn infants. The American Heart Association and the American Academy of Pediatrics have developed a program called the Neonatal Resuscitation Program that addresses the needs of neonatal clients in the delivery room (AHA & AAP, 2000).

When a premature or infant at high risk is born at a level I or II perinatal center, a transport team with specialized equipment and training is required to move the infant to a regional center. Problems that develop during neonatal transport may be serious. Thermal stress, equipment failure, and other unexpected events may occur.

Neonatal Transport Team

Neonatal transport teams were developed to provide access to limited health care resources. They are composed of highly trained personnel experienced in the care of premature and infants at high risk. These teams extend the care of the level III perinatal center to the community with their expertise and specially designed equipment (Figure 21-29).

Members of the neonatal transport team assist the referring unit with stabilization of the infant before transport. Infants must have the following before being transported: normal temperature, normal blood sugar level, and blood pressure within the normal range; stable airway, either breathing easily on their own or with an endotracheal tube in place; normal blood gas values, normal electrolyte values, and acid-base balance. When infection is suspected, treatment must begin before transport.

Parents should have the opportunity to see and touch their infant before transport. Small mementos of the infant are important. A lock of hair, the infant's footprints, or a picture may be given to the parents. Mothers should be encouraged to continue with plans for breastfeeding if that was their intent before delivery. Mothers should be encouraged to begin expressing breast milk as soon as possible after delivery and be referred to a lactation consultant or support group if the infant will not be able to breastfeed shortly after birth.

Back Transport

Level III nurseries often are located far from the parent's home. The location may make access difficult for some parents. Distance, traffic, weather, and parking costs are barriers to the nursery. When the infant no longer needs the expertise and support services offered by the level III nursery return transport should be considered as the infant's condition improves.

Return transport, or back transport, refers to transporting the infant back to the referral hospital for care until the infant is ready to go home. Return transport provides a number of advantages. The costs incurred at a community hospital are frequently lower than those at a tertiary center. If the infant is nearer the parents' home, they may have the opportunity to visit more frequently. Close proximity makes parent teaching easier and increases parents' familiarity with the care of their infant.

The infant's pediatrician can assume primary care and facilitate discharge planning.

DISCHARGE PLANNING

Preparations for discharge of a high-risk preterm infant should begin on admission to the ICU. Many factors must be considered, and the discharge process often can be traumatic for the family. Providing a smooth transition for the infant and the parents is essential (Figure 21-30).

Criteria to be met before discharge include the infant's ability to maintain temperature in an open crib, steady weight gain, ability to breastfeed or bottle-feed, and absence of apnea or appropriate monitoring devices available at home. In some instances the infant may be discharged before being able to take all feedings orally. In these cases, the parents must be able to demonstrate the ability to provide alternate feeding strategies.

As the infant approaches being discharged, parents should be encouraged to assume more responsibility for the infant's care. In many units a special area is set aside for families to stay at the hospital for 24 to 48 hours before discharge and care for their babies with the support of the nursing staff. This opportunity allows the family to become comfortable with caring for the infant, when they

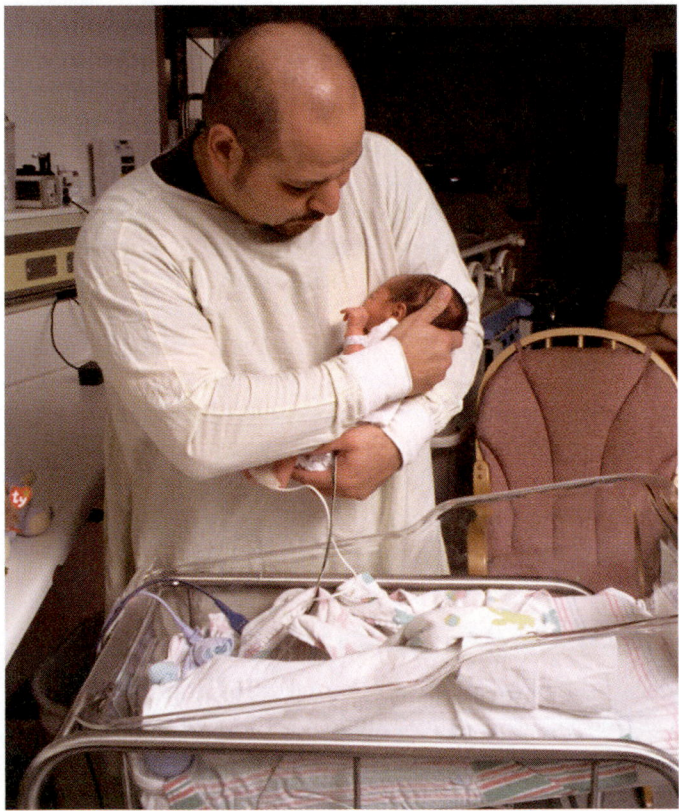

Figure 21-30 Parents need to develop comfort and confidence with their newborn before discharge.

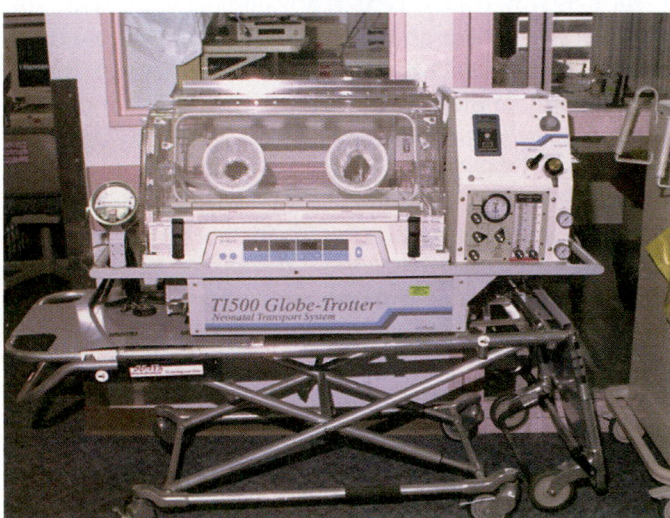

Figure 21-29 Transport incubator.

Nursing Tip

Changing Role of the NICU Nurse

One of the gaps in the care of the preterm or high-risk infant has been in the lack of support to families in making the transition from the hospital to the home with their infants. As infants have been discharged from NICUs younger, smaller, and with more complex care needs, the challenge to families has increased. NICUs are beginning to explore the efficacy and efficiency of having nurses from the intensive care environment work with the parents in preparation for discharge and then make home visits after the infant's discharge. The nurse, who is already familiar with the infant and the infant's care needs and with the parents (and they with the nurse), can provide support, consultation, and teaching to facilitate the family's adjustment to their new circumstances.

have someone readily available to answer questions, and for the nurse to identify and address possible areas of concern before the infant's discharge. A particular focus at this time should be for the nurse and parents to discuss how each aspect of caregiving will be managed in the home environment. It is important to remember that parents may need some help in adapting the caregiving procedures they see in the nursery to the situation they will face at home. When possible, a home visit before the infant's discharge will be invaluable in assisting parents to make this transition.

In addition to the routine care of the infant, discharge teaching should include discussions on how to evaluate the infant's signs and symptoms of illness. The nurse may need to teach the parents how to take a temperature and

ensure that the parents have a thermometer in the home. Guidelines on when to call the clinic or pediatrician and when to go to the emergency room also are helpful. It is helpful to speak with parents about who they have available as a personal support system. Are extended family members, friends, or members of a church or other religious community available? If so it may be appropriate to involve that person in the teaching process in the hospital.

The discharge process is a multidisciplinary team effort. Involvement of the primary nurse or advanced practice nurse, neonatologist, social services, respiratory services, occupational therapists, physical therapists, and appropriate consultants is essential for a smooth transition. Follow-up needs should be reviewed and their importance emphasized.

Resources are available in the community for parents of infants at high risk. Early childhood intervention programs provide for many of the follow-up services needed and are generally available nationwide. These programs also provide for transition from one stage of development to another. Support programs are common in urban areas, often through tertiary care centers and religious organizations. Ideally parents should have access to professional advice by telephone. Many nurseries also provide routine telephone follow-up after discharge.

Financial planning must be addressed with the family early in the clinical course. Due to advances in technology, smaller and sicker infants are surviving. Insurance provisions often are used up while the infant is hospitalized. Assisting the family with the process of obtaining financial aid is critical, and social services plays an integral part in this process.

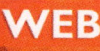

COLLABORATIVE CARE

Potential Discharge Needs for a Premature Infant

- Pediatrician capable of complex care
- Developmental follow-up
- Ophthalmologist
- Pulmonary specialists
- Speech and language therapists
- Occupational therapists
- Nutritionist

WEB ACTIVITIES

••• Search the Internet for Web sites offering information on some of the disorders discussed in this chapter, such as NEC, GER, BPD, and ROP.

••• Visit the Internet to find support groups for parents of infants who are SGA, LGA, and premature. Do these sites have chat rooms? Information exchanges? Literature for sale?

••• Compare the statistics of your state on low-birth-weight incidence, teenage pregnancy, and infant mortality and morbidity rates with the goals outlined in "Healthy People 2010."

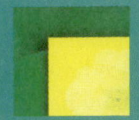

CASE STUDY/CARE PLAN
INFANT BORN AT 28 WEEKS' GESTATION

Nurses caring for preterm neonates can individualize care to make the infant's growth and development easier by modifying the environment and initiating interventions that make the infant's self-regulatory action easier or have a calming effect on the infant. This requires careful monitoring of both the infant and the environment and continual adaptation of care. The following case study illustrates not only the nursing process, but within each diagnosis a specific illustration of the dynamic adaptation of the nursing interventions to the changes in the neonate and the environment.

At 2:08 a.m.: Kevin was born at 28 weeks' gestational age. His birth weight was 987 g and his Apgar scores were 5 (minus 1 for heart rate, 2 for color, 1 for respirations, 1 for muscle tone) at 1 minute; 8 (minus 1 for color, 1 for respirations) at 5 minutes. After being stabilized in the delivery room, Kevin was transported to the NICU in an incubator with free flow oxygen. On admission to the NICU, he was placed on a warmer bed, and oxygen therapy with nasal continuous positive airway pressure (NCPAP) was initiated. Routine cardiopulmonary monitoring and continuous pulse oximetry was begun. An umbilical venous catheter was placed to allow for the delivery of nutrients. Kevin's mother (Mrs. Jones) is a 29-year-old who had experienced two spontaneous abortions before the pregnancy with Kevin. Kevin's father (Mr. Jones), a 32-year-old engineer, was in the delivery room with his wife. Both parents deeply wanted a child and were highly anxious about Kevin's condition and prognosis.

10:00 a.m.: Kevin was lying in a supine position, wearing only a diaper. His heart rate and respiratory rate were labile (HR 148-176 with excursions to 190+; RR 32-54 with excursions 72), with excursions in response to any loud, sharp, or unexpected noise in the environment. He also demonstrated repeated apneic periods of 15 to 20 seconds. He demonstrated frequent periodic twitching and tremors in both lower extremities. His brow was furrowed in a "frown" expression, and his color darkened and paled in response to activity around him. Kevin's parents came into the NICU. It was Kevin's mother's first time to see him, although the father was in the during the night.

Assessment

This preterm neonate is developmentally immature and unable to regulate and stabilize autonomic, motor, and sensory activity. He has exhibited signs of distress in response to environmental stimuli. Developmentally, it is crucial for him to conserve energy to maintain vital function and to grow.

Nursing Diagnosis

Disorganized infant behavior related to excessive environmental stimuli.

Expected Outcomes	The infant will exhibit physiologic stability as evidenced by the autonomic responses of heart rate, respirations, skin color, and a decrease in the motor signs of distress.
Planning	Developmental care will be instituted. This entails careful monitoring and response to infant behavior and environmental events.
NOC	Preterm Infant Organization
NIC	Envronmental Management

Nursing Interventions	Rationales
1. The nurse will modify the environment by moving the infant to an isolette with a cover and moving the isolette to a quiet area of the nursery.	1. This helps to isolate the neonate from some of the noise and light in the environment.
2. The nurse will swaddle and position the infant in a flexed position if the infant shows signs of distress.	2. These positions and swaddling help the infant to self regulate and minimize the startle response that is very energy taxing.

Evaluation	Vital signs will be monitored and the infant will be carefully observed for signs of distress. (The following shows the dynamic monitoring and adaptation of the nursing process related to this diagnosis).

(continues)

Nursing Diagnosis

Neurobehavioral stability related to gestational immaturity.

Expected Outcomes	The baby will increase physiologic stability as measured by: no HR excursions over 170 and no RR excursions over 60. Periodic breathing expected. No apneic pauses. No mottling is present. Skin remains pink. Reduced tremors of lower extremities. Hands remain in a relaxed posture. Face is relaxed.
Planning	Environment and caregiving activities will be evaluated for stimulating effect and timing.
NOC	Vital Signs
NIC	Vital Signs Monitoring

Nursing Interventions	**Rationales**
1. Advocate for moving the infant to an isolette.	1. To reduce environmental stimuli to the baby.
2. Provide isolette cover.	2. To reduce bright lights.
3. Create a quiet zone around the baby. Place signs around the isolette. Remind staff and visitors to lower their voices and minimize noise levels around the baby.	3. Reduced noise levels reduce stimuli.
4. Swaddle the infant to provide containment and flexion for extremities. Position the baby in a side-lying position with limbs flexed. Provide support with blanket rolls.	4. This is a soothing position and makes the infant feel more secure, simulating the containment of the uterine environment.

Evaluation	Infant maintained HR between 154 and 162, with no excursions above 172; RR between 36 and 48, with no excursions above 54. Oxygen saturation stable between 97% and 99%. Apneic periods decreased; no tremors of lower extremities noted. Color, pink.

Assessment

In a period of 15 hours (6:45 a.m.–9:15 p.m.) Kevin was approached for multiple caregiving activities. These included an examination by the resident, morning assessments by the primary care nurse, feeding by gavage, medical rounds, and a blood draw. Kevin was being handled or receiving some care for 45 minutes of each hour of the 15 hours, with no more than 15 minutes between any two activities to allow for recovery.

Nursing Diagnosis

Inability to maintain physiologic stability related to fatigue.

Expected Outcomes	Following caregiving events the infant will demonstrate: • A rapid return to stable baseline HR, RR, and oxygen saturation • Decrease in apneic episodes • Continued baseline tone in the extremities and face
Planning	The caregiving activities will be planned and grouped to avoid nonessential stimulation and allow the infant rest periods to stabilize. Reduce unnecessary noise or activity near the infant.
NOC	Vital Signs
NIC	Vital Signs Monitoring

Nursing Interventions	**Rationales**
1. The nurse will group essential caregiving activities to allow for rest and recuperative periods. This also involves negotiating with other providers who care for the infant. The nurse will modify the environment to reduce noise and activity and allow rest time after feeding.	1. The excessive stimulation has created distress for this infant that is energy taxing and has disrupted autonomic function. The reduction of stimuli will allow the infant to restabilize vital functions.

(continues)

Nursing Interventions	Rationales
2. Assess need and timing for each caregiving event.	2. Avoids unnecessary stimulation for handling.
3. Collaborate with the resident so that only one physical examination is performed in the early morning.	3. Minimize unnecessary simulation.
4. If infant tolerance allows based on cues exhibited, schedule feeding around the physical examination so that there is at least 1 hour of rest for the infant before medical rounds.	4. Allows for rest and energy exposure.
5. Negotiate with house staff to limit discussion at the bedside, stand away from the incubator when possible, and keep the handling of the baby to only the essentials.	5. Decreases unnecessary stimuli.

Evaluation   The nurse continually monitors the infant for signs of stress and autonomic functioning. The process of limiting caregiving episodes and providing rest periods between caregiving or other interventions was effective in reducing the signs of stress in the infant. Following medical rounds, Kevin's HR was 156 bpm; RR, 42 rpm; color, normal; tone, normal. No apneic episodes were noted.

Kevin's parents are obviously distressed and fearful. On further discussion, neither parent has cared for babies and had no information about understanding the developmental issues with a preterm infant.

Assessment

The infant born at 28 weeks' conceptional age differs in important ways from the full-term infant the parents may have experienced in the past and whom they were preparing to parent. The preterm infant lacks the ability to express pleasure, distress, interest, and comfort with the same robust behaviors that are available to the full-term infant. The behaviors of the preterm infant that do communicate the infant's comfort, tolerance, and distress may not be recognized by parents. From the parents' first visits to the nursery the nurse can begin to teach them to recognize their baby's individual strengths, vulnerabilities, and ways of responding.

Nursing Diagnosis

Fear related to lack of experience.

Expected Outcomes
- Parents will recognize positive signs in Kevin's condition.
- Parents will identify behaviors that indicate stress or comfort and stability in Kevin.
- Parents will identify Kevin's responses to environmental stimuli.
- Parent's will identify the importance of their role in Kevin's recovery and development.

Planning   Nurses will use the time that the parents come to see Kevin to teach them about his development, the reason for medical and nursing interventions, and encourage them to begin to care for Kevin in a manner that does not overstimulate him.

NOC   Coping

NIC   Coping Enhancement

Nursing Interventions	Rationales
1. Stand quietly with the parents and talk about what they are seeing. Explain some of the equipment and how you will be caring for Kevin. Talk about the purpose of swaddling, and how correct positioning can help aid breathing and improve motor stability.	1. Teaching the parents as care is given to Kevin allows spontaneous interaction, and the parents can ask questions.
2. When speaking with the parents, emphasize their importance to their baby—how much Kevin needs them.	2. Parents often feel displaced by the more knowledgeable health care professionals.

(continues)

Nursing Interventions	Rationales
3. Support the parents in touching the baby's hand or face gently. Talk about some of the baby's individual characteristics, emphasizing strengths and qualities the parents would identify as normal.	3. These activities make parent-infant attachment easier.
4. When the parents seem ready, introduce the idea of kangaroo care, emphasizing the importance of their closeness and touch for the baby.	4. This makes attachment easier.
5. When the parents are present during caregiving activities, use the opportunity to point out some of the baby's responses that indicate comfort, stress, or self-comforting behaviors.	5. This makes the parents' understanding of infant behavior easier.

Evaluation The parents continue to express concern about Kevin's progress but also are able to identify and take pleasure in indicators that show that he is progressing, that is, weight gain, more stable vital signs, better color, more self-comforting behaviors. Parents initiate opportunities to touch or hold Kevin and begin to ask about caregiving activities. Parents begin to express preferences about how things are done for their baby.

Key Concepts

- The smallest of changes in the care and management of infants who are preterm and have low birth weights may have profound effects on health.

- In addition to the technical care responsibilities of the nurse caring for infants at high risk is the responsibility of educating the parents and family and helping them to bond with their infant.

- In addition to the technical care of the preterm infant, it is the responsibility of the bedside nurse to educate the parents and family. It is also the nurse's responsibility to aid the parents in bonding with their infant.

- The preterm infant's status may change very rapidly; therefore, it is the nurse's assessment skills and ability to recognize changes in the infant's behavior that are crucial in identifying the disease process early in the course.

- Over the past decade there have been remarkable changes in the management of preterm infants. Improvement in mortality and morbidity has been seen in infants as early as 24 weeks' gestation.

- Neonatology encompasses the care of the very fragile preterm infant and also caring for the ill term infant. The bedside nurse may care for an infant as small as 500 grams or an infant as large as 4000 grams.

- Premature infants have special needs for care to assist with normal development.

- The environment of the NICU is a factor that can enhance or detract from development of the high-risk neonate.

- Even high-risk and preterm infants provide cues for caregivers when these infants experience stress.

- The purpose of developmental care is to support the infant's neurobehavioral development and subsystems.

- The survival of smaller and younger gestation infants brings with it many ethical dilemmas that the caregivers and family must face. It is important for the nurse to identify and come to terms with these issues in order to assist the family in adjusting to the reality of their preterm infant.

Review Questions and Activities

1. Identify non-reassuring fetal heart rate patterns using electronic fetal monitoring and discuss the physiology and nursing interventions for each pattern.

2. What are the characteristics of a reassuring fetal heart pattern?

3. What are the goals of short-term fluid therapy?
   a. Prevention of hypoglycemia, limitation of negative fluid balance, and provision of protein sparing carbohydrates
   b. Prevention of hypoglycemia, provision of enough fluids to give a positive fluid balance, and to provide carbohydrates
   c. Provision of adequate glucose and fluids to prevent dehydration
   d. Replacement of insensible water losses

   The correct answer is a.

4. The major routes of water losses include:
   a. Urine and stool

b. Gastrointestinal losses

c. Evaporative from skin and lungs

d. Answers a and c

The correct answer is d.

5. To be classified as symmetric IUGR, what must the infant be?
   a. Less than the 10th percentile in birth weight
   b. Less than the 10th percentile in birth weight and length
   c. Diagnosed in utero by Doppler ultrasonography
   d. Less than the 10th percentile in birth weight, length, and head circumference

   The correct answer is d.

6. What is the purpose of serial X-rays in clients with necrotizing enterocolitis?
   a. Assessment of lung volume
   b. Assessment for pneumotosis or free air in the bowel
   c. To irradiate the infant
   d. To check for pneumonia

   The correct answer is b.

7. What causes compromise of the respiratory system of an infant born at 26 weeks' gestation?
   a. The infant's chest wall is stiff and very compliant
   b. The alveoli's inability to expand easily and lack of surfactant
   c. The infant's intercostal muscles are underdeveloped
   d. The infant's skin is translucent

   The correct answer is b.

8. Which are the common signs and symptoms of a patent ductus arteriosus in preterm infants?
   a. Murmur, widened pulse pressures, and increased heart size
   b. Weak pulses, normal blood pressure, and deterioration in ventilatory status
   c. Murmur, narrowed pulse pressure, and pulmonary edema
   d. Clammy skin and thready pulse

   The correct answer is a.

9. Which is the most common form of lung disease in the newborn?
   a. Meconium aspiration
   b. Retained fetal lung fluid
   c. Hyaline membrane disease
   d. Asthma

   The correct answer is b.

10. What are the components of sound or noise in the NICU?

11. Identify three strategies for reducing sound levels in the NICU.

12. Identify three strategies for protecting infants from excessive light in the NICU.

13. Identify three strategies for maintaining body temperature in preterm infants.

14. Identify three behaviors in preterm infants that may indicate pain or stress.

References

Als, H. (1982). Toward a synactive theory of development: Promise for the assessment and support of infant individuality. *Infant Mental Health Journal, 3*(4), 237–238.

American Academy of Pediatrics (AAP). (2000). *Changing concepts of sudden infant death syndrome: Implications for infant sleeping environment and sleep position.* American Academy of Pediatrics. Policy Statement RE9946. *Pediatrics, 105*(3), 650–656.

American Heart Association and American Academy of Pediatrics. (2000). Neonatal Revisitation Textbook. Dallas, TX: Authors.

Appleton, S. (1997). Touch or handling. *Midwives, 110*(1317), 246.

Ballard, J. L., Khoury, J. C., Wedig, K., Wang, L., Ellers-Walsman, B. L., & Lipp, R. (1991). New Ballard Score expanded to include extremely premature infant. *The Journal of Pediatrics, 119*, 417–423.

Bernstein, S., Heimler, R., & Sasidharan, P. (1998). Approaching the management of the neonatal intensive care unit graduate through history and physical assessment. *Pediatric Clinics of North America, 45*(1), 79–105.

Bildner, J., & Krechel, S. (1996). Increasing staff awareness of postoperative pain management in the NICU. *Neonatal Network, 15*(1), 11–16.

Blackburn, S. T. (2003). *Maternal, fetal and neonatal physiology: A clinical perspective* (2nd ed.). Philadelphia: W. B. Saunders.

Bossi, E., & Koerner, F. (1995). Retinopathy of prematurity. *Intensive Care Medicine, 21*(3), 241–246.

Bozzette, M. (1993). Observation of pain behavior in the NICU: An exploratory study. *Journal of Perinatal and Neonatal Nursing, 7*(1), 76–87.

Casey, P. M. (1999). Respiratory distress. In J. D. Deacon & P. O'Neill (Eds.), *Core curriculum for neonatal intensive care nursing* (2nd ed., pp. 118–150). Philadelphia: W. B. Saunders.

Chen, J. V., Wu, T. S., & Chanlai, S. P. (1995). Recombinant human erythropoietin in the treatment of anemia of prematurity. *American Journal of Perinatology, 12*(5), 314–318.

Consensus Committee to Establish Recommended Standards for Newborn ICU Design. (1999). Recommended Standards for Newborn ICU Design. Physical and Developmental Environment of the High-Risk Infant Project. Washington, DC.

Corff, K., Seideman, R., Venkataraman, P., Lutes, L., & Yates, B. (1995). Facilitated tucking: A nonpharmacologic comfort measure for pain in preterm neonates. *Journal of Obstetric, Gynecologic, and Neonatal Nursing, 24*(2), 143–147.

Craig, K., Whitfield, M., Grunau, R., Linton, J., & Hadjistavropoulos, H. (1993). Pain in the preterm neonate: Behavioural and physiological indices. *Pain, 52*, 287–299.

Davis, P., Turner-Gomes, S., Cunningham, K., Way, C., Roberts, R. & Schmidt, B. (1995). Precision and accuracy of clinical and radiological signs in premature infants at risk for patent ductus arteriosus. *Archives of Pediatrics and Adolescent Medicine, 149*(10), 1136–1141.

de Onis, M., Blossner, M., & Villar, J. (1998). Levels and patterns of intrauterine growth retardation in developing countries. *European Journal of Clinical Nutrition, 52*(Suppl. 1), S5–15.

Dollison, E. J., & Beckstrand, J. (1995). Adhesive tape versus pectin-based barrier use in preterm infants. *Neonatal Network, 14*(4), 35–39.

Engebretson, J., & Wardell, D. (1997). Development of a pacifier for low-birth weight infants on nutritive sucking. *Journal of Obstetric, Gynecologic, and Neonatal Nursing, 6*(6), 660–664.

Field, T., Scafidi, F., & Schanberg, S. (1987). Massage of preterm newborns to improve growth and development. *Pediatric Nursing, 13*(6), 385–387.

Field, T., Schanberg, S., Scafidi, F., & Bauer, C. R., Vegan-Lahr, N., Garcia, R., et al. (1986). Tactile/kinesthetic stimulation effects on preterm neonates. *Pediatrics, 77*(5), 654–658.

Franck, L., & Gregory, G. (1993). Clinical evaluation and treatment of infant pain in the neonatal intensive care unit. In N. Schechter, C. Berde, & M. Yaster (Eds.), *Pain in infants, children, and adolescents* (pp. 519–535). Baltimore: Williams & Wilkins.

Gardosi, J. (1997). Customized growth curves. *Clinical Obstetrics and Gynecology, 40*(4), 715–722.

Goldenberg, R. L., & Cliver, S. P. (1997). Small for gestational age and intrauterine growth restriction: Definitions and standards. *Clinical Obstetrics and Gynecology, 40*(4), 704–714.

Gordon, M., & Montgomery, L. A. (1996). Minimizing epidermal stripping in the very low birth weight infant: Integrating research and practice to affect infant outcome. *Neonatal Network, 14*(1), 37–44.

Grunau, R., Whitfield, M., & Petrie, J. (1994). Pain sensitivity and temperament in extremely low birth weight premature toddlers and preterm and full-term controls. *Pain, 58*, 341–346.

Hansen, A. R., & Snyder, E. Y. (1998). Medical management of neonatal post hemorrhagic hydrocephalus. *Neurosurgery Clinics of North America, 9*(1), 95–104.

Harrison, L., & Woods, S. (1991). Early parental touch and premature infants. *Journal of Obstetric, Gynecologic, and Neonatal Nursing, 20*(4), 299–306.

Hodgkinson, K., Bear, M., Thorn, J., & Van Blaricum, S. (1994). Measuring pain in neonates: Evaluating an instrument and developing a common language. *The Australian Journal of Advanced Nursing, 12*(1), 17–22.

Johnston, C., Stevens, B., Craig, K., & Grunau, R. (1993). Developmental changes in pain expression in premature, full-term, two- and four-month-old infants. *Pain, 52*, 201–208.

Johnston, C., Stevens, B., Yang, F., & Horton, L. (1995). Differential response to pain by very premature neonates. *Pain, 61*, 471–479.

Jorgensen, K. (1993). *Developmental care of the premature infant: A concise overview.* S. Weymouth, MA: Developmental Care Division of Children's Medical Ventures.

Kenner, C., Amlung, S. R., & Flandermeyer, A. A. (1998). *Protocols in neonatal nursing.* Philadelphia: W. B. Saunders.

Kok, J. H., den Ouden, A. L., Verloove-Vanhorick, S. P., & Brand, R. (1998). Outcome of very preterm small for gestational age infants: The first nine years of life. *British Journal of Obstetrics and Gynaecology, 105*(2), 162–168.

Lotas, M., & Walden, M. (1996). Individualized developmental care for very low birth weight infants: A critical review. *Journal of Obstetric, Gynecologic, and Neonatal Nursing, 25*(8), 681–687.

Lott, J. W. (1994). *Neonatal infection: Assessment, diagnosis, and management.* Santa Rosa, CA: NICU Ink.

Masterson, J., Zucker, C., & Schulze, K. (1987). Prone and supine positioning effects on energy expenditure and behaviour of low birth weight neonates. *Pediatrics, 80*(5), 689–692.

McCain, G. (1992). Facilitating inactive awake states in preterm infants: A study of three interventions. *Nursing Research, 41*(3), 157–160.

McIntosh, N., van Veen, I., & Brameyer, H. (1994). Alleviation of the pain of heel prick in preterm infants. *Archives of Disease in Childhood, 70*, F177–F181.

Merenstein, G. B., & Gardner, S. L. (2002). *Handbook of neonatal intensive care* (5th ed.). St. Louis, MO: Mosby.

Moise, A. A., & Hansen, T. N. (1998). In T. N. Hansen, T. R. Cooper, & L. E. Weisman (Eds.), *Contemporary diagnosis and management of neonatal respiratory diseases* (2nd ed., pp. 79–95). Newton, PA: Handbooks in Health Care.

Nelson, D., Heitman, R., & Jennings, C. (1986). Effects of tactile stimulation on premature infant weight gain. *Journal of Obstetric, Gynecologic, and Neonatal Nursing, 15*(3), 262–267.

Nyquist, K. H., & Lutes, L. M. (1998). Co-bedding twins: A developmentally supportive care strategy. *Journal of Obstetric, Gynecologic, and Neonatal Nursing, 27*(4), 450–456.

Paterson, L. (1990). Baby massage in the neonatal unit. *Nursing, 4*(23), 19–21.

Perez-Woods, R., Malloy, M., & Tse, A. (1992). Positioning and skin care of the low birth weight neonate. *NAACOG's Clinical Issues in Perinatal and Women's Health, 3*(1), 97–113.

Porter, F. (1993). Pain assessment in children: Infants. In N. Schechter, C. Berde, & M. Yaster (Eds.), *Pain in infants, children, and adolescents* (pp. 87–96). Baltimore: Williams, & Wilkins.

Robertson, A., & Philbin, M. (1996). Studies of sound and auditory development. Paper presented at the Physical and Developmental Environment of the High Risk Neonate, January 31, 1996. Clearwater Beach: University of South Florida College of Medicine.

Roland, E. H., & Hill, A. (1997). IVH and post hemorrhagic hydrocephalus. *Clinics in Perinatology, 24*(3), 589–605.

Russell, J. (1993). Touch and infant massage. *Paediatric Nursing, 5*(3), 8, 10–11.

Schaap, A. H., Wolf, H., Bruinse, H. W., den Ouden, A. L., Smolders-de Hass, H., van Ertbruggen, I., et al. (1997). Influence of obstetric management on outcome of extremely preterm growth retarded infants. *Archives of Disease in Childhood, Fetal and Neonatal Education, 77*(2), F95–99.

Schwoebel, A., & Sakraida, S. (1997). Hyperbilirubinemia: New approaches to an old problem. *The Journal of Perinatal & Neonatal Nursing, 11*(3), 78–97.

Seaman, S. L. (1995). Renal physiology part II: Fluid and electrolyte regulation. *Neonatal Network, 14*(5), 5–11.

Shapiro, C., & Askin, D. F. (1999). Ophthalmologic disorders. In J. D. Deacon & P. O'Neill (Eds.), *Core curriculum for neonatal intensive care nursing* (2nd ed., pp. 597–615). Philadelphia: W. B. Saunders.

Sherear, D. M., & Devon, M. Y. (1997). Fetal growth in multifetal gestation. *Clinical Obstetrics and Gynecology, 40*(4), 764–770.

Stevens, B., & Johnston, C. (1994). Physiological responses of premature infants to a painful stimulus. *Nursing Research, 43*(4), 226–231.

Stevens, B., Johnston, C., & Horton, L. (1993). Multidimensional pain assessment in premature neonates: A pilot study. *Journal of Obstetric, Gynecologic, and Neonatal Nursing, 22*(6), 531–541.

Stevens, B., Johnston, C., & Horton, L. (1994). Factors that influence the behavioral pain responses of premature infants. *Pain, 59,* 101–109.

Stevens, B., Johnston, C., Petryshen, P., & Taddio, A. (1996). The premature infant pain profile: Development and validation. *The Clinical Journal of Pain, 12*(1), 13–22.

Victor, L., & Person, J. (1994). Implementation of kangaroo care: Apparent-health care team approach to practice change. *Critical Care Nursing Clinics of North America, 6*(4), 891–895.

Whitley, S., & Cowan, M. (1991). Developmental intervention in the newborn intensive care unit. *NAACOG's Clinical Issues in Perinatal and Women's Health Nursing, 2*(1), 84–110.

Zenk, K. E., Sills, J. H., & Koeppel, R. M. (2000). *Neonatal medication and nutrition: A comprehensive guide.* Santa Rosa, CA: NICU Ink.

Elmore, S., Betrus, P., & Burr, R. (1994). Light, social zeitgebers, and the sleep-wake cycle in the entrainment of human circadian rhythms. *Research in Nursing and Health, 17,* 471–478.

Lopes, J., Braz, R., Moreira, M., & Motta, M. (1997). A randomized trial of the effects of ambient light on the incidence of retinopathy of prematurity. *Pediatric Research, 41,* 954A.

Murray, Michelle (1997). *Antepartal and intrapartal fetal monitoring.* Albuquerque, NM: Learning Resources International Inc.

Rushforth, J., & Levene, M. (1994). Behavioral response to pain in healthy neonates. *Archives of Disease in Childhood, 70,* F174–F176.

Sanders, R. (1996). *Structural fetal anomalies: The total picture.* St. Louis, MO: Mosby.

Simpson, K. R., & Creehan, P. A. (1996). *Perinatal nursing.* Philadelphia: Lippincott.

Stevens, B., Johnston, C., & Grunau, R. (1995). Issues of assessment of pain and discomfort in neonates. *Journal of Obstetrics, Gynecologic, and Neonatal Nursing, 24*(9), 849–855.

Suggested Readings

American Academy of Pediatrics (AAP). (1997). Noise: A hazard for the fetus and newborn. American Academy of Pediatrics Policy Statement (RE9728). *Pediatrics, 100*(4).

American Academy of Pediatrics (AAP) and American College of Obstetricians and Gynecologists (ACOG). (1997). *Guidelines for perinatal care* (4th ed.). Washington, DC: Authors.

Association of Women's Health, Obstetrics, and Neonatal Nurses (AWHONN). (1999). *Clinical competencies and education guide: Limited ultrasound examinations in obstetrics and gynecology/infertility settings.* Chicago: Author.

Bakewell-Sachs, S., & Porth, S. (1995). Discharge planning and home care of the technology dependent infant. *Journal of Obstetric, Gynecologic, and Neonatal Nursing, 24*(1), 77–83.

Resources

AmnioNet, http://www.amnionet.com (ultrasound and amniocentesis)

Center for Prenatal Diagnosis, http://www.cpdx.com

Fetal Ultrasound, http://www.fetal.com

Unversity College London Hospitals, http://www.medphys.ucl.ac.uk. Search for "medical graphics." On the Medical Graphics and Imaging Group page, click on "fetal studies."

University of Pennsylvania School of Medicine, http://www.med.upenn.edu

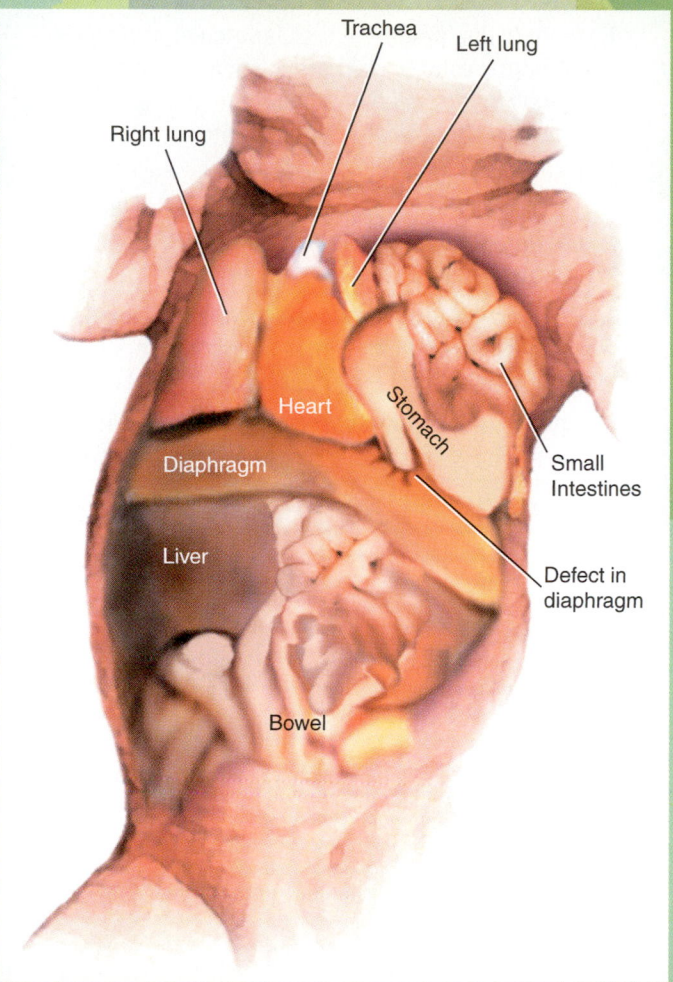

CHAPTER 22

Trachea
Left lung
Right lung
Heart
Stomach
Diaphragm
Small Intestines
Liver
Defect in diaphragm
Bowel

CARE OF NEWBORNS AT RISK RELATED TO CONGENITAL AND ACQUIRED CONDITIONS

During a pregnancy, a family dreams of giving birth to the perfect child (or what they consider to be a normal child) both physically and mentally. The birth of a child with a congenital or acquired anomaly challenges those dreams and forces families to deal with a crisis for which they may be completely unprepared. As a nurse, you must tend to not only the physical needs of the infant and the family's need for knowledge, but also the psychologic needs of the family as they strive to control the emotional upheaval that may result from this birth. You must also closely examine your own feelings and attitudes toward birth anomalies, so that you can effectively and sensitively guide families through the adaptation process.

Key Terms

ABO incompatibility
Acquired disorder
Anencephaly
Brachial palsy
Choanal atresia
Cleft lip
Cleft palate
Clubfoot (talipes
    equinovarus)
Congenital disorder
Congenital heart defect
Developmental dysplasia
    of the hip (DDH)
Diaphragmatic hernia
ECMO
Encephalocele
Epispadias
Erythroblastosis fetalis
Esophageal atresia
Exstrophy of the bladder
Facial palsy
Gastroschisis
Genetic disorder
Hydrocephaly
Hydrops fetalis
Hyperbilirubinemia
Hypocalcemia
Hypoglycemia

Hypomagnesemia
Hypospadias
Imperforate anus
Infant of a diabetic
    mother (IDM)
Intracranial hemorrhage
Jaundice
Kernicterus
Macrosomia
Maternal sensitization
Meningocele
Microcephaly
Myelomeningocele
Omphalocele
Pathologic jaundice
Phototherapy
Physiologic jaundice
Polycythemia
Rh incompatibility
Sepsis
Spina bifida
STORCH
Subarachnoid
    hemorrhage
Subdural hemorrhage
Tracheoesophageal
    fistula

Competencies

Upon completion of this chapter, the reader should be able to:

1. Identify the incidence, risk, anatomic anomalies, pathophysiologic markers, clinical manifestations, and potential complications of congenital or acquired defects in the neonate.

2. Develop a plan of care with specific nursing diagnoses and appropriate interventions for the neonate who is born with a congenital or acquired anomaly.

3. Design an educational plan to meet the needs of the parents and family of a neonate with a congenital or acquired anomaly.

4. Develop a therapeutic relationship to better meet the needs of the family of a neonate who is born with a congenital or acquired anomaly.

The hope and expectation of every pregnant woman is to deliver a healthy, normal infant who will grow and develop into a mature adult who will someday make a contribution to society. Numerous factors, including heredity and the environment, can affect the outcome of a pregnancy. Some abnormalities or disorders can occur in a single or a few genes from either parent, from factors influencing the intrauterine environment, or from a combination of these.

A congenital disorder is an anomaly that results from genetic, prenatal, or environmental factors, or a combination of these, and is present at birth. A genetic disorder is an inherited defect that is transmitted from generation to generation. An acquired disorder is a condition that results from environmental factors rather than genetic circumstances.

This chapter describes the most common congenital and acquired disorders in the neonate and the immediate nursing care that is required, using the nursing process. In addition, the psychosocial impact of the disorders on the parents and family is presented. Both the perinatal and the neonatal team must anticipate and be ever aware of the needs, not only of the compromised neonate, but also of the infant's family. Parents should always be kept informed of their infant's condition and involved in care as soon and as often as possible.

CONGENITAL ANOMALIES

Congenital anomalies are abnormalities present at birth as a result of either genetic or prenatal environmental factors or both. Genetic anomalies are the result of hereditary factors and are transmitted from generation to generation.

Congenital defects occur in 3% to 4% of all live births (Wardinsky, 1994) but this number increases if one includes congenital defects that may not be diagnosed until later in childhood, such as developmental dysplasia of the hip (DDH). Major congenital defects are the leading cause of death in infants less than 1 year of age in the United States and account for 20% of all neonatal deaths.

Central Nervous System Anomalies

As one of the most complex systems of the body, the central nervous system (CNS) is subject to a multitude of congenital anomalies. The stages in the development of the nervous system must proceed in a predetermined order or a defect occurs. These stages can be affected by both genetic and environmental factors, or a combination of both.

The most common anomalies of the CNS occur during the primary neurulation period, which is during the first 3 to 4 weeks of gestation. These anomalies, termed "neural tube defects," occur as a result of failure of the neural tube to close. There has been a steady decline in the number of children born with all forms of neural tube defects as the result of prenatal diagnosis (via abnormal triple screen and/or obstetrical ultrasound) and elective termination of affected pregnancies (Finberg & Kleinman, 2002). Recent evidence suggests that the nutrient folic acid promotes neural tube closure. Therefore, women considering conception are encouraged to begin taking folic acid supplements before conception and to continue with them until 12 weeks' gestation (Rayburn, Stanley, and Garrett, 1996). In 1993, the American Academy of Pediatrics recommended that folic acid be administered to all women of childbearing age.

Encephalocele

Encephalocele is a herniation of the brain and meninges through an opening in the skull (Figure 22-1). This neural tube defect is readily visible at birth. Skin generally covers the encephalocele, but it may break open, increasing the risk for infection. Treatment consists of surgical intervention to replace brain contents and repair the defect. If hydrocephalus or enlargement of the head without enlargement of the facial structures is present, a ventricular shunting procedure is generally performed 7 to 10 days after the encephalocele has been repaired. The shunt is formed by placing a flexible tube into the ventricular system of the brain, which diverts the abnormal accumulation of cerebrospinal fluid (CSF) into another area of the body, most often the abdominal cavity, where it can be absorbed. (Refer to the section on hydrocephaly in this chapter for nursing care of the infant with a shunt.)

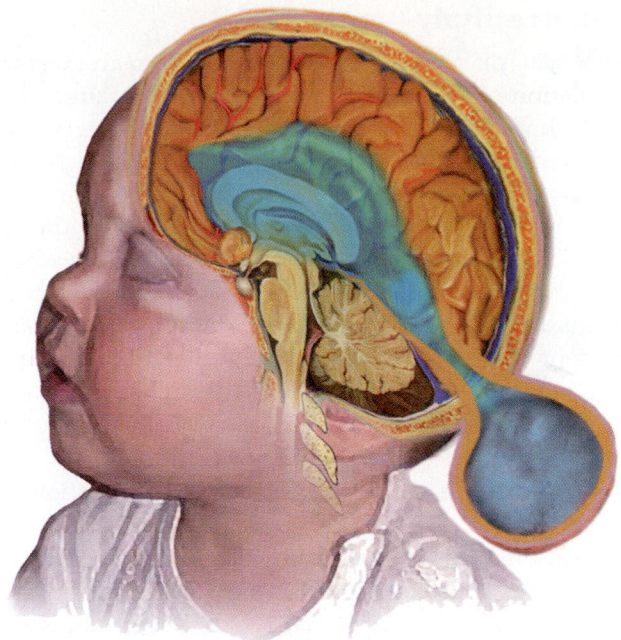

Figure 22-1   Infant with encephalocele.

Anencephaly

In **anencephaly**, there is a complete or partial absence of the cerebral hemispheres and skull. The exact cause of anencephaly is unknown; it occurs in 1 of 1,000 live births (Paidas & Cohen, 1994). These infants are frequently stillborn or die within the first few days of life because they do not have any cerebral function. Nursing interventions are directed toward providing comfort measures until the infant dies from respiratory or cardiac failure. The families require a great deal of emotional and spiritual support in grieving the impending death of their newborn.

Microcephaly

Microcephaly is the condition in which there is a normal-sized head that contains a small brain. This condition can be either congenital or acquired. Congenital microcephaly may be seen in conjunction with a chromosomal abnormality; an intrauterine infection, such as rubella, cytomegalovirus, or toxoplasmosis; and maternal exposure to X-rays. The acquired form of microcephaly may result from maternal herpes, ischemic insults, or hypothyroidism. Diagnostic evaluation includes a **STORCH** titer for syphilis, toxoplasmosis, other infections, rubella, cytomegalovirus, and herpes, and skull X-rays films. There is no treatment for this disorder, which generally results in mental retardation. Nursing care is predominantly supportive. The parents must be supported while they learn to cope with and accept this disorder in their newborn.

Hydrocephaly

Hydrocephaly is a condition that results from an excess accumulation of CSF in the ventricles of the brain and the subarachnoid space as a result of an imbalance between CSF production and absorption (Figure 22-2). Normal growth and development of the brain is altered because of the increased intracranial pressure (ICP) from the CSF fluid. This condition occurs in 3 to 4 of 1000 newborns (Jackson & Harvey, 2004). Cesarean section may be necessary because of the enlarged head. This disorder is readily apparent at birth. The infant is born with an enlarged head, bulging fontanelles, separated skull sutures, and a prominent forehead with depressed eyes that are rotated downward, causing the "setting sun" sign.

Nursing care includes continuous observation and assessment of neurologic status of the infant. Ongoing observations must be carefully documented. The head should be supported while holding, turning, or positioning the infant. A flotation mattress or sheepskin is used under the infant to prevent skin breakdown and infection. Signs of increased ICP should be continuously assessed, and serial head circumference measurements should be plotted.

Surgical intervention includes the placement of a shunt from the ventricle in the brain to the peritoneum to allow for drainage of excess CSF. Postoperatively, the infant is positioned on the side opposite the shunt to prevent pressure and kinking of the shunt. The infant's bed is left in a flat position to prevent rapid loss of CSF and decompression. The long-term prognosis depends on the cause of hydrocephalus, the extent of tissue damage, and the success of the shunt procedure. Parents should be taught the care of the infant and shunt, including positioning and skin care, before discharge. They need to be educated on the signs of increased intracranial pressure, shunt malfunction, skin breakdown, and infection.

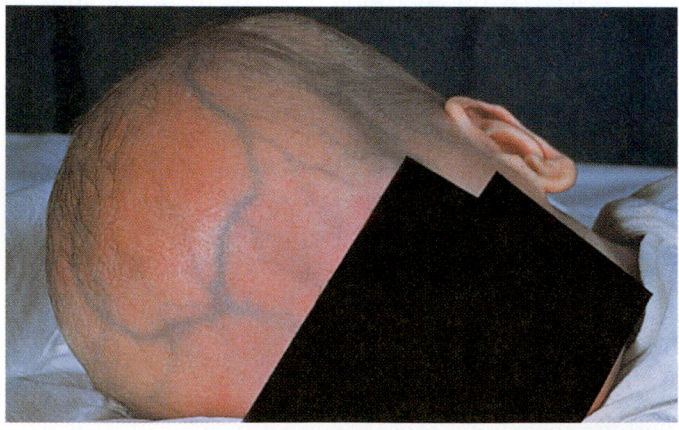

Figure 22-2 Hydrocephalus. *(Courtesy of Armed Forces Institute of Pathology.)*

Nursing Alert

Clinical Manifestations of Increased Intracranial Pressure

- Widening sutures
- Bulging anterior fontanelle
- Lethargy
- Irritability
- High-pitched, shrill cry
- Poor feeding
- Poor sucking
- Decreased level of consciousness
- "Setting sun" sign
- Opisthotonos (spasm of the head and feet)

Spina Bifida

Spina bifida is a common CNS defect that results from failure of the spinal cord to close. There are two categories: spina bifida occulta and spina bifida cystica. Spina bifida occulta is the failure of the spinal column to close when neither the cord nor the meninges herniate through the defect (Figure 22-3). This condition occurs in 10% to 30% of all live births (Kenner, Amlung, & Flandermeyer, 1998).

Spina bifida cystica, which includes meningocele and myelomeningocele, has an incidence of 1 in 1,000 live births (Kenner et al., 1998). In a **meningocele**, there is an external sac that protrudes through the defect that contains meninges and CSF. However, the spinal cord and nerve roots are in their normal position. **Myelomeningocele** is the most common form of spina bifida cystica and occurs in 1 of 1,000 live births (Ball & Bindler, 2003). In a myelomeningocele, the sac contains both meninges and CSF, as in meningocele, but it also contains neural tissue. Myelomeningocele may arise at any point in the vertebral column from C-1 to the coccyx but is most common in the lumbar, lumbosacral, and sacral segments.

Spina bifida may be diagnosed in utero through the testing of amniotic fluid. Elevated levels of alpha-fetoprotein (AFP) found in the amniotic fluid confirm the diagnosis of an open neural tube defect, such as spina

Nursing Tip *Signs of Shunt Infection*

Observe for signs of infection, such as fever, a decrease in responsiveness, poor feeding, and seizures.

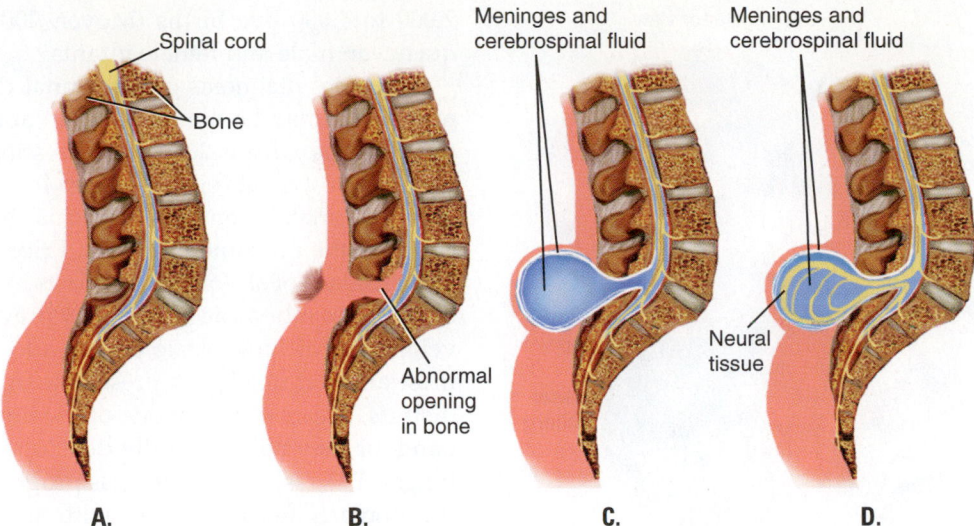

Figure 22-3   Spina bifida. A. Normal spine; B. Spina bifida occulta; C. Spina bifida with meningocele; D. Spina bifida with myelomeningocele.

bifida. The open defect allows leakage of CSF into the amniotic fluid, causing the elevated AFP levels. An ultrasound examination may also be performed to visualize the defect. If the diagnosis of spina bifida is not made in utero, it is usually apparent at birth. The head should be carefully examined for signs of hydrocephalus, and serial head-circumference measurements done. A computerized tomographic (CT) scan or magnetic resonance imaging (MRI) study may be performed to define the type and severity of hydrocephalus. Electromyography may assist in assessing the motor function of the lower extremities. In addition, an abdominal sonogram or intravenous pyelogram may be performed to rule out hydronephrosis (Avery, Fletcher, & MacDonald, 2000).

Whenever possible, the spinal lesion should be closed within the first few hours of life. Prompt surgery is performed to prevent infection and halt any further loss of existing neurologic function. Since a high percentage of infants with neural tube defects develop hydrocephalus, a ventriculoperitoneal shunt is placed after the neural tube defect has been repaired.

Immediate nursing care includes placing the infant in a prone or side-lying position with rolled towels to prevent pressure on the sac and to protect the sac from tearing. The infant's position should be changed every hour to prevent pressure on a specific area. The sac should be covered with a moist, sterile gauze dressing, and the skin around the defect should be cleansed and dried to prevent skin breakdown. The nurse should administer prescribed prophylactic antibiotic agents. The infant's bladder should be emptied, using Credé's method, at regular intervals to prevent stasis of urine in the bladder resulting from the loss of normal nerve innervation.

Postoperatively, nursing care involves assessing the infant for signs and symptoms of infection, increased ICP, and bowel and bladder assessment. The infant is placed in a prone or lateral position to keep pressure off the incisional area. Manual emptying of the bladder to stimulate urination is continued. Passive range of motion (ROM) exercises should be performed with the lower extremities; a physical therapist should be consulted for appropriate exercises. A number of orthopedic problems, such as foot deformities, dislocated hips, and kyphoscoliosis, can occur. Therefore, orthopedic status must be continually monitored and vigorous physical therapy must be initiated.

Respiratory System Anomalies

The upper respiratory system begins forming early in the fourth week of gestation; formation of the lower respiratory system begins in the middle of that week. Malformations in the respiratory system can be life-threatening; therefore, recognition of these anomalies in the delivery room is imperative for proper treatment. The first few minutes of life are the most crucial, so ensuring adequate oxygenation during this period is necessary to the long-term positive outcome for the newborn.

Choanal Atresia

Choanal atresia is a condition in which there is a bony or membranous separation between the nose and the pharynx (Figure 22-4). Ninety percent of atresias are bony, and 10% are membranous. The incidence of choanal atresia is 1 in 5,000 to 7,000 births (Avery et al., 2000). Unilateral atresia is much more common than bilateral atresia, and the female-to-male ratio for affected infants is 2:1. Twenty to fifty percent of clients with choanal atresia have other anomalies; therefore, genetic consultation for these clients is recommended, along with a thorough search for additional anomalies (Fanaroff & Martin, 2001). The most common anomalies are coloboma of the eyes, heart defects, renal anomalies, growth and mental retardation, ear

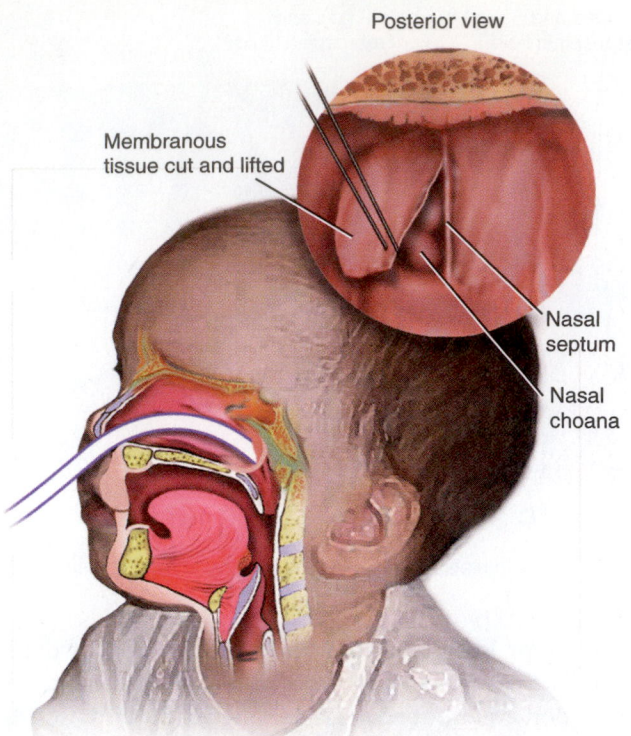

Figure 22-4 Choanal atresia, separation between the nose and pharynx.

2,000 to 4,000 live births (Moyer, 2001) with equal frequency in male and female infants.

Prenatal diagnosis of congenital diaphragmatic hernia (CDH) may be made using an antenatal ultrasound technique as early as 26 weeks' gestation (Fanaroff & Martin, 2001). Surgical repair in utero has been completed at some perinatal centers, but this has not markedly changed the outcome (Holland, Price, & Bensaro, 1998). The presence of abdominal contents in the thoracic cavity during the embryonic period may prevent the normal development of lung tissue on the affected side. At birth, most affected newborns present with severe respiratory distress, because at least one of the lungs is unable to expand, or may not have fully developed (i.e., hypoplastic lungs). The respiratory distress progressively worsens as the stomach and bowels fill with air. Breath sounds are usually diminished or absent on the affected side and, instead, bowel sounds are audible in the chest. In 85% to 90% of cases, the hernia is on the left side because the liver fills the defects on the right side (Holland et al., 1998). Physical examination of the newborn reveals a large or asymmetric chest and a flat, relatively small abdomen.

deficits, and gastroesophageal reflux (referred to by the acronym "CHARGE") (Coniglio, Manzione, & Hengerer, 1988).

Infants are nose breathers for the first 3 months of life. Choanal atresia may be immediately recognizable at birth by signs of respiratory distress, especially if the atresia is bilateral. One method that may be used in the delivery room to assess the infant for choanal atresia is passing a catheter through each nostril to check for patency. If the catheter does not pass bilaterally, the diagnosis of choanal atresia is made. Infants with choanal atresia may be cyanotic at rest, but their color improves when they open their mouth to cry. Nasal discharge is present.

If it is determined that the infant has bilateral choanal atresia, surgical intervention is an immediate necessity. Prognosis is excellent if there are no other concomitant related medical conditions. Unilateral choanal atresia is often not detected until the infant's nostril becomes blocked with secretions, such as during a cold.

Diaphragmatic Hernia

Congenital **diaphragmatic hernias** occur during gestational life when the diaphragm fails to close during the seventh or eighth week. The defect allows the abdominal organs to be displaced into the left side of the chest through an opening in the diaphragm (Figure 22-5). It occurs in 1 in

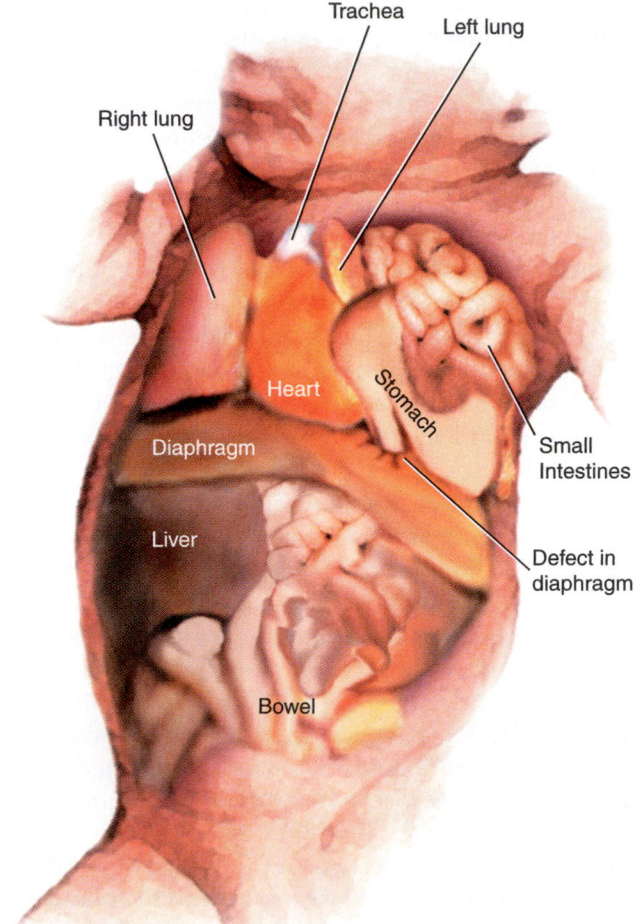

Figure 22-5 Diaphragmatic hernia.

Before surgery to repair the hernia is attempted, the infant's medical condition must be stabilized. Medical measures are taken to reverse hypoxia, hypercarbia, and metabolic acidosis. A nasogastric tube is inserted for gastric decompression. Mechanical ventilation with 100% oxygen is used to maintain functional respiratory status. If the infant's respiratory status does not improve, extracorporeal membrane oxygenation (ECMO) therapy may be required before the hernia repair (Avery et al., 2000). **ECMO** is a cardiopulmonary bypass therapy that allows the infant's lungs to rest and heal by exchanging blood gases through a membrane oxygenator outside the body.

Preoperative nursing interventions include: positioning the newborn on the affected side with the head and chest elevated to allow for better expansion of the normal lung; placement of a gastric tube and connection to continuous low suction to keep the stomach and intestines decompressed; maintenance of oxygen and ventilatory support; and medication administration. Close and careful monitoring is essential at all times.

Once the infant is medically stable, surgical repair is performed. Postoperatively, maintenance of respiratory function is a high priority. Ventilatory support continues with careful monitoring for possible complications, such as pneumothorax and acid-base imbalances. Prognosis depends on the degree of pulmonary development and success of the closure. If the infant required mechanical ventilation during the first 18 to 24 hours of life, the survival rate is approximately 50%. If the infant with a diaphragmatic hernia did not experience any respiratory distress within the first 24 hours of life, survival rates reach 100% (Holland et al., 1998).

Cardiovascular System Anomalies

By the end of the third week of gestation, a functional cardiovascular system is in place to support further development of the embryo. Partitioning of the heart, a complex process, is completed by the end of the seventh week of gestation. Many women are not even aware that they are pregnant during this period. Formation of the cardiovascular system can be altered as a result of the presence of many factors, including genetic and environmental factors and some maternal medical conditions. A thorough maternal history and careful physical examination are important in the diagnosis of congenital heart disease.

Congenital Heart Defects

Congenital heart defects (CHD) are anatomic abnormalities in the heart that are present at birth (Figure 22-6). The incidence of CHD is approximately 1% of births (Hoffman, 1995). There are more than 100 different types of cardiac anomalies; ventricular septal defects are the most com-

mon and constitute more than 20% of all CHDs. Transposition of the great arteries and coarctation of the aorta are the most common life-threatening anomalies. CHDs are the second major cause of death in the first year of life (premature birth is the first).

The causes of CHDs are unknown, but both genetic and environmental factors are thought to influence their development. Infants with Down, Marfan, or Turner's syndromes frequently have related cardiac anomalies. Other factors linked to CHDs include maternal alcoholism; maternal rubella infection; maternal diabetes mellitus; maternal use of certain medications, including anticonvulsants, estrogen, progesterone (Provera), lithium (Lithane), warfarin (Coumadin), or isotretinoin (Accutane); and exposure to X-rays. Prematurity, low birth weight, and congenital infections can also increase the risk for CHDs.

Client Education

Congenital Heart Defects

Teach parents about the heart condition:

- **Provide pictures and diagrams of the heart and then demonstrate the defect.**
- **Provide written material on the specific heart defect.**

Instruct parents on medication administration:

- **Provide a written schedule of times when the medication(s) should be administered.**
- **Instruct on the purpose, dose, correct administration, and side effects of the medication(s). Inform parents about when to notify the physician.**
- **Allow parents to demonstrate their knowledge of medication administration (after instructions have been provided) to validate their understanding.**

Educate parents about detecting these signs and symptoms and reporting them to the physician:

- **Increased respiratory rate**
- **Breathing difficulties (such as nasal flaring or retractions)**
- **Excessive sweating**
- **Poor sucking**
- **Weight loss**
- **Poor feeding**
- **Cyanosis**

Patent Ductus Arteriosus

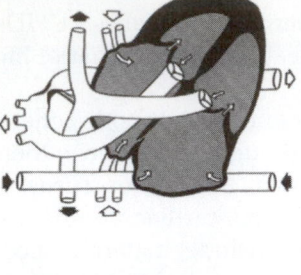

The patent ductus arteriosus is a vascular connection that, during fetal life, short-circuits the pulmonary vascular bed and directs blood from the pulmonary artery to the aorta. Functional closure of the ductus normally occurs soon after birth. If the ductus remains patent after birth, the direction of blood flow in the ductus is reversed by the higher pressure in the aorta.

Ventricular Septal Defects

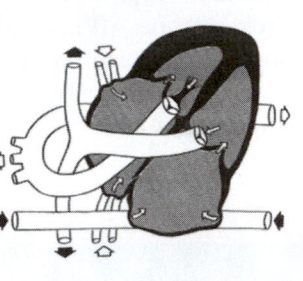

A ventricular septal defect is an abnormal opening between the right and left ventricle. Ventricular septal defects vary in size and may occur in either the membranous or muscular portion of the ventricular septum. Due to higher pressure in the left ventricle, a shunting of blood occurs from the left to right ventricle during systole. If pulmonary vascular resistance produces pulmonary hypertension, the shunt of blood is then reversed from the right to the left ventricle, with cyanosis resulting.

Truncus Arteriosus

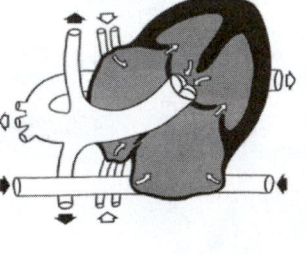

Truncus arteriosus is a retention of the embryologic bulbar trunk. It results from the failure of normal septation and division of this trunk into an aorta and pulmonary artery. This single arterial trunk overrides the ventricles and receives blood from them through a ventricular septal defect. The entire pulmonary and systemic circulation is supplied from this common arterial trunk.

Subaortic Stenosis

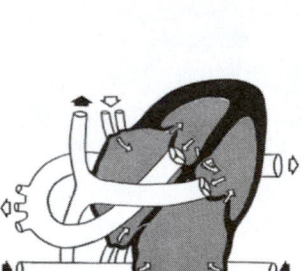

In many instances, the stenosis is valvular with thickening and fusion of the cusps. Subaortic stenosis is caused by a fibrous ring below the aortic valve in the outflow tract of the left ventricle. At times, both valvular and subaortic stenosis exist in combination. The obstruction presents an increased work load for the normal output of the left ventricular blood and results in left ventricular enlargement.

Coarctation of the Aorta

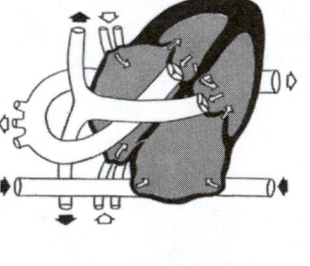

Coarctation of the aorta is characterized by a narrowed aortic lumen. It exists as a preductal or postductal obstruction, depending on the position of the obstruction in relation to the ductus arteriosus. Coarctations exist with great variation in anatomical features. The lesion produces an obstruction to the flow of blood through the aorta, causing an increased left ventricular pressure and work load.

Tetralogy of Fallot

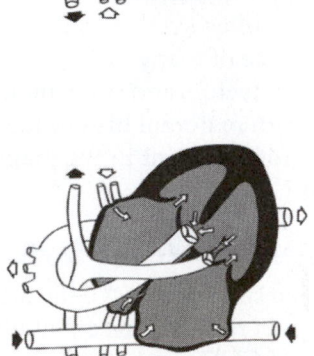

Tetralogy of Fallot is characterized by the combination of four defects: 1) pulmonary stenosis, 2) ventricular septal defect, 3) overriding aorta, and 4) hypertrophy of right ventricle. It is the most common defect causing cyanosis in patients surviving beyond two years of age. The severity of symptoms depends on the degree of pulmonary stenosis, the size of the ventricular septal defect, and the degree to which the aorta overrides the septal defect.

Complete Transposition of Great Vessels

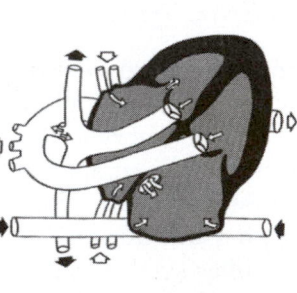

This anomaly is an embryologic defect caused by a straight division of the bulbar trunk without normal spiraling. As a result, the aorta originates from the right ventricle and the pulmonary artery from the left ventricle. An abnormal communication between the two circulations must be present to sustain life.

Atrial Septal Defects

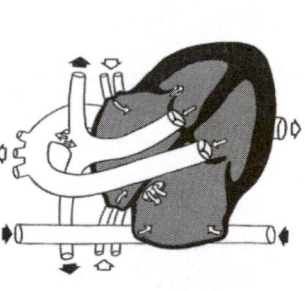

An atrial septal defect is an abnormal opening between the right and left atria. Basically, three types of abnormalities result from incorrect development of the atrial septum. An incompetent foramen ovale is the most common defect. The high ostium secundum defect results from abnormal development of the septum secundum. Improper development of the septum primum produces a basal opening known as an ostium primum defect, frequently involving the atrioventricular valves. In general, left to right shunting of blood occurs in all atrial septal defects.

Tricuspid Atresia

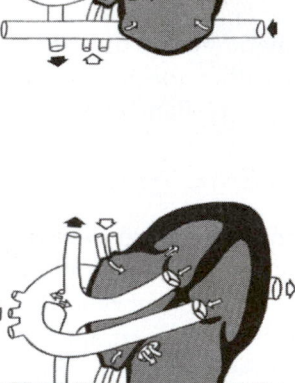

Tricuspid valvular atresia is characterized by a small right ventricle, large left ventricle, and usually a diminished pulmonary circulation. Blood from the right atrium passes through an atrial septal defect into the left atrium, mixes with oxygenated blood returning from the lungs, flows into the left ventricle, and is propelled into the systemic circulation. The lungs may receive blood through one of three routes: 1) a small ventricular septal defect, 2) patent ductus arteriosus, and 3) bronchial vessels.

Anomalous Venous Return

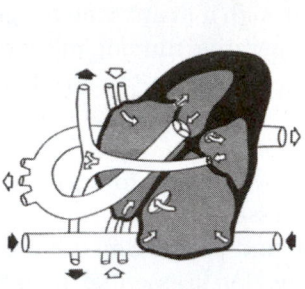

Oxygenated blood returning from the lungs is carried abnormally to the right side of the heart by one or more pulmonary veins emptying directly, or indirectly through venous channels, into the right atrium. Partial anomalous return of the pulmonary veins to the right atrium functions the same as an atrial septal defect. In complete anomalous return of the pulmonary veins, an interatrial communication is necessary for survival.

Figure 22-6 Congenital heart abnormalities. *(Used with permission of Ross Products, Division of Abbott Laboratories, Columbus, Ohio.)*

Table 22-1	Physiologic Signs of Cardiac Defects
PHYSIOLOGIC SIGN	**CARDIAC DEFECT**
Increase in pulmonary blood flow	Atrial septal defects Ventricular septal defects Patent ductus arteriosus
Obstruction to pulmonary blood flow	Coarctation of aorta Subaortic stenosis
Decrease in pulmonary blood flow	Tetralogy of Fallot Tricuspid atresia
Mixed blood flow	Complete transposition of great vessels Anomalous venous return Truncus arteriosus

CHDs are now categorized physiologically rather than as cyanotic or acyanotic (Wong, Perry, & Hockenberry-Eaton, 2002). The four physiologic signs and the associated defects are listed in Table 22-1.

Assessment begins with a thorough review of the maternal history for risk factors that could predispose the infant to a congenital heart defect. The admitting nurse must carefully assess the infant's cardiovascular and respiratory functions and promptly report any abnormal findings. The infant is assessed for signs and symptoms of respiratory distress, including cyanosis, and congestive heart failure (CHF). In addition, a thorough assessment of the cardiac rate, rhythm, and sounds should be conducted. Signs of CHF to look for include tachycardia, tachypnea, gallop rhythm, diminished peripheral pulses, diaphoresis, edema, and hepatomegaly. Newborns exhibiting these signs require prompt diagnosis and appropriate therapy in a neonatal intensive care unit. Diagnostic tests used to obtain specific information about the defect and the need for surgical intervention include arterial blood gas analysis, chest X-ray studies, electrocardiogram (ECG), echocardiogram, and cardiac catheterization.

Nursing interventions include continuous monitoring of the infant's cardiac and respiratory status, maintaining a thermoneutral environment, administering oxygen as ordered, administering medications as prescribed, offering comfort measures to minimize crying when it precipitates cyanosis, and gavage feeding of the infant if necessary to decrease the workload of the heart. In addition, the nurse should inform the parents of the newborn's condition and management.

Before discharge, parents need detailed instruction and experience in providing care. Parents should be taught about their infant's heart defect, medication ad-

ministration, and how to observe for signs and symptoms. In addition, home-based care should be instituted.

Gastrointestinal System Anomalies

Proper formation of the gastrointestinal (GI) system is necessary for the infant to support adequate nutrition and growth after delivery. During the fourth week of gestation, a primitive gut is formed. Many intricate steps are involved in the development of the complete GI tract, during which it is exposed to the possibility of formation of various anomalies. These malformations can occur anywhere in the GI tract and may be simple or complex. Knowledge of the signs and symptoms of GI anomalies is crucial because the nurse is often the first person to detect a problem.

Cleft Lip and Palate

Cleft lip or palate are terms that indicate a congenital opening in the lip or palate, or both, that results from failure of the maxillary and premaxillary processes to fuse during the 7th to 12th week of intrauterine life. This facial malformation is frequently seen in conjunction with other syndromes that occur in relation to avitaminosis or viral infections during the first trimester. Clefts of the lip or palate occur in approximately 1 in 600 to 700 Caucasian newborns. The incidence is double that rate in Asians and half that rate in Blacks. Cleft lip occurs more often in males and is generally located on the left side (Avery et al., 2000). The cleft deformity ranges from minor notching to complete separation of the entire lip and nasal floor (Figure 22-7). The defect may involve the lip, both the lip and palate, or only the palate, and may be unilateral or bilateral. Rarely is the defect located in the midline. The defect tends to occur more often in families in which a close relative also has the anomaly. Environmental factors, such as exposure to radiation or toxic substances, also play a part in contributing to the multifactorial nature of the defect.

Diagnosis of cleft lip may be made from physical appearance of the infant at birth. To determine if a cleft palate is present, the examiner inserts a gloved finger inside the newborn's mouth to feel the soft and hard palate.

Initial care of the child with a cleft lip or palate focuses on feeding. Feeding problems arise because of the infant's inability to create adequate suction and difficulty in swallowing. The infant with a cleft lip is unable to hold onto and form a seal around the nipple. When feeding the infant, the bottle should be held while the infant's cheeks are grasped together to close the cleft. The infant should be bubbled or burped at frequent intervals, because air may be swallowed. If a cleft palate is present, the infant is

Cleft Lip

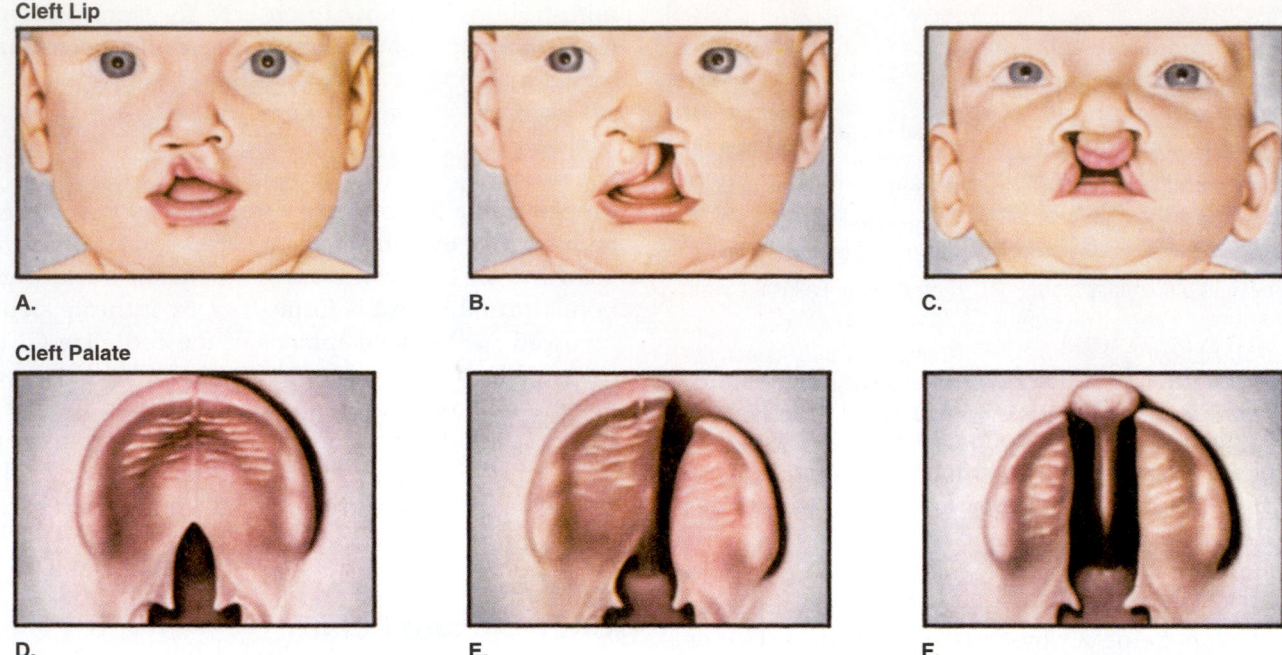

A.   B.   C.

Cleft Palate

D.   E.   F.

Figure 22-7   Cleft lip. A. Unilateral incomplete; B. Unilateral complete; C. Bilateral complete. Cleft Palate. D. Incomplete; E. Unilateral complete; F. Bilateral complete. *(Used with permission of Ross Products, Division of Abbott Laboratories, Columbus, OH.)*

unable to form a vacuum to maintain the suction necessary for feeding. The infant must be fed in an upright position, and the flow of milk should be directed to one side of the mouth to avoid choking. The degree of feeding difficulty depends on the size and type of defect; it is greatest in the child with a cleft palate. Infants with large clefts may need O_2 saturation monitoring during their first feeds to ensure adequate oxygenation while feeding. Newborns with less severe defects and intact lips can often successfully breastfeed because the breast may fill the cleft. Devices available for use with infants with cleft lip and palate include special nipples, compressible bottles, and syringe feeders.

Education, counseling, and emotional support for the parents is an important aspect of nursing care. This defect can be quite disfiguring. Parents need to be encouraged to ask questions and verbalize their anxieties and fears. Provide the parents with pamphlets that show photographs of infants both before and after surgical repairs. Parents must be taught to feed their infant in an upright position and to aim the nipple toward the intact part of the palate, while gently squeezing the bottle.

Surgical repair of the cleft lip is performed at approximately 3 months of age. Repair of the cleft palate is generally postponed until the infant is between 9 and 12 months of age. This delay allows time for the anatomic changes that normally occur in the palate contour (increase of the palate arch). Early surgery of a cleft palate seems to have a negative effect on facial growth, but the

trend is toward closure during infancy because improved speech results. Preoperative teaching with parents should include information about the type of surgery being performed, postoperative care that the child will require, and how to use any appliances the infant needs. These chil-

 **COLLABORATIVE CARE**

Children with Congenital Anomalies

Children born with cleft lips and palates require multidisciplinary care throughout their growth period. Many of the following disciplines will need to be involved in the support of the family and their care:

- Specialized nurses
- Pediatrician or nurse practitioner
- Speech pathologist
- Otolaryngologist
- Plastic surgeon
- Orthodontist
- Social worker
- Child life specialist
- Support groups
- Lactation consultant

dren require multidisciplinary care through adolescence, including nursing care and specialist care, such as a pediatrician, audiologist, speech pathologist, otolaryngologist, plastic surgeon, orthodontist, and social worker (Avery et al., 2000).

Esophageal Atresia and Tracheoesophageal Atresia

Esophageal atresia (EA) and tracheoesophageal fistula (TEF) are uncommon anomalies in which the esophagus and trachea do not separate in a normal way. **Esophageal atresia** is a condition in which the esophagus ends in a blind pouch or narrows into a thin cord and is not connected to the stomach. During the 34th to 36th days of gestation, the trachea and esophagus ordinarily separate into two distinct tubes. Failure of this separation causes a **tracheoesophageal fistula** (TEF). TEF occurs in 1 in 4,500 births (Holland et al., 1998). The exact cause is unknown. These may be life-threatening anomalies of the esophagus and may occur together or singly (Figure 22-8).

Atresia is the congenital absence or closure of a normal body opening. EA can occur with or without a fistula (TEF) into the trachea. The most common esophageal atresia has a fistula between the distal esophagus and the trachea. This type occurs in 86% of newborns born with *an esophageal defect*. Other types include esophageal atresia without a fistula (7.7%), H-type tracheoesophageal fistula without esophageal atresia (4.2%), esophageal atresia with a proximal fistula (0.8%), and atresia with proximal and distal fistulae (0.7%) (Holland et al., 1998) (Figure 22-8). Infants born with this anomaly must be examined for other congenital anomalies, because 30% to 70% of affected infants have other malformations. CHD is the most common accompanying anomaly. Other potentially accompanying anomalies include vertebral malformations, atresias of the small intestine, imperforate anus, and genitourinary defects; the acronym for this syndrome is VATER, which stands for vertebral, anal, tracheoesophageal atresia or fistula, and renal anomalies. Some experts use the acronym VACTERL to delineate the same group of symptoms. The "C" stands for congenital heart defect and the "L" for limb deformities (Kenner & Lott, 2003).

Infants with EA and TEF may appear to be well immediately after birth. However, soon afterward, they present with copious oral secretions or are unable to swallow oral feedings. Signs and symptoms of esophageal atresia (with or without TEF) include drooling, choking, coughing, cyanosis, and regurgitation of food. Abdominal distention is a prominent feature in an infant with a distal fistula, because air is forced into the stomach.

Diagnosis of esophageal atresia is confirmed if a nasogastric catheter cannot be passed any further than 10

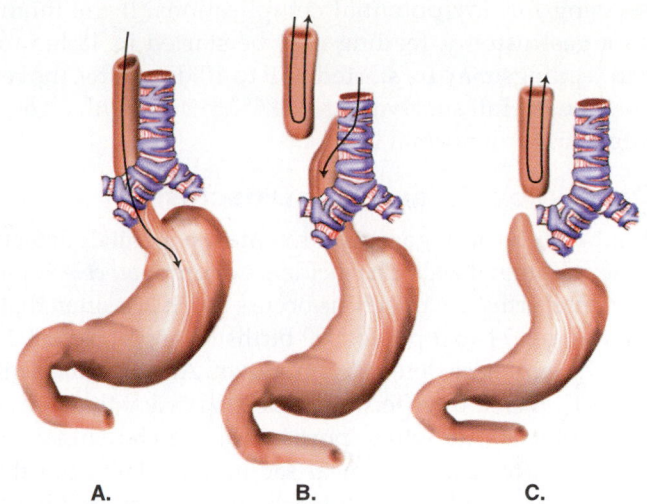

Figure 22-8   A. Normal esophagus; B. Tracheoesophageal fistula (esophagus ends in blind pouch, connects to trachea by fistula); C. Congenital esophageal atresia (esophagus has two blind pouch ends with no communication to the trachea).

cm past the infant's nares, through the esophagus, and into the stomach. If a radiopaque catheter is used, an X-ray film reveals that the tube coils in the blind end (pouch) of the esophagus.

If the infant is stable, immediate primary surgical repair is done. If the infant is medically unstable, surgery is delayed until the infant's clinical status is stable and he or she can tolerate the surgical procedure.

After diagnosis is made and before surgery, nursing care of these infants includes positioning the infant in a 30-degree upright position to prevent gastroesophageal reflux; these infants should not be given anything orally. A catheter is placed in the upper esophageal pouch and connected to continuous low suction to remove secretions and prevent aspiration. The infant needs intravenous fluids to maintain fluid and electrolyte balance. Supplemental oxygen and intubation may be required if the infant experiences respiratory distress. Parents must be educated about the defect, the management plan, supported during this acute period, and kept informed about the care of the infant before and after surgery. Clarify and reinforce the physician's explanations about the malformation and the impending surgical repair. Encourage parents to ask questions and explain that the surgery is done in staged repairs. The first repair is provision of a gastrostomy and ligation of the fistula; the second is repair of the atresia, done several days later.

Surgery consists of closure of the fistula and anastomosis of the esophageal segments. Postoperative care involves the careful and continuous monitoring of the infant's cardiovascular and respiratory status and assessing for any potential complications. If the infant has a gastrostomy, feeding may be started in 48 hours. Oral feedings may be started in 5 to 10 days after the repair. The overall survival rate is 85% to 90%, with a good prognosis for a normal life.

Omphalocele and Gastroschisis

Omphalocele and gastroschisis are congenital defects in the abdominal wall. The incidence of omphalocele is 1 in 5,000 live births; gastroschisis occurs much less often than omphalocele, 1 to 3 per 10,000 births (Wong et al., 2002). The cause of these defects is unknown. An **omphalocele** is a defect covered by a peritoneal sac, located at the base of the umbilicus into which portions of the abdominal organs herniate. The peritoneal sac may contain both the small and large intestine, stomach, liver, spleen, and bladder. The peritoneal sac covering the defect may rupture during or after birth. Omphalocele develops during the 10th to 12th weeks of gestation and is often seen in conjunction with other cardiac, genitourinary, neurologic, or chromosomal anomalies.

This defect may be detected on an antenatal sonogram. If omphalocele is present, a vaginal delivery is still permitted, because the outcome is not any different than if the infant is delivered by cesarean section. If the diagnosis has not been made by sonogram, the defect is easily recognizable at the time of birth.

Gastroschisis is a condition in which the bowel herniates through an abdominal wall defect to the right of the umbilicus. In contrast to omphalocele, the contents are not contained in a sac, but instead the contents lie openly on the abdomen. Gastroschisis occurs in 1 to 3 in 10,000 live births (Hockenberry, Wilson, Winkelstein, & Kline, 2003). This condition is often seen in small for gestational age and preterm newborns and is rarely associated with other anomalies. Generally, there is a greater loss of fluid in the infant with gastroschisis than in the infant with omphalocele, unless the omphalocele is not covered by a layer of peritoneum. In utero, the intestine was allowed to float freely in amniotic fluid, so it may appear edematous and may be covered with black necrotic tissue.

Surgery is indicated for both omphalocele and gastroschisis. Preoperative care is similar for infants born with either defect. Immediate care is directed toward maintaining body heat and fluid and electrolyte balance and protecting the exposed abdominal organs. The exposed organs should be covered with a warm, sterile, saline-soaked gauze, which, in turn, should be covered with plastic wrap to contain body heat and prevent further trauma. The newborn should be positioned in the lateral position; the bowel should be supported to prevent injury. A nasogastric tube is inserted for gastric decompression. Intravenous fluids, volume expanders, and antibiotics are ordered by the physician.

The surgical procedure to replace the organs in the abdominal cavity varies, depending on how large the defect is. If the defect is large, the surgery may need to be done in stages. A staged repair is done with a polymeric silicone (Silastic) pouch, which is used to suspend the viscera above the infant. Daily reduction maneuvers are done to return the suspended organs to the abdominal cavity. This staged reduction is generally done over 7 to 10 days. The infant then returns to surgery for closure of the abdominal wall (Kenner & Lott, 2003). If the defect is small, surgery to return the organs back into the abdominal cavity is performed as soon after birth as possible.

Parental support is extremely important. Parents need to be encouraged to hold their infant's hand and have as much physical contact as possible. The parents may experience a great deal of difficulty in accepting these disfiguring anomalies and in bonding with their newborn. The nurse must keep the parents informed about their newborn's condition, prognosis, physical appearance, and management plan. The nurse should assist and counsel parents who are trying to cope with this crisis.

Imperforate Anus

Imperforate anus refers to a group of congenital anomalies involving the rectum and anus. These anomalies result when the membrane separating the rectum from the anus fails to absorb during the seventh or eighth week of gestation. The condition occurs in 1 in 5,000 births and is more common in males (Holland et al., 1998). The anomalies are classified by location, either high or low. In the low type, there may be stenosis of the anal opening or a thin transparent membrane may cover the normal anal opening. In the high type, the rectum ends in a blind pouch or there is no connection between the anus and the rectum (Figure 22-9). The necessary treatment and the prognosis are determined by the type of defect.

Approximately 20% to 75% of infants with an imperforate anus have accompanying anomalies. These anomalies are of the VATER or VACTERL variety as described earlier in this chapter.

Visual inspection of the anal opening may lead the examiner to the diagnosis of imperforate anus. Additional clinical findings may include failure to pass a meconium stool and the inability of the rectum to allow insertion of a thermometer or a gloved small finger.

Surgery is done in stages if the anomaly is the high type. The infant requires a temporary colostomy in the interim. If the anomaly is of the low classification and a thin transparent membrane covers the anal opening, treatment consists of membrane excision, followed by daily dilation. Parents are taught the dilation procedure.

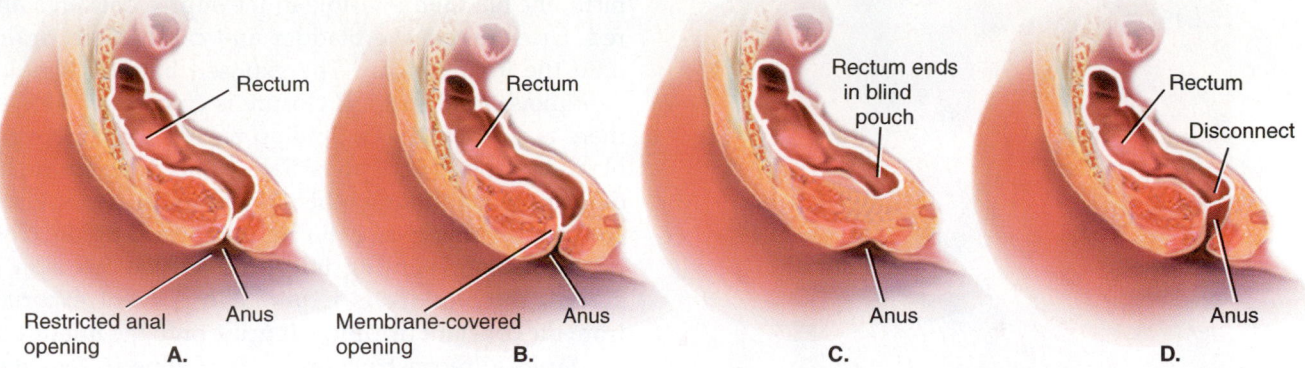

Figure 22-9   Imperforate anus. A. Anal opening is present but constricted; B. Anus and rectum are normal but the anal opening is covered by a thin membrane; C. Rectum ends in a blind pouch; D. Rectum and anal canal are present but not connected.

Assessing Newborn Intestinal Elimination

1. Newborns usually pass their first stool (meconium) by 8–24 hours. Meconium is passed for the first few days and is typically black or green in color, sticky, and tarlike.

2. By the second and third day the newborn passes transitional stools, which are of thinner consistency than meconium, greenish-brown to yellowish-brown in color, and less sticky.

3. By the 5th day of life, the newborn typically passes 4–6 stools per day (frequency may vary from 1 stool per 2 days to 10 stools per day).

4. Breastfed newborns have yellowish (sometimes greenish) stools, which are more liquid in consistency and frequent, while bottlefed infants tend to have more formed, pale stools.

Warning signs:

- If no stool is passed for 24 hours, consider imperforate anus

- Watery, green, excessive mucus, foul odor, and flatus may be evidence of intestinal problems or infection.

Genitourinary System Anomalies

The urinary system begins to form during the fourth week of gestation, whereas first indications of the genitals appear during the fifth week. Defects in the genitourinary system are often not life-threatening but may be of great concern to the family, especially if the defect has involved formation of the genitalia. The anomalies can be surgically repaired with varying outcomes in regard to function and appearance. Some of the malformations may be a symptom of a much more complex disease.

Hypospadias

Hypospadias is a congenital anomaly in which the urethral meatus is located on the ventral surface of the glans penis instead of at the tip (Figure 22-10). This anomaly is fairly common, occurring in approximately 8 of 1,000 male births (Rudolph, Rudolph, Hostetter, Lister, & Siegel, 2003). The exact cause is unknown, but it may be that hypospadias is inherited as a multifactorial problem. The sibling of an affected infant has an increased risk (14%) of also having this anomaly (Avery et al., 2000). Surgical repair is generally completed during the first year of life. The infant should not be circumcised before surgical repair because the foreskin is used, if necessary, for plastic surgery.

Epispadias

In **epispadias**, the urethral meatus is located on the dorsal surface of the penis (Figure 22-11). This is a rare anomaly, which occurs in only 1 of 100,000 live births (Avery et al.,

Reflections from a Father

When my first son was born, I was absolutely on "cloud nine." The pregnancy, the birth, and our growth together as a couple had all been more than I could have ever hoped for. But when I looked at my son more closely, I noticed that his penis did not look right, because the opening was on the top rather than at the tip. I must admit that I was quite relieved to learn that this condition is easily repaired and will have no lasting negative effects on my son's growth and development.

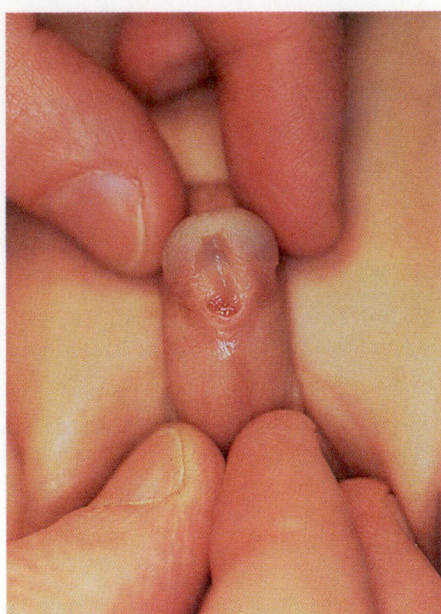

Figure 22-10 Hypospadias. *(Courtesy of Dr. James Mandell, Children's Hospital Boston.)*

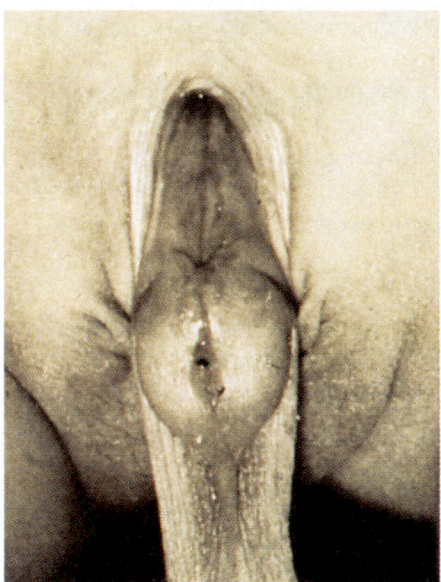

Figure 22-11 Epispadias. *(Courtesy of Dr. James Mandell, Chief Children's Hospital Boston.)*

2000). This condition often occurs with exstrophy of the bladder. Surgical repair is necessary and, as in infants with hypospadias, circumcision should not be done before the repair.

Exstrophy of the Bladder

Exstrophy of the bladder is an anomaly in which the anterior wall of the bladder and the lower portion of the abdominal wall are absent, causing the bladder to lie open and exposed on the lower abdomen. This defect is rare and occurs in only 1 of 25,000 live births (Avery et al., 2000). At

birth, the bladder is visible in the suprapubic area and is red. Urine enters the bladder and can be seen draining onto the infant's skin. The exposed bladder should be kept moist until surgical closure is completed. However, there is a difference of opinion on whether to cover the bladder or not; some physicians prefer to keep the bladder exposed, although others prefer to use a moist, sterile covering. Nursing care during this period before closure is aimed at preventing infection. Meticulous skin care around the bladder is required to prevent excoriation from the constant dripping of urine onto the infant's skin.

Surgical reconstruction is often done in two stages. The first stage is done within the first few hours after birth. The bladder and abdominal wall are surgically closed. The second surgical procedure involves creating a urethra, which is performed before the child goes to school, if possible.

Parents need support and education. They need understanding and guidance on how to accept their infant with such an obvious anomaly. They must be taught how to care for their infant at home until the final stage of the surgery is completed.

Ambiguous Genitalia

Even though parents may know the probable gender of their fetus from an ultrasonographic examination, gender is not certain until birth occurs. In rare cases, the gender of the newborn remains unclear at the time of birth. In these situations, it is imperative for the staff and physicians to be extremely cautious but to reassure the parents that the gender of their infant will be determined as soon as possible. Evaluation of the newborn with ambiguous genitalia must be treated as a medical emergency for many reasons. First, the ambiguous genitalia may be the result of several types of congenital adrenal hyperplasia that are life-threatening. Second, if the uncertainty of gender assignment is handled poorly, it can provoke long-term consequences for both the parents and the child (Avery et al., 2000).

Gender assignment should be achieved as soon as possible, preferably no later than age 2. However, gender determination within 3 to 6 months after birth is helpful in cases in which reconstructive surgery is necessary (Kenner & Lott, 2003). Gender determination should only be done after careful review and consideration. The process of review should be initiated with a thorough maternal and family history, physical examination of the infant, and laboratory and radiographic studies. The mother should be asked about drugs that she took during the pregnancy, family history of a previous sibling who died during the first 10 days of life, or siblings who experienced precocious puberty. Positive responses from these questions might indicate congenital adrenal hyperplasia (Avery et al., 2000). The laboratory and radiographic evaluation consists of measurement of circulating hormones, analysis of the chromosomes (results are usually available in 2 to 3 days), and visualization of the internal organs (Kenner & Lott, 2003).

Parental involvement is a critical consideration that the nurse must include in her plan of care. Parents require a great deal of support as they learn to deal with this situation. The nurse is responsible for coordination of care to ensure that the parents understand all the information they are given by various members of the health care team. Knowledge and understanding of basic neonatal embryology and sexual ambiguity can be beneficial to the nurse in identifying newborns with this disorder (Kenner & Lott, 2003).

Assessing Newborn Urinary Elimination

1. Newborns usually void during delivery or immediately following delivery.
2. Urinary function may be suppressed for several hours after birth.
3. Newborns usually void 10–15 times each day by 2–3 days of life.

Warning signs:

■ Failure to void within 24 hours
■ Concentrated, red, or rusty reddish brown urine

Musculoskeletal System Anomalies

Similar to many of the other systems, formation of the musculoskeletal system begins in the fourth week of gestation. This system includes development of the joints, muscles, and skeleton. Malformations are often relatively minor and, with proper recognition and treatment, the outcome is usually favorable.

Developmental Dysplasia of the Hip

Developmental dysplasia of the hip (DDH) was previously termed "congenital hip dislocation." DDH includes malformations of the hip involving varying degrees of deformity that may be present at birth, ranging from subluxation to complete dislocation. There are two basic types of DDH: developmental dislocation and teratogenesis. The more common of the two is the developmental dislocation, which is embryologically normal but is the result of mechanical forces in utero and the influence of maternal hormones, mainly estrogen, which relaxes tissues in preparation for birth. The infant's hip is generally dislocated in the perinatal period. The less common type of DDH, in which the hip is dislocated in the embryologic period of gestation, has a teratogenic cause, seen in conjunction with malformation of the pelvis and hip (Avery et al., 2000). Some affected infants show normal hip movement at birth, so the initial examination may be normal, but they later demonstrate abnormal hip development. Therefore, dysplastic hip screenings should be done at 2

weeks and 2, 4, 6, 9, and 12 months of age (Kenner & Lott, 2003).

DDH occurs in 10 of 1,000 live births (Finberg & Kleinman, 2002). The cause is considered to be multifactorial, with genetic, hormonal, and environmental influences that predispose the hip joint to dislocation. The condition is approximately six times more common in girls than in boys. It is usually, but not always, unilateral, with the left hip being more commonly involved.

DDH must be detected in the neonatal period to enable early treatment and prevent complications. Ortolani's maneuver and Barlow's test are useful in making the diagnosis of DDH. These tests should be completed only by an experienced practitioner. Ortolani's maneuver determines whether one or both hips are dislocated (Figure 22-12). A positive result on Ortolani's maneuver is elicited when the hip is flexed at a 90-degree angle the leg is gently abducted, and an audible clunk is heard. In infants with DDH, Ortolani's maneuver elicits positive results until 8 weeks of age or longer (Avery et al., 2000). Barlow's test determines whether the hip can be dislocated on manipulation. Positive results on Barlow's test occur when the examiner flexes both hips and knees and slightly adducts the hips; a posterior-directed force on the

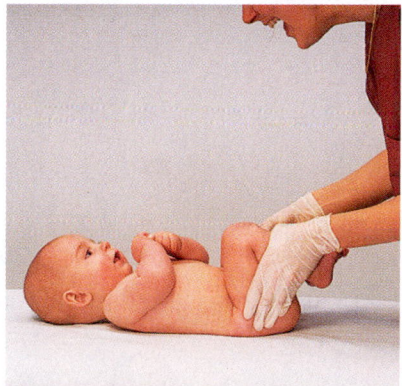

A.

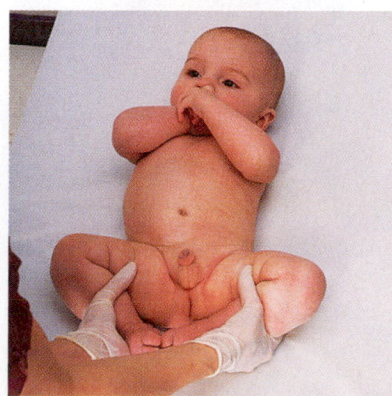

B.

Figure 22-12 Ortolani's maneuver. A. Hand placement; B. Hip abduction.

knees causes the hip to dislocate (Finberg & Kleinman, 2002).

Secondary signs of DDH develop after 6 weeks of life, when the hip migrates laterally and superiorly (Figure 22-13). These signs are asymmetrical gluteal folds (higher on the affected side); limited abduction of the affected hip; and a femur that appears to be shorter on the affected side (Galeazzi's sign) (Avery et al., 2000).

Treatment should be started as soon as possible after diagnosis to prevent any further deformity. Regardless of the type of hip dysplasia, the hips must be maintained in a flexed and abducted position. Methods used to maintain this position include triple diapering and an orthopedic splint, such as the Pavlik harness (Figure 22-14). The harness may be worn for the first 1–2 months of life. Frequently, a spontaneous relocation of the hip will occur in 3 to 4 weeks as a result of wearing the Pavlik harness (Fa-

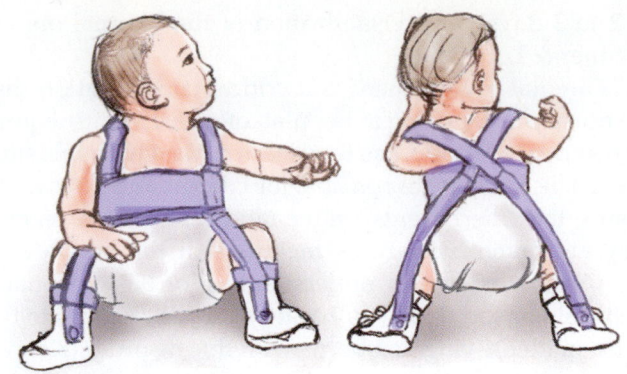

Figure 22-14 Infant in a Pavlik harness, used to treat developmental dysplasia of the hip.

naroff & Martin, 2001). The harness is effective in 90% of cases. However, if the harness is ineffective in attempting to stabilize the hip, a spica cast may be applied to the hip or surgery may be necessary.

Parental support and teaching is an important part of the treatment plan. Parents must be educated about the disorder, treatment management, and care of the infant in a harness or cast. Care should be directed toward preparing the parents for home care and assisting them in feeling comfortable holding and caring for their infant in an orthopedic device. The infant requires extensive follow-up with the orthopedist, and the nurse should stress keeping these follow-up visits.

Clubfoot

Clubfoot (talipes equinovarus) is the most common congenital deformity of the foot, in which portions of the foot and ankle are twisted out of a normal position (Figure 22-15). The foot is fixed in plantar flexion (downward) and is deviated medially (inward). Clubfoot is a musculoskeletal disorder that occurs twice as often in boys as in girls, with an overall incidence of 1 in 1,000 births (Fanaroff & Martin, 2001). The exact cause is unknown. This is a structural

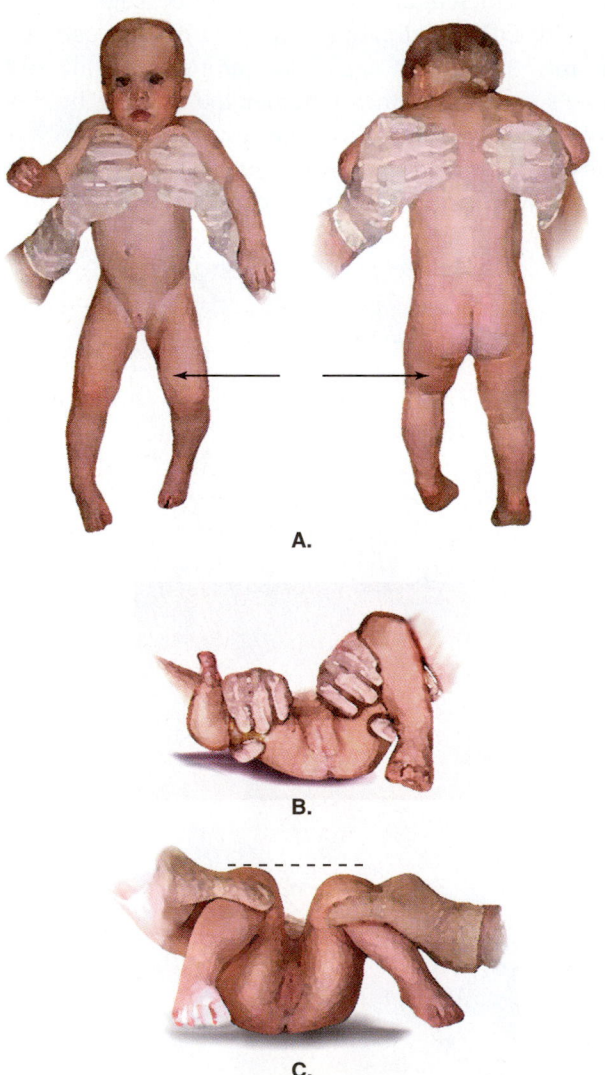

Figure 22-13 Assessing for DDH. A. Thighs and gluteal folds show asymmetry; B. Flexion shows limited hip abduction; C. Knee height shows uneven level caused by shortened femur.

Reflections from Families

Having our daughter in a Pavlik harness was a real challenge at first—especially the positioning, the diaper and clothing changes, and handling questions from curious observers. But then our 7-year-old son said, "Hey, it looks like a slingshot to me," and since then, we've had a more light-hearted view of the treatment and a more positive outlook about our daughter's future.

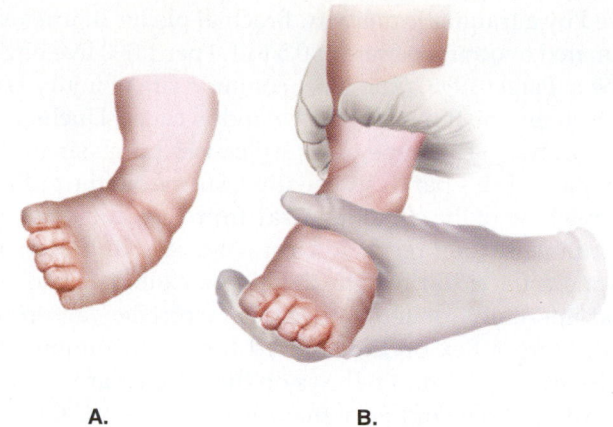

A.   **B.**

Figure 22-15   A. Talipes equinovarus (clubfoot); B. If the foot can be moved toward midline, the twisting is positional rather than congenital.

deformity that is easily recognized by its resistance to manual correction (Avery et al., 2000).

Treatment is most successful when begun soon after birth, before the muscles and bones of the leg develop abnormally, causing shortening of the tendons. Nonsurgical treatment consists of gentle repeated manipulations of the foot, with serial castings done every few days for the first 1 to 2 weeks, then every week or two until correction of the foot is satisfactorily completed. Correction is usually completed in 6 to 8 weeks. To maintain the correction from serial castings, braces are usually worn for another 6 months, or longer. If conservative measures are unsuccessful in correcting the foot, surgical intervention is required during infancy.

Infants with this deformity are frequently placed in a cast while they are still in the newborn nursery. Nursing care is aimed toward supporting and educating the parents about this anomaly; nursing interventions include teaching the parents cast care, how to assess the toes to ensure adequate vascular circulation, how to handle the infant in a cast, and adhering to the follow-up treatment plan.

ACQUIRED DISORDERS

Conditions that result from environmental factors are referred to as acquired disorders. Although some disorders may be detected soon after birth, others may not become evident for several days. The longer an acquired disorder goes undetected and untreated, the greater the possibility of complications or long-term sequelae. Neonatal admission nurses must learn to carefully screen the maternal history for risk factors and must maintain up-to-date assessment skills. In addition, the nursing staff must remember to keep the parents of these neonates informed about the condition, treatment modalities, prognosis, and possible outcomes for infants with the disorder.

Trauma and Birth Injuries

In a difficult or traumatic delivery, certain birth injuries may occur. The injuries range from mild to life-threatening. A complete and thorough assessment of the neonate soon after birth allows the nurse to identify injuries sustained and develop an appropriate plan of care. In addition to meeting the specific needs of the neonate with a birth injury, nurses must also see to parental needs. The parents should be informed of their infant's condition, his or her special needs during the hospital stay and after discharge, and the possible outcomes.

A review of mortality rates indicates a steady decline in fetal deaths caused by birth injuries. Between 1981 and 1993, injury-related deaths decreased from 23.8 to 3.7 per 100,000 live births. Despite the significant decrease in mortality rates, birth injuries still rank as an important risk factor for neonatal morbidity (Fanaroff & Martin, 2001).

Fractures

Fractures often occur as the result of a difficult labor, breech deliveries, or large infants or when fetal distress is present and a rapid delivery is necessary. Common sites of fractures include the clavicle; long bones, such as the humerus and femur; and the skull. Fractures may not be detected immediately after birth because the infant may not display any signs of pain or the deformity may not be apparent. Definitive diagnoses for all fractures are determined by X-ray studies. During birth, the bone most often fractured is the clavicle. Fractured clavicles occur in at least 1.7% to 2.9% of term deliveries and more frequently on the right side (Avery et al., 2000). The break often occurs in the middle third of the bone; it is usually the result of dystocia in a vertex delivery. The newborn may be asymptomatic if the fracture is not displaced, and the fracture may not be detected until the infant is 2 to 3 weeks old. At that time, the infant develops a callus and mass over the fractured clavicle. Signs and symptoms of a fractured clavicle may include decreased mobility or immobility of the affected arm, crepitus along the involved clavicle, absence of the Moro reflex on the affected side, and crying by the infant when the arm is moved. Other than gentle handling to minimize pain, there is no medical or surgical treatment. The prognosis for complete recovery is good. Health care providers and the parents must be taught not to lift the infant up by the arms. If a fractured clavicle is suspected, the scarf sign should not be assessed on that side. Immobilization of the affected arm by immobilizing it close to the body (i.e., pinning sleeve to shirt or using a sling) may provide pain relief. The immobilization may be discontinued in 8 to 10 days when there is callus formation.

The second most often fractured bone is the humerus. These fractures result from a difficult delivery of the arms or shoulders during a vertex or breech delivery. The fracture is generally detected during delivery when the obstetrician hears and feels the humerus snap (Avery et al., 2000). Signs and symptoms are the same as those of a fractured clavicle, with the exception that crepitus is not evident. The fractured arm should be immobilized in the adducted position with a splint or cast for 2 to 4 weeks, or until healing occurs.

Fractures of the femur also occur as the result of a difficult delivery. Deformity of the thigh, swelling, or immobility may be noted. Treatment involves traction, suspension, and casting for approximately 3 to 4 weeks (Fanaroff & Martin, 2001).

The newborn's skull is extremely flexible and can withstand a great deal of molding; therefore, skull fractures are rare. The types of fractures that may occur are linear fractures and depressed fractures. Linear fractures, the most common, account for 70% of all skull fractures. This skull fracture generally has no signs or symptoms and does not require any special treatment, unless an intracranial hemorrhage has occurred. In depressed fractures, the skull becomes indented from the pressure exerted on the head by the pelvis or by forceps during delivery. Depressed fractures may require surgery if brain tissue is involved. Skull X-ray studies and CT scans are done to determine the site of fracture and to identify any potential complications.

The parents of newborns with fractures are often fearful of hurting their infant. To allay some of their fears, they should be taught how to handle and feed their infant and change diapers. Parents also should be taught the importance of follow-up care that includes additional X-ray films and CT scans, which may be necessary for several months after discharge to make sure that reunion of the bone occurs (Moe & Paige, 1998).

Facial Palsy or Paralysis

Facial palsy or paralysis results from pressure exerted on the seventh cranial nerve during a difficult vaginal delivery or from pressure of forceps, which causes paralysis on one side of the infant's face. The incidence of facial palsy in the newborn varies from 0.05% to 1.8% (Avery et al., 2000). In 75% of cases, the facial paralysis occurs on the left side (Moe & Paige, 1998). Usual signs of facial paralysis include inability to close the eye on the affected side, absence of wrinkles in the forehead during crying, and drawing of the mouth to one side when crying. No medical treatment is required, and the condition usually resolves within 3 weeks.

Brachial Paralysis or Palsy

Brachial palsy is a paralysis of the muscles involving the upper extremity that occurs as a result of injury to the brachial plexus during a prolonged and difficult labor, fol-

lowed by a traumatic delivery. Brachial plexus injuries are estimated to occur at a rate of 0.5 to 1.9 per 1,000 live births (Moe & Paige, 1998). The most common site of injury is at the fifth and sixth cranial nerve and is called Duchenne-Erb paralysis. This type of injury causes paralysis in the upper arm. Erb's paralysis usually results from the pulling or stretching of the shoulder away from the head during a difficult vertex or breech delivery. Clinical manifestations include a flaccid arm with the elbow extended and the hand internally rotated, an intact grasp reflex, absent or weak Moro reflex on the affected limb, and diminished or absent deep tendon reflexes on the affected arm.

Another type of injury that can occur from C-8 to T-1 is called Klumpke's palsy. This injury causes paralysis to the lower arm and hand. The incidence of Klumpke's paralysis is less than 2% of all cases. Treatment of brachial plexus injuries may include immobilization for 1 to 5 days, passive ROM exercises, and proper positioning of the affected arm and hand. In 88% to 92% of cases, full recovery is seen during the first year of life. Parents must be taught how to do passive ROM exercises and must be informed that these exercises are done to prevent further complications caused by contractures (Moe and Paige, 1998). If the brachial plexus is completely torn, the infant will need referral to a specialty clinic that treats these injuries.

Intracranial Hemorrhage

Intracranial hemorrhage (ICH) is a collection of blood within the cranium. It results from birth trauma and is more likely to occur in the large, full-term newborn and spontaneously in the premature newborn, who is at highest risk for the development of ICH. There are different types of hemorrhage; the newborn can have one or more of these types. The most common types are subdural and subarachnoid hemorrhage.

Subdural hemorrhage (hematoma) is a collection of blood in the subdural space of the brain that results from lacerations of the large veins and sinuses that are frequently seen in conjunction with a tear in the dura. Subdural hemorrhages occur less frequently now than in the past; they now account for less than 10% of all ICHs in the newborn because of improvements in obstetric monitoring and care. Subdural hemorrhages are a life-threatening condition because of their inaccessibility for aspiration by subdural tap (Fanaroff & Martin, 2001). Surgical evacuation of subdural clots may be necessary on an emergency basis.

Signs and symptoms include a decreased level of consciousness, seizures, and asymmetry of motor function. Diagnosis depends on results of a CT scan of the brain. If a subdural hemorrhage is confirmed, the prognosis is poor if the laceration is of the tentorium or falx; this diagnosis carries a mortality rate of 45%. The majority of infants with this type of laceration develop other complications, such as hydrocephalus. If the hemorrhage is of a lesser degree, 50% of the infants are neurologically normal at follow-up visits (Avery et al., 2000).

Subarachnoid hemorrhage is the most common type of neonatal ICH. This type of hemorrhage in the full-term newborn is usually the result of trauma; in the premature infant, the hemorrhage results from hypoxia. Bleeding is of venous origin and is the result, more commonly, of smaller hemorrhages rather than massive ones. Diagnosis is confirmed by results of lumbar puncture and a CT scan of the brain. Signs of a subarachnoid hemorrhage include irritability, decreased level of consciousness, and seizures. Seizures are treated with anticonvulsant medications (Moe & Paige, 1998).

The nursing care of the newborn with ICH is generally supportive. Care includes monitoring of ventilatory and neurologic status; intravenous therapy to maintain fluid and electrolyte balance; observation and management of seizures; and prevention of increased ICP. The newborn should be handled minimally to promote rest and reduce stressors (Wong et al., 2002).

Because follow-up care varies, depending on the type and extent of hemorrhage, parent teaching must be individualized according to the prognosis for the infant's condition. Referral to local support groups may be beneficial.

Infants of Diabetic Mothers

Diabetes mellitus and gestational diabetes mellitus are increasing throughout the population. Gestational diabetes occurs in approximately 2% to 3% of pregnant women (Sills & Rapaport, 1994).

The infant of a diabetic mother (IDM) presents with a number of clinical problems. A better understanding of maternal and fetal metabolism, resulting in stricter metabolic control, improved fetal surveillance, early delivery, and neonatal intensive care, has increased the survival rates for IDMs over the past few years (Fanaroff & Martin, 2001). In recent years, perinatal mortality rates have decreased by 6% in IDMs, from more than 10% to less than 4% (Fanaroff & Martin, 2001).

The fetus is at risk for many problems when the mother has diabetes mellitus. Alteration in glucose metabolism affects the fetus in utero and the infant immediately after birth. One factor that determines how the fetus is affected is the severity and duration of the maternal diabetes. A positive outcome for the health of the fetus requires maintenance of normoglycemia in the pregnant woman with diabetes. Even with good control of the mother's glucose levels, problems can occur. Common problems observed in infants of diabetic mothers include macrosomia, respiratory distress syndrome, hypoglycemia, hypocalcemia, hypomagnesemia, hyperbilirubinemia, polycythemia, and congenital anomalies.

Macrosomia

Macrosomia is defined as a fetal weight above the 90th percentile for gestational age or a birth weight of more than 4,000 g (8 lb, 12.8 oz). Macrosomia is a common characteristic of infants of diabetic mothers. The probability of insulin-dependent women giving birth to a macrosomatic infant is 20% to 30% (Avery et al., 2000). Women with gestational diabetes have the same likelihood of bearing a macrosomatic infant as a woman with preexisting diabetes. The macrosomatic infant has a round chubby face, chubby body, and a plethoric appearance, which is related to polycythemia. The infant's internal organs (liver, spleen, and heart) are enlarged and amount of body fat is greater than normal. Much of this fat is deposited in the shoulders and intrascapular area. The IDM has normal brain growth, and the characteristic disproportion between head and shoulder size greatly contributes to dystocia and trauma during birth (Avery et al., 2000).

Insulin is the hormone central to the development of macrosomia. Late in pregnancy, when the mother's pancreas does not release enough insulin to meet the increasing needs, she becomes hyperglycemic. These high levels of maternal blood glucose cross through the placenta to the fetus, and the fetal pancreas responds by releasing large amounts of insulin. This increased production of insulin by the fetus stimulates the growth of insulin-sensitive tissues (i.e., adipose, muscle, and connective tissue), which causes macrosomia (Fanaroff & Martin, 2001).

Respiratory Distress Syndrome

IDMs are at greater risk of developing respiratory distress syndrome (RDS) than normal full-term newborns. Fetal hyperinsulinemia adversely affects fetal lung maturation by inhibiting the development of enzymes necessary for the synthesis of the phospholipid components of surfactant.

Hypoglycemia

The most common problem in an IDM at birth is hypoglycemia (i.e., blood glucose levels of less than 40 mg/dL). The infant's blood glucose level is high at the time of birth because of maternal hyperglycemia. Because of this elevated level of fetal blood glucose, the fetal pancreas responds by producing large quantities of insulin, causing a state of hyperinsulinemia. Even though there is a cessation of the maternal glucose supply when the cord is clamped, the infant is still in a hyperinsulinemic state. Hypoglycemia usually occurs during the first 3 hours after birth. The blood glucose level in the newborn is checked by heel stick after birth and again at frequent intervals, especially during the first 24 hours of life. Most IDMs are asymptomatic. Signs of hypoglycemia can include jitteriness and tremors, apnea, cyanosis, a high-pitched cry, lethargy, and tachypnea. Treatment includes providing early feedings (within 30 minutes after birth if bowel sounds are present) or the administration of intravenous glucose.

Hypocalcemia and Hypomagnesemia

Hypocalcemia and hypomagnesemia are metabolic problems seen in IDMs. **Hypocalcemia** is a blood calcium level of less than 7 mg/dL. It is one of the most common clinical problems that affect IDMs. Approximately 10% to 20% of IDMs experience hypocalcemia during the neonatal period. The cause is believed to be related to decreased concentrations of parathyroid hormone during the first four days of life (Avery et al., 2000). Many infants with hypocalcemia are asymptomatic, but some may exhibit jitteriness, a high-pitched cry, irritability, seizures, and twitching. These symptoms may be indistinguishable from those of hypoglycemia, except that they generally occur between 24 and 36 hours after birth versus hypoglycemia, which occurs during the first 1 to 3 hours of life. To restore normal calcium levels, therapy is initiated by providing early feedings, intravenous calcium, or oral calcium supplements.

Reduced serum magnesium levels may occur in pregnant diabetic women and their infants. **Hypomagnesemia** is a serum magnesium level of less than 1.6 mg/dL. Hypomagnesemia in the newborn is believed to result from increased maternal losses of magnesium in the urine, which are characteristic of diabetes. Magnesium deficiency may inhibit fetal parathyroid hormone secretion, which is associated with hypocalcemia (Barron, Lindheimer, & Davison, 2000).

Hyperbilirubinemia

Hyperbilirubinemia , or jaundice, is a common finding in all newborns. Hyperbilirubinemia is an excess of bilirubin in the blood, which causes jaundice. Bilirubin is formed from the breakdown of hemoglobin in the red blood cells. Jaundice results from deposits of the yellow pigment in bilirubin. Excess amounts of bilirubin are evidenced by a yellowish discoloration of the neonate's skin, mucous membranes, and sclera, termed **jaundice**. Jaundice proceeds in a cephalopedal progression, first appearing on the head and face and then progressing to the trunk and extremities. If jaundice is present, it may be observed by blanching the skin on the infant's forehead or over the bridge of the nose. If the skin blanches to a yellow hue, jaundice is present. In dark-skinned infants, the nurse may more easily detect jaundice by observing the color of the sclera and the buccal mucosa.

Hyperbilirubinemia may result from either physiologic or pathologic factors. Even though hyperbilirubinemia is a common clinical finding in the newborn, the normal physiologic jaundice process must be distinguished from the abnormal pathologic jaundice condition.

Polycythemia

Many infants with hyperbilirubinemia also have **polycythemia**, which results from an increased number of red blood cells, and plays a significant role in hyperbilirubinemia. An increased rate of erythrocyte breakdown results from changes in erythrocyte membrane composition, which, in turn, result from changes in maternal glucose availability (Avery et al., 2000). This increased red blood cell breakdown, along with bruising suffered by the macrosomatic infant at birth, may contribute to high bilirubin levels.

Congenital Anomalies

The incidence of congenital malformations is two to four times higher in IDMs than in infants born to mothers who do not have diabetes (Avery et al., 2000). The most common anomalies are cardiac and skeletal malformations and neural tube defects. In most anomalies related to diabetic pregnancies, the structural abnormalities have occurred before the eighth embryonic week. This reinforces the importance of women with diabetes monitoring their glucose levels before conception and delaying pregnancy until their glycosylated hemoglobin level is within the normal range (Fanaroff & Martin, 2001).

The incidence of congenital heart lesions in IDMs can be as much as five times that of infants of normoglycemic mothers. The most common lesions in the IDM are atrial or ventricular septal defects, transposition of the great vessels, and coarctation of the aorta (Fanaroff & Martin, 2001).

Skeletal malformations may include delayed ossification, osseous defects, caudal regression syndrome, and femur agenesis or hypoplasia. CNS anomalies include hydrocephalus, meningomyelocele, and anencephaly (Kenner et al., 1998).

These infants may also present with abdominal distention, failure to pass meconium stool, and bile-stained vomitus, caused by a transient delay in the development of the left side of the colon. This condition is known as neonatal small left colon, or lazy colon syndrome. Normal bowel function develops in early infancy (Fanaroff & Martin, 2001).

Jaundice

Physiologic Jaundice

Physiologic jaundice occurs in approximately 50% to 60% of full-term newborns and up to 80% of preterm newborns during the first week of life. It is a transient elevation of unconjugated bilirubin, which occurs after 24 hours of age, and is a normal physiologic process. The mean unconjugated bilirubin level in cord blood is 1.8 mg/dL. The full-term infant reaches peak bilirubin concentration levels of 6 to 7 mg/dL between 48 and 72 hours after birth. Increased bilirubin levels resolve without any intervention, declining to less than 2 mg/dL by 6 to 7 days after birth. Ethnic variability may also influence bilirubin levels during the first week of life. Asian and Native Americans have average peak serum bilirubin levels that are twice the level of other ethnic groups.

Pathologic Jaundice

Jaundice that is evident in the first 24 hours of life, a bilirubin level that rises more than 0.5 mg/dL per hour, or true hemolysis is considered pathologic jaundice. The most common cause of pathologic jaundice is blood group incompatibility, specifically ABO and Rh incompatibility. Other less common situations that may be seen in conjunction with pathologic jaundice in the newborn are maternal or fetal infections, swallowed maternal blood, maternal diabetes, fetal enzyme deficiencies, fetal enclosed hemorrhage (e.g., cephalhematoma or bruising), fetal polycythemia, fetal small-bowel obstruction, and fetal hypothyroidism.

Kernicterus

A possible complication of pathologic jaundice is kernicterus, also termed "bilirubin encephalopathy." Kernicterus is the excess accumulation of unbound, unconjugated bilirubin, which is deposited in brain tissues, particularly the basal ganglia. The excess bilirubin crosses the blood-brain barrier, causing yellow staining of the brain tissue, similar to its effect on the skin. Kernicterus causes varying degrees of neurologic damage. There is not a direct correlation between serum bilirubin levels and the severity of brain tissue damage. However, in the full-term healthy infant whose total serum bilirubin exceeds 25 mg/dL, the risk for kernicterus increases. Premature infants or infants with other medical complications are at risk for kernicterus at much lower serum bilirubin levels. Perinatal conditions can also influence the bilirubin-binding capacity of hemoglobin and increase the risk for kernicterus at lower serum bilirubin levels; these include hypoxia, acidosis, hypothermia, hypoglycemia, sepsis, and administration of certain medications (e.g., salicylates, sodium benzoate). Kernicterus usually becomes evident during the first 6 days of life. Early signs, which may be absent or present, include lethargy, poor feeding, temperature instability, hypotonia, and a high-pitched cry. Permanent neurologic sequelae in these children include ataxia, opisthotonos, deafness, seizures, and mental retardation (Blackburn, 1995).

ABO Incompatibility

ABO incompatibility occurs as a result of the mother and fetus having different blood groups. The mixing of maternal and fetal blood leads to hemolysis of fetal red blood cells. ABO incompatibility is the most common and mildest type of hemolytic disease; it rarely causes severe hemolytic problems, which would require an exchange transfusion. The incompatibility occurs when the fetal blood is type A, B, or AB and the mother is type O. The incompatibility arises because the mother does not have the fetal red blood cell antigen A or B and produces antibodies that cross the placenta to the fetus. This problem may occur in the first pregnancy, because mothers with type O blood already have naturally occurring anti-A and anti-B antibodies in their blood. There is no way of preventing ABO incompatibility.

Laboratory studies may be helpful in establishing a diagnosis of ABO incompatibility. Positive results on direct Coombs' test occur in 3% of cases, but positive results in both direct and indirect Coombs' test occur in 80% of cases. The direct Coombs' test measures the presence of antibodies on the red blood cell surface, and the indirect test is a measurement of antibodies in the serum (Kenner et al., 1998).

Rh Incompatibility

Rh incompatibility is a hemolytic disease caused by the incompatibility of Rh factors in maternal and fetal blood. Rh incompatibility, or isoimmunization, occurs when the woman is Rh-negative and the fetus is Rh-positive. If both parents are Rh-negative, there is no hemolytic incompatibility with the infant and the infant is Rh-negative. Isoimmunization occurs when fetal blood cells escape and pass through the placenta into the maternal circulation. The fetal blood cells may pass into the maternal circulation as early as 8 weeks' gestation or during an abortion, amniocentesis, ectopic pregnancy, hydatidiform mole, abdominal trauma, or when the placenta separates during delivery. The woman may form protective antibodies against the fetal blood cells. The process by which the maternal immunologic system forms antibodies against fetal blood cells is termed maternal sensitization. Usually, the woman becomes sensitized during the first pregnancy but does not form enough antibodies to adversely affect the infant. However, during subsequent pregnancies, antibodies form rapidly, resulting in lysis or destruction of fetal red blood cells.

Erythroblastosis fetalis is a condition in which there is vast destruction of fetal red blood cells by maternal antibodies, resulting in fetal anemia and hyperbilirubinemia. The severity of this condition depends on how well the infant can compensate for the destruction of red blood cells. However, the destruction of fetal red blood cells may be so severe that a marked hemolytic anemia develops and the blood does not have sufficient capacity to carry oxygen to the tissues. Fetal death or birth of an infant with hydrops fetalis may result from this condition (Ensher & Clark, 1994). **Hydrops fetalis** is the most severe form of fetal hemolytic disease: there is severe anemia resulting in hypoxia, cardiac decompensation, and hepatosplenomegaly.

The signs of Rh incompatibility in the newborn are jaundice, pallor, and enlargement of the liver and spleen. Jaundice becomes evident within the first 4 to 5 hours after birth and peaks when the infant is 3 or 4 days old (Avery et al., 2000).

Management of Rh incompatibilities focuses on prevention of the disease by administering Rho (D) immune globulin (RhoGAM) to the mother after delivery or abortion, if the infant was Rh-positive. This agent should be administered within 72 hours after delivery; this treatment should prevent the woman from producing antibodies to the fetal blood cells that entered her bloodstream during the delivery.

Management of Newborn Jaundice

The goal of managing the newborn with jaundice is to keep the serum bilirubin below neurotoxic levels. The most common treatment modalities are phototherapy and exchange transfusions.

Phototherapy is the use of ultraviolet light in the treatment of jaundice in the newborn (Figure 22-16). Phototherapy works by encouraging the liver to excrete bile in the form of unconjugated bilirubin. Blue or fluorescent bulbs are commonly used in phototherapy. The adverse effects of using phototherapy include dermal rash, lethargy, abdominal distention, possible eye damage, dehydration, thrombocytopenia, hypocalcemia, secretory diarrhea, and "bronze baby" syndrome (Kenner et al., 1998).

The prolonged exposure to ultraviolet light may cause retinal damage; therefore, it is extremely important to keep the infant's eyes shielded with eye patches when under the light. However, try to keep as much of the infant's skin exposed as possible. During oral feedings, the light and eye patches can be removed to provide sensory stimulation and interaction with the parents or care provider.

Infants undergoing phototherapy require close monitoring of their body temperature, fluid and electrolyte balance, and serum bilirubin concentration (lights should be turned off while drawing blood). The serum bilirubin levels must be checked frequently to ensure that phototherapy is effective.

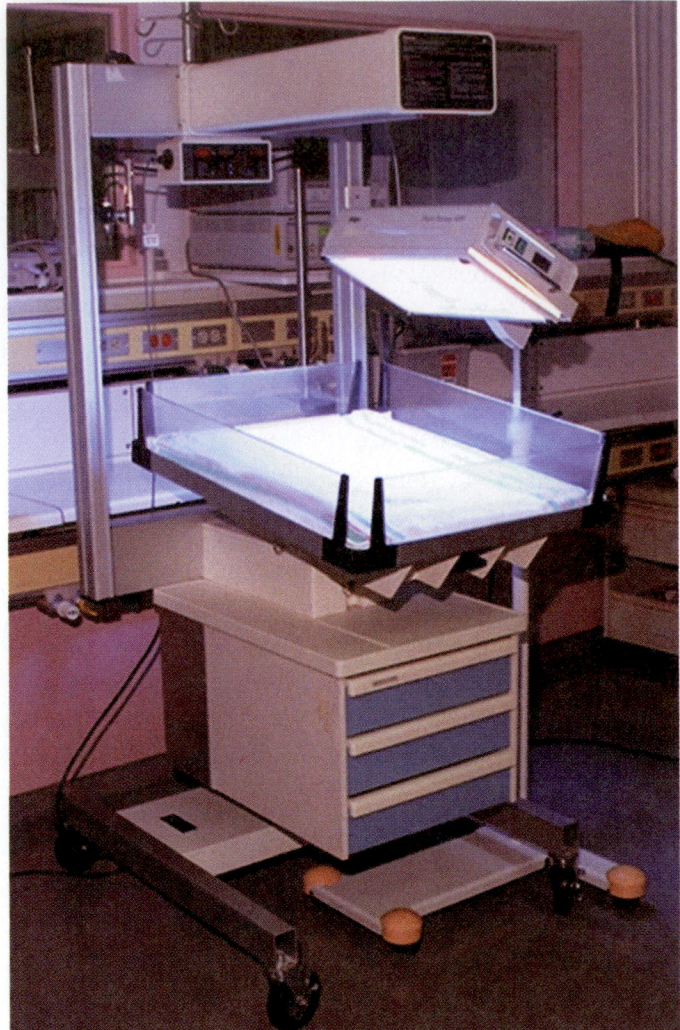

A.

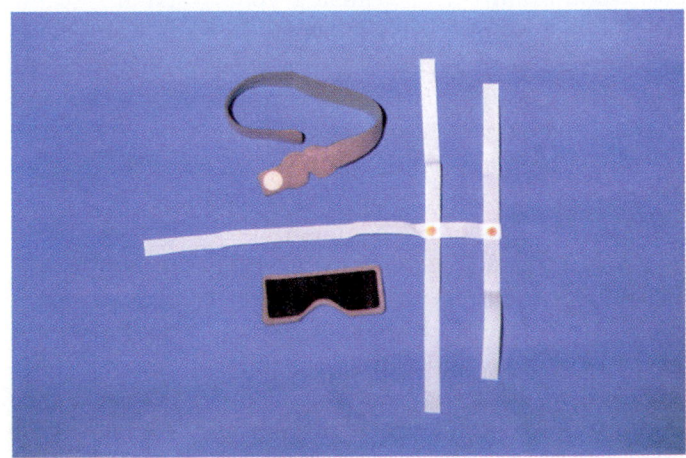

B.

Figure 22-16 A. Phototherapy, setup for jaundiced newborn; B. Phototherapy equipment, including bilateral eye patches.

If the infant is to receive phototherapy at home, the nurse is responsible for teaching the parents to record the infant's temperature, weight, and fluid intake; to weigh diapers; and to note the frequency of stools. Another method of phototherapy uses a fiber-optic blanket and is more convenient for home use.

If phototherapy is ineffective and the serum bilirubin level is rising to a level that may be neurotoxic, an exchange transfusion may be necessary. Exchange transfusions should lower the bilirubin level by 50% to 60%. During an exchange transfusion, the infant's antibody-coated red blood cells and excess bilirubin are removed and replaced by donor blood that contains noncoated red blood cells. Only small amounts of the infant's blood are removed and replaced at a time. The procedure is repeated until the infant's total blood volume has been diluted with the fresh blood. Exchange transfusions are considered safe, but complications may arise. The nurse must be alert for the following complications: bradycardia, arrhythmias, infection, thrombosis, hypocalcemia, and fluid overload.

NEONATAL INFECTIONS

Neonatal infections cause more than 30% of all neonatal deaths. Approximately 50% of neonatal mortalities that occur during the first 24 hours of life are attributed to infection (Kenner & Lott, 2003). Infection in the neonate can be caused by a variety of agents. Infection may be passed through the placenta to the baby during pregnancy or from exposure to organisms present in the vagina during birth or from the environment. Organisms that initially infect the mother and then are passed on transplacentally to the fetus are referred to by the acronym TORCH (toxoplasmosis, other [gonorrhea, syphilis, varicella, parvovirus, HBV, and HIV], rubella, cytomegalovirus, and herpes simplex virus. Major complications from infections include respiratory distress, shock, acidosis, disseminated intravascular coagulation (DIC), and meningitis (Kenner & Lott, 2003).

Sepsis

Sepsis is a systemic bacterial, viral, or parasitic infection that invades the bloodstream of the newborn. It occurs either during or after birth in approximately 1 of 1,000 full-term births (Ensher & Clark, 1994). Bacterial sepsis in the newborn is divided into two categories: early onset or late onset. Early-onset sepsis occurs during the first few days of life and is generally caused by obstetric complications, such as prolonged or premature rupture of membranes, chorioamnionitis, peripartum maternal fever, fetal distress, or aspiration by the newborn. The microorganisms that usually cause the early-onset infection are from the maternal vaginal tract and include group B *Streptococcus species*, *Haemophilus influenza*, *Listeria monocytogenes*, *Escherichia coli*, and *S. pneumoniae*. Infants with early-onset sepsis have a high mortality rate.

Late-onset sepsis generally occurs after the first week of life. Bacteria that cause the late-onset sepsis include organisms acquired either from the mother's genital tract or by contact from humans and equipment (Merenstein & Gardner, 2002). The bacteria that commonly cause late-onset sepsis include *Staphylococcus aureus*, *S. epidermidis*, *Pseudomonas* organisms, and group B beta-hemolytic streptococci. The most common organism for causing sepsis in the newborn is the group B *Streptococcus* species, which is acquired from the mother.

It is often difficult to distinguish sepsis in the neonate from other medical conditions because the symptoms of both early- and late-onset sepsis are vague and nonspecific. Because of the high mortality rate of sepsis, it is imperative for the nurse to observe and report to the physician any subtle changes that occur in the neonate's status.

The most accurate method of confirming bacterial sepsis is isolation of the bacteria from either the blood, CSF, or urine. Generally, the CSF is tested in the symptomatic newborn, because meningitis is a frequent cause or complication of sepsis (Merenstein & Gardner, 2002). Other tests include a complete blood cell (CBC) count with differential, C-reactive protein, erythrocyte sedimentation rate, total platelet count, and cultures (blood, urine, or CSF). A chest X-ray study detects pneumonia.

After obtaining the appropriate laboratory samples, antibiotic therapy is initiated. A broad-spectrum antibiotic, such as ampicillin in combination with an aminoglycoside, is commonly administered, pending culture and sensitivity results. Once the causative organism is determined and the antibiotic sensitivities are known, the least toxic antibiotic is administered for an appropriate period of time (Merenstein & Gardner, 2002).

Before the advent of antibiotic therapy, the mortality rate from bacterial sepsis was 95% to 100%, but now, with antibiotics, the mortality rate has been reduced to less than 50%. The most common complications of bacterial sepsis are meningitis and septic shock. Bacterial meningitis affects 1 in 2,500 live births (Wong et al., 2002). The outcome of neonatal sepsis is influenced by early recognition, antibiotic therapy, and supportive care (Merenstein & Gardner, 2002) (Table 22-2).

Table 22-2 Common Drugs to Treat Sepsis in the Term Infant			
MEDICATION	**DOSE**	**ROUTE**	**IV DILUTION/RATE**
Ampicillin	75–150 mg/kg/24 h q 12 h	IM/IV	30 mg/mL over 15–30 min
Cefotaxime (Claforan)	50 mg/kg/24 h q 12 h	IM/IV	20–60 mg/mL over 10–30 min
Ceftriazone (Rocephin)	25–50 mg/kg/24 h q 24 h	IM/IV	10–40 mg/mL over 10–30 min
Gentamicin	2.5 mg/kg/dose q 12 h	IM/IV	1–2 mg/mL over 30–60 min

FAMILY EXPERIENCES

The nursing care of the family with a newborn who has a congenital disorder is extremely demanding and must involve a multidisciplinary team approach, including such specialists as nurse practitioners, surgeons, social workers, dieticians, physical therapists, and neurologists. The care must address the surgical and rehabilitative needs of the infants and the educational, psychosocial, and financial needs of the family.

In the early postpartum period, it is particularly challenging to work with the parents. At this time, parents are going through the shock and disappointment of having had a "less-than-perfect" child. They must first be given the time, opportunity, and support to go through the grief process. This process involves the parents experiencing shock, denial, anger, and depression before accepting the newborn and reorganizing the family. Nurses can best make parental passage through the process easier by being accessible and keeping the lines of communication open between the parents and staff. Nurses should educate the family about the disorder and their infant's present and future health care needs. When they are ready, parents should be encouraged to touch and become involved in their infant's care.

NURSING PROCESS

Although not all congenital disorders can be predicted in the perinatal period, the nursing process provides a framework for nurses caring for families after the birth of an infant with an anomaly.

Assessment

Nursing assessment begins with a thorough review of the mother's history, including the family, past medical, psychosocial, previous obstetrical, and present prenatal history. Histories are reviewed to identify potential risk factors that alert the health care team to the possibility of a disorder in the fetus. As soon as the infant is delivered, the neonatal team must perform a physical assessment of the infant and its adaptation to extrauterine life. Initially, care is directed toward stabilization of the newborn and transport to the neonatal intensive care unit (NICU). Once the neonate with a disorder is stabilized in the NICU, attention is turned toward assessing the needs of the parents and family. Certain variables that may influence a family's ability to cope with the birth of an infant with a congenital or acquired disorder include age of the parents, culture, religion, and the support systems available to them. The nurse formulating the plan of care should assess the effect of these variables on the family and use that knowledge when providing information and communicating.

Nursing Diagnoses

Newborn

Care is individualized based on the disorder, the threat to survival, and family structure and coping abilities, but several general aspects of nursing care are common to most cases. Initially, nursing care is directed toward the stabilization and maintenance of life support. At this time, potential nursing diagnoses are:

- Ineffective thermoregulation related to stress of condition and or birth defect
- Infective breathing pattern related to oropharyngeal secretions and/or structural anomalies
- Decreased cardiac output related to decreased circulating oxygen secondary to a congenital cardiovascular defect

Should the infant survive the initial neonatal period, surgical correction of the birth defect is scheduled as soon as the infant's condition is stabilized. Postoperatively, potential nursing diagnoses are:

- Risk for infection related to the immature immune system, lack of normal flora, environmental hazards, and open wounds
- Impaired skin integrity related to structural anomalies and immobility
- Imbalanced nutrition: less than body requirements, related to NPO status that is required by the structural anomaly
- Pain related to procedures and treatments

Parents and Family

- Grieving related to realization of present or future loss for family and/or child and birth of a newborn with a defect
- Ineffective coping (depression) related to perceived parental role failure and loss of a "perfect infant"
- Deficient knowledge related to cause, management, and care of a newborn with a birth defect
- Anxiety related to unpredictable outcomes or prognosis of impaired infant
- Impaired parenting related to inadequate bonding, secondary to parent-child separation or failure to accept impaired child

Outcome Identification

Newborn

Sample targeted outcomes for the infant born with an anomaly might include:

- Maintaining a core body temperature of 97°F to 99.5°F
- Maintaining adequate gas exchange to support life
- Demonstrating signs of adequate circulating oxygen
- Exhibiting no signs of infection
- Maintaining and/or demonstrating no further breakdown in skin integrity
- Receiving adequate nutrients to support growth
- Remaining free of, or displaying less frequent signs of, episodic pain

Parents and Family

Anticipated outcomes of nursing care for the family might include that parents will:

- Verbalize their feelings and concerns regarding their newborn's medical problems, prognosis, and outcome
- Demonstrate an understanding of their infant's needs while participating in care
- Show the beginnings of attachment and the development of a parent-infant bond

Planning

Newborn

After delivery, the infant born with a congenital or acquired anomaly is cared for in a NICU. There the infant is placed under a radiant heater, connected to a cardiac monitor, and oxygen is administered to maintain respiratory function. Care is directed toward stabilization and preparation for surgery if indicated.

Parents and Family

In addition to meeting the infant's needs, the nurse must also recognize and deal with the educational, emotional, and psychosocial needs of the parents and family. The nurse must function as educator, support person, and facilitator to the parents and family during all aspects of care for the infant born with a defect or disorder. The parents' feelings and reactions are carefully assessed, as is their ability to absorb and understand information regarding their infant's condition. Families need constant information, guidance, and support from the nursing staff to make decisions regarding the course of action to be taken.

Nursing Intervention

Preoperative interventions for the infant include temperature regulation, maintenance of respiratory and cardiovascular function, and management of fluid and electrolyte balance. Depending on the type of defect present, other potential nursing interventions may include the management of open lesions and gastric decompression with the insertion of an oral gastric tube.

Postoperatively, the infant returns to the NICU and must be continuously monitored and frequently assessed for changes in condition or the development of complications. Vital functions are maintained with oxygen or mechanical ventilation and monitored with a pulse oximeter and measurement of arterial blood gas levels. Other nursing interventions include maintaining a neutral thermal environment, administration of intravenous fluids and strict measurement of intake and output, daily weight, hourly vital signs, and blood glucose monitoring. The nurse also provides care of the surgical site, administers antibiotics, and provides pain relief for the promotion of comfort.

It is crucial that the nursing staff encourage and facilitate parent-infant bonding by encouraging parental involvement in the care of the infant. Touching, talking to, and holding the infant during visitation should be encouraged by the nurse.

Another important aspect of nursing care is the referral to appropriate community and national agencies for financial and psychologic support. Nurses should familiarize themselves with available community services that provide support, assistance, and education to families with special needs or problems.

Evaluation

Newborn

The effectiveness of nursing interventions is determined by continuous assessment of the infant's condition and the evaluation of care. The following guidelines provide the basis by which to evaluate care and measure the degree of accomplishment of the expected outcomes.

- Assess and monitor vital signs including body temperature hourly. Measure blood glucose levels at frequent intervals.

- Assess respiratory function at frequent intervals: respiratory rate, breath sounds, skin color, and signs and symptoms of respiratory distress (nasal flaring, grunting, retractions).

- Continuous pulse oximetry and frequent blood sampling for arterial blood gas (ABG) values provides valuable information about the oxygenation and ventilation status in the newborn.

- Assess cardiovascular function and perfusion at frequent intervals: heart rate, blood pressure, rhythm, presence of murmur, capillary refill, skin color, and peripheral pulses.

- Observe for signs and symptoms of infection.

- Assess for signs of skin breakdown.

- Strictly monitor infant's intake and output of fluids, maintain patency of infant's peripheral lines, and take body weight daily.

- Observe infant's response to pain and pain relief interventions.

Parents and Family

- Document all phone calls from parents and family received in the unit regarding infant's condition and progress.

- Observe and document all visits from parents and family to the NICU.

- Observe and document parent-infant interactions (i.e., talking to, holding, touching).

- Document all parent teaching done (including CPR training).

- Assess level of understanding of teaching done (i.e., return demonstration, question-and-answer).

CASE STUDY/CARE PLAN
INFANT OF A MOTHER WITH GESTATIONAL DIABETES

Rudy is a 4,200 g (9 lb, 4 oz) male infant born via cesarean section at 38 weeks' gestation. His mother is a 27-year-old gravida 1, para 0, in whom gestational diabetes was detected at 28 weeks' gestation. His Apgar scores were: 7 at 1 minute (1 point off each for color, tone, and irritability); and 8 at 5 minutes (1 point off each for color and tone). Initial physical examination reveals the following: large for gestational age; blood glucose level, 38 mg/dL; heart rate, 156; respirations, 64/min with nasal flaring; gestational age, 37 weeks by Ballard scale; and apparent congenital anomalies or birth trauma, none.

Assessment

- 4200 g male
- IDM, LGA
- Apgar 7, 8
- HR 156, R 64

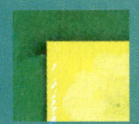

Nursing Diagnosis

Risk for injury related to hyperinsulinemia, secondary to gestational diabetes as evidenced by hypoglycemia.

Expected Outcome	Infant will maintain blood glucose levels that are within normal limits.
Planning	Discuss preferred feeding methods with parents.
NOC	Blood glucose level
NIC	Teaching: Disease process

Nursing Interventions	**Rationales**
1. Monitor glucose levels: at birth, on admission to the nursery, every 2 hours for the first 8 hours, and then every 4 hours for 24 hours. If glucose levels are abnormal, the testing should be repeated every 30 to 60 minutes until the infant has been stabilized.	1. Hypoglycemia may be present without any observable signs.

(continues)

Nursing Interventions	Rationales
2. Observe for signs of hypoglycemia (i.e., jitteriness and tremors, lethargy, apnea, cyanosis, tachypnea, and high-pitched cry).	2. These signs may indicate hypoglycemia, which generally develops 1 to 3 hours after birth.
3. Feed newborn early by providing glucose, breast milk, or formula.	3. Prevents or treats hypoglycemia that may develop 1 to 2 hours after birth.
4. Provide a neutral thermal environment.	4. Avoids cold stress, which increases metabolism, thereby causing rapid consumption of glucose.

Evaluation   Blood glucose levels are stabilized and remain above 40 mg/dL. No signs of hypoglycemia are evident. Axillary temperature remains between 97°F and 99.5°F (36.4°C and 36.7°C).

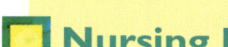

Nursing Diagnosis

Impaired gas exchange related to immature pulmonary system, secondary to maternal gestational diabetes.

Expected Outcome   Infant will demonstrate a normal respiratory status as evidenced by: a normal respiratory rate, rhythm, and depth; normal clear breath sounds; and arterial blood gas levels within the normal range.

Planning   Explain assessments and care to parents so that they will know what to expect.

NOC   Respiratory status: Gas exchange

NIC   Respiratory monitoring

Nursing Interventions	Rationales
1. Observe for signs of respiratory distress (i.e., nasal flaring, grunting, retractions, apnea, cyanosis).	1. IDMs are at greater risk of developing respiratory distress because fetal hyperinsulinemia adversely affects fetal lung maturity.
2. Assess respiratory rate and effort and suction nasopharynx as needed.	2. Maintaining a clear airway will make respiratory efforts easier.
3. Position infant on side with a rolled towel to the back.	3. Makes drainage of mucus easier.
4. Auscultate breath sounds every 3 to 4 hours as needed; assess infant for cyanosis, noting its relationship to activity.	4. Breath sounds and effectiveness of perfusion will indicate potential respiratory distress.
5. Provide a neutral thermal environment.	5. Prevents cold stress, which can increase the consumption of oxygen, leading to respiratory distress.

Evaluation   Respiratory rates are within normal limits (30 to 60 breaths per minute). No signs of respiratory distress are evident.

Nursing Diagnosis

Risk for injury related to hypocalcemia, secondary to maternal gestational diabetes.

Expected Outcome   Infant will maintain a calcium level between 7 mg/dL and 11 mg/dL.

Planning   Help parents understand the relationship between maternal gestational diabetes and the newborn's condition and required care.

NOC   Risk control

NIC   Risk identification

Nursing Interventions	Rationales
1. Monitor serum calcium levels.	1. Approximately 10% to 20% of IDMs experience hypocalcemia.
2. Observe for signs of hypocalcemia (i.e., muscle twitching and jitteriness, irritability, seizures, and vomiting).	2. Hypocalcemia, generally occurs between 24 and 36 hours after birth.
3. Administer calcium supplements as ordered by physician.	3. Treats or prevents hypocalcemia.

Evaluation   No signs of hypocalcemia are evident and serum calcium levels remain above 7 mg/dL.

WEB ACTIVITIES

••• Search the Internet for some of the disorders discussed in this chapter, such as spina bifida. Are there support groups for families experiencing these conditions? What type of information is available? Do they also direct information to health care professionals?

••• Search the Internet for government statistics on survival rates and quality-of-life issues for infants with the anomalies discussed in this chapter.

Key Concepts

- Genetic disorders are inherited defects passed down through generations; acquired disorders result from environmental factors.

- The most common anomalies affecting the CNS occur during the first 3 to 4 weeks' gestation, and many are detectable through prenatal diagnosis.

- Respiratory system anomalies are often life-threatening and require immediate intervention in the delivery room.

- There are more than 100 types of congenital heart defects, many with no known cause.

- Families need explicit instructions in feeding and caring for a newborn with a gastrointestinal anomaly, because special equipment, formulas, or techniques may be required.

- Many musculoskeletal anomalies, once detected, can be aggressively treated and have good prognoses.

- Birth injuries or trauma are often not evident at birth but are detected in the first few hours or days following delivery.

- Macrosomia, or fetal weight above the 90th percentile, is a common characteristic of infants born to mothers with diabetes.

- Jaundice, or an elevated serum bilirubin level, occurs in more than half of all full-term newborns during the first week of life.

- Neonatal infections can have many causes and many characteristic complications, including respiratory distress, shock, acidosis, DIC, meningitis, and death.

Review Questions and Activities

Match the terms in Column I with a definition or statement from Column II.

Column I

_____ congenital disorder

_____ spina bifida

_____ meningocele

_____ myelomeningocele

_____ gastroschisis

_____ intracranial hemorrhage

_____ subdural hemorrhage

_____ phototherapy

Column II

a. Collection of blood within the cranium

b. Collection of blood in the subdural space of the brain

c. Results from genetic or prenatal environmental factors, or both

d. Contains meninges and CSF

e. Results from failure of the spinal cord to close

f. Exposure to an ultraviolet light

g. Abdominal wall defect to the right of the umbilicus, through which the abdominal organs herniate

h. Contains meninges, CSF, and neural tissue

The correct answers are:

c—congenital disorder

e—spina bifida

d—meningocele

h—myelomeningocele

g—gastroschisis

a—intracranial hemorrhage

b—subdural hemorrhage

f—phototherapy

Identify the following statements as true or false:

1. Hypocalcemia is defined as a calcium level of more than 7 mg/dL.

   The correct answer is true.

2. Hypoglycemia is defined as a blood glucose level of less than 60 mg/dL.

   The correct answer is false.

3. Physiologic jaundice generally occurs during the first 24 hours after birth.

   The correct answer is false.

4. Ortolani's maneuver and Barlow's test are useful in detecting clubfoot.

   The correct answer is false.

5. Hypospadias is a congenital anomaly in which the urethral meatus is located on the ventral surface of the glans penis.

   The correct answer is true.

6. Prenatal diagnosis of congenital diaphragmatic hernia can be made by antenatal ultrasound examination as early as 26 weeks' gestation.

   The correct answer is true.

7. Myelomeningocele is the most common form of spina bifida cystica.

   The correct answer is true.

8. Clinical manifestations of increased ICP include: widening sutures; bulging anterior fontanelle, high-pitched shrill cry, and the "setting sun" sign.

   The correct answer is true.

9. Differentiate physiologic from pathologic jaundice.

10. Provide four planning and implementation nursing actions for the infant at risk for injury related to hyperinsulinemia.

11. List five signs of respiratory distress in the newborn.

12. List seven signs of hypoglycemia in a newborn.

13. Describe the nursing care for an infant who is receiving phototherapy.

References

Avery, G., Fletcher, M., & MacDonald, M. (Eds.). (2000). *Neonatology: Pathophysiology and management of the newborn* (5th ed.). Philadelphia: Lippincott.

Ball, J., & Birdler, R. (2003). *Pediatric nursing: Caring for children* (3rd ed.). Stamford, CT: Appleton & Lange.

Barron, W. H., Lindheimer, M. D., & Davison, J. M. (2000). *Medical disorders during pregnancy* (3rd ed.). St. Louis, MO: Mosby.

Blackburn, S. (1995). Hyperbilirubinemia and neonatal jaundice. *Neonatal Network, 14*, 7.

Coniglio, J., Manzione, J., & Hengerer, A. (1988). Anatomic findings and management of choanal atresia and the CHARGE association. *Annals of Otology, Rhinology, and Laryngology, 97*, 448.

Ensher, G., & Clark, D. (1994). *Newborns at risk: Medical care and psychoeducational intervention* (2nd ed.). Baltimore: Aspen.

Fanaroff, A., & Martin, R. (2001). *Neonatal-perinatal medicine: Diseases of the fetus and newborn* (7th ed.). St. Louis, MO: Mosby.

Finberg, L., & Kleinman, R. (2002). *Saunders' manual of pediatric practice* (2nd ed.). Philadelphia: W. B. Saunders.

Hockenberry, M., Wilson, D., Winklestein, M., & Kline, N. (2003). *Wong's nursing care of infants and children* (7th ed.). St. Louis, MO: Mosby.

Hoffman, J. (1995). Incidence of congenital heart disease: I. Postnatal incidence. *Pediatric Cardiology 6*(4), 103.

Holland, R., Price, F. N., & Bensaro, D. D. (1998). Neonatal surgery. In G. Merenstein, & S. Gardner. *Handbook of neonatal intensive care* (4th ed.). St. Louis, MO: Mosby.

Jackson, P., & Harvey, J. (2004). Hydrocephalus. In P. Jackson & J. Vessey (Eds.). *Primary care of the child with a chronic condition* (4th ed.). St. Louis, MO: Mosby.

Kenner, C., Amlung, S., Flandermeyer, A. (1998). *Protocols in neonatal nursing*. Philadelphia: W. B. Saunders.

Kenner, C., & Lott, J. W. (2003). *Comprehensive neonatal nursing: A physiologic perspective* (3rd ed.). Philadelphia: W. B. Saunders.

Merenstein, G., & Gardner, S. (2002). *Handbook of neonatal intensive care* (5th ed.). St. Louis, MO: Mosby.

Moe, P., & Paige, P. (1998). Neurologic disorders. In G. Merenstein, & S. Gardner. *Handbook of neonatal intensive care*. St Louis, MO: Mosby.

Mayer, V. (2001). *Late versus early surgical correction for congenital diaphragmatic hernia in newborn infants*. The Cochrane Library, Issue 1. Oxford: Update software.

Paidas, M., & Cohen, A. (1994). Disorders of the central nervous system. *Seminars in Perinatology, 18*(4), 226–282.

Rayburn, W. F., Stanley, J. R., & Garrett, M. E. (1996). Periconceptual folate intake and neural tube defects. *Journal of the American College of Nutrition, 15*(2), 121.

Rudolph, C., Rudolph, A., Hostetter, M., Lister, G., & Siegel, N. (2003). *Rudolph's pediatrics* (21st ed.). Stamford, CT: Appleton & Lange.

Sills, I., & Rapaport, R. (1994). New-onset IDDM presenting with diabetic ketoacidosis in a pregnant adolescent. *Diabetes Care, 17*(8), 904–905.

Wardinsky, T. (1994). Visual clues to diagnosis of birth defects and genetic disease. *Journal of Pediatric Health Care, 8*(2), 63–73.

Wong, D., Perry, S., & Hockenberry-Eaton, M. (2002). *Maternal child nursing care* (2nd ed.). St. Louis, MO: Mosby.

Suggested Readings

Howell, K. (1998). Understanding gastroschisis: An abdominal wall defect. *Neonatal Network, 17*(8), 17–25, 34–37.

McClain, B., & Anand, K. (1996). Neonatal pain management. In J. Deshpande, & J. Tobias, (Eds.), *The pediatric pain handbook*. St. Louis, MO: Mosby.

Milas, M., Carlson, J., & Fink, S. (1996). Sources of support reported by mothers and fathers in infants hospitalized in an NICU. *Neonatal Network, 15*(3), 45.

Resources

Association of Women's Health, Obstetric, and Neonatal Nurses (AWHONN), 2000 L St. NW, Suite 740, Washington, DC, 20036, 800-673-8499, http://www.awhonn.org

National Association of Neonatal Nurses, 4700 W. Lake Avenue, Glenview, IL 60025-1485, 800-451-3795, http://www.nann.org

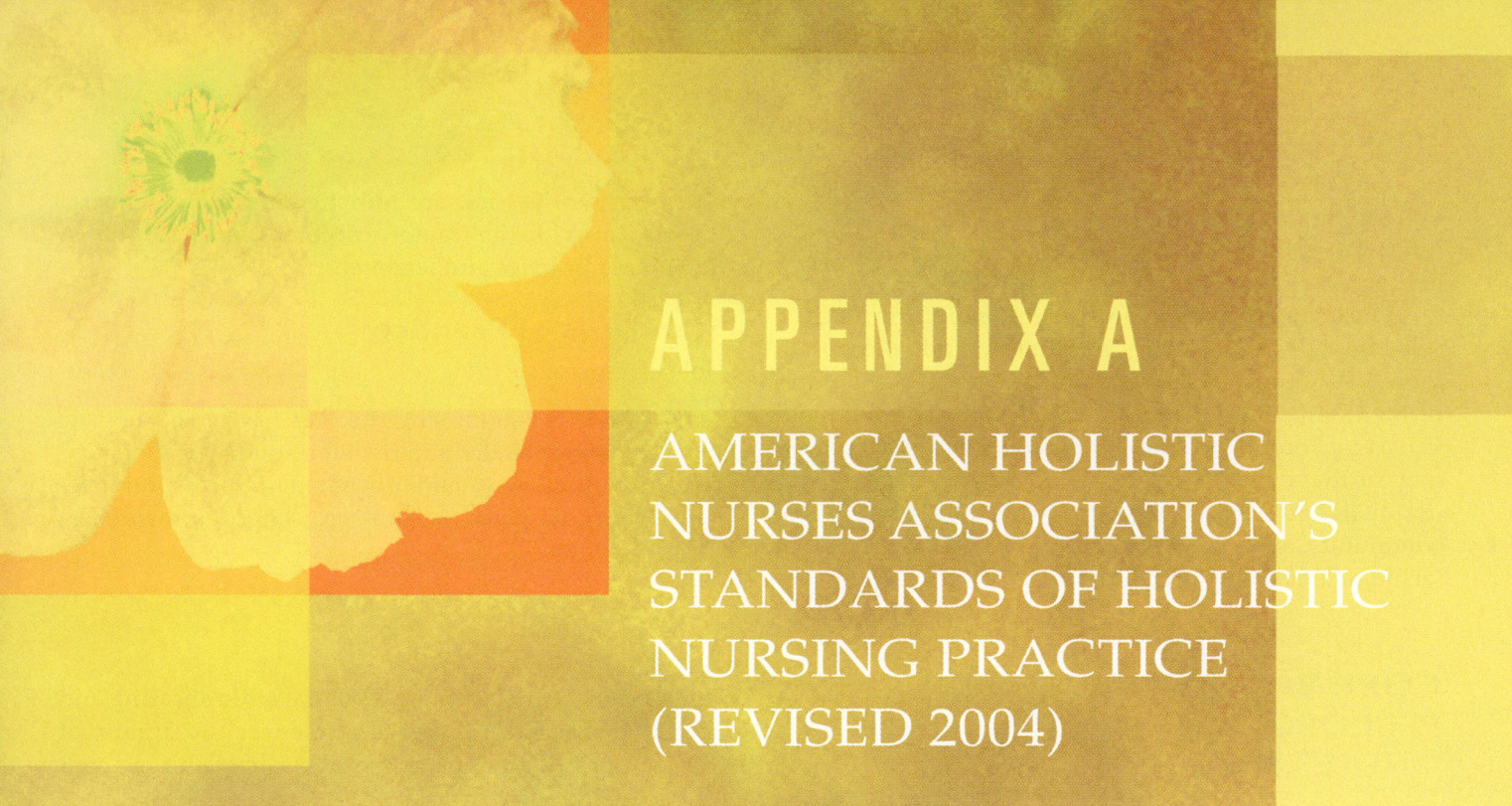

GUIDELINES

The AHNA Standards of Holistic Nursing Practice:

- are used in conjunction with the American Nurses Association Standards of Practice and the specific specialty standards where holistic nurses practice.
- contain five core values that are followed by a description and standards of practice action statements. Depending on the setting or area of practice, holistic nurses may or may not use all of these action statements.
- draw on modalities derived from a number of explanatory models, of which biomedicine is only one model.
- reflect the diverse nursing activities in which holistic nurses are engaged.
- serve holistic nurses in personal life, clinical and private practice, education, research, and community service.

AHNA HOLISTIC NURSING DESCRIPTION

Holistic nursing embraces all nursing which has enhancement of healing the whole person from birth to death as its goal. Holistic nursing recognizes that there are two views regarding holism: that holism involves identifying the interrelationships of the bio-psycho-social dimensions of the person, recognizing that the whole is greater than the sum of its parts; and that holism involves understanding the individual as a unitary whole in mutual process with the environment. Holistic nursing responds to both views, believing that the goals of nursing can be achieved within either framework.

The holistic nurse is an instrument of healing and a facilitator in the healing process. Holistic nurses honor the individual's subjective experience about health, health beliefs, and values. to become therapeutic partners with individuals, families, and communities, holistic nursing practice draws on nursing knowledge, theories, research,

©2004 American Holistic Nurses Association. Permission is given to duplicate this document for teaching purposes by an educational institution. Written consent is required for duplication by an author or publisher. AHNA, P.O. Box 2130, Flagstaff, AZ 86003-2130; phone (800) 278-2462, fax (928) 526-2752; www.ahna.org.

expertise, intuition, and creativity. Holistic nursing practice encourages peer review of professional practice in various clinical settings and integrates knowledge of current professional standards, laws, and regulations governing nursing practice.

Practicing holistic nursing requires nurses to integrate self-care, self-responsibility, spirituality, and reflection in their lives. This may lead the nurse to greater awareness of the interconnectedness with self, others, nature, and God/Life Force/Absolute/Transcendent. This awareness may further enhance the nurses' understanding of all individuals and their relationships to the human and global community, and permits nurses to use this awareness to facilitate the healing process.

CORE VALUE 1: HOLISTIC PHILOSOPHY, THEORIES, AND ETHICS

Holistic nursing practice is based on the philosophy and theory of holism and the foundation of ethical practice.

1.1 Holistic Philosophy

Holistic nurses develop and expand their conceptual framework and overall philosophy in the art and science of holistic nursing to model, practice, teach, and conduct research in the most effective manner possible.

Standards of Practice

Holistic nurses:

1.1.1 recognize the person's capacity for self-healing and the importance of supporting the natural development and unfolding of that capacity.

1.1.2 support, share, and recognize expertise and competency in holistic nursing practice that is used in many diverse clinical and community settings.

1.1.3 participate in person-centered care by being a partner, coach, and mentor who actively listens and supports others in reaching personal goals.

1.1.4 focus on strategies to bring harmony, unity, and healing to the nursing profession.

1.1.5 communicate with traditional health care practitioners about appropriate referrals to other holistic practitioners when needed.

1.1.6 interact with professional organizations in a leadership or membership capacity at local, state, national, and international levels to further expand the knowledge and practice of holistic nursing and awareness of holistic health issues.

1.2 Holistic Theories

Nursing theories that are holistic, and other relevant theories, provide the framework for all aspects of holistic nursing practice and leadership.

Standards of Practice

Holistic nurses:

1.2.1 strive to use nursing theories to develop holistic nursing practice and transformational leadership.

1.2.2 interpret, use, and document information relevant to a person's care according to a theoretical framework.

1.3 Holistic Ethics

Holistic nurses hold to a professional ethic of caring and healing that seeks to preserve wholeness and dignity of themselves and all persons/families/communities in all practice settings.

Standards of Practice

Holistic nurses:

1.3.1 identify the ethics of caring and its contribution to unity of self, others, nature, and God/Life Force/Absolute/Transcendent as central to holistic nursing practice.

1.3.2 integrate the standards of holistic nursing practice with applicable state laws and regulations governing nursing practice.

1.3.3 engage in activities that respect, nurture, and enhance the integral relationship with the earth, and advocate for the well-being of the global community's economy, education, and social justice.

1.3.4 advocate for the rights of patients to have educated choices into their plan of care.

1.3.5 participate in peer evaluation to ensure knowledge and competency in holistic nursing practice.

1.3.6 protect the personal privacy and confidentiality of individuals, especially with health care agencies and managed care organizations.

CORE VALUE 2: HOLISTIC EDUCATION AND RESEARCH

Holistic nursing practice is guided by, and developed through, holistic education and research.

2.1 Holistic Education

Holistic nurses acquire and maintain current knowledge and competency in holistic nursing practice.

Standards of Practice

Holistic nurses:

2.1.1   participate in activities of continuing education and related fields that have relevance to holistic nursing practice.

2.1.2   identify areas of knowledge from nursing and various fields such as biomedical, epidemiology, behavioral medicine, cultural and social theories.

2.1.3   continually develop and standardize holistic nursing guidelines, protocols and practice to promote competency in holistic nursing practice and assure quality of care to individuals.

2.1.4   use the results of quality care activities to initiate change in holistic nursing practice.

2.1.5   may seek certification in holistic nursing as one means of advancing the philosophy and practice of holistic nursing.

2.2 Holistic Nursing and Related Research

Holistic nurses provide care and guidance to persons through nursing interventions and holistic therapies consistent with research findings and other sound evidence.

Standards of Practice

Holistic nurses:

2.2.1   use available research and evidence from different explanatory models to mutually create a plan of care with a person.

2.2.2   use expert clinical judgment to select appropriate interventions.

2.2.3   discuss holistic application to clinical situations where rigorous research has not been done.

2.2.4   create an environment conducive to systematic inquiry into healing and health issues by engaging in research or supporting and utilizing the research of others.

2.2.5   disseminate research findings at meetings and through publications to further develop the foundation and practice of holistic nursing.

2.2.6   provide consultation services on holistic nursing interventions to persons and communities based on research.

CORE VALUE 3: HOLISTIC NURSE SELF-CARE

Holistic nursing practice requires the integration of self-care and personal development activities into one's life.

3.1 Holistic Nurse Self-Care

Holistic nurses engage in holistic self-assessment, self-care, and personal development, aware of being instruments of healing to better serve self and others.

Standards of Practice

Holistic nurses:

3.1.1   recognize that a person's body-mind-spirit has healing capacities that can be enhanced and supported through self-care practices.

3.1.2   identify and integrate self-care strategies to enhance their physical, psychological, sociological, and spiritual well-being.

3.1.3   recognize and address at-risk health patterns and begin the process of change.

3.1.4   consciously cultivate awareness and understanding about the deeper meaning, purpose, inner strengths, and connections with self, others, nature, and God/ Life Force/Absolute/Transcendent.

3.1.5   use clear intention to care for self and to seek a sense of balance, harmony, and joy in daily life.

3.1.6   participate in the evolutionary holistic process with the understanding that crisis creates opportunity in any setting.

CORE VALUE 4: HOLISTIC COMMUNICATION, THERAPEUTIC ENVIRONMENT, AND CULTURAL DIVERSITY

Holistic nursing practice honors and includes holistic communication, therapeutic environment, and cultural diversity as foundational concepts.

4.1 Holistic Communication

Holistic nurses engage in holistic communication to ensure that each person experiences the presence of the nurse as authentic and sincere; there is an atmosphere of shared humanness that includes a sense of connectedness and attention reflecting the individual's uniqueness.

Standards of Practice

Holistic nurses:

4.1.1   develop an awareness of the most frequently encountered challenges to holistic communication.

4.1.2   increase therapeutic and cultural competence skills to enhance their effectiveness through listening to themselves and others.

4.1.3 explore with each person those strategies that can assist her/him, as desired, to understand the deeper meaning, purpose, inner strengths, and connections with self, others, nature, and God/Life Force/Absolute/Transcendent.

4.1.4 recognize that holistic communication and awareness of individuals is a continuously evolving multi-level exchange that offers itself through dreams, images, symbols, sensations, meditations, and prayers.

4.1.5 respect the person's health trajectory which may be incongruent with conventional wisdom.

4.2 Therapeutic Environment

Holistic nurses recognize that each person's environment includes everything that surrounds the individual, both the external and the internal (physical, mental, emotional, and spiritual) as well as patterns not yet understood.

Standards of Practice

Holistic nurses:

4.2.1 promote environments conducive to experiencing healing, wholeness, and harmony, and care for the person in as healthy an environment as possible.

4.2.2 work toward creating organizations that value sacred space and environments that enhance healing.

4.2.3 integrate holistic principles, standards, policies, and procedures in relation to environmental safety and emergency preparedness.

4.2.4 recognize that the well-being of the ecosystem of the planet is a prior determining condition for the well-being of the human.

4.2.5 promote social networks and social environments where healing can take place.

4.3 Cultural Diversity

Holistic nurses recognize each person as whole body-mind-emotion-spirit being and mutually create a plan of care consistent with cultural background, health beliefs and practices, sexual orientation, values, and preferences.

Standards of Practice

Holistic nurses:

4.3.1 assess and incorporate the person's cultural practices, values, beliefs, meanings of health, illness, and risk behaviors in care and health education.

4.3.2 use appropriate community resources and experts to extend their understanding of different cultures.

4.2.3 assess for discriminatory practices and change as necessary.

4.2.4 identify discriminatory health care practices as they impact the person and engage in effective nondiscriminatory practices.

CORE VALUE 5: HOLISTIC CARING PROCESS

Holistic nursing practice is guided by the holistic caring process, whether used with individuals, families, population groups, or communities. This circular process involves the following six steps, which may occur simultaneously.

5.1 Assessment

Holistic nurses assess each person holistically using appropriate conventional and holistic methods while the uniqueness of the person is honored.

Standards of Practice

Holistic nurses:

5.1.1 use an assessment process including appropriate traditional and holistic methods to systematically gather information.

5.1.2 value all types of knowing including intuition when gathering data from a person and validate this intuitive knowledge with the person when appropriate.

5.2 Patterns/Challenges/Needs

Holistic nures identify and prioritize each person's actual and potential patterns/challenges/needs and life processes related to health, wellness, disease, or illness, which may or may not facilitate well being.

Standards of Practice

Holistic nurses:

5.2.1 assist the person to access inner wisdom that can provide opportunities to enhance and support growth, development, and movement towards health and well-being.

5.2.2 collect data and collaborate with the person and health care team members as appropriate to identify and record a list of actual and potential patterns/challenges/needs.

5.2.3 use collected data to formulate an etiology of the person's identified actual or potential patterns/challenges/needs.

5.2.4 make referrals to other holistic practitioners or traditional therapists when appropriate.

5.3 Outcomes

Holistic nurses specify appropriate outcomes for each person's actual or potential patterns/challenges/needs.

Standards of Practice

Holistic nurses:

5.3.1 honor the person in all phases of her/his healing process regardless of expectations or outcomes.

5.3.2 identify and partner with the person to specify measurable outcomes and realistic goals.

5.4 Therapeutic Care Plan

Holistic nurses engage each person to mutually create an appropriate plan of care that focuses on health promotion, recovery, restoration, or peaceful dying so that the person is as independent as possible.

Standards of Practice

Holistic nurses:

5.4.1 partner with the person in a mutual decision process to create a health care plan for each pattern/challenge/need or opportunity to enhance health and well-being.

5.4.2 help a person identify areas for education to make decisions about life choices in a conscious, informed manner that empowers the person to maintain her/his uniqueness and independence.

5.4.3 offer self-assessment tools, word associations, storytelling, dreams, journals as appropriate.

5.4.4 use skills of cultural competence and communicate acceptance of the person's values, beliefs, culture, religion, and socioeconomic background.

5.4.5 assist the person in recognizing at-risk patterns/challenges/needs for potential or existing health situations (e.g., personal habits, personal and family health history, age-related risk factors), and also assist in recognizing opportunities to enhance well-being.

5.4.6 engage the person in problem-solving dialogue in relation to living with changes secondary to illness and treatment.

5.5 Implementation

Holistic nurses prioritize each person's plan of holistic care, and holistic nursing interventions are implemented accordingly.

Standards of Practice

Holistic nurses:

5.5.1 implement the mutually created plan of care within the context of assisting the person towards the higher potential of health and well-being.

5.5.2 support and promote the person's capacity for the highest level of participation and problem-solving in the plan of care and collaborate with other health team members when appropriate.

5.5.3 use holistic nursing skills in implementing care including cultural competency and all ways of knowing.

5.5.4 advocate that the person's plan, choices, and unique healing journey be honored.

5.5.5 provide care that is clear about and respectful of the economic parameters of practice, balancing justice with compassion.

5.6 Evaluation

Holistic nurses evaluate each person's response to holistic care regularly and systematically and the continuing holistic nature of the healing process is recognized and honored.

Standards of Practice

Holistic nurses:

5.6.1 collaborate with the person and with other health care team members when appropriate in evaluating holistic outcomes.

5.6.2 explore with the person her/his understanding of the cause of any significant deviation between the responses and the expected outcomes.

5.6.3 mutually create with the person and other team members a revised plan if needed.

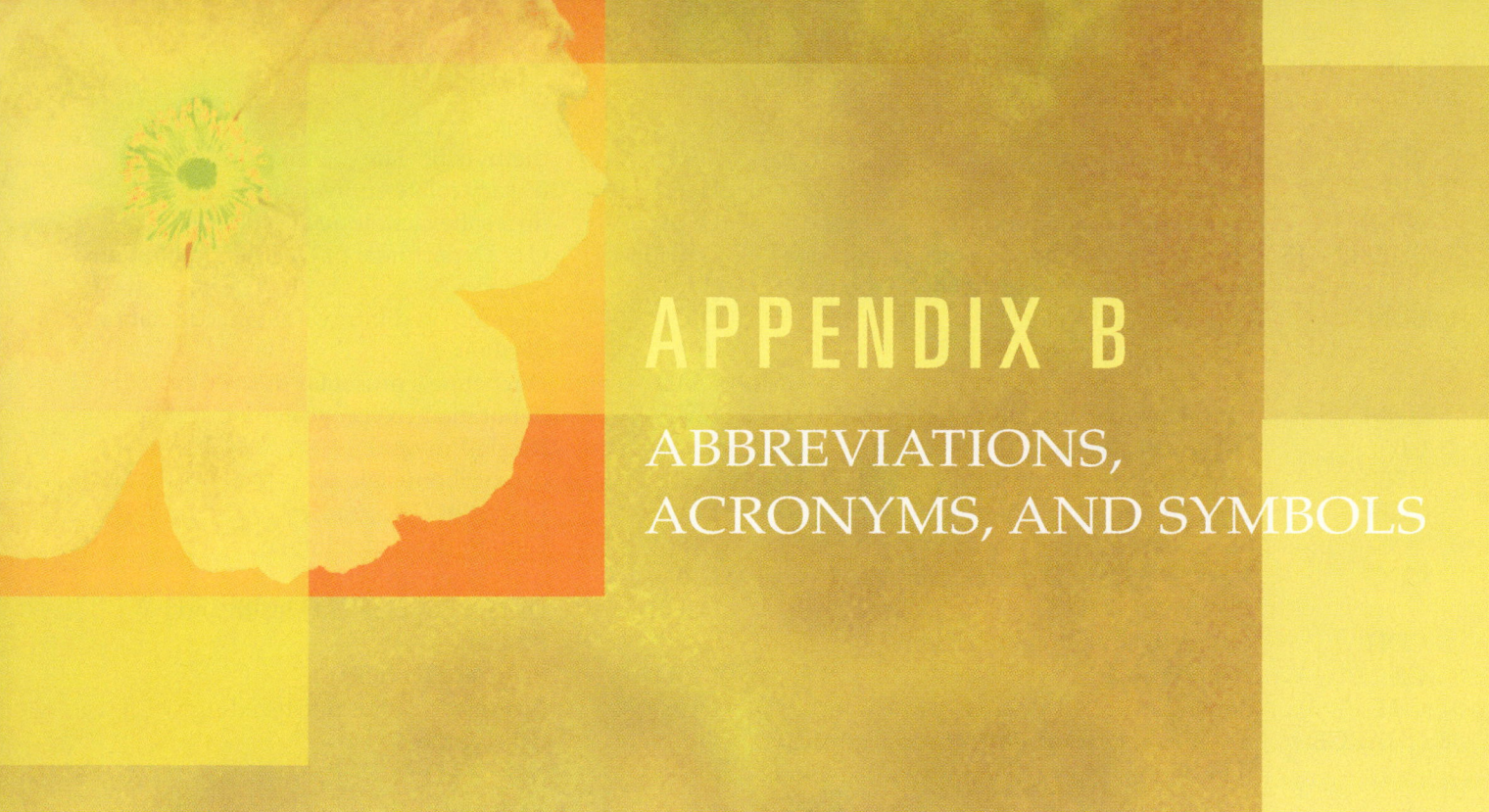

APPENDIX B

ABBREVIATIONS, ACRONYMS, AND SYMBOLS

AA	Alcoholics Anonymous		ANAD	anorexia nervosa and associated disorders
AA	arachidonic acid		ANDMCN	American Nursing Division of Maternal Child Nursing
AANA	American Association of Nurse Anesthetists		ANRED	anorexia nervosa and related eating disorders
AAP	American Academy of Pediatrics			
ABC	airway breathing circulation		ANS	autonomic nervous system
ABG	arterial blood gas		AOA	U.S. Administration on Aging
ACE	angiotensin-converting enzyme		APIB	Assessment of Premature Infant Behavior
ACOG	American College of Obstetricians and Gynecologists		APN	advanced practice nurse
ACS	American Cancer Society		APS	Adult Protective Services
ACTG	AIDS Clinical Trial Group		ARBD	alcohol-related birth defects
ADH	antidiuretic hormone		AROM	artificial rupture of membranes
ADOPE	age, diabetes, obesity, postterm, excessive		ART	assistive reproduction technology
AFDC	Aid to Families with Dependent Children		AUB	abnormal uterine bleeding
AFP	alpha-fetoprotein		AWHONN	Association of Women's Health, Obstetric, and Neonatal Nurses
AFV	amniotic fluid volume			
AGA	appropriate for gestational age		AZT	zidovudine
AHCPR	Agency for Health Care Policy and Research			
AHNA	American Holistic Nurses Association		BBT	basal body temperature
AHPA	American Herbal Products Association		β-hCG	β-human chorionic gonadotropin
AHRQ	Agency for Healthcare Research and Quality		BINS	Bayley Infant Neurodevelopmental Screen
AI	adequate intake		BMC	bone mineral content
AICR	American Institute for Cancer Research		BMD	bone mineral density
AIDS	acquired immunodeficiency syndrome		BMR	basal metabolic rate
AMA	American Medical Association		BNE	Board of Nursing Examiners
ANA	American Nurses Association		BP	blood pressure
			bpm	beats per minute

BPP	biophysical profile	DES	diethylstilbestrol
BRP	bed rest bathroom privileges	DFE	dietary folate equivalent
BSE	breast self-examination	DHA	docosahexaenoic acid
BUBBLE-HE	breasts, uterus, bladder, bowel, lochia, episiotomy, Homan's sign, emotional status	DHHS	U.S. Department of Health and Human Services
BUN	blood urea nitrogen	DIC	disseminated intravascular coagulation
		dL	deciliter
Ca	calcium	DMD	Duchenne's muscular dystrophy
CAM	complementary and alternative medicine	DMPA	depot medroxyprogesterone acetate (Depo-Provera)
CB	childbirth classes	DNA	deoxyribonucleic acid
CBC	complete blood count	DO	Doctor of Osteopathy
CCES	Council of Childbirth Education Specialists	DRI	Dietary Reference Intake
CDC	U.S. Centers for Disease Control and Prevention	DRV	daily reference value
		DSHEA	Dietary Supplement Health and Education Act
CDH	congenital diaphragmatic hernia	DTR	deep tendon reflex
CF	cystic fibrosis	DUB	dysfunctional uterine bleeding
C-H	crown-heel	DV	daily value
CHARGE	coloboma, heart disease, choanal atresia, retardation (physical and mental), genital hypoplasia, ear anomalies	EA	esophageal atresia
CHD	congenital heart defect	ECG	electrocardiogram
CHD	coronary heart disease	ECI	early childhood intervention
CHF	congestive heart failure	ECMO	extracorporeal membrane oxygenation
CHO	carbohydrate	EDB	expected date of birth
CIMS	Coalition for Improved Maternity Services	EDC	expected date of confinement
		EDD	expected date of delivery
CIS	Communities in Schools	EDNP	energy-dense, nutrient-poor
cm	centimeter	EEG	electroencephalogram
CMV	cytomegalovirus	EFM	electronic fetal monitoring
CNM	Certified Nurse Midwife	EFNEP	Expanded Food and Nutrition Education Program
CNS	central nervous system		
CO$_2$	carbon dioxide	EIP	early intervention program
COC	combined oral contraceptive	ELISA	enzyme-linked immunosorbent assay
COPD	chronic obstructive pulmonary disease	EMLA	eutectic mixture of local anesthetics
CPAP	continuous positive airway pressure	ER	estrogen receptors
CPD	cephalopelvic disproportion	ERT	estrogen replacement therapy
CPR	cardiopulmonary resuscitation	ESPGN	European Society of Pediatric Gastroenterology and Nutrition
CPS	Canadian Paediatric Society		
C-R	crown-rump	ET	embryo transfer
CRNA	Certified Registered Nurse Anesthetist		
CRS	congenital rubella syndrome	FAE	fetal alcohol effects
CSF	cerebrospinal fluid	FAS	fetal acoustic stimulation
CST	contraction stress test	FAS	fetal alcohol syndrome
CT	complementary therapy	FCMC	family-centered maternity care
CT	computerized tomography	FDA	U.S. Food and Drug Administration
CVD	cardiovascular disease	FFN	fetal fibronectin
CVS	chorionic villus sampling	FH	familial hypercholesterolemia
		FHR	fetal heart rate
D & C	dilation and curettage	FHT	fetal heart tone
D & E	dilation and evacuation	FMC	fetal movement counting
DDH	developmental dysplasia of the hip	FOBT	fecal occult blood test
DDT	dichlorodiphenyltrichloroethane	FOC	frontal-occipital circumference

FPAL	full-term deliveries, preterm deliveries, abortions, living children		HTLV-1	human T-cell leukemia virus type 1
FSE	fetal scalp electrode		HVAF	home visiting for at-risk families
FSH	follicle-stimulating hormone		IBFAN	International Breastfeeding Association
ftc	footcandle		ICEA	International Childbirth Education Association
g	gram		ICH	intracranial hemorrhage
G6PD	glucose-6-phosphate dehydrogenase		ICSI	intracytoplasmic sperm injection
GAO	General Accounting Office		ICU	intensive care unit
GBS	group B *Streptococcus*		IDDM	insulin-dependent diabetes mellitus
GC	gonorrhea screening		IDM	infant of a diabetic mother
GCT	genetic counseling team		IF	intrinsic factor
GFR	glomerular filtration rate		IFSP	Individual Family Service Plan
GI	gastrointestinal		IgA	immunoglobulin A
GIFT	gamete intra-fallopian transfer		IgE	immunoglobulin E
gm	gram		IgG	immunoglobulin G
GNP	gross national product		IICP	increased intracranial pressure
GnRH	gonadotropin releasing hormone		ILCA	International Lactation Consultants Association
			ILP	interstitial lymphocytic pneumonia
H & H	hematocrit and hemoglobin		IM	intramuscular
HbeAg	hepatitis B e antigen		IMR	infant mortality rate
HBIG	hepatitis B immune globulin		in	inch
HBsAg	hepatitis B surface antigen		IOM	Institute of Medicine
HC/AC	head-abdomen circumference		IQ	intelligence quotient
HCADA	Houston Council on Alcoholism and Drug Abuse		ISONG	International Society of Nurses in Genetics
hCG	human chorionic gonadotropin		ITP	idiopathic thrombocytopenic purpura
Hct	hematocrit		IUD	intrauterine device
HDL	high-density lipoprotein		IUFD	intrauterine fetal demise
HDN	hemolytic disease of the newborn		IUGR	intrauterine growth restriction
HEENT	head, ears, eyes, nose, and throat		IUPC	intrauterine pressure catheter
HELLP	hemolysis, elevated liver enzymes, low platelets		IV	intravenous
			IVF	in vitro fertilization
Hep C	hepatitis C		IVH	intraventricular hemorrhage
HexA	hexosaminidase		IWL	insensible water loss
HFA	Healthy Families Alexandria			
Hgb	hemoglobin		JCAHO	Joint Commission on Accreditation of Healthcare Organizations
HGH	human growth hormone		JOGNN	*Journal of Obstetric, Gynecologic, and Neonatal Nursing*
HGP	Human Genome Project			
HGPRT	hypoxanthine-guanine phosphoribosyl-transferase			
HHCC	Home Health Care Classification		KC	kangaroo care
HIV	human immunodeficiency virus		kg	kilogram
HMG	hydroxymethylglutaryl			
HMO	health maintenance organization		LAM	lactational amenorrhea method
HNC	holistic nurse certification		lb	pound
HNC	Holistic Nurse Certified		LBW	low birth weight
hPL	human placental lactogen		LDL	low-density lipoprotein
HPV	human papillomavirus		LDR	labor, delivery, recovery
HRT	hormone replacement therapy		LDRP	labor, delivery, recovery, postpartum
HSV	herpes simplex virus		LEEP	loop electrosurgical excision procedure
HT	Healing Touch		LGA	large for gestational age
HTI	Healing Touch International		LH	luteinizing hormone

LLI	LaLeche League International	NHANES	National Health and Nutrition Examination Society
LMA	left-mentum-anterior	NIC	Nursing Intervention Classification
LMP	last menstrual period	NICU	neonatal intensive care unit
LMP	left-mentum-posterior	NIDCAP	Newborn Individualized Developmental
LMT	left-mentum-transverse		Care Assessment Program
LOA	left-occiput-anterior	NIH	National Institutes of Health
LOP	left-occiput-posterior	NIHF	nonimmune hydrops fetalis
LOT	left-occiput-transverse	NIPS	Neonatal Infant Pain Scale
LSA	left-sacrum-anterior	NLN	National League for Nursing
LSP	left-sacrum-posterior	NMDS	nursing minimum data set
LST	left-sacrum-transverse	NRC	National Research Council
LTV	long-term variability	NSAID	nonsteroidal anti-inflammatory drug
		NST	nonstress test
μg	microgram	NTD	neural tube defect
m	meter	NVP	nausea and vomiting of pregnancy
MAI	Maternal Attachment Inventory		
MCV	mean corpuscular volume	O_2	oxygen
Mg	magnesium	OAM	Office of Alternative Medicine
mg	milligram	OCA	oral contraceptive agents
MI	myocardial infarction	OCP	oral contraceptive pill
mL	milliliter	OI	osteogenesis imperfecta
mmHg	millimeters of mercury	OMAR	Office of Medical Applications and Research
MNF	multiple neurofibromatosis	OMH	Office of Minority Health
MPA/E2C	medroxy progesterone and estradiol cypionate	ORWH	Office of Research on Women's Health
MPS	mucopolysaccharide accumulation	OSHA	U.S. Occupational Safety and Health Administration
MRFIT	Multiple Risk Factor Intervention Trial	OTC	over-the-counter
MRI	magnetic resonance imaging	oz	ounce
MSAFP	maternal serum alpha-fetoprotein		
MSDS	Material Safety Data Sheet	P	phosphorus
MVU	Montevideo Unit	PAI	Prenatal Attachment Inventory
		PaO_2	partial pressure of oxygen
NAACOG	Nurses Association of the American College of Obstetricians and Gynecologists	PAT	Pain Assessment Tool
		PBB	polybromated biphenyl
NANBH	non-A, non-B hepatitis	PCA	patient-controlled analgesia
NANDA	North American Nursing Diagnosis Association	PCB	polychlorinated biphenyl
		PCO_2	partial pressure of carbon dioxide
NANN	National Association of Neonatal Nurses	PCOS	polycystic ovary syndrome
NAS	National Academies of Science	PCP	*Pneumocystis carinii* pneumonia
NBAS	Neonatal Behavioral Assessment Scale	PCR	polymerase chain reaction
NCAST	Nursing Child Assessment Satellite Training	PDA	patent ductus arteriosus
		PDR	*Physicians' Desk Reference*
NCCAM	National Center for Complementary and Alternative Medicine	PEEP	positive end expiratory pressure
		PEPI	postmenopausal estrogen/progestin interventions
NCEA	National Center for Elder Abuse	PG	phosphatidylglycerol
NCHPEG	National Coalition for Health Professional Education in Genetics	PGE_2	prostaglandin E_2
		PGIS	Perinatal Grief Intensity Scale
NCHS	National Center for Health Statistics	PHS	Public Health Service
NCPAP	nasal continuous positive airway pressure	PID	pelvic inflammatory disease
		PIH	pregnancy-induced hypertension
NCPCA	National Committee to Prevent Child Abuse	PIPP	Premature Infant Pain Profile
NE	niacin equivalent		
NEC	necrotizing enterocolitis		

PKU	phenylketonuria
PLISSIT	permission, limited information, specific suggestions, intensive therapy
PMI	point of maximum impulse
PMS	premenstrual syndrome
PNI	psychoneuroimmunology
PO$_2$	partial pressure of oxygen
POS	point of service
PPHN	persistent pulmonary hypertension of the newborn
PPO	preferred provider organization
PPROM	preterm premature rupture of membranes
PPT	partial prothrombin time
PROM	premature rupture of membranes
PT	prothrombin time
PTL	preterm labor
PTSD	post-traumatic stress disorder
PTT	partial thromboplastin time
PTU	propylthiouracil
PUBS	percutaneous umbilical blood sampling
PUPPP	pruritic urticarial papules and plaques of pregnancy
PVR	pulmonary vascular resistance
RBC	red blood cell
RD	registered dietitian
RDA	recommended daily allowance
RDI	Reference Daily Intake
RDS	respiratory distress syndrome
REEDA	redness, edema, ecchymosis, discharge, approximation
Rh	rhesus factor
RH$_o$GAM	Rh$_o$(D) immune globulin
RMA	right-mentum-anterior
RMP	right-mentum-posterior
RMT	right-mentum-transverse
RNA	ribonucleic acid
ROA	right-occiput-anterior
ROM	range of motion
ROM	rupture of membranes
ROP	retinopathy of prematurity
ROP	right-occiput-posterior
ROT	right-occiput-transverse
RSA	right-sacrum-anterior
RSP	right-sacrum-posterior
RST	right-sacrum-transverse
RUQ	right upper quadrant
Rx	treatment; prescription
SC disease	sickle cell-hemoglobin C disease
SCD	sickle-cell disease
SDA	specific dynamic action
SGA	small for gestational age
SIDS	sudden infant death syndrome

sIgA	secretory immunoglobulin A
SLE	systemic lupus erythematosus
SOAP	subjective, objective, assessment, plan
SQ	subcutaneous
SS disease	sickle cell disease
STD	sexually transmitted disease
STORCH	syphilis, toxoplasmosis, other infections, rubella, cytomegalovirus, herpes
STV	short-term variability
SVE	sterile vaginal examination
TB	tuberculosis
TC	total cholesterol
TCM	traditional Chinese medicine
TEF	tracheoesophageal fistula
TENS	transcutaneous electrical nerve stimulation
THF	tetrahydrofolate
TNM	tumor, nodal involvement, and metastasis
TOLAC	trial of labor after cesarean
TORCH	toxoplasmosis, other (gonorrhea, syphilis, varicella, parvovirus, HBV, and HIV), rubella, cytomegalovirus, and herpes simplex virus
TPR	temperature, pulse, respirations
TRH	thyrotropin-releasing hormone
TSD	Tay-Sachs disease
TSH	thyroid-stimulating hormone
TT	Therapeutic Touch
TTN	transient tachypnea of the newborn
UAP	unlicensed assistive personnel
UA	urinalysis
UC	uterine contraction
uE$_3$	unconjugated estrogen
UIL	upper intake level
UNAIDS	Joint United Nations Programme on HIV/AIDS
UNICEF	United Nations Children's Fund
US	ultrasonography
USDA	United States Department of Agriculture
USDA/FCS	United States Department of Agriculture, Food, and Consumer Service
USDHHS	United States Department of Health and Human Services
USFDA	United States Food and Drug Administration
USP	United States Pharmacopoeia
USPSTF	United States Preventive Services Task Force
UTI	urinary tract infection
VACTERL	vertebral, anal, congenital heart defect, tracheoesophageal atresia or fistula, renal anomalies, and limb deformities

VATER	vertebral, anal, tracheoesophageal atresia or fistula, and renal anomalies
VBAC	vaginal birth after cesarean
VDRL	Venereal Disease Research Laboratory
VLBW	very low birth weight
VNA	Visiting Nurse Association
VNS	Visiting Nurse Service
VPS	ventricular peritoneal shunt
VSD	ventricular septal defect

VZIG	varicella-zoster immune globulin
WABA	World Alliance for Breastfeeding Action
WBC	white blood cell
WHO	World Health Organization
WIC	Women, Infants, and Children's Program
YRBSS	Youth Risk Behavior Surveillance System
ZDV	zidovudine

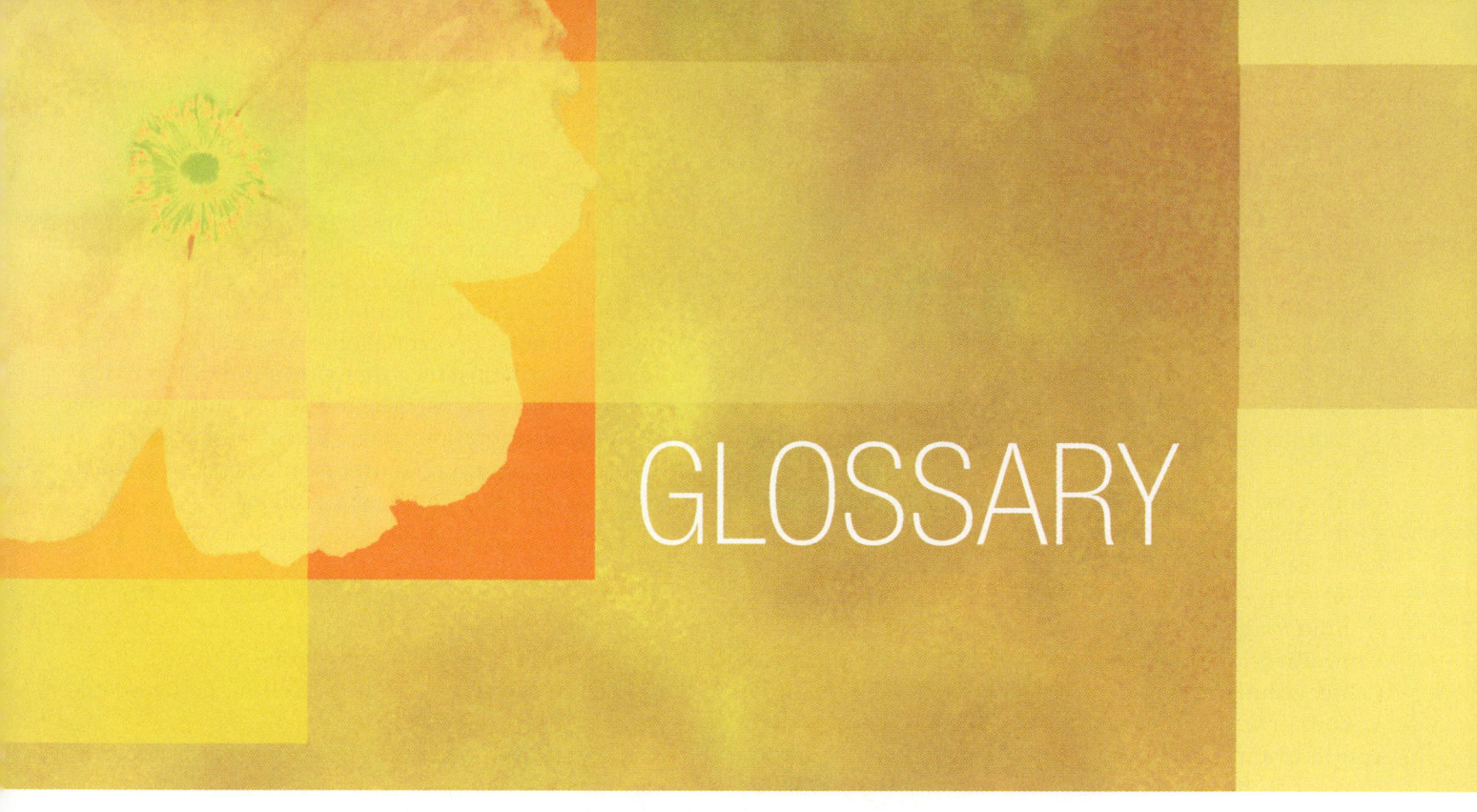

GLOSSARY

A

ABO incompatibility Condition that occurs when the blood types of the mother and the fetus do not match.

Abortion Expulsion of the products of conception (termination of pregnancy) before fetal viability.

Abruptio placentae Premature placental separation from the uterine wall; separation may be partial or complete, involve small or large areas, and be hidden.

Acceleration An increase in fetal heart rate above the baseline level, with a return to baseline within 10 minutes.

Accretion Growth in size, especially by addition or accumulation.

Acme Peak or time of greatest intensity of a uterine contraction.

Acquaintance rape Sexual assault that occurs when a perpetrator with whom the victim has had a previous relationship uses deceit and coercion to obtain sex.

Acquired disorder Condition resulting from environmental factors rather than genetic circumstances.

Acquired immunodeficiency syndrome/human immunodeficiency syndrome (AIDS/HIV) Retrovirus that causes progressive and severe impairment of the body's natural immunologic function (HIV), resulting in serious opportunistic infections, various cancers, and eventual death (AIDS).

Acrocyanosis The transient bluish skin color of an infant's feet or hands after delivery.

Active phase The second phase of the first stage of labor during which the cervix dilates from 4 to 8 cm.

Acupressure Application of pressure along certain meridians of the skin.

Acupuncture Insertion of needles into the skin along certain meridians.

Adolescence Period of life beginning with the appearance of secondary sex characteristics and ending with the cessation of growth, approximately 11 to 18 years of age; passage from childhood to maturity.

Adolescent pregnancy Pregnancy in girls ages 11 to 19.

Adult maltreatment syndrome *ICD-9* diagnostic code category for the adult who is abused.

Advanced reproductive age Women between ages 45 and 50 who are perimenopausal or postmenopausal.

Afterpains Abdominal cramping caused by the uterus contracting or involuting.

Agonists Drugs that block or reduce the action of a substance in the human body.

Air-block syndrome Term used to encompass pneumomediastinum and pulmonary interstitial emphysema in ventilated infants.

Allantois Small diverticulum of the yolk sac.

Allele Alternative expression of a gene at a given locus.

Allopathy Traditional or established medical or surgical procedures, both invasive and noninvasive, used in the diagnosis and treatment of mental or physical illness.

Alpha-fetoprotein (AFP) Protein produced by the developing fetus that can be used as a marker for neural tube defects (increased AFP) and Down syndrome (decreased AFP).

Alternative therapies Therapies used instead of conventional biomedicine.

Alveoli Secretory units of the mammary gland in which milk production takes place.

Amenorrhea Absence of menstruation for 3 or more months in women who have established menstrual cycles.

Amniohook A plastic instrument with a blunt hook at the distal end used for amniotomy.

Amniocentesis Prenatal diagnostic procedure that consists of withdrawal of a small sample of amniotic fluid for genetic analysis of embryonic cells.

Amnioinfusion An instillation of an isotonic, glucose-free solution into the uterus to cushion the umbilical cord or thin out meconium.

Amnion Inner membrane of the two fetal membranes; it forms the sac in which the fetus and the amniotic fluid are contained.

Amniotic fluid Fluid surrounding the developing fetus during pregnancy; formed from maternal serum and fetal urine.

Amniotic fluid embolism Life-threatening condition in which amniotic fluid and particulate matter such as lanugo, vernix caseosa, meconium, or other fetal cells enter the maternal circulation and obstruct the pulmonary circulation, resulting in classic embolic symptoms.

Amniotomy Artificial rupture of the fetal membranes (AROM) using a plastic amniohook or sometimes a fetal scalp electrode.

Amylophagia Ingestion of nonfood substances, such as laundry starch or cornstarch.

Analgesia Relief of pain.

Anal wink reflex Drawing together of the buttocks in response to a stroking motion. The buttocks come together at the exact anatomic position of the anal opening.

Anencephaly Complete or partial absence of the cerebral hemispheres and the skull overlying the brain.

Anesthesia Absence of sensation.

Anesthesiologist Physician who has completed a postgraduate residency in anesthesia.

Aneuploidy Abnormal chromosome pattern in which the total number of chromosomes is not a multiple of the haploid number (n = 23).

Anorexia nervosa Condition of self-starvation motivated by excessive concern with weight and an irrational fear of becoming fat.

Anovulatory Lack of ovulation.

Anovulatory cycle Menstrual cycle in which no ovum is discharged.

Anterior fontanel The diamond-shaped open space formed by the anterior and posterior sagittal and frontal sutures on an infant's skull.

Anticipatory grieving Emotional responses based on the perception of potential or expected loss.

Antioxidant A substance that slows down the oxidation of hydrocarbons, oils, and so on, and thus helps to check deterioration.

Antiretroviral therapy Course of medications used to suppress HIV replication and viral load.

Apgar score A scoring system used to evaluate newborns at 1 minute, 5 minutes, and 10 minutes after delivery. The total score is achieved by assessing heart rate, respiratory effort, muscle tone, reflex irritability, and skin color, and assigning a score of 0 to 2 in each of the five categories. The highest possible score is 10.

Apnea Cessation of respirations for more than 20 seconds.

Areola Pigmented ring of tissue surrounding the nipple.

Asphyxia Interference with gas exchange resulting in decreased oxygen delivery (hypoxemia), accumulation of carbon dioxide (hypercapnia), development of respiratory and metabolic acidosis, and inadequate perfusion of the tissues and major organs (ischemia).

Assault Intentional act of inflicting physical injury on another person.

Asymmetric intrauterine growth restriction Fetal growth in which the length and head circumference are at higher percentiles than the measurement for weight based on standardized graphs.

Atony Lack of uterine muscle tone.

Attachment Process of connecting with another human being over time.

Auditory brain evoked response A hearing screen designed for newborns that records electrical potentials arising from the auditory nervous system.

Augmentation of labor Stimulation of uterine contractions after labor has already started.

Autonomy An individual's right to hold a particular view, make choices, and undertake actions based on values and beliefs.

Autosome The 22 pairs of chromosomes that do not greatly influence sex determination at conception; excludes the sex chromosomes, X and Y.

Ayurvedic medicine Traditional medicine of India meaning knowledge of life or science of longevity.

B

Ballottement Rebounding of the floating fetus against the examiner's fingers.

Barrier to service utilization Any deterrent, either real or perceived, that prevents or delays use of available health care.

Basal metabolism Energy used to support body functions while the body is at rest.

Baseline fetal heart rate The fetal heart rate between contractions and accelerations.

Beat-to-beat variability Short-term variability in the fetal heart rate from one beat to the next.

Behavioral medicine Branch of medicine that focuses on behavior and cognitive, emotional, motivational, and biobehavioral interactions.

Behavioral state Continuum of levels of consciousness, encompassing quiet sleep, drowsiness, wakeful attentiveness, and hyperalert, agitated, or crying states.

Beneficence The practice of doing good, which may include prevention of harm, removal of evil, or promotion of good.

Biischial diameter Distance between the two ischial tuberosities.

Bilirubin Product of red cell destruction, which may be by natural or hemolytic process.

Binge eating An eating disorder of periodic binge eating (several thousand calories) not normally followed by vomiting, use of laxatives, or excessive exercise.

Bioavailability Rate at which a nutrient enters the bloodstream and is circulated to specific organs or tissues.

Biomedicine The scientific-based professional medicine taught in medical schools and generally practiced in the United States and Canada.

Biophysical profile (BPP) Noninvasive dynamic assessment of the fetus and the fetal environment.

Birth rate Number of births per 1,000 population.

Blastocyst Mammalian conceptus in the postmorula stage; consists of the trophoblast and an inner cell mass and develops into the embryo.

Blended family Family formed through remarriage.

Bloody show Release or expulsion of the thick, tenacious mucous plug that is inside the cervical canal 24–48 hours before the onset of labor.

Body mass index (BMI) Ratio that defines the relationship between height and weight. BMI is calculated by the formula: BMI = weight (kg)/height (m^2) × 100, or weight (lb) × 700/height (in^2).

Boggy Term used to describe a fundus that is soft, atonic, and nonpalpable; bogginess is a warning sign of uterine atony and possible postpartum hemorrhage.

Botanicals All parts of plants that have medicinal value: roots, rhizomes, leaves, stems, and flowers.

Brachial palsy Paralysis of the muscles involving the upper extremity; occurs as a result of a prolonged and difficult labor followed by a traumatic delivery.

Braxton Hicks contractions Intermittent painless contractions of the uterus observed throughout pregnancy; also known as false labor.

Breech presentation Fetal descent in which the fetal buttocks, legs, feet, or combination of these parts is found first in the maternal pelvis.

Bronchopulmonary dysplasia (BPD) Chronic lung disease in the neonate defined as an oxygen or impairment at 36 weeks' corrected gestational age.

Brow presentation Fetal descent in which the area between the anterior fontanel and the fetal eyes descend into the maternal pelvis first.

Bulimia nervosa Condition characterized by binge eating, or excessive consumption of calories over a short period of time; purging by self-induced vomiting; use of laxatives or diuretics, or both; excessive exercise; or periods of severe caloric restriction.

C

Calorie Amount of energy needed to raise the temperature of 1 kilogram of water (about 4 cups) from 1°C.

Calorimetry Measurement of the quantity of heat; used for measuring the energy produced by food when oxidized in the body.

Cancer Uncontrolled growth or spread of abnormal cells, resulting from malfunction of genes that control cell growth and cell division.

Capacitation Process by which the spermatozoon (sperm) is capable of penetrating the ovum.

Caput succedaneum Soft tissue edema or swelling from birth trauma that crosses suture lines; localized between the skin and the periosteum.

Carcinoma in situ Cancer that involves only the cells of the organ in which it began and has not spread to any other tissue.

Carotenoids Pigments in fruits and vegetables, which include alpha carotene, beta carotene, lycopene, lutein, and many other compounds.

Case management, care coordination Process of coordinating care and services to ensure that clients receive appropriate care and services in a timely manner.

Categorical imperative Supreme rule that governs actions.

Cephalhematoma Subperiosteal hemorrhage from birth trauma that causes a swelling that does not cross suture lines.

Cephalopelvic disproportion (CPD) Abnormal relationship in which the maternal pelvis will not permit the descent of the fetal head for delivery.

Cerclage Suturing to manage an incompetent cervix.

Certified registered nurse anesthetist (CRNA) Advanced practice nurse who has graduated from an accredited program of nurse anesthesia education and has passed the National Certification Examination.

Cervical cancer   Neoplasm of the uterine cervix.

Cervical cap   Barrier contraceptive device that is held in place by suction over the cervix.

Cervical dilation   Widening of the cervical opening that occurs from myometrial contractions in labor, which allow the cervix to accommodate passage of the fetal head through the birth canal.

Cervical infection   Inflammation of the cervix caused by a microorganism or foreign body.

Cesarean section   Birth of the fetus through a surgical incision in the mother's abdomen.

Chadwick's sign   Dark blue or purple coloration in the mucous membranes of the cervix, vagina, and vulva during pregnancy.

Chi   Concept in Asian medicine that refers to the subtle material or energy that influences physiologic function and maintains the health and vitality of the individual.

Chi gong   The Asian practice of "working the chi," or exercises to maintain health and vitality.

Child abuse   Physical or mental injury, sexual abuse, exploitation, negligent treatment, or maltreatment of a child.

Childbirth education   Originally, specific techniques for breathing, relaxation, and positioning to prepare women for labor that reduce the need for medication and unnecessary medical interventions.

Chloasma   Brownish pigmentation of the face commonly called "the mask of pregnancy."

Choanal atresia   A bony or membranous separation between the nose and the pharynx.

Chorioamnionitis   An infection of the amniotic fluid that can be transferred to the infant before delivery, which places the infant at risk for a life-threatening condition.

Chorion   Outermost portion of the fetal membrane composed of trophoblast and mesoderm lining; develops villi and becomes vascularized; forms the fetal portion of the placenta.

Chorionic villi   Vascular protrusions along the chorion.

Chorionic villus sampling (CVS)   Procedure that obtains fetal cells in the first trimester of the developing pregnancy.

Chorioretinitis   Inflammation of the membrane of the retina of the eye.

Chromosome   Filament-like nuclear structure consisting of chromatin that stores genetic information as base sequences in DNA and whose chromosome number is constant in each species.

Chronic grief   Prolonged and recurrent sorrow felt by parents whose child has a serious physical anomaly or mental disability but does not die at birth.

Chronic hypertension   Hypertension that occurs before the 20th week of gestation, or continues beyond the 42nd postpartum day.

Civil law   Protects individuals by punishing wrongs against the individual.

Clastogen   Agent capable of producing chromosome breakage.

Cleansing breath   Initial breath taken at the beginning of uterine contraction activity or other conscious breathing technique; helps replenish the oxygen deficit.

Cleft lip   Congenital fissure or elongated opening of the lip.

Cleft palate   Congenital fissure in the palate.

Clubfoot (talipes equinovarus)   Congenital deformity in which portions of the foot and ankle are twisted out of normal position.

Coarctation of the aorta   A congenital condition characterized by the narrowing of the arterial walls of the aorta. This condition may be diagnosed in infancy by diminished femoral pulses as compared to radial pulses, a systolic blood pressure >90 mmHg, and a difference of 10 mmHg or more lowered systolic blood pressure between the infant's arm and thigh.

Code   Definition of professional obligations and responsibilities expected of practitioners by society.

Cognitive development   Age-related development of intellectual reasoning and perception.

Cohabitation   Couple living together without entering into marriage.

Coitus interruptus   Contraceptive method involving removal of the penis from the vagina before ejaculation.

Colostrum   A yellowish, protein-rich fluid secreted from the breast during pregnancy and for 3 to 4 days following delivery.

Communal family   Group of individuals, couples, or families living together and jointly carrying out family functions.

Complementary therapies   Therapies used in addition to or as an adjunct to biomedicine for the promotion of health and well-being.

Congenital disorder   Anomaly present at birth; results from genetic or prenatal environmental factors, or both.

Congenital heart defect   A structural abnormality or defect of the heart that is present at birth.

Containment   Developmental technique using the caregiver's hands or cloth boundaries to support an infant's arms and legs close to the body.

Contraception   Prevention of pregnancy.

Contracted maternal pelvis Abnormalities in pelvic measures or shapes that fall short of the measures or shapes required for an average delivery.

Contraction Tightening and shortening of the uterine muscles during labor, causing effacement and dilation of the cervix.

Contraction stress test (CST) Evaluation of uterine contractions for the purpose of assessing fetal response.

Corona radiata Layer of cells surrounding the zona pellucida of the ovum.

Corpus luteum Yellow glandular mass in the ovary formed by an ovarian follicle that has matured and discharged its ovum.

Cost-benefit analysis Process of measuring and comparing the cost of doing something against the outcome in monetary terms.

Cost containment Reduction of expenses by working more efficiently.

Cost-effectiveness analysis Process of comparing the cost of doing something and measuring the outcomes in nonmonetary terms.

Cotyledons Subdivisions along the uterine surface of the placenta.

Couvade Physical symptoms experienced by an expectant father during pregnancy; also the ritualistic behaviors he performs during labor and birth.

Criminal law Addresses public concerns and punishes the wrongs that threaten a group or society.

Crisis Situation in which the balance in an individual or family life is disrupted and new coping strategies must be developed.

Critical thinking Formal and structured type of reasoning used in nursing as the foundation for sound clinical judgment.

Crowning The point at which the fetal head is visible at the vulvar opening.

Cultural competence continuum Progressive description of the ability of an individual or institution to respond to the individual culturally specific needs of the people.

Cultural competency Process of integrating cultural awareness in the delivery of culturally appropriate clinical care.

Culture An individual's way of looking at life, encompassing the person's feelings, beliefs, attitudes, and practices in dealing with family, community, and society.

Cyanosis The bluing of the skin or mucous membranes that results from the inability of the circulatory system to properly oxygenate the tissues. Cyanosis in infancy may be noted centrally on the chest and face or peripherally in the fingers and toes.

Cytogenetics The study of chromosomes, with special focus on chromosome abnormalities.

Cytotrophoblast Inner layer of the trophoblast; also referred to as Langhan's layer.

D

Daily Reference Values (DRVs) Standards for daily intake of total fat, saturated fat, cholesterol, total carbohydrate, dietary fiber, and protein.

Date rape Assault between a dating couple without the consent of one of the participants.

Deceleration Slowing of the fetal heart rate in response to parasympathetic activity.

Decidua Term applied to the endometrium during pregnancy.

Decidua basalis Portion on which the implanted ovum rests.

Decidua capsularis Portion directly overlying the implanted ovum.

Decidua parietalis Decidua exclusive of the area occupied by the implanted ovum.

Deletion Loss of chromosomal material.

Deontology Form of ethical reasoning that focuses on duty; right actions are those that fulfill duty.

Dermatome Area of the body innervated by a specific spinal nerve.

Descent Progression of the fetal head into the pelvis.

Desire phase First phase of human sexual response in which an individual develops a motivation or intention to be sexual.

Developmental care Infant care protocol designed to promote optimal physical, cognitive, and emotional development in the first weeks or months of life.

Developmental crisis Adjustment of an individual to new stages of development.

Developmental dysplasia of the hip (DDH) Malformation of the hip involving varying degrees of deformity, ranging from subluxation to complete dislocation.

Developmental tasks Competencies in psychosocial development related to identity formation, sexual identity, vocational identity, and autonomy and independence.

Diaphragm Barrier contraceptive device that fits over the cervix.

Diaphragmatic hernia Condition in which the diaphragm fails to close during the seventh or eighth week, allowing the abdominal organs to be displaced into the left chest.

Diastasis recti   Muscle separation midline in the abdomen due to pregnancy.

Dietary Guidelines for Americans   Guidance on diet and health for the general population with practical recommendations that meet nutritional requirements, promote health, support an active lifestyle, and reduce the risk of chronic disease.

Dilation   The widening of the external os of the uterine cervix from closed to a maximum of 10 cm, at which time the cervix is said to be fully dilated.

Dilemma   Choice between two equally unsatisfactory alternatives.

Diploid   Cell that contains two copies of each chromosome; the diploid number (2n) in humans is 46.

Disease prevention   Activities taken to prevent the onset of a disease or disorder.

Disseminated intravascular coagulation (DIC)   Hemorrhagic disorder that occurs following the uncontrolled activation of clotting factors and fibrinolytic enzymes throughout small blood vessels, resulting in tissue necrosis and bleeding.

Dizygotic   Derived from two separate zygotes (e.g., fraternal twins).

Doctrine of the golden mean   Virtues at the midpoint between extremes of less desirable characteristics.

Dominant   Allele that is phenotypically expressed in single copy (heterozygote) as well as double copy (homozygote).

Doppler blood studies   Measurement of blood flow velocity and direction in major fetal and uterine structures; also known as umbilical vessel velocimetry.

Dosha   Term used in Ayurvedic medicine to refer to metabolic types of people.

Doula   A woman who is employed by the pregnant woman to assist her through labor by helping her cope with the pain.

Ductus arteriosus   Fetal shunt that connects the pulmonary artery to the descending aorta.

Ductus venosus   Fetal shunt passing through the liver that connects the umbilical vein to the inferior vena cava.

Due care   Legal and ethical standard of performance by which nursing professionals are expected to abide.

Duration   Period from the beginning of one contraction to the end of the same contraction.

Dyad   Group of two people.

Dysfunctional grieving   Extended, unsuccessful use of intellectual and emotional responses by which individuals, families, or communities attempt to work through the process of modifying self-concept based on the perception of loss.

Dysfunctional labor pattern   Labor that does not proceed normally.

Dysfunctional uterine bleeding (DUB)   Any significant deviation from the usual menstrual pattern; also known as abnormal uterine bleeding (AUB).

Dysmenorrhea   Painful menses or cramping associated with menstruation.

Dysmotility   Low rate of gastrointestinal peristalsis.

Dyspareunia   Painful sexual intercourse.

Dystocia   Failure of labor to progress.

E

Early detection   The use of screening techniques to identify the stages of a disease, when early treatment may reduce its development.

Early onset deceleration   Slowing of the fetal heart rate corresponding to the onset of a uterine contraction and a slow return to the baseline soon after the contraction ends, like a mirror image; caused by fetal head compression.

Eclampsia   Seizures in a pregnant woman.

ECMO (extracorporeal membrane oxygenation)   A type of cardiopulmonary bypass therapy.

Ecologic environment   Combined societal context in which a family resides.

Ectopic pregnancy   Implantation of a fertilized ovum in a location other than the endometrial lining of the uterus.

EDB   Estimated date of birth.

EDC   Estimated date of confinement or "due date."

EDD   Expected date of delivery.

Effacement   Shortening and thinning of the cervix that occurs during the labor process.

Elderly primigravida   A woman over age 35 who is pregnant for the first time.

Elective abortion   Voluntary termination of pregnancy before fetal viability at the request of the client.

Embryo   Period of human development from the second week until the eighth week after fertilization; period characterized by cell differentiation and hyperplasic growth.

Embryo transfer (ET)   Transfer of an externally fertilized egg in embryonic stage by transcervical or other methods.

Emergency childbirth   Childbirth that occurs too rapidly for the mother to get to the hospital.

Emergency contraception   Postcoital prevention of pregnancy.

Empowering   A therapeutic approach that encourages the family to actively participate in the solution to their problems and acknowledge that capacity.

Empowerment   Process of assisting clients to care for themselves.

Enablement   Process of assisting clients in locating needed services and resources.

Enabling   The approach to interventions that allows competencies to develop in the client.

Encephalocele   Herniation of the brain and meninges through a skull defect.

Endometrial cancer   Malignant neoplasm of the uterine lining.

Endometriosis   Chronic disorder caused by implantation of endometrial tissue outside the uterus.

Endometritis   Infection of the uterine lining.

Endometrium   Cellular lining of the uterus that is shed monthly at the time of menses.

En-face positioning   Face-to-face positioning between parent and newborn.

Engorgement   Process of swelling of the breast tissue due to vascular congestion following delivery and preceding lactation.

Engrossment   Process characterized by intense paternal interest in the newborn.

Enhancement   Process of building on a client's existing strengths to increase capacity for problem solving and self-care.

Epidural   Technique used to produce analgesia or anesthesia of the lower body by placing opioid and/or local anesthetic within the epidural space, which then diffuses into the nerve roots as they exit the dura.

Episiotomy   Surgical incision made to enlarge the vaginal opening for delivery of the baby's head.

Epispadias   Condition in which the urethral meatus is located on the dorsal surface of the penis.

Erythema toxicum   A transient, red, irregular rash appearing shortly after birth first on the infant's face and then spreading to the chest and extremities. The cause of the rash is unknown and no special treatment is required.

Erythroblastosis fetalis   Vast destruction of fetal red blood cells by maternal antibodies, resulting in fetal anemia.

Esophageal atresia   Condition in which the esophagus ends in a blind pouch or narrows into a thin cord and is not connected to the stomach.

Estrogen   Female sex hormone produced primarily by the ovary and stored in fat cells.

Estrogen deficiency vulvovaginitis   Vulvovaginal burning related to estrogen decline.

Ethic of care   Perspective that recognizes the personal concerns and vulnerabilities of clients in health and illness.

Ethics   Branch of philosophy that provides rules and principles that can be used for resolving ethical dilemmas.

Ethnic group   Community of people who share the same cultural and social beliefs, which have been passed from one generation to another.

Euploid   Cell (and, by extension, an individual) whose chromosome number is a multiple of 23.

Evidence-based practice   Systematic approach to finding, appraising, and judiciously using research results as a basis for clinical decisions.

Excitement phase   Phase of the human sexual response in which physical and emotional changes take place in the person to increase interest in intercourse.

Exstrophy of the bladder   Anomaly in which the anterior wall of the bladder and lower portion of the abdominal wall are absent, causing the bladder to lie open and exposed on the lower abdomen.

Extended family   Family that includes generations beyond the parents and their children such as grandparents or aunts and uncles; two or more nuclear families together.

External cephalic version   Procedure by which the physician manipulates the fetus externally through the maternal abdomen to turn the fetus from an abnormal presentation (usually breech) to a cephalic presentation.

Extrauterine life   Life outside of the uterus following birth.

Extremely low birth weight (ELBW)   Weight of 1,000 grams or less at birth.

F

Face presentation   Fetal descent in which hyperextension of the fetal head and neck allows the fetal face to descend into the maternal pelvis, as opposed to flexion, which results in fetal vertex presentation.

Facial palsy   Paralysis of one side of the face.

Facilitated tucking   Gentle handling of an infant by providing boundary support.

False discharge   Fluid appearing on the nipple or areolar surface that is not secreted by the breast tissue.

Family   Group of adults and children linked by biological, kinship, or social bonds.

Family boundaries   The demarcations between individuals within a family and between the family and the rest of society.

Family dynamics   Concept from psychology that refers to patterns in the interrelationships within the family.

Family planning   Cognitive decisions and behavioral practices that enable individuals to conceive a wanted pregnancy and avoid an unwanted or badly timed pregnancy.

Family structure   Configuration of the family unit, including who is in the family and their relationship to each other.

Femicide   Homicide of women.

Fern test   Procedure done to determine presence of amniotic fluid.

Fertility rate   Number of births per 1,000 women ages 15 to 44.

Fertilization   Process by which the male's sperm unites with the female's ovum.

Fetal alcohol effects   Detectable effects of maternal alcohol consumption.

Fetal alcohol syndrome   A collection of deformities and disabilities seen in offspring of women who use alcohol heavily in pregnancy.

Fetal attitude   Relationship of fetal body parts to one another.

Fetal circulation   The pathway of blood circulation in the fetus.

Fetal distress   Nonreassuring fetal heart rate responses to the intrauterine environment. Distress reflects hypoxia and respiratory or metabolic acidosis.

Fetal fibronectin (fFN) testing   Screening procedure for the prediction of preterm labor.

Fetal heart rate (FHR)   The number of times the fetal heart beats per minute.

Fetal lie   Relationship of the fetal long axis to that of the maternal long axis or spinal cord.

Fetal movement counting (FMC)   Daily maternal assessment of fetal activity by counting the number of fetal movements within a specified time period.

Fetal position   Relationship of the fetal presenting part to the left or right side of the maternal pelvis.

Fetal presentation   Anatomic part of the fetus that is either in, or closest to, the birth canal.

Fetal tissue sampling   Direct biopsy of fetal tissue.

Fibroadenoma   Painless solid breast mass or tumor.

Fibrocystic changes   Hormonal age-related changes most commonly involving cyst formation and thickening of breast tissue.

Fibroid tumor   Benign tumor arising in the myometrium that can protrude into the uterine cavity, bulge through the outer uterine layer, and grow within the myometrium.

Fidelity   Quality of being faithful.

Fimbriae   Fine, hair-like structures.

First stage of labor   Begins with regular contractions and ends when the cervix is completely dilated. The first stage of labor is divided into three phases: latent, active, and transition.

Flexion   Occurs when the fetal head meets resistance from the pelvic floor and wall at the cervix, causing the fetal head to flex the chin against the fetal chest.

Focal point   Internal or external point of reference that serves as a centering factor. This is used to focus cognitive attention away from the discomforts of labor.

Follicle-stimulating hormone (FSH)   Hormone produced by the anterior pituitary whose function is to stimulate the ovary to prepare a mature ovum for release.

Follicular phase   Phase of the ovarian cycle in which a follicle becomes mature and prepared for ovulation.

Follow-up services   Health care services provided following hospital discharge.

Fontanel   Point of intersection where the skull bones are united by membranes that allows the head to mold during the birthing process.

Food Guide Pyramid   Translation of the *Dietary Guidelines for Americans* into practical eating portions and, if foods are chosen carefully, they also meet the recommended daily allowances (RDA) and Dietary Reference Intakes (DRI).

Foramen ovale   An opening in the septum between the right and the left atria of the fetal heart.

Forceps   Metal instruments used on the fetal head to assist in delivery.

Foremilk   Thin, watery breast milk secreted at the beginning of a feeding.

Fourth stage of labor   First 4 hours after delivery of the placenta.

FPAL   Acronym for the four digits of parity: *full-term* deliveries (37–40 weeks gestation); *premature* or *preterm* deliveries (between 20 and 36 weeks' gestation); *abortions*, spontaneous or induced (termination of pregnancy before 20 weeks' gestation); and *living children* born to the client who are alive at time of data collection.

Frequency   Period of time from the beginning of one contraction to the beginning of the next contraction.

Fundus   Top portion of the uterus; massaged with the hands after delivery to ascertain and maintain firmness.

G

Galactopoiesis   Maintenance of established lactation.

Galactorrhea   White discharge from the nipples.

Gamete   Mature reproductive cell; spermatozoon or ovum.

Gametogenesis   Series of mitotic and meiotic divisions that occurs in the gonads that leads to the production of gametes; in males, *spermatogenesis*, and in females, *oogenesis*.

Gastroesophageal reflux (GER)   Spontaneous passage of acidic gastric contents from the stomach into the esophagus.

Gastroschisis   Abdominal wall defect to the right of the umbilicus through which the abdominal organs have herniated.

Gavage feeding   Feedings given through a tube that is passed through the nose or the mouth into the stomach.

Gene   Segment of nucleic acid that contains genetic information necessary to control a certain function, such as the synthesis of a polypeptide (structural gene); also referred to as a site, or locus, on a chromosome.

General anesthesia   Loss of sensation from the entire body secondary to loss of consciousness produced by intravenous and/or inhalation anesthetic agents.

Genetic counseling   Process by which genetic information is given to clients and their families.

Genetic disorder   Inherited defect transmitted from generation to generation.

Genotype   Genetic constitution of an individual at any given locus.

Geophagia   Ingestion of nonfood substances such as dirt or clay.

Gestational diabetes   Diabetes diagnosed in pregnancy.

Glycosuria   The presence of sugar (glucose) in the urine.

Goals   Broad statements of a desired outcome.

Gonadal   Pertaining to the ovaries in the female and the testes in the male.

Gonadotropin releasing hormone (Gn-RH)   Neurohormone released by the hypothalamus that acts on the pituitary to stimulate the release of follicle-stimulating hormone, luteinizing hormone, thyroid stimulating hormone, and prolactin.

Goodell's sign   Marked softening of the cervix in early pregnancy.

Graafian follicle   Fully mature ovum and surrounding elements just before ovulation.

Gravida   Number of pregnancies, regardless of duration or outcome.

Gravidity   Number of times a woman has been pregnant.

Grief   Intense and personal experience in response to a loss.

Grief work   Work that includes acceptance of painful emotions, active review of the experience and events, and testing new patterns of interaction and integration of the loss into daily living.

GTPAL   A five-digit number that indicates (1) the number of conceptions; (2) the number of full-term deliveries; (3) the number of premature or preterm deliveries; (4) the number of abortions; and (5) the number of children born to the client who are alive at the time of data collection.

H

Habituation   A newborn's ability to alter response to a repeated stimulus by decreasing and finally eliminating the response after repetitions of the stimulus.

Haploid   Cell that contains one copy of each chromosome; the haploid number (n) in humans is 23.

Harm   Interference with the mental or physical well-being of others.

Healing   Restoring to health.

Health care informatics   Integration of computer science, information science, and various health care professionals involved in collecting, processing, and managing data.

Health maintenance   Preventing, or detecting early, particular health deviations through routine periodic exams and screenings.

Health promotion   Process, action, program, or endeavor to obtain the goal of complete physical, mental, and social well-being.

Health protection   Includes provision of safe childbearing through adequate prenatal and postnatal care, safe delivery, and effective family planning for child spacing and desired family size; it also includes prevention, early diagnosis, and appropriate treatment for infections, cancer, cardiovascular and respiratory disease, diabetes, and other chronic illnesses.

Heavy metal   A chemical substance, such as lead or mercury, that may be a by-product of industry.

Hegar's sign   Softening of the isthmus of the uterus in pregnancy.

HELLP syndrome   A severe manifestation of PIH with *h*emolysis, *e*levated *l*iver enzymes, and *l*ow *p*latelets.

Heme iron   Iron from animal sources, which constitutes about half of the iron available from animal sources.

Hemizygous   Condition in which an allele is present in a single copy.

Hemochromatosis   Rare genetic defect in iron metabolism in which excess iron is deposited in tissues, causing skin pigmentation, hepatic cirrhosis, and decreased carbohydrate tolerance, which eventually ends in multiple organ failure.

Hemolytic disease of the newborn   Destruction of the neonate's red blood cells due to isoimmunization (RH or ABO incompatibility) or inadequate vitamin K, which leads to the inability to produce clotting factors and consequent risk of hemorrhage.

Hemosiderosis   Iron storage disorder resulting in iron toxicity.

Herbicide   Chemical designed to kill unwanted plant life such as weeds.

Herbs   Leafy plants that do not have woody stems.

Heterozygote   Individual who has two different alleles at a given locus on a pair of homologous chromosomes.

Hindmilk   Thicker, high-fat breastmilk secreted at the end of a feeding.

Holism   Philosophy of integration of body, mind, and spirit within a dynamic environment.

Home care   Provision of technical, psychologic, and other therapeutic support in the client's home environment rather than in an institution.

Home care nursing   Delivery of nursing care in the home environment.

Home visit   Visit occurring in the family's place of residence or in any such facility where a family may be housed, such as a homeless shelter, group home, church, or halfway house.

Homologous   Refers to chromosomes with matching genes.

Homozygote   Individual who has a pair of identical alleles at a given locus.

Homozygous   Individual possessing a pair of identical alleles of a given gene.

Human chorionic gonadotropin (hCG)   Hormone secreted by the corpus luteum of the ovary after conception.

Human immunodeficiency virus/acquired immunodeficiency syndrome (HIV/AIDS)   Retrovirus that causes progressive and severe impairment of the body's natural immunologic function (HIV), resulting in serious opportunistic infections, various cancers, and eventual death (AIDS).

Human placental lactogen (hPL)   Hormone produced by the syncytiotrophoblast cell as early as 3 weeks after ovulation and is detectable in the maternal serum at 4 weeks after fertilization.

Hyaline membrane disease (HMD)   Surfactant deficiency characterized by collapsed alveoli and low lung volume.

Hydramnios   Excess of amniotic fluid.

Hydrocele   Collection of serous fluid in the scrotum.

Hydrocephalus   Increased circulating cerebrospinal fluid, resulting in an increase in the size of the fetal head.

Hydrocephaly   Condition that results from an excess accumulation of cerebrospinal fluid (CSF) in the ventricles of the brain, caused by an imbalance between CSF production and absorption.

Hydrops fetalis   Severe form of fetal hemolytic disease; severe anemia results in hypoxia, cardiac decompensation, and hepatosplenomegaly.

Hyperbilirubinemia   Elevated level of bilirubin in the blood.

Hyperemesis gravidarum   Severe vomiting during pregnancy.

Hyperglycemia   Blood glucose level greater than 125 mg/dL in the term infant and greater than 150 mg/dL in the preterm infant.

Hyperkalemia   Infant's serum potassium greater than 7 mg/dL.

Hypernatremia   Infant's serum sodium greater than 155 mg/dL.

Hyperthermia   Dangerous elevation in body temperature due to fever or external heat sources.

Hypertonic contractions   Elevated uterine resting tone or contractions that are either too strong in intensity or more frequent than 5 in 10 minutes.

Hypertonic labor   Uterine activity characterized by uterine irritability, poor resting tone, and contractions

occurring at a frequency of closer than every 2 minutes.

Hyperventilation   A change in the oxygen-carbon dioxide exchange; a consequence of breathing too rapidly and too deeply.

Hypocalcemia   Low level of calcium in the blood (less than 7 mg/dL).

Hypochromic anemia   Anemia characterized by red blood cells lacking in color.

Hypoglycemia   A less than normal amount of glucose in the blood; in the newborn, a plasma glucose level of less than 40 mg/dL.

Hypomagnesemia   An abnormally low amount of magnesium in the blood.

Hyponatremia   Infant's serum sodium less than 125 mg/dL.

Hypophyseal-pituitary-ovarian axis   Transport mechanism of gonadotropin releasing hormone from the hypothalamus that stimulates the release of gonadotropins from the anterior pituitary that, in turn, causes stimulation of the ovaries to release estrogen and progesterone.

Hypospadias   Congenital anomaly in which the urethral meatus is located on the ventral surface of the glans penis instead of at the end.

Hypothalamic-pituitary-gonadal axis   Triad of the hypothalamus, pituitary, and ovaries that must function in synchrony in order for conception to occur.

Hypothalamic-pituitary-ovarian axis   Transport mechanism of gonadotropin releasing hormone (Gn-RH) from the hypothalamus that stimulates the release of gonadotropins from the anterior pituitary, which then causes stimulation of the ovaries to release estrogen and progesterone.

Hypothermia   Rectal or axillary temperature below 97°F.

Hypotonic labor   Abnormal labor pattern in which uterine contractions are inadequate in terms of frequency, intensity, or duration.

Hypovolemia   Decreased circulating blood volume.

I

Imperforate anus   A group of anomalies of the rectum and anus.

Implantable contraception   Contraceptive surgically implanted into the client.

Implantation   Embedding of the fertilized ovum into the endometrium.

Impotence   Inability of the male to achieve or maintain an erection.

Incest   Sexual relations between blood relatives or surrogate family members.

Incompetent cervix   Used to describe painless dilation of the cervix, which causes the pregnancy to be lost.

Induced abortion   Termination of pregnancy brought on intentionally by medical or surgical intervention. Induced abortions may be classified as therapeutic, performed for physical or mental health reasons, or as elective, performed at the request of the client.

Infant of a diabetic mother (IDM)   Infant born to a mother who has diabetes mellitus.

Infertility   Diminished or absent ability to produce an offspring despite regular unprotected intercourse for 1 year.

Informed consent   Information regarding treatment procedures given to clients, and their consent is secured.

Injectable contraception   Contraceptive administered by intramuscular injection.

Insensible water loss (IWL)   Evaporation of water through the skin and mucous membranes.

Insoluble fiber   Fiber that resists absorption into the body.

Integrated medicine   Provision of health care services combining both biomedical and complementary medicine.

Intensity   Strength of the contraction at its peak.

Interdisciplinary team   Health care delivered by individuals from various disciplines who share responsibility, authority, and decision-making.

Interspinous diameter   Transverse diameter between the two ischial spines of the pelvis.

Intracranial hemorrhage   Collection of blood within the cranium.

Intrathecal   Technique used to produce analgesia of the lower body by placing a small amount of opioid drug into the cerebrospinal fluid.

Intrauterine growth restriction (IUGR)   Term to describe an infant whose birth weight, length, and head circumference are less than the 10th percentile based on standardized graphs.

Intrauterine pressure catheter (IUPC)   A fetal monitoring device that accurately monitors internal uterine pressure during labor.

Intraventricular hemorrhage (IVH)   Hemorrhage into the ventricles of the brain; common in preterm infants.

Invasive breast cancer   Cancer that has extended beyond the local epithelium and has the potential to spread from the breast to other parts of the body.

Invasive cancer   Cancer that has spread or infiltrated beyond the original site or organ.

Inversion of the uterus   Turning of the uterus inside out, resulting in serious hemorrhage and shock.

Involution   Reduction in size of the uterus following childbirth.

Ionizing radiation   Energy in wave or particle form (such as X-ray) that is capable of releasing ions from irradiated tissue.

J

Jaundice   Accumulation of bilirubin that produces a yellow discoloration of the newborn's skin, mucous membranes, and sclera.

Justice   Division of benefits and burdens in society.

K

Kangaroo care   Skin-to-skin contact between mother and infant.

Karyotype   Chromosome constitution of an individual represented by a laboratory-made display, in which chromosomes are arranged by size and centromere position.

Kernicterus   Excess accumulation of unbound, unconjugated bilirubin deposited in brain tissues, especially the basal ganglia.

Ketoacidosis   Acidosis with the accumulation of ketone bodies in the body's tissues and fluids.

Kleihauer-Betke test   A test used to note evidence of fetal cells in maternal circulation, which is of special significance for Rh-negative pregnant women.

L

Labor   Physiologic process by which the fetus, placenta, and membranes are expelled through the uterus; also known as parturition.

Labor augmentation   Process of stimulating more effective uterine activity through the use of oxytocin.

Labor induction   Stimulation of uterine contractions before the onset of labor for the purpose of accomplishing delivery.

Laceration   A tear in the perineum, vagina, or cervix caused by childbirth.

Lactation consultant   Specially trained health care provider whose primary focus is providing assistance to help new mothers establish breastfeeding.

Lactation discharge   Any secretory breast discharge occurring as a physiologic response to the normal hormonal stimulation of pregnancy, postpartum, or after weaning.

Lactogenesis   The process of milk production 2–5 days postpartum.

La Leche League   International organization that promotes breastfeeding.

Langhan's layer   Inner layer of the trophoblast; also referred to as the cytotrophoblast.

Lanugo   Downy hair that is present on the fetus between the 13th week and birth.

Large for gestational age (LGA)   Term to describe an infant whose birth weight is 2 standard deviations above the mean weight for gestational age or above the 90th percentile.

Latching-on   Proper attachment of the infant to the breast for feeding.

Latent phase   First phase of the first stage of labor, from 0–4 cm of cervical dilation.

Late onset deceleration   Slowing of the fetal heart rate that commences after the onset of the contraction. The fetal heart rate returns to baseline after the contraction has ended. This ominous pattern is caused by uteroplacental insufficiency and occurs in conjunction with diminished or absent variability.

Laws   Rules governing human behavior that represent the minimum standard of mortality.

Leopold's maneuvers   Method of abdominal palpation to determine the presentation and position of the fetus.

Let-down reflex   Milk ejection from the breast triggered by nipple stimulation or emotional response to the infant.

Letting-go phase   Final phase of maternal adjustment characterized by role attainment and relationship adjustment.

Leydig cells   Interstitial tissue cells of the testes that produce testosterone.

Liability   Accountability for professional conduct according to standards that have been set.

Libido   Conscious or unconscious sexual desire.

Life expectancy   Average number of years for which a group of individuals of the same age are expected to live.

Lightening   Movement of the presenting part of the fetus into the true pelvis.

Linea nigra   Dark line of pigmentation that extends from the symphysis pubis to the umbilicus, in the midline of the abdomen, during pregnancy.

LMP   Last menstrual period.

Local anesthetic   Class of drugs that produces reversible blockade of electrical impulses along nerve fibers.

Local infiltration anesthesia   Loss of sensation in a small area owing to blockade of neural impulses as a result of infiltration of tissue with an anesthetic drug such as lidocaine.

Localized breast cancer   Cancer that has not metastasized, is usually less than 2 cm in size, is considered noninvasive beyond the breast, and has the best outcome.

Lochia   Normal uterine discharge of blood, mucus, and tissue following childbirth.

Long-term variability (LTV)   Type of fetal heart rate variability measured in minute intervals from the baseline and rated as decreased, 0–5 bpm; average, 6–25 bpm; or marked, >25 bpm (on a 3-point scale).

Low birth weight (LBW)   Weight of 2,500 grams or less at birth.

Low-lying placenta   A condition in which the exact relationship of the placenta to the cervical os is not determined, or when apparent placenta previa occurs before the third trimester of pregnancy.

Luteal phase   Phase of the ovarian cycle after ovulation when the corpus luteum secretes hormones to prepare the uterine endometrium for implantation until the placenta matures and assumes the function of providing nutrients for the embryo.

Luteinizing hormone (LH)   Anterior pituitary hormone whose surge occurs immediately before ovulation and is responsible for release of the ovum.

M

Macrocephaly   A head circumference that measures more than 38 cm at delivery and remains 38 cm or larger at 48 hours of life.

Macro-environment   Elements that define the caregiving milieu, that is, conditions that define the surrounding space in which caregiving occurs.

Macronutrients   Any of the chemical elements, such as carbon, required in relatively large quantities for growth.

Macrosomia   Infant with a birth weight above the 90th percentile for gestational age or birth weight greater than 4 kg (8 lb, 12.8 oz).

Magnetic resonance imaging (MRI)   Noninvasive diagnostic tool that provides high-resolution cross-sectional images of fluid-filled soft tissues.

Malposition   Fetal position other than occiput anterior, including occiput transverse, occiput posterior, and oblique, or acynclytic, positions.

Malpractice   Negligence involving the actions of professionals.

Malpresentation   Fetal presentation other than vertex, including breech, transverse, compound, shoulder, face, and brow.

Mammogenesis   Mammary growth.

Managed care   Health care plan with a selected list of providers and institutions from which the recipient is entitled to receive health care that is reimbursed by the insurer.

Marginal placenta previa   The placenta lies within 2–3 cm of the cervical os.

Mastectomy   Excision (removal) of the breast.

Mastitis   Infection in the breast, usually confined to a milk duct, characterized by influenza-like symptoms and redness and tenderness in the infected breast.

Material principles of justice   Guidelines that can be used to justify the distribution of benefits.

Maternal-infant bonding Formation of an emotional attachment between mother and newborn.

Maternal role attainment Process by which a women acquires knowledge of maternal behavior that aids in transforming her maternal identity.

Maternal sensitization Process by which the maternal immunologic system forms antibodies against fetal blood cells.

Maternal serum-alpha-fetoprotein (MS-AFP) Screening of maternal blood (MS) for the presence and volume of alpha-fetoprotein (AFP).

Mature milk Breast milk that contains 10% solids for energy and growth.

Meconium Initial stool developed in the fetus; it is viscid, sticky, dark in color, sterile, and odorless.

Meconium staining Staining of the newborn's skin and nails; results from fetal passage of stool in utero.

Medicalization of childbirth Treatment of childbirth as a medical event rather than a natural process.

Medical model Biomedical approach to health care oriented to treating specific diagnoses and focused on physical problems.

Meiosis Process by which germ cells divide and decrease their chromosomal number by half.

Menarche Initiation of the first menses.

Meningocele Spinal cord defect in which an external sac protrudes through the defect and contains meninges and cerebrospinal fluid.

Menopause Natural or surgically imposed cessation of menses.

Menses Monthly bleeding from the lining of the uterus.

Menstrual phase Phase of the menstrual cycle when a woman experiences vaginal bleeding.

Meridian In Asian medicine, the channels or pathways in the body through which Chi travels.

Mesenchyme Meshwork of embryonic connective tissue that forms the connective tissue of the body, blood vessels, and lymph vessels.

Metastatic breast cancer Breast cancer that is found in parts of the body in addition to the breasts.

Microcephaly Condition in which there is a normal-sized head that contains a small brain.

Microcytic anemia Anemia characterized by red blood cells of small size.

Micro-environment Elements that are specifically related to the individual infant's environment or care experiences.

Micronutrients Any of the chemical elements, such as iron, required in minute quantities for growth.

Midpelvis Second of three pelvic planes.

Milia Small, white pimples that appear on the infant's face and chin after delivery.

Mitosis Process in which body cells duplicate themselves and then separate into two new daughter cells.

Mittelschmerz Abdominal pain occurring at the time of ovulation.

Modified-paced breathing Controlled pacing of the increased respiratory rate needed for adequate oxygenation as labor progresses.

Molding Overlapping of the fetal skull bones that helps the fetal head adapt to the size and shape of the maternal pelvis.

Mongolian spots The dark purple-blue or blue-green diffuse skin color noted on the buttocks of an infant.

Monosomy Aneuploid condition of having a chromosome represented by a single copy in a somatic cell; that is, the absence of a chromosome from a given pair.

Monozygotic Derived from one zygote (e.g., identical twins).

Montevideo units A numerical method of calculating adequacy of contraction strength.

Morbidity rate Ratio of the number of cases of a disease or a condition to a given population.

Mortality rate Ratio of the number of deaths in various categories to a given population.

Morula Solid mass of cells formed by cleavage of a fertilized ovum.

Mosaicism Condition that results in an individual (mosaic) with two or more genetically different cell populations.

Mottling A transient skin condition in infancy noted by a lacy framework of blue or red blood vessels surrounding whitened areas of skin in a "cobblestone" appearance; also called cutis marmorata.

Moxibustion In Asian medicine, the burning of herbs near the skin in order to affect movement of Chi.

Multifactorial Resulting from interactions between genetic and environmental factors.

Multipara A woman who has given birth following two or more pregnancies of at least 20 weeks' gestation each.

Multiple gestation Carrying more than one fetus during the same pregnancy.

Mutation Abrupt genetic alteration in an individual, which is transmitted to the offspring.

Myelomeningocele Spinal cord defect in which part of the spinal cord is herniated into an external sac, which contains meninges, neural tissue, and cerebrospinal fluid.

N

Naegele's rule Method for calculating the "due date" from the date of last menstrual period.

Necrotizing enterocolitis (NEC) An acquired disease process characterized by necrosis of the mucosal and submucosal layers of the gastrointestinal tract.

Neglect Withholding of essential components of daily living such as food, clothing, medications, and shelter.

Negligence Unintentional wrong caused by failure to act as a reasonable person would under similar circumstances.

Neonatal abstinence syndrome A collection of symptoms that may include sneezing, vomiting, diarrhea, irritability, and seizures seen in newborns withdrawing from prenatal exposure to narcotics.

Neonatal death A live-born infant who dies before completing 28 days of life, regardless of gestational age.

Nephrocalcinosis Renal calcifications of unknown etiology; may be associated with premature infants who require furosemide therapy, fluid retention, and calcium supplementation.

Nesting Burst of energy experienced by many women 24–48 hours before the onset of labor.

Neurohormonal Pertaining to hormones formed by neurosecretory cells and liberated by nerve impulses.

Neutral thermal environment A set of environmental conditions created to maintain normal body temperature and minimize oxygen consumption and caloric expenditure.

Neutropenia Decreased number of neutrophils.

Nipple discharge Fluid produced by and accumulating within a secretory unit of the breast exiting through the nipple.

Nitrazine test A test for the presence of anmiotic fluid. Nitrazine paper is sensitive to pH and turns blue when in contact with the alkaline amniotic fluid.

Nondisjunction Failure of homologous chromosomes, or chromatids, to separate properly during anaphase meiosis I and II, or mitosis, resulting in daughter cells with unequal chromosome numbers; meiotic nondisjunction may result in gametes with abnormal chromosome number, which on fertilization may produce aneuploidy; miotic nondisjunction that occurs in a developing embryo may result in mosaicism.

Nonheme iron Dietary iron from foods other than meats, in which the iron is not bound in the hemoglobin molecule; comprises half of the iron found in animal sources and all of the iron found in plant sources, including grains and cereals.

Nonimmune hydrops fetalis (NIHF) Severe edema of the fetus that is not the result of isoimmunization.

Nonmaleficence Acting to prevent harm to others.

Nonperiodic fetal heart rate changes Transient changes in fetal heart rate not associated with contractions, although they can occur during a contraction.

Nonstress test (NST) Evaluation of fetal heart rate in response to an increase in either spontaneous or stimulated fetal activity.

Nuchal cord Umbilical cord encircling the fetal neck.

Nuclear family Unit composed of two generations, parents and their children.

Nutrition Facts Food Label Labeling on processed packaged foods that lists credible health and nutrient content claims, standardized serving sizes, and percent daily values (DVs) based on a 2,000-calorie diet.

O

Obesity Body weight of 20% or more over ideal body weight.

Objectives Specific short-term achievements expected to result in the accomplishment of a goal. These are generally written in specific measurable outcomes.

Obstetrical conjugate Anterior-posterior diameter of the pelvic inlet plane; indirect measurement estimated from the sacral promontory to the back of the symphysis pubis.

Oligohydramnios Condition in which the amount of amniotic fluid is significantly less than the amount expected for the third trimester of pregnancy (less than 500 mL) or less than 5 cm total of a four-quadrant sonographic assessment.

Oliguria Diminished urine production in relation to fluid intake.

Omphalocele Defect covered by a peritoneal sac at the base of the umbilicus, into which portions of the abdominal organs herniate.

Opioid Type of drug that binds to opioid receptors and produces a degree of analgesia; also known as a narcotic.

Opsonization Action of opsonins (substances that coat foreign antigens) to facilitate phagocytosis.

Organogenesis Development of organs.

Orgasmic phase Phase of the human sexual response after the plateau phase in which immense sexual tension is released.

Osteopenia Bone mass below normal levels.

Osteoporosis Progressive bone loss, increased bone fragility, and increased risk for bone fractures, which occurs in postmenopausal women.

Ovarian cancer Malignant neoplasm of the ovary.

Overshoot A rebound increase in fetal heart rate following a variable deceleration.

Ovulation Release of a mature ovum in preparation for conception.

Ovulation prediction Contraceptive method involving female prediction of fertile period through the use of basal body temperature charts and/or cervical mucus changes.

Oxytocin   Hormone produced by the posterior pituitary that stimulates uterine contractions and the release of milk from the mammary glands.

P

Paced breathing   Deep breathing that is consciously paced to no less than half the woman's normal respiratory rate; used during pregnancy and during the early phase of labor to promote relaxation.

Pagophagia   Ingestion of nonfood substances such as ice and ice frost.

Pap smear   A screening device for cervical cancer; the results identify women at risk.

Para   Number of births after 20 weeks' gestation, whether live or stillbirth.

Parenteral   Administration of drug via intramuscular or intravenous routes.

Parity   Number of past pregnancies that have reached a gestation of viability regardless of whether the infant or infants were alive or stillborn.

Partial previa   A class of placenta previa in which the placenta is within 3 cm of the cervical os but does not completely cover it.

Parturient   Woman giving birth.

Parturition   Physiologic process by which the fetus, placenta, and membranes are expelled through the uterus; also called labor.

Patent ductus arteriosus (PDA)   Continued patency of the ductus arteriosus (blood vessel connecting the pulmonary artery with the aorta) after the first 24 hours of life.

Paternalism   Interference in the liberty of a person, in which the interference is justified by promoting the well-being of that individual.

Pathologic discharge   Results from pathologic conditions affecting the hypothalamic-pituitary axis, prolactin levels, or breast diseases that affect both breasts.

Pathologic grief   Distortion of the normal bereavement process, including stoic responses to a death.

Pathologic jaundice   Jaundice of the newborn caused by the excessive breakdown of red blood cells as a result of hematologic incompatibility.

Patterned-paced breathing   Similar to modified-paced breathing but with the addition of a rhythmic pattern.

PCBs and PBBs   Polychlorinated biphenyls and polybromated biphenyls, respectively, chemicals now banned but once produced in industry, that are highly stable and thus last for extended periods of time in the environment and human body. Exposure is hazardous in pregnancy, causing spontaneous abortion, growth deficits, and other problems in fetuses.

Pedigree (genogram)   Diagram that describes family relationships and gender, disease status, or other relevant information about a family.

Pelvic inflammatory disease (PID)   Inflammation of the uterus, fallopian tubes, or ovaries caused by ascent of vaginal flora or bacteria.

Pelvic inlet   First of three pelvic planes encountered by the fetal head during the delivery process; often termed the brim of the true pelvis.

Pelvic outlet   Third of the pelvic planes defined by the ischial tuberosities and the tip of the coccyx.

Pelvic relaxation   The loss of muscle support of the pelvic organs.

Percutaneous umbilical blood sampling (PUB)   Evaluation technique that provides direct access to the fetal circulation and involves direct aspiration of fetal blood.

Perimenopause   Time period before the cessation of menses.

Perinatal asphyxia profound   Metabolic acidosis at birth associated with Apgar scores of 3 or less that persist after 5 minutes and is associated with multisystem organ dysfunction and neurologic manifestations.

Perinatal education   Education offered during the childbearing years to expectant families that provides insight and information about pregnancy, preparation for childbearing, family adaptation, and newborn care and development.

Periodic fetal heart rate changes   Changes in the fetal heart rate associated with uterine contraction.

Periventricular leukomalacia (PVL)   Symmetric, nonhemorrhagic lesion within the periventricular white matter of the brain.

Perpetrator   Person accused of a criminal offense.

Persistent pulmonary hypertension in the newborn (PPHN)   A condition caused by a sustained elevation in pulmonary vascular resistance after birth, preventing transition to the normal extrauterine circulatory pattern.

Pesticide   Chemical designed to kill insects, rodents, or other unwanted small life forms harmful to crops or human habitation.

Phenotype   Any observable or measurable expression of gene function.

Phototherapy   Special ultraviolet light used in the treatment of jaundice in the newborn.

Physiologic anemia of pregnancy   Disproportionate increase of the plasma volume compared with the red blood cell volume, resulting in a lower-than-normal hemoglobin and hematocrit level during pregnancy.

Physiologic discharge   Result of physiologic conditions affecting all breast tissue equally, involving secretory tissue in each breast and resulting in milky white or multicolored fluid.

Physiologic jaundice Benign form of jaundice that usually occurs after the third day of life and is caused by the normal breakdown of superfluous red blood cells.

Phytochemicals Plant-based chemicals.

Phytotherapy The therapeutic use of plants, often referring to herbal remedies.

Pica Psychobehavioral disorder that manifests as persistent ingestion of substances having little or no nutritional value or the craving of unnatural articles as food during pregnancy.

Placenta percreta Abnormal placental attachment that completely penetrates the uterine myometrium.

Placenta previa Implantation of the placenta in the uterus that ranges from completely covering the cervical os (complete previa) to lying next to the os (marginal previa).

Placental stage The third stage of labor that begins as soon as the fetus is delivered and lasts until the placenta is delivered.

Plateau phase Phase of human sexual response occurring just before orgasm.

Plethora Deep rosy red color of the skin often seen with polycythemia, hyperoxia, or overheating.

Plumbism Ingestion of nonfood substances such as lead paint flakes.

Pneumatosis intestinalis Intraluminal gas in the bowel wall commonly seen with necrotizing enterocolitis (NEC).

Polycystic ovary syndrome Endocrine disorder characterized by long-term anovulation and an excess of androgens circulating in the blood; characterized by formation of cysts in the ovaries, a process related to the failure of the ovary to release an ovum.

Polycythemia Increased number of red blood cells.

Polydactyly Presence of more than five fingers or five toes on an infant's hand or foot. The extra digits may or may not include bone and are characteristics of family members.

Polygenic Referring to a trait whose phenotypic expression results from the cooperation of various genes.

Polyhydramnios Condition in which the amount of amniotic fluid in the uterus is increased to 2 or more liters within the third trimester.

Position statement Formalized statement by a professional organization to express the opinion of its membership.

Postconceptional age An infant's age from conception described in weeks.

Posterior fontanel The triangular-shaped open space between the sagittal suture and the lambdoidal suture.

Posthemorrhagic hydrocephalus Excess accumulation of cerebrospinal fluid in the brain.

Postnatal circulation The normal extrauterine circulatory pattern of blood flow through the heart, lungs, and body.

Post-term infant An infant determined to be greater than 42 weeks' gestational age by exam.

Postterm pregnancy A pregnancy that is greater than 42 postmenstrual weeks.

Prana Term used in Ayurvedic medicine referring to vital energy.

Precipitate labor Labor that progresses rapidly and ends with the delivery occurring less than 3 hours after the onset of uterine activity.

Precipitous delivery Unduly rapid progression of labor or occurrence of a delivery in which no physician is in attendance.

Precocious Developing maturity very early or rapidly.

Preconception care Consultation with health care professionals by a client before pregnancy to facilitate optimal pregnancy outcomes.

Pre-eclampsia Toxemia of pregnancy characterized by hypertension, edema, and proteinuria.

Pregnancy-induced hypertension (PIH) One of the three signs of pre-eclampsia (proteinuria, edema, and hypertension).

Premature ovarian failure Failure of ovarian estrogen production and ovulation after menarche and before age 40, in which the woman experiences the symptoms of menopause.

Premature rupture of membranes (PROM) Spontaneous rupture of the amniotic membranes before the onset of labor.

Prematurity Delivery at 37 weeks' or less gestation.

Premenstrual syndrome Cyclic cluster of behavioral, emotional, and physical symptoms that occurs during the luteal phase of the menstrual cycle and are of sufficient severity to interrupt normal activity.

Presenting part The part of the fetus that lies closest to the internal os of the cervix.

Preterm An infant born at less than 38 weeks' gestation.

Preterm birth Birth occurring before 37 weeks of gestation.

Preterm infant An infant determined to be younger than 37 weeks' gestational age by exam.

Preterm labor Labor that ensues before 37 completed weeks of gestation.

Preterm premature rupture of membranes (PPROM) Spontaneous rupture of the amniotic membranes before the onset of labor (PROM), which occurs before 37 completed weeks of gestation.

Prima facie A conditional duty that can be overridden by a more stringent duty.

Primary amenorrhea   Absence of menarche until age 16 or absence of the development of secondary sex characteristics and menarche until age 14.

Primary apnea   A self-limited condition characterized by absence of respiration; occurs in the early stage of asphyxia.

Primary dysmenorrhea   Painful menses from uterine causes but without pelvic pathology; usually occurs within 3 years of the onset of menstrual cycling.

Primary powers   Involuntary uterine contractions.

Primipara   Term for a woman who has given birth from her first pregnancy of at least 20 weeks' gestation.

Proactive   Development of capacity to deal with stressors before a crisis.

Proband   Clinically identified person who displays the characteristics or features of the disease; also referred to as *index case*, or *propositus* (fem: *proposita*).

Progesterone   Antiestrogenic hormone produced by the corpus luteum of the ovary that assists in maintenance of pregnancy through implantation.

Prolactin   Hormone from the pituitary gland that triggers milk production in response to tactile stimulation of the breast.

Proliferative phase   Phase of the menstrual cycle in which the endometrium becomes prepared for implantation.

Prostaglandins   Class of hormones found in many tissues that affects vasodilatation, constriction, and uterine smooth muscle.

Pseudomenstruation   Pinkish-white mucoid vaginal discharge noted shortly after birth owing to the maternal transfer of estrogen.

Puberty   Period in which the secondary sex characteristics begin to develop and the capability of sexual reproduction is attained; onset of the process of physical maturity.

Pudendal block   Technique using local anesthesia to block transmission through the pudendal nerves.

Puerpera   Term assigned to the woman during the puerperium.

Puerperal sepsis   Postpartum infection.

Puerperium   Postpartum period; the period of time lasting from delivery of the placenta to approximately 6 weeks after delivery; also known as the fourth trimester.

Pulmonary vascular resistance   Resistance in the pulmonary vascular bed against which the right ventricle must eject blood.

Pushing stage   Second stage of labor that begins when the cervix is completely dilated and effaced and ends when the fetus is expelled.

Pustular melanosis   A skin condition that develops *in utero* with blister formation that resolves after delivery with the peeling of the outer layer of skin, leaving behind a scale of darker, pigmented skin.

Q

Quickening   First fetal movement felt by the mother; usually noticed at about 18 to 20 weeks' gestation.

R

Race   Group of people defined by similar physical features, such as skin color, facial features, and texture of body hair.

Rape   Nonconsensual sexual penetration of another by force or threat of force.

Reactive nonstress test   Presence of at least two spontaneous fetal heart rate accelerations of at least 15 bpm and at least 15 seconds duration each within a 10-minute window.

Recessive   Allele whose phenotypic expression occurs in homozygous or hemizygous conditions.

Recommended Dietary Allowances (RDAs)   Average daily nutrient intake levels recommended for healthy Americans.

Reconstituted family   Family formed through remarriage.

Recovery stage   Fourth stage of labor defined as the first 4 hours after delivery of the placenta.

Reducing agent   Any substance that reduces another substance, or brings about reduction, and is itself oxidized in the process.

Reference Daily Intakes (RDIs)   Standards that address the vitamin and mineral content of foods.

Refractory period   Period of time after orgasm when the human is incapable of further sexual activity.

Regional anesthesia   Loss of sensation from a large area of the body owing to a blockade of neural impulses.

Relactation   Reinstitution of lactation after it has been discontinued.

Relinquishment   The pregnant woman's decision to "give up" or relinquish her rights to parent her child.

Renal solute load   The sum of solutes that must be excreted by the kidneys.

Reproductive loss   Any loss related to reproductive function that may result in the process of grieving, including monthly menstruation for the infertile couple, miscarriage, preterm birth, birth of a child with an anomaly, death of one or more of a multiple gestation, intrauterine fetal death, neonatal death, relinquishment, and sudden infant death syndrome.

Residual urine   Urine remaining in the bladder after elimination.

Resolution phase   Phase of human sexual response when the physiologic changes in the body that occur as a result of sexual activity return to normal.

Respiratory distress syndrome (RDS)   A membrane disease, also known as hyaline membrane disease, causing breathing difficulty in infants.

Resting tone   Firmness of the uterus between contractions.

Resuscitation   Basic emergency procedure used for life support consisting of airway management, positive pressure ventilation, chest compressions, medication, and thermal support.

Retinopathy of prematurity (ROP)   Proliferation of abnormal blood vessels in the newborn retina.

Rh incompatibility   Hemolytic disease caused by the incompatibility of Rh factors in maternal and fetal blood; also known as isoimmunization.

Risk assessment   Process of examining the risk factors that may place an individual at risk for disease.

Risk-benefit analysis   Determination of the risk of a given procedure versus its potential benefits.

Role attainment   Completing the developmental tasks of a new social role.

Role mastery   Successful attainment of developmental tasks.

Role transition   Process of adopting new behaviors to accomplish change and developmental tasks.

Rooting reflex   Normal response of the newborn to move toward whatever touches the area around the mouth.

S

Saltatory pattern   Marked long-term variability; a baseline that is chaotic and jumps up and down multiple times each minute.

Screening   A test or examination to detect the most characteristic signs of a disorder or disease that may require further investigation.

Secondary amenorrhea   Absence of menses for at least 6 months or for three cycles after previously experiencing menstrual cycles.

Secondary apnea   An abnormal condition that occurs in the late stages of asphyxia in which respiration is absent and does not resume spontaneously without resuscitation.

Secondary dysmenorrhea   Painful menses accompanied by a pathologic process.

Secondary powers   A woman's intentional effort to push out the fetus.

Second stage of labor   Begins when the cervix is completely dilated and effaced and ends when the fetus is expelled.

Secretory phase   Phase of the menstrual cycle that occurs after ovulation and before menstruation.

Seminiferous tubules   Tubules that carry semen from the testes.

Sepsis   Systemic bacterial, viral, or parasitic infection that invades the bloodstream.

Serial monogamy   Practice of having one sexual partner at a time but several partners during a lifetime.

Seroconversion   Conversion of blood serum from negative to positive for any infecting agent.

Sexual dysfunction   Related to a disorder of one of the phases of human sexual response.

Sexual maturation   Establishment of menstruation and ovulation in females and the development of spermatogenesis in males.

Short bowel syndrome   Occurs with extensive resection of the gastrointestinal tract. This loss of absorptive surface results in diarrhea, dehydration, and poor growth.

Short-term variability   Type of fetal heart rate variability measured in beat-to-beat changes in the baseline as either present or absent. It is only measurable with internal mode of fetal monitoring.

Shoulder   An acceleratory phase preceding or following a variable deceleration.

Shoulder dystocia   Condition in which fetal shoulder width prevents the fetal shoulders from being freely delivered beneath the maternal symphysis pubis; related to large fetal size and/or small size of maternal pelvis.

Shoulder presentation   Fetal descent in which the shoulder precedes the fetal head in the maternal pelvis alone or along with the fetal arm and hand.

Situational crisis   Event or situation that occurs in a personal or a family life that requires the adaptation or acquisition of new coping mechanisms.

Sleep-wake cycle   Stages of newborn sleep pattern.

Small for gestational age (SGA)   Term to describe an infant whose birth weight is smaller than expected for the gestational age.

Social assets   Assets or benefits to one's health that are related to one's social position and socioeconomic status.

Soluble fiber   Fiber that binds bile acids and coats the intestines, thus inhibiting absorption.

Solvent   Organic compound widely used in industry to clean and manufacture mechanical or electronic components, which is hazardous to fetal well-being.

Somite   One of the paired segments along the neural tube of the embryo.

Spermatogenesis   Entire process of development and maturation of sperm cells.

Spermatozoon   Male gamete or sex cell; spermatozoa (plural).

Sperm capacitation   Process by which the tail is removed from the sperm, enabling it to penetrate and fertilize an egg.

Spermicide   Chemical method of contraception.

Spina bifida   Congenital defect in which the spinal canal does not close and protrudes from the back.

Spinnbarkeit   Stringy, elastic character of cervical mucus at the time of ovulation.

Spontaneous abortion   Expulsion of products of conception that occurs naturally; commonly referred to as miscarriage.

Stalking   Course of conduct directed at a specific person that involves repeated visual or physical proximity; nonconsensual communication; violence toward property; verbal, written, or implied threats; or a combination thereof.

Standards of care   Documents developed by members of a profession to establish a mutually adopted level of practice.

Station   Relationship between the ischial spines and the presenting part of the fetus in the birth canal.

Sterilization   Surgical procedure resulting in permanent loss of reproductive capability.

STORCH   An acronym used to describe a titer for syphilis, toxoplasmosis, other, rubella, cytomegalovirus, and herpes.

Stranger rape   Nonconsensual sexual experience between a victim and assailant who are strangers.

Stress incontinence   Involuntary discharge of urine with a cough, sneeze, or laughter owing to the loss of muscular support at the neck of the urethra.

Stressor   Illness or change in family structure or circumstances that may result in change.

Striae   Stretch marks.

Striae gravidarum   Pinkish or darkened streaks resulting from stretching of the skin during pregnancy that occurs predominantly on the breasts and abdomen.

Subarachnoid hemorrhage   Collection of blood in the subarachnoid space of the brain.

Subdural hemorrhage   Collection of blood in the subdural space of the brain.

Subinvolution   Failure of the uterus to return to a nonpregnant state; occurs when the process of involution is prolonged or stopped owing to hemorrhage, infection, or retained placental parts.

Sudden infant death syndrome (SIDS)   An unexpected baby death in which a thorough postmortem examination, medical history, and case study demonstrate adequate care before death.

Supine hypotension   Condition of reduced blood flow to the right atrium when the pregnant woman lies in a supine position.

Surfactant   Complete lipoprotein that reduces the surface tension of pulmonary fluids, allowing the exchange of gases in the alveoli of the lungs.

Symmetric intrauterine growth restriction   Term to describe fetal growth in which weight, length, and head circumference are all less than the 10th percentile based on standardized graphs.

Sympathomimetic   A drug that stimulates the sympathetic nervous system.

Syncytiotrophoblast   Outer layer of the trophoblast.

Syndactyly   Condition in which fingers or toes are joined together by skin or bone; often called "webbing."

Systemic vascular resistance   Resistance against which the left ventricle must eject its stroke volume with each heartbeat.

T

Tachycardia   A rapid heart rate. In a neonate, especially one that is above 160 bpm.

Tachypnea   A rapid respiratory rate. In a neonate, especially one that is equal to or above 70 respirations/minute.

Taking-hold phase   Second phase of maternal adjustment characterized by an increased readiness to be involved with the newborn.

Taking-in phase   Initial, early period of maternal adjustment characterized by basic maternal needs for food, care, and comfort.

Tanner Stages   Five stages of female and male physiologic development.

Teratogen   Environmental substance that can cause physical defects in the developing embryo and fetus.

Term infant   An infant who is determined to be between 37 and 42 weeks' gestational age by exam.

Testosterone   The most potent naturally occurring androgen (male) hormone that is made in the testes, ovary, and adrenal cortex.

Thelarche   Beginning of the development of the breasts at puberty, with prominence of glandular tissue behind the nipples; the first sign of puberty.

Therapeutic abortion   Pregnancy is terminated because of health risks to the mother in continuation of the pregnancy or for fetal disease.

Thermoregulation   The control of heat production and heat loss, specifically the maintenance of body temperature through physiologic mechanisms activated by the hypothalamus.

Third stage of labor   Begins when the fetus is delivered and lasts until the placenta is delivered.

Thrombocytopenia   Decreased platelet count (<100,000/mL).

Thyrotoxicosis   A disorder of the thyroid gland; hyperthyroidism.

TORCH   A syndrome of infections that includes *t*oxoplasmosis, *o*ther infections including hepatitis, *rubella, cytomegalovirus,* and *herpes,* of which all have been linked to fetal or neonatal harm.

Tort   Civil wrong that may be caused either intentionally or unintentionally.

Total parenteral nutrition (TPN)   Intravenous fluid that provides daily requirements of carbohydrates, protein, electrolytes, vitamins, and minerals.

Tracheoesophageal fistula   Condition in which the trachea and esophagus are abnormally connected.

Transient tachypnea of the newborn   Mild, self-limited, respiratory disorder characterized by increased respiratory rate and mild cyanosis; thought to be related to delayed resorption of fetal lung fluid.

Transition   The third phase of the first stage of labor during which the cervix dilates from 8 to 10 cm.

Transitional milk   Milk produced at the end of colostrum production and immediately before mature milk comes in the breast.

Translocation   Misplacement of genetic material from one chromosome to another.

Transverse lie   Involves the fetus assuming a more horizontal position in the uterus.

Trisomy   Aneuploid condition caused by the presence of an extra chromosome, which is added to a given chromosome pair and results in a total number of 47 chromosomes per cell; Down syndrome is the most common human autosomal trisomy.

Trophoblast cells   Peripheral cells of the blastocyst that attach the fertilized ovum to the uterine wall and develop into the placenta and membranes.

True labor   Rhythmic contraction and relaxation of the uterus with progressive effacement and dilation of the cervix.

Tubal ligation   Surgical method of permanent female sterilization in which the fallopian tubes are severed and tied.

Turtle sign   Deviation or interruption in fetal descent in which the fetal head pulls back instead of completing the external rotation process and progressing forward to the maternal perineum.

Type I diabetes mellitus   Insulin-dependent diabetes.

Type II diabetes mellitus   Non–insulin-dependent diabetes.

U

Ultrasonography   Use of high-frequency (>20,000 Hz) sound waves to detect differences in tissue density and to visualize outlines of structures within the body.

Umbilical cord compression   Pressure from a fetal body part or the uterine wall applied directly to the umbilical cord in utero, resulting in decreased circulation and oxygenation of the fetus for a period of time.

Umbilical cord prolapse   Condition in which a length of umbilical cord precedes the presenting part through the cervix and birth canal.

Undulating variability   A fetal heart rate variability waveform pattern that is repetitive and uniform in appearance.

Universalizability   Rule used to guide actions that could be followed in all other similar situations.

Upper intake level (UL)   Maximum level of daily nutrient intake.

Urge incontinence   Occurs when the urge to void is present but the bladder is unable to empty normally.

Uterine atony   Inability of the uterus to contract.

Uterine rupture   Separation of the uterine wall that may allow protrusion of fetal parts into the abdomen.

Uteroplacental insufficiency   Decline in placental function leading to fetal hypoxia and acidosis; evidenced by late onset fetal heart rate decelerations.

Utilitarianism   Type of ethical thinking focusing on the consequences of actions; actions are right if they bring about the best possible outcomes and the least bad effects for the greatest number of persons.

V

Vaginal infection   Inflammation of the vagina caused by a microorganism or foreign body.

Vaginal ring   Contraceptive device that delivers steroids through the vaginal mucosa.

Vaginismus   Painful spasms of the muscles of the introitus that prevent penetration.

Variability   Fluctuations in the fetal heart rate.

Variable deceleration   Slowing of the fetal heart rate not necessarily associated with uterine contractions, caused by umbilical cord compression.

Varicocele   Varicose veins in the spermatic cord.

Vasa previa   Involves the cord vessels crossing the cervical os and results in significant compression and possible rupture from the pressure of the fetal head during descent.

Vasectomy   Surgical method of permanent male sterilization in which the vas deferens are severed and tied.

Vegan   Vegetarian who consumes no animal products.

Velamentous insertion of the cord   Condition in which the umbilical cord joins the placenta at the edge.

Ventricular peritoneal shunt (VPS)   A tunneled, external ventricular drain for excess spinal fluid that empties into the peritoneal cavity, where the excess spinal fluid is reabsorbed.

Veracity   Truthfulness.

Vertex   Crown of the fetal head.

Vertical transmission   Transmission of HIV by the mother to the fetus or neonate during pregnancy, delivery, and postnatally, during breastfeeding.

Very low birth weight (VLBW)   Weight of 1,500 grams or less at birth.

Virtue   Character trait that is valued.

Virtue ethics   The way in which personal characteristics of the moral agent or person guide moral action.

Vitalism   Term used in 19th century Europe and America referring to a type of vital energy or life force.

W

Weaning   Process of discontinuing breastfeeding and accustoming an infant to another feeding method.

Wet nurse   Woman employed to breastfeed infants who are not her own.

Wharton's jelly   Soft, jelly-like substance of the umbilical cord.

Wife rape   Forced sexual experience with a common law or legally married spouse.

Z

Zona pellucida   Transparent, noncellular layer surrounding the ovum.

Zygote   Cell resulting from the union of the ovum and spermatozoon.

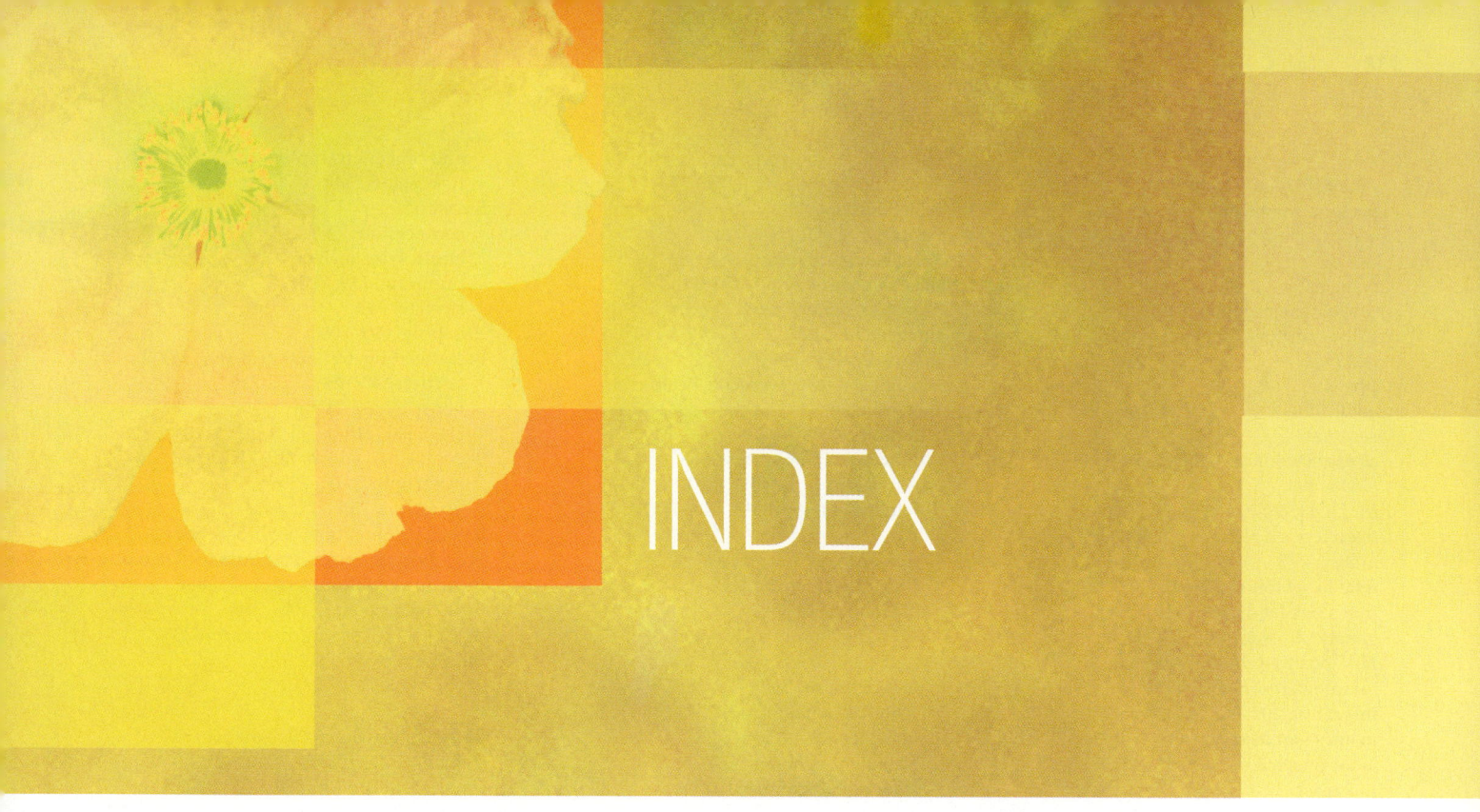

INDEX

('F' indicates a figure, 'T' indicates a table)

618.2   Littleton, Lynna Y.
LIT   Maternity nursing care
2005   114455
c.3

618.2
LIT
2005
c.3

J. C. O Neal Sr. Library & Technology Center
J. F. Drake State Technical College
3421 Meridian Street, North
Huntsville, AL 35811
256-551-5208

618.2   Littleton, Lynna Y.
LIT   Maternity nursing care
2005   114455
c.3